HANDBOOK OF
OBESITY

HANDBOOK OF OBESITY

Clinical Applications
Third Edition

Edited by
GEORGE A. BRAY
Pennington Biomedical Research Center
Baton Rouge, Louisiana, USA

CLAUDE BOUCHARD
Pennington Biomedical Research Center
Baton Rouge, Louisiana, USA

informa
healthcare

New York   London

Informa Healthcare USA, Inc.
52 Vanderbilt Avenue
New York, NY 10017

International Standard Book Number-10: 1-4200-5144-X (Hardcover)
International Standard Book Number-13: 978-1-4200-5144-5 (Hardcover)

Library of Congress Cataloging-in-Publication Data

Handbook of obesity : clinical applications / edited by George Bray, Claude Bouchard. — 3rd ed.
   p. ; cm.
  Includes bibliographical references and index.
  ISBN-13: 978-1-4200-5144-5 (hardcover : alk. paper)
  ISBN-10: 1-4200-5144-X (hardcover : alk. paper)
  1. Obesity—Handbooks, manuals, etc. I. Bray, George A. II. Bouchard, Claude.
  [DNLM: 1. Obesity—therapy—Statistics. 2. Anti-Obesity Agents—therapeutic use—Statistics. 3. Obesity—prevention & control—Statistics. WD 210 H2362 2008]
  RC628.H289 2008
  616.3'98—dc22

                                               2008008242

For Corporate Sales and Reprint Permissions call 212-520-2700 or write to: Sales Department, 52 Vanderbilt Avenue, 16th floor, New York, NY 10017.

**Visit the Informa Web site at
www.informa.com**

**and the Informa Healthcare Web site at
www.informahealthcare.com**

Preface

Welcome to the third edition of the *Handbook of Obesity: Evaluation and Treatment*. When the second edition of this book was published, it was printed in two separate volumes. Volume I dealt with etiology and pathophysiology, and Volume II with clinical applications. This division made it easier to focus on one aspect of obesity at a time when revising this complex body of work. The growth of activity in the therapeutic arena made the second volume, Clinical Applications, the obvious one to tackle first for the third edition.

The new edition of the second volume has been divided into five parts. The first part deals with evaluation of the overweight or obese patient. Included in this section are chapters on evaluation of individual patients, a critical evaluation of the waist circumference in evaluating central adiposity, and genetic strategies in evaluating overweight and obese people. In addition, there are chapters on the usefulness of waist circumference and how to handle it in the health care setting. The other five chapters in Part I deal with cultural differences associated with the approach to obesity, the effects of bias and discrimination, with the issues around weight loss and regain as an example of the false hope syndrome, with the impact of voluntary weight loss on reducing the risk of morbidity and mortality, and finally with approaching the overweight patient in the primary care setting.

Part II focuses on prevention of obesity. This is the obvious first line of defense in our effort to curtail the obesity pandemic. We have included five chapters in this part. There is a chapter on preventing obesity in children and one on preventing obesity in adults, followed by chapters that deal with ways to modify the obesogenic environment, strategies for reengineering the built environment, and the relationship of the food industry to obesity.

The largest number of chapters in this volume is in Part III, which is devoted to the medical management of obesity. It covers behavior, diet, exercise, and pharmacology. Part III begins with a chapter on behavioral approaches to obesity, followed by one on the behavioral techniques that can be used to prevent regain of weight once it is lost. This is followed by a chapter on diets and their use and one on the role of exercise in treatment and prevention of obesity. The next group of chapters is on pharmacological approaches. Sibutramine and orlistat, the only two drugs approved by the U.S. Food and Drug Administration, each have separate chapters. Next is a chapter on the cannabinoid CB1 receptor antagonists, one of which has been approved in Europe but not in the United States. Pramlintide is the subject of a separate chapter, followed by chapters on neuropeptide Y, melanocortin-4 receptor agonists, serotonin receptors, and the potential for histamine H3 receptors in the treatment of obesity. Part III ends with three chapters that cover herbal preparations, the potential for gene therapy, and approaches to patients with the metabolic syndrome.

Surgical treatment of obesity was presented in a single chapter in the second edition, but growth of the field has been such that the topic is now addressed in a separate Part IV with five chapters. These chapters cover operative procedures, the Swedish Obese Subjects (SOS) study as a long-term follow-up for operated patients, the laparoscopic procedures for this surgery, newer surgical strategies, and liposuction.

Part V covers a number of special issues. These include binge eating, the challenges from obesity in pediatric patients, issues in treating overweight patients in the clinic, the economic aspects of obesity, and the role of the government in dealing with this problem.

We are indebted to a number of people for this volume. In particular, Ms. Nina Laidlaw, who assisted us through all the phases of the development of this third edition, deserves special recognition. She managed all aspects of our relations with the authors with patience and elegance. She reviewed all manuscripts in detail to ensure compliance with all requirements of the Publisher and made sure that all permissions had been obtained for the reproduction of material from other publications. We are also grateful for the high-quality support given to us by Ms. Carole Lachney at the Pennington Biomedical Research Center. At Informa Healthcare, Inc., Ms. Sherri Nizoliek has taken the principal role during the development of the manuscript. We are both indebted to each of them. But in the end, without the excellent writing from each of the authors and their collaborators, we would not have the superb chapters that make up this volume. We thank all of them.

George A. Bray
Claude Bouchard

Contents

Contributors

Stephen D. Anton   Department of Aging and Geriatric Research and Department of Clinical and Health Psychology, University of Florida, Gainesville, Florida, U.S.A.

Louis J. Aronne   Department of Medicine, Weill Medical College of Cornell University, New York, New York, U.S.A.

Arne Astrup   Department of Human Nutrition, Faculty of Life Sciences, University of Copenhagen, Frederiksberg C, Denmark

Michael J. Barker   Department of Surgery, Brody School of Medicine, East Carolina University, Greenville, North Carolina, U.S.A.

John E. Blundell   Institute of Psychological Sciences, University of Leeds, Leeds, U.K.

George A. Bray   Pennington Biomedical Research Center, Baton Rouge, Louisiana, U.S.A.

Kelly D. Brownell   Rudd Center for Food Policy and Obesity, Department of Psychology, Yale University, New Haven, Connecticut, U.S.A.

Henry Buchwald   Department of Surgery, University of Minnesota, Minneapolis, Minnesota, U.S.A.

Tim Church   Laboratory of Preventive Medicine Research, Pennington Biomedical Research Center, Baton Rouge, Louisiana, U.S.A.

Deborah A. Cohen   Rand Corporation, Santa Monica, California, U.S.A.

Stephen R. Daniels   Department of Pediatrics, The Children's Hospital, University of Colorado School of Medicine, Aurora, Colorado, U.S.A.

Garry Egger   School of Health and Applied Sciences, Southern Cross University, Lismore, Australia, and Centre for Health Promotion and Research, Sydney, Australia

Ngozi E. Erondu   Clinical Research, Metabolism, Merck Research Laboratories, Rahway, New Jersey, U.S.A.

I. Sadaf Farooqi University of Cambridge Metabolic Research Laboratories, Institute of Metabolic Science, Addenbrooke's Hospital, Cambridge, U.K.

Tung M. Fong Department of Metabolic Disorders, Merck Research Laboratories, Rahway, New Jersey, U.S.A.

Luigi Fontana Division of Geriatrics and Nutritional Sciences, Center for Human Nutrition, Washington University School of Medicine, St. Louis, Missouri, U.S.A., and Division of Food Science, Human Nutrition and Health, Istituto Superiore di Sanità, Rome, Italy

John P. Foreyt Baylor College of Medicine, Houston, Texas, U.S.A.

Gary D. Foster Center for Obesity Research and Education, School of Medicine, Temple University, Philadelphia, Pennsylvania, U.S.A.

Ken Fujioka Nutrition and Metabolic Research and Center for Weight Management, Department of Diabetes and Endocrinology, Scripps Clinic, La Jolla, California, U.S.A.

Ira Gantz Clinical Research, Metabolism, Merck Research Laboratories, Rahway, New Jersey, U.S.A.

Timothy P. Gill Institute of Obesity, Nutrition and Exercise, The University of Sydney, New South Wales, Australia

Frank Greenway Pennington Biomedical Research Center, Baton Rouge, Louisiana, U.S.A.

M.R.C. Greenwood Departments of Nutrition and Internal Medicine, University of California, Davis, California, U.S.A.

Edward W. Gregg Division of Diabetes Translation, National Center for Chronic Disease Prevention and Health Promotion, Centers for Disease Control and Prevention, Atlanta, Georgia, U.S.A.

Scott M. Grundy Center for Human Nutrition, University of Texas Southwestern Medical Center at Dallas, Dallas, Texas, U.S.A.

Jason C.G. Halford Laboratory for the Study of Human Ingestive Behaviour, School of Psychology, University of Liverpool, Liverpool, U.K.

David Heber Center for Human Nutrition, UCLA School of Medicine, Los Angeles, California, U.S.A.

C. Peter Herman Department of Psychology, University of Toronto, Toronto, Ontario, Canada

Marie-France Hivert Endocrinology and Metabolism Division, Department of Internal Medicine, Université de Sherbrooke, Sherbrooke, Quebec, Canada

Rolf Hohlweg Department of Patent Information, Novo Nordisk Library, Novo Nordisk A/S, Bagsværd, Denmark

W. Philip T. James International Obesity TaskForce, London, U.K.

Samira S. Jones Department of Nutrition, University of California, Davis, California, U.S.A.

Alexandra G. Kazaks Department of Nutrition, University of California, Davis, California, U.S.A.

Nicole C. Kesty Medical Affairs, Amylin Pharmaceuticals, Inc., San Diego, California, U.S.A.

Samuel Klein Division of Geriatrics and Nutritional Science and Center for Human Nutrition, Washington University School of Medicine, St. Louis, Missouri, U.S.A.

Robert E. Kramer Section of Pediatric Gastroenterology, Hepatology, and Nutrition, The Children's Hospital, University of Colorado School of Medicine, Aurora, Colorado, U.S.A.

Shiriki Kumanyika School of Medicine, University of Pennsylvania, Philadelphia, Pennsylvania, U.S.A.

Robert F. Kushner Feinberg School of Medicine, Northwestern University, Chicago, Illinois, U.S.A.

Janet D. Latner Department of Psychology, University of Hawaii at Manoa, Honolulu, Hawaii, U.S.A.

Rui Li Division of Diabetes Translation, National Center for Disease Prevention and Health Promotion, Centers for Disease Control and Prevention, Atlanta, Georgia, U.S.A.

Tim Lobstein Child Obesity Research Program, International Association for the Study of Obesity, London, U.K., and SPRU–Science and Technology Policy Research, University of Sussex, Brighton, U.K.

Christine Mack In Vivo Pharmacology, Amylin Pharmaceuticals, Inc., San Diego, California, U.S.A.

Angela P. Makris Center for Obesity Research and Education, School of Medicine, Temple University, Philadelphia, Pennsylvania, U.S.A.

Kjell Malmlöf Department of Anatomy, Physiology and Biochemistry, Faculty of Veterinary Medicine, SLU, Uppsala, Sweden

James B. Meigs General Medicine Division, Department of Medicine, Massachusetts General Hospital and Harvard Medical School, Boston, Massachusetts, U.S.A.

Paul E. O'Brien Centre for Obesity Research and Education, Monash University, The Alfred Hospital, Melbourne, Victoria, Australia

Stephen O'Rahilly University of Cambridge Metabolic Research Laboratories, Institute of Metabolic Science, Addenbrooke's Hospital, Cambridge, U.K.

David G. Parkes In Vivo Pharmacology, Amylin Pharmaceuticals, Inc., San Diego, California, U.S.A.

Michael G. Perri Department of Clinical and Health Psychology, University of Florida, Gainesville, Florida, U.S.A.

Janet Polivy Department of Psychology, University of Toronto at Mississauga, Mississauga, Ontario, Canada

Walter J. Pories Department of Surgery, Brody School of Medicine, East Carolina University, Greenville, North Carolina, U.S.A.

Rebecca M. Puhl Rudd Center for Food Policy and Obesity, Department of Psychology, Yale University, New Haven, Connecticut, U.S.A.

Karin Rimvall Section of Diabetes and Obesity, AstraZeneca R&D, Mölndal, Sweden

Jonathan D. Roth   In Vivo Pharmacology, Amylin Pharmaceuticals, Inc., San Diego, California, U.S.A.

Donna H. Ryan   Pennington Biomedical Research Center, Baton Rouge, Louisiana, U.S.A.

Lars Sjöström   SOS Secretariat, Sahlgrenska University Hospital, Göteborg, Sweden

Judith S. Stern   Department of Nutrition, University of California, Davis, California, U.S.A.

Alison Strack   Department of Pharmacology, Merck Research Laboratories, Rahway, New Jersey, U.S.A.

Boyd Swinburn   School of Exercise and Nutrition Sciences, Deakin University, Melbourne, Victoria, Australia

James E. Tillotson   Friedman School of Nutrition Science and Policy, Tufts University, Boston, Massachusetts, U.S.A.

Søren Toubro   Reduce aps - Research Clinic of Nutrition, Hvidovre Hospital, Hvidovre, University of Copenhagen, Copenhagen, Denmark

Luc F. Van Gaal   Department of Diabetology, Metabolism and Clinical Nutrition, Antwerp University Hospital and Faculty of Medicine, Antwerp, Belgium

Christian Weyer   Clinical Research, Amylin Pharmaceuticals, Inc., San Diego, California, U.S.A.

G. Terence Wilson   Graduate School of Applied and Professional Psychology, Rutgers University, Piscataway, New Jersey, U.S.A.

Rena R. Wing   Department of Psychiatry and Human Behavior, Brown Medical School, The Miriam Hospital, Weight Control and Diabetes Research Center, Providence, Rhode Island, U.S.A.

Catherine E. Woteki   Scientific Affairs, Mars, Incorporated, McLean, Virginia, U.S.A.

Ping Zhang   Division of Diabetes Translation, National Center for Disease Prevention and Health Promotion, Centers for Disease Control and Prevention, Atlanta, Georgia, U.S.A.

Sergei Zolotukhin   Division of Cellular and Molecular Therapy, Department of Pediatrics, Cancer and Genetics Research Complex, University of Florida, Gainesville, Florida, U.S.A.

1

Classification and Evaluation of the Overweight Patient

GEORGE A. BRAY

Pennington Biomedical Research Center, Baton Rouge, Louisiana, U.S.A.

INTRODUCTION

Since the major cause of death in the United States and most other countries is cardiovascular disease, the approach to obesity should be designed to reduce the risks of this problem. This chapter will discuss a classification of obesity that is based on anatomic, etiologic, and functional considerations. I will then use the natural history of the development of obesity to identify the factors associated with its progression and to suggest a stepped approach to evaluating the overweight patient. This discussion is done in the context of obesity as a disease of energy storage (1) whose etiology is a cumulatively greater energy intake than is needed for daily activities. The excess energy is stored in the form of fat, carbohydrate, or protein. The pathology is enlarged fat cells. The extent to which these enlarged cells produce detrimental health consequences depends on two major factors. The first is the mass of fat, which leads to changes in body configuration and resulting reactions (e.g., stigma, osteoarthritis, or sleep apnea). The second is the location of the fat cells. The principal detrimental metabolic consequences occur when fat cells enlarge. Increased intra-abdominal or visceral fat may accentuate this problem (2). Production of adipocytokines, inflammatory markers, vascular factors, and leptin from enlarged visceral fat cells causes the primary metabolic derangements, such as diabetes, atherogenic dyslipidemia (decreased HDL cholesterol and increased triglycerides), and release of inflammatory markers such as interleukin 6 (IL-6) and tumor necrosis factor α (TNF-α) or procoagulant factors such as plasminogen activator inhibitor 1 (PAI-1) (3,4).

CLINICAL CLASSIFICATION

Anatomy of Adipose Tissue and Fat Distribution

Obesity is a disease and its pathology lies in the increased size and number of fat cells. An anatomic classification of obesity from which a pathologic classification arises is based on the number of adipocytes, on the regional distribution of body fat, or on the characteristics of localized fat deposits (5).

Size and Number of Fat Cells

The number of fat cells can be estimated from the total amount of body fat and the average size of a fat cell (6). Because fat cells differ in size in different regions of the body, a reliable estimate of the total number of fat cells should be based on the average fat cell size from more than one location. In adults, the upper limits of the total of normal fat cells range from 40×10^9 to 60×10^9. The number of fat cells increases most rapidly during late childhood and puberty, but may increase even in adult life (7) and can be affected by thiazolidinedione. The number of fat cells can increase three- to fivefold when obesity occurs in childhood or adolescence.

Hypertrophic obesity

Enlarged fat cells are the pathologic sign of obesity (5). Enlarged fat cells tend to correlate with an android or truncal fat distribution (8), and are often associated with metabolic disorders such as glucose intolerance, dyslipidemia, hypertension, and coronary artery disease. These derangements occur because large fat cells secrete more peptides and metabolites, such as IL-6, TNF-α, leptin, and PAI-1. The exception is adiponectin, whose secretion decreases as fat cells enlarge (9).

Hypercellular obesity

An increase in the number of fat cells usually occurs when obesity develops in childhood. Whether it begins in early or middle childhood, this type of obesity tends to be severe. Increased numbers of fat cells may also occur in adult life, and this is to be expected when the body mass index (BMI) is >40 kg/m^2.

Fat Distribution

Measurement

Measuring fat distribution is important because increased visceral fat predicts the development of health risks better than total body fat. The concept that android or male fat distribution was associated with diabetes and heart disease was originally suggested by Vague in 1948 (10) and is now widely accepted. The distribution of body fat can be estimated by a variety of techniques. The ratio of waist circumference to hip circumference (WHR) was used in the pioneering studies that brought scientific recognition in the 1980s to the relationship of centrally located fat to the risk of developing heart disease, diabetes, and other chronic problems associated with obesity (11–13). However, the preferred method is waist circumference, measured according to National Heart, Lung, and Blood Institute/North American Association for the Study of Obesity (NHLBI/NAASO) guidelines (14). The subscapular skinfold has also been used to estimate central fat in epidemiologic studies, but is not clinically valuable. The sagittal diameter, measured as the distance between the surface of the mid-abdominal skin and the table beneath a recumbent subject, has been used as an index of central fat, but is not more valuable than the waist circumference. More precise estimates of visceral fat can be obtained by computed tomography (CT) (6) or magnetic resonance imaging. Using this technique and its association with dyslipidemia, Pouliot and colleagues and Lean and colleagues (11,12) showed that waist circumference was as good as or better than WHR or sagittal diameter in estimating visceral fat. Recent studies show that waist circumference is as good as CT in estimating onset of diabetes (13,15). For practical purposes, waist circumference should be used to evaluate the contribution of fat distribution to the health risk from obesity (15,16).

Lipomas and Lipodystrophy

Lipomas

Localized fat accumulations include single lipomas, multiple lipomas, liposarcomas, and lipodystrophy (5). Lipomas vary in size from 1 cm to more than 15 cm. They can occur in any body region, and represent encapsulated accumulations of fat. Multiple lipomatosis is an inherited disease transmitted as an autosomal dominant trait. Von Recklinghausen's syndrome, Maffucci's syndrome, and Madelung's deformity are lipomatous syndromes.

Liposarcomas are relatively rare, representing less than 1% of lipomas. They tend to affect the lower extremities and consist of four types: well-differentiated myxoid, poorly differentiated myxoid, round cell or adenoid, and mixed (5).

Weber-Christian disease and Dercum's disease are idiopathic accumulations of fat. Dercum's disease, also called adiposis dolorosa, is named after the painful nodules in the subcutaneous fat of middle-aged women. Weber-Christian disease, on the other hand, is a relapsing febrile disease occurring in younger women. All of these forms of localized fat deposits are relatively rare (5).

Lipodystrophy

Lipodystrophy is a loss of body fat in one or more regions of the body (17). It can have genetic causes or it can be acquired. Table 1 shows the various types of lipodystrophy. The clinical features include regional or general decrease in adipose tissue, severe insulin resistance, often with diabetes, markedly elevated triglycerides, and fatty liver. Acanthosis nigricans is also common. Human beings and animals with no body fat (18) show marked insulin resistance, which can be relieved when small amounts of fat are transplanted into fat-deficient animals, or when they are treated with leptin (19).

Familial partial lipodystrophy is a genetic defect due to an alteration in the laminin A/C gene (5). The protein normally produced by this gene is thought to be involved in the entry of molecules into the nucleus. When the aberrant base substitution in the DNA is in one end of the molecule, the disease manifests itself as muscular dystrophy or congestive heart failure. When the molecular substitution is at the other end of the molecule, lipodystrophy is the result.

Drug-induced lipodystrophies appeared when patients with HIV were treated with proteases (5). The proteases reduce the viral burden, but also cause a central distribution of body fat. The mechanism for this central location of fat is currently under intense study.

Table 1 A Summary of Some of the Features of Lipodystrophy

Type	Gene	Chr	Product	Clinical	Laboratory
Total lipodystrophy (Beradinelli-Seip syndrome)				Poor infant feeding; failure to thrive; hepatomegaly; hirsutism; acanthosis nigricans, rapid growth; hollowed cheeks; early puberty	High TG
Type 1	BSCL-1	9q34	Acylglycerol-phosphoacyl transferase 2		
Type II	GNG3LG1	11q13	Seipin		
Partial lipodystrophy (Dunnigan Type)				Profound insulin resistance, diabetes, acanthosis nigricans, high TG, low leptin and adiponectin	High TG, low leptin, low adiponectin
Type I					
Type II		1q21	Lamin A		
Type III			PPAR-γ		
AIDS lipodystrophy					

Etiologic Classification

A number of specific etiologies that cause obesity are described below.

Neuroendocrine Obesity

Hypothalamic obesity

Overweight due to hypothalamic injury is rare in humans (20,21), but it can be regularly produced in animals by injuring the ventromedial or paraventricular region of the hypothalamus or the amygdala (22). These brain regions are responsible for integrating metabolic information on nutrient stores provided by leptin with afferent sensory information on food availability. When the ventromedial hypothalamus is damaged, hyperphagia develops, the response to leptin is eliminated, and overweight follows. Hypothalamic overweight in humans may be caused by trauma, tumor, inflammatory disease, surgery in the posterior fossa, or increased intracranial pressure (23). The symptoms usually present in one or more of three patterns: (*i*) headache, vomiting, and diminished vision due to increased intracranial pressure; (*ii*) impaired endocrine function affecting the reproductive system with amenorrhea or impotence, diabetes insipidus, and thyroid or adrenal insufficiency; or (*iii*) neurologic and physiologic derangements, including convulsions, coma, somnolence, and hypothermia or hyperthermia. As noted earlier, ghrelin, a peptide released from the stomach that can stimulate food intake, is decreased in overweight individuals and increased in Prader-Willi syndrome. In a group of 16 adolescents with hypothalamic obesity, most due to craniopharyngioma,

ghrelin averaged 1345 pg/mL, which was similar to that in 16 overweight adolescents (1399 pg/mL), both of which values were significantly lower than in 16 normal-weight controls (1759 pg/mL) (Table 2) (24).

Cushing's syndrome

Obesity is one of the cardinal features of Cushing's syndrome (Table 3) (25).

Thus the differential diagnosis of obesity from Cushing's syndrome and pseudo-Cushing's syndrome is clinically important for therapeutic decisions (25,26). Pseudo-Cushing's is a name used for a variety of conditions that distort the dynamics of the hypothalamic-pituitary-adrenal

Table 2 Hypothalamic Obesity

Hypothalamic lesions that cause obesity
- tumors
- inflammation
- trauma

Clinical features of hypothalamic obesity
1. Endocrine disturbances
   - amenorrhea/impotence
   - impaired growth
   - diabetes insipidus
   - thyroid/adrenal insufficiency
2. Intracranial pressure
   - papilledema
   - vomiting
3. Neurologic disturbances
   - thirst
   - somnolence

Table 3 Clinical Findings with Cushing's Syndrome (Percentage of Patients)

Sign	Series 1	Series 2	Series 3
Obesity	97	86	97
Amenorrhea	71	72	86
Asthenia	50	58	83
Hypertension	85	88	84
Virilism	69	84	73
Edema of lower extremities	28	66	60
Plethora	50	78	89
Hemorrhagic manifestations	23	68	60

Source: Adapted from Ref. 158.

axis and can confuse the interpretations of biochemical tests for Cushing's syndrome. Pseudo-Cushing's includes such things as depression, anxiety disorder, obsessive-compulsive disorder, poorly controlled diabetes mellitus, and alcoholism. Four different biochemical tests can be used to separate these entities. The first is a urinary free cortisol, which is the initial screening test, and is considered abnormal if it is more than twice the upper limit of normal (27,28). Patients with pseudo-Cushing's syndrome can have values that are elevated fourfold, and thus other tests may be needed. The next test is the overnight suppression of cortisol at 8 AM with a 1-mg dose of dexamethasone given orally at midnight. The dividing line is 3.6 μg/dL, but the lower the value the more likely it is to exclude Cushing's syndrome. If the overnight dexamethasone test is equivocal, a nighttime cortisol level may be drawn. This distinguishes Cushing's syndrome from pseudo-Cushing's syndrome with 95% accuracy if the value is <7.5 μg/dL. The final test is a dexamethasone-CRH test. This test can be helpful, but is also cumbersome to perform because of the timing. If tests are equivocal, then they may be repeated, but it may be advisable to wait for a few weeks in case the patient is an individual with intermittent Cushing's syndrome. For the differential diagnosis and treatment of Cushing's syndrome, the reader is referred elsewhere (25,29,30).

Hypothyroidism

Patients with hypothyroidism frequently gain weight because of a generalized slowing of metabolic activity. Some of this gain is fat. However, the weight gain is usually modest and marked obesity is uncommon. Hypothyroidism is common, particularly in older women. In this group, measurement of thyroid-stimulating hormone (TSH) is a valuable diagnostic tool (31).

Polycystic ovary syndrome

The polycystic ovary syndrome (PCOS) was originally described in the first half of the 20th century by Stein and Levinthal and bore their name for many years. It was characterized by polycystic ovaries and thus its name. The criteria for establishing the diagnosis of this syndrome emerged from a conference at National Institutes of Health in 1990 and one in Rotterdam in 2003. The diagnosis can be made if two of the following three features are present and other causes are eliminated. Those features are polycystic ovaries on ultrasound examination, elevated testosterone, and chronic anovulation manifested as prolonged menstrual periods—oligomenorrhea. Clinical studies show that 80% to 90% of women with oligomenorrhea have PCOS. The syndrome has a prevalence in the population of 6% to 8%.

Better understanding of the syndrome has come from studies of families where more than one woman has PCOS. In these families, the presence of hyperandrogenemia appears to be the central feature. In some women, there is the additional presence of polycystic ovaries. Overweight appears in about half of the women and seems to exaggerate the appearance of the other features, including the insulin resistance that is so characteristic of the syndrome. The insulin resistance and the overweight make diabetes a common association (32).

The mechanism for the abnormalities seems to be an increase in the normal pulsatile release of luteinizing hormone (LH) from the pituitary due to the high androgens. LH is normally released in a pulsatile fashion responsive to the gonadotrophin-releasing hormone released from the hypothalamus and is inhibited by estrogen from the ovary. The high androgen blocks this feedback of estrogen and allows the excessive secretion of LH. An animal model of PCOS in nonhuman primates occurs when androgens are given to young female monkeys. One concept for the origin of the human condition is that there is early exposure to androgens in the mother with subsequent impairment of the androgen-feedback system.

Insulin resistance is another characteristic feature of the polycystic ovarian syndrome. In the family study noted above, it occurred even when the individuals were not overweight, and it, too, probably reflects the influence of increased androgen on the responses of the insulin signaling system. For the pathophysiology of the syndrome, effective treatment might result from inhibiting androgen production or action or enhancing insulin sensitivity. Metformin, an insulin-sensitizing drug, improves ovulation. A similar result of reduced insulin resistance is produced by blocking androgen production with spironolactone, flutamide, or buserelin (Table 4) (33,34).

Growth hormone deficiency

Lean body mass is decreased and fat mass is increased in adults and children who are deficient in growth hormone, compared with those who have normal growth hormone secretion. However, the increase in fat does not produce clinically significant obesity. Growth hormone replacement reduces body fat and visceral fat (35). Acromegaly produces the opposite effects with reduced body fat and

Table 4 Features of the Polycystic Ovary Syndrome

Clinical and metabolic components of the polycystic ovary syndrome	
Menstrual abnormalities	Amenorrhea or oligomenorrhea
	Anovulation
	Infertility
	Increased risk of miscarriage
	Dysfunctional bleeding
Hyperandrogenism	Hirsutism
	Seborrhea and acne
	Male pattern of balding
	Elevated plasma androgens
Hypothalamic-pituitary abnormalities	Increased LH or LH/FSH ratio
	Increased prolactin
Metabolic abnormalities	Obesity (10–80%)
	Insulin resistance, even in nonobese women
	Acanthosis nigricans

particularly visceral fat. Treatment of acromegaly, which lowers growth hormone, increases body fat and visceral fat. Growth hormone selectively decreases visceral fat. The gradual decline in growth hormone with age may be one reason for the increase in visceral fat with age.

Drug-Induced Weight Gain

Several drugs can cause weight gain, including a variety of psychoactive agents (36) and hormones (Table 5). The degree of weight gain is usually limited to 10 kg or less, but occasionally patients treated with high-dose cortico-steroid, with psychoactive drugs, or with valproate may gain more.

Some phenothiazines and many of the "atypical" antipsychotics are particularly prone to causing weight gain. This increase in weight is primarily fat and is associated with an increase in respiratory quotient, suggesting that there is an increase in carbohydrate utilization, which might stimulate food intake. Metabolic rate does not change (37). A recent multicenter trial compared change in body weight among other outcomes during treatment of schizophrenia with antipsychotics. Olanzapine produced the most weight gain (9.4 $\pm$ 0.9 lb) compared to smaller weight gains with the newer antipsychotics, such as quetiapine (1.1 $\pm$ 0.9 lb), risperidone (0.8 $\pm$ 0.9 lb), and ziprasidone (-1.6 ± 1.1), compared to the older perphenazine (-2.0 ± 1.1) (38).

Some antidepressants also can cause weight gain. The tricyclic antidepressant amitriptyline is a common culprit and may also increase the preference for carbohydrates. Lithium also has been implicated in weight gain. Two antiepileptic drugs, valproate and carbamazepine, which act on the N-methyl-D-aspartate (glutamate) receptor, cause weight gain in up to 50% of patients.

Glucocorticoids cause fat accumulation on the neck and trunk, similar to that seen in patients with Cushing's syndrome. These changes occur mostly in patients taking >10 mg/day of prednisone or its equivalent. Megestrol acetate is a progestin used in women with breast cancer and in patients with AIDS to increase appetite and induce weight gain. The increase in weight is caused by fat. The serotonin antagonist cyproheptadine is associated with weight gain. Insulin probably produces weight gain

Table 5 Drugs That Produce Weight Gain and Alternatives

Category	Drugs that cause weight gain	Possible alternatives
Neuroleptics	Thioridazine, olanzepine, quetiapine, resperidone, clozapine	Molindone, haloperidol, ziprasidone
Antidepressants		
Tricyclics	Amitriptyline, nortriptyline	Protriptyline
Monoamine oxidase inhibitors	Imipramine	Bupropion, nefazodone
	Mitrazapine	
Selective serotonin reuptake inhibitors	Paroxetine	Fluoxetine, sertraline
Anticonvulsants	Valproate, carbamazepine, gabapentin	Topiramate, lamotrigine, zonisamide
Antidiabetic drugs	Insulin	Acarbose,
	Sulfonylureas	Miglitol, sibutramine
	Thiazolidinediones	Metformin, orlistat
Anti-serotonin	Pizotifen	
Antihistamines	Cyproheptidine	Inhalers, decongestants
β-Adrenergic blockers	Propranolol	ACE inhibitors, calcium channel blockers
α-Adrenergic blockers	Terazosin	
Steroid hormones	Contraceptives	Barrier methods
	Glucocorticoids	Nonsteroidal anti-inflammatory agents
	Progestational steroids	

by stimulating appetite, with intermittent hypoglycemia as the most likely mechanism.

Insulin stimulates appetite, probably through hypoglycemia. Weight gain occurs not only in patients with diabetes treated with insulin but also in patients treated with sulfonylureas, which enhance endogenous insulin release, and with glitazones, which act on the peroxisome proliferator–activated receptor γ (PPAR-γ) receptor to increase insulin sensitivity (7). In one clinical trial, 48 adults with diabetes not being treated with thiazolidinediones were randomized to receive either a placebo or pioglitazone and 42 completed the trial. The average age was close to 54 years; the subjects weighed 92 kg and had 35% body fat. Body weight decreased by 0.7 kg in the placebo group and increased by 3.6 kg in the glitazone group ($p < 0.0001$) and essentially all of the weight gain was fat (3.5 kg, $p < 0001$). Multislice measurements of visceral fat showed no significant change from baseline to 12 weeks of treatment (5.7 $\pm$ 2.2 to 5.5 $\pm$ 2.3 kg in the glitazone group, $p = 0.058$; 5.9 $\pm$ 1.9 to 5.8 $\pm$ 2.0 kg in the placebo group, $p = 0.075$). After six months, the visceral fat masses for both the placebo and the glitazone-treated group were not different from baseline or from each other. Stratifying the group into those who received sulfonylurea treatment and those who did not had no effect on the response to pioglitazone. Thus glitazones cause significant increases in body fat, almost all of which is subcutaneous.

Metformin is the one antidiabetic drug that does not cause weight gain. In the large United Kingdom Prospective Diabetes Study (39), patients with diabetes who received conventional treatment with metformin gained 3.1 kg in 10 years, not significantly different than what would be expected in the population as a whole. In contrast, those treated with chlorpromazine gained 5.7 kg, those treated with glibenclamide gained 4.8 kg, and the patients treated with insulin gained 7.1 kg. The effect of insulin was dose-dependent. In individuals with type 1 diabetes who were treated intensively in the Diabetes Control and Complications Trial (40), weight gain was 5.1 kg, in contrast to the lower weight gain of 2.4 kg in those receiving insulin in a conventional manner (39,40).

Cessation of Smoking

Weight gain is very common when people stop smoking and is at least partly mediated by nicotine withdrawal. Weight gain of 1 to 2 kg in the first few weeks is often followed by an additional 2- to 3-kg weight gain over the next four to six months. Average weight gain is 4 to 5 kg, but can be much greater (41). Researchers have estimated that smoking cessation increases the odds ratio of overweight to 2.4-fold in men and 2.0-fold in women, compared with nonsmokers.

This weight gain is the result of increased food intake and reduced energy expenditure.

Sedentary Lifestyle

A sedentary lifestyle lowers energy expenditure and promotes weight gain in both animals and humans. Restriction of physical activity in rats causes weight gain, and animals in zoos tend to be heavier than those in the wild. In an affluent society, energy-sparing devices in the workplace and at home reduce energy expenditure and may enhance the tendency to gain weight (42). In children there is a graded increase in BMI as the number of hours of television watching increases (43).

A number of additional observations illustrate the importance of decreased energy expenditure in the pathogenesis of weight gain. The highest frequency of overweight occurs in men in sedentary occupations. Estimates of energy intake and energy expenditure in Great Britain suggest that reduced energy expenditure is more important than increased food intake in causing obesity (42). A study of middle-aged men in the Netherlands found that the decline in energy expenditure accounted for almost all the weight gain (44). According to the Surgeon General's Report on Physical Activity (45), the percentage of adult Americans participating in physical activity decreases steadily with age, and reduced energy expenditure in adults and children predicts weight gain. In the United States, and possibly other countries, the amount of time spent watching television is related to the degree of obesity in children; the number of automobiles is related to the degree of obesity in adults. Finally, the fatness of men in several affluent countries (the Seven Country Study) was inversely related to levels of physical activity (46).

Diet

The amount of energy intake relative to energy expenditure is the central reason for the development of obesity. However, diet composition also may be variably important in its pathogenesis. Dietary factors become important in a variety of settings.

Overeating

Voluntary overeating (repeated ingestion of energy exceeding daily energy needs) can increase body weight in normal-weight men and women. This has been demonstrated repeatedly in experimental settings (47–52). The most convincing, however, is the study by Bouchard and colleagues (53) where they gave identical twins an extra 1000 kcal/day for 84 days under observed conditions. The similarity of weight gain for each pair was closer than for weight gain between pairs of twins. This study shows two important things. First, there is a significant difference in weight gain between individuals, and second, that the genetic influences keep the twins relatively close together in the amount of weight they gained. When these men stopped overeating, they lost most or all of the excess weight. The use of overeating protocols to study the consequences of food ingestion has shown the importance of genetic factors in the pattern of weight gain (53).

Overfeeding has also been practiced culturally among both women and men prior to marriage. Pasquet and Apfelbaum (54) reported data on nine young men who participated in the traditional fattening ceremony called Guru Walla in the northern Cameroon, who overate during a five-month period and gained 19 kg in body weight and 11.8 kg of body fat. Before fattening, these men ate on average 12.9 MJ/day (3086 kcal/day); this increased to 28.2 MJ/day (6746 kcal/day). Over the 2.5 years following the overfeeding interval, the men returned to their prefattening body weight (54).

A second form of overeating with clinical implications I have called progressive hyperphagic overweight (55). A number of patients who begin to become overweight in childhood have unrelenting weight gain. This can only mean that month by month and year by year their intake is exceeding their energy expenditure. Since more energy is required as we get heavier, this must mean that they have steadily increasing intakes of food. These individuals usually surpass 140 kg (300 lb) by 30 years of age, for a weight gain of about 4.5 kg/yr (10 lb/yr). These patients gain about the same amount of weight year after year. Because approximately 22 kcal are required to maintain each extra kilogram of body weight in an obese individual, the energy requirements in these patients must increase year by year, with the weight gain being driven by excess energy intake.

Japanese sumo wrestlers are an example of conscious overeaters. During their training they eat large quantities of food twice a day for many years. While in training they have a very physically active schedule and they have low visceral fat relative to total weight during training. When their active careers end, however, the wrestlers tend to remain overweight and have a high probability of developing diabetes mellitus (56).

Dietary fat intake

Epidemiologic data suggest that a high-fat diet is associated with obesity. The relative weight in several populations, for example, is directly related to the percentage of fat in the diet (57,58). A high-fat diet introduces palatable, often high-fat foods into the diet, with a corresponding increase in energy density (i.e., lesser weight of food for the same number of calories). This makes overconsumption more likely. Differences in the storage capacity for various macronutrients also may be involved. The capacity to store glucose as glycogen in liver and muscle is

limited, and needs to be replenished frequently. This contrasts with fat stores, which are more than 100 times the daily intake of fat. The small storage capacity for glucose as glycogen in liver and muscle, as opposed to very large storage for fat in adipocytes, makes eating carbohydrates to provide glucose a more important physiologic need that may lead to overeating when dietary carbohydrate is limited and carbohydrate oxidation cannot be reduced sufficiently (59).

Dietary carbohydrate and fiber

When the consumption of sugar and body weight is examined there is usually an inverse relationship. However, there are recent data to suggest that the consumption of sugar-sweetened beverages in children may enhance the risk of more rapid weight gain. Both the baseline consumption and the change in consumption over two years were positively related to the increase in BMI over two years. That is, children who drank more sugar-sweetened beverages gained more weight, and those who increased their beverage consumption had an even greater increase (60).

A second relationship between obesity and carbohydrate intake may be through the glycemic index or glycemic load. Glycemic index is defined by the peak blood glucose of a test food relative to a standard load of glucose or white bread (61). A high glycemic index is a high glucose peak. Glucose load is the product of the glycemic index of a food multiplied by the amount of carbohydrate in the food. In a review of six studies, Roberts documented that the consumption of higher-glycemic-index foods was associated with higher energy intake than when the foods had a lower glycemic index. The low-glycemic-index foods are the fruits and vegetables that tend to have fiber. Potatoes, white rice, and white bread are high-glycemic-index foods. Legumes, whole wheat, and so on, are low-glycemic-index foods. This means that the higher-fiber foods (low glycemic index) that release carbohydrate more slowly stimulate food intake less than the foods in which the glucose is rapidly released, as it is in the high-glycemic-index foods (62).

In addition to the relation of energy intake to glycemic index, recent data support the idea that diets with higher fiber intake are associated with lower weight. The Seven-Country Study initiated by Keys and associates more than 40 years ago has been a fertile source for epidemiologic data (46). A recent reexamination of this group has shown that the fiber intake within each of the participating countries was inversely related to body weight. Men eating more fiber had lower body weight. Epidemiologic data suggest that countries where there is higher fiber consumption have a lower prevalence of obesity (46).

Fiber intake may also be inversely related to the development of heart disease (63) and diabetes (64).

Dietary calcium

Nearly 20 years ago McCarron and colleagues (65) reported that there was a negative relationship between BMI and dietary calcium intake in the data collected by the National Center for Health Statistics. More recently, Zemel and colleagues (66) found that there was a strong inverse relationship between calcium intake and the risk of being in the highest quartile of BMI. These studies have prompted a reevaluation of studies measuring calcium intake or giving calcium orally. In the prospective trials, subjects receiving calcium had a greater weight loss than those who were receiving placebos. Increasing calcium from 0 to nearly 2000 g/day was associated with a reduction in BMI of about 5 BMI units (67). These data might suggest that low calcium intake was playing a role in the current epidemic of overweight.

The relationship of calcium and body weight is complicated and confusing, because a patent for the effects of dairy products for producing weight loss has been issued to one of the proponents of this approach. Such a relationship, where monetary gain is associated with the publication of positive studies, raises concerns over the interpretation of the published studies. Moreover, there is inconsistency in both animal and human studies. In one small clinical trial, increasing dietary intake of calcium by adding 800 mg/day of supplemental calcium to a diet containing 400 to 500 mg/day was claimed to augment weight loss and fat loss on reducing diets (68). In two small studies in African-American adults, Zemel and colleagues (69) claimed that substitution of calcium-rich foods in isocaloric diets reduced adiposity and improved metabolic profiles during a 24-week trial. In another small study the Zemel group randomized 34 subjects to receive a control calcium diet with 400 to 500 mg/day ($N = 16$) or a yogurt-supplemented diet ($N = 18$) for 12 weeks. In this small, short-duration study, fat loss was greater on the yogurt diet (-4.43 kg) than the control diet (-2.75 kg). On the basis of these data the investigators claim that yogurt enhances central fat loss (70). In a large multicenter trial that enrolled nearly 100 subjects, the same authors claim that a hypocaloric diet with calcium supplemented to the level of 1400 mg/day did not significantly improve weight loss or body composition when compared to a diet with lower calcium intake (600 mg/day), whereas a diet with three servings per day of dairy products augmented weight and fat loss (70).

In contrast to these three papers from the patent holder's group are a number of studies that do not show an effect of calcium supplementation on body weight (71–74). In a group of 90 women eating a hypocaloric diet, calcium was increased from 800 to 1400 mg/day for 48 weeks. There was no significant effect of the calcium supplement on body fat or weight (74). In the study by Bowen and colleagues (73), the effect of a hypocaloric diet was compared in subjects with 500 or 2400 mg/day supplements of calcium. In the third study (75), a supplement of 1000 mg/day of elemental calcium added to a hypocaloric diet did not enhance weight loss. The evidence of benefit is thus equivocal and limited to small trials. Since there are no major concerns regarding adverse events, and calcium can be beneficial to bone health, there would be no disadvantage in increasing calcium and vitamin D intake modestly.

Frequency of eating

The relationship between the frequency of meals and the development of overweight is unsettled. Many anecdotal reports argue that overweight persons eat less often than normal-weight persons, but documentation is scanty. However, frequency of eating does change lipid and glucose metabolism. When normal subjects eat several small meals a day, serum cholesterol concentrations are lower than when they eat a few large meals a day. Similarly, mean blood glucose concentrations are lower when meals are frequent (76). One explanation for the effects of frequent small meals compared with a few large meals could be the greater insulin secretion associated with larger meals.

Restrained eating

A pattern of conscious limitation of food intake is called restrained eating (77). It is common in many, if not most, middle-aged women of normal weight. It also may account for the inverse relationship of body weight to social class; women of upper socioeconomic status (SES) often use restrained eating to maintain their weight. In a weight loss clinic, higher restraint scores were associated with lower body weights (78). Weight loss was associated with a significant increase in restraint, indicating that people with higher levels of conscious control maintain lower weight. Greater increases in restraint correlate with greater weight loss, but also with higher risk of lapse or loss of control and overeating.

Binge-eating disorder

Binge-eating disorder is a psychiatric illness characterized by uncontrolled episodes of eating, usually in the evening (79). The patient may respond to treatment with drugs that modulate serotonin. Individuals with binge-eating disorder showed more objective bulimic and overeating episodes and more concerns about their shape and body weight, and were disinhibited on the three-factor eating inventory when compared with patients with the night-eating syndrome (80).

Night-eating syndrome

Night-eating syndrome is the consumption of at least 25% of energy between the evening meal and the next morning, and awakening during the night to eat three or more times per week (81,82). In a study of 399 patients in psychiatric outpatient clinics, 12.5% met the criteria for the night-eating syndrome (83). In a comparison of overweight individuals (average BMI 36.1 kg/m^2) with the night-eating syndrome who ate on average 35.9% of their food after the evening meal and who awakened to eat an average 1.5 times/night with comparably overweight individuals (BMI 38.7 kg/m^2) who did not have these features, Allison and colleagues (84) showed that glucose and insulin were higher at night, as expected from the eating pattern, and ghrelin was lower. Plasma cortisol, melatonin, leptin, and prolactin did not differ, but there was a trend toward higher TSH. Patients with the night-eating syndrome were also more depressed (84).

Psychologic and Social Factors

Psychologic factors in the development of obesity are widely recognized, although attempts to define a specific personality type that causes obesity have been unsuccessful. One condition linked to weight gain is seasonal affective disorder, which refers to the depression that occurs during the winter season in some people living in the north, where days are short. These patients tend to increase body weight in winter. This can be effectively treated by providing higher-intensity artificial lighting in the winter (85).

Socioeconomic and Ethnic Factors

Obesity is more prevalent in lower socioeconomic groups in the United States and other developed countries. The inverse relationship of SES and overweight is found in both adults (particularly women) and children. In the Minnesota Heart Study (86), for example, the SES and BMI were inversely related. People of higher SES were more concerned with healthy weight control practices, including exercise, and tended to eat less fat. In the NHLBI Growth and Health Study (87), SES and overweight were strongly associated in Caucasian 9- and 10-year-old girls and their mothers, but not in African-American girls. The association of SES and overweight is much stronger in Caucasian women than in African-American women. African-American women of all ages are more obese than are Caucasian women. African-American men are less obese than white men, and socioeconomic factors are much less evident in men. The prevalence of obesity in Hispanic men and women is higher than in Caucasians. The basis for these ethnic differences is unclear. In men, the socioeconomic effects of obesity are weak or absent.

This gender difference, and the higher prevalence of overweight in women, suggests important interactions of gender with many factors that influence body fat and fat distribution. The reason for this association is not known.

Genetic and Congenital Disorders

Monogenic causes of excess body fat or fat distribution

The rare syndromes are listed in Table 6. These include leptin deficiency, a leptin receptor defect, a defect in the processing of pro-opiomelanocortin (POMC), a defect in pro-convertase 1 (PC 1), a defect in TSH-β, and a defect in PPAR-γ. Although these defects are relatively rare, they show the powerful effects that some genes have on the deposition of body fat. More important, they show that the information obtained from the study of genetic defects in animals can be directly applied to humans. Discovery of the basis for the five single-gene defects that produce overweight in animals was followed by the recognition that these same defects, though rare, also produce overweight in human beings.

Mutations occur in the melanocortin receptor (88–91). Several forms of this receptor transmit signals for activation of the adrenal gland by ACTH (melanocortin-1 receptor), activation of the melanocyte (melanocortin-2 receptor), and suppression of food intake by α-MSH (melanocortin-3 receptor and melanocortin-4 receptor). Genetic engineering to eliminate the MC4-R in the mouse brain produces massive overweight. Several reports claim that a genetic defect in this receptor is the culprit in some overweight human beings. These individuals are of either sex and are massively obese. A much rarer form of overweight in human beings has been reported when production of POMC, the precursor for peptides that act on the melanocortin receptors, is defective (92). These people have red hair and endocrine defects and are moderately obese.

The rare humans with leptin deficiency correspond to the obese (ob/ob) mouse animal model (93–95). Leptin is a 167-amino-acid protein, produced in adipose tissue and the placenta and possibly other tissues, that signals the brain through leptin receptors about the size of adipose stores. In three families, consanguineous marriages led to expression of the recessive leptin-deficient state. These very fat children are hypogonadal, but are not hypothermic or endocrine deficient. They lose weight when treated with leptin. During treatment of these and other children, several important responses, in addition to reduced food intake, reduced appetite, and reduced fat mass and insulin, have been noted. There was a rapid increase in thyrotropin (TSH), free thyroxine, and triiodothyronine, a resumption of normal pubertal development, and improvement in function and number of CD4+ T cells (96). In 13 heterozygotes from three families with the frameshift mutation

Table 6 Monogenic Human Obesities

	Melanocortin-4 receptor deficiency	Leptin deficiency	Leptin receptor deficiency	POMC deficiency	Prohormone convertase-1
Frequency	0.5–1% adults Up to 6% severely overweight children Prevalence 1:2000	$N = 9$	$N = 3$	$N = 7$	$N = 2$ (adult and child)
Appearance			Pale skin Reddish hair		
Growth	Accelerated	Normal	Retarded ↓ IGF-1		
Lean body mass	↑	Normal or ↓			
Bone density	↑				
Food intake	Normal to ↑↑↑	↑↑↑↑	↑↑↑ (aggressive when food deprived)	↑↑	
Metabolic rate	Normal	Normal	Normal		
Insulin	↑↑	↑↑↑	SI ↑		↑ Proinsulin
Immune function		T-cells abnormal			
Thyrotropin		Slightly low	Hypothalamic Hypothyroidism		
Cortisol			Normal	Low Low ACTH	Low
Reproduction		Impaired	Impaired		Impaired
Growth hormone	Normal		Low basal and stimulation ↓ IGF-1 ↓ IGFBP3		
Heterozygotes	Overweight but less than homozygotes	Overweight			

Abbreviation: POMC, pro-opiomelanocortin.
Source: Adapted from Ref. 159.

(deletion of a glycine residue 133), leptin levels were significantly lower than in controls. In contrast to all other populations so far studied where leptin is related to body fatness, there was no correlation in the heterozygotes of leptin with BMI. However, 76% of the heterozygotes had a BMI >30 kg/m^2, compared to only 26% of the controls. Thus the effects of leptin on body weight are gene dose dependent (97).

A defect in the leptin receptor has also been described (98). Among 300 hyperphagic subjects with severe early-onset obesity, nonsense or missense mutations were identified in eight (3%). Although obese and hyperphagic, neither of these phenotypes was as severe as in leptin-deficient individuals. The LepR-deficient subjects also showed delayed puberty due to hypogonadotrophic hypogonadism and alterations in immune function. Serum leptin levels were within the range predicted by the elevated fat mass in these subjects, and clinical features were less severe than in those with congenital leptin deficiency. They do not respond to leptin because they lack the leptin receptor. In experimental animals, the replacement of the leptin receptor using gene-transfer technologies reverses the obesity by restoring sensitivity to leptin (99).

The PPAR-γ is important in the control of fat cell differentiation (100). Defects in the PPAR-γ receptor in humans have been reported to produce modest degrees of overweight that begin later in life. The activation of this receptor by thiazolidinediones, a class of antidiabetic drugs, is also a cause for an increase in body fat.

The final human defect that has been described is in prohormone convertase-1 (101,102). In one family a defect in this gene and in a second gene was associated with overweight. Members of the family with only the PC-1 defect were not obese, suggesting that it was the interaction of two genes that leads to overweight.

Polygenic causes of excess body fat

The more common genetic factors involved in obesity regulate the distribution of body fat, the metabolic rate and its response to exercise and diet, and the control of feeding and food preferences. Several approaches are being used to identify these genes. The first is studies of genetic linkage of families where obesity is prevalent.

The second is in screening the genome with genetic markers in conditions where there are clear-cut phenotypes related to obesity. The third is using animal models that can be examined by breeding to pinpoint areas of the human genome where defects are likely to be found. The final approach is the candidate-gene approach using physiologic clues for obesity to examine possible genetic relationships. It is with the candidate-gene approach that the defects in the melanocortin receptor described above were identified. There are presently more than 25 sites on the genome that have been identified as possible links in the development of obesity. One interesting example is the angiotensinogen gene with substitution of a methionine for threonine at position 235 (M235T). The Heritage Family Study is a study of the response to physical activity in two generations—parents and children. The angiotensinogen M235T polymorphism is associated with body fatness in women.

One of the areas of greatest progress in the past few years has been through the development of animals that express or fail to express genes that may be important for controlling energy expenditure. The list of these so-called transgenic animals is well outside the scope of this review. However, a few general points may be made. Alteration in any one of three genes can produce massive obesity in animals. The first of these is the leptin gene, discussed above. The second is the melanocortin-4 receptor gene, also noted above. When this gene is knocked out, animals become very obese. The third gene is one involved with control of brain levels of γ-aminobutyric acid (GABA). Like other neurotransmitters, GABA can be taken back up into the cell from which it was secreted. When the transporter that controls this process is overly active, the animals become fat, suggesting that GABA plays a role in whether obesity develops or not.

Genetic and congenital disorders

Several congenital forms of overweight exist that are more abundant than most of the single-gene defects (Table 7). Prader-Willi syndrome results from an abnormality on chromosome 15 q 11.2 that is usually transmitted paternally (103). This chromosomal defect produces a "floppy" baby who usually has trouble feeding. Overweight in these children begins at about 2 years and is associated with overeating, hypogonadism, and mental retardation (103). The levels of plasma ghrelin, a peptide that stimulates food intake, are very high in children with Prader-Willi syndrome (104–106). Obestatin is not elevated or correlated with insulin in children with Prader-Willi syndrome (107).

Bardet-Biedl syndrome (108,109) is a rare variety of congenital overweight. It is named after the two physicians who described it in separate publications in the 1920s. It is a recessively inherited disorder that can be

Table 7 Pleiotropic Syndromes of Human Obesity

Bardet-Biedl syndrome	*BBS-1*
	BBS-2
	BBS-3 (ARL6)
	BBS-4
	BBS-5
	BBS-6
	BBS-7
	BBS-8
Albright hereditary osteodystrophy	*GNAS1*
Fragile X syndrome	*FMR1*
Cohen syndrome	*COH1*
Alstrom syndrome	*ALMS1*
Ulnar mammary syndrome	
Syndromes with chromosomal deletions or rearrangement	
Prader-Willi syndrome	*IPW; MKRN3; PWCR1; SNRP; MAGEL2; NDN*
Single-minded	*SIM1*
WAGR with obesity	*WT1; PAX6*
Borjeson-Forssman-Lehman syndrome (X-linked)	*PHF-6*

Source: Adapted from Ref. 159.

diagnosed when four of the six cardinal features are present. These six cardinal features are: (*i*) progressive tapetoretinal degeneration; (*ii*) distal limb abnormalities; (*iii*) overweight; (*iv*) renal involvement (110); (*v*) hypogenitalism in men; and (*vi*) mental retardation. Eight different genes can produce this syndrome, resulting in the so-called Bardet-Biedl syndromes 1 through 8 (BBS-1 through BBS-8). The protein for the BBS-4 version is involved as a subunit in transport machinery that recruits pericentriolar material 1 (PCM-1) to the satellites during cell division. Loss of this protein produces mislocation of the protein with cell death (111). The genetic defect in one form of Bardet-Biedl syndrome (BBS-6) has been identified on chromosome 20q12 as a chaperonin-like protein that is involved in folding proteins (112). It is allelic with McKusick-Kaplan syndrome (MKKS). This latter syndrome is characterized by polydactyly, hydrometrocolpus, and heart problems, but without overweight.

NATURAL HISTORY OF OBESITY

Individuals can become overweight at any age, but this is more common at certain ages. At birth, those who will and those who will not become obese later in life can rarely be distinguished by weight (113), except for the infants of diabetic mothers, for whom the likelihood of obesity later in life is increased (114). Thus, at birth, a large pool of individuals will eventually become overweight, and a smaller group will never become overweight. I have labeled these pools "pre-overweight" and "never overweight."

Several surveys suggest that one-third of overweight adults become overweight before age 20 years, and two-thirds do so after that (5). Thus, 75% to 80% of adults will become overweight at some time. Between 20% and 25% of this subpopulation will display their overweight before age 20 years, and 50% will do so after age 20 years. Some of these overweight individuals will develop clinically significant problems such as diabetes, hypertension, gall-bladder disease, or metabolic syndrome. These are the overweight people who likely have central adiposity.

Overweight in the United States and elsewhere, particularly in women, is more prevalent in those with less education. The inverse relationship between SES and overweight is found in both adults and children. In the Minnesota Heart Study (86), for example, SES and BMI were inversely related. People of higher SES were more concerned with healthy weight control practices, including exercise, and tended to eat less fat. In the NHLBI Growth and Health Study (87), SES and overweight were strongly associated in Caucasian 9- and 10-year-old girls and their mothers, but not in African-American girls. The association of SES and overweight is much stronger in Caucasian women than in African-American women. African-American women of all ages are more overweight than are Caucasian women. African-American men are less overweight than Caucasian men, and socioeconomic factors are much less evident in men. The prevalence of overweight in Hispanic men and women is higher than in Caucasians. The basis for these ethnic differences is unclear. In men, the socioeconomic effects of overweight are weak or absent. This gender difference and the higher prevalence of overweight in women suggest important interactions of gender with many factors that influence body fat and fat distribution. The reason for this association is not known.

Because most pre-overweight people will become overweight, it is important to have as much insight as possible into the risk factors. Table 8 lists a number of predictors for overweight. These predictors fall into two broad groups: demographic and metabolic. When an individual becomes overweight, in turn, s/he may show clinical signs of diabetes, hypertension, gallbladder disease, or dyslipidemia.

Table 8 Predictors of Weight Gain

Infant of diabetic mother or mother who smoked
Overweight parents
Overweight in childhood
Lower education or income group
Cessation of smoking
Sedentary lifestyle
Low metabolic rate
Lack of maternal knowledge of child's sweets-eating habits
Recent marriage
Multiple births

Overweight Developing Before Age 10 Years

Prenatal Factors

Caloric intake by the mother may influence body size, shape, and later body composition. Birth weights of identical and fraternal twins have the same correlation ($r = 0.63$), indicating that birth weight in the middle range is a poor predictor of future obesity (113). However, those infants above the 99th percentile at birth may be at future risk. In the first years of life, the correlation of body weight among identical twins begins to converge, rapidly approaching $r = 0.9$, whereas dizygotic twins diverge during this same period ($r = 0.5$). Infants born to diabetic mothers have a higher risk of being overweight as children and adults (114). Infants who are small-for-dates, short, or have a small head circumference are at higher risk of developing abdominal fatness and other comorbidities associated with obesity later in life (115). Similarly, infants born to mothers who smoke during pregnancy are at a higher risk of obesity in the first three decades of life.

Infancy Through Age 3 Years

Genetic defects

Infancy and early childhood are important times to identify genetic defects in which obesity is a primary component. These were discussed in detail earlier in this chapter.

Breast-feeding

Several recent papers have suggested that breast-feeding may reduce the prevalence of overweight in later life. In a large German study of more than 11,000 children, von Kries and colleagues (116) showed that the duration of breast-feeding as the sole source of nutrition was inversely related to the incidence of overweight, defined as a weight above the 95th percentile, when children entered the first grade. In this study the incidence was 4.8% in children with no breast-feeding, falling in a graded fashion to 0.8% in children who were solely fed from the breast for 12 months or more. A second large report (117) also showed that breast-feeding reduced the incidence of overweight, but not obese, adolescents. The third report, with fewer subjects and more ethnic heterogeneity, failed to show this effect (118). However, the potential that breast-feeding can reduce the future risk of overweight is another reason to recommend breast-feeding for at least 6 to 12 months (Table 9) (119,120). In a study of breast-feeding by diabetic mothers, Rodekamp and colleagues (121) concluded that it is the first week of life that has the most influence on subsequent changes in weight.

The composition of human breast milk changed over the last 50 years of the 20th century (122), with an increasing proportion of linoleic acid derived largely

Table 9 Effect of Breast-Feeding on the Prevalence of Overweight when Children Enter School at Age 5 to 6 years

Duration of breast-feeding	Prevalence of obesity (%)
None	4.5
3 mo	3.8
3–5 mo	2.3
6–12 mo	1.7
>12 mo	0.8

Source: From Ref. 116.

from vegetable fats relative to a stable amount of the omega-3 (n-3) fatty acid α-linolenic acid. This suggests the possibility that this changing proportion of n-6 and n-3 fatty acids may affect prostacyclin production, which in turn could influence the proliferation of new fat cells in the early months of life.

Body weight triples and body fat normally doubles in the first year of life. This increase in body fat and how long the infant was breastfed in the first year of life are important predictors of overweight later in life. Birth weight and weight gain over the first six months of life are positively associated with being overweight at age 5 and 14 years (123). In infants and young children with overweight parents, an infant above the 85th percentile at age 1 to 3 years has a fourfold increased risk of adult overweight if either parent is overweight, compared with non-overweight infants. If neither parent is overweight, this infantile overweight does not predict overweight in early adult life (124). These observations are similar to the older observations suggesting that the risk for overweight in adults was 80% for children with two overweight parents, 40% for those with one overweight parent, and less than 10% if neither parent was overweight (55).

Childhood Obesity from Age 3 to 10 Years

The ages between 3 and 10 are high-risk years for developing obesity. *Adiposity rebound* describes the inflection point between a declining BMI and an increasing BMI that occurs between age 5 and 7 years. The earlier this rebound occurs, the greater the risk of overweight later in life. About half of overweight grade-school children remain overweight as adults. Moreover, the risk of overweight in adulthood is at least twice as great for overweight children as for non-overweight children. The risk is 3 to 10 times higher if the child's weight is above the 95th percentile for age. Parental overweight plays a strong role in this group as well. Nearly 75% of overweight children age 3 to 10 years remained overweight in early adulthood if they had one or more overweight parents, compared with 25% to 50% if neither parent was overweight. Overweight 3- to 10-year-olds with an overweight parent thus constitute an ideal group for

behavioral therapy. When body weight progressively deviates from the upper limits of normal in this age group, I label it "progressive obesity" (5); this is usually severe and lifelong, and is associated with an increase in the number of fat cells.

Sleep adequacy is also a predictor of future weight gain. Children who sleep less are more likely to be overweight later in life. An analysis of factors at age 2 years identified a number of variables that predicted weight status at age 5 to 6 years in 4289 German children (125). Overall prevalence of overweight was 11%. High early weight gain accounted for only 25% of the children. Obese parents and high early weight gain accounted for a likelihood ratio of 3.6 with a corresponding positive predictive value of 40% and was found in 4% of the children.

Overweight Developing in Adolescence and Adult Life

Adolescence

Weight in adolescence becomes a progressively better predictor of adult weight status. In a 55-year follow-up of adolescents, the weight status in adolescence predicted later adverse health events (126). Adolescents above the 95th percentile had a 5- to 20-fold greater likelihood of overweight in adulthood. In contrast with younger ages, parental overweight is less important, or has already had its effect. While 70% to 80% of overweight adolescents with an overweight parent were overweight as young adults, the numbers were only modestly lower (54%–60%) for overweight adolescents without overweight parents. Despite the importance of childhood and adolescent weight status, however, it remains clear that most overweight individuals develop their problem in adult life (5,55).

Adult Women

Most overweight women gain their excess weight after puberty. This weight gain may be precipitated by a number of events, including pregnancy, oral contraceptive therapy, and menopause.

Pregnancy

Weight gain during pregnancy, and the effect of pregnancy on subsequent weight gain, are important events in the weight-gain history of women (127). A few women gain considerable weight during pregnancy, occasionally >50 kg. The pregnancy itself may leave a legacy of increased weight, as suggested by one study that evaluated women prospectively between the ages of 18 and 30 years (128). Women who remained nulliparous (*n* = 925) were compared with women who had a single pregnancy of 28 weeks' duration during that period and who were at least

12 months postpartum. The primiparas gained 2 to 3 kg more weight and had a greater increase in WHR compared with the nulliparous women during this period. The overall risk of weight gain associated with childbearing after age 25 years, however, is quite modest for most American women (129).

Oral contraceptives

Oral contraceptive use may initiate weight gain in some women, although this effect is diminished with the low-dose estrogen pills. One study evaluated 49 healthy women initiating treatment with a low-dose oral contraceptive (30-mg ethinyl estradiol plus 75-mg gestodene). Anthropometric measurements before and after the initiation of this formulation were used to compare 31 age- and weight-matched women (130). Baseline BMI, percent fat, percent water, and WHR did not change significantly after six cycles in the birth control pill users. A similar number of women gained weight in both groups (30.6% of users, 35.4% of controls). The typical weight gain in the pill-user group was only 0.5 kg, but the small weight gain in these women was attributable to the accumulation of fat, not body water. Approximately 20% of women in both groups lost weight.

Menopause

Weight gain and changes in fat distribution occur after menopause. The decline in estrogen and progesterone secretion alters fat cell biology so that central fat deposition increases.

Estrogen replacement therapy does not prevent the weight gain, although it may minimize fat redistribution (131). A prospective study of 63 early postmenopausal women compared 34 who initiated continuous estrogen and progesterone therapy to the remaining women who refused it. Body weight and fat mass increased significantly in both the treatment (71.5–73.5 kg) and the control groups (73.2–75.6 kg). However, WHR increased significantly only in the control group (0.80–0.85). Caloric and macronutrient intake did not change in either group. A two-year trial with estrogen in postmenopausal women also showed an increase in body fat (132).

Adult Men

The transition from an active lifestyle during the teens and early 20s to a more sedentary lifestyle thereafter is associated with weight gain in many men. The rise in body weight continues through the adult years until the sixth decade. After ages 55 to 64, relative weight remains stable and then begins to decline. Evidence from the Framingham Study and studies of men in the armed services suggests that men have become progressively heavier for height during the past century.

Weight Stability and Weight Cycling

Body weight varies throughout the day as food is eaten and then metabolized. Body weight also varies from day to day, week to week, and over longer intervals. Understanding these fluctuations and their relationship to more significant weight cycling related to dieting and regain (yo-yo dieting) is important in understanding obesity (133). Adults under age 55 years tend to gain weight, and those over 55 tend to lose it (134). The youngest adults gain the most weight, and the oldest adults lose the most. Women have significantly greater variation in their weight over 10 years than do men. A 25% weight gain was found in 2.9% of men aged 25 to 44, compared with 6.5% of women in the same age group. In the middle-age range, from 45 to 64 years, the numbers with weight gain of 25% had dropped by nearly half: 1.8% of men, compared with 2.9% of women in the same age group. Weight loss of 25% or more in Americans age 65 to 74 years was higher in women (6.5%) than in men (2.2%). The likelihood of a significant weight gain was substantially higher in the overweight than in those of normal weight in the younger age groups (134). Because the incidence of significant weight gain is more common in young adults, these individuals are a prime target for preventive measures.

Weight cycling associated with dieting is popularly known as yo-yo dieting (133). Weight cycling refers to the downs and ups in weight that often happen to people who diet, lose weight, stop dieting, and regain the weight they lost and sometimes more. The possibility that loss and regain is more detrimental than staying heavy has been hotly debated. In a review of the literature between 1964 and 1994, a group of experts concluded that most studies did not support any adverse effects on metabolism associated with weight cycling. Also, little or no data supported the contention that it is more difficult to lose weight a second time after regaining weight from a previous therapeutic approach. Most researchers agree that weight cycling neither necessarily increases body fat, nor adversely affects blood pressure, glucose metabolism, or lipid concentrations.

CLINICAL EVALUATION OF OVERWEIGHT PATIENTS

Overweight is now recognized as a risk factor for cardiovascular disease and as a contributing factor in the development of other diseases, most notably diabetes and gall bladder disease. In this context, it is important to evaluate and treat the obesity and other risk factors so as to reduce the overall likelihood for developing disease and to reduce the social consequences of being obese.

This section addresses the clinical evaluation of the overweight patient (1,14,135). It then reviews criteria for successful outcomes of treatment and goals of preventing progression from being at risk for overweight to becoming overweight, then developing the clinical sequelae of overweight. Both clinical and laboratory information are needed for this evaluation. To make this evaluation effective, it must be done in the context of a sympathetic office practice concerned with the care and treatment of overweight patients. For additional insights into care of the obese patient in a primary care setting, the reader is referred to the chapter by Kushner and Aronne (chap. 8).

Information from the Clinical Interview

The clinician or therapist who sees an overweight patient needs to obtain certain basic information which is relevant to assessing the patient's risk (Table 10) (14,135–142). This includes an understanding of the events that led to the development of obesity, what the patient has done to deal with the problem, and how successful and unsuccessful the patient was in these efforts. Several of these items are listed in Table 10. The family constellation is important for identifying attitudes about obesity and the possibility of finding rare genetic causes. Information about the amount of weight gain (>20 lb or >10 kg) since age 18 to 20 years and the rate of weight gain is important because this is related to the risk of developing complications from obesity (143). The type and regularity of physical activity is also important because physical inactivity increases cardiovascular risk, particularly in overweight individuals (144). Information about comorbid conditions such as diabetes, hypertension, heart disease,

Table 10 Clinical Information from Interview

	Yes	No
Are members of your family overweight?		
Do your parents or grandparents have diabetes?		
Do you have diabetes?		
Do you have high blood pressure?		
Do you take thyroid hormone?		
Have you gained 20 lb or more (10 kg) since age 20 yr?		
Do you fall asleep easily during the day?		
Do you exercise regularly?		
Do you have gallstone or gall bladder disease?		
Do you take medications regularly? If so, specify		
Are you depressed?		
FOR WOMEN: Do you have normal menstrual periods?		

sleep apnea, and gall gladder disease also needs to be elicited. Because a number of drugs can cause significant weight gain, a history of medication use for mental health problems, depression, convulsive disorders, and diabetes, and for the use of steroids for asthma should be elicited as well. Information about whether the patient/client is ready to put in the effort needed to lose weight can help the physician decide with the patient whether this is the right time to proceed with treatment. Information about possible etiologies for obesity also needs to be obtained, for example, altered menstrual history in women, suggesting polycystic ovary syndrome, or purplish abdominal striae, suggesting Cushing's syndrome.

Clinical Evaluation

Step 1: Physical Measurements

Vital signs

As part of any clinical encounter the nurse or physician should measure several vital signs including height, weight (calculate BMI), waist circumference, pulse, blood pressure and, if indicated by the patient's complaints, temperature.

BMI

Accurate measurement of height and weight, which are used to calculate the BMI, is the initial step in the clinical assessment of the patient (141,145). This index is calculated as the body weight (kg) divided by the stature [height (m)] squared (wt/ht^2), or body weight (lb) × 703 divided by the height (stature) squared {[wt (lb) × 703]/ [ht (in)]^2}. Table 11 lists BMI values for height in centimeters or inches and weight in kilograms or pounds. BMI correlates well with body fat and is relatively unaffected by height.

Step 2: Measure Waist Circumference

Waist circumference is the most practical clinical alternative approach to assessing visceral fat. Waist circumference is measured with a flexible tape placed horizontally at the level of the superior iliac crest (141,145). Tracking the change in waist circumference is a good tool for following the progress of weight loss. It is particularly valuable when patients become more physically active. Physical activity may slow loss of muscle mass and thus slow weight loss while fat continues to be mobilized. Changes in waist circumference can help in making this distinction. As with BMI, the relationship of central fat to risk factors for health varies among populations as well as within them.

Current classifications of obesity are based on BMI and waist circumference. The one recommended by the World

Table 11 Body Mass Index (Using Either Pounds and Inches or Kilograms and Centimeters)

Body mass index (kg/m²) — The italics are for pounds and inches; the bold is for kilograms and centimeters.

Inches	19	20	21	22	23	24	25	26	27	28	29	30	31	32	33	34	35	36	37	38	39	40	Cm
58	*91* **41**	*95* **43**	*100* **45**	*105* **48**	*110* **50**	*115* **52**	*119* **54**	*124* **56**	*129* **58**	*134* **61**	*138* **63**	*143* **65**	*148* **67**	*153* **69**	*158* **71**	*162* **73**	*167* **76**	*172* **78**	*177* **80**	*181* **82**	*186* **84**	*191* **86**	147
59	*94* **43**	*99* **45**	*104* **47**	*109* **50**	*114* **52**	*119* **54**	*124* **56**	*128* **59**	*133* **61**	*138* **63**	*143* **65**	*148* **68**	*153* **70**	*158* **72**	*163* **74**	*168* **77**	*173* **79**	*178* **81**	*183* **83**	*188* **86**	*193* **88**	*198* **90**	150
60	*97* **44**	*102* **46**	*107* **49**	*112* **51**	*118* **53**	*123* **55**	*128* **58**	*133* **60**	*138* **62**	*143* **65**	*148* **67**	*153* **69**	*158* **72**	*164* **74**	*169* **76**	*174* **79**	*179* **81**	*184* **83**	*189* **85**	*194* **88**	*199* **90**	*204* **92**	152
61	*100* **46**	*106* **48**	*111* **50**	*116* **53**	*121* **55**	*127* **58**	*132* **60**	*137* **62**	*143* **65**	*148* **67**	*153* **70**	*158* **72**	*164* **74**	*169* **77**	*174* **79**	*180* **82**	*185* **84**	*190* **86**	*195* **89**	*201* **91**	*206* **94**	*211* **96**	155
62	*104* **47**	*109* **50**	*115* **52**	*120* **55**	*125* **57**	*131* **60**	*136* **62**	*142* **65**	*147* **67**	*153* **70**	*158* **72**	*164* **75**	*169* **77**	*175* **80**	*180* **82**	*186* **85**	*191* **87**	*196* **90**	*202* **92**	*207* **95**	*213* **97**	*218* **100**	158
63	*107* **49**	*113* **51**	*118* **54**	*124* **56**	*130* **59**	*135* **61**	*141* **64**	*146* **67**	*152* **69**	*158* **72**	*163* **74**	*169* **77**	*175* **79**	*180* **82**	*186* **84**	*192* **87**	*197* **90**	*203* **92**	*208* **95**	*214* **97**	*220* **100**	*225* **102**	160
64	*110* **49**	*116* **51**	*122* **54**	*128* **58**	*134* **60**	*140* **63**	*145* **66**	*151* **68**	*157* **71**	*163* **73**	*169* **76**	*174* **79**	*180* **81**	*186* **84**	*192* **87**	*198* **89**	*204* **92**	*209* **94**	*215* **97**	*221* **100**	*227* **102**	*233* **105**	162
65	*114* **50**	*120* **52**	*126* **55**	*132* **58**	*138* **60**	*144* **63**	*150* **66**	*156* **68**	*162* **71**	*168* **73**	*174* **76**	*180* **79**	*186* **81**	*192* **84**	*198* **87**	*204* **89**	*210* **92**	*216* **94**	*222* **97**	*228* **100**	*234* **102**	*240* **105**	165
66	*117* **52**	*124* **54**	*130* **57**	*136* **60**	*142* **63**	*148* **65**	*155* **68**	*161* **71**	*167* **73**	*173* **76**	*179* **79**	*185* **82**	*192* **84**	*198* **87**	*204* **90**	*210* **93**	*216* **95**	*223* **98**	*229* **101**	*235* **103**	*241* **106**	*247* **109**	168
67	*121* **54**	*127* **56**	*134* **59**	*140* **62**	*147* **65**	*153* **68**	*159* **71**	*166* **73**	*172* **76**	*178* **79**	*185* **82**	*191* **85**	*198* **87**	*204* **90**	*210* **93**	*217* **96**	*223* **99**	*229* **102**	*236* **104**	*242* **107**	*248* **110**	*255* **113**	170
68	*125* **55**	*131* **58**	*138* **61**	*144* **64**	*151* **66**	*158* **69**	*164* **72**	*171* **75**	*177* **78**	*184* **81**	*190* **84**	*197* **87**	*203* **90**	*210* **92**	*217* **95**	*223* **98**	*230* **101**	*236* **104**	*243* **107**	*249* **110**	*256* **113**	*263* **116**	173
69	*128* **57**	*135* **60**	*142* **63**	*149* **66**	*155* **69**	*162* **72**	*169* **75**	*176* **78**	*182* **81**	*189* **84**	*196* **87**	*203* **90**	*209* **93**	*216* **96**	*223* **99**	*230* **102**	*237* **105**	*243* **108**	*250* **111**	*257* **114**	*264* **117**	*270* **120**	175
70	*132* **58**	*139* **61**	*146* **64**	*153* **67**	*160* **70**	*167* **74**	*174* **77**	*181* **80**	*188* **83**	*195* **86**	*202* **89**	*209* **92**	*216* **95**	*223* **98**	*230* **101**	*236* **104**	*243* **107**	*250* **110**	*257* **113**	*264* **116**	*271* **119**	*278* **123**	178
71	*136* **60**	*143* **63**	*150* **67**	*157* **70**	*165* **73**	*172* **76**	*179* **79**	*186* **82**	*193* **86**	*200* **89**	*207* **92**	*215* **95**	*222* **98**	*229* **101**	*236* **105**	*243* **108**	*250* **111**	*258* **114**	*265* **117**	*272* **120**	*279* **124**	*286* **127**	180
72	*140* **62**	*147* **65**	*155* **68**	*162* **71**	*169* **75**	*177* **78**	*184* **81**	*191* **84**	*199* **87**	*206* **91**	*213* **94**	*221* **97**	*228* **100**	*235* **104**	*243* **107**	*250* **110**	*258* **113**	*265* **117**	*272* **120**	*280* **123**	*287* **126**	*294* **130**	183
73	*144* **64**	*151* **67**	*159* **70**	*166* **74**	*174* **77**	*182* **80**	*189* **84**	*197* **87**	*204* **90**	*212* **94**	*219* **97**	*227* **100**	*234* **104**	*242* **107**	*250* **111**	*257* **114**	*265* **117**	*272* **121**	*280* **124**	*287* **127**	*295* **131**	*303* **134**	185
74	*148* **65**	*155* **68**	*163* **72**	*171* **75**	*179* **79**	*187* **82**	*194* **86**	*202* **89**	*210* **92**	*218* **96**	*225* **99**	*233* **103**	*241* **106**	*249* **110**	*256* **113**	*264* **116**	*272* **120**	*280* **123**	*288* **127**	*295* **130**	*303* **133**	*311* **137**	188
75	*152* **67**	*160* **71**	*168* **74**	*176* **78**	*184* **81**	*192* **85**	*200* **88**	*208* **92**	*216* **95**	*224* **99**	*232* **102**	*240* **106**	*247* **110**	*255* **113**	*263* **117**	*271* **120**	*279* **124**	*287* **127**	*295* **131**	*303* **134**	*311* **138**	*319* **141**	190
76	*156* **69**	*164* **72**	*172* **76**	*180* **79**	*189* **83**	*197* **87**	*205* **90**	*213* **94**	*221* **97**	*230* **101**	*238* **105**	*246* **108**	*254* **112**	*262* **116**	*271* **119**	*279* **123**	*287* **126**	*295* **130**	*303* **134**	*312* **137**	*320* **141**	*328* **144**	193
BMI	**19**	**20**	**21**	**22**	**23**	**24**	**25**	**26**	**27**	**28**	**29**	**30**	**31**	**32**	**33**	**34**	**35**	**36**	**37**	**38**	**39**	**40**	BMI

The BMI is shown as bold underlined numbers at the top and bottom. To determine your BMI, select your height in either inches or cm and move across the row until you find your weight in pounds or inches. Your BMI can be read at the top or bottom. The italics are for pounds and inches; the bold is for kilograms and centimeters.

Abbreviation: BMI, body mass index.

Source: Courtesy of George A. Bray.

Table 12 Classification of Overweight and Obesity as Recommended by the NHLBI Guidelines

	BMI (kg/m²)	Obesity Class	Disease risk[a] relative to normal weight and waist circumference	
			Men < 102 cm Women < 88 cm	>102 cm >88 cm
Underweight	<18.5		—	—
Normal[b]	18.5–24.9		—	—
Overweight	25.0–29.9		Increased	High
Obesity	30.0–34.9	1	High	Very high
	35.0–39.9	2	Very high	Very high
Extreme obesity	≥40.0	3	Extremely high	Extremely high

[a]Disease risk for type 2 diabetes, hypertension, and CVD.
[b]Increased waist can also be a marker for increased risk in normal weight individuals.

Health Organization (139) and the NHLBI (135) is shown in Table 12.

BMI has a curvilinear relationship to risk. Several levels of risk can be identified using the BMI. These cut-points are derived from data collected on Caucasians. It is now clear that different ethnic groups have different percentages of body fat for the same BMI. Thus, the same BMI presumably carries a different risk in each of these populations. The variations in percentage of body fat for Caucasians, African-Americans, Asians, and Latinos for the same BMI and age are shown in Table 13 (146). For Japanese, a BMI of 23 or 24 kg/m² has the same percent fat as that of a BMI of 25 in Caucasians or 28 to 29 in African-Americans. On the basis of these differences and the observations that the risk for diabetes and hypertension had doubled when the BMI was 25 kg/m², a taskforce from the Asia-Oceania section of the International Association for the Study of Obesity has proposed an alternative table, where obesity is defined as a BMI >25 kg/m² and high-risk waist circumference at >90 cm for men and >80 cm for women (Table 14).

Data from Hispanics and African-Americans suggest that increased body fat carries a greater risk of diabetes, but has less impact on heart disease. After treatment begins, regular measurement of body weight is one important way to follow the progress of any treatment program.

Other Physical Aspects of Obesity

A number of physical features of an obese individual may help identify a specific cause for the individual's problem. Features of the hypothalamic syndrome were presented in Table 2. Cushing's syndrome has been described in Table 3. Polycystic ovarian disease is a common cause of obesity in younger women, and its features are shown in Table 4. Among the various genetic diseases that produce obesity, Prader-Willi is the most common. It includes hypotonia, mental retardation, and sexual immaturity, and can usually be recognized clinically. Bardet-Biedl syndrome, with its polydactyly and retinal disease, is distinctive. Obesity and red hair in a child might suggest a defect in the processing of POMC. Detection

Table 13 Variations in Percent Body Fat for Caucasians, African-Americans, and Asians

	Females			Males		
	African-American	Asian	Caucasian	African-American	Asian	Caucasian
Age 20–39 yr						
BMI						
18.5	20	25	21	8	13	8
25	32	35	33	20	23	21
30	38	40	39	26	28	26
Age 40–59 yr						
18.5	21	25	23	9	13	11
25	34	36	35	22	24	23
30	39	41	41	27	29	29

Source: Adapted from Ref. 146.

Table 14 Classification of Obesity as Recommended by the Asia-Pacific Task Force

| | | Risk of comorbidties | |
| | | Waist circumference | |
Classification	BMI (kg/m^2)	<90 cm (men) <80 cm (women)	≥90 cm (men) ≥80 cm (women)
Underweight	<18.5	Low (but increased risk of other clinical problems)	Average
Normal range	18.5–22.9	Average	Increased
Overweight:	≥23		
At risk	23–24.9	Increased	Moderate
Obese I	25–29.9	Moderate	Severe
Obese II	≥30	Severe	Very severe

of acanthosis nigricans should suggest significant insulin resistance. This is a clinical finding of increased, very dark pigmentation in the folds of the neck, along the exterior surface of the distal extremities, and over the knuckles. It may signify increased insulin resistance or malignancy, and these possibilities should be evaluated.

Laboratory Tests

The third part of the evaluation is the laboratory tests. At the present time, laboratory tests often come in batteries that provide a larger number of tests than may be needed, but unbundling these tests is more expensive than it is worth. It is thus important to focus attention on the laboratory tests that are most relevant to decision-making about the overweight patient. Because diabetes, gall bladder disease, heart disease, sleep apnea, and cancer have a relationship to obesity, these are important conditions to evaluate with laboratory tests.

Plasma Glucose

With over 7% of the adult American population having diabetes and in the face of an epidemic, measurement and, if needed, confirmation of a high glucose or a two-hour value in a glucose tolerance test is the first order of business (Table 15).

Table 15 Diagnostic Criteria for Diabetes

	Fasting glucose	2-hr value from glucose tolerance test
Diagnostic category	mg/dL	mg/dL
Normal	<100	≤140
IGT	100–125	140–199
Diabetes	≥126	≥200

Abbreviation: IGT, impaired glucose tolerance.

Plasma Lipids

A low HDL cholesterol and a high triglyceride level provide one combination of laboratory values that are included in the diagnosis of the metabolic syndrome. These are thus important values to determine. LDL cholesterol is the pivotal lipoprotein in decisions about prevention and treatment of coronary heart disease and other vascular diseases. In the presence of diabetes, these values are lowered (Table 16).

TSH

TSH is important as an index of hypothyroidism, which can occur in up to 4% of older women and may be a factor in weight gain at this time in life.

Prostate-Specific Antigen

Prostate cancer is one of the male cancers associated with obesity. Although prostate-specific antigen (PSA) is a common screening test in men, the relationship of obesity to prostate cancer highlights its value when screening overweight men.

Mammography

Breast cancer is increased in obese women. The presence of obesity may suggest the need for mammography on a regular basis.

Ultrasound of the Gall Bladder

The high prevalence of gall stones in obese men and women would suggest the desirability of an ultrasound, especially if there are any complaints of indigestion.

Metabolic Syndrome

Metabolic syndrome is a complex of traits that enhance the risk of cardiovascular disease. It includes a variety of

Table 16 LDL Cholesterol Goals and Cutpoints for Therapeutic Lifestyle Changes and Drug Therapy

Risk category	LDL goal (mg/dL)	LDL level at which to initiate therapeutic lifestyle changes (mg/dL)	LDL level at which to consider drug therapy
CHD or CHD risk equivalents (10 yr risk >20%)	<100	≥100	≥130 mg/dL (100–129 mg/dL: drugs optional)
2+ risk factors(10-yr risk ≤20%)	<130	≥130	10-yr risk 10–20%, ≥130 mg/dL; 10-yr risk <10%, ≥160 mg/dL
0–1 risk factors	<160	>160	≥190 mg/dL (160–189 mg/dL: LDL-lowering drugs optional)

factors, including central obesity, hypertension, insulin resistance, dyslipidemia, and diabetes mellitus. In an effort to provide a definition of this syndrome, the Adult Treatment Panel III of the National Cholesterol Education Program (13) has provided the following defining features (Table 17). The syndrome is associated with abdominal obesity, measured in this definition by waist circumference (16). The recognition that the differences in ethnic populations have different relations of abdominal fat and its risks indicates that these definitions, like BMI itself, may need ethnic sensitivity in their interpretation. For example, measurements of insulin resistance suggest that individuals of Asian descent (Chinese, Japanese, and South Indians) may have more abdominal fat for a given BMI and body fat than Caucasians.

Clinical Plan

Once the work-up for etiologic and complicating factors is complete, the risk associated with elevated BMI, fat distribution, weight gain, and level of physical activity can be evaluated. Several algorithms have been developed for this purpose (136), but the one we will use was developed by the NHLBI (135).

The BMI provides the first assessment of risk. Individuals with a BMI <25 kg/m^2 are at very low risk but,

nonetheless, nearly half of those in this category at ages 20 to 25 will become overweight by age 60 to 69 years. Thus, a large group of pre-overweight individuals need to prevent further weight gain. Risk rises with a BMI >25 kg/m^2. The presence of complicating factors further increases this risk. Thus, an attempt at a quantitative estimate of these complicating factors is important.

Treatments for obesity can be risky, as evidenced by the results from various treatments attempted over the past 100 years (Table 18). In many cases, treatment for obesity needs to be chronic, hence the emphasis on risk-benefit and safety.

Each treatment listed in Table 18 has been associated with a therapeutic disaster. This must temper enthusiasm for new treatments unless the risk is very low. Because obesity is stigmatized, any treatment approved by the FDA will be used for cosmetic purposes by pre-overweight people who suffer the stigma of obesity. Thus, drugs to treat obesity must have very high safety profiles.

With a risk score based on BMI and waist circumference, treatment goals can be delineated. The BMI is divided into five-unit intervals. Risk, goals, and potential treatment strategies are noted opposite each of these intervals. Low levels of comorbid risk factors reduce the impact of any BMI, whereas high levels of comorbid

Table 17 Clinical Features of the Metabolic Syndrome

Risk factor	Defining level
Abdominal obesity (Waist circumference)	
Men	>102 cm (>40 in)
Women	>88 cm (>35 in)
HDL cholesterol	
Men	<40 mg/dL
Women	<50 mg/dL
Triglycerides	≥150 mg/dL
Fasting glucose	≥100 mg/dL
Blood pressure (SBP/DBP)	≥130/≥85 mmHg

Table 18 Disasters with Drug Treatments for Obesity

Date	Drug	Outcome
1893	Thyroid	Hyperthyroidism
1933	Dinitrophenol	Cataracts, neuropathy
1937	Amphetamine	Addiction
1967	Rainbow pills (digitalis, diuretics)	Death
1971	Aminorex	Pulmonary hypertension
1997	Fenfluramine + phentermine	Valvular insufficiency
1998	Phenylpropanolamine	Strokes
2003	Ma huang	Heart attacks, strokes

risk augment the effect of BMI. Using the BMI, selection of treatments is more rational.

Is the Patient Ready to Lose Weight?

Before initiating any treatment, the physician must know that the patient is ready to make changes. A series of questions developed by Brownell (147) in *The Dieting Readiness Test* can be used to assess this.

When physicians counsel patients who are ready to lose weight, accommodation of their individual needs, as well as ethnic factors, age, and other differences is essential. The approach outlined above is not rigid and must be used to help guide clinical decision-making, not to serve as an alternative to considering individual factors in developing a treatment plan. Because of increasing complications of obesity, more aggressive efforts at therapy should be directed at people in each of the successively higher risk classifications.

Do the Patient and Doctor Have Realistic Expectations?

The doctor and the assistant who see an elevated BMI should take a moment to make sure the patient knows the BMI and waist circumference and how to interpret them. If the patient knows the BMI, it means that the physician or assistant also knows the BMI. However, a recent survey showed that only 42% of obese patients seen for a routine checkup were told they needed to lose weight (148). We need to do better for our patients. The realities of treatment for obesity are often at odds with a patient's expectations. Patients were asked to give the weights they wanted to achieve in several categories, from their dream weight to a weight loss that would leave them disappointed. These can be grouped as in Table 19 (149). When we compare the goals of these patients with reported outcomes, we find that many treatments will leave patients disappointed. Note that only the surgical intervention produced a "dream" weight loss. None of the other treatments produced weight loss that would allow patients to achieve their dream weight, which was on average 38% below

Table 19 Patients' Expectations for Weight Loss at the Beginning of a Weight Loss Study

Outcome	Weight (lb)	Reduction (%)
Initial	218	0
Dream	135	38
Happy	150	31
Acceptable	163	25
Disappointed	180	17

Source: From Ref. 149.

baseline. Nearly half failed to achieve even a weight loss outcome that would disappoint them. The desire to lose weight from a cosmetic standpoint almost always conflicts with the reality of weight loss. This mismatch between patient expectations and the realities of weight loss provides clinicians and their patients with an important challenge as they begin treatment. A weight loss goal of 5% to 15% can be achieved by most patients and will improve many of the risk factors associated with obesity.

One complaint about treatments for obesity is that they frequently fail. By this, patients mean that weight loss stops well short of their desired level. An alternative interpretation may be better (155). Overweight is not curable. However, it can be treated in many ways, but in all cases weight loss reaches a "plateau." When treatment is stopped, weight is regained. This is similar to what happens in patients with hypertension who stop taking their antihypertensive drugs, and in patients with high cholesterol who stop taking their hypocholesterolemic drugs. In each case, blood pressure or cholesterol rises. Like overweight, these chronic diseases have not been cured, but rather palliated. When treatment is stopped, the risk factor recurs.

Patients who are ready to lose weight and have a reasonable expectation for their weight loss goals are ready to begin. An ideal outcome is a return of body weight to normal range, with no weight gain thereafter (156).

However, this is rarely achieved and is unrealistic for most patients. Rather, they need guidance in accepting a realistic goal (142). A satisfactory outcome is a maintenance of body weight over the ensuing years. A good outcome would be a loss of 5% to 15% of initial body weight and regain no faster than the increase in body weight of the population (156). Patients who achieve this should be applauded. An excellent outcome would be weight loss of more than 15% of body weight. An unsatisfactory outcome is a loss of less than 5% with regain above the population weight.

Treatment Strategies by Age Group

Once a patient has been evaluated and is ready to lose weight, an appropriate treatment strategy is selected. The potential treatments can be grouped by age.

Age 1 to 10 Years

Table 20 shows the strategies available for overweight children. A variety of genetic factors can enhance obesity in this age group. This age group also contains a high percentage of pre-overweight individuals. Identifying individuals at highest risk for becoming overweight in adult life allows us to focus on preventive strategies. Among these strategies is the need to develop patterns

Table 20 Therapeutic Strategies for Age 1 to 10 Years

| Age | Predictors of overweight | Therapeutic strategies | | |
		Pre-overweight at risk	Preclinical overweight	Clinical overweight
1–10	Positive family history Genetic defects (dysmorphic Prader-Willi syndrome; Bardet-Biedl; Cohen) Hypothalamic injury Low metabolic rate Diabetic mother	Family counseling Reduce inactivity	Family behavior therapy Exercise Low-fat/low-energy-dense diet	Treat comorbidities Exercise Low-fat/low-energy-dense diet

of physical activity and good eating habits, including a lower fat intake, lower energy-density diet, and smaller portion sizes. Table 8 lists some predictors for developing overweight. Some of these are evident in children; others are not evident until adult life. For growing children, medications should be used to treat the comorbidities directly. Drugs for weight loss are generally inappropriate until the patient reaches adult height, and surgical intervention should only be considered after consultation with medical and surgical experts.

Age 11 to 50 Years

Table 21 outlines the available strategies for overweight and obese adults. Because nearly two-thirds of pre-overweight individuals move into the overweight and obese categories in this age range, this age is quantitatively the most important. Preventive strategies should be used for patients with predictors of weight gain (Table 8). These should include advice on lifestyle changes, including increased physical activity, which would benefit almost all adults, and good dietary practices, including a diet lower in saturated fat.

For patients in the overweight category, behavior strategies should be added to these lifestyle strategies. This is particularly important for overweight adolescents,

because good 10-year data show that intervention for this group can reduce the degree of overweight in adult life (157). Data on the efficacy of behavior programs carried out in controlled settings show that weight losses average nearly 10% in trials lasting more than 16 weeks. The limitation is the likelihood of regaining weight once the behavior treatment ends, although a long-term behavior therapy study did provide long-term weight loss (151).

Medication should be seriously considered for clinically overweight individuals in this group. Two strategies can be used. The first is to use drugs to treat each comorbidity, that is, individually treating diabetes, hypertension, dyslipidemia, and sleep apnea. Alternatively, or in addition, patients with a BMI >30 kg/m^2 could be treated with antiobesity drugs. Current drugs include appetite suppressants that act on the central nervous system and orlistat, which blocks pancreatic lipase. The availability of these agents differs from country to country, and any physician planning to use them should be familiar with the local regulations. Most of the drugs on the market were reviewed and approved more than 20 years ago, and are approved for short-term use only (155). The basis for the short-term use is twofold. First, almost all the studies of these agents are short term. Second, the regulatory agencies are concerned about the potential for abuse, and thus have restricted most of them to

Table 21 Therapeutic Strategies for Age 11 to −50 Years

| Age | Predictors of overweight | Therapeutic strategies | | |
		Pre-overweight at risk	Preclinical overweight	Clinical overweight
11–50	Positive family history of diabetes or obesity Endocrine disorders (PCO) Multiple pregnancies Marriage Smoking cessation Medication	Reduce sedentary lifestyle Low-fat/low-energy-dense diet Portion control	Behavior therapy Low-fat/low-energy-dense diet Reduce sedentary lifestyle	Treat comorbidities Drug treatment for overweight Reduce sedentary lifestyle Low-fat/low-energy-dense diet Behavior therapy Surgery

prescription use with limitations. The withdrawal of fen-fluramine and dexfenfluramine from the market in 1997 following in the development of valvular heart disease further compounds the concern of health authorities about the safety of these drugs. Because of the regulatory limitations and the lack of longer-term data on safety and efficacy, the use of the drugs approved for short-term treatment must be carefully justified. They may be useful in initiating treatment and in helping a patient who is relapsing.

Sibutramine (Meridia®, Reductil®) is approved in most countries for long-term use. The evidence shows that weight loss of 10% or more can be produced with this drug. The side-effect profile includes dry mouth, asthenia, insomnia, and constipation. It also produces a small increase in heart rate of between 2 and 5 beats per minute, and a small rise in blood pressure of between 2 and 4 mmHg. Clinical data show no evidence of valvulopathy. Blood pressure should be followed carefully, and the drug may be inappropriate in patients with stroke, congestive heart failure, or recent myocardial infarction. It should not be used with other serotonergic drugs or drugs that inhibit monoamine oxidase.

Orlistat (Xenical®), a drug that blocks intestinal lipase, has been approved for long-term use in most countries. In clinical trials lasting up to two years, orlistat was associated with a mean weight loss of up to 10% at the end of one year in patients who were prescribed a 30% fat diet. As might be expected, because the drug blocks pancreatic lipase in the intestine, fecal fat loss is increased. Major side effects reported early were markedly reduced over time, implying that patients learned to use the drug effectively in relation to dietary intake of fat. The effective use of this medication requires that physicians and their staffs provide good dietary control counseling to patients.

Age over 51 Years

Table 22 shows the proposed treatments for this age group. By age 50 years, almost all of the people who will become overweight have done so. Thus, preventive strategies are no longer important, and the focus is on treatment for those who are overweight or obese. The basic treatments and treatment considerations are similar to those of the younger group. However, in this age group, the argument may be stronger for directly treating comorbidities and paying less attention to weight loss. For patients in this group who wish to lose weight, however, the considerations for patients between age 11 and 50 years still apply. Surgery should only be considered for individuals with class II or III obesity, or who are severely overweight. This form of treatment requires skilled surgical intervention, and should only be carried out in specialized centers.

Quality of Life

Quality of life is important for all patients. This has effects in many areas. From the health care perspective, a reduction in comorbidities is a significant improvement. Remission of Type 2 diabetes or hypertension can reduce costs of treating these conditions, as well as delay or prevent the development of disease. Weight loss can reduce the wear and tear on joints and slow the development of osteoarthritis. Sleep apnea usually resolves.

Psychosocial improvement is of great importance to patients. Studies of patients who achieved long-term weight loss from surgical intervention show improved social and economic function of previously disabled overweight patients. Loss of 5% or more of initial weight almost always translates into improved mobility, improvement in sleep disturbances, increased exercise tolerance, and heightened self-esteem. A focus on these, rather than cosmetic outcomes, is essential.

THE REALITIES OF OVERWEIGHT

Overweight is a chronic, stigmatized disease that is increasingly prevalent, with more than 60% of the American population now overweight (BMI >25 kg/m^2). This represents more than 100 million people. The prevalence

Table 22 Therapeutic Strategies for Age over 51 Years

Age	Predictors of overweight	Therapeutic strategies		
		Pre-overweight at risk	Preclinical overweight	Clinical overweight
51–75	Menopause Declining growth hormone Declining testosterone Smoking cessation Medication	Few individuals remain in this subgroup	Behavior therapy Low-fat/low-energy-dense diet Reduce sedentary lifestyle	Treat comorbidities Drug treatment for overweight Reduce sedentary lifestyle Low-fat/low-energy-dense diet Behavior therapy Surgery

of obesity (BMI >30 kg/m^2) has risen more than 100% in the last 30 years and continues to increase. The social disapproval of obesity and the lengths people go to prevent or reverse it fuels a $80 billion/yr set of industries. Nearly 65% of American women consider themselves overweight, and even more (66% to 75%) want to weigh less. The figures for men are somewhat less. More than 50% of the women with a BMI <21 kg/m^2 (normal weight) want to weigh less. This individual perception of a "desirable" weight for them indicates the degree of both the stigmatization for those who are not "thin" and the drive to lose weight.

The cultural expectations for thinness are evident in the decreasing weight of the Miss America pageant contestants from 1950 to 1980 and in the centerfold models of *Playboy* magazine. This has now leveled off with quite thin contestants. The stigma of obesity is also evident in the general public disapproval of corpulence, and in the disapproving moral attitudes of many health care professionals. For example, mental health workers are more likely to assign negative psychological symptoms to the obese than to normal-weight people. Nursing, medical, and ancillary health care personnel also carry these negative stereotypes. Sensitivity training for health care professionals dealing with overweight patients is important in any office or clinic offering treatment for obesity.

Overweight has many causes. The natural history of obesity indicates that it occurs gradually. Although overweight in childhood carries a serious adverse prognosis, particularly if the parents are overweight, nearly two-thirds of overweight adults developed their problem in adult life.

Results from most long-term clinical studies of treatment for overweight patients show a high prevalence of weight regain. In the Institute of Medicine report "Weighing the Options" (135), for those who achieved weight loss, more than one-third of the weight typically was regained within one year, and nearly all within five years. Despite this gloomy report, many long-term successes have occurred. A study of secondary prevention in successful weight maintainers showed no differences between those who regained weight in reported level of energy expenditure from exercise. However, those who successfully maintained weight loss showed greater control of fat intake, which included avoiding fried foods and substituting low-fat foods for high-fat foods. Several other programs have also reported long-term weight loss or prevention, especially in children (149).

Overweight, central or abdominal fat, weight gain after age 20 years, and a sedentary lifestyle all increase health risks and increase economic costs of obesity. Intentional weight loss by overweight individuals, on the other hand, reduces these risks. Although data are not yet available, researchers widely believe that long-term intentional weight loss lowers overall mortality, particularly from diabetes, gallbladder disease, hypertension, heart disease, and some types of cancer.

REFERENCES

1. Bray GA. Obesity is a chronic, relapsing neurochemical disease. Int J Obes Relat Metab Disord 2004; 28(1):34–38.
2. Despres JP. Intra-abdominal obesity: an untreated risk factor for type 2 diabetes and cardiovascular disease. J Endocrinol Invest 2006; 29(3 suppl):77–82.
3. Bastard JP, Maachi M, Lagathu C, et al. Recent advances in the relationship between obesity, inflammation, and insulin resistance. Eur Cytokine Netw 2006; 17(1):4–12.
4. Lewis GF, Carpentier A, Adeli K, et al. Disordered fat storage and mobilization in the pathogenesis of insulin resistance and type 2 diabetes. Endocr Rev 2002; 23(2): 201–229.
5. Bray GA. The Metabolic Syndrome and Obesity. Totowa, NJ: Humana Press Inc, 2007.
6. Smith SR, Lovejoy JC, Greenway F, et al. Contributions of total body fat, abdominal subcutaneous adipose tissue compartments, and visceral adipose tissue to the metabolic complications of obesity. Metabolism 2001; 50(4): 425–435.
7. Smith SR, De Jonge L, Volaufova J, et al. Effect of pioglitazone on body composition and energy expenditure: a randomized controlled trial. Metabolism 2005; 54(1):24–32.
8. Bjorntorp P, Bengtsson C, Blohme G, et al. Adipose tissue fat cell size and number in relation to metabolism in randomly selected middle-aged men and women. Metabolism 1971; 20(10):927–935.
9. Frayn KN, Karpe F, Fielding BA, et al. Integrative physiology of human adipose tissue. Int J Obes Relat Metab Disord 2003; 27(8):875–888.
10. Vague J. The degree of masculine differentiation of obesities: a factor determining predisposition to diabetes, atherosclerosis, gout, and uric calculous disease. Am J Clin Nutr 1956; 4(1):20–34.
11. Pouliot MC, Despres JP, Lemieux S, et al. Waist circumference and abdominal sagittal diameter: best simple anthropometric indexes of abdominal visceral adipose tissue accumulation and related cardiovascular risk in men and women. Am J Cardiol 1994; 73(7):460–468.
12. Lean ME, Han TS, Morrison CE. Waist circumference as a measure for indicating need for weight management. BMJ 1995; 311(6998):158–161.
13. Expert Panel on Detection, Evaluation, and Treatment of High Blood Cholesterol in Adults. Executive Summary of the Third Report of the National Cholesterol Education Program (NCEP) Expert Panel on Detection, Evaluation, and Treatment of High Blood Cholesterol in Adults (Adult Treatment Panel III). JAMA 2001; 285(19):2486–2497.
14. National Institutes of Health, National Heart, Lung, and Blood Institute, North American Association for the Study of Obesity. The Practical Guide. Identification, Evaluation, and Treatment of Overweight and Obesity in Adults.

Bethesda: National Institutes of Health, 2000. NIH Publication Number 00–4084.

15. Fujimoto WY, Jablonski KA, Bray GA, et al. Diabetes Prevention Program Research Group. Body size and shape changes and the risk of diabetes in the diabetes prevention program. Diabetes 2007; 56(6):1680–1685.

16. Wajchenberg BL. Subcutaneous and visceral adipose tissue: their relation to the metabolic syndrome. Endocr Rev 2000; 21(6):697–738.

17. Reitman ML, Gavrilova O. A-ZIP/F-1 mice lacking white fat: a model for understanding lipoatrophic diabetes. Int J Obes Relat Metab Disord 2000; 24(suppl 4):S11–S14.

18. Garg A. Lipodystrophies. Am J Med 2000; 108(2): 143–152.

19. Oral EA, Simha V, Ruiz E, et al. Leptin-replacement therapy for lipodystrophy. N Engl J Med 2002; 346(8): 570–578.

20. Srinivasan S, Ogle GD, Garnett SP, et al. Features of the metabolic syndrome after childhood craniopharyngioma. J Clin Endocrinol Metab 2004; 89(1):81–86.

21. Muller HL, Bueb K, Bartels U, et al. Obesity after childhood craniopharyngioma—German multicenter study on pre-operative risk factors and quality of life. Klin Padiatr 2001; 213(4):244–249.

22. King BM. The rise, fall, and resurrection of the ventromedial hypothalamus in the regulation of feeding behavior and body weight. Physiol Behav 2006; 87(2):221–244.

23. Bray GA, Gallagher TF Jr. Manifestations of hypothalamic obesity in man: a comprehensive investigation of eight patients and a review of the literature. Medicine (Baltimore) 1975; 54(4):301–330.

24. Kanumakala S, Greaves R, Pedreira CC, et al. Fasting ghrelin levels are not elevated in children with hypothalamic obesity. J Clin Endocrinol Metab 2005; 90(5): 2691–2695.

25. Findling JW, Raff H. Cushing's syndrome: important issues in diagnosis and management. J Clin Endocrinol Metab 2006; 91(10):3746–3753.

26. Orth DN. Cushing's syndrome. N Engl J Med 1995; 332 (12):791–803 (erratum in N Engl J Med 1995; 332(22): 1527).

27. Papanicolaou DA, Yanovski JA, Cutler GB, et al. A single midnight serum cortisol measurement distinguishes Cushing's syndrome from pseudo-Cushing states. J Clin Endocrinol Metab 1998; 83 (4):1163–1167.

28. Newell-Price J, Trainer P, Besser M, et al. The diagnosis and differential diagnosis of Cushing's syndrome and pseudo-Cushing's states. Endocr Rev 1998; 19(5): 647–672.

29. Arnaldi G, Angeli A, Atkinson AB, et al. Diagnosis and complications of Cushing's syndrome: a consensus statement. J Clin Endocrinol Metab 2003; 88(12):5593–5602.

30. Findling JW, Raff H. Screening and diagnosis of Cushing's syndrome. Endocrinol Metab Clin North Am 2005; 34(2):385–402, ix–x.

31. Doucet J, Trivalle C, Chassagne P, et al. Does age play a role in clinical presentation of hypothyroidism? J Am Geriatr Soc 1994; 42(9):984–986.

32. Palmert MR, Gordon CM, Kartashov AI, et al. Screening for abnormal glucose tolerance in adolescents with polycystic ovary syndrome. J Clin Endocrinol Metab 2002; 87(3):1017–1023.

33. Gambineri A, Patton L, Vaccina A, et al. Treatment with flutamide, metformin, and their combination added to a hypocaloric diet in overweight-obese women with polycystic ovary syndrome: a randomized, 12-month, placebo-controlled study. J Clin Endocrinol Metab 2006; 91(10): 3970–3980.

34. Welt CK, Gudmundsson JA, Arason G, et al. Characterizing discrete subsets of polycystic ovary syndrome as defined by the Rotterdam criteria: the impact of weight on phenotype and metabolic features. J Clin Endocrinol Metab 2006; 91(12):4842–4848.

35. Lonn L, Johansson G, Sjostrom L, et al. Body composition and tissue distributions in growth hormone deficient adults before and after growth hormone treatment. Obes Res 1996; 4(1):45–54.

36. Allison DB, Mentore JL, Heo M, et al. Antipsychotic-induced weight gain: a comprehensive research synthesis. Am J Psychiatry 1999; 156(11):1686–1696.

37. Graham KA, Perkins DO, Edwards LJ, et al. Effect of olanzapine on body composition and energy expenditure in adults with first-episode psychosis. Am J Psychiatry 2005; 162(1):118–123.

38. Lieberman JA, Stroup TS, McEvoy JP, et al. Clinical Antipsychotic Trials of Intervention Effectiveness (CATIE) Investigators. Effectiveness of antipsychotic drugs in patients with chronic schizophrenia. N Engl J Med 2005; 353(12):1209–1223.

39. UK Prospective Diabetes Study (UKPDS) Group. Intensive blood-glucose control with sulphonylureas or insulin compared with conventional treatment and risk of complications in patients with type 2 diabetes (UKPDS 33). Lancet 1998; 352(9131):837–853 (erratum in Lancet 1999; 354(9178):602).

40. DCCT Research Group. Weight gain associated with intensive therapy in the diabetes control and complications trial. Diabetes Care 1988; 11(7):567–573.

41. Flegal KM, Troiano RP, Pamuk ER, et al. The influence of smoking cessation on the prevalence of overweight in the United States. N Engl J Med 1995; 333(18):1165–1170.

42. Prentice AM, Jebb SA. Obesity in Britain: gluttony or sloth? BMJ 1995; 311(7002):437–439.

43. Crespo CJ, Smit E, Troiano RP, et al. Television watching, energy intake, and obesity in US children: results from the third National Health and Nutrition Examination Survey, 1988–1994. Arch Pediatr Adolesc Med 2001; 155(3): 360–365.

44. Kromhout D. Changes in energy and macronutrients in 871 middle-aged men during 10 years of follow-up (the Zutphen study). Am J Clin Nutr 1983; 37(2):287–294.

45. U.S. Department of Health and Human Services. Physical Activity and Health: A Report of the Surgeon General. Atlanta: Centers for Disease Control and Prevention, National Center for Chronic Disease Prevention and Health Promotion, 1996.

46. Kromhout D, Bloemberg B, Seidell JC, et al. Physical activity and dietary fiber determine population body fat levels: the Seven Countries Study. Int J Obes Relat Metab Disord 2001; 25(3):301–306.

47. Levitsky DA, Obarzanek E, Mrdjenovic G, et al. Imprecise control of energy intake: absence of a reduction in food intake following overfeeding in young adults. Physiol Behav 2005; 84(5):669–675.

48. Tappy L. Metabolic consequences of overfeeding in humans. Curr Opin Clin Nutr Metab Care 2004; 7(6):623–628.

49. Teran-Garcia M, Despres JP, Couillard C, et al. Effects of long-term overfeeding on plasma lipoprotein levels in identical twins. Atherosclerosis 2004; 173(2):277–283.

50. Redden DT, Allison DB. The Quebec Overfeeding Study: a catalyst for new hypothesis generation. Obes Rev 2004; 5(1):1–2.

51. McDevitt RM, Bott SJ, Harding M, et al. De novo lipogenesis during controlled overfeeding with sucrose or glucose in lean and obese women. Am J Clin Nutr 2001; 74(6):737–746.

52. Schutz Y. Human overfeeding experiments: potentials and limitations in obesity research. Br J Nutr 2000; 84(2): 135–137.

53. Bouchard C, Tremblay A, Despres JP, et al. The response to long-term overfeeding in identical twins. N Engl J Med 1990; 322(21):1477–1482.

54. Pasquet P, Apfelbaum M. Recovery of initial body weight and composition after long-term massive overfeeding in men. Am J Clin Nutr 1994; 60(6):861–863.

55. Bray GA. The Obese Patient. Philadelphia: WB Saunders, Co., 1976.

56. Nishizawa T, Akaoka I, Nishida Y, et al. Some factors related to obesity in the Japanese sumo wrestler. Am J Clin Nutr 1976; 29(10):1167–1174.

57. Bray GA, Popkin BM. Dietary fat intake does affect obesity! Am J Clin Nutr 1998; 68(6):1157–1173.

58. Astrup A. The role of dietary fat in the prevention and treatment of obesity. Efficacy and safety of low-fat diets. Int J Obes Relat Metab Disord 2001; 25(suppl 1):S46–50.

59. Sparti A, Windhauser MM, Champagne CM, et al. Effect of an acute reduction in carbohydrate intake on subsequent food intake in healthy men. Am J Clin Nutr 1997; 66(5): 1144–1150.

60. Vartanian LR, Schwartz MB, Brownell KD. Effects of soft drink consumption on nutrition and health: a systematic review and meta-analysis. Am J Public Health 2007; 97(4):667–675.

61. Jenkins DJ, Jenkins AL, Wolever TM, et al. Low glycemic index: lente carbohydrates and physiological effects of altered food frequency. Am J Clin Nutr 1994; 59(3 suppl): 706S–709S.

62. Roberts SB, Pi-Sunyer FX, Dreher M, et al. Physiology of fat replacement and fat reduction: effects of dietary fat and fat substitutes on energy regulation. Nutr Rev 1998; 56(5 pt 2):S29–S41.

63. Wolk A, Manson JE, Stampfer MJ, et al. Long-term intake of dietary fiber and decreased risk of coronary heart disease among women. JAMA 1999; 281(21):1998–2004.

64. Salmeron J, Manson JE, Stampfer MJ, et al. Dietary fiber, glycemic load, and risk of non-insulin-dependent diabetes mellitus in women. JAMA 1997; 277(6):472–477.

65. McCarron DA, Morris CD, Henry HJ, et al. Blood pressure and nutrient intake in the United States. Science 1984; 224(4656):1392–1398.

66. Zemel MB, Shi H, Greer B, et al. Regulation of adiposity by dietary calcium. FASEB J 2000; 14(9):1132–1138.

67. Davies KM, Heaney RP, Recker RR, et al. Calcium intake and body weight. J Clin Endocrinol Metab 2000; 85(12): 4635–4638.

68. Zemel MB, Thompson W, Milstead A, et al. Calcium and dairy acceleration of weight and fat loss during energy restriction in obese adults. Obes Res 2004; 12(4):582–590.

69. Zemel MB, Richards J, Milstead A, et al. Effects of calcium and dairy on body composition and weight loss in African-American adults. Obes Res 2005; 13(7): 1218–1225.

70. Zemel MB, Richards J, Mathis S, et al. Dairy augmentation of total and central fat loss in obese subjects. Int J Obes (Lond) 2005; 29(4):391–397.

71. Shapses SA, Heshka S, Heymsfield SB. Effect of calcium supplementation on weight and fat loss in women. J Clin Endocrinol Metab 2004; 89(2):632–637.

72. Barr SI. Increased dairy product or calcium intake: is body weight or composition affected in humans? J Nutr 2003; 133(1):245S–248S.

73. Bowen J, Noakes M, Clifton PM. Effect of calcium and dairy foods in high protein, energy-restricted diets on weight loss and metabolic parameters in overweight adults. Int J Obes (Lond) 2005; 29(8):957–965.

74. Thompson WG, Rostad Holdman N, Janzow DJ, et al. Effect of energy-reduced diets high in dairy products and fiber on weight loss in obese adults. Obes Res 2005; 13(8): 1344–1353.

75. Shapses SA, Von Thun NL, Heymsfield SB, et al. Bone turnover and density in obese premenopausal women during moderate weight loss and calcium supplementation. J Bone Miner Res 2001; 16(7):1329–1336.

76. Jenkins DJ, Wolever TM, Vuksan V, et al. Nibbling versus gorging: metabolic advantages of increased meal frequency. N Engl J Med 1989; 321(14):929–934.

77. Lawson OJ, Williamson DA, Champagne CM, et al. The association of body weight, dietary intake, and energy expenditure with dietary restraint and disinhibition. Obes Res 1995; 3(2):153–161.

78. Williamson DA, Lawson OJ, Brooks ER, et al. Association of body mass with dietary restraint and disinhibition. Appetite 1995; 25(1):31–41.

79. Yanovski SZ, Gormally JF, Leser MS, et al. Binge eating disorder affects outcome of comprehensive very-low-calorie diet treatment. Obes Res 1994; 2(3):205–212.

80. Allison KC, Grilo CM, Masheb RM, et al. Binge eating disorder and night eating syndrome: a comparative study of disordered eating. J Consult Clin Psychol 2005; 73(6): 1107–1115.

81. Stunkard AJ, Grace WJ, Wolff HG. The night-eating syndrome: a pattern of food intake among certain obese patients. Am J Med 1955; 19(1):78–86.

82. Stunkard A. Two eating disorders: binge eating disorder and the night eating syndrome. Appetite 2000; 34(3):333–334.

83. Lundgren JD, Allison KC, Crow S, et al. Prevalence of the night eating syndrome in a psychiatric population. Am J Psychiatry 2006; 163(1):156–158.

84. Allison KC, Ahima RS, O'Reardon JP, et al. Neuroendocrine profiles associated with energy intake, sleep, and stress in the night eating syndrome. J Clin Endocrinol Metab 2005; 90(11):6214–6217.

85. Partonen T, Lonnqvist J. Seasonal affective disorder. Lancet 1998; 352(9137):1369–1374.

86. Jeffery RW, Forster JL, Folsom AR, et al. The relationship between social status and body mass index in the Minnesota Heart Health Program. Int J Obes 1989; 13(1):59–67.

87. Obarzanek E, Schreiber GB, Crawford PB, et al. Energy intake and physical activity in relation to indexes of body fat: the National Heart, Lung, and Blood Institute Growth and Health Study. Am J Clin Nutr 1994; 60(1):15–22.

88. Hinney A, Schmidt A, Nottebom K, et al. Several mutations in the melanocortin-4 receptor gene including a nonsense and a frameshift mutation associated with dominantly inherited obesity in humans. J Clin Endocrinol Metab 1999; 84(4):1483–1486.

89. Vaisse C, Clement K, Guy-Grand B, et al. A frameshift mutation in human MC4R is associated with a dominant form of obesity. Nat Genet 1998; 20(2):113–114.

90. Yeo GS, Farooqi IS, Aminian S, et al. A frameshift mutation in MC4R associated with dominantly inherited human obesity. Nat Genet 1998; 20(2):111–112.

91. Farooqi IS, Yeo GS, Keogh JM, et al. Dominant and recessive inheritance of morbid obesity associated with melanocortin 4 receptor deficiency. J Clin Invest 2000; 106(2):271–279.

92. Krude H, Biebermann H, Luck W, et al. Severe early-onset obesity, adrenal insufficiency and red hair pigmentation caused by POMC mutations in humans. Nat Genet 1998; 19(2):155–157.

93. Montague CT, Farooqi IS, Whitehead JP, et al. Congenital leptin deficiency is associated with severe early-onset obesity in humans. Nature 1997; 387(6636):903–908.

94. Ozata M, Ozdemir IC, Licinio J. Human leptin deficiency caused by a missense mutation: multiple endocrine defects, decreased sympathetic tone, and immune system dysfunction indicate new targets for leptin action, greater central than peripheral resistance to the effects of leptin, and spontaneous correction of leptin-mediated defects. J Clin Endocrinol Metab 1999; 84(10):3686–3695 (erratum in J Clin Endocrinol Metab 2000; 85(1):416).

95. Strobel A, Issad T, Camoin L, et al. A leptin missense mutation associated with hypogonadism and morbid obesity. Nat Genet 1998; 18(3):213–215.

96. Farooqi IS, Matarese G, Lord GM, et al. Beneficial effects of leptin on obesity, T cell hyporesponsiveness, and neuroendocrine/metabolic dysfunction of human congenital leptin deficiency. J Clin Invest 2002; 110(8):1093–1103.

97. Farooqi IS, Keogh JM, Kamath S, et al. Partial leptin deficiency and human adiposity. Nature 2001; 414(6859):34–35.

98. Farooqi IS, Wangensteen T, Collins S, et al. Clinical and molecular genetic spectrum of congenital deficiency of the leptin receptor. N Engl J Med 2007; 356(3):237–247.

99. Kalra SP, Kalra PS. Gene-transfer technology: a preventive neurotherapy to curb obesity, ameliorate metabolic syndrome and extend life expectancy. Trends Pharmacol Sci 2005; 26(10):488–495.

100. Ristow M, Muller-Wieland D, Pfeiffer A, et al. Obesity associated with a mutation in a genetic regulator of adipocyte differentiation. N Engl J Med 1998; 339(14):953–959.

101. Jackson RS, Creemers JW, Ohagi S, et al. Obesity and impaired prohormone processing associated with mutations in the human prohormone convertase 1 gene. Nat Genet 1997; 16(3):303–306.

102. Snyder EE, Walts B, Perusse L, et al. The human obesity gene map: the 2003 update. Obes Res 2004; 12(3):369–439.

103. Gunay-Aygun M, Cassidy SB, Nicholls RD. Prader-Willi and other syndromes associated with obesity and mental retardation. Behav Genet 1997; 27(4):307–324.

104. Cummings DE, Clement K, Purnell JQ, et al. Elevated plasma ghrelin levels in Prader Willi syndrome. Nat Med 2002; 8(7):643–644.

105. Theodoro MF, Talebizadeh Z, Butler MG. Body composition and fatness patterns in Prader-Willi syndrome: comparison with simple obesity. Obesity (Silver Spring) 2006; 14(10):1685–1690.

106. Festen DA, de Weerd AW, van den Bossche RA, et al. Sleep-related breathing disorders in prepubertal children with Prader-Willi syndrome and effects of growth hormone treatment. J Clin Endocrinol Metab 2006; 91(12):4911–4915.

107. Park WH, Oh YJ, Kim GY, et al. Obestatin is not elevated or correlated with insulin in children with Prader-Willi syndrome. J Clin Endocrinol Metab 2007; 92(1):229–234.

108. Grace C, Beales P, Summerbell C, et al. The effect of Bardet-Biedl syndrome on the components of energy balance. Int J Obes Related Metab Disord 2001; 25(suppl 2):S42.

109. Green JS, Parfrey PS, Harnett JD, et al. The cardinal manifestations of Bardet-Biedl syndrome, a form of Laurence-Moon-Biedl syndrome. N Engl J Med 1989; 321(15):1002–1009.

110. O'Dea D, Parfrey PS, Harnett JD, et al. The importance of renal impairment in the natural history of Bardet-Biedl syndrome. Am J Kidney Dis 1996; 27(6):776–783.

111. Kim JC, Badano JL, Sibold S, et al. The Bardet-Biedl protein BBS4 targets cargo to the pericentriolar region and is required for microtubule anchoring and cell cycle progression. Nat Genet 2004; 36(5):462–470.

112. Katsanis N, Beales PL, Woods MO, et al. Mutations in MKKS cause obesity, retinal dystrophy and renal malformations associated with Bardet-Biedl syndrome. Nat Genet 2000; 26(1):67–70.

113. Wilson RS. Twin growth: initial deficit, recovery, and trends in concordance from birth to nine years. Ann Hum Biol 1979; 6(3):205–220.

114. Blank A, Grave GD, Metzger BE. Effects of gestational diabetes on perinatal morbidity reassessed. Report of the International Workshop on Adverse Perinatal Outcomes of Gestational Diabetes Mellitus, December 3–4, 1992. Diabetes Care 1995; 18(1):127–129.

115. Barker DJ, Hales CN, Fall CH, et al. Type 2 (non-insulin-dependent) diabetes mellitus, hypertension and hyperlipidaemia (syndrome X): relation to reduced fetal growth. Diabetologia 1993; 36(1):62–67.

116. von Kries R, Koletzko B, Sauerwald T, et al. Breast feeding and obesity: cross sectional study. BMJ 1999; 319(7203):147–150.

117. Gillman MW, Rifas-Shiman SL, Camargo CA, et al. Risk of overweight among adolescents who were breastfed as infants. JAMA 2001; 285(19):2461–2467.

118. Hediger ML, Overpeck MD, Kuczmarski RJ, et al. Association between infant breastfeeding and overweight in young children. JAMA 2001; 285(19):2453–2460.

119. Bergmann KE, Bergmann RL, Von Kries R, et al. Early determinants of childhood overweight and adiposity in a birth cohort study: role of breast-feeding. Int J Obes Relat Metab Disord 2003; 27(2):162–172.

120. Rogers I, EURO-BLCS Study Group. The influence of birthweight and intrauterine environment on adiposity and fat distribution in later life. Int J Obes Relat Metab Disord 2003; 27(7):755–777.

121. Rodekamp E, Harder T, Kohlhoff R, et al. Long-term impact of breast-feeding on body weight and glucose tolerance in children of diabetic mothers: role of the late neonatal period and early infancy. Diabetes Care 2005; 28(6):1457–1462.

122. Ailhaud G, Guesnet P. Fatty acid composition of fats is an early determinant of childhood obesity: a short review and an opinion. Obes Rev 2004; 5(1):21–26.

123. Mamun AA, Lawlor DA, O'Callaghan MJ, et al. Family and early life factors associated with changes in overweight status between ages 5 and 14 years: findings from the Mater University Study of Pregnancy and its outcomes. Int J Obes (Lond) 2005; 29(5):475–482.

124. Whitaker RC, Wright JA, Pepe MS, et al. Predicting obesity in young adulthood from childhood and parental obesity. N Engl J Med 1997; 337(13):869–873.

125. Toschke AM, Beyerlein A, von Kries R. Children at high risk for overweight: a classification and regression trees analysis approach. Obes. Res 2005; 13(7): 1270–1274.

126. Must A, Jacques PF, Dallal GE, et al. Long-term morbidity and mortality of overweight adolescents. A follow-up of the Harvard Growth Study of 1922 to 1935. N Engl J Med 1992; 327(19):1350–1355.

127. Smith DE, Lewis CE, Caveny JL, et al. Longitudinal changes in adiposity associated with pregnancy. The CARDIA Study. Coronary Artery Risk Development in Young Adults Study. JAMA 1994; 271(22):1747–1751.

128. Brown JE, Kaye SA, Folsom AR. Parity-related weight change in women. Int J Obes Relat Metab Disord 1992; 16(9):627–631.

129. Williamson DF, Madans J, Pamuk E, et al. A prospective study of childbearing and 10-year weight gain in US white women 25 to 45 years of age. Int J Obes Relat Metab Disord 1994; 18(8):561–569.

130. Reubinoff BE, Grubstein A, Meirow D, et al. Effects of low-dose estrogen oral contraceptives on weight, body composition, and fat distribution in young women. Fertil Steril 1995; 63(3):516–521.

131. Aloia JF, Vaswani A, Russo L, et al. The influence of menopause and hormonal replacement therapy on body cell mass and body fat mass. Am J Obstet Gynecol 1995; 172(3):896–900.

132. Haarbo J, Christiansen C. Treatment-induced cyclic variations in serum lipids, lipoproteins, and apolipoproteins after 2 years of combined hormone replacement therapy: exaggerated cyclic variations in smokers. Obstet Gynecol 1992; 80(4):639–644.

133. National Task Force on the Prevention and Treatment of Obesity. Weight cycling. JAMA 1994; 272(15): 1196–1202.

134. Williamson DF. Descriptive epidemiology of body weight and weight change in U.S. adults. Ann Intern Med 1993; 119(7 pt 2):646–649.

135. NHLBI Obesity Education Initiative Expert Panel on the Identification, Evaluation, and Treatment of Overweight and Obesity in Adults. Clinical guidelines on the identification, evaluation, and treatment of overweight and obesity in adults—the evidence report. Obes Res 1998; (6 suppl 2):51S–209S.

136. Bray GA, Gray DS. Obesity. Part II—Treatment. West J Med 1988; 149(5):555–571.

137. US Department of Health and Human Services. Screening for obesity. In: Guide to Clinical Preventive Services. 2nd ed. Washington D.C.: DHEW, 1989:219–229.

138. American Obesity Association and Shape Up America! Guidance for Treatment of Adult Obesity. Available at: http://www.shapeup.org/profcenter/eguide/eguide.php. Accessed August 28, 2007.

139. World Health Organization. Obesity: Preventing and Managing the Global Epidemic. Geneva: World Health Organization, 1998.

140. AACE/ACE Obesity Task Force. AACE/ACE position statement on the prevention, diagnosis, and treatment of obesity (1998 Revision). Endocr Pract 1998; 4(5): 297–350.

141. US Department of Health and Human Services. Body measurements. In: Clinician's Handbook of Preventive Services: Put Prevention into Family Practice. Washington D.C.: US Department of Health and Human Services, 1994:141–146.

142. Institute of Medicine, Thomas P, ed. Weighing the Options: Criteria for Evaluating Weight-Management Programs. Washington D.C.: National Academy Press, 1995.

143. Willett WC, Manson JE, Stampfer MJ, et al. Weight, weight change, and coronary heart disease in women. Risk within the 'normal' weight range. JAMA 1995; 273(6):461–465.

144. Blair SN, Kohl HW, Paffenbarger RS, et al. Physical fitness and all-cause mortality. A prospective study of healthy men and women. JAMA 1989; 262(17): 2395–2401.

145. Roche A, Heymsfield SB, Lohman T. Human Body Composition. Champaign, IL: Human Kinetics, 1996.

146. Gallagher D, Heymsfield SB, Heo M, et al. Healthy percentage body fat ranges: an approach for developing guidelines based on body mass index. Am J Clin Nutr 2000; 72(3):694–701.

147. Brownell KD. Dieting readiness. Weight Control Digest 1990; 1:1–9.

148. Galuska DA, Will JC, Serdula MK, et al. Are health care professionals advising obese patients to lose weight? JAMA 1999; 282(16):1576–1578.

149. Foster GD, Wadden TA, Vogt RA, et al. What is a reasonable weight loss? Patients' expectations and evaluations of obesity treatment outcomes. J Consult Clin Psychol 1997; 65(1):79–85.

150. Pories WJ, MacDonald KG Jr., Morgan EJ, et al. Surgical treatment of obesity and its effect on diabetes: 10-y follow-up. Am J Clin Nutr 1992; 55(2 suppl):582S–585S.

151. Bjorvell H, Rossner S. A ten-year follow-up of weight change in severely obese subjects treated in a combined behavioural modification programme. Int J Obes Relat Metab Disord 1992; 16(8):623–625.

152. Weintraub M, Sundaresan PR, Madan M, et al. Long-term weight control study. I (weeks 0 to 34). The enhancement of behavior modification, caloric restriction, and exercise by fenfluramine plus phentermine versus placebo. Clin Pharmacol Ther 1992; 51(5):586–594.

153. Garrow JS, Gardiner GT. Maintenance of weight loss in obese patients after jaw wiring. Br Med J (Clin Res Ed) 1981; 282(6267):858–860.

154. Davis BR, Blaufox MD, Oberman A, et al. Reduction in long-term antihypertensive medication requirements. Effects of weight reduction by dietary intervention in overweight persons with mild hypertension. Arch Intern Med 1993; 153(15):1773–1782.

155. Bray G. Drug treatment of obesity: don't throw the baby out with the bath water. Am J Clin Nutr 1998; 67(1): 1–2.

156. Rossner S. Factors determining the long-term outcome of obesity treatment. In: Bjorntorp P, Brodoff BN, eds. Obesity. Philadelphia: JB Lippincott, 1992:712–719.

157. Epstein LH, Valoski A, Wing RR, et al. Ten-year follow-up of behavioral, family-based treatment for obese children. JAMA 1990; 264(19):2519–2523.

158. Nelson D. Cushing's Disease. In: Endocrinology; deGroot LJ, ed. Philadelphia: W.B. Saunders; 1995, p. 1661.

159. Farooqi IS, O'Rahilly S. Monogenic obesity in humans. Annu Rev Med 2005; 56:443–458.

2

Waist Girth: A Critical Evaluation of Usefulness

MARIE-FRANCE HIVERT

Endocrinology and Metabolism Division, Department of Internal Medicine, Université de Sherbrooke, Sherbrooke, Quebec, Canada

JAMES B. MEIGS

General Medicine Division, Department of Medicine, Massachusetts General Hospital and Harvard Medical School, Boston, Massachusetts, U.S.A.

OVERVIEW: THE PROBLEM OF OBESITY

Obesity has reached epidemic proportions worldwide. Recent World Health Organization (WHO) projections estimate that globally in 2005 approximately 1.6 billion adults older than 15 years were overweight and at least 400 million adults were obese (1). The WHO also underlines that this pandemic, once considered a problem only in high-income countries, is now dramatically on the rise in low- and middle-income countries, particularly in urban settings (1). In the United States, the latest National Health and Nutrition Examination Surveys (NHANES; 2003–2004) data demonstrate that two-thirds of the adult population have a body mass index (BMI) of 25 kg/m^2 or higher and 32.2% are obese (BMI > 30 kg/m^2) (2).

The health risks related to overweight and obesity may be defined by BMI, but increasing importance has been given to the central fat accumulation. Waist circumference (WC) has dramatically risen in the American population over the past decades. In men, the mean WC went from 89 cm in 1960 to 99 cm in 2000, while in women, mean WC went from 77 to 94 cm during the same period (3). Unfortunately, the same trends have been observed in U.S. children and adolescents (4).

Abdominal obesity was included as one of the five criteria defining the metabolic syndrome by the National Cholesterol Education Program–Adult Treatment Panel III (NCEP-ATP III) in 2001. They defined excess abdominal adiposity as a WC >102 cm in men and >88 cm in women (5). More recently, the International Diabetes Federation (IDF) proposed that the abdominal obesity was the essential criteria for the definition of metabolic syndrome, and they lowered the WC cutoffs for individuals of European origin (men >94 cm and women >80 cm), with different cutoffs for different ethnic populations (6).

In this chapter, we will review the scientific evidence linking visceral adiposity (measured directly by imaging) to adverse metabolic profiles and outcomes, the reliability of WC as a surrogate marker for visceral adiposity, the predictability of WC for clinical endpoints, and the usefulness of WC for clinical evaluation.

METABOLIC CONSEQUENCES OF VISCERAL ADIPOSITY ASSESSED DIRECTLY BY IMAGING

There is abundant evidence that visceral adipose tissue (VAT) is related to many adverse metabolic markers. Radiological imaging is the most accurate way to evaluate the distribution of adipose tissue (7). Visceral adipose tissue can be estimated by magnetic resonance imaging (MRI) or by computerized tomography (CT). By definition, VAT should include all the adipose tissue distributed in the three body cavities containing viscera: intrathoracic, intra-abdominal, and intrapelvic (8). In humans, most investigators using imaging to evaluate VAT volume have included intra-abdominal plus intrapelvic adipose tissue or only the intra-abdominal compartment. Multiple slice imaging offers the opportunity to estimate the actual volume of adipose tissue in the different compartments, although many investigators choose to do single slice imaging to reduce cost, time, and exposure to radiation. The most often used imaging to evaluate VAT area is a single-slice CT at the level of L4-L5 because of relative availability and rapidity compared to MRI (Fig. 1).

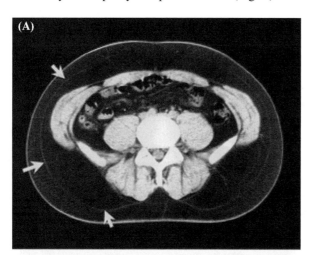

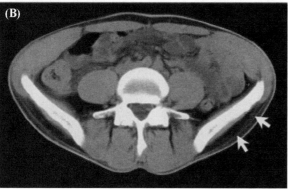

Figure 1 Abdominal axial CT scans of an obese (**A**) and a thin subject (**B**). Subcutaneous adipose tissue is divided into superficial and deep subcutaneous adipose tissue by a fascial plane (*white arrows*). *Source*: Adapted from Ref. 8.

Visceral Adiposity and Lipid Profiles

Accumulation of VAT has been associated with adverse lipid profiles in many different populations. For instance, in a cohort of 137 men with a wide range of age and BMI, Hunter et al. showed that CT-assessed intra-abdominal fat was positively related to total cholesterol, HDL, LDL, IDL, VLDL, and triglyceride levels, even after adjusting for age, fat mass, and fat-free mass (9). Conversely, BMI and waist-to-hip ratio (WHR) were related to lipid profile, but the relationship disappeared after adjustment for intra-abdominal fat, indicating that these two variables obtain their significant relationship through intra-abdominal fat (9). Splitting a cohort of 178 nonobese women into four age groups, DeNino et al. have shown that both VAT and subcutaneous adipose tissue (SAT) increase with age strata and that the observed unfavorable changes in plasma lipids with age were strongly associated with the increase in visceral adiposity (10).

In more selected populations, excess visceral fat has been related to low HDL cholesterol in premenopausal (11) and peri- or postmenopausal women (12). Postmenopausal women with increased visceral fat also display high triglycerides (13,14) and high apo B levels (14). Visceral fat was shown to be associated with an adverse lipid in cohorts of children and adolescents (15–18) as well as in elderly (19). In obese men (20) and women (21), visceral obesity is related to high triglycerides. An adverse lipid profile has been related to visceral fat in populations with a high prevalence of the metabolic syndrome (22), in glucose intolerant individuals (23), in patients with type 2 diabetes (24), and in women with polycystic ovarian syndrome (25). Heterozygotes for familial hypercholesterolemia have shown to have increased triglycerides and even more elevated LDL if they have accumulated intra-abdominal fat (26).

Visceral Adiposity and Insulin Resistance

The link between central obesity and insulin resistance has been well investigated with the help of adipose tissue imaging. Epidemiological studies have related increased VAT to high fasting insulin in various populations: from adolescents (18) to elderly (27) and among people of various ethnicities (14,28,29). The HEalth, RIsk factors, exercise Training And GEnetics (HERITAGE) Family Study found that common genes and/or nongenetic factors influence both abdominal visceral fat and fasting insulin level (30). Longitudinal follow-up of children for over three years has demonstrated that the change in fasting insulin levels was associated to change in both visceral and subcutaneous abdominal fat (31).

Surrogate markers of insulin sensitivity, such as the quantitative insulin sensitivity check index (QUICKI), have been correlated with abdominal adipose tissue (32). Many investigators have used the oral glucose tolerance test (OGTT) to evaluate the association between visceral adiposity and insulin resistance. Visceral adipose tissue is related to decreased glucose tolerance assessed by OGTT in both men and women with a wide range of BMI (12,33–37). The OGTT performed by obese women with a higher degree of VAT (matched for BMI to women with lower VAT) showed greater plasma glucose area under the curve and higher two-hour insulin levels (34).

In the Insulin Resistance Atherosclerosis Study (IRAS) of Hispanic and African-American families, insulin sensitivity was assessed by the frequently sampled intravenous glucose tolerance test with minimal model analyses (38). Visceral adipose tissue, SAT, and their joint interaction were all associated with insulin resistance, but VAT was the strongest correlate. Subcutaneous adipose tissue was associated with acute insulin response but explained a minor part of the effect on insulin secretion. Finally, VAT was an important determinant of the disposition index and was shown to be the fat depot with a stronger association with insulin resistance than SAT (38).

The gold standard to evaluate insulin sensitivity is the euglycemic hyperinsulinemic clamp study. Once again, the association between visceral adiposity and insulin resistance has been investigated in both genders (10,33,39–41), in various ethnic backgrounds (42–45), and from adolescence (17,46) to postmenopausal status (13,47,48), although sometimes with conflicting results. Association of increased VAT to elevated insulin resistance assessed by clamp has been demonstrated in patients with obesity (48–50), type 2 diabetes (44,51,52) and in offspring of parents with diabetes (53). Some authors state that subcutaneous truncal fat is as important as visceral fat in determining insulin resistance (reviewed in Ref. 54), but not all investigators have found significant relationships between SAT and clamp-measured insulin resistance (48–50). When partitioning SAT into deep and superficial (delimitated by fascia, see Fig. 2), both VAT and deep SAT, but not superficial SAT, are strongly correlated to fasting insulin levels (55) and to insulin-stimulated glucose utilization (33). These observations have led some investigators to hypothesize that deep SAT might be more metabolically active than superficial SAT and might explain some of the discordant findings from the different clamp studies.

Visceral Adiposity and Other Metabolic Markers

Central obesity and the metabolic syndrome are also characterized by a proinflammatory state. Many plasma inflammatory proteins have been identified in the process of trying to understand the pathophysiology of links between adiposity and cardiovascular and metabolic risk.

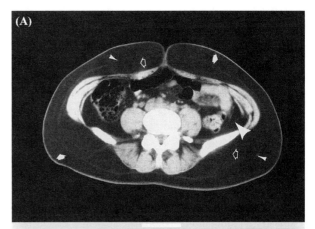
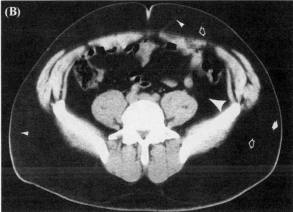

Figure 2 Representative cross-sectional abdominal CT scans of a lean (**A**) and an obese (**B**) research volunteer are shown with demarcations of VAT (*large arrowheads*), deep subcutaneous (*open arrows*), and superficial subcutaneous (*closed arrows*) AT depots. The fascia (*small arrowhead*) within subcutaneous abdominal AT was used to distinguish superficial from deep depot. In the two CT scans shown, the area of superficial subcutaneous AT was similar (144 vs. 141 cm^2), whereas areas for deep subcutaneous (126 vs. 273 cm^2) and VAT (84 vs. 153 cm^2) were quite different. Insulin-stimulated glucose metabolism was 6.1 and 4.0 mg/min/kgFFM in lean and obese volunteers, respectively. *Abbreviations*: VAT, visceral adipose tissue; AT, adipose tissue; FFM, fat-free mass. *Source*: Adapted from Ref. 33.

C-reactive protein (CRP) was one of the first inflammatory markers associated with metabolic syndrome. Accumulation of VAT measured by imaging was associated with elevated CRP in healthy individuals (56,57), in type 2 diabetic patients (58), and in offspring of parents with diabetes (53). Longitudinal follow-up of patients with diabetes showed that change in CRP was correlated with change in both visceral and subcutaneous abdominal fat area (58).

Adiponectin is a protein produced by adipocytes and, in contrast to most of the adipokines, its plasma concentration is decreased in individuals with obesity, insulin resistance, and diabetes. In studies with CT-measured adipose tissue, low adiponectin level has been associated with increased visceral fat in both lean and obese individuals of various ethnic backgrounds (42,59–61) and offspring of parents with diabetes (53). In one study partitioning the distribution of adipose tissue by CT, visceral fat was related to adiponectin while subcutaneous fat was related to leptin (62). MRI allows an even more refined subdivision of abdominal adipose tissue masses. Plasma adiponectin levels are inversely related to intra-peritoneal, posterior subcutaneous, and anterior subcutaneous abdominal adipose tissue, with the stronger correlation being accorded to posterior subcutaneous subdivision in multiple regression models analysis (63).

Obesity and metabolic syndrome are also characterized by an alteration of the fibrinolytic cascade. For instance, plasminogen activator inhibitor 1 (PAI-1) is positively correlated to VAT in healthy men and women (64–66) as well as in obese (67) and diabetic patients (68).

Visceral adiposity may also reflect increased systemic oxidative stress. Urinary 8-epi-PGF2 alpha, a biomarker of systemic oxidative stress, is associated with overall obesity (18) and has been correlated with VAT (69), and plasma levels of group IIA phospholipase A_2 were higher in men with increased VAT. These two factors were strong correlates of oxidized LDL levels (70).

Nonalcoholic fatty liver disease has been associated with abdominal obesity and metabolic syndrome and is often associated with elevated inflammatory markers. The association between hepatic steatosis and increased plasma biomarkers of inflammation or endothelial dysfunction (CRP, von Willebrand factor, fibrinogen, PAI-1) may be mediated by the measured VAT (71). Abnormal liver enzyme tests were correlated with VAT in the Swedish Obese Subjects study (72), especially in women. Increased hepatic fat (evaluated by MRI) and elevated alanine transaminase have been associated with VAT in both obese children (73) and adolescents (74).

Visceral Adiposity and the Metabolic Syndrome

So far we have examined the association of adipose tissue measured by CT or MRI with separate components of the metabolic syndrome. Increased VAT has also been associated with clustering of metabolic risk factors, including abnormal glucose tolerance, lipid profile, and elevated blood pressure (36,75,76). In 2000, Kelley et al. showed that when partitioning the adipose tissue measurements, VAT and deep SAT follows a highly congruent pattern of association with levels of glucose and insulin area under the OGTT curve, mean arterial blood pressure, apo B, HDL cholesterol, and triglyceride, while superficial SAT had markedly weaker associations with all these parameters (33). In another study, von Eyben et al. compared four

different measurements of adiposity: BMI, body fat percentage measured using a dual energy X-ray absorptiometry (DEXA) scanner, WHR, and intra-abdominal adipose tissue area measured using CT scanning. Only intra-abdominal adipose tissue area was significantly associated with levels of systolic blood pressure, diastolic blood pressure, fasting blood glucose, HDL cholesterol, serum triglyceride, and PAI-1 (64). Clustering of impaired glycemic and lipid profiles has been correlated with visceral adiposity in diverse age groups from obese adolescents (17) to peri- and postmenopausal women (12,14).

Ribeiro-Filho et al. showed a strong correlation in obese women between VAT and metabolic syndrome, defined as presence of abdominal obesity and at least two of hypertension, dyslipidemia, and glucose intolerance and/or hyperinsulinemia (34). In logistic regression analysis, VAT and WC were both independent correlates of metabolic syndrome, while the BMI and SAT were not (34).

In a cohort of healthy men and women with a wide range of age and BMI, Carr et al. showed that in multivariate models, insulin sensitivity, intra-abdominal fat, and abdominal subcutaneous fat area were all associated with NCEP-ATP III metabolic syndrome (77). They also demonstrated that intra-abdominal fat determined by CT was associated with all five of the metabolic syndrome criteria independently of insulin sensitivity and SAT (77). Goodpaster et al. showed that CT-measured VAT was associated with NCEP-ATP III metabolic syndrome in a large cohort of older men and women with a wide BMI range (78). Greater amount of VAT was associated with a higher prevalence of metabolic syndrome in all three BMI categories (normal weight, overweight, and obese), but the association was weaker among obese men and women (Fig. 3). The odd ratios predicting metabolic syndrome were lower or nonsignificant for the association between subcutaneous abdominal adipose tissue (78).

Recently, Kuk et al. showed that VAT volume is strongly associated with the metabolic syndrome defined by either the NCEP-ATP III or IDF criteria (79). They measured abdominal adipose tissue volume and multiple levels of single axial images of 85 men and found that total VAT volume and VAT measures at the levels T12-L1 or L1-L2 were strongly associated with either definition of metabolic syndrome. Subcutaneous abdominal adipose tissue was only weakly associated with metabolic syndrome (79).

CLINICAL OUTCOMES ASSOCIATED WITH VISCERAL ADIPOSITY ASSESSED DIRECTLY BY IMAGING

Visceral Adiposity and Diabetes

In the preceding sections, we reviewed evidence linking visceral adiposity with an adverse metabolic and

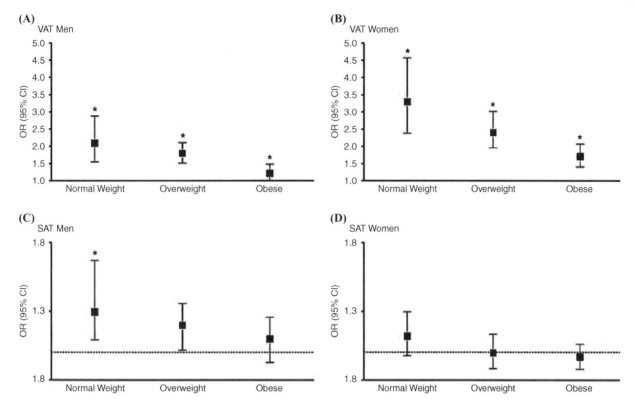

Figure 3 ORs, adjusted for age and race, and 95% CIs of having metabolic syndrome with increasing VAT and SAT by 50 cm^2 in normal-weight, overweight, and obese men and women. The dashed line represents an OR of 1. Asterisk denotes significant ($p < 0.05$) OR. Note the different scales for VAT and SAT. *Abbreviations*: OR, odds ratio; CI, confidence interval; VAT, visceral adipose tissue; SAT, subcutaneous abdominal adipose tissue. *Source*: Adapted from Ref. 78.

cardiovascular risk profile. Visceral fat is also associated with adverse disease outcomes. The correlation between measured VAT and diabetes has been investigated in a few cohort and case-control studies. Increased VAT has been associated with impaired glucose tolerance (IGT) or diabetes mellitus (DM) diagnosed by an OGTT in cohorts of men (80) and women (12). Goodpaster et al. have shown that elderly people with IGT or DM had higher VAT and SAT than normal glucose tolerant individuals (27). The association between VAT and diabetes has been reproduced in various ethnic backgrounds, including Asian Indians (81) and Japanese-Americans (82–84).

Very few longitudinal studies have explored the link between radiological measurements of VAT and IGT or diabetes incidence (85). Prospective follow-up over up to 10 years of second and third generation of Japanese-Americans demonstrated that intra-abdominal adipose tissue predicted the incidence of new diabetes, even after adjustment of potential cofactors (86). In this study, significant positive associations between intra-abdominal fat area and incidence of diabetes remained even after adjustment for any of the other adiposity measures (subcutaneous abdominal fat, non-intra-abdominal fat, total fat, or BMI) (86).

Visceral Adiposity and Cardiovascular Diseases

Visceral adipose tissue measured by imaging has been correlated with many cardiovascular risk factors, but few studies have examined directly the association of visceral fat and cardiovascular disease (CVD) outcomes. Some data suggest an association of intra-abdominal adipose tissue with subclinical atherosclerosis determined by electron beam CT–assessed coronary artery calcium scores (87,88). In obese individuals with a recent diagnosis of DM, increased VAT was shown to be related to arterial stiffness by pulse wave velocity, but not to the carotid artery intimal-medial thickness, plaque index, or to coronary and aortic calcification (89). In patients heterozygous for familial hypercholesterolemia, greater amounts of VAT were associated with a more severe coronary stenosis index score evaluated by angiography (26). Several cross-sectional studies have shown that patients with coronary artery disease have greater visceral fat volumes than patients without it (22,36,90).

Again, longitudinal data are sparse. In one study, Fujimoto et al. followed 175 Japanese-American men for up to 10 years for coronary heart disease (CHD) events (91). In univariate analysis, the risk of developing CHD was significantly associated with intra-abdominal fat, glucose levels (fasting and 2-hour OGTT), HDL, triglycerides, blood pressure (diastolic and systolic), and diabetes at baseline. In regression models adjusted for age and BMI, intra-abdominal fat remained significantly associated with incidence of CHD (91).

Increased visceral fat has also been associated with increased risk of all-cause mortality. In a cohort of middle-aged men followed for two years, visceral fat, abdominal subcutaneous fat, liver fat, and WC were significant individual predictors of mortality after controlling for age and length of follow-up. In a model including all three fat measures (subcutaneous, visceral, and liver fat), age, and length of follow-up, only visceral fat [odds ratio (OR) per SD, 1.93; 1.15 to 3.23] was a significant predictor of mortality (92).

WC AS A SURROGATE MARKER FOR VAT

We have seen that VAT is associated with many metabolic risk factors, metabolic syndrome, diabetes, and CVDs. In the clinical setting, measurement of VAT by CT or MRI is not used outside of research protocols. In clinical practice, we can use anthropometric measurements such as WC or WHR to estimate central adiposity. WC is generally measured in the horizontal plane, midway between the inferior margin of the ribs and the superior border of the iliac crest (93).

WC Vs. Imaging by CT or MRI to Estimate Central Adiposity

WC has long been recognized to be a strong correlate of VAT (94,95). In a cohort of unselected men and women, linear regression analysis for correlates of VAT area identified WC as the only independent variable in a model comprising age, sex, WC, WHR, and BMI (96). When using MRI to subdivide abdominal adipose tissue compartments, WC was the anthropometric index (compared to WHR and BMI) that was the strongest predictor of intra-peritoneal adipose tissue in both men (97) and women (98). Longitudinal follow-up of premenopausal women has shown that change in VAT assessed by CT was strongly correlated with change in waist girth, hip girth, sagittal diameter, and body fat mass ($r = 0.80–0.91$), but less strongly correlated with WHR (99).

In another study of Caucasian men and women, WC and abdominal sagittal diameter were the anthropometric measures most strongly associated with visceral and total abdominal fat, while WHR was a weaker correlate (100). This study also compared truncal and abdominal fat mass estimated by DEXA to the CT-measured fat area and concluded that the DEXA measurements did not offer

better prediction than simpler anthropometric measures such as WC (100).

WC has been shown to be a strong correlate of intra-abdominal adipose tissue in diverse race/ethnic groups, including black, white (101), and Hispanic people (14), and to be the strongest predictor of VAT in general populations in countries all around the world, including Canada (in a French-Canadian population) (102), Japan (103), Italy (104), and the Netherlands (105).

The association of WC with the level of VAT seems to vary according to age (106), but significant correlations have been found from childhood (107) to older age (108). In black and white youth aged 8 to 17 years, across a broad range of overall obesity (BMI 14–50 kg/m^2), WC was strongly correlated with VAT ($r = 0.88$) even after adjustment for BMI ($r = 0.83$), while BMI showed no correlation after adjustment for WC (109).

In obese individuals there appears to be a weaker correlation of WC with measured VAT compared with lean individuals (110). Lemieux et al. showed that the same WC (95 cm) was associated with an increased VAT area (130 cm^2) in both normal-weight and overweight individuals (106). In obese women (BMI ~ 38 kg/m^2), WC and WHR showed moderate ($r = 0.56$ and 0.58, respectively) but stronger correlations with VAT than BMI ($r = 0.33$) (34).

Some weight loss studies have found good correlations between change in visceral fat and change in WC (111) or sagittal diameter (112), but WHR seems to be a poor correlate to measure loss of VAT by intentional means (113,114).

In patients with type 2 diabetes, WHR has been shown to be moderately related ($r = 0.46$) to intra-abdominal fat volume measured by MRI (slightly more than BMI with $r = 0.38$) (115). A case-control study in Asian Indians showed that WC was associated with VAT in both type 2 diabetes and normal controls, but the correlations were stronger in nondiabetics ($r = 0.571$ in controls vs. $r = 0.338$ in diabetics) (81).

Overall, the data support the idea that WC shows correlation to VAT that can be qualified as good to excellent in lean individuals, but only moderate in more obese populations, probably caused by the increased subcutaneous abdominal adipose tissue.

WC Vs. Visceral Adipose Tissue Assessed Directly by Imaging as a Correlate of Adverse Metabolic Risk

One would expect that extent of VAT measured directly with imaging would be more strongly associated with adverse metabolic profiles than is WC. However, a few cross-sectional studies have shown that both have similar

Table 1 Partial Correlation Coefficients Between Metabolic CHD Risk Factors and VAT Area and WC

	VAT area	WC
Total cholesterol	0.04	0.12
LDL cholesterol	0.04	0.10
HDL cholesterol	−0.39[a]	−0.37[a]
Log HDL$_2$ cholesterol	−0.28[a]	−0.2[b]
LDL/HDL cholesterol	0.20[b]	0.13
Log triglyceride	0.25[a]	0.21[b]
Fasting insulin	0.42[a]	0.42[a]
Fasting glucose	0.28[a]	0.24[b]
2-hr glucose	0.25[a]	0.23[b]

Analysis adjusted for age and race.
[a]$p < 0.001$
[b]$p < 0.01$
Abbreviations: CHD, coronary heart disease; VAT, visceral adipose tissue; WC, waist circumference.
Source: Adapted from Table 2 in Ref. 12.

associations with metabolic risk. In peri- and postmenopausal women, partial correlation coefficients were similar between VAT area or WC and various metabolic risk factors (Table 1) (12). In a small Danish cohort (46 men and women), investigators evaluated the predicting power of intra-abdominal adipose tissue and different anthropometric measurements (116). They calculated area under the receiver operating characteristic (ROC) curves for measurements of obesity with regard to combinations of at least two of three nonobese components of the metabolic syndrome (hypertension, hypertriglyceridemia, and impaired fasting glucose). Area under the ROC curve was the highest for intra-abdominal fat measured by CT (0.83), but the areas for WC and BMI were very close to the former (0.77 for both) and better predictors than all the other anthropometric measures (Fig. 4) (116).

However, for prediction of incident disease, WC does not perform as well as directly measured visceral fat. In a prospective follow-up of Japanese-Americans, a number of regression models were tested to assess the effects of body fat distribution on IGT incidence (85). After adjustment for insulin sensitivity, insulin secretion, BMI, fasting plasma glucose, age, and sex, intra-abdominal fat was associated with risk of IGT. Replacing BMI by WC did not alter the model (85). In a similar population followed for incidence of CHD over 10 years, intra-abdominal fat, but not WC, was significantly associated with CHD incidence in multiple logistic regression models that included potential confounding variables (91). In the prospective follow-up of 291 men (predominantly Caucasian), logistic regression was used to determine the independent association between fat depots and all-cause mortality (92). Visceral fat (OR per SD, 1.83) and WC (OR per SD, 1.41) were both significant individual predictors of mortality after controlling for age and follow-up time. Using a

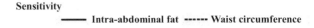

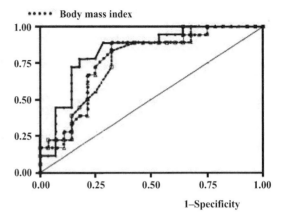

Figure 4 Receiver operating characteristic curves for intra-abdominal fat, waist circumference, and body mass index with regard to combinations of at least two of three metabolic risk factors: systolic blood pressure of 130 mmHg or higher, serum triglyceride concentration of more than >1.7 mmol/L, and fasting capillary blood glucose concentration of 5.6 mmol/L or more. *Source*: Adapted from Ref. 116.

model controlling for all CT fat measures (subcutaneous, visceral, and liver) in addition to age and follow-up time, only visceral fat was a significant predictor of mortality (92). Thus, when fat imaging is available, it appears to be preferable to WC as an indicator of obesity-associated disease risk, but the two may be equivalent when considering associations with metabolic risk factors.

WC AS A PREDICTOR OF METABOLIC RISK

WC and Metabolic Risk Factors

We have seen that WC is a reasonable proxy measure for visceral fat, especially when overall body fat is not extremely high, but that when considered simultaneously, directly measured visceral fat is more strongly associated with adverse disease risk than WC. Since direct visualization of fat distribution by CT or MRI may not be available in many settings, we now consider the performance of WC versus other anthropometric measures as a marker of adverse metabolic and CVD risk.

Correlations between central adiposity measured by anthropometry with cardiovascular risk factors have been reported in many studies (117–123). In the United States, data from the NHANES have shown a continuous increase in WC over the period 1988 to 2004 (124). In the NHANES III data, correlations with metabolic syndrome–related risk factors tended to be slightly better with WC than with BMI in overweight Americans (Table 2) (125). Low sensibilities of the recommended cutoffs (men ≥

Table 2 Correlation of WC or BMI with Lipid Profiles, Blood Pressure, and Glucose

	Men		Women	
	WC (cm)	BMI (kg/m^2)	WC (cm)	BMI (kg/m^2)
WC	—	0.891	—	0.880
LDL cholesterol	0.132[a]	0.067	0.221[a]	0.131
HDL cholesterol	−0.284	−0.285	−0.269	−0.281
Blood pressure	—	—	—	—
Diastolic	0.312[b]	0.291	0.308[a]	0.281
Systolic	0.273[a]	0.155	0.319[a]	0.181
Glucose	0.208[a]	0.168	0.259[a]	0.200

Comparisons of two dependent correlation coefficients between correlations of risk factors with WC or BMI by z-test.
[a]$p < 0.001$
[b]$p < 0.01$
Abbreviations: WC, waist circumference; BMI, body mass index.
Source: Adapted from Table 2 in Ref. 126

102 cm and women ≥ 88 cm) to predict cardiovascular risk factors (125) led to evaluation of various cutoffs for WC (126). NHANES III data showed that WC cutoffs corresponding to roughly equivalent risk for adverse levels of metabolic syndrome–related risk factors at BMI = 25 were 90 cm for men and 83 cm for women and at BMI = 30 were 100 cm in men and 93 cm in women. However, in children in NHANES III, BMI was more strongly correlated with adverse risk factors than was WHR (127).

The somewhat superior cross-sectional association of WC with risk factors has been seen in various other countries. In the Canadian Heart Health Surveys, WC showed better ROC curves predicting adverse levels of cardiovascular risk factors compared with WHR and BMI (128). In China, WC contributed more to metabolic syndrome–related cardiovascular risk factor levels than BMI (129). However, the Australian National Survey in 2000 showed that WHR was most strongly associated with type 2 diabetes, dyslipidemia, and hypertension (130), and the 1998 Health Survey for England showed that BMI and WHR were the major components of population attributable risk for elevated levels of the 10-year Framingham CHD Risk Score (131).

WC and Type 2 Diabetes

Anthropometric measurements of central adiposity have been correlated with diabetes prevalence in many cross-sectional studies (132–134). In the IRAS study, WC was significantly associated with insulin sensitivity (estimated by intravenous glucose tolerance test) even after adjustment for age, sex, height, BMI, glucose tolerance status, ethnicity, and clinics (135). Evaluating the best anthropometric measurements for screening of type 2 diabetes using OGTT, WHR was found to be superior to BMI

based on ROC curves in a general population (136). In NHANES III, risk of type 2 diabetes was associated with WC after adjustment for BMI, age, smoking, and alcohol consumption in white, Hispanic, and black women (137). Cross-sectional relationships between type 2 diabetes and WC have been confirmed in New Zealand (138), China (139), and Turkey (140).

Increased WC also predicts diabetes incidence. In a follow-up over 13.5 years of Swedish middle-aged men, WHR predicted development of DM, even after accounting for BMI (141). The Health Professional Follow-Up Study of over 27,000 men compared BMI, WC, and WHR as predictors of diabetes incidence over 13 years (142). Age-adjusted relative risk for the highest compared to the lowest quintiles were 12.0 for WC, 6.9 for WHR, and 7.9 for BMI. Adjustment for BMI substantially attenuated relative risk for WC and WHR. In ROC curve analysis, WC and BMI were better predictors of diabetes incidence than WHR (Fig. 5) (142). Prospective follow-up of large cohorts of women have also shown a positive association between WC and diabetes incidence, independent of BMI (143). In the Nurses' Health Study, the relative risk of diabetes incidence was evaluated comparing low (10th percentile) versus high (90th percentile) levels of adiposity (144). After controlling for age, family history of diabetes, smoking, exercise, dietary factors, and BMI, relative risk of developing diabetes was 3.1 for a high WHR and 5.1 for a high WC (144). The MONItoring trends and determinants in CArdiovascular disease (MONICA) survey followed middle-aged men and women for over 9.2 years and confirmed that abdominal obesity had an additive effect on prediction of diabetes incidence and recommended that WC should be measured in addition to BMI in both sexes (145). Follow-up of the Heart Outcomes Prevention Evaluation (HOPE) study also showed that WC was more strongly

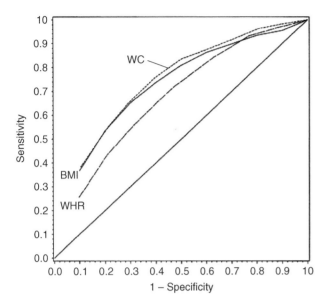

Figure 5 Receiver operating characteristic curves for BMI, WC, and WHR deciles ($n = 27,270$). *Abbreviations*: BMI, body mass index; WC, waist circumference; WHR, waist-to-hip ratio. *Source*: Adapted from Ref. 142.

associated than BMI and WHR with an increased risk of developing diabetes (146).

Anthropometric prediction of diabetes incidence appears to be similar even in different race/ethnic groups. The Atherosclerosis Risk in Communities (ARIC) study followed a large black and white cohort of middle-aged men and women for over nine years for incident diabetes (147). WC had the highest area under the ROC curve compared to BMI and WHR, although differences were small (147). WC has been shown to be a good predictor of diabetes incidence in various countries, including Turkey (148), Taiwan (149), and Jamaica (150). In contrast, in Pima Indians, BMI showed better correlations with diabetes incidence than other anthropometric measurements (151).

WC and CVDs or Mortality

Prediction of CVD incidence by anthropometry is of interest for obvious clinical reasons. CVD outcomes have been correlated with increased WC or WHR. In INTERHEART, a large (more than 25,000 cases and controls) international study of acute myocardial infarction and age-sex matched controls, BMI had a modest association with myocardial infarction, which was substantially reduced after adjustment for WHR and was nonsignificant after further adjustment for other risk factors (Fig. 6) (152). WHR and WC were significantly associated with myocardial infarction, even after adjustment for BMI and other risk factors, with WHR having the

highest OR and the best area under the ROC curve (152). In Sweden, a cohort of middle-aged women was followed up for 12 years: WHR was significantly associated with incidence of myocardial, angina pectoris, strokes, and death even after accounting for standard CVD risk factors (153). In this study, associations were stronger for WHR than for other anthropometric variables. In middle-aged Swedish men of anthropometric measures only, WHR was significantly associated with the 13-year incidence of ischemic heart disease and stroke, although in this study, controlling for standard CVD risk factors attenuated risk associated with central adiposity (154). A recent prospective study in Turkey showed that WC was independently related to incidence of CHDs in both men and women (148,155). In the Melbourne Collaborative Cohort Study of about 17,000 men and 24,000 women followed for about 11 years, compared with BMI and fat mass estimated by bioimpedance, WC, and WHR were better predictors of mortality, especially in women (156). In the Framingham Study, central adiposity as estimated by the ratio of waist/height was associated with incidence of cardiovascular events and mortality over 24 years of follow-up (157). BMI also showed similar associations, but in a model including BMI as covariate, the waist/height ratio was still an independent predictor of strokes, cardiac failure, and cardiovascular mortality in men, and of overall mortality in both men and women. In the IOWA study, over 30,000 women were followed for about 12 years. In multivariable adjusted relative risk, WHR was the best predictor of overall and CVD mortality (158). This, observational data consistently demonstrate that central adiposity measured either by WC or WHR is a strong correlate of increased CVD risk even after adjusting for BMI and other CVD risk factors.

WC IN CLINICAL PRACTICE

Practical Consideration for Clinical Use

The vast body of data reviewed leaves no doubt that abdominal obesity confers increased metabolic and CVD risk and may also add prognostic value to measurement of BMI. The question now is, Will measuring WC (with or without hip circumference) change our clinical management of our patients beyond measurement of BMI?

First of all, we should keep in mind that WC is very strongly related to total adiposity. In the Quebec Family Study and the HERITAGE Family Study, WC correlations to BMI and total fat mass were in the ranges of $r = 0.86$ to 0.96 (159). Visceral fat is strongly related to WC ($r = 0.77$, range 0.69–0.83) but is equally well correlated to BMI ($r = 0.72$, range 0.69–0.77) and total fat mass ($r = 0.73$, range 0.71–0.79) (159). Those correlations are often not controlled for in the studies relating WC to VAT.

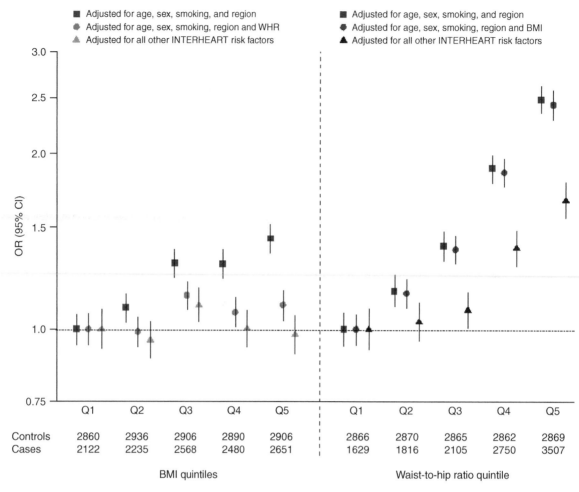

Figure 6 Association of BMI and WHR with myocardial infarction risk. *Abbreviations*: BMI, body mass index; WHR, waist-to-hip ratio. *Source*: Adapted from Ref. 152.

Studies interpretations should take these facts into account.

The WHO MONICA Project showed that BMI explained most of the variance of WC (75% in women and 77% in men), while it explained only a much smaller part of the variance of the WHR (18% in women and 31% in men) suggesting that WHR may be reflecting other biological information beyond central adiposity. The major part of the WHR variance remained unexplained (70% in women and 51% in men) by the usual determinants (height, BMI, age, population source), leading to the conclusion that WHR is difficult to interpret biologically while WC reflect mainly the degree of excess body fat. (160). However, the very high correlation in many studies between BMI and WC leaves open the question as to whether measurement of WC would change management for most patients once BMI has been measured and treatment decisions made based on this common estimate of total body fatness.

As reviewed above, NHANES III data suggested that WC might offer a better predicting power than BMI to detect at least one obesity-associated risk factor (high LDL, low HDL, high blood pressure, high fasting plasma glucose) (126). The better sensitivity afforded by WC means that if anthropometric measurements are used to determine who needs blood screening tests, some people would be missed using BMI cutoffs compared to WC. NHANES III data suggest that the cutoff values for WC (90 cm for men and 83 cm for women) that are equivalent to a BMI of 25 kg/m² might represent appropriate action levels for counseling patients to limit further weight gain. However, if BMI is known then the same advice might be given, and if the measurement is performed in clinic then patient may undergo blood testing in any case (since WC or BMI are not perfect measures of hyperglycemia or dyslipidemia), so whether WC per se adds useful clinical information remains an open question. Certainly, measurement of WC is inexpensive and relatively easy to do

Table 3 Selected Values for Waist Circumference, Specific for Nationality or Ethnicity

Country/ethnic group		WC as measure of central obesity
Europids	Male	≥94 cm
	Female	≥80 cm
South Asians (based on a Chinese, Malay, and Asian Indian population)	Male	≥90 cm
	Female	≥80 cm
Chinese	Male	≥90 cm
	Female	≥80 cm
Japanese	Male	≥85 cm
	Female	≥90 cm

Abbreviation: WC, waist circumference.

and may change treatment or screening advice in some patients not otherwise recognized to be at high risk by BMI measurement alone.

Recommendations for Measurement of WC

Abundant data support the contention that increased adverse health risks are associated with excess body fat, especially visceral fat, which can be quantified by measures of BMI, WC, or WHR. WC might be more sensitive for metabolic and cardiovascular risk screening, especially for individuals in the upper end of the spectrum of normal BMI. For diabetes screening, it is unclear if WC should be part of a clinical protocol, as few data allow us to recommend to measure WC over BMI when deciding to perform an OGTT. Certainly, the level of overweight or obesity should be measured by one of the anthropometric measurements. The success of weight loss interventions should be assessed by change in both WC and BMI. Additional research is required to determine the true marginal information value of WC measurement, which WC cut-points are optimal in various race/ethnic groups (Table 3) to identify obesity risk above and beyond measurement of BMI, and whether therapies that reduce WC above and beyond reduction in BMI offer unique metabolic or CVD risk benefits.

REFERENCES

1. World Health Organization. Obesity and overweight. Available at: http://www.who.int/mediacentre/factsheets/fs311/en/.
2. Ogden CL, Carroll MD, Curtin LR, et al. Prevalence of overweight and obesity in the United States, 1999–2004. JAMA 2006; 295(13):1549–1555.
3. Okosun IS, Chandra KM, Boev A, et al. Abdominal adiposity in U.S. adults: prevalence and trends, 1960–2000. Prev Med 2004; 39(1):197–206.
4. Li C, Ford ES, Mokdad AH, et al. Recent trends in waist circumference and waist-height ratio among US children and adolescents. Pediatrics 2006; 118(5): e1390–e1398.
5. Expert Panel on Detection, Evaluation, and Treatment of High Blood Cholesterol in Adults. Executive summary of the third report of the National Cholesterol Education Program (NCEP) expert panel on detection, evaluation, and treatment of high blood cholesterol in adults (Adult Treatment Panel III) [see comment]. JAMA 2001; 285(19): 2486–2497.
6. International Diabetes Federation. IDF worldwide definition of the metabolic syndrome. Available at: http://www.idf.org/home/index.cfm?node=1429.
7. Snijder MB, van Dam RM, Visser M, et al. What aspects of body fat are particularly hazardous and how do we measure them? Int J Epidemiol 2006; 35(1):83–92.
8. Shen W, Wang Z, Punyanita M, et al. Adipose tissue quantification by imaging methods: a proposed classification. Obes Res 2003; 11(1):5–16.
9. Hunter GR, Kekes-Szabo T, Snyder SW, et al. Fat distribution, physical activity, and cardiovascular risk factors. Med Sci Sports Exerc 1997; 29(3):362–369.
10. DeNino WF, Tchernof A, Dionne IJ, et al. Contribution of abdominal adiposity to age-related differences in insulin sensitivity and plasma lipids in healthy nonobese women. Diabetes Care 2001; 24(5):925–932.
11. Despres JP, Moorjani S, Ferland M, et al. Adipose tissue distribution and plasma lipoprotein levels in obese women. Importance of intra-abdominal fat. Arteriosclerosis 1989; 9(2):203–210.
12. Nicklas BJ, Penninx BW, Ryan AS, et al. Visceral adipose tissue cutoffs associated with metabolic risk factors for coronary heart disease in women. Diabetes Care 2003; 26(5):1413–1420.
13. Rendell M, Hulthen UL, Tornquist C, et al. Relationship between abdominal fat compartments and glucose and lipid metabolism in early postmenopausal women. J Clin Endocrinol Metab 2001; 86(2):744–749.
14. Hernandez-Ono A, Monter-Carreola G, Zamora-Gonzalez J, et al. Association of visceral fat with coronary risk factors in a population-based sample of postmenopausal women. Int J Obes 2002; 26(1):33–39.

15. Choi YJ, Jo YE, Kim YK, et al. High plasma concentration of remnant lipoprotein cholesterol in obese children and adolescents. Diabetes Care 2006; 29(10): 2305–2310.

16. Asayama K, Dobashi K, Hayashibe H, et al. Threshold values of visceral fat measures and their anthropometric alternatives for metabolic derangement in Japanese obese boys. Int J Obes 2002; 26(2):208–213.

17. Bacha F, Saad R, Gungor N, et al. Obesity, regional fat distribution, and syndrome X in obese black versus white adolescents: race differential in diabetogenic and atherogenic risk factors. J Clin Endocrinol Metab 2003; 88(6): 2534–2540.

18. Caprio S, Hyman LD, McCarthy S, et al. Fat distribution and cardiovascular risk factors in obese adolescent girls: importance of the intra-abdominal fat depot. Am J Clin Nutr 1996; 64(1):12–17.

19. Weltman A, Despres JP, Clasey JL, et al. Impact of abdominal visceral fat, growth hormone, fitness, and insulin on lipids and lipoproteins in older adults. Metabolism 2003; 52(1):73–80.

20. Rissanen J, Hudson R, Ross R. Visceral adiposity, androgens, and plasma lipids in obese men. Metabolism 1994; 43(10):1318–1323.

21. Lerario AC, Bosco A, Rocha M, et al. Risk factors in obese women, with particular reference to visceral fat component. Diabetes Metab 1997; 23(1):68–74.

22. Onat A, Avci GS, Barlan MM, et al. Measures of abdominal obesity assessed for visceral adiposity and relation to coronary risk. Int J Obes 2004; 28(8):1018–1025.

23. Pascot A, Despres JP, Lemieux I, et al. Deterioration of the metabolic risk profile in women. Respective contributions of impaired glucose tolerance and visceral fat accumulation. Diabetes Care 2001; 24(5):902–908.

24. Banerji MA, Buckley MC, Chaiken RL, et al. Liver fat, serum triglycerides and visceral adipose tissue in insulin-sensitive and insulin-resistant black men with NIDDM [see comment]. Int J Obes 1995; 19(12):846–850.

25. Lord J, Thomas R, Fox B, et al. The central issue? Visceral fat mass is a good marker of insulin resistance and metabolic disturbance in women with polycystic ovary syndrome. BJOG 2006; 113(10):1203–1209.

26. Nakamura T, Kobayashi H, Yanagi K, et al. Importance of intra-abdominal visceral fat accumulation to coronary atherosclerosis in heterozygous familial hypercholesterolaemia. Int J Obes 1997; 21(7):580–586.

27. Goodpaster BH, Krishnaswami S, Resnick H, et al. Association between regional adipose tissue distribution and both type 2 diabetes and impaired glucose tolerance in elderly men and women. Diabetes Care 2003; 26(2): 372–379.

28. Leonetti DL, Bergstrom RW, Shuman WP, et al. Urinary catecholamines, plasma insulin and environmental factors in relation to body fat distribution. Int J Obes 1991; 15(5):345–357.

29. Ross R, Fortier L, Hudson R. Separate associations between visceral and subcutaneous adipose tissue distribution, insulin and glucose levels in obese women. Diabetes Care 1996; 19(12):1404–1411.

30. Hong Y, Rice T, Gagnon J, et al. Familial clustering of insulin and abdominal visceral fat: the HERITAGE Family Study. J Clin Endocrinol Metab 1998; 83(12): 4239–4245.

31. Huang TT, Johnson MS, Gower BA, et al. Effect of changes in fat distribution on the rates of change of insulin response in children. Obes Res 2002; 10(10):978–984.

32. Ouyang P, Sung J, Kelemen MD, et al. Relationships of insulin sensitivity with fatness and fitness and in older men and women. J Womens Health (Larchmt)2004; 13(2):177–185.

33. Kelley DE, Thaete FL, Troost F, et al. Subdivisions of subcutaneous abdominal adipose tissue and insulin resistance. Am J Physiol Endocrinol Metab 2000; 278(5): E941–E948.

34. Ribeiro-Filho FF, Faria AN, Kohlmann NE, et al. Two-hour insulin determination improves the ability of abdominal fat measurement to identify risk for the metabolic syndrome. Diabetes Care 2003; 26(6):1725–1730.

35. Seidell JC, Bjorntorp P, Sjostrom L, et al. Visceral fat accumulation in men is positively associated with insulin, glucose, and C-peptide levels, but negatively with testosterone levels. Metabolism 1990; 39(9):897–901.

36. Yamashita S, Nakamura T, Shimomura I, et al. Insulin resistance and body fat distribution [see comment]. Diabetes Care 1996; 19(3):287–291.

37. Sparrow D, Borkan GA, Gerzof SG, et al. Relationship of fat distribution to glucose tolerance. Results of computed tomography in male participants of the Normative Aging Study. Diabetes 1986; 35(4):411–415.

38. Wagenknecht LE, Langefeld CD, Scherzinger AL, et al. Insulin sensitivity, insulin secretion, and abdominal fat: the Insulin Resistance Atherosclerosis Study (IRAS) Family Study. Diabetes 2003; 52(10):2490–2496.

39. Abate N, Garg A, Peshock RM, et al. Relationships of generalized and regional adiposity to insulin sensitivity in men. J Clin Invest 1995; 96(1):88–98.

40. Goodpaster BH, Thaete FL, Simoneau JA, et al. Subcutaneous abdominal fat and thigh muscle composition predict insulin sensitivity independently of visceral fat. Diabetes 1997; 46(10):1579–1585.

41. Gan SK, Kriketos AD, Poynten AM, et al. Insulin action, regional fat, and myocyte lipid: altered relationships with increased adiposity. Obes Res 2003; 11(11):1295–1305.

42. Katsuki A, Suematsu M, Gabazza EC, et al. Decreased high-molecular weight adiponectin-to-total adiponectin ratio in sera is associated with insulin resistance in Japanese metabolically obese, normal-weight men with normal glucose tolerance. Diabetes Care 2006; 29(10):2327–2328.

43. Banerji MA, Faridi N, Atluri R, et al. Body composition, visceral fat, leptin, and insulin resistance in Asian Indian men. J Clin Endocrinol Metab 1999; 84(1):137–144.

44. Banerji MA, Lebowitz J, Chaiken RL, et al. Relationship of visceral adipose tissue and glucose disposal is independent of sex in black NIDDM subjects. Am J Physiol 1997; 273(2 pt 1):E425–E432.

45. Raji A, Seely EW, Arky RA, et al. Body fat distribution and insulin resistance in healthy Asian Indians and Caucasians. J Clin Endocrinol Metab 2001; 86(11): 5366–5371.

46. Bacha F, Saad R, Gungor N, et al. Are obesity-related metabolic risk factors modulated by the degree of insulin resistance in adolescents? Diabetes Care 2006; 29 (7):1599–1604.

47. Sites CK, Calles-Escandon J, Brochu M, et al. Relation of regional fat distribution to insulin sensitivity in postmenopausal women. Fertil Steril 2000; 73(1):61–65.

48. Brochu M, Starling RD, Tchernof A, et al. Visceral adipose tissue is an independent correlate of glucose disposal in older obese postmenopausal women. J Clin Endocrinol Metab 2000; 85(7):2378–2384.

49. Ross R, Freeman J, Hudson R, et al. Abdominal obesity, muscle composition, and insulin resistance in premenopausal women. J Clin Endocrinol Metab 2002; 87(11): 5044–5051.

50. Ross R, Aru J, Freeman J, et al. Abdominal adiposity and insulin resistance in obese men. Am J Physiol Endocrinol Metab 2002; 282(3):E657–E663.

51. Miyazaki Y, Glass L, Triplitt C, et al. Abdominal fat distribution and peripheral and hepatic insulin resistance in type 2 diabetes mellitus. Am J Physiol Endocrinol Metab 2002; 283(6):E1135–E1143.

52. Gastaldelli A, Miyazaki Y, Pettiti M, et al. Metabolic effects of visceral fat accumulation in type 2 diabetes. J Clin Endocrinol Metab 2002; 87(11):5098–5103.

53. Salmenniemi U, Ruotsalainen E, Vanttinen M, et al. High amount of visceral fat mass is associated with multiple metabolic changes in offspring of type 2 diabetic patients. Int J Obes 2005; 29(12):1464–1470.

54. Garg A. Regional adiposity and insulin resistance. J Clin Endocrinol Metab 2004; 89(9):4206–4210.

55. Smith SR, Lovejoy JC, Greenway F, et al. Contributions of total body fat, abdominal subcutaneous adipose tissue compartments, and visceral adipose tissue to the metabolic complications of obesity. Metabolism 2001; 50(4):425–435.

56. Saijo Y, Kiyota N, Kawasaki Y, et al. Relationship between C-reactive protein and visceral adipose tissue in healthy Japanese subjects. Diabetes Obes Metab 2004; 6(4):249–258.

57. Sites CK, Toth MJ, Cushman M, et al. Menopause-related differences in inflammation markers and their relationship to body fat distribution and insulin-stimulated glucose disposal. Fertil Steril 2002; 77(1):128–135.

58. Iwasaki T, Nakajima A, Yoneda M, et al. Relationship between the serum concentrations of C-reactive protein and parameters of adiposity and insulin resistance in patients with type 2 diabetes mellitus. Endocr J 2006; 53(3):345–356.

59. Kantartzis K, Rittig K, Balletshofer B, et al. The relationships of plasma adiponectin with a favorable lipid profile, decreased inflammation, and less ectopic fat accumulation depend on adiposity. Clin Chem 2006; 52(10):1934–1942.

60. Kim C, Park J, Park J, et al. Comparison of body fat composition and serum adiponectin levels in diabetic obesity and non-diabetic obesity. Obesity 2006; 14(7): 1164–1171.

61. Cote M, Mauriege P, Bergeron J, et al. Adiponectinemia in visceral obesity: impact on glucose tolerance and plasma lipoprotein and lipid levels in men. J Clin Endocrinol Metab 2005; 90(3):1434–1439.

62. Park KG, Park KS, Kim MJ, et al. Relationship between serum adiponectin and leptin concentrations and body fat distribution. Diabetes Res Clin Pract 2004; 63(2):135–142.

63. Farvid MS, Ng TW, Chan DC, et al. Association of adiponectin and resistin with adipose tissue compartments, insulin resistance and dyslipidaemia. Diabetes Obes Metab 2005; 7(4):406–413.

64. von Eyben FE, Mouritsen E, Holm J, et al. Intra-abdominal obesity and metabolic risk factors: a study of young adults. Int J Obes 2003; 27(8):941–949.

65. Cigolini M, Targher G, Bergamo Andreis IA, et al. Visceral fat accumulation and its relation to plasma hemostatic factors in healthy men. Arterioscler Thromb Vasc Biol 1996; 16(3):368–374.

66. Janand-Delenne B, Chagnaud C, Raccah D, et al. Visceral fat as a main determinant of plasminogen activator inhibitor 1 level in women. Int J Obes 1998; 22(4):312–317.

67. Mertens I, Van der Planken M, Corthouts B, et al. Is visceral adipose tissue a determinant of von Willebrand factor in overweight and obese premenopausal women? Metabolism 2006; 55(5):650–655.

68. Kitagawa N, Yano Y, Gabazza EC, et al. Different metabolic correlations of thrombin-activatable fibrinolysis inhibitor and plasminogen activator inhibitor-1 in non-obese type 2 diabetic patients. Diabetes Res Clin Pract 2006; 73(2):150–157.

69. Fujita K, Nishizawa H, Funahashi T, et al. Systemic oxidative stress is associated with visceral fat accumulation and the metabolic syndrome. Circ J 2006; 70(11): 1437–1442.

70. Paradis ME, Hogue MO, Mauger JF, et al. Visceral adipose tissue accumulation, secretory phospholipase A2-IIA and atherogenecity of LDL. Int J Obes 2006; 30(11): 1615–1622.

71. Targher G, Bertolini L, Scala L, et al. Non-alcoholic hepatic steatosis and its relation to increased plasma biomarkers of inflammation and endothelial dysfunction in non-diabetic men. Role of visceral adipose tissue. Diabetic Med 2005; 22(10):1354–1358.

72. Torgerson JS, Lindroos AK, Sjostrom CD, et al. Are elevated aminotransferases and decreased bilirubin additional characteristics of the metabolic syndrome? Obes Res 1997; 5(2):105–114.

73. Fishbein MH, Mogren C, Gleason T, et al. Relationship of hepatic steatosis to adipose tissue distribution in pediatric nonalcoholic fatty liver disease. J Pediatr Gastroenterol Nutr 2006; 42(1):83–88.

74. Burgert TS, Taksali SE, Dziura J, et al. Alanine aminotransferase levels and fatty liver in childhood obesity: associations with insulin resistance, adiponectin, and visceral fat. J Clin Endocrinol Metab 2006; 91(11): 4287–4294.

75. Zamboni M, Armellini F, Milani MP, et al. Body fat distribution in pre- and post-menopausal women: metabolic and anthropometric variables and their inter-relationships. Int J Obes 1992; 16(7):495–504.

76. Peiris AN, Sothmann MS, Hoffmann RG, et al. Adiposity, fat distribution, and cardiovascular risk. Ann Intern Med 1989; 110(11):867–872.

77. Carr DB, Utzschneider KM, Hull RL, et al. Intra-abdominal fat is a major determinant of the National Cholesterol Education Program Adult Treatment Panel III criteria for the metabolic syndrome. Diabetes 2004; 53(8):2087–2094.

78. Goodpaster BH, Krishnaswami S, Harris TB, et al. Obesity, regional body fat distribution, and the metabolic syndrome in older men and women. Arch Intern Med 2005; 165(7):777–783.

79. Kuk JL, Church TS, Blair SN, et al. Does measurement site for visceral and abdominal subcutaneous adipose tissue alter associations with the metabolic syndrome? Diabetes Care 2006; 29(3):679–684.

80. Pascot A, Despres JP, Lemieux I, et al. Contribution of visceral obesity to the deterioration of the metabolic risk profile in men with impaired glucose tolerance. Diabetologia 2000; 43(9):1126–1135.

81. Anjana M, Sandeep S, Deepa R, et al. Visceral and central abdominal fat and anthropometry in relation to diabetes in Asian Indians. Diabetes Care 2004; 27(12):2948–2953.

82. Shuman WP, Morris LL, Leonetti DL, et al. Abnormal body fat distribution detected by computed tomography in diabetic men. Invest Radiol 1986; 21(6):483–487.

83. Newell-Morris LL, Treder RP, Shuman WP, et al. Fatness, fat distribution, and glucose tolerance in second-generation Japanese-American (Nisei) men. Am J Clin Nutr 1989; 50(1):9–18.

84. Liao D, Shofer JB, Boyko EJ, et al. Abnormal glucose tolerance and increased risk for cardiovascular disease in Japanese-Americans with normal fasting glucose. Diabetes Care 2001; 24(1):39–44.

85. Hayashi T, Boyko EJ, Leonetti DL, et al. Visceral adiposity and the risk of impaired glucose tolerance: a prospective study among Japanese Americans. Diabetes Care 2003; 26(3):650–655.

86. Boyko EJ, Fujimoto WY, Leonetti DL, et al. Visceral adiposity and risk of type 2 diabetes: a prospective study among Japanese Americans [see comment]. Diabetes Care 2000; 23(4):465–471.

87. Snell-Bergeon JK, Hokanson JE, Kinney GL, et al. Measurement of abdominal fat by CT compared to waist circumference and BMI in explaining the presence of coronary calcium. Int J Obes 2004; 28(12):1594–1599.

88. Arad Y, Newstein D, Cadet F, et al. Association of multiple risk factors and insulin resistance with increased prevalence of asymptomatic coronary artery disease by an electron-beam computed tomographic study. Arterioscler Thromb Vasc Biol 2001; 21(12):2051–2058.

89. Hegazi RA, Sutton-Tyrrell K, Evans RW, et al. Relationship of adiposity to subclinical atherosclerosis in obese patients with type 2 diabetes. Obes Res 2003; 11(12):1597–1605.

90. Tirkes AT, Gottlieb RH, Voci SL, et al. Risk of significant coronary artery disease as determined by CT measurement of the distribution of abdominal adipose tissue. J Comput Assist Tomogr 2002; 26(2):210–215.

91. Fujimoto WY, Bergstrom RW, Boyko EJ, et al. Visceral adiposity and incident coronary heart disease in Japanese-American men. The 10-year follow-up results of the Seattle Japanese-American Community Diabetes Study. Diabetes Care 1999; 22(11):1808–1812.

92. Kuk JL, Katzmarzyk PT, Nichaman MZ, et al. Visceral fat is an independent predictor of all-cause mortality in men. Obesity 2006; 14(2):336–341.

93. Alberti KG, Zimmet P, Shaw J. Metabolic syndrome—a new world-wide definition. A Consensus Statement from the International Diabetes Federation. Diabetic Med 2006; 23(5):469–480.

94. Weits T, van der Beek EJ, Wedel M, et al. Computed tomography measurement of abdominal fat deposition in relation to anthropometry. Int J Obes 1988; 12(3):217–225.

95. Seidell JC, Oosterlee A, Deurenberg P, et al. Abdominal fat depots measured with computed tomography: effects of degree of obesity, sex, and age. Eur J Clin Nutr 1988; 42(9):805–815.

96. Onat A, Avci GS, Barlan MM, et al. Measures of abdominal obesity assessed for visceral adiposity and relation to coronary risk. Int J Obes 2004; 28(8):1018–1025.

97. Chan DC, Watts GF, Barrett PH, et al. Waist circumference, waist-to-hip ratio and body mass index as predictors of adipose tissue compartments in men. QJM 2003; 96(6):441–447.

98. Tai ES, Lau TN, Ho SC, et al. Body fat distribution and cardiovascular risk in normal weight women. Associations with insulin resistance, lipids and plasma leptin. Int J Obes 2000; 24(6):751–757.

99. Lemieux S, Prud'homme D, Tremblay A, et al. Anthropometric correlates to changes in visceral adipose tissue over 7 years in women. Int J Obes 1996; 20(7):618–624.

100. Clasey JL, Bouchard C, Teates CD, et al. The use of anthropometric and dual-energy X-ray absorptiometry (DXA) measures to estimate total abdominal and abdominal visceral fat in men and women. Obes Res 1999; 7(3):256–264.

101. Hill JO, Sidney S, Lewis CE, et al. Racial differences in amounts of visceral adipose tissue in young adults: the CARDIA (Coronary Artery Risk Development in Young Adults) study. Am J Clin Nutr 1999; 69(3):381–387.

102. Rankinen T, Kim SY, Perusse L, et al. The prediction of abdominal visceral fat level from body composition and anthropometry: ROC analysis. 1999; 23(8):801–809.

103. Miyatake N, Takenami S, Fujii M. Evaluation of visceral adipose accumulation in Japanese women and establishment of a predictive formula. Acta Diabetol 2004; 41(3):113–117.

104. Armellini F, Zamboni M, Perdichizzi G, et al. Computed tomography visceral adipose tissue volume measurements of Italians. Predictive equations. Eur J Clin Nutr 1996; 50(5):290–294.

105. Han TS, McNeill G, Seidell JC, et al. Predicting intra-abdominal fatness from anthropometric measures: the influence of stature. Int J Obes 1997; 21(7):587–593.

106. Lemieux S, Prud'homme D, Bouchard C, et al. A single threshold value of waist girth identifies normal-weight and overweight subjects with excess visceral adipose tissue. Am J Clin Nutr 1996; 64(5):685–693.

107. Brambilla P, Bedogni G, Moreno LA, et al. Crossvalidation of anthropometry against magnetic resonance

imaging for the assessment of visceral and subcutaneous adipose tissue in children. Int J Obes 2006; 30(1):23–30.

108. Snijder MB, Visser M, Dekker JM, et al. The prediction of visceral fat by dual-energy X-ray absorptiometry in the elderly: a comparison with computed tomography and anthropometry. Int J Obes 2002; 26(7):984–993.

109. Lee S, Bacha F, Gungor N, et al. Waist circumference is an independent predictor of insulin resistance in black and white youths. J Pediatr 2006; 148(2):188–194.

110. Busetto L, Baggio MB, Zurlo F, et al. Assessment of abdominal fat distribution in obese patients: anthropometry versus computerized tomography. Int J Obes 1992; 16(10):731–736.

111. Ross R, Rissanen J, Hudson R. Sensitivity associated with the identification of visceral adipose tissue levels using waist circumference in men and women: effects of weight loss. Int J Obes 1996; 20(6):533–538.

112. van der Kooy K, Leenen R, Seidell JC, et al. Abdominal diameters as indicators of visceral fat: comparison between magnetic resonance imaging and anthropometry. Br J Nutr 1993; 70(1):47–58.

113. van der Kooy K, Leenen R, Seidell JC, et al. Waist-hip ratio is a poor predictor of changes in visceral fat. Am J Clin Nutr 1993; 57(3):327–333.

114. Pare A, Dumont M, Lemieux I, et al. Is the relationship between adipose tissue and waist girth altered by weight loss in obese men? Obes Res 2001; 9(9):526–534.

115. Poll L, Wittsack HJ, Willers R, et al. Correlation between anthropometric parameters and abdominal fat volumes assessed by a magnetic resonance imaging method in patients with diabetes. Diabetes Technol Ther 2004; 6(6):844–849.

116. von Eyben FE, Mouritsen E, Holm J, et al. Computed tomography scans of intra-abdominal fat, anthropometric measurements, and 3 nonobese metabolic risk factors. Metabolism 2006; 55(10):1337–1343.

117. Haffner SM, Stern MP, Hazuda HP, et al. Do upper-body and centralized adiposity measure different aspects of regional body-fat distribution? Relationship to non-insulin-dependent diabetes mellitus, lipids, and lipoproteins. Diabetes 1987; 36(1):43–51.

118. Folsom AR, Burke GL, Ballew C, et al. Relation of body fatness and its distribution to cardiovascular risk factors in young blacks and whites. The role of insulin. Am J Epidemiol 1989; 130(5):911–924.

119. Seidell JC, Cigolini M, Charzewska J, et al. Fat distribution in European women: a comparison of anthropometric measurements in relation to cardiovascular risk factors. Int J Epidemiol 1990; 19(2):303–308.

120. Seidell JC, Cigolini M, Charzewska J, et al. Fat distribution in European men: a comparison of anthropometric measurements in relation to cardiovascular risk factors. Int J Obes 1992; 16(1):17–22.

121. Lemieux S, Prud'homme D, Tremblay A, et al. Anthropometric correlates to changes in visceral adipose tissue over 7 years in women. Int J Obes 1996; 20(7):618–624.

122. Seidell JC, Perusse L, Despres JP, et al. Waist and hip circumferences have independent and opposite effects on cardiovascular disease risk factors: the Quebec Family Study. Am J Clin Nutr 2001; 74(3):315–321.

123. Kissebah AH, Vydelingum N, Murray R, et al. Relation of body fat distribution to metabolic complications of obesity. J Clin Endocrinol Metab 1982; 54(2):254–260.

124. Li C, Ford ES, McGuire LC, et al. Increasing trends in waist circumference and abdominal obesity among US adults. Obesity 2007; 15(1):216–224.

125. Okosun IS, Liao Y, Rotimi CN, et al. Predictive values of waist circumference for dyslipidemia, type 2 diabetes and hypertension in overweight White, Black, and Hispanic American adults. J Clin Epidemiol 2000; 53(4): 401–408.

126. Zhu S, Wang Z, Heshka S, et al. Waist circumference and obesity-associated risk factors among whites in the third National Health and Nutrition Examination Survey: clinical action thresholds [see comment]. Am J Clin Nutr 2002; 76(4):743–749.

127. Gillum RF. Distribution of waist-to-hip ratio, other indices of body fat distribution and obesity and associations with HDL cholesterol in children and young adults aged 4–19 years: the third National Health and Nutrition Examination Survey. Int J Obes 1999; 23(6):556–563.

128. Dobbelsteyn CJ, Joffres MR, MacLean DR, et al. A comparative evaluation of waist circumference, waist-to-hip ratio and body mass index as indicators of cardiovascular risk factors. The Canadian Heart Health Surveys. Int J Obes 2001; 25(5):652–661.

129. Thomas GN, Ho SY, Lam KS, et al. Impact of obesity and body fat distribution on cardiovascular risk factors in Hong Kong Chinese. Obes Res 2004; 12(11):1805–1813.

130. Dalton M, Cameron AJ, Zimmet PZ, et al. Waist circumference, waist-hip ratio and body mass index and their correlation with cardiovascular disease risk factors in Australian adults. J Intern Med 2003; 254(6):555–563.

131. Nanchahal K, Morris JN, Sullivan LM, et al. Coronary heart disease risk in men and the epidemic of overweight and obesity. Int J Obes 2005; 29(3):317–323.

132. Freedman DS, Rimm AA. The relation of body fat distribution, as assessed by six girth measurements, to diabetes mellitus in women [see comment]. Am J Public Health 1989; 79(6):715–720.

133. Hartz AJ, Rupley DC, Rimm AA. The association of girth measurements with disease in 32,856 women. Am J Epidemiol 1984; 119(1):71–80.

134. Hartz AJ, Rupley DC Jr., Kalkhoff RD, et al. Relationship of obesity to diabetes: influence of obesity level and body fat distribution. Prev Med 1983; 12(2):351–357.

135. Karter AJ, Mayer-Davis EJ, Selby JV, et al. Insulin sensitivity and abdominal obesity in African-American, Hispanic, and non-Hispanic white men and women. The Insulin Resistance and Atherosclerosis Study. Diabetes 1996; 45(11):1547–1555.

136. Sosenko JM, Kato M, Soto R, et al. A comparison of adiposity measures for screening non-insulin dependent diabetes mellitus. Int J Obes 1993; 17(8):441–444.

137. Okosun IS. Ethnic differences in the risk of type 2 diabetes attributable to differences in abdominal adiposity in American women. J Cardiovasc Risk 2000; 7(6):425–430.

138. Turley M, Tobias M, Paul S. Non-fatal disease burden associated with excess body mass index and waist

circumference in New Zealand adults. Aust N Z J Public Health 2006; 30(3):231–237.

139. Rosenthal AD, Jin F, Shu XO, et al. Body fat distribution and risk of diabetes among Chinese women. Int J Obes 2004; 28(4):594–599.

140. Satman I, Yilmaz T, Sengul A, et al. Population-based study of diabetes and risk characteristics in Turkey: results of the Turkish diabetes epidemiology study (TURDEP). Diabetes Care 2002; 25(9):1551–1556.

141. Ohlson LO, Larsson B, Svardsudd K, et al. The influence of body fat distribution on the incidence of diabetes mellitus. 13.5 years of follow-up of the participants in the study of men born in 1913. Diabetes 1985; 34(10):1055–1058.

142. Wang Y, Rimm EB, Stampfer MJ, et al. Comparison of abdominal adiposity and overall obesity in predicting risk of type 2 diabetes among men [see comment]. Am J Clin Nutr 2005; 81(3):555–563.

143. Kaye SA, Folsom AR, Sprafka JM, et al. Increased incidence of diabetes mellitus in relation to abdominal adiposity in older women. J Clin Epidemiol 1991; 44(3): 329–334.

144. Carey VJ, Walters EE, Colditz GA, et al. Body fat distribution and risk of non-insulin-dependent diabetes mellitus in women. The Nurses' Health Study. Am J Epidemiol 1997; 145(7):614–619.

145. Meisinger C, Doring A, Thorand B, et al. Body fat distribution and risk of type 2 diabetes in the general population: are there differences between men and women? The MONICA/KORA Augsburg cohort study. Am J Clin Nutr 2006; 84(3):483–489.

146. Dagenais GR, Auger P, Bogaty P, et al. Increased occurrence of diabetes in people with ischemic cardiovascular disease and general and abdominal obesity. Can J Cardiol 2003; 19(12):1387–1391.

147. Stevens J, Couper D, Pankow J, et al. Sensitivity and specificity of anthropometrics for the prediction of diabetes in a biracial cohort. Obes Res 2001; 9(11):696–705.

148. Onat A, Uyarel H, Hergenc G, et al. Determinants and definition of abdominal obesity as related to risk of diabetes, metabolic syndrome and coronary disease in Turkish men: a prospective cohort study. Atherosclerosis 2007; 191(1):182–190.

149. Sheu WH, Chuang SY, Lee WJ, et al. Predictors of incident diabetes, metabolic syndrome in middle-aged adults: a 10-year follow-up study from Kinmen, Taiwan. Diabetes Res Clin Pract 2006; 74(2):162–168.

150. Sargeant LA, Bennett FI, Forrester TE, et al. Predicting incident diabetes in Jamaica: the role of anthropometry. Obes Res 2002; 10(8):792–798.

151. Tulloch-Reid MK, Williams DE, Looker HC, et al. Do measures of body fat distribution provide information on the risk of type 2 diabetes in addition to measures of general obesity? Comparison of anthropometric predictors of type 2 diabetes in Pima Indians. Diabetes Care 2003; 26(9):2556–2561.

152. Yusuf S, Hawken S, Ounpuu S, et al. Obesity and the risk of myocardial infarction in 27,000 participants from 52 countries: a case-control study [see comment]. Lancet 2005; 366(9497):1640–1649.

153. Lapidus L, Bengtsson C, Larsson B, et al. Distribution of adipose tissue and risk of cardiovascular disease and death: a 12 year follow up of participants in the population study of women in Gothenburg, Sweden. Br Med J (Clin Res Ed) 1984; 289(6454):1257–1261.

154. Larsson B, Svardsudd K, Welin L, et al. Abdominal adipose tissue distribution, obesity, and risk of cardiovascular disease and death: 13 year follow up of participants in the study of men born in 1913. Br Med J (Clin Res Ed) 1984; 288(6428):1401–1404.

155. Onat A, Sari I, Hergenc G, et al. Predictors of abdominal obesity and high susceptibility of cardiometabolic risk to its increments among Turkish women: a prospective population-based study. Metabolism 2007; 56(3):348–356.

156. Simpson JA, MacInnis RJ, Peeters A, et al. A comparison of adiposity measures as predictors of all-cause mortality: the Melbourne Collaborative Cohort Study. Obesity 2007; 15(4):994–1003.

157. Kannel WB, Cupples LA, Ramaswami R, et al. Regional obesity and risk of cardiovascular disease; the Framingham Study. J Clin Epidemiol 1991; 44(2):183–190.

158. Folsom AR, Kushi LH, Anderson KE, et al. Associations of general and abdominal obesity with multiple health outcomes in older women: the Iowa Women's Health Study. Arch Intern Med 2000; 160(14):2117–2128.

159. Bouchard C. BMI, fat mass, abdominal adiposity and visceral fat: where is the 'beef'? Int J Obes (Lond) 2007; 31(10):1552–1553.

160. Molarius A, Seidell JC, Sans S, et al. Waist and hip circumferences, and waist-hip ratio in 19 populations of the WHO MONICA Project. Int J Obes 1999; 23(2):116–125.

3

Genetic Evaluation of Obese Patients

I. SADAF FAROOQI and STEPHEN O'RAHILLY

University of Cambridge Metabolic Research Laboratories, Institute of Metabolic Science, Addenbrooke's Hospital, Cambridge, U.K.

INTRODUCTION

The recent rapid rise in the prevalence of obesity has been driven by environmental factors such as the increased availability of palatable energy-dense foods and the reduced requirement for physical activity during working and domestic life. These marked changes in our environment, acting over a relatively short time frame ($\sim$40–50 years for Western populations), have contributed to an increase in mean body mass index (BMI) in many Western populations. Yet, despite the obesogenic environment, body weight remains relatively constant over long periods of time for most people. Body weight, and more specifically fat mass, is maintained by homeostatic mechanisms that allow compensatory changes in energy intake and energy expenditure in response to fluctuations in energy balance (1,2). Elegant studies in monozygotic twins versus dizygotic twins have demonstrated that the regulation of body weight is highly heritable, most notably seen in monozygotic twins reared apart (3–5). Furthermore, Stunkard and colleagues showed that adopted children have body weights that are very similar to those of their biological parents in comparison with their adoptive parents with whom they share the childhood environment (6). It is likely that these genetic influences, which exert their effects across the whole spectrum of body weight, are determined by variation in the genes that encode molecules involved in energy homeostasis. As with other common, complex diseases, the genetic determinants of interindividual variation in fat mass are likely to be multiple and interacting (7).

Genome-wide association studies have proved to be an extremely valuable tool for unraveling the etiology of complex diseases. Frayling et al. recently found an obesity susceptibility gene as a by-product of a genome-wide association study for type 2 diabetes (8). They found that single nucleotide polymorphisms in the fat mass and obesity associated gene were strongly associated with type 2 diabetes, but the association was abolished after adjusting for BMI, indicating that the association with type 2 diabetes was due to obesity, a finding that has been replicated in multiple studies (9). It is likely that genome-wide approaches in larger cohorts and/or those with early-onset disease will result in the identification of other common variants that contribute to obesity risk in populations. Ultimately, these findings may guide a more rational targeted approach to prevention and/or treatment of genetically susceptible individuals.

ASSESSMENT OF INDIVIDUALS WITH SEVERE OBESITY

Obesity is frequently considered to be a "modern" disease—a reflection of the excesses of Western urbanized society. However, artifacts dating from the Paleolithic Stone Age clearly represent subjects with an excess of body fat, and descriptions of obese individuals have emerged in manuscripts and medical texts from many of the ancient civilizations from Mesopotamia to Arabia and from China to India (10). This historical evidence suggests that there has always been a subset of individuals who have harbored the propensity to store excess energy as fat. It is clear that with the rising global prevalence of obesity, the proportion of people with severe obesity has increased. Genetic factors are likely to play a major role in the obesity of these individuals. On the basis of current findings from the study of patients with single gene defects resulting in obesity (monogenic obesity syndromes), the early onset of obesity (<10 years of age) is a hallmark clinical feature of the genetic obesity syndromes.

DEFINITIONS OF SEVERE OBESITY

Obesity is defined as an excess of body fat, which is associated with an increased risk of morbidity and/or premature mortality. In adults, obesity is defined as a BMI >30 kg/m^2 and severe obesity as a BMI >40 kg/m^2. In children, the relationship between BMI and body fat varies considerably with age and with pubertal maturation; however, when adjusted for age and gender, BMI is a reasonable proxy for fat mass. BMI centile charts using national BMI reference data have now been published in several countries and facilitate the graphical plotting of serial BMI measurements in individual patients (11). However, such charts are often based on arbitrary statistical measures and not on biological data related to the risk of later morbidity. Cole et al. developed age- and gender-specific cutoff lines from BMI data derived from six countries, which extrapolate risk from the adult experience to children (12). The International Obesity Task Force (IOTF) has recommended the use of these age- and gender-specific BMI cutoffs (overweight as ~91st percentile or greater and obesity as ~99th percentile or greater) for the comparison of obesity prevalence in different populations. Although there is no accepted definition for severe or morbid obesity in childhood, a BMI SD >2.5 (weight off the chart) is often used in specialist centers, and the crossing of major weight percentile lines upward is an early indication of risk of severe obesity (13).

CLINICAL HISTORY, EXAMINATION, AND INVESTIGATION

The assessment of severely obese children and indeed adults should be directed at screening for potentially treatable endocrine and neurological conditions and identifying genetic conditions so that appropriate genetic counseling and in some cases treatment can be instituted. Much of the information needed can be obtained from a careful medical history and physical examination (14), which should also address the potentially hidden complications of severe obesity such as sleep apnea (13). In addition to a general medical history, a specific weight history should be taken carefully establishing the age of onset (clinical photographs are helpful here) and the presence (or less likely the absence) of hyperphagia (Fig. 1). A careful family history to identify potential consanguineous relationships, the presence of other subjects with severe early-onset obesity and the ethnic and geographical origin of family members should be taken.

The history and examination can then guide the appropriate use of diagnostic tests, which will affect the management of the patient (Figs. 1 and 2).

GENETIC OBESITY SYNDROMES

Classically, patients affected by genetic obesity syndromes have been identified as a result of their association with developmental delay, dysmorphic features, and/or other developmental abnormalities. More recently, several single gene disorders resulting from disruption of the hypothalamic leptin–melanocortin signaling pathway have been identified (15). In these disorders, obesity itself is the predominant presenting feature, although frequently accompanied by characteristic patterns of neuroendocrine dysfunction, which will only become apparent on investigation. For the purposes of clinical assessment, it remains useful to categorize the genetic obesity syndromes as those with dysmorphism and/or developmental delay and those without these features (Fig. 3).

OBESITY WITH DEVELOPMENTAL DELAY

There are about 30 Mendelian disorders with obesity as a clinical feature but often associated with mental retardation, dysmorphic features, and organ-specific developmental abnormalities (i.e., pleiotropic syndromes) (16).

Prader-Willi Syndrome

The Prader-Willi syndrome (PWS) is the most common syndromal cause of human obesity, with an estimated prevalence of about 1 in 25,000 (17). It is an autosomal dominant disorder characterized by hypotonia, mental retardation, short stature, hypogonadotropic hypogonadism, and hyperphagia (increased food intake) and obesity (18,19). Children with PWS display diminished growth, reduced lean body mass, and increased fat mass—body composition abnormalities resembling those seen in growth hormone (GH) deficiency, and GH treatment in these children decreases body fat and increases linear

- Age of onset—use of growth charts and family photographs. Early onset (<5 years of age) suggests a genetic cause.
- Duration of obesity—short history suggests endocrine or central cause.
- A history of damage to the CNS (e.g., infection, trauma, hemorrhage, radiation therapy, seizures) suggests hypothalamic obesity with or without pituitary growth hormone deficiency or pituitary hypothyroidism. A history of morning headaches, vomiting, visual disturbances, and excessive urination or drinking also suggests that the obesity may be caused by a tumor or mass in the hypothalamus.
- A history of dry skin, constipation, intolerance to cold, or fatigue suggests hypothyroidism. Mood disturbance and central obesity suggest Cushing's syndrome. Frequent infections and fatigue may suggest ACTH deficiency due to POMC mutations.
- Hyperphagia—often denied but sympathetic approach needed and specific questions, such as waking at night to eat and demanding food very soon after a meal suggest hyperphagia. If severe, especially in children, suggests a genetic cause for obesity.
- Developmental delay—milestones, educational history, behavioral disorders. Consider craniopharyngeoma or structural causes (often relatively short history) and genetic causes.
- Visual impairment and deafness can suggest genetic causes.
- Onset and tempo of pubertal development—onset can be early or delayed in children and adolescents. Primary hypogonadotropic hypogonadism or hypogenitalism associated with some genetic disorders.
- Family history—consanguineous relationships, other children affected, family photographs useful. Severity may differ due to environmental effects.
- Treatment with certain drugs or medications. Glucocorticoids, sulfonylureas, oral contraceptives, antidepressants, and antipsychotics.

Figure 1 Clinical assessment—key points in the medical history. *Abbreviations*: CNS, central nervous system; ACTH, adrenocorticotropic hormone; POMC, pro-opiomelanocortin.

- Document weight and height compared to normal centiles. Calculate BMI and WHR (in adults). In children, obtain parental heights and weights where possible.
- Short stature or a reduced rate of linear growth in a child with obesity suggests the possibility of growth hormone deficiency, hypothyroidism, cortisol excess, pseudohypoparathyroidism, or a genetic syndrome such as Prader-Willi syndrome.
- Obese children and adolescents are often tall (on the upper centiles), however, accelerated linear growth (height SDS >2) is a feature of MC4R deficiency.
- Body fat distribution—central distribution with purple striae suggests Cushing's syndrome. Selective fat deposition (60%), a feature of leptin and leptin receptor deficiency.
- Dysmorphic features or skeletal dysplasia.
- Hair colour—red hair (if not familial) may suggest mutations in POMC in White Caucasians.
- Pubertal development/secondary sexual characteristics. Most obese adolescents grow at a normal or excessive rate and enter puberty at the appropriate age; many mature more quickly than children with normal weight, and bone age commonly is advanced. In contrast, growth rate and pubertal development are diminished or delayed in growth hormone deficiency, hypothyroidism, cortisol excess, and a variety of genetic syndromes. Conversely, growth rate and pubertal development are accelerated in precocious puberty and in some girls with PCOS.
- Acanthosis nigricans.
- Varus deformities in severe childhood obesity (often where coexistent vitamin D deficiency).

Figure 2 Clinical assessment—key points in the examination. *Abbreviations*: BMI, body mass index; WHR, waist-to-hip ratio; MC4R, melanocortin 4 receptor; POMC, pro-opiomelanocortin; PCOS, polycystic ovary syndrome.

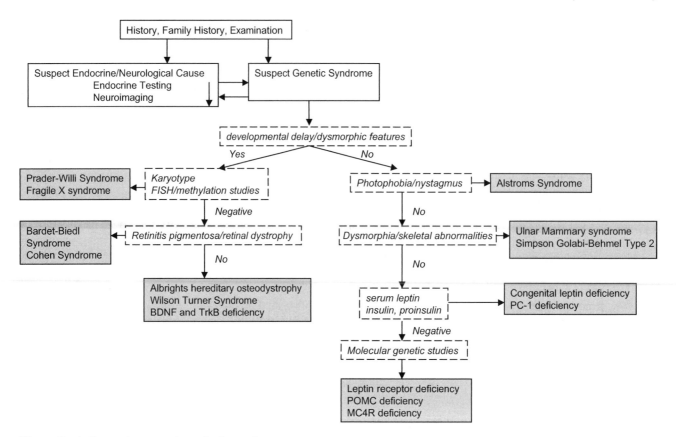

Figure 3 A diagnostic approach to obesity syndromes.

growth, muscle mass, fat oxidation, and energy expenditure (20,21). One suggested mediator of the obesity phenotype in PWS patients is the enteric hormone ghrelin, which is implicated in the regulation of mealtime hunger in rodents and humans and is also a potent stimulator of GH secretion. Several groups have shown that children and adults with PWS have fasting plasma ghrelin levels that are 4.5-fold higher in PWS subjects than equally obese controls and thus may be implicated in the pathogenesis of hyperphagia in these patients (22). However, somatostatin suppresses ghrelin but not appetite in PWS patients (23).

It is clear that chromosomal abnormalities are principally responsible for PWS either through deletion of the paternal "critical" segment 15q11.2-q12 or through loss of the entire paternal chromosome 15 with presence of two maternal homologues (uniparental maternal disomy) (24). The opposite, i.e., maternal deletion or paternal uniparental disomy, causes another characteristic phenotype, the Angelman syndrome (AS). This indicates that both parental chromosomes are differentially imprinted and that both are necessary for normal embryonic development. Most chromosomal abnormalities in PWS occur sporadically. Deletions account for 70% to 80% of cases; the majority are interstitial deletions, many of which can be visualized

by prometaphase banding examination. A minority consists of unbalanced translocations, which are easily detected by routine chromosome examination (25). The remainder of cases are the result of maternal uniparental disomy. In most of these latter cases, cytogenetic examinations yield normal results. There are distinct differences in DNA methylation of the parental alleles at the D15S9 locus, providing further evidence for the association of methylation with genomic imprinting and that DNA methylation can be used as a reliable postnatal diagnostic tool in PWS (26).

Within the 4.5 Mb PWS region in 15q11-q13, where there is a lack of expression of paternally imprinted genes, several candidate genes have been studied and their expression shown to be absent in the brains of PWS patients (27). These include necdin, small nuclear ribonucleoprotein polypeptide N (SNRPN), Ring Zinc finger 127 polypeptide gene, the MAGE-like 2 (Magel2) gene, and the Prader-Willi critical region 1 gene (28). The rhythmicity of Magel2 expression in the suprachiasmatic nucleus reveal Magel2 to be a clock-controlled circadian output gene whose disruption results in some of the phenotypes, characteristic of PWS, such as neonatal growth retardation, excessive weight gain after weaning, and increased adiposity (29,30). However, the precise role of these genes and the mechanisms by which they lead to a pleiotropic obesity syndrome remains elusive.

Albright Hereditary Osteodystrophy

Albright hereditary osteodystrophy (AHO) is an autosomal dominant disorder due to germ line mutations in GNAS1 that decrease expression or function of Gs (α) protein (31). Maternal transmission of GNAS1 mutations leads to AHO (characterized by short stature, obesity, skeletal defects, and impaired olfaction) plus resistance to several hormones (e.g., parathyroid hormone) that activate Gs in their target tissues (pseudohypoparathyroidism type IA), while paternal transmission leads only to the AHO phenotype (pseudopseudohypoparathyroidism). Studies in both mice and humans demonstrate that GNAS1 is imprinted in a tissue-specific manner, being expressed primarily from the maternal allele in some tissues and biallelically expressed in most other tissues, thus multihormone resistance occurs only when Gs (α) mutations are inherited maternally (32).

Fragile X Syndrome

Fragile X syndrome is characterized by moderate-to-severe mental retardation, hyperactive behavior, macroorchidism, large ears, prominent jaw, and high-pitched jocular speech associated with mutations in the FMR1 gene (33). Expression is variable, with mental retardation being the most common feature. Behavioral characteristics such as hyperkinesis, autistic-like behavior, and apparent speech and language deficits may help point toward the diagnosis of the fragile X syndrome. It has been suggested that a reasonable estimate of frequency is 0.5 per 1000 males.

Bardet-Biedl Syndrome

Bardet-Biedl syndrome (BBS) is a rare (prevalence < 1/ 100,000) autosomal recessive disease characterized by obesity, mental retardation, dysmorphic extremities (syndactyly, brachydactyly, or polydactyly), retinal dystrophy or pigmentary retinopathy, hypogonadism, and structural abnormalities of the kidney or functional renal impairment. BBS is a genetically heterogeneous disorder that is now known to map to at least twelve loci (34). Although BBS had been originally thought to be a recessive disorder, clinical manifestation of some forms of BBS requires recessive mutations in one of the six loci plus an additional mutation in a second locus. Recently, primary cilium dysfunction has been shown to underlie the pathogenesis of BBS, with the identification of a complex composed of seven highly conserved BBS proteins that is required for ciliogenesis (35). BBS may be caused by defects in vesicular transport to the cilium (36). Multifocal electroretinogram (ERG) testing can demonstrate areas of retinal dysfunction in carriers of the BBS mutations in the presence of a normal appearing fundus.

BDNF and TrkB Deficiency

Brain-derived neurotrophic factor (BDNF) regulates the development, survival, and differentiation of neurons through its high-affinity receptor, tropomyosin-related kinase B (TrkB). Recently, BDNF has been implicated in the regulation of body weight. We reported a child with severe obesity, impaired short-term memory, and developmental delay who had a de novo missense mutation impairing the function of TrkB, the tyrosine kinase receptor that mediates the effects of both BDNF and the neurotrophin NT4/5 (37). We have also identified a patient with a de novo chromosomal inversion 46,XX, inv(11)(p13p15.3), which encompasses the BDNF locus and disrupts BDNF expression (38). The clinical features include severe hyperphagia and obesity and a complex neurobehavioral phenotype including impaired cognitive function and memory as well as distinctive hyperactive behavior. Although to date only two such patients have been identified, these diagnoses should be considered in patients with developmental delay and severe obesity.

OBESITY WITHOUT DEVELOPMENTAL DELAY

Energy homeostasis is tightly regulated with the hypothalamus playing a pivotal role in integrating signals from adipose tissue stores, such as leptin and short-term, meal-related signals from the gut (PYY, GLP-1, CCK, and ghrelin), which act on first-order neurons in the arcuate nucleus of the hypothalamus (39). Leptin stimulates the expression of pro-opiomelanocortin (POMC), which is cleaved by prohormone convertases to yield the melanocortin peptides, which act as suppressors of feeding through the melanocortin 4 receptor (MC4R), which is expressed on second-order neurons in the paraventricular nucleus (40). Targeted disruption of MC4R in rodents leads to increased food intake, obesity, severe early hyperinsulinemia, and increased linear growth (41). Mutations in several of these molecules cause severe obesity in humans (Fig. 3).

LEPTIN AND LEPTIN RECEPTOR DEFICIENCY

Serum leptin is a useful test in patients with severe early-onset obesity, as an undetectable serum leptin is highly suggestive of a diagnosis of congenital leptin deficiency due to homozygous loss of function mutations in the gene encoding leptin. Serum leptin concentrations are appropriate for the degree of obesity in leptin receptor-deficient patients and as such an elevated serum leptin concentration is not necessarily a predictor of leptin receptor deficiency (42). Among patients with hyperphagic obesity of early onset from consanguineous families, the prevalence of leptin mutations is approximately 1% and of leptin receptor mutations is 2% to 3%. Leptin receptor mutations have been found in some nonconsanguineous families, where both parents are unrelated but happen to carry rare alleles in heterozygous form.

The clinical phenotypes associated with congenital leptin and leptin receptor deficiencies are similar. Leptin and leptin receptor–deficient subjects are of normal birth weight but exhibit rapid weight gain in the first few months of life, resulting in severe obesity. Body composition measurements show that these disorders are characterized by the preferential deposition of fat mass giving a distinct clinical appearance with excessive amounts of subcutaneous fat over the trunk and limbs. Patients are hyperinsulinemic, consistent with the severity of obesity, and some adults have developed type 2 diabetes in the third to fourth decade.

All affected subjects in these families are characterized by intense hyperphagia with food-seeking behavior and aggressive behavior when food is denied, and energy intake at an ad libitum meal is markedly elevated (43). While measurable changes in resting metabolic rate or total energy expenditure have not been demonstrated, abnormalities of sympathetic nerve function in leptin-deficient adults suggest that defects in the efferent sympathetic limb of thermogenesis may contribute to the phenotype observed.

Leptin and leptin receptor deficiency are associated with hypothalamic hypothyroidism and hypogonadotropic hypogonadism. Complete leptin deficiency is associated with a moderate degree of hypothalamic hypothyroidism characterized by low free thyroxine and high serum thyroid stimulating hormone (TSH), which is bioinactive. In leptin-deficient children, plasma-free thyroxine concentrations are often within the normal range, but four children had significantly elevated TSH levels; the pulsatility of TSH secretion, studied in a single adult with congenital leptin deficiency, was characterized by a markedly disorganized secretory pattern (44). Two subjects homozygous for a nonsense mutation in the leptin receptor were diagnosed with hypothyroidism in childhood and thyroid hormone replacement therapy commenced.

Normal pubertal development does not occur in adults with leptin or leptin receptor deficiency, with biochemical evidence of hypogonadotropic hypogonadism. However, there is some evidence for the delayed but spontaneous onset of menses in leptin and leptin receptor-deficient adults.

Leptin- and leptin receptor-deficient children have normal linear growth in childhood and normal IGF1 levels. However, because of the absence of a pubertal growth spurt the final height of adult subjects is reduced. In the first reported leptin receptor-deficient family, short stature and abnormal serum levels of GH, IGFBP3 were noted in childhood. However, assessment of the GH/IGF axis is difficult in obese children and adults as obesity itself is associated with abnormalities in basal and dynamic tests of the GH/IGF axis. Thus, while impaired linear growth has been reported in some cases of leptin receptor deficiency, this does not appear to be a common characteristic of this disease (45).

We demonstrated that children with leptin deficiency had profound abnormalities of T cell number and function, consistent with high rates of childhood infection and a high reported rate of childhood mortality from infection in obese Turkish subjects.

RESPONSE TO LEPTIN ADMINISTRATION IN LEPTIN DEFICIENCY

Although leptin deficiency appears to be rare, it is entirely treatable with daily subcutaneous injections of recombinant human leptin with beneficial effects on the degree of hyperphagia, fat mass and hyperinsulinemia, reversal of the immune defects, and infection risk, and permissive effects on the appropriate development of puberty (Fig. 4). Such treatment is currently available to patients on a named patient basis.

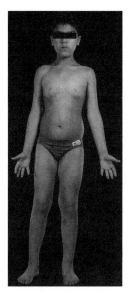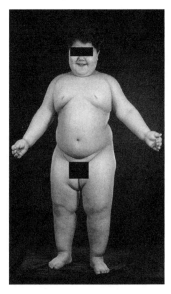

Figure 4 Leptin therapy reduces body weight in congenital leptin deficiency.

The major effect of leptin is on appetite with normalization of hyperphagia. Leptin treatment was associated with reduced hunger scores with no change in satiety in adults with leptin deficiency. We were unable to demonstrate a major effect of leptin on basal metabolic rate (BMR) or free-living energy expenditure, but, as weight loss by other means is associated with a decrease in BMR, the fact that energy expenditure did not fall in our leptin-deficient subjects is notable. The administration of leptin permitted progression of appropriately timed pubertal development in the single child of appropriate age and did not cause the early onset of puberty in the younger children. In adults with leptin deficiency, leptin induced the development of secondary sexual characteristics and pulsatile gonadotrophin secretion. In the three previously reported children there were small, but sustained, increases in free T_4, free T_3, and TSH that occurred within one month of leptin therapy. These observations are fully consistent with an effect of leptin at the hypothalamic level. A fourth patient had substantial elevation of TSH before treatment, such that thyroxine therapy was commenced. However, replacement therapy was stopped when thyroid function tests normalized after leptin treatment (46).

DISORDERS AFFECTING POMC AND POMC PROCESSING

Children who are homozygous or compound heterozygous for mutations in the POMC gene (Fig. 5) present in neonatal life with adrenal crisis due to adrenocorticotropic hormone (ACTH) deficiency, as POMC is a precursor of ACTH in the pituitary, and require long-term corticosteroid replacement (47,48). Such children have pale skin, and white Caucasians have red hair because of the lack of

melanocyte-stimulating hormone (MSH) function at melanocortin 1 receptors in the skin. Although red hair may be an important diagnostic clue in patients of Caucasian origin, its absence in patients originating from other ethnic groups should not result in this diagnostic consideration being excluded as children from different ethnic backgrounds may have a less obvious phenotype such as dark hair with red roots (49).

POMC deficiency results in hyperphagia and early-onset obesity because of loss of melanocortin signaling at the MC4R (47,48). The clinical features are comparable to those reported in patients with mutations in the receptor for POMC-derived ligands, MC4R (see below).

The significantly higher prevalence of obesity/overweight in the carriers provides compelling support for the idea that loss of one copy of POMC is sufficient to markedly predispose to obesity. This is particularly relevant as a variety of heterozygous point mutations in POMC have been described which significantly increase obesity risk but are not invariably associated with obesity. R236G disrupts a dibasic cleavage site between β-MSH and β-endorphin, resulting in a β-MSH/β-endorphin fusion protein that binds to MC4R but has reduced ability to activate the receptor. Its presence in both obese probands and controls in several ethnic groups suggests that this mutation is not a highly penetrant cause of inherited obesity but may increase the risk of obesity in carriers. A rare missense mutation in the region encoding β-MSH, Tyr221Cys has impaired ability to bind to and activate signaling from the MC4R, and obese children carrying the Tyr221Cys variant are hyperphagic and showed increased linear growth, which are features of MC4R deficiency. These observations support a role for β-MSH in the control of human energy homeostasis. Selective MC4R agonists of melanocortin analogues may be feasible therapies for such patients in the future.

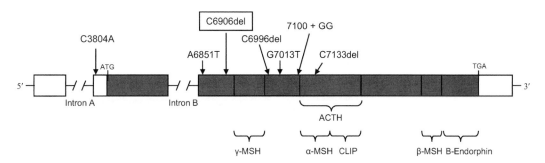

Figure 5 Structure of the POMC gene and location of all homozygous and compound heterozygous mutations identified to date. Untranslated (*white*) and translated regions (*filled*) indicated. Proband 1–compound heterozygote for G7013T and C7133del; Proband 2–C3804A (homozygous); Proband 3–compound heterozygote for A6851T and 6996del; Proband 4–C3804A (homozygous); Proband 5–compound heterozygote for 7100 + GG and C3804A; Proband 6–C6906del (homozygous). *Abbreviation*: POMC, pro-opiomelanocortin.

Table 1 PC1 Deficiency—Clinical Features and Affected Prohormone Conversion

Obesity	POMC-MSH
Hypogonadotropic hypogonadism	ProGnRH-GnRH
Hypoadrenalism	POMC-ACTH
Reactive hypoglycemia/impaired glucose tolerance	Proinsulin-insulin
Intestinal malabsorption	Proglucagon-GLP1 and GLP2

Abbreviations: PC1, prohormone convertase; ACTH, adrenocorticotropic hormone; POMC, pro-opiomelanocortin; MSH, melanocyte-stimulating hormone.

PC1 Deficiency

Many biologically inactive prohormones and neuropeptides are cleaved by serine endoproteases to release biologically active peptides. The prohormone convertases (PC1 and 2) are expressed in neuroendocrine tissues and act on a range of substrates including proinsulin, proglucagon, and POMC. Compound heterozygous or homozygous mutations in this gene cause small bowel enteropathy and complex neuroendocrine effects because of a failure to process a number of prohormones as well as severe early-onset obesity (clinical features and biochemical findings summarized in Table 1).

MC4R Deficiency

MC4R deficiency is a codominantly inherited obesity syndrome, which was first described in 1998. Since then, many different heterozygous MC4R mutations have been reported in obese people from various ethnic groups. The prevalence of such mutations has varied from 0.5% in obese adults to 6% in patients with severe childhood obesity (50). Recent studies provide an important indication of the true population prevalence of this disorder: 0.5% to 2.5% of people with a BMI >30 kg/m^2 being found to harbor pathogenic mutations in MC4R in the U.K. and European populations, confirming that MC4R deficiency is the most common obesity syndrome described to date. In an unselected U.K. population, the prevalence of MC4R mutation carriers was 0.1%, suggesting that MC4R deficiency is one of the most common genetic diseases in the U.K. population, with a higher prevalence than more familiar diseases such as cystic fibrosis. While we found a 100% penetrance of early-onset obesity in heterozygous probands, others have described obligate carriers who were not obese. Given the large number of potential influences on body weight, it is perhaps not surprising that both genetic and environmental modifiers will have important effects in some pedigrees. Indeed, we have now studied several families in whom the probands were homozygotes and in all of these, the homozygotes were more obese than heterozygotes. Interestingly, in these families, some heterozygous carriers were not obese. Taking account of all of these observations, codominance, with modulation of expressivity and penetrance of the phenotype, is the most appropriate descriptor for the mode of inheritance.

The clinical features of MC4R deficiency include hyperphagia, which invariably starts in the first year of life. Of particular note is the finding that the severity of receptor dysfunction seen in in vitro assays can predict the amount of food ingested at a test meal by the subject harboring that particular mutation, showing that melanocortinergic tone is an important determinant of human appetite (50).

Alongside the increase in fat mass, MC4R-deficient subjects also have an increase in lean mass and a marked increase in bone mineral density, thus they often appear "big-boned." They exhibit accelerated linear growth in early childhood, which does not appear to be due to dysfunction of the GH axis and may be a consequence of the disproportionate early hyperinsulinemia seen in these patients (50). Despite this early hyperinsulinemia, obese adult subjects who are heterozygous for mutations in the MC4R gene are not at increased risk of developing glucose intolerance and type 2 diabetes compared with controls of similar age and adiposity.

We recently studied the metabolic complications of obesity in adults with MC4R deficiency. The main findings were that MC4R deficiency was associated with a lower prevalence of hypertension and significantly lower systolic and diastolic blood pressure values than equally obese subjects with a normal MC4R genotype. These observations suggest that despite severe obesity, MC4R-deficient adults may be protected from developing hypertension and raises the possibility that the MC4R mediates blood pressure through modulation of sympathetic nervous system activity.

We also demonstrated impaired fat oxidation in MC4R-deficient patients, which may contribute to the development of obesity as has been shown in rodent models.

While, at present, there is no specific therapy for MC4R deficiency, it is highly likely that these patients would respond well to pharmacotherapy that overcame the reduction in the hypothalamic melanocortinergic tone that exists. As most patients are heterozygotes with one functional allele intact, it is possible that small molecule MC4R agonists might, in future, be appropriate treatments for this disorder.

CONCLUSIONS

As the prevalence of obesity is rising, we are seeing a greater proportion of patients with severe obesity. It is important to have a practical approach to the investigation and management of these vulnerable patients who have considerably increased morbidity and mortality. There have been major advances in our understanding of the molecular basis for a number of complex obesity syndromes, such as BBS, which have provided novel insights into processes essential for human hypothalamic function and the regulation of body weight. We now realize that there is a whole group of monogenic obesity syndromes involving the leptin-melanocortin pathway, where obesity itself is the presenting feature.

The practical implications of these findings for genetic counseling, prognostication, and even therapy have already emerged, and given the rapid pace of genetic and molecular technologies, it is very likely that new genes, proteins, and mechanisms will emerge to explain a variety of previously unrecognized obesity syndromes in the near future. As more is learned about these genes and more syndromes are described, it is likely that the need to evaluate severely obese patients in recognized centers will grow and close collaboration with academic centers with experience in this field is needed to ensure that the benefits of laboratory research are made available to the patients that need them. The clinical evaluation of the severely obese patient will become increasingly sophisticated and require the development of expertise in the recognition of these emerging syndromes together with the incorporation of novel biochemical and molecular genetic diagnostics. These approaches will need to be combined with the more traditional nutritional and behavioral approaches to optimize treatment for individual patients.

Discovery of the causative genetic defect has led to dramatically successful mechanism-based therapy in a few individuals. Finally, mutations in one gene, the MC4R, may be responsible for thousands of patients with obesity in the United Kingdom alone. Knowledge of the specific molecular mechanisms in this and other genetic disorders should lead to better mechanism-directed pharmacotherapy in the future.

REFERENCES

1. Bouchard C, Tremblay A, Després JP, et al. The response to long-term overfeeding in identical twins. N Engl J Med 1990; 322(21):1477–1482.
2. Bouchard C, Tremblay A, Després JP, et al., Overfeeding in identical twins: 5-year postoverfeeding results. Metabolism 1996; 45(8):1042–1050.
3. Maes HH, Neale MC, Eaves LJ. Genetic and environmental factors in relative body weight and human adiposity. Behav Genet 1997; 27(4):325–351.
4. Allison DB, Kaprio J, Korkeila M, et al., The heritability of body mass index among an international sample of mono-zygotic twins reared apart. Int J Obes Relat Metab Disord 1996; 20(6):501–506.
5. Stunkard AJ, Harris JR, Pedersen NL, et al. The body-mass index of twins who have been reared apart. N Engl J Med 1990; 322(21):1483–1487.
6. Stunkard AJ, Sørensen TI, Hanis C, et al. An adoption study of human obesity. N Engl J Med 1986; 314(4):193–198.
7. Comuzzie AG. The emerging pattern of the genetic contribution to human obesity. Best Pract Res Clin Endocrinol Metab 2002; 16(4):611–621.
8. Frayling TM, Timpson NJ, Weedon MN, et al. A common variant in the FTO gene is associated with body mass index and predisposes to childhood and adult obesity. Science 2007; 316(5826):889–894.
9. Dina C, Meyre D, Gallina S, et al. Variation in FTO contributes to childhood obesity and severe adult obesity. Nat Genet 2007; 39(6):724–726.
10. Beller A. Fat and Thin: A Natural History of Obesity. New York: Farrar, Straus and Giroux, 1977.
11. Cole TJ, Freeman JV, Preece MA. Body mass index reference curves for the UK, 1990. Arch Dis Child 1995; 73(1):25–29.
12. Cole TJ, Bellizzi MC, Flegal KM, et al. Establishing a standard definition for child overweight and obesity worldwide: international survey. BMJ 2000; 320(7244): 1240–1243.
13. Dietz WH, Robinson TN. Clinical practice. Overweight children and adolescents. N Engl J Med 2005; 352(20): 2100–2109.
14. Farooqi IS. The severely obese patient—a genetic work-up. Nat Clin Pract Endocrinol Metab 2006; 2(3):172–177.
15. Farooqi IS. Genetic and hereditary aspects of childhood obesity. Best Pract Res Clin Endocrinol Metab 2005; 19(3):359–374.
16. Farooqi IS, O'Rahilly S. Monogenic obesity in humans. Ann Rev Med 2005; 56:443–458.
17. Butler M. Prader-Willi syndrome: current understanding of cause and diagnosis. Am J Med Genet 1990; 35(3): 319–332.
18. Bray GA, Dahms WT, Swerdloff RS, et al. The Prader-Willi syndrome: a study of 40 patients and a review of the literature. Medicine (Baltimore) 1983; 62(2):59–80.
19. Goldstone AP. Prader-Willi syndrome: advances in genetics, pathophysiology and treatment. Trends Endocrinol Metab 2004; 15(1):12–20.
20. Carrel AL, Allen DB. Prader-Willi syndrome: how does growth hormone affect body composition and physical function? J Pediatr Endocrinol Metab 2001; 14(suppl 6): 1445–1451.
21. Carrel AL, Myers SE, Whitman BY, et al. Growth hormone improves body composition, fat utilization, physical strength and agility, and growth in Prader-Willi syndrome: a controlled study. J Pediatr 1999; 134(2):215–221.
22. Haqq AM, Farooqi IS, O'Rahilly S, et al., Serum ghrelin levels are inversely correlated with body mass index, age, and insulin concentrations in normal children and are markedly increased in Prader-Willi syndrome. J Clin Endocrinol Metab 2003; 88(1):174–178.

23. Tan TM, Vanderpump M, Khoo B, et al. Somatostatin infusion lowers plasma ghrelin without reducing appetite in adults with Prader-Willi syndrome. J Clin Endocrinol Metab 2004; 89(8):4162–4165.

24. Ohta T, Gray TA, Rogan PK, et al. Imprinting-mutation mechanisms in Prader-Willi syndrome. Am J Hum Genet 1999; 64(2):397–413.

25. Carrozzo R, Rossi E, Christian SL, et al. Inter- and intra-chromosomal rearrangements are both involved in the origin of 15q11-q13 deletions in Prader-Willi syndrome. Am J Hum Genet 1997; 61(1):228–231.

26. Clayton-Smith J, Driscoll DJ, Waters MF, et al. Difference in methylation patterns within the D15S9 region of chromosome 15q11-13 in first cousins with Angelman syndrome and Prader-Willi syndrome. Am J Med Genet 1993; 47(5):683–686.

27. Swaab DF, Purba JS, Hofman MA. Alterations in the hypothalamic paraventricular nucleus and its oxytocin neurons (putative satiety cells) in Prader-Willi syndrome: a study of five cases. J Clin Endocrinol Metab 1995; 80(2):573–579.

28. MacDonald HR, Wevrick R. The necdin gene is deleted in Prader-Willi syndrome and is imprinted in human and mouse. Hum Mol Genet 1997; 6(11):1873–1878.

29. Kozlov SV, Bogenpohl JW, Howell MP, et al. The imprinted gene Magel2 regulates normal circadian output. Nat Genet 2007; 39(10):1266–1272.

30. Bischof JM, Stewart CL, Wevrick R. Inactivation of the mouse Magel2 gene results in growth abnormalities similar to Prader-Willi syndrome. Hum Mol Genet 2007; 16(22):2713–2719.

31. Weinstein LS, Chen M, Liu J. Gs(alpha) mutations and imprinting defects in human disease. Ann N Y Acad Sci 2002; 968:173–197.

32. Weinstein LS, Yu S, Liu J. Analysis of genomic imprinting of Gs alpha gene. Methods Enzymol 2002; 344:369–383.

33. de Vries BB, Robinson H, Stolte-Dijkstra I, et al. General overgrowth in the fragile X syndrome: variability in the phenotypic expression of the FMR1 gene mutation. J Med Genet 1995; 32(10):764–769.

34. Katsanis N. The oligogenic properties of Bardet-Biedl syndrome. Hum Mol Genet 2004; 13(Spec No 1):R65–R71.

35. Mykytyn K, Sheffield VC. Establishing a connection between cilia and Bardet-Biedl Syndrome. Trends Mol Med 2004; 10(3):106–109.

36. Gerdes JM, Liu Y, Zaghloul NA, et al. Disruption of the basal body compromises proteasomal function and perturbs intracellular Wnt response. Nat Genet 2007; 39(11):1350–1360.

37. Yeo GS, Connie Hung CC, Rochford J, et al. A de novo mutation affecting human TrkB associated with severe obesity and developmental delay. Nat Neurosci 2004; 7(11):1187–1189.

38. Gray J, Yeo GS, Cox JJ, et al., Hyperphagia, severe obesity, impaired cognitive function, and hyperactivity associated with functional loss of one copy of the brain-derived neurotrophic factor (BDNF) gene. Diabetes 2006; 55(12):3366–3371.

39. Schwartz MW, Woods SC, Porte D Jr., et al. Central nervous system control of food intake. Nature 2000; 404(6778):661–671.

40. Cone RD. Anatomy and regulation of the central melanocortin system. Nat Neurosci 2005; 8(5):571–578.

41. Huszar D, Lynch CA, Fairchild-Huntress V, et al., Targeted disruption of the melanocortin-4 receptor results in obesity in mice. Cell 1997; 88(1):131–141.

42. Farooqi IS, Wangensteen T, Collins S, et al. Clinical and molecular genetic spectrum of congenital deficiency of the leptin receptor. N Engl J Med 2007; 356(3):237–247.

43. Farooqi IS, Matarese G, Lord GM, et al. Beneficial effects of leptin on obesity, T cell hyporesponsiveness, and neuro-endocrine/metabolic dysfunction of human congenital leptin deficiency. J Clin Invest 2002; 110(8):1093–1103.

44. Mantzoros CS, Ozata M, Negrao AB, et al., Synchronicity of frequently sampled thyrotropin (TSH) and leptin concentrations in healthy adults and leptin-deficient subjects: evidence for possible partial TSH regulation by leptin in humans. J Clin Endocrinol Metab 2001; 86(7):3284–9321.

45. Farooqi IS, Wagenstein T, Collins S, et al. Clinical and molecular genetic spectrum of congenital deficiency of the leptin receptor. N Engl J Med 2007; 356(3):237–247.

46. Gibson WT, Farooqi IS, Moreau M, et al. Congenital leptin deficiency due to homozygosity for the {Delta}133G Mutation: report of another case and evaluation of response to four years of leptin therapy. J Clin Endocrinol Metab 2004; 89(10):4821–4826.

47. Krude H, Biebermann H, Luck W, et al. Severe early-onset obesity, adrenal insufficiency and red hair pigmentation caused by POMC mutations in humans. Nat Genet 1998; 19(2):155–157.

48. Krude H, Biebermann H, Schnabel D, et al. Obesity due to proopiomelanocortin deficiency: three new cases and treatment trials with thyroid hormone and ACTH4-10. J Clin Endocrinol Metab 2003; 88(10):4633–4640.

49. Farooqi IS, Drop S, Clements A, et al. Heterozygosity for a POMC-null mutation and increased obesity risk in humans. Diabetes 2006; 55(9):2549–2553.

50. Farooqi IS, Keogh JM, Yeo GS, et al. Clinical spectrum of obesity and mutations in the melanocortin 4 receptor gene. N Engl J Med 2003; 348(12):1085–1095.

4

Cultural Differences as Influences on Approaches to Obesity Treatment

SHIRIKI KUMANYIKA

School of Medicine, University of Pennsylvania, Philadelphia, Pennsylvania, U.S.A.

INTRODUCTION

The significance of cultural influences in the etiology of obesity has been well documented, particularly in the area of societal standards of female attractiveness (1–3). Among the major chronic conditions that affect morbidity and mortality, obesity is unique in having a sociocultural significance unrelated to its presumed effects on long-term health, and biomedical definitions of obesity compete with sociocultural definitions (4). This chapter addresses the related issue of the potential influence of cultural factors on obesity treatment approaches and outcomes. The spectrum of cultural influences on obesity treatment goes far beyond body image or physical attractiveness variables. From the client perspective, this spectrum also includes perceptions and priorities in the domains of general health, food and eating, and physical activity as well as behavioral change variables. The latter include how food, activity, and weight interrelate with mechanisms for coping with stress, attitudes toward health systems and health professionals and a host of social and economic context variables in which these attitudes and behaviors are shaped. From the programmatic perspective, cultural influences and the contexts relevant to these influences affect treatment models, professional orientations, program content and form, and provider attitudes and behaviors. The respective intersections of these types of cultural influences on obesity treatment are shown in Figure 1. This figure also serves as a conceptual outline of the issues addressed in this chapter.

The goal of this chapter is to facilitate understanding of how the incorporation of cultural and related contextual considerations into program design and implementation might improve obesity treatment outcomes, particularly long-term treatment outcomes. The chapter focuses primarily on treatment of adults. The term "obesity treatment" is defined broadly to refer to the various types of health behavior change interventions that focus on weight reduction or weight control (5). The discussion is framed primarily in terms of situations in which clients and providers have different sociocultural backgrounds, e.g., ethnic minority clients are being treated by providers who are not from the same ethnic group. The concepts are applicable to cross-cultural issues in obesity treatment more generally. One underlying theme is that cultural processes are inextricably linked to other aspects of social contexts. Another is that all obesity treatment situations are "cross-cultural" to the extent that obesity treatment paradigms of the providers are not aligned with the sociocultural and contextual realities of obesity and weight control in the general population.

The section "Culture, Environment, and Ethnic Minority Populations" of the chapter provides some background

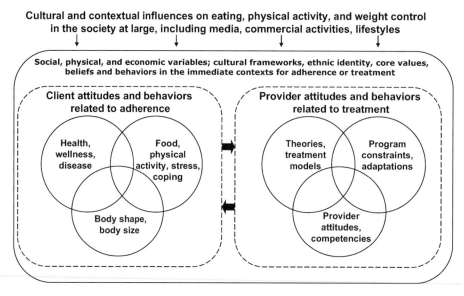

Figure 1 Schematic representation of the cultural influences in obesity treatment.

on what is meant by cultural and cross-cultural differences and on why these considerations are of increasing interest to the field of obesity treatment. This section also describes differences in obesity prevalence and contributing factors in U.S. ethnic minority groups compared to the majority U.S. population. As explained, cultural influences on obesity treatment can and should be explored for many specific ethnic groups or subgroups. Here most examples are drawn from literature relating to African-Americans. The section "Behavior Change Paradigms" examines the status of cultural considerations in relevant health and behavior change paradigms. The section "Treatment Providers" focuses on the cultural variables that influence those who provide obesity treatment. The sections "Cultural Adaptation Strategies" and "Summary and Conclusion" highlight ways that cultural factors have been addressed in obesity treatment programs and comment on future directions for the field.

CULTURE, ENVIRONMENT, AND ETHNIC MINORITY POPULATIONS

Culture and Cultural Differences

Cultural processes influence all human behavior and dialectically shape social institutions and social interactions among populations, groups, and individuals. "Culture" has many definitions, but all embody the underlying concept of implicit and explicit norms, attitudes, and beliefs that are inherited and shared by members of a particular society or societal subgroup (6,7). These norms, attitudes, and beliefs act as guidelines for "how to view

the world, how to experience it emotionally, and how to behave in it in relation to other people, to supernatural forces or gods, and to the natural environment" (7). Cultural perspectives are identifiable and transmitted from one generation to the next through distinctive symbols, language, and rituals. Of particular relevance to cross-cultural treatment issues, cultural influences on behavior seem universal, natural, and nonnegotiable to those influenced by a given culture (7). In fact, the influence of culture often becomes evident only when cultural differences are encountered, e.g., in interaction between individuals or groups that have contrasting beliefs, expectations, or values related to a particular issue; that is, one might not perceive that one is operating within a culture until one has to operate outside of it.

Table 1 lists examples of culturally influenced values and beliefs (8–14). Some of these variables, such as worldview or spirituality, are overarching and form the context for other elements as well. Differences between cultures on specific topics, sometimes termed "cultural distance," are often a matter of degree or emphasis. However, the sum total of cultural differences may result in qualitatively different ways of approaching life and day-to-day transactions. Furthermore, cultural norms, e.g., what is considered usual, expected, or appropriate, result from the interaction of cultural values and beliefs with environmental or ecological influences in the social structure including the availability of commodities such as food and health care.

The extent to which subgroups (e.g., different ethnic groups) within a society remain distinctive depends on social, economic, and political circumstances and on intergroup relations and is also influenced by the nature

Table 1 Examples of Culturally Influenced Values and Beliefs

1. Worldwide—how a person views himself or relation to the environment; the types of explanatory models used to understand day-to-day occurrences and to make sense of life experiences
2. Spirituality—beliefs in God, in the supernatural, sense of destiny and control over one's life; view of life, death, and afterlife
3. Harmony—view of oneself as interdependent with the environment; desire to dominate the environment; responsibility of the individual to humanity; sense of interconnectedness or discreteness of the various aspects of one's life; consumption and sharing of resource
4. Health and reproduction—concepts of wellness and optimal performance; disease and illness; food and sustenance; procreation
5. Interdependence—of people, individuals' freedoms and responsibilities, social orientation vs. individualistic orientation; definition of family (e.g., nuclear family; extended family; biological vs. socially defined kinship); definitions of self-reliance; expectations for caregiving; gender roles
6. Rhythm—sense of rhythmic nature to life; role of seasons; orientation to rhythms music, dance in behavior, and overall approach to life
7. Affect and cognition—importance of rationality; importance of emotion; degree to which emotion and thinking are considered separate; role of emotions and rationality in social relation in social relations
8. Individualism and communalism—separateness of self; uniqueness of individuals; social conformity; importance of individual expression; degree of interdependence with others
9. Linearity—value of order and step-by-step progression; acceptance of chaos and unpredictability
10. Vitality—energy of living; fullness of participation in all aspects of life
11. Interpersonal relationship—views about conflict and aggression; value for cooperation; ways of conveying approval/disapproval or social support
12. Status orientation—value of education and material possessions
13. Work orientation—work ethic; industriousness; work as self-definition; work as economic necessity
14. Approaches to technology—attitudes toward computers; attraction to new inventions; support of research and development activities
15. Communication styles—relative value of oral and written communication; directness of communication; body language
16. Time perspective—orientation to clock time or to events; future orientation or present orientation; history as a basis for reflection

Source: From Refs. 8–11,14.

and impact of cultural and structural changes affecting the society at large (15). Understanding how cultural influences relate to the potential for reducing obesity-related health disparities affecting U.S. racial/ethnic minority populations relative to whites requires consideration of these broader contextual variables.

The Obesity-Promoting Environment

There is a general concern within the field of behavior change that the available methods are not sufficient to produce long-term improvements in lifestyle risk factors related to diet and physical activity, including obesity as well as cigarette smoking (16). The need for effective long-term weight control strategies continues to be urgent in light of persistent upward trends in obesity prevalence (17,18). At the ecological level, these upward trends, observed in both adults and children, can be linked to cultural norms and social structural factors, which encourage and maintain chronic overconsumption of calories and physically inactive lifestyles (9,20). The most obvious trends are those related to food portion sizes (e.g., super-sizing of food packaging and restaurant portions), use of automobiles, television watching, use of computers, and

sedentary forms of recreation (21–23). These trends are driven by a synergism between cultural values (e.g., for individual choice, free-market activity, and consumerism) and societal processes (production, availability, and aggressive marketing of large quantities of high-calorie foods; and technological advances that yield labor-saving devices and electronic communications) that have both social and economic benefits for people in the society at large (24). Thus, in the United States and in other countries where similar trends and cultural shifts have occurred, obesity treatment occurs in a context where there are strong societal forces promoting weight gain and potentially counteracting individual attempts to lose weight (25).

Thus, we are now attempting to treat obesity in situations in which both being overweight and the eating and activity behaviors that lead to being overweight, although not normal in a physiological sense, are normative; that is, those who do not maintain adequate weight control now outnumber those who do. The difficulty of maintaining self-control over behaviors related to eating and physical activity has increased from prior times partly because people are bombarded with consumption stimuli via the mass media, and partly because they are receiving mixed signals about eating, physical activity, and weight.

Both the social structure and many current cultural norms favor day-to-day (e.g., not just on occasional holidays and at celebrations) behaviors that are highly obesity promoting, whereas obesity itself is still viewed as problematic.

Obesity in Ethnic Minority Populations in the United States

Minority Populations

Last (26) defines an ethnic group as follows:

> A social group characterized by a distinctive social and cultural tradition, maintained within the group from generation to generation, a common history and origin; and a sense of identification with the group. Members of the group have distinctive features in their way of life, shared experiences, and often a common genetic heritage. These features may be reflected in their health and disease experience (26, p. 63).

Ethnicity is often a more appropriate designation than "race," which purports to describe a biologically homogeneous group (26,27). Variations in cultural perspectives of different ethnic groups have always been of some interest for biomedicine in comparisons across societies (28,29). Cultural issues are receiving more attention in the United States as the population becomes more diverse (27,30). There is considerable ethnic, socioeconomic, and sociocultural diversity within the broad minority population categories used by the U.S. Census Bureau. From a sociopolitical perspective, what these groups have in common is being "nonwhite" or "Hispanic," whereas the majority population is defined as whites who do not indicate Hispanic ethnicity (27). Stated from a behavioral intervention perspective, minority populations are viewed as sufficiently different from the U.S. mainstream population to trigger cultural considerations in treatment, i.e., are not necessarily well served by programs designed with the majority or white population in mind (31). The more distant the language and cultural characteristics of the population from that of the majority, the greater the implied need for special considerations. However, if only by virtue of residence in the U.S. society, members of ethnic minority populations are also—to varying degrees—participants in the general U.S. culture and are influenced by mainstream cultural variables through media, workplace interactions, and other forms of social exchange.

Ethnicity and "minority" status are additive or synergistic rather than alternative cultural influences; minority status relates to social, economic, and political circumstances of the group in question. There are many cultural and contextual similarities among U.S. minority populations and between minority populations and whites. Both the similarities and the differences must be considered when examining cultural influences.

As already noted, not all social and behavioral differences among ethnic minority population and the majority are attributable to cultural values and beliefs. There are also differences in sociodemographic indicators such as the percentage who are foreign born, fertility rates, life expectancy, household and family structure, educational achievement, occupations, neighborhood characteristics, income distribution, health insurance coverage, and interactions with the health system (27,30,32,33). It is therefore difficult to separate ethnic differences that are culturally determined from those due to sociodemographic factors, particularly those related to social structural factors that affect minority populations differentially, such as poverty or discrimination. Moreover, there are culturally determined difference in attitudes and behaviors according to factors such as gender, age, geographic region, religious affiliation, and occupation within all populations. Each individual is, therefore, potentially influenced by a range of interrelated cultural and social structural variables. Behaviors of individuals in ethnic minority populations reflect a blend of the cultural perspectives to which they are exposed.

Obesity Prevalence and Contributing Factors

The prevalence of obesity in adults is generally higher in ethnic minority populations compared to non-Hispanic whites, especially among women (17,34,35). This is evident in National Health and Nutrition Examination Survey (NHANES) estimates based on weight and height measurements for non-Hispanic whites and blacks and Mexican-Americans (17) (Fig. 2) and also in estimates based on self-reported data from the National Health Interview Survey (NHIS) (35) (Fig. 3), although the estimates based on self-reported data underestimate prevalence. The NHIS data provide estimates for Hispanics overall and for American-Indians/Alaska Natives, Asian-Americans, and Native Hawaiians and other Pacific Islanders. The high obesity prevalence in ethnic minority populations is associated with a high burden of diabetes and other obesity-related diseases (36–42). Asian-Americans have the lowest prevalence of obesity, although lower BMI cutoffs have been recommended for obesity interventions in people of Asian descent (43). Obesity-related comorbidities are observed in Asian descent populations at BMI levels below 25, associated with relatively higher percent body fat compared to non-Asian descent populations with the same BMI level (42,43).

The excess risk of obesity in ethnic minority populations also applies to children and adolescents (17,44,45). For example, in the 2003–2004 NHANES data for 2- to 19-year-olds, 22% of Mexican-American boys compared

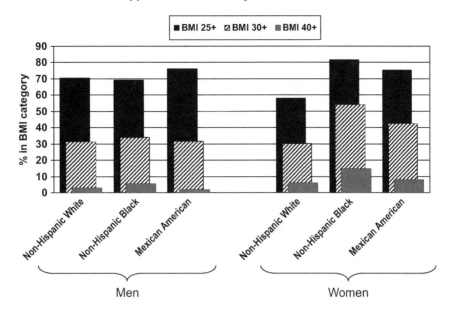

Figure 2 Age-adjusted prevalence of overweight or obesity, obesity, and extreme obesity in U.S. men and women ages 20 years and over, National Health and Nutrition Examination Survey, 2003–2004. *Source*: From Ref. 17.

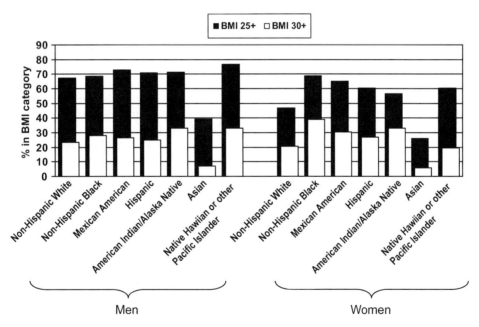

Figure 3 Prevalence of overweight or obesity and obesity in U.S. men and women ages 18 years and over, National Health Interview Survey, 2002–2004. *Source*: From Ref. 35.

to 18% of non-Hispanic white boys were obese and 24% of non-Hispanic black girls compared to 15% of non-Hispanic white girls were obese (17). Obesity in children and adolescents is now clearly recognized as associated with health problems during childhood, including childhood onset of type 2 diabetes, as well as increasing the risk of obesity and related health problems during

adulthood (46). Excess obesity in minority populations has led to explicit questions about ethnic group differences in the factors that predispose to obesity and about the ability to effectively prevent and treat obesity in minority populations. It is possible that the prevalence of a biological predisposition to gain weight is higher in the ethnic groups that exhibit such a high prevalence of obesity. However, to date, this biological predisposition has not been identified (3,47). What has been established, for example, from comparisons of Pima Indians and of African-descent individuals living in different environments (48,49) is that the predisposition to obesity is only expressed under permissive environmental circumstances.

Table 2 lists examples of culturally influenced variables that are specifically relevant to obesity treatment (50). As shown, these include variables that determine usual eating and physical activity patterns and assumptions about how food and activity relate to health as well as eating and physical activity related attitudes and behaviors that are specific to weight. As discussed elsewhere (3), cultural attitudes that favor a larger body image or at least do not support a strong drive to become thin can be documented for several ethnic minority populations (51). Overweight and obesity are especially likely to be socially normative in those minority populations where it affects the majority of adults or of women, and where the link between obesity and poor health outcomes is not always recognized (52–54). That illnesses associated with thinness or wasting (e.g., cancer, tuberculosis, or AIDS) are prominent in the health profiles of minority populations (55) may perpetuate the sense that being heavy is healthier than being thin, particularly among low-income women (53,54,56).

Several aspects of body image, dieting and dieting motivations appear to differ by ethnicity (57–59). However, there are also striking similarities in the prevalence of dieting across ethnic groups (60–63). That is, although there are clear body image differences that alter the motivation and context for obesity treatment, there is substantial diversity in these attitudes within minority communities as well as substantial evidence of strong weight loss motivations—even if of a differential quality than in the white population (63–67). In an analysis of national survey data (63), Hispanic men and women were somewhat more likely than non-Hispanic white men and women to report trying to lose weight. Body image may be the most dissimilar across ethnic groups in women who are not overweight or obese—a lesser tendency of normal weight women in ethnic minority compared to white populations to think that they are overweight. In most or all populations and even where there are positive cultural values for large body size, those who are overweight or obese seem to be less satisfied with their weight than those who are lean (64,65). Wolfe (68) has criticized the amount of attention given to cultural attitudes of black women suggesting that it diverts attention from the many societal factors that predispose black women to gain weight and the need to address these in attempts to control obesity.

As shown in Table 2, there are many culturally influenced attitude and behaviors related to food and activity that have implications for weight but that are not driven primarily by body image or weight concerns. Norms about food, activity, and health are defined and continually reinforced within cultures—for example, the concept of what constitutes having enough food, or feasting when food is abundant to anticipate possible food shortages; how food should be flavored; what combinations of food can be eaten together; what physical activities are appropriate for children but not for adults or for males but not females; the importance of inactivity (e.g., rest); or how one should cope with stress and restore physical and mental balance (51,69–71). The cultural embeddedness of food and the role of food as a carrier of ethnic identity and vehicle for social expression and social interactions are subjects of a large anthropological literature (51, 72–74) that, when taken seriously, can be very daunting to anyone who seeks to change food habits. Nevertheless, weight and health risk reduction considerations can only

Table 2   Examples of General and Weight-Specific, Culturally Influenced Attitudes and Perceptions Relevant to Weight Management

Food, activity, and health in general	Related to body size and weight
Medicinal or health promoting properties of food; health-related food restrictions	Ideal, acceptable, and undesirable body sizes and shapes
Symbolic meanings and social uses of food	Definitions of thinness and fatness
Food and flavor preference and aversions	Perceived determinants of weight status
Fasting and food deprivation	Importance of personal body size and shape and relationship to self-concept
Food portions; leaving food on plate; satiety	Functional and health effects (positive and negative) of being at a given weight
Overeating; food and coping style	Priority given to weight management
Physiological effects and health benefits of physical activity, exercise, and rest	Ways to loose or gain weight or influence body shape, including role of diet and exercise
Food-related social roles	Standards of personal attractiveness
Role constraints related to gender, age, social position, and work	Perceived social pressure to lose or gain weight
Preferred types of leisure time activity	Inclination toward low-fat diets, diet pills, or purging

Source: Adapted from Ref. 50.

be viewed logically as superimposed onto these more basic attitudes and as competing with other day-to-day survival and quality-of-life priorities. Priority on weight reduction relative to other health or survival concerns may be lower for the medically obese in ethnic or socioeconomic status groups for which body size and shape are less central to self-image or social acceptance or where some aspects of large body size (shapeliness, muscularity, strength) improve social acceptance or status (3). As discussed below, there may also be less congruency between basic attitudes and beliefs related to food and activity in minority populations with those assumed necessary for effective weight management.

Compared to the U.S. white population, minority populations are experiencing social and economic transitions from relative poverty, food shortages, and lifestyles that involved significant physical labor to circumstances in which there are more than sufficient amounts of food readily available to even the poorest segment of society and limited demand for physical work (75–78). Although cultural perspectives change, they may follow societal changes after a considerable time lag. Thus, the food and activity-related cultural perspectives of ethnic minority populations may still be primed to promote survival under prior circumstances—simplistically, to feasting and resting from hard work rather than restricting food and seeking extra physical work or exercise (79). Such perspectives would heighten the vulnerability to obesity in the current environment in which food and activity-related survival needs have been reversed from prior times. For example, low food security—defined as worrying about having access to sufficient food—has been associated with an excess of overweight in women, and the prevalence of overweight was generally highest among women in the lowest income categories (80).

National surveys do not necessarily show higher energy intakes in minority populations compared to whites (81,82). It is unclear whether this is due to ethnic differences in bias in dietary reports. In any case, conclusive evidence of differences in energy balance requires data on both energy intake and energy expenditure, and data for minority populations are indicative of higher levels of physical inactivity (83), implying lower total caloric energy expenditure. Excess obesity could, therefore, result even if energy intakes in minority populations were not high in comparison to those of less obese populations. Physical activity questionnaires may have differential validity in populations with different leisure time and occupational activity lifestyles. However, in black women, for example, the finding of lower activity compared to white women has been corroborated in studies using objective measures of physical activity (84,85).

Those with the least latitude in personal choices have the greatest lifestyle constraints (86). Thus, when the society at large has an overabundance of obesity-promoting forces, the potential deleterious effects may be intensified in minority populations. U.S. communities continue to be ethnically segregated (87). Constraints of particular importance in ethnic minority neighborhoods may include too few supermarkets and neighborhood or workplace physical fitness facilities, too many fast food establishments or food vendors selling high-fat foods at low prices, and high neighborhood crime rates that discourage outdoor activities (88–90). Media exposure may also be particularly detrimental (91,92). For example, a recent analysis of food advertising on prime-time television found that the shows oriented to blacks had significantly more food commercials per 30-minute segment and that more of these commercials were for high-calorie, low-nutrient density foods (91). These authors also noted that more of the characters on the black-oriented shows were overweight—perhaps reflecting the prevalence of obesity in the community but also reinforcing the concept that obesity is normative. That is, the high prevalence of obesity in minority populations is in itself an important contextual factor potentially influencing obesity treatment.

Finally, the reproductive and health status profiles of minority populations may predispose to weight gain and physical inactivity. Fertility rates are higher in minority women than white women (30), predisposing to pregnancy-related weight gain. The amount of weight that is gained and retained with each pregnancy may also be higher (93). In addition, the high prevalence of obesity-related health problems such as diabetes or osteoarthritis may interact with age-related social role perceptions to limit, or be perceived as limiting, participation in physical activity.

In summary, living circumstances, social and economic resources, eating and activity practices, and related attitudes vary among ethnic groups, leading to potential differences in weight loss motivations and in the way that obesity treatment programs will be received and adhered to. Relevant factors include the psychosocial receptivity to food restriction, body image issues, the congruency between behavior change recommendations and accustomed habits, feasibility of recommended changes, and social network and community support for lower calorie eating or increased physical activity.

BEHAVIOR CHANGE PARADIGMS

All paradigms reflect and are grounded in culture. However, the currently dominant biomedical paradigm in the United States is allopathic, technology-centered, and clinical (28,94). As such, it does not readily incorporate cultural considerations in its explanatory framework, at least not directly, even for conditions such as obesity that are clearly culture bound in many respects (4). However, the awareness of cultural issues in U.S. health care generally has increased with ongoing globalization and population diversity and with the resulting interactions and overlap among cultures (94–96). This general phenomenon, together with the particularly high burden of obesity and related diseases in minorities and some evidence that obesity treatments are less effective in minority populations than in whites, has led to some acknowledgment of the importance of attention to cultural influences in obesity treatment (97). It is therefore useful to examine the extent to which current obesity treatment or lifestyle change theories and treatment models, which are still grounded in the dominant paradigm, accommodate cross-cultural issues.

The relevant conceptualizations for these paradigms relate primarily to theories of long-term maintenance of behavior change and involve two related themes. One theme is that individual behavior and, consequently, behavior change, occur within contexts that constitute critical influences on treatment outcomes. Cultural variables are implicit and explicit elements of these contexts. The other theme is that the client's adherence perspectives, including cultural norms and values and social-structural constraints, should be used to tailor behavioral change programs for greater effectiveness with subgroups and individuals. Both themes are discussed in more detail in the following text.

Contextualization of Learning and Behavior

Social Cognitive Theory

Bandura, whose theoretical guidance has been a critical underpinning of obesity treatment, has commented on the relationship of cultural factors to Social Cognitive Theory (SCT) (98). He is critical of the apparent divergence between microanalytic and macroanalytic inquiry into the processes of human functioning. The microanalysts focus on "the inner workings of the mind in processing, representing, retrieving, and using the coded information to manage various task demands, and locating where the brain activity for these events occurs ... [with] these cognitive processes generally studied disembodied from interpersonal life, purposeful pursuits, and self-reflectiveness" (98, p. 5). In contrast, the macroanalysts focus on the "workings of socially situated factors in human development, adaptation, and change ... [and] human functioning is analyzed as socially interdependent, richly contextualized, and conditionally orchestrated within the dynamics of various societal subsystems and their complex interplay" (98, p. 5). He observes that because sociostructural influences operate through psychological mechanisms to produce behavioral effects, "comprehensive theory must merge the analytic

dualism by integrating personal and social foci of causation within a unified causal structure" (98, p. 5).

In an attempt to make this link, Bandura promotes the notion of "human agency," which embodies the endowments, belief systems, self-regulatory capacities, and distributed structures and functions through which personal influence is exercised. In short, he introduces a theoretical view of the human being as an agent who can intentionally make things happen by his or her actions. For example, he proposes that efficacy beliefs are the foundation of human agency, and that cross-cultural research attests to their universal functional value. Bandura also notes that "cultural embeddedness shapes the ways in which efficacy beliefs are developed, the purposes to which they are put, and the sociostructural arrangements through which they are best exercised" (98, p. 16). People from cultures that are individualistic "feel most efficacious and perform best under an individually oriented system, whereas those from collectivistic cultures judge themselves most efficacious and work most productively under a group-oriented system" (98, p. 16). Congruency between the person's psychological orientation and the structure of the social system is thought to provide for the greatest personal efficacy (98). If that is true, it follows then that attention to cultural issues in obesity treatment programs has as its goal the fostering of such congruency. However, providers from the individualistically oriented U.S. society may have difficulty in understanding the efficacy orientations of ethnic minority participants who are grounded in a collectivistic culture. Fisher et al. suggest that the tendency of those with an individualistic perspective to view social support as "a 'crutch' that psychologically mature individuals do not need" (99, p. 54), in itself a value judgment, may interfere with appropriate programming in minority communities.

Social Ecological Theory

Stokols, a proponent of Social Ecological Theory, emphasizes the critical influence of the context in which behaviors occur on the potential for behavior change (100). Referring to cardiovascular risk reduction programs such as the Multiple Risk Factor Intervention Trial (MRFIT) and the Minnesota Heart Health Program, he suggests that the "modest impact of these interventions reveals some potential limitations that are inherent in behavior change models of health promotion" (100, p. 284). These limitations center around insufficient attention to economic, social, and cultural constraints that may impede a person's efforts to modify his/her health practices. Strategies to enhance the health promoting capacity of the environment are advised in conjunction with those that are geared to facilitating behavior change at the individual level, that is, strategies that "enhance the fit between people and their surroundings." Similar to the concepts discussed by Bandura, Stokols notes that "instances of people-environment fit occur in settings where participants enjoy a high degree of control over their surroundings and are free to initiate goal directed efforts to modify the environment in accord with their preferences and plans" (100, p. 290).

Social Ecological Theory may be viewed by some as relating primarily to community-based treatment programs, whereas obesity treatment paradigms are dominated by practice in clinical settings. However, as Bandura's analysis (98) reminds us, the concept of enhancing person-environment fit as a goal of treatment applies generally. If one accepts that effective human functioning depends on a level of efficacy that requires a reasonable person-environment fit, the result of a mismatch between a treatment program and the needs and perspectives of the client may be either psychological stress (because of the high psychosocial cost of adherence) or nonadherence (to avoid the stress).

Context Dependency of Learning

Bouton (101) offers some insights as to how context influences behavioral adoption and long-term maintenance, drawing on both human and animal experiments, as follows. All learned behaviors, both old and new, are dependent upon the context in which they are learned, and the cues that lead to a given behavioral response are associated with that context. Consistent with the discussion above, Bouton points out that context can be defined broadly, to include physical and psychosocial stimuli and presumably—although not mentioned by Bouton—cultural forces. Furthermore, when behaviors are unlearned or relearned, this "extinction" or "counterconditioning" does not involve permanent removal of a prior behavior or habit. Rather, both old and new behaviors persist as possible responses to a given cue or set of cues, and the context is what "selects" or determines the response that occurs. Bouton's elaboration on this theoretical perspective offers a plausible explanation for the problem of lapse and relapse in the treatment of obesity as well as for other areas of lifestyle change. For example, he points out that the second response learned to a given stimulus seems to be more context dependent than the original learning, rendering the old or first-learned behaviors likely to occur and reoccur whenever the context does not preclude their occurrence. Relapse can then be thought of not as failure of the new behaviors but as success of the old ones. Using this logic, eating and physical activity behaviors targeted in obesity treatment can be viewed as strongly cued and reinforced by the conditions under which they were initially learned. This initial learning presumably takes place in family and community settings. The behaviors can, therefore, be expected to respond to reference group cultural

values and norms. In contrast, new behaviors developed during treatment would be viewed as secondary learning, inherently weaker responses, and tied to cues present only in association with treatment and the associated values and norms. Leaving the treatment setting ("returning home" physically or psychologically) would then clearly favor the original behaviors, leading to lapses and, potentially, to continued reinforcement of the original behavior (relapses) (101).

Bouton extends this reasoning to a discussion of how one might prevent lapses and relapses (101). One approach would be to avoid contexts that will retrieve the original behavior. Although this may be advised, such cue avoidance is almost always impossible—especially in the long term—given that the context in question includes, for example, a person's deep-seated cultural values and beliefs related to eating, as well as day-to-day social- or work-related behaviors and interactions within which eating occasions and activities occur. The other approaches suggested by Bouton involve providing a broader contextualization of the new learning, for example: placing cues to the treatment context in the larger environment (phone calls at home; mailings) or actually conducting the therapy in multiple environments, or extending the temporal context of treatment over longer period of time. Bouton also suggests that deliberately switching contexts during treatment may ultimately lead to more robust learning, although the initial effect may be to make learning more difficult. As will be discussed, the strategies that are used increasingly in tailoring treatment and cultural adaptation are very consistent with the realization that a person's usual context of daily living cannot be avoided and may be counter to the treatment context.

Bouton's perspective on context is consistent with Bandura's discussion of human agency in SCT (98) and with Social Ecological Theory (100), as discussed above, in expressing the principle that elicited changes must by definition be linked to the person's usual operational cultural context in order to be maintained over the long term. Several major SCT constructs are indicative of the need to contextualize learning, both physically and affectively (101,102). However, those who design and implement SCT-based programs may not emphasize these cultural aspects. Culturally based provider attitudes may promote the belief that potentially problematic contextual cues can be overcome by sheer self-control.

Tailoring Treatment Programs

"Focal Points" for Intervention

Rakowski defines "tailoring" as a deliberate attempt to account for important individual or subgroup variables when developing program messages or intervention strategies (103). This concept has particular relevance to theories that incorporate contextual factors as primary intervention variables as opposed to theories that tend to subordinate the importance of contextual issues in favor of greater emphasis on self-control. As reviewed by Rakowski (103), the concept of tailoring has evolved to a high level of specificity with respect to how tailoring can be approached and why it might work where other approaches have failed (103). Many of the relevant variables are culturally determined, although this is implicit rather than directly argued. According to Rakowski, key principles are the need for prior knowledge of the constellation of variables that predict individual variation in a given behavior, and the context specificity of these variables to the interaction of behavior, population, and setting. He designates the particular combination of these three elements as "focal points" for intervention, giving as an example, "blood pressure control [behavioral focus] among blue collar smokers [population focus] in a worksite intervention [setting]" (103, p. 285).

Rakowski's discussion of tailoring highlights the importance of needs assessment and process evaluation in the development and conduct of interventions. This approach is at the other extreme from one in which professionals design a program and then expect clients to fit themselves to it. Defining an initial focal point is one stage of tailoring; the second stage would involve further tailoring to individuals within this focal point based on additional variables. The definition of the focal points themselves is dynamic to the extent that subgroups initially thought to be relatively homogeneous on certain broad characteristics might subsequently be found to comprise several focal points, for example, the increasingly recognized heterogeneity within the major ethnic minority populations (104). Kreuter et al. (104) emphasize the importance of attending to heterogeneity within cultural groups or subgroups identified as focal points for intervention by differentiating "tailoring" to individuals, based on data obtained from individual assessments, from "targeting" population groups, where targeting is based on group characteristics and implicitly assumes within group homogeneity. Similarly, increasing levels of differentiation are also possible for behavioral foci and settings. Evaluation of intervention process variables and assessments of the relationship of process to outcome can ultimately inform tailoring to refine program strategies and improve effectiveness.

Table 3 lists variables identified by Rakowski as potentially important for tailoring within a given focal point, selected to illustrate the multiple types of cultural influences that are relevant. The selected variables relate either to characteristics of target populations or to the performance demand characteristics of the behavior. Rakowski stresses the importance of basing both the selection and refinement of focal points and the tailoring

Table 3 Culturally Relevant Variables Important for Tailoring Behavioral Interventions

Client or population characteristics
  Age, race/ethnicity, gender and socioeconomic variables
  Risk perception/perceived threat of illness
  Readiness for change; stage of change
  Self-efficacy perception
  Attitudes about the health practice or illness
  Information processing style
  Attribution of causality for illness
  Availability of family/friend support; social support systems
  Reliance on medical professionals to determine one's health actions
  Tendency to avoid (approach) the health care system
  Level of acculturation to mainstream
Required psychosocial resources and performance
  Demands
  Holding a positive self-image
  Social support to assist the change process
  Optimism/long-range time perspective
  Sense of timing/scheduling
  Tolerance of discomfort

Source: Adapted from Ref. 103.

of intervention strategies on theoretical frameworks, and cites an array of available theories, including SCT and the Transtheoretical Model. However, he cautions that formal theories may not have incorporated key relevant considerations. For example, current theoretical frameworks that do not include culturally based explanatory models of disease causation would provide inadequate guidance for tailoring interventions in situations where a health problem is attributed to irreversible aging.

Cultural Sensitivity

"Surface structure" and "deep structure"

Resnicow et al. define "cultural sensitivity" as "the extent to which ethnic/cultural characteristics, experiences, norms, values, behavioral patterns and beliefs of a target population as well as relevant historical, environmental, and social forces are incorporated in the design, delivery, and evaluation of targeted health promotion materials and programs" (105, p. 11). These authors differentiate between "culturally tailored" interventions, which may involve adaptation of existing materials and programs for racial/ethnic subpopulations, and "culturally based" interventions. Culturally based intervention, a relatively recent term, refers to "programs and messages that combine culture, history, and core values as a medium to motivate behavior change" (105, p. 11), for example, programs for American-Indians that focus on ancestral spiritual systems.

Resnicow et al. conceptualize cultural sensitivity in two primary dimensions using the terminology, from sociology and linguistics, of surface structure and deep structure. Cultural sensitivity at the level of surface structure involves attention to relatively superficial characteristics, e.g., depicting people from the same ethnic group in illustrations, incorporating preferences for settings, brands, clothing, or music, or having ethnically matched staff. These superficial characteristics are viewed as important for improving program fit with the culture or experience of the population served and can increase the face validity of the program. Deep structure is much more difficult to characterize and grasp. Sensitivity at this level requires an understanding of a range of contextual variables, including core cultural values, historical factors, and others. These authors comment that cultural sensitivity at these different levels has different effects on outcome; deep structure relates more to the salience of the program, whereas surface structure relates more to receptivity to the program.

Resnicow et al. emphasize the importance of focus groups and pretesting in the early stages of implementation of culturally tailored or culturally based programs (105). Focus groups provide for elicitation of surface structure variables as well as a potential opportunity for exploration of deep structure. Pretesting to assess the actual responses of members of the proposed audience to the materials or messages is particularly critical, because cultural content and cultural tailoring are highly vulnerable to nuances of connotation or context that can cause a well-intended message to be received negatively rather than positively.

PEN-3 model

Airhihenbuwa's PEN-3 model provides a conceptual framework for designing health programs in which cultural considerations are at the core of rather than peripheral or latent considerations in program design (12). In the terminology of Resnicow et al. (105), this would refer to culturally based programming. Airhihenbuwa's premise is that "it is more effective to adapt preventive health programs to fit community needs and cultural contexts than the reverse . . ." (12, p. 26). This, again, expresses the principle of client-program fit and attention to context but in a completely client-centered tone.

The PEN-3 model is shown schematically in Figure 4. The three domains of the model relate to the foci of health education, the understanding of health-related beliefs, and the classification of relevant cultural influences in ways that can guide the selection of program emphases and strategies. In the health education domain, Airhihenbuwa suggests that a central focus on cultural variables cannot be achieved by focusing only on individuals; rather, extended family and neighborhood foci should be included. One could argue that even in individually

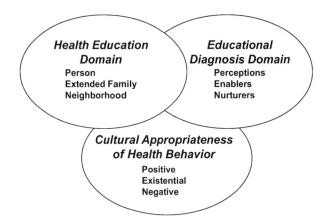

Figure 4 The PEN-3 model. *Source*: From Ref. 12.

focused, clinic-based programs it is more efficient to include the family and community in the treatment perspective to the greatest extent possible because of their relationship to the contextual cues of culturally defined behaviors of the primary client. This is particularly true for ethnic groups in which individuals consider themselves to be very interdependent with others and have a communal orientation. One can also argue, using obesity as a case in point, that behavioral programs restricted to clinical environments become increasingly less culturally appropriate as the relevance of culture to the focal points of intervention (to use Rakowski's term) increases.

The second domain for consideration in PEN-3 is educational diagnosis, i.e., the identification of factors that influence health actions of the individual, family, or community. Airhihenbuwa notes that this dimension of PEN-3 evolved from the confluence of three of the principal theoretical frameworks in the health behavior change field: the Health Belief Model, the Theory of Reasoned Action, and the PRECEDE framework (12). Culture does not have a central role in educational diagnosis in these models, but PEN-3 identified cultural elements that are implied in these other models, as follows:

Perceptions comprise the knowledge, attitudes, values, and beliefs, within a cultural context, that may facilitate or hinder personal, family, and community motivation to change. . . . Enablers are cultural, societal, systematic, or structural influences or forces that may enhance or be barriers to change, such as the availability of resources, accessibility, referrals, employers, government officials, skills, and types of services (e.g., traditional medicine) . . . (12, pp. 31–32).

Nurturers reflect the "degree to which health beliefs, attitudes, and actions are influenced and mediated, or nurtured, by extended family, kin, friends, peers, and the community" (12, p. 33).

The third dimension of PEN-3 provides specific guidance for the development of culturally appropriate health programs by offering a schema in which culturally based beliefs, norms, and actions can be classified as positive (known to be beneficial to health), existential (exotic to the outside observer but having no harmful health consequences), and negative (known to be harmful to health). Airhihenbuwa notes that the designation given to a particular belief or practice will vary depending on the targeted behavioral outcome. That is, a belief could be positive in relation to one behavior and negative or existential in relation to another. This aspect of the PEN-3 framework can help health professionals, particularly if from outside of the community or culture in question, to avoid overemphasizing negative behaviors without sufficient reinforcement of positive behaviors, to avoid viewing behaviors that are existential or neutral as harmful simply because they are unusual, and to avoid underestimating the cultural anchoring of certain behaviors. Airhihenbuwa recommends segmentation of beliefs and practices with respect to whether they are historically rooted in cultural traditions over the long term or are more recent and short term. For example, the home setting may be most appropriate for addressing traditional or relatively recent beliefs and practices, whereas media strategies may only work for those beliefs and practices that are not traditionally entrenched.

TREATMENT PROVIDERS

Obesity treatment is ultimately a social exchange between one or more clients and one or more providers who are usually health care professionals. From the foregoing discussion, it is clear that cultural variables and related contextual factors are highly relevant to lifestyle change from the client's perspective. This section addresses cultural influences from the provider perspective. For example, what factors support or limit the receptivity of those who provide obesity treatment to recognizing the importance of cultural variables in treatment? What does professional competence in this domain require?

Cultural Competence

The topic of cultural competence, i.e., "the ability of a system, agency, or professional to work effectively in cross-cultural situations" (95), has become prominent in the health care literature as the challenge of delivering effective health care to an increasingly diverse population has emerged (11,95,106–108). Unlike the terms "compliance" and "adherence," which emphasize client variable

as potential barriers to the success of treatment, "cultural competence" puts the focus on what the provider brings to the treatment relationship and requires self-reflection among health professionals. Providers vary in age (e.g., reflecting both generation effects and life stage), ethnicity, regional background, disciplines, language skills, and gender. There are also wide variations in socioeconomic status, political opinions, values, moral codes, and worldviews among health professionals. These culturally influenced attributes are not eliminated by professional training, and they influence the treatment process. Moreover, because of the social stigma that has been attached to it, obesity constitutes a special case with respect to potential providers; that is, in treating obesity, professionals have the additional challenge of managing their own culturally influenced attitudes about obesity and obese people (109). This does not apply to conditions such as diabetes or hypertension, for example.

The three critical domains of cultural competence are awareness of one's own cultural values and biases, knowledge of client views and perspectives, and skills for designing and delivering culturally appropriate interventions (95). Examples of specific competencies within each of these domains as they relate to nutrition counseling are presented in Table 4. The steps in developing cultural competence follow directly from the nature of the competencies themselves, e.g., increasing one's personal readiness to engage in cross-cultural interactions through self-reflection and learning how to value and be comfortable with differences; learning about other cultures, how one is viewed by people from other cultures, and how to find common ground with people from other cultures; improving both verbal and nonverbal communication styles in cross-cultural interactions, and overcoming associated fears; and learning how to maintain alertness to cross-cultural issues and information (110).

A workshop conducted within the clinical trials component of the Women's Health Initiative (WHI) is an example of the increased recognition of the need for cultural competence among health professionals involved in behavioral change interventions (111). The WHI was a set of interrelated clinical trials involving about 68,000 older women (ages 50–79) recruited from throughout the United States and including nearly 28,000 from ethnic minority populations. Participant adherence to lifestyle change or medication regimens was of paramount importance to the scientific integrity of this large-scale and costly study. The workshop curriculum was designed to increase knowledge of the demographic and cultural characteristics among and within the diverse groups of women in the WHI, to increase awareness of how diversity affected the interpersonal interactions with study staff, including the potential effect of staff behavior on participant adherence and retention, and to improve effective

Table 4 Multicultural Nutrition Counseling Competencies

Domain	Competencies
Self-awareness	• Knowing how personal cultural background and experiences as well as attitudes, values, and biases influence nutrition counseling
	• Knowing the limits of one's own cultural competencies and abilities
	• Being aware of and sensitive to one's own cultural heritage and also valuing and respecting differences
	• Being comfortable with differences between self and clients related to ethnicity, culture, beliefs, and food practices
	• Valuing personal cultural heritage and world view as a significant starting point for understanding those who are culturally different
	• Believing that cultural differences do not have to affect interactions negatively
	• Being aware of personally held stereotypes and preconceived notions toward culturally different groups
	• Being knowledgeable about cultural differences in communication styles and able to anticipate how one's own style might influence the counseling process
Food and nutrition counseling knowledge	• Understanding cultural influences on food selection, preparation, and storage
	• Having knowledge about cultural eating patterns and family traditions, e.g., core foods
	• Being familiar with latest research findings about food practices and related health problems of various ethnic groups
	• Having specific knowledge of cultural values, beliefs, and eating practices of population served, including culturally different clients
	• Having knowledge of diversity in food practices within ethnic groups
	• Using the principle of "starting where the client is" with respect to recommending changes in eating patterns
Nutrition counseling skills	• Being able to evaluate new techniques, research, and knowledge for validity and applicability in working with culturally diverse populations
	• Taking responsibility for orienting the client to the counseling process with respect to goals and expectations
	• Having an explicit knowledge of the general characteristics of counseling and how they may clash with expectations of different cultural groups
	• Having the ability to gain trust and respect of individuals who are culturally different
	• Being aware of institutional or agency factors that may be barriers to accessing treatment
	• Being able to identify additional resources that may be useful to the client
	• Understanding how ethnicity, culture, and economics may affect food practices, related health problems, and the appropriateness of various counseling strategies

Source: Adapted from Ref. 95.

listening and communication skills. Five cultural domains identified as particularly relevant to the conduct of the WHI were explored during this workshop.

Ard et al. (112) have proposed a model for achieving cultural appropriateness in behavioral modification trials that involve African-Americans. As in the WHI, Ard et al. (112) address the need to achieve similar levels of intervention effectiveness in ethnic minority and white participants within the same treatment context. These authors suggest that focus groups be used to probe for content related to sociocultural issues or ethnicity-specific variables that might influence the targeted behaviors rather than only obtaining reactions to proposed intervention strategies. They point out that eliciting reactions to proposed strategies may not be sufficiently informative if the focus group participants have little first-hand experience with the type

of program being offered. A focus on the proposed intervention as such also may fail to identify potential contextual or attitudinal influences on adherence. In addition, Ard et al. (112) suggest that assessment of acculturation to the relevant beliefs and practices of the majority culture may also be useful, particularly to identify intra-group differences influenced by socioeconomic status.

Professional Culture

As cultures are least visible to those who operate within them, it may be especially difficult for providers to recognize that their professional and organizational cultures have a significant impact on the treatment interaction. Professions create cultures (113) that may act as barriers to both the motivation and ability to provide services in a culturally competent manner. Professional cultures define the ethics of professional conduct, expectations that professionals have about each other and about clients, and systems of rewards and sanctions that help them to gain and maintain public confidence and trust (114,115). Professionals place a high premium on lifelong commitment (116), invest heavily in their training, and incorporate their identity as professionals into their self-concepts. Professionals also develop jargon and learn a communication style that makes them at ease with each other, often in a way that excludes or creates discomfort for others, including their clients (117). These styles are not easy to change. Professionals embrace paradigms to help make sense of their domain, the nature of their knowledge, and the directions of their research agendas (118). Thus, a professional will use and defend his or her dominant paradigm, often blocking other venues for treatment and understanding.

Professionals, by definition, rely on expert knowledge or skill to claim authority for their roles in diagnosis and treatment and tend to minimize the importance of possible causal factors that fall outside of their areas of expertise (115). Relevant here, to the extent that obesity has been claimed by the domains of clinical medicine and psychology (119,120), the importance of social-contextual factors in obesity causation and treatment will be deemphasized even where acknowledged. "Medicalization" of obesity has also led to a preference for using treatment approaches that have been tried and tested for other medical conditions and to comparing the costs and benefits of obesity treatment with those for other conditions. These professional biases may limit the ability to understand and manage obesity as a unique entity. The training of professionals to keep an appropriate emotional distance in the treatment encounter is also relevant, since—in a cross-cultural interaction—expression of emotion may be necessary for establishing trust and rapport (106).

Understanding the cultural perspective that the provider brings to the treatment encounter also requires an understanding of the culture of the organization in which the professional works (121). Organizations work hard to create a distinctive culture, viewing this as contributing to both organizational identity and higher effectiveness (122). For example, organizational culture may be expressed in the form of preferred communications (123), hierarchical structures, and decision-making processes (124) as well as in time horizons, market approaches, and style of teamwork (125). Organizations have bureaucratic rules and processes and legal requirements (126,127). In addition, to survive financially, they must attain goals that have very little to do with any specific treatment and use methods that have a high level of productivity. To be successful within an organization, providers must be able to absorb and function within the culture of their organization. For example, they master and abide by the administrative processes and show productivity by organizational standards. These elements directly or indirectly influence the way the provider views obesity as a condition, the treatment options, and the clients themselves (i.e., as potential "treatment successes" or "treatment failures").

The intersection of these personal, professional (including paradigmatic), and organizational elements culminates in expectations about patient/client compliance or adherence. Providers have guidance to offer, and the goal of treatment is for patients to follow that guidance. However, Anderson and Funnell (128) argue that adherence is a dysfunctional concept in relation to the treatment of chronic diseases such as diabetes, because it takes the value of following the health professional's advice as the central value apart from the context in which the patient must follow such advice. Their arguments, summarized in Table 5, are also relevant to obesity treatment, as follows: the health professional has needs, expectations, and values with respect to adherence that are inappropriate, because health professionals have no control over the client behaviors in question. These professional expectations and needs may be carryovers from the model of acute-illness care in which it makes sense to expect a patient to give short-term priority to following, directly, a health professional's life-saving advice. In contrast, chronic disease management, and particularly management of conditions such as obesity that may not even be considered by the client to be "diseases," is primarily a function of day-to-day decisions made by the patient. As noted previously, these decisions are, of necessity, made in the context of other life decisions, regardless of the provider's expectations about adherence.

Thus, in the social interaction that is obesity treatment, several forces are at work that tend to be incompatible, and it is within the realm of the professional, not the client, to find solutions for bridging these forces and creating "win-win" scenarios. This implies that the professional not only grasps the contextual limitations and possibilities of the clients, but also can negotiate substantial amounts of flexibility within his or her own professional and social contexts (129). To use Bandura's conceptualization (98), professionals have to learn the art of human agency as well.

CULTURAL ADAPTATION STRATEGIES

Overview

To be theoretically sound, cultural adaptation strategies should link culturally influenced variables to specific

Table 5 Problematic Aspects of the Concept of Adherence or Compliance

Professional expectations
  High investment made to develop helping skills to improve patients' health
  Expectation, from training, that patients should follow advice directly
  Awareness of potential health consequences to individuals of their failure to adopt or refrain from certain health practices
  Need to feel competent and effective in chosen profession
  Strongly held beliefs
  Strong belief that patients should strive to prevent disease progression and complications
  Strong belief that patients who do not comply will later regret this
  Perceived obligation to convey seriousness of disease
  Limited control over what patients do on a day-to-day basis
  Sense of responsibility for outcome without leverage to affect outcome
  Inadvertent frustration with patients who do not maximize their adherence
  Blaming patients to compensate for feelings of ineffectiveness (e.g., labeling those who are noncompliant as "disobedient")
  Patients may blame provider for not appreciating the impact of recommendations on their lives

Source: From Ref. 128.

aspects of treatment process and outcomes. Examples of such possible links from the client and provider perspective are presented in Table 6. For example, body image and other attitudes may have an influence primarily through effects on the motivation to seek treatment initially or to continue with treatment. Outreach to increase enrollment in a program might then employ persuasive strategies to increase awareness of the possible health or functional status benefits of modest weight loss (e.g., on blood pressure, breathing difficulties, or knee problems) as separate from potentially less salient social or physical attractiveness issues. Cultural sensitivity in the way treatment is delivered would be helpful in ensuring that participants fully engage

in the process (quality of participation). The distinction between factors affecting initial adoption versus long-term behavior changes is informed by Rothman's proposition that different theoretical models are needed to explain initial adoption and maintenance (130). For example, whereas initial adoption is related primarily to a desire to achieve a favorable outcome and expectations that these outcomes will be achieved, once adopted, behaviors may be maintained by satisfaction with the outcomes that result.

Thus, offering behavior change content in ways that are relevant to the patient's lifestyle issues and accessible from the perspective of language and learning style would be expected to facilitate short-term behavior changes.

Table 6 Potential Links Between Culturally Influenced Client Variables and Treatment Process and Outcomes[a]

Influences from and interactions between primary reference culture(s) and mainstream culture	Relevant treatment process and outcome variables
Body image	Motivation to seek treatment
Social pressure to lose weight	Enrollment in treatment
Weight-related health concern	Remaining in treatment (vs. dropping out)
Perceived appeal of program	Quality of participation in treatment program
Reactions to treatment setting	Regular attendance
Interactions with provider	Ability to establish trust and rapport
Interactions with other participants	Active engagement in program (passive participation)
Preferred language	Adoption of weight management behaviors
Baseline knowledge, attitudes, and practices	Learning and skill acquisition while in program
Prior relevant experience	Adherence to recommended short-term behavior changes
Perceived relevance of program content	Achievement of short-term weight reduction (vs. no loss, or gain)
Experience of program	Long-term behavior change
Worldview	Motivation for long-term behavior change
Health lifestyle	Feasibility of long-term behavior change
Contextual congruence	Maintenance of long-term behavior changes
Perceived benefits of weight loss	Continued or maintained weight loss (vs. relapse and regain)

[a]Cultural influences on these pathways may be magnified or reduced by other relevant variables that influence feasibility or appropriateness of the program (see text).
Source: Adapted from Ref. 50.

Contextual factors such as the worldview, the general salience of health considerations in making lifestyle choices, and the structural constraints would be most relevant at the level of maintaining long-term change. Ultimately then, the rewards of having lost weight must be sufficiently reinforcing (positively) within the applicable context to motivate continued practice of the altered eating and activity patterns or, rather, according to Bouton, to drown out the inherently strong reinforcement for the prior, original, and culturally embedded behavior pattern. Clinical programs may be able to maintain changes by providing continued reinforcement through continued treatment. On the other hand, given the nature of obesity and its determinants, a better alternative might be to reframe obesity treatment within health promotion paradigms. Health promotion paradigms are broader than clinical paradigms, are more inclusive of contextual issues, and are ahead of clinical paradigms in articulating specific frameworks for addressing cultural variables (100,131–133).

Examples of Cultural Adaptations

In spite of the high prevalence of obesity in ethnic minority populations, expert panels developing clinical guidelines for obesity treatment have noted the dearth of evidence relating to efficacy or effectiveness of various approaches in ethnic minority populations (134,135). For example, the U.S. Preventive Services Task Force guidelines state:

> The data supporting the effectiveness of interventions to promote weight loss are derived mostly from women, especially white women.... The USPSTF believes that, although the data are limited, these interventions may be used with obese men, physiologically mature older adolescents, and diverse populations, taking into account cultural and other individual factors (135, p. 931).

Table 7 lists variables within each of several aspects of program design or implementation that might be foci for adaptations to improve cultural relevance or sensitivity. The reference in Table 7 to "school culture" is taken from the aforementioned Wilcox et al. (111) WHI workshop summary. Participation in clinical trials was viewed as involving skills that are usually learned in school, including "self-discipline, observing and reporting events, setting long-term goals, and reading and completing forms" (111, p. 285). The WHI authors noted that these demands may be stressful for study participants who lack these skills. This may also apply to clients who have a strong cultural preference for a different style of learning. The emphasis on active discovery learning and nondidactic approaches in programs that have been culturally adapted for ethnic

Table 7 Culturally Influenced Programmatic Variables as Possible Targets for Cultural Adaptation

Selection and interpretation of theoretical framework
    Emphasis on contextual factors
    Emphasis on cognition over emotion
    Conceptualization of obesity
Provider behavior
    Type of provider
    Role perception, expectations, and needs in the treatment setting
    Perception of the ideal client
    Cultural competency (Table 3)
    Cultural distance from clients
Delivery system and setting
    Research, clinical, or commercial setting
    Emphasis on functionality or familiarity
    Psychological and physical accessibility
    Resources available
Focus of treatment
    Individual
    Family unit
    Community
Treatment goals
    Expected amount and rate of weight loss
    Inclusion of treatment goals other than weight loss
    Protocol or client-driven goal setting
Program content
    Food selections and recipes
    Activity choices
    Assumptions and messages about body size and shape
    Attention to emotions and spirituality
    Language used
Format and mode of contact
    Group, individual, or both
    Didactic or interactive process
    Program duration
    Sequencing of information
    School culture (see text)
    Face to face, telephone, mail

minority populations may reflect the recognition of the need to minimize the school culture that is common in conventional programs.

The typical approach to cultural adaptation has involved ethnicity or culture-specific approaches in which a weight loss program is specially designed for and offered to the group in question. Several examples of the approaches used in such programs or studies are listed in Table 8. Each focuses on a single ethnic minority population, e.g., African-Americans (136,139,141–143,145,146,148); Mexican Americans (137,144), Caribbean Latinos (52), Pima Indians (140), or Native Hawaiians (138,147). One strategy for increasing the cultural sensitivity of those providing treatment is to involve peer counselors (140–142) instead of or in addition to professional counselors. Some studies

Table 8 Examples of Types of Cultural Adaptations in Weight Loss or Lifestyle Change Programs in Adults in Specific Ethnic Groups

First author and yr (reference) (ethnic group focus)	Program description highlighting components of cultural adaptation
Lasco, 1989 (136) (African-American)	CHAPP was a 10-wk nutrition and exercise program designed by a community coalition on the basis of data from a needs assessment. Numerous supports were provided, e.g., child care, transportation, and a home visit to build family support. Ancillary topics and activities were included in response to participants' requests (e.g., a class on makeup, a wardrobe and fashion analysis, and a theater party). Participant feedback and suggestions were solicited and incorporated.
Cousins, 1992 (137) (Mexican-Americans)	*Cuidando el Corazon* was a 1-yr weight loss program for Mexican-American women who were married with at least one preschool child. Bilingual manual with nutrition, exercise, and behavior information and modified to reflect cultural values of the population; family condition included content on parenting skills to encourage healthful eating; a cookbook with fat-modified traditional Mexican-American foods, and behavior modification strategies illustrated in simple terms. Spouses were encouraged to attend classes; separate classes were held for preschool children.
Shintani, 1994 (138) (Native Hawaiians)	The Waianae Diet Program used a traditional Hawaiian diet (low in fat and very high in complex carbohydrates) to reduce weight and cardiovascular disease risk factors in Native Hawaiians. Participants were encouraged to eat to satiety; calories were not restricted. Program themes included family support, role modeling, and a whole-person approach.
Agurs-Collins, 1997 (139) (African-Americans)	Weight loss and exercise program for older African-American adults with type 2 diabetes. Program was offered at an African-American university hospital. Program materials depicted African-American individuals, families, and community settings. Recipes used in dietary instruction were provided by participants. Program format allowed time for participants to discuss and problem-solve regarding social context issues such as church meals.
Venkat-Narayan, 1997 (140) (Pima Indians)	Pima Pride was a lifestyle change program for Pima Indians in Arizona. Main emphasis was self-directed learning through monthly small group meetings led by a member of the community. Discussion focused on attitudes about current lifestyle in the community. Local speakers were invited to address Pima culture and history. Newsletters sometimes carried poetry, stories, and folklore contributed by group members.
McNabb, 1997 (141) (African-Americans)	PATHWAYS was a church-based weight loss program for African-American women with type 2 diabetes (14 wk). Program was adapted from a successful clinical program for delivery in a community setting by trained lay volunteers and emphasized health rather than appearance motivations for weight loss. Interactive, guided discovery approach to learning activities; small-group instruction.
Vazquez, 1998 (52) (Caribbean Latinos)	*Buena Alimentación, Buena Salud* (Good Eating, Good Health) was a nutrition intervention program designed for Caribbean Latinos with type 2 diabetes (12 wk). Intervention was developed by a multidisciplinary bilingual team of health professionals in collaboration with Latino community based on results of a planning survey and focus group interviews. Intervention was designed based for cultural sensitivity in relation to 12 concepts. Resulting features included involving bilingual/bicultural staff; offering the program in Spanish; emphasis on health risks of obesity; using a group setting; using interactive rather than didactic sessions; recommending modifications to traditional recipes; making intervention sessions into social events; and introducing the concept of empowerment.
Ard, 2000 (124) (African-Americans)	Clinical program based on the Duke University Rice Diet, involving commonly available foods, daily dietary counseling, nutrition education, and an exercise prescription, with the following cultural adaptations for African-American patients: • Costs of program were reduced • Ethnic recipes were used in cooking classes • Changes in ideas about exercise were targeted • Open invitation to family members to attend weekly classes Most classes were conducted by an African-American instructor.
Keyserling, 2000 (142) (African-American)	*New Leaf . . . Choices for Healthy Living with Diabetes was* designed for African-American women with type 2 diabetes. Cultural relevance and acceptability of program components were assessed in a series of focus groups. Recipes build on positive aspects of the Southern regional diet, e.g., the use of dry peas and beans. Simplified counseling materials in both individually tailored and nontailored formats. Telephone counseling provided by community diabetes advisers (African-American women with type 2 diabetes acting as per counselors). Active discovery learning approach was used in group sessions.

(Continued)

Table 8 Examples of Types of Cultural Adaptations in Weight Loss or Lifestyle Change Programs in Adults in Specific Ethnic Groups (*Continued*)

First author and yr (reference) (ethnic group focus)	Program description highlighting components of cultural adaptation
Oexmann, 2000 (143) (African-American)	"Lighten Up," a church-based program for African-American men, women, and children (8-wk group program) was developed and implemented in collaboration with the local faith community using: Bible study combined with a health message. Eight educational sessions based on the spiritual fruits of love, knowledge, peace, faith, kindness, joy, self-control, and Godliness. All sessions were opened and closed with prayer. Participants brought food items from home for practice in label-reading skills.
Poston et al., 2003 (144) (Mexican-Americans)	Bilingual, Mexican-American instructor with culturally specific recipes and intervention materials and culturally tailored rationales for dietary and exercise modification.
Mayer-Davis, 2004 (145) (African-American)	POWER, Adapted Diabetes Prevention Program intervention, a modified program based on pilot study and focus groups. Program was based on regular group sessions. Written materials were simplified and reduced in amount. Regional and culturally appropriate foods and recipes were included. Safe places to walk in the community were identified. Chair exercises were suggested for some participants.
Fitzgibbon et al., 2005 (146) (African-American)	People, places, and language in recruitment and intervention materials were geared to African-Americans. Healthy ways of preparing traditional African-American foods were demonstrated. Family and social support were emphasized and family issues discussed. Child care was provided. There were active food demonstrations and the sessions conducted in familiar places at convenient times, as well as use of narratives that involved well-known or historical African-American women.
Bradshaw et al., 2005 (147) (Native Hawaiians)	Multi-focal, holistic approach that included a blend of convention medical approaches with complementary healing methods; emphasizing small changes over time, and individualized evaluation and instruction.

Abbreviations: CHAPP, Community Health Assessment and Promotion Project; POWER, pounds off with empowerment.

provide for explicit attention to family issues through home visits (136) or by framing treatment as for families rather than individuals (137). Changing the setting in which treatment is offered is another common strategy. Churches may be used as the physical setting for program delivery (141) or as both a physical setting and psychosocial setting (143) through the direct incorporation of spiritual content. A strong "process orientation" is also evident in some programs, e.g., a deliberate attempt to be flexible and incorporate participant suggestions during the course of the program (136). A commonly reported change in program format cited in programs described as culturally adapted is the use of active discovery learning and non-didactic methods (52,138,141). Programs with an opportunity to provide individualized instruction allowed for tailoring as well as targeting, using the distinction made by Kreuter et al. (104).

Three studies were identified as culturally based (Resnicow's terminology) in that core cultural traditions or values were used as the basis for the intervention. In one case, the cultural tradition was a very low-fat, high-carbohydrate diet based on traditional foods of ethnic groups in Hawaii (138). Another program in Native Hawaiians incorporated traditional healing approaches (147). The third example, "Pima Pride," involved discussion focused on attitudes about current lifestyles in the

community and invited local speakers to address Pima Indian culture and history (140). This intervention was used as the control condition for comparison with a conventional structured lifestyle change program but had comparable, if not better, effects than the active intervention. Fitzgibbon also addressed deep structure issues in her study with black women (146).

Kreuter et al (104) have developed a taxonomy of commonly used strategies for cultural adaptation that facilitates a conceptual understanding of the approaches used in these studies, as follows:

- *Peripheral strategies* that seek to improve cultural appropriateness by packaging materials or programs for greater appeal to a particular group, e.g., formatting and labeling printed materials in ways designed to appeal to the group, or using familiar music. They likened this to Resnicow's concept of addressing *"surface characteristics" to improve appeal and acceptance of messages.*

- *Evidential strategies* that seek to enhance relevance by drawing particular attention to information about the importance of a health issue for the target group. An example would be emphasizing the higher than average mortality from obesity related diseases when undertaking treatment with African-Americans.

- *Linguistic strategies* that render programs or materials more accessible by offering them in the preferred or native language of the group.
- *Constituent involving strategies* that improve program relevance by directly incorporating experiences of members of the target group in program design and delivery, e.g., through hiring professional staff or lay educators from the ethnic group or target community.
- *Sociocultural strategies* that position the discussion of health issues within the broader social and cultural context of the target group, to add salience and meaning to the information and messages within the program. They liken this to Resnicow's concept of addressing deep structure.

The focus here is on the types of cultural adaptations that have been implemented from a conceptual perspective, i.e., not with respect to the weight losses achieved. As reviewed elsewhere (97), many culturally adapted programs reported in the literature have generally been of relatively low intensity and short duration. These approaches would not necessarily be expected to lead to large initial weight changes, and in many cases they were not continued long enough to determine whether larger effects would have resulted with continued counseling. Overall, based on these and similar studies in the literature, there is not a clear advantage of culturally specific approaches when retention or weight outcomes are compared with those reported for ethnic minority participants in standard obesity treatment programs (97).

More research is needed to clarify how cultural adaptations can be designed and implemented to improve obesity treatment outcomes in ethnic minority populations above and beyond what is possible using standard approaches, and in both ethnically mixed and ethnicity specific settings. Ideally, as suggested above, to understand the value added by cultural adaptations requires a comparison condition without the adaptation. This type of comparison has been relatively infrequent and limited with respect to the types of cultural adaptations evaluated. Ard et al. (149) assessed the effect of group composition (all African-American or mixed) in a substudy within the Weight Loss Maintenance trial of dietary and lifestyle change strategies for blood pressure control and found no difference in weight loss between the two conditions. Whether this lack of effect was related to the background of extensive overall cultural adaptation of the intervention approach (150) (discussed below) cannot be determined. Fitzgibbon compared culturally tailored interventions in African-American women with and without the addition of an active faith component in a 12-week pilot study (151). Results suggested a benefit of adding the faith component. Yanek (152) attempted a comparison of two church-based interventions in African-Americans, one with and one without a spiritual component, but participants' spontaneous addition of a spiritual component negated the ability to make this comparison; this highlights the potential challenges of actually conducting effective trials in which cultural aspects are artificially suppressed in order to create an experimental axis.

A second type of approach to incorporating cultural considerations into the intervention design—an approach that is not ethnicity specific—has emerged from multiethnic studies of weight loss for chronic disease prevention and control and in which effective treatment of high risk ethnic minority populations has been made a priority. The Diabetes Prevention Program (DPP) (153) and the PREMIER trial (150) are both excellent examples of cultural adaptations undertaken within the context of an ethnically diverse study population. The DPP lifestyle intervention—which was delivered to individuals rather than in groups—included materials and strategies designed for cultural tailoring to African-Americans, Hispanic Americans, American-Indians, and Asian-Americans, who in the aggregate comprised 45% of the approximately 1000 participants assigned to the lifestyle intervention (Table 9). The PREMIER interventions, which involved group counseling supplemented by individual counseling, were designed with specific attention to cultural issues of African-Americans (150). Cultural adaptation aspects of the intervention development and staff training were guided by a "Minority Implementation Committee" composed of

Table 9 Examples of Strategies Used to Address the Needs of an Ethnically Diverse Population in the Diabetes Prevention Program

---

- Matching of ethnicity of case manager to that of the participant in some cases
- Ability of case manager to tailor the intervention content and pace for the participant
- Core curriculum available in both English and Spanish
- Inclusion of ethnic foods and cooking methods in intervention materials, menus, and cooking classes
- Availability of alternative methods of self-monitoring
- Availability of diverse options for case manager use in facilitating maintenance
- Ethnic tailoring of type of physical activity
- Ample opportunity for other types of individual tailoring, as needed

---

Source: From Ref. 153.

investigators, staff, and external consultants with relevant experiences and expertise. In addition, after the pilot study of the first six sessions, a series of focus groups to assess participant experiences included special focus groups with African-American participants (150,154).

The effectiveness of these approaches cannot be directly evaluated in that there was no comparison condition without cultural tailoring. The DPP reported somewhat lower attainment of the weight loss goal in all of the ethnic minority groups, although this finding was statistically significant only for African-Americans (155). However, the favorable outcome for reduction in diabetes incidence applied to all ethnic subgroups in the DPP (156). Tailoring on cultural issues as such may be inadequate for equalizing weight losses among ethnic groups if the social and environmental context for weight loss is less favorable, e.g., if the relevant physical and economic environmental influences make it relatively more difficult to lose weight or maintain weight loss, as discussed previously.

SUMMARY AND CONCLUSION

Cultural issues arise in conjunction with health programs in general, including weight management programs, because of the belief that attending to cultural factors will allow for services that are better aligned with the client's needs and circumstances and thus more sensitive and effective. In addition, cultural influences on obesity treatment are of particular interest because of the disproportionate prevalence of obesity in U.S. ethnic minority populations. Culture influences obesity and weight change through several attitudinal and behavioral pathways that converge in food intake and energy output. Differences in weight related attitudes and practices can be readily documented among U.S. ethnic groups. In particular, compared to middle-class whites, some population groups with a higher prevalence of obesity have more tolerant views about obesity.

Cultural perspectives on obesity treatment should be viewed along all relevant dimensions, such as age, gender, and socioeconomic status. Moreover, both clients and providers bring cultural issues to the treatment setting, and the cultural competence of providers is a critical element of cultural sensitivity. Inasmuch as the treatment setting is the professional's domain, so should the building of cultural bridges be considered a primary responsibility of the treatment provider. However, there is a sense that adequately addressing cultural influences ultimately will require a paradigm expansion in the obesity treatment—moving away from more narrowly conceived clinical treatment models to broader health promotion paradigms—or at least a stronger and clearer

articulation of the existing paradigmatic guidance on this issue.

The validity of attending to cultural and contextual influences in the design and delivery of obesity treatment can be established on a theoretical basis. However, success in cultural adaptations is inherently difficult to define and evaluate. We do not yet have many examples of scientifically rigorous models of culturally adapted weight management programs applied over long duration and we are far from knowing how culturally adapted programs can best be packaged to improve overall treatment outcomes in specific populations. Some components of possible cultural adaptations have been outlined, and these can be formatively evaluated. Other salient cultural influences may be difficult to articulate and assess because they are tied to subtle symbolic meanings learned through affective rather than rational mechanisms. In addition, if a certain level of cultural appropriateness is a minimum standard for any program, then it is difficult to conduct studies in ethnic minority populations in which no cultural adaptations have been made. The time course for effectiveness of cultural adaptations may be long, that is, far out into the maintenance phase of behavior change rather than observable in the short term. Finally, addressing cultural issues alone will not necessarily address environmental and social context issues that may limit adherence. "Cultural" adaptations should be framed broadly to consider the dialectic pattern of the culture-structure interactions that shape all our lives.

REFERENCES

1. Rodin J. Cultural and psychosocial determinants of weight concerns. Ann Intern Med 1993; 119:643–645.
2. Sobal J, Maurer D. Weighty Issues. Fatness and Thinness as Social Problems. Hawthorne, NY: Gruyte, 1999.
3. Brown PJ, Konner M. An anthropological perspective on obesity. Ann NY Acad Sci 1987; 499:29–46.
4. Ritenbaugh C. Obesity as a culture-bound syndrome. Cult Med Psychiatry 1982; 6:347–361.
5. Thomas PR, ed. Weighing the Options Criteria for Evaluating Weight-Management Programs. Washington: National Academy Press, 1995.
6. Kuhn TS. The Structure of Scientific Revolutions. Chicago: University of Chicago Press, 1995.
7. Helman CF. Culture Health, and Illness. An Introduction for Health Professionals. Boston: Wright, 1990.
8. Mithun JS. The role of the family in acculturation and assimilation in America. A psychocultural dimension. In: McCready WC, ed. Culture, Ethnicity, and Identity. Current Issues In Research. New York: Academic Press, 1983:209–232.
9. Baldwin JA, Hopkins R. African-American and European-American cultural differences as assessed by the worldviews paradigm. An empirical analysis. West J Black Stud 1990; 14:38–52.

10. Sue DW, Sue D. Counseling the Culturally Different: Theory and Practice. 2nd ed. New York: John Wiley and Sons, 1990:27–48.

11. Leininger M. Becoming aware of type of health practitioners and cultural imposition. J Transcult Nurs 1991; 2:32–39.

12. Airhihenbuwa CO. Developing Culturally Appropriate Health Programs. Health and Culture. Beyond the Western Paradigm. Thousand Oaks, CA: Sage Publications, 1995: 25–43.

13. Huff RM, Kline MV, eds. Promoting Health in Multi-cultural Populations. A Handbook for Practitioners. Thousand Oaks, CA: Sage Publications, 1999.

14. Williams J, Tharp M. African Americans: ethnic roots, cultural diversity. In: Tharp M, ed. Marketing and Consumer Identity in Multicultural America. Thousand Oaks, CA: Sage Publications, 2001:161–211.

15. Page JB. The concept of culture: a core issue in health disparities. J Urban Health 2005; 82(2, suppl 3):iii35–iii43.

16. Wing RR, Vorhees CC, Hill DR. Maintenance of behavior change in cardiorespiratory risk reduction. Health Psychol 2000; 19(suppl 1):1–88.

17. Ogden CL, Carroll MD, Curtin LR, et al. Prevalence of overweight and obesity in the United States, 1999–2004. JAMA 2006; 295:1549–1555.

18. Wang Y, Beydoun MA. The obesity epidemic in the United States—gender, age, socioeconomic, racial/ethnic, and geographic characteristics: a systematic review and meta-regression analysis. Epidemiol Rev 2007; 29:6–28.

19. World Health Organization. Obesity: Preventing and Managing the Global Epidemic. Report of a WHO Consultation. Geneva World Health Organization, WHO Technical Report Series 894, 2000.

20. Egger G, Swinburn B. An 'ecological' approach to the obesity pandemic. BMJ 1997; 315:477–480.

21. Nestle M, Jacobson MF. Halting the obesity epidemic. A public health policy approach. Public Health Rep 2001; 115:12–24.

22. French SA, Story M, Jeffery RW. Environmental influences on eating and physical activity. Annu Rev Public Health 2001; 22:309–335.

23. Jeffery RW, Utter J. The changing environment and population obesity in the United States. Obes Res 2003; 11(suppl):12S–22S.

24. Kumanyika SK. Minisymposium on obesity: overview and some strategic considerations. Annu Rev Public Health 2001; 22:293–308.

25. Kumanyika S, Jeffery RW, Morabia A, et al. Public Health Approaches to the Prevention of Obesity (PHAPO) Working Group of the International Obesity Task Force (IOTF). Obesity prevention: the case for action. Int J Obes Relat Metab Disord 2002; 26:425–436.

26. Last J. A Dictionary of Epidemiology. 4th ed. New York: Oxford University Press, 2001.

27. Pollard K, O'Hare W. America's racial and ethnic minorities. Popul Bull 1999; 54:1–34.

28. Kleinman A, Eisenberg L, Good B. Culture, illness and care. Clinical lessons from anthropologic and cross cultural research. Ann Intern Med 1978; 88:251–258.

29. McElroy A, Jezewski MA. Cultural variation in the experience of health and illness. In: Albrecht GL, Fitzpatrick R, Scrimshaw SC, eds. Handbook of Social Studies in Health and Medicine. Thousand Oaks CA: Sage Publications, 2000:191–209.

30. Riche MF. America's Diversity and Growth. Signposts for the 21st Century. Population Bulletin 2000; 55(2). Population Reference Bureau. Retrieved on September 26, 2007 from http://www.prb.org/Source/ACFD2C.pdf.

31. Kumanyika SK. Minority populations. In: Burke LE, Ockene IS, eds. Compliance in Healthcare and Research Armonk, NY: Futura, 2001:195–218.

32. Council on Economic Advisers for the President's Initiative on Race (1998). Changing America. Indicators of Social and Economic Well-being by Race and Hispanic Origin. Available at: http://www.accessgpo.Gov/eop/ca/index.html. Accessed October 16, 2001.

33. Kreider RM, Simmons T. Marital Status: 2000. U.S. Census 2000. Retrieved on September 26, 2007 from www.census.gov/prod/2003pubs/c2kbr-30.pdf.

34. Will JC, Denny C, Serdula M, et al. Trends in body weight among American Indians. Findings from a telephone survey, 1985–1996. Am J Public Health 1999; 89: 395–398.

35. Adams PF, Schoenborn CA. Health behaviors of adults: United States, 2002–04. National Center for Health Statistics. Vital Health Stat 10 2006; (230):1–140.

36. Ellis JL, Campos-Outcalt D. Cardiovascular diseases risk factors in Native Americans a literature review. Am J Prev Med 1994; 10:295–307.

37. Howard BV, Lee ET, Cowan LD, et al. Coronary heart diseases prevalence and its relation to risk factors in American Indians. The Strong Heart Study. Am J Epidemiol 1995; 142:254–268.

38. Must A, Spadano J, Coakley EH, et al. The disease burden associated with overweight and obesity. JAMA 1999; 282:1523–1529.

39. Sahyoun NR, Hochberg MC, Helmick CG, et al. Body mass index, weight change and incidence of self-reported, physician diagnosed arthritis among women. Am J Public Health 1999; 89:391–394.

40. Ostir GV, Markides KS, Freeman DH, et al. Obesity and health conditions in elderly Mexican Americans: the Hispanic EPESE. Ethn Dis 2000; 10:31–38.

41. Diabetes 2001. Vital Statistics. Alexandria, VA: Americans Diabetes Association, 2001.

42. Smith SC Jr., Clark LT, Cooper RS, et al. Discovering the full spectrum of cardiovascular disease: Minority Health Summit 2003 Report of the obesity, metabolic syndrome, and hypertension writing group. Circulation 2005; 111: e134–e139.

43. WHO Expert Consultation. Appropriate body-mass index for Asian populations and its implications for policy and intervention strategies. Lancet 2004; 363:157–163.

44. Story M, Evans M, Fabsitz RR, et al. The epidemic of obesity in American Indian communities and the need for childhood obesity-prevention programs. Am J Clin Nutr 1999; 69:747S–754S.

45. Kumanyika S, Grier S. Targeting interventions for ethnic minority and low-income populations. Future Child 2006; 16:187–207.

46. Daniels SR. The consequences of childhood overweight and obesity. Future Child 2006; 16:47–67.

47. Goran MI, Weinsier RL. Role of environmental vs. metabolic factors in the etiology of obesity. Time to focus on the environment. Obes Res 2000; 8:407–409.

48. Ravussin E, Valencia ME, Esparza J, et al. Effects of a traditional lifestyle on obesity in Pima Indians. Diabetes Care 1994; 17:1067–1074.

49. Luke A, Cooper RS, Prewitt TE, et al. Nutritional consequences of the African diaspora. Annu Rev Nutr 2001; 21:47–71.

50. Kumanyika SK, Morssink CB. Cultural appropriateness of weight management programs. In: Dalton S, ed. Overweight and Weight Management. Sudbury, MA: Jones and Barlett Publishers, 1997:69–106.

51. Counihan C, Van Esterik P, eds. Food and Culture: A Reader. New York: Routledge, 1997.

52. Vazquez IM, Millen B, Bissett L, et al. A preventive nutrition intervention in Caribbean Latinos with type 2 diabetes Am J Health Promot 1998; 13:116–119.

53. Allan JD, Mayo K, Michel Y. Body size values of white and black women. Res Nurs Health 1993; 16:323–333.

54. Baturka N, Hornsby PP, Schorling JB. Clinical implications of body image among rural African-American women. J Gen Intern Med 2000; 15:235–241.

55. National Center for Health Statistics. Health, United States, 2006, with Chartbook on the Health of Americans. Hyattsville, MD, 2006.

56. Jain A, Sherman SN, Chamberlain DL, et al. Why don't low-income mothers worry about their preschoolers begin overweight? Pediatrics 2001; 107:1138–1146.

57. Faith MS, Manibay E, Kravitz M, et al. Relative body weight and self-esteem among African Americans in four nationally representative samples. Obes Res 1998; 6:430–437.

58. Flynn KJ, Fitzgibbon M. Body images and obesity risk among black females. Ann Behav Med 1998; 20:13–24.

59. Lynch E, Liu K, Spring B, et al. Association of ethnicity and socioeconomic status with judgments of body size: the Coronary Artery Risk Development in Young Adults (CARDIA) Study. Am J Epidemiol 2007; 165:1055–1062.

60. Williamson DF, Serdula MK, Anda RF, et al. Weight loss attempts in adults: goals, duration and rate of weight loss. Am J Public Health 1992; 82:1251–1257.

61. Serdula MK, Williamson DF, Anda RF, et al. Weight control practices in adults results of a multistage telephone survey. Am J Public Health 1994; 84:1821–1824.

62. Cachelin FM, Striegel-Moore R, Elder KA. Realistic weight perception and body size assessment in a racially diverse community sample of dieters. Obes Res 1998; 6: 62–68.

63. Bish CL, Blanck HM, Serdula MK, et al. Diet and physical activity behaviors among Americans trying to lose weight: 2000 behavioral risk factor surveillance system. Obes Res 2005; 13:596–607.

64. Smith DE, Thompson JK, Raczynski JM, et al. Body image among men and women in a biracial cohort. The CARDIA Study. Int J Eat Disord 1999; 25:71–82.

65. Sherwood NE, Harnack L, Story M. Weight-loss practices, nutrition beliefs, and weight loss program preferences of urban American Indian women. J Am Diet Assoc 2000; 100:442–446.

66. Diaz VA, Mainous AG III, Pope C. Cultural conflicts in the weight loss experience of overweight Latinos. Int J Obes (Lond) 2007; 31:328–333.

67. Barnes AS, Goodrick GK, Pavlik V, et al. Weight loss maintenance in African-American women: focus group results and questionnaire development. J Gen Intern Med 2007; 22:915–922 (Epub April 6, 2007).

68. Wolfe WA. Obesity and the African-American woman. A cultural tolerance of fatness or other neglected factors? Ethn Dis 2000; 10:446–453.

69. Matthews HF. Rootwork. Description of an ethnomedical system in the American South. South Med J 1987; 80: 885–891.

70. Airhihenbuwa CO, Kumanyika S, Agurs TD, et al. Perceptions and beliefs about physical activity, exercise, and rest among African Americans. Am J Health Promot 1995; 9:426–429.

71. Airhihenbuwa CO, Kumanyika S, Agurs TD, et al. Cultural aspects of Africans American eating patterns. Ethn Health 1996; 1:245–260.

72. Murcott A. Sociological and social anthropological approaches to food and eating. World Rev Nutr Diet 1988; 55:1–40.

73. Mintz SW. Tasting Food, Tasting Freedom. Excursions into Eating, Culture and the Past. Boston: Beacon Press, 1997.

74. Kittler PG, Sucher KP. Food and Culture in America: A Nutrition Handbook. 2nd ed. Washington : West/Wadsworth, 1998.

75. Sobal J, Stunkard AJ. Socioeconomic status and obesity: a review of the literature. Psychol Bull 1989; 105: 260–275.

76. Kumanyika SK, Golden PM. Cross-sectional differences in health status in U.S. racial/ethnic minority groups. Potential influences of temporal changes, disease, and lifestyle transition. Ethn Dis 1991; 1:50–59.

77. Kumanyika S. Nutrition and chronic disease prevention: priorities for U.S. minority groups. Nutr Rev 2006; 64 (2 pt 2):S9–S14.

78. Gillum RF. The epidemiology of cardiovascular disease in black Americans. New Engl J Med 1996; 335:1597–1599.

79. Kumanyika SK, Teff K. Biobehavioral consequences of interactions between environment and culture. In: Progress in Obesity Research: Vol 10. Proceedings of the 10th International Congress on Obesity. Oxford: Blackwell, 2007.

80. Townsend MS, Peerson J, Love B, et al. Food insecurity is positively related to overweight in women. J Nutr 2001; 121:1738–1745.

81. Kumanyika SK, Krebs-Smith SM. Preventive nutrition issues in ethnic and socioeconomic groups in the United States. In: Bendich A, Deckelbaum RJ, eds. Preventive Nutrition. Vol 2. Totowa, NJ: Humana Press, 2001: 325–356.

82. Kant AK, Graubard BI, Kumanyika SK. Trends in black–white differentials in dietary intakes of U.S. adults, 1971–2002. Am J Prev Med 2007; 32:264–272.

83. Centers for Disease Control and Prevention (CDC). Trends in leisure-time physical inactivity by age, sex,

and race/ethnicity—United States, 1994–2004. MMWR Morb Mortal Wkly Rep 2005; 54:991–994.

84. Kushner RF, Racette SB, Neil K, et al. Measurement of physical activity among black and white obese women. Obes Res 1995; 3:261s–265s.

85. Hunter GR, Weinsier RL, Darnell BE, et al. Racial differences in energy expenditure and aerobic fitness in premenopausal women. Am J Clin Nutr 2000; 71:500–506.

86. Cockerham WC, Rütten A, Abel T. Conceptualizing contemporary health lifestyle: moving beyond Weber. Sociol Q 1997; 38:321–342.

87. Population Reference Bureau. Segregation in Cities and Suburbs. Old Trends and New. February 2004. Retrieved on September 26, 2007 from http://www.prb.org/CPIPR/NewReleases/Fischer2004.aspx.

88. Diez-Roux AV, Nieto FJ, Caulfield L, et al. Neighborhood differences in diet: the atherosclerosis risk in communities (ARIC) study. J Epidemiol Community Health 1999; 53:55–63.

89. Taylor WC, Floyd MF, Whitt-Glover MC, et al. Environmental justice: a framework for collaboration between the public health and parks and recreation fields to study disparities in physical activity. J Phys Act Health 2007; 4(suppl 1):S50–S63.

90. Eyler AA, Matson-Koffman D, Vest JR, et al. Environmental, policy, and cultural factors related to physical activity in a diverse sample of women: The Women's Cardiovascular Health Network Project—summary and discussion. Women Health 2002; 36:123–134.

91. Tirodkar MA, Jain A. Food messages on African American television shows. Am J Public Health 2003; 93:439–441.

92. Henderson VR, Kelly B. Food advertising in the age of obesity: content analysis of food advertising on general market and African American television. J Nutr Educ Behav 2005; 37:191–196.

93. Smith DE, Lewis CE, Caveny JL, et al. Longitudinal changes in adiposity associated with pregnancy. The CARDIA Study. JAMA 1994; 271:1747–1751.

94. Pachter LM. Culture and clinical care. Folk illness beliefs and behaviors and their implications for health care delivery. JAMA 1994; 271:690–694.

95. Harris-Davis E, Haughton B. Model for multicultural nutrition counseling competencies. J Am Diet Assoc 2000; 100:1178–1185.

96. Office of Minority Health. Assuring Cultural Competence in Health Care. Recommendations for National Standards and on Outcomes-Focused Research Agenda. Available at: http://www.Omhrc.gov/cls/finalculturalla.htm. Accessed October 16, 2001.

97. Kumanyika SK. Obesity treatment in minorities. In: Wadden TA, Stunkard AJ, eds. Handbook of Obesity Treatment. New York: Guilford Publications, 2002: 416–446.

98. Bandura A. Social cognitive theory. An agentic perspective. Annu Rev Psychol 2001; 52:1–26.

99. Fisher EB, Auslander W, Sussman L, et al. Community organization and health promotion in minority neighborhoods. In: Becker DM, Hill DR, Jackson JS, et al., eds.

Health Behavior Research in Minority Populations. Washington: U.S. Government Printing Office, 1992: 53–72. NIH Publication No. 92-2965.

100. Stokols D. Translating social ecologic theory into guidelines for community health promotion. Am J Health Promot 1996; 10:282–298.

101. Bouton ME. A learning theory perspective on lapse, relapse, and the maintenance of behavior change. Health Psychol 2000; 19(suppl 1):57–63.

102. Baranowski T, Perry CL, Parcel GS. How individuals, environments, and health behavior interact. Social cognitive theory. In: Glanz K, Lewis FM, Rimer BK, eds. Health Behavior and Health Education: Theory, Research, and Practice. 2nd ed. San Francisco: Jossey Bass, 1997: 153–178.

103. Rakowski W. The potential variances of tailoring in health behavior interventions. Ann Behav Med 1999; 21:284–289.

104. Kreuter MW, Lukwago SN, Bucholtz RD, et al. Achieving cultural appropriateness in health promotion programs: targeted and tailored approaches. Health Educ Behav 2003; 30:133–146.

105. Resnicow K, Baranowski T, Ahluwalia JS, et al. Cultural Sensitivity in Public health. Defined and demystified. Ethn Dis 1999; 9:10–12.

106. Kavanagh KH, Kennedy PH. Promoting Cultural Diversity. Strategies for Health Care Professionals. Newbury Park, CA: Sage Publications, 1992.

107. Huff RM. Cross cultural concepts of health and disease. In: Huff RM, Kline MV, eds. Promoting Health in Multicultural Populations. A Handbook for Practitioners. Thousand. Oaks, CA: Sage Publications, 1999:23–39.

108. Yutrenzka BA. Making a case for training in ethnic and cultural diversity in increasing treatment efficiency. J Consult Clin Psychol 1995; 63:197–206.

109. Harvey EL, Hill AJ. Health professionals' views of overweight people and smokers. Int J Obes Relat Metab Disord 2001; 25:1253–1261.

110. Kumanyika SK, Morssink CB. Working effectively in cross-cultural and multicultural settings. In: Owen AL, Splett PL, Owen GM, eds. Nutrition in the Community The Art and Science of Delivering Services. 4th ed. New York: McGraw Hill, 1998:542–567.

111. Wilcox S, Shumaker SA, Bowen DJ, et al. Promoting adherence and retention to clinical trails in special populations. A women's health initiative workshop. Control Clin Trials 2001; 22:279–289.

112. Ard JD, Carter-Edwards L, Svetkey LP. A new model for developing and executing culturally appropriate behavior modification clinical trials for African Americans. Ethn Dis 2003; 13:279–285.

113. Leicht KT, Fennell ML. The changing organizational context of professional work. Annu Rev Sociol 1997; 23:215–231.

114. Abbot A. The Systems of Professions; An Essay on the Division of Expert Labor. Chicago: University of Chicago Press, 1989.

115. Freidson E. Professionalism Reborn; Theory, Prophecy, and Policy. Chicago: University of Chicago Press, 1994.

116. Brierely J. The measurement of organizational commitment and professional commitment. J Soc Psychol 1996; 136:265–267.

117. Anderson JM, Dyck I, Lynam J. Health care professional and women speaking; constraints in everyday life and the management of chronic illness. Health 1997; 1:57–79.

118. Glanz K, Lewis FM, Rimer BK, eds. Health Behavior and Health Education: Theory, Research, and Practice. 2nd ed. San Francisco: Jossey-Bass, 1997.

119. Conrad P, Kern R, eds. The Sociology of Health and Illness; Critical Perspectives. New York: St. Martin's Press, 1997.

120. Sobal J. The medicalization and demedicalization of obesity. In: Maurer D, Sobal J, eds. Eating Agendas Food and Nutrition as Social Problems. Social Problems and Social Issues. Hawthorne, NY: Aldine de Gruyter, 1995:67–90.

121. Martin J. Cultures in Organization: Three Perspectives. New York: Oxford University Press, 1992.

122. Peters T, Waterman R. In Search of Excellence. New York: Harper & Rowe, 1983.

123. Mohan ML. Organizational Communication and Cultural Visions: Approaches for Analysis. Albany: State University of New York Press, 1993.

124. Mumby DK. Communication and Power in Organizations: Discourse, Ideology, and Domination. Norwood, NJ: Ablex Publishing Co., 1988.

125. Hofstede G. Culture's Consequences: International Differences in Work-Related Values. Newbury Park, CA: Sage Publications, 1980.

126. Downs A. Inside Bureaucracy. Chicago: Waveland Press, 1994.

127. Caiden Gerald E. Excessive bureaucratization: the J-curve theory of bureaucracy and Max Weber through the looking glass. In: Farazmand A, ed. Handbook of Bureaucracy. New York: Marcel Dekker, 1994:66–72.

128. Anderson RM, Funnel M. Compliance and adherence are dysfunctional concepts in diabetes care. Diabetes Educ 2000; 26:597–601.

129. Kidd KE, Altman DG. Adherence in social context. Control Clin Trials 2000; 21:184S–187S.

130. Rothman AJ. Towards a theory-based analysis of behavioral maintenance. Health Psychol 2000; 191:64–69.

131. Frankish JC, Lovato CY, Shannon WJ. Models, theories, and principles of health promotion with multicultural populations. In: Huff RM, Kline MV, eds. Promoting Health in Multicultural Populations. A Handbook for Practitioners. Thousand Oaks, CA: Sage Publications, 1999:41–72.

132. Kumanyika S. Obesity prevention concepts and frameworks. In: Kumanyika S, Brownson RC, eds., Handbook of Obesity Prevention. A Resource for Health Professionals. New York: Springer, 2007:85–114.

133. Teufel-Shone NI. Promising strategies for obesity prevention and treatment within American Indian communities. J Transcult Nurs 2006; 17:224–229.

134. National Heart, Lung, and Blood Institute Obesity Education Initiative. Clinical guidelines on the identification evaluation, and treatment of overweight and Obesity in adults. Obes Res 1998; 6(suppl 2):51S–209S.

135. US Preventive Services Task Force. Screening for obesity in adults: recommendations and rationale. Ann Intern Med 2003; 139:930–932.

136. Lasco RA, Curry RH, Dickson VJ, et al. Participation rates, weight loss, and blood pressure changes among obese women in a nutrition-exercise program. Public Health Rep 1989; 104:640–646.

137. Cousins JH, Rubovits DS, Dunn JK, et al. Family versus individually-oriented intervention for weight loss in Mexican American women. Public Health Rep 1992; 107:549–555.

138. Shintani T, Beckham S, Kanawaliwali-O'Connor H, et al. The Waianae Diet Program. A culturally-sensitive, community-based obesity and clinical intervention program for the Native Hawaiian population. Hawaii Med J 1994; 53:136–147.

139. Agurs-Collins TD, Kumanyika SK, Ten Have TR, et al. A randomized controlled trial of weight reduction and exercise for diabetes management in older African American subjects. Diabetes Care 1997; 20:1503–1511.

140. Venkat-Narayan KM, Hoskin M, Kozak D, et al. Randomized clinical trial of lifestyle interventions in Pima Indians: a pilot study. Diabet Med 1998; 15:66–72.

141. McNabb W, Quinn M, Kerver J, et al. The Pathways church-based weight loss program for urban African Americans. Diabetes Care 1997; 20:1518–1523.

142. Keyserling TC, Ammerman AS, Samuel-Hodge CD, et al. A diabetes management program for African American women with type 2 diabetes. Diabetes Educ 2000; 26: 796–805.

143. Oexmann MJ, Thomas JC, Taylor KB, et al. Short-term impact of a church-based approach to lifestyle change on cardiovascular risk in African Americans. Ethn Dis 2000; 10:17–23.

144. Poston WS, Reeves RS, Haddock CK, et al. Weight loss in obese Mexican Americans treated for 1-year with orlistat and lifestyle modification. Int J Obes Relat Metab Disord 2003; 27:1486–1493.

145. Mayer-Davis EJ, D'Antonio AM, Smith SM, et al. Pounds off with empowerment (POWER): a clinical trial of weight management strategies for black and white adults with diabetes who live in medically underserved rural communities. Am J Public Health 2004; 94(10):1736–1742.

146. Fitzgibbon ML, Stolley MR, Schiffer L, et al. A combined breast health/weight loss intervention for Black women. Prev Med 2005; 40:373–383.

147. Beckham S, Bradley S, Washburn A. One health center's response to the obesity epidemic. An overview of three innovative, culturally appropriate, community-based strategies. Hawaii Med J 2005; 64:151–158.

148. Ard J, Rosati R, Oddone EZ. Culturally-sensitive weight loss program produces significant reduction in weight, blood pressure, and cholesterol in eight weeks. J Natl Med Assoc 2000; 92:515–523.

149. Ard JD, Kumanyika S, Stevens VJ, et al. Effect of group racial composition on weight loss in African Americans. Obesity 2008; 16:306–310.

150. Funk KL, Elmer PJ, Stevens VJ, et al. PREMIER—a trial of lifestyle interventions for blood pressure control:

intervention design and rationale. Health Promot Pract 2006 Jun 27(Epub ahead of print).

151. Fitzgibbon ML, Stolley MR, Ganschow P, et al. Results of a faith-based weight loss intervention for black women. J Natl Med Assoc 2005; 97:1393–1402.

152. Yanek LR, Becker DM, Moy TF, et al. Project Joy: faith based cardiovascular health promotion for African American women. Public Health Rep 2001; 116(suppl 1): 68–81.

153. Diabetes Prevention Program (DPP) Research Group. The Diabetes Prevention Program (DPP): description of lifestyle intervention. Diabetes Care 2002; 25:2165–2171.

154. Ard JD, Durant RW, Edwards LC, et al. Perceptions of African-American culture and implications for clinical trial design. Ethn Dis 2005; 15:292–299.

155. Wing RR, Hamman RF, Bray GA, et al. Achieving weight and activity goals among diabetes prevention program lifestyle participants. Obes Res 2004; 12:1426–1434.

156. Knowler WC, Barrett-Connor E, Fowler SE, et al. Reduction in the incidence of type 2 diabetes with lifestyle intervention or metformin. New Engl J Med 2002; 346:393–403.

5

Bias, Discrimination, and Obesity

REBECCA M. PUHL and KELLY D. BROWNELL

Rudd Center for Food Policy and Obesity, Department of Psychology, Yale University, New Haven, Connecticut, U.S.A.

INTRODUCTION

Obese individuals are highly stigmatized in our society, with bias and discrimination as common outcomes (1,2). Given the prevalence of overweight and obesity in the American population, the number of children and adults potentially faced with stigmatization is immense. The consequences of being denied jobs, disadvantaged in education, marginalized by health care professionals, or victimized by peers because of one's weight can have a profound impact on quality of life. Obese individuals can suffer terribly from this, both from direct discrimination and from less overt behaviors (e.g., teasing and social exclusion) that arise from weight-related stigma.

Despite a long-standing awareness of the problem of weight discrimination dating back at least 30 years (3,4) this topic has only recently begun to receive focused attention in the obesity field. The accumulation of work over the past decade provides clear evidence of weight bias in areas of health care, employment, education, and even close interpersonal relationships, thus painting a picture of obese persons as acceptable targets of stigma in multiple domains of living (1,2). The purpose of this chapter is to summarize existing literature, examine the emotional and physical health consequences of bias, and highlight existing stigma reduction strategies with attention to research needs in this important area of study.

WEIGHT BIAS IN HEALTH CARE SETTINGS

Obese individuals are vulnerable to weight bias from multiple providers in health care settings. Negative attitudes towards obese patients have been reported among physicians, nurses, dietitians, psychologists, and medical students (5–14). Even health professionals who specialize in obesity are not immune to negative attitudes (15). Attitudes documented in self-report studies by health professionals include perceptions that obese patients are noncompliant, unsuccessful, unpleasant, unintelligent, overindulgent, weak-willed, and lazy (1). Attributions about the causes of obesity may reinforce negative attitudes, as several studies have demonstrated that physicians hold assumptions that obesity can be prevented by self-control (5), that patient noncompliance explains failure at weight loss (7), and that obesity is caused by emotional problems (16).

Experimental research has also assessed weight bias among health professionals. Study participants are typically randomly assigned to read case descriptions of hypothetical patients varying in weight categories, followed by questions requesting their professional judgments about the patient. For example, in one study psychologists were randomly assigned to one of two conditions—in one condition they read about an obese patient and in the other condition they read about a nonobese patient. The patient descriptions were identical in each condition except for the patient's body weight. Psychologists more frequently assigned negative attributes, more severe psychological symptoms, and more pathology to obese clients than to non-overweight clients (17,18). In another study, medical students were presented with cases where patient were depicted as average weight or obese, and students perceived the obese patients to be less attractive, more depressed, and less likely to comply with diet and lifestyle recommendations than average-weight patients (19).

Obese patients report frequent weight bias from providers. In a recent self-report study, we assessed 2449 overweight and obese adult women to examine their experiences of weight bias (20). We provided participants with a list of 22 different individuals (such as peers, family members, coworkers, employers, strangers, and health care providers), and asked them how often each individual had stigmatized them because of weight. Participants reported doctors to be the second most frequent source of bias that they confronted (behind family members who were the most frequently cited sources); 69% reported that they had experienced weight bias by a doctor on one occasion, and 52% reported that this had happened multiple times. Other health care professionals were also frequent sources of bias: 46% of women reported weight bias by nurses, 37% by dietitians, and 21% by mental health professionals (20).

Negative attitudes by providers raise concerns about the quality of health care that obese patients receive. A number of studies have documented that obese people delay seeking preventive health services such as pelvic exams, mammograms, and additional cancer screenings (21–25), and other research shows a positive relationship between body mass index (BMI) and appointment cancellations (26). These findings are not a result of low access to care, but instead point directly to bias (27). When a sample of 498 obese women were asked about the reasons for canceling, delaying, and avoiding health services, they attributed these decisions to disrespectful treatment and negative attitudes from providers, unsolicited advice to lose weight, embarrassment of being weighed, and medical equipment that was too small to be functional for their body size. The percentage of patients who reported these barriers to heath care increased with BMI (27).

WEIGHT BIAS IN EMPLOYMENT SETTINGS

Both laboratory and field studies show widespread weight bias in all aspects of the employment process (28–32). Research addressing employer attitudes and hiring decisions suggests that overweight people face prejudice even prior to initial job interviews. Studies have manipulated perceptions of employee weight with written vignettes, videos, or photographs and then ask individuals to evaluate a fictional applicant's qualifications. Overweight employees are evaluated more negatively and are rated as less likely to be hired than average-weight employees, despite identical qualifications (33). Though this bias has been demonstrated within a variety of employment positions, it appears that overweight applicants are especially denigrated in sales positions and are perceived to be unfit for jobs involving face-to-face interactions (28,34,35). Population-based studies support the findings of this experimental research, and indicate that obese individuals are less likely to be employed than thinner individuals. For example, a recent Canadian study of over 75,000 adults found that obesity was associated with lower workforce participation independent of associated comorbidity and sociodemographic variables (36).

Once an overweight person is employed, weight bias can continue from coworkers and employers. Overweight employees are viewed as sloppy, lazy, less competent, poor role models, lacking in self-discipline, disagreeable, and emotionally unstable (29,37). In our study of 2449 overweight and obese adult women, 54% of participants reported experiencing weight bias from coworkers, and 38% stated that this had occurred multiple times. In addition, 43% of respondents reported weight bias from employers, with 26% reporting this form of bias on multiple occasions (20).

Negative attitudes may be a primary reason for inequities faced by overweight employees in wages, promotions, and termination, as suggested by studies showing lower promotion prospects for obese individuals than for average-weight employees with identical qualifications (38,39). Obese men are also more likely to hold low-paying jobs and are underrepresented in professional positions compared to average-weight men (40). There is also evidence of lower wages for obese women doing the same work performed by average-weight counterparts (41), and overweight women are more likely to have low-paying jobs compared to thinner women (40).

Finally, legal case documentation reveals a growing number of cases in which obese employees have been fired or suspended because of their weight (42–45). Many terminated employees held jobs in which body weight was unrelated to job responsibilities (computer analyst, office manager, lecturer, etc.) and received excellent job performance ratings.

There are no federal laws that prohibit weight discrimination in employment settings, and only one state (Michigan) prohibits discrimination based on weight. Thus, victims of weight-based employment discrimination have few options if they wish to seek redress in court (45). These obstacles will likely remain until weight is included as a protected category of antidiscrimination statutes.

VULNERABILITY OF YOUTH TO WEIGHT BIAS

Self-report, prospective, and experimental studies have examined various forms of weight bias towards overweight and obese youth (46). Most of this research has examined biased attitudes, stereotypes, and peer victimization and demonstrates that weight bias is a common experience for obese children. For example, a study of 4746 middle and high school students found that 30% of girls and 24% of boys reported weight-based teasing from peers. For students at or above the 95th BMI percentile, rates of victimization increased to 63% of girls and 58% of boys (47). A prospective study of 8210 children documented that 36% of obese boys and 34% of obese girls reported being victims of weight-based teasing and various forms of bullying (48). A Canadian study of youth aged 11 to 16 years ($N = 5749$) found that overweight and obese adolescents in all age groups (with the exception of 15- to 16-year-old boys) were more likely to be victims of bullying behaviors than average-weight peers, and BMI was positively associated to increased verbal, physical, and relational peer victimization (49). A similar study of 10 to 14-year-olds ($N = 156$) demonstrated weight-based teasing to be more severe, frequent, and upsetting among overweight children compared to non-overweight children (50). Children who reported the most teasing expressed more weight concerns, loneliness, lower confidence in physical appearance, and higher preferences for isolating activities, independent of the sex and weight status of children.

Anti-fat attitudes are established early in childhood, which likely sets the stage for later peer rejection and teasing described above. Biased attitudes toward overweight peers have been demonstrated in preschool children as young as age three, and by age four children can attribute excess body weight as the reason for their negative attitudes (51). Research with preschoolers found that 3-year-olds ascribed to overweight peers negative characteristics of being mean, stupid, loud, ugly, lazy, sad, and lacking in friends (52). Stigmatizing attitudes appear to increase throughout childhood (51,53), and by elementary school, children believe that overweight peers are ugly, selfish, lazy, and stupid, and that they lie, get teased, and have few friends (53). Among adolescents, qualitative research has demonstrated that overweight high school students report being stereotyped by peers as being lazy, unclean, eating too much, unable to perform certain physical activities (e.g., dancing), not having feelings, and unable to "get a boyfriend" (54).

In addition to peer victimization, obese children are also vulnerable to bias from educators. In a study examining attitudes toward obesity among 115 middle and high school teachers, 1/5 of respondents reported beliefs that obese persons are untidy, less likely to succeed than thinner persons, more emotional, and more likely to have family problems (55). Over 50% believed that obesity is often caused by a form of compensation for lack of love or attention, and 43% strongly agreed that *most people feel uncomfortable when they associate with obese people*. Similarly, in a study examining beliefs about obesity among 227 elementary school principals, over 50% cited lack of self-control and psychological problems as primary contributors to obesity (56).

Other work found that physical education teachers ($N = 105$) reported overweight students to have poorer social, reasoning, physical, and cooperation skills than non-overweight students (57). Participants also reported lower expectations for overweight students across a range of performance areas. These findings support a recent study showing strong implicit weight bias among 180 university students training to become physical educators; they expressed more negative attitudes than did a matched sample of psychology students and other health professionals (58). Physical education students also showed more negative explicit beliefs that obese individuals lack willpower, and those who were near completion of training expressed stronger weight bias than those who were beginning their training.

Educational discrimination appears to continue at the college level. There are cases of obese students being dismissed from college on the basis of weight despite good academic performance (59). Research also shows that obese students receive poorer evaluations and lower college acceptances than average-weight students with comparable application rates and school performance (60).

CONSEQUENCES OF WEIGHT BIAS

Given the multiple domains in which weight bias occurs and the pervasiveness of anti-fat attitudes, it is important to consider the consequences of being exposed to this negative stigmatization. A range of adverse outcomes is associated with weight bias for overweight and obese individuals, affecting emotional well-being, social relationships, and physical health.

Weight bias has clear and powerful implications for emotional well-being. Weight-based teasing and victimization is related to poorer body image, lower self-esteem, and higher risk of depression (50,61–68). Obese youth who experience weight-based victimization from peers are two to three times more likely to engage in suicidal thoughts and behaviors (64). Neumark-Sztainer and colleagues (47) found that 51% of girls who were targets of weight-based teasing from peers and family members had thought about committing suicide, compared to 25% of those who had not been teased. Among boys, 13% who were teased by family members about their weight reported attempting suicide compared to 4% who were not teased (47).

Interpersonal relationships are also negatively affected by weight bias (69). Obese children are liked less and rejected more often by peers than average-weight students (70). A large-scale study assessed adolescents ($N = 90,118$) from the National Longitudinal Study of Adolescent Health, and reported that overweight adolescents were more likely to be socially isolated and less likely to be nominated by their peers as friends than average-weight students (71). Other work with adolescents ($N = 9943$) found that obese students spent less time with friends than thinner peers, after controlling for variables such as grade level, race, and socioeconomic status (72). Among adults, weight has been negatively associated with frequency of dating (73), and experimental research shows that overweight women are rated more negatively by men in interpersonal conversations than thinner women (74–76).

Weight bias may also reinforce unhealthy behaviors that contribute to obesity. For example, overweight youth who are teased about their weight are more likely to engage in unhealthy weight control and binge eating behaviors compared to overweight youth who are not targets of weight-based teasing (47). Prospective research has demonstrated that weight-based teasing predicted binge eating at five years of follow-up among both males and females, even after controlling for factors like age, race, and socioeconomic status (77). Our own studies also illustrate a relationship between experiences of weight bias and unhealthy eating behaviors among adults. After assessing experiences of weight bias and coping strategies in a sample of overweight and obese women ($N = 2449$), findings showed that 79% of participants reported that they had coped with weight bias by eating more food and 75% reported that they refused to keep dieting in response to bias (20). In addition, further analyses with a subsample from this study ($N = 1013$) showed that participants who internalized weight bias and believed that weight-based stereotypes were true reported more frequent binge eating compared to those who reported stereotypes to be false (78).

There is also evidence to suggest that obese individuals may avoid physical activity because of weight bias. Overweight youth who are victimized by their peers are less likely to participate in physical activity and physical education classes (79,80). Adults who experience weight bias have less desire to exercise, and as a result, engage in decreased levels of strenuous and moderate exercise (81). It may be that overweight individuals feel heightened vulnerability to negative attitudes or teasing in public settings where exercise occurs, and therefore make attempts to avoid potentially embarrassing or stigmatizing situations. More work is needed to determine the impact of weight bias on participation in physical activities.

It is possible that weight bias may affect important health outcomes. A recent study found that adolescents who reported unfair treatment because of their physical appearance had elevated ambulatory blood pressure compared to those who did not report unfair treatment, even after accounting for typical determinants of blood pressure including BMI, gender, race, physical activity, posture, consumption, and mood (82).

This area of research has received very little attention, but warrants additional research given the potential for stigma to worsen health outcomes among individuals whose weight already poses increased health risks. Figure 1 outlines possible links between weight bias and important health outcomes. Investigating and documenting these relationships will be extremely important in efforts to understand and reduce the medical impact of weight bias.

IMPROVING ATTITUDES: WHAT WE KNOW AND DON'T KNOW

Despite abundant research documenting weight bias toward children and adults, little empirical work has tested strategies to reduce stigma and improve attitudes. Attributions about the causes of obesity have been the target of several experimental studies testing strategies to reduce weight bias. For example, research with students in grades 3 to 6 ($N = 184$) found that children attributed less blame to an obese child whose weight was attributed to external (e.g., medical) causes compared to a target whose obesity was attributed to personally controllable factors (83). However, causal information had little effect on overall attitudes, especially among older children. Another study of elementary school children ($N = 99$) found that children were less likely to blame an obese peer for being heavy if they were provided with information suggesting the target had little responsibility for her obesity, although this information did not change their liking of the peer (84). In a similar experiment, 74 children (grades 4–6) receiving a brief presentation about the uncontrollability of body size were compared to a control group involving normal classroom activities (85). Children in the intervention group attributed less personal control to obesity following the intervention, but did not change negative weight-based stereotypes. Experimental work in adolescents shows similar findings (86,87). Perceptions about the causes of obesity may be more modifiable than weight-based attitudes or stereotypes among youth.

With adults, experimental work has yielded mixed findings in attempts to improve attitudes through targeting attributions of causality. One study found that emphasizing external, noncontrollable causes for obesity (e.g.,

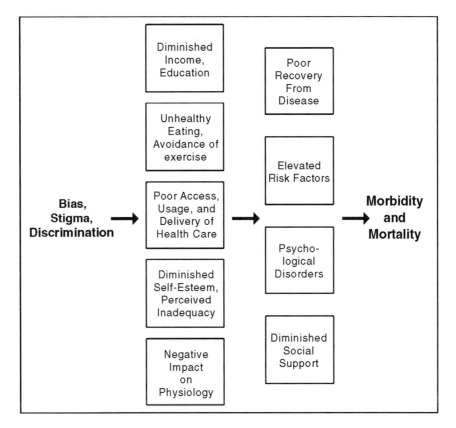

Figure 1 Conceptual scheme of potential links between weight bias and health outcomes. *Source*: From Ref. 2.

biological and genetic factors) had little impact on improving negative attitudes or behaviors in adults (88), whereas two other experimental studies provided participants with information about biological, genetic, and noncontrollable reasons for obesity and found reductions in negative attitudes (89,90).

Several other approaches have been tested with adults. Two experimental studies have attempted to improve attitudes by inducing empathy toward obese individuals, which involved having participants read stories about weight discrimination or watch videos of obese women designed to evoke empathy. Both of these interventions were unsuccessful in changing negative attitudes compared to control groups (88,91). Other research reduced negative weight-based stereotypes among medical students by combining strategies of empathy induction and education about the noncontrollable causes of obesity, as well as role-play exercises, although no control group was used for comparison (92).

More recent experimental research has pointed to new avenues for bias reduction. Hague and White (93) tested a web-based educational intervention among 258 student teachers and schoolteachers who enrolled in an online course about obesity (93). The course covered topics such as the causes of obesity, consequences of weight stigma, social pressures to be thin, strategies to reduce weight bias

in school settings, and ways to help students cope with stigma. Participants were randomly assigned to either a control group or one of four intervention groups that manipulated the perceived credibility and body size of the course presenter who provided the online lectures. Attitudes improved in intervention groups, and exposure to a credible overweight presenter improved attitudes more than a credible non-overweight presenter. While these results suggest that Internet-based interventions may have potential to reduce bias, it is unclear how the content of the course topics affected attitude changes.

Other recent experimental work has tested a "social consensus" framework of attitude change, which highlights the importance of social norms and suggests that stigmatizing attitudes are a function of one's perceptions of other people's stereotypical beliefs. In this research, participants completed self-report measures of their attitudes towards obese persons prior to and following manipulated feedback depicting the attitudes of other students (90). In a first experiment, university students ($N = 60$) who received feedback suggesting that their peers held more favorable beliefs about obese people than they did reduced their negative weight-based stereotypes and increased positive attitudes toward obese persons. They also attributed obesity less to personal control. In a second experiment ($N = 55$), participants who received feedback that other students had more favorable attitudes toward obese individuals were more likely to improve their attitudes about obese people if this feedback came from an in-group source with whom participants identified (e.g., students who belonged to their university) versus an out-group source (e.g., students from a different college).

In a third experiment of 200 university students, this social consensus approach was compared to four other conditions that provided (1) written materials about the uncontrollable causes of obesity, (2) written materials about the controllable causes of obesity, (3) information on supposed scientific prevalence rates of stereotypical traits in obese people, or (4) no information (control group). Perceptions of others' attitudes significantly affected the students' attitudes about obese people as well as their beliefs about the causes of obesity. Receiving social consensus feedback was equally or more effective in improving attitudes toward obese people compared to the other conditions, including providing information about the uncontrollable causes of obesity and supposed scientific evidence about characteristic traits of obese individuals (both of which also improved participants' attitudes towards obese people). These experiments indicate that learning about the unbiased attitudes of others can be effective in improving attitudes toward obese people.

Taken together, there is too little work to identify the most effective methods of reducing weight bias. It will be important to conduct additional comparisons of existing methods, and to test whether attitude change is sustained over time and translates into less biased behaviors toward obese individuals.

Table 1 Domains of Research Needs to Advance Work on Weight Bias

Domain	Research needs
General methodological issues	• Include behavioral measures to assess bias, in addition to self-reported attitudes. • Increase use of randomized designs and ecologically valid settings. • Evaluate the reliability and validity of measures assessing weight discrimination. • Develop new assessment methods to examine experiences of weight bias in different populations (e.g., children versus adults; cross-cultural assessment tools).
Weight bias in health settings	• Assess how negative professional attitudes influence different health care outcomes. • Compare weight bias across different specialty groups of providers. • Examine the impact of different forms of weight bias in health settings (e.g., lack of appropriate equipment versus negative provider attitudes) on obese patients. • Assess whether improvements in provider attitudes lead to increased utilization of health care and higher quality of care reported by obese patients.
Weight bias in employment settings	• Increase research attention to hiring, promotion, and benefits discrimination against obese employees. • Examine which occupations are most vulnerable to weight bias. • Compare prevalence rates of weight discrimination in employment settings to discrimination based on gender, age, or race.
Weight bias among youth	• Identify the nature and severity of stigma toward youth by educators and parents. • Assess whether reductions in weight stigma improve social, emotional, and academic outcomes among obese youth. • Assess endorsement of stigma across variables of ethnicity, gender, age, and weight among youth. • Examine the impact of different forms of weight bias (e.g., verbal teasing, physical aggression, social exclusion) on obese youth. • Develop and test curricula to promote weight acceptance in schools.
Consequences of weight bias	• Determine the impact of weight bias on self-esteem, body image, depression, anxiety, and suicidality. • Identify the influence of weight bias on unhealthy lifestyle behaviors (e.g., binge eating, exercise avoidance). • Assess how weight bias influences other physical health outcomes (e.g., cardiovascular health). • Examine how internalization of stigma affects health outcomes among overweight youth and adults.
Prevention/intervention	• Identify theoretical components to guide stigma reduction strategies. • Develop and test of stigma reduction strategies on anti-fat attitudes. • Test experimental comparisons of different methods to reduce weight bias. • Identify the most effective modes of delivery for stigma reduction messages. • Assess whether interventions lead to sustained attitude changes over time. • Assess whether interventions lead to changes in behavior and attitudes. • Examine coping strategies used by obese persons to combat aversive stigma experiences.

FUTURE DIRECTIONS FOR RESEARCH

Despite the accumulation of research on the topic of weight bias, important questions remain unanswered. More work is needed to improve upon previous methodologies, to address additional research questions, to determine the nature and extent of consequences of weight bias, and to test interventions to reduce bias. Table 1 outlines areas of research which we believe are necessary directions in which to take these efforts.

CONCLUSION

The medical consequences of obesity are of immediate concern, but we cannot ignore the negative psychological, social, and physical outcomes that obese people face as a result of bias, stigma, and discrimination. These adverse experiences are pervasive, rarely challenged in our society, and have a detrimental impact on quality of life. Given the number of people affected, the inherent unfairness of prejudice, and the consequences of discrimination in key areas of living, such as employment, education, and health care, much more needs to be done.

The obesity field can and must play a central role in these efforts. While there has been increasing research attention to topics of bias and discrimination, many gaps in our knowledge remain. Without more focused work in this area to understand the nature and extent that weight bias compromises emotional and physical health, and to identify effective methods of improving societal attitudes, most obese individuals will be left to cope with the negative consequences of stigmatization on their own. This is especially concerning given that so many overweight and obese children are vulnerable to victimization on a daily basis, without sufficient support, coping strategies, or intervention. The national obesity research agenda must include attention to weight bias so that efforts can begin to change societal conditions that have created and perpetuated this social justice issue which has also become a public health problem.

REFERENCES

1. Puhl R, Brownell KD. Obesity, bias, and discrimination. Obes Res 2001; 9:788–805.
2. Brownell KD, Puhl R, Schwartz MB, et al., eds. Weight Bias: Nature, Consequences, and Remedies. New York: Guilford Publications, 2005.
3. Allon N. The stigma of overweight in everyday life. In: Woldman BB, ed. Psychological Aspects of Obesity. New York: Random House, 1982:130–174.
4. Jarvie GJ, Lahey B, Graziano W, et al. Childhood obesity and social stigma: what we know and what we don't know. Dev Rev 1983; 3:237–273.
5. Maroney D, Golub S. Nurses' attitudes toward obese persons and certain ethnic groups. Percept Mot Skills 1992; 75:387–391.
6. Price JH, Desmond SM, Krol RA, et al. Family practice physicians' beliefs, attitudes, and practices regarding obesity. Am J Prev Med 1987; 3:339–345.
7. Hoppe R, Ogden J. Practice nurses' beliefs about obesity and weight related interventions in primary care. Int J Obes Relat Metab Disord 1997; 21:141–146.
8. Bagley CR, Conklin DN, Isherwood RT, et al. Attitudes of nurses toward obesity and obese patients. Percept Mot Skills 1989, 68:954.
9. Kristeller JL, Hoerr RA. Physician attitudes toward managing obesity: differences among six specialty groups. Prev Med 1997; 26:542–549.
10. Chambliss HO, Finley CE, Blair SN. Attitudes toward obese individuals among exercise science students. Med Sci Sports Exerc 2004; 36:468–474.
11. Oberrieder H, Walker R, Monroe D, et al. Attitude of dietetics students and registered dietitians toward obesity. J Am Diet Assoc 1995; 95:914–916.
12. Harvey E, Summerbell C, Kirk S, et al. Dietitians' views of overweight and obese people and reported management practices. J Hum Nutr Diet 2002; 15:331–347.
13. Davis-Coelho K, Waltz J, Davis-Coelho B. Awareness and prevention of bias against fat clients in psychotherapy. Prof Psychol Res Pr 2000; 31:682–684.
14. Fabricatore AN, Wadden TA, Foster GD. Bias in health care settings. In: Brownell KD, Puhl R, Schwartz MB, et al., eds. Weight Bias: Nature, Consequences, and Remedies. New York: Guilford Publications, 2005:29–41.
15. Schwartz MB, O'Neal H, Brownell KD, et al. Weight bias among health professionals specializing in obesity. Obes Res 2003; 11:1033–1039.
16. Maiman LA, Wang VL, Becker MH, et al. Attitudes toward obesity and the obese among professionals. J Am Diet Assoc 1979; 74:331–336.
17. Hassel TD, Amici CJ, Thurston NS, et al. Client weight as a barrier to non-biased clinical judgment. J Psychol Christ 2001; 20:145–161.
18. Young LM, Powell B. The effects of obesity on the clinical judgements of mental health professionals. J Health Soc Behav 1985; 26:233–246.
19. Wigton RS, McGaghie WC. The effect of obesity on medical students' approach to patients with abdominal pain. J Gen Intern Med 2001; 16:262–265.
20. Puhl R, Brownell KD. Confronting and coping with weight stigma: an investigation of overweight and obese adults. Obesity 2006; 14:1802–1815.
21. Ostbye T, Taylor DH, Yancy WS, et al. Associations between obesity and receipt of screening mammography, Papanicolaou tests, and influenza vaccination: results from the Health and Retirement Study (HRS) and the Asset and Health Dynamics Among the Oldest Old (AHEAD) Study. Am J Pub Health 2005; 95:1623–1630.
22. Fontaine KR, Faith MS, Allison DB, et al. Body weight and health care among women in the general population. Arch Fam Med 1998; 7:381–384.

23. Wee CC, McCarthy EP, Davis RB, et al. Obesity and breast cancer screening. J Gen Int Med 2004; 19:324–331.

24. Meisinger C, Heier M, Loewel H. The relationship between body weight and health care among German women. Obes Res 2004; 12(9):1473–1480.

25. Wee CC, Phillips RS, McCarthy EP. BMI and cervical cancer screening among White, African-American, and His-panic women in the United States. Obes Res 2005; 13(7): 1275–1280.

26. Olson CL, Schumaker HD, Yawn BP. Overweight women delay medical care. Arch Fam Med 1994; 3:888–892.

27. Amy NK, Aalborg A, Lyons P, et al. Barriers to routine gynecological cancer screening for White and African-American obese women. Int J Obes (Lond) 2006; 30(1): 147–155.

28. Bellizzi JA, Hasty RW. Territory assignment decisions and supervising unethical selling behavior: the effects of obe-sity and gender as moderated by job-related factors. J Personal Selling Sales Manage 1998; XVIII(2):35–49.

29. Roehling MV. Weight-based discrimination in employ-ment: psychological and legal aspects. Pers Psychol 1999; 52:969–1017.

30. Decker WH. Attributions based on managers' self-presentation, sex, and weight. Psychol Rep 1987; 61: 175–181.

31. Klessen ML, Jasper CR, Harris RJ. The role of physical appearance in managerial decisions. J Bus Psychol 1993; 8:181–198.

32. Rothblum ED, Miller CT, Garbutt B. Stereotypes of obese female job applicants. Int J Eat Disord 1988; 7:277–283.

33. Kutcher EJ, Bragger JD. Selection interviews of over-weight job applicants: can structure reduce the bias? J Appl Soc Psychol 2004; 34:1993–2022.

34. Everett M. Let an overweight person call on your best customers? Fat chance. Sales Mark Manage 1990; 142:66–70.

35. Pingitoire R, Dugoni R, Tindale S, et al. Bias against overweight job applicants in a simulated employment interview. J Appl Psychol 1994; 79:909–917.

36. Klarenbach S, Padwal R, Chuck A, et al. Population-based analysis of obesity and workforce participation. Obesity 2006; 14:920–927.

37. Paul RJ, Townsend JB. Shape up or ship out? Employment discrimination against the overweight. Employee Respon-sibilities Rights J 1995; 8:133–145.

38. Bordieri JE, Drehmer DE, Taylor DW. Work life for employees with disabilities: recommendations for promo-tion. Rehab Couns Bull 1997; 40:181–191.

39. Brink TL. Obesity and job discrimination: mediation via personality stereotypes? Percept Mot Skills 1988; 66:494.

40. Pagan JA, Davila A. Obesity, occupational attainment, and earnings. Soc Sci Q 1997; 78:756–770.

41. Register CA, Williams DR. Wage effects of obesity among young workers. Soc Sci Q 1990; 71:130–141.

42. Frisk AM, Hernicz CB. Obesity as a disability: an actual or perceived problem? Army Law 1996; 3:3–19.

43. Perroni PJ. Cook v. Rhode Island, Department of Mental Health, Retardation, and Hospitals: the First Circuit tips the scales of justice to protect the overweight. New Engl Law Rev 1996; 30:993–1018.

44. Post R. Prejudicial appearances: the logic of American anti-discrimination. Calif Law Rev 2000; 88:1–40.

45. Theran EA. Legal theory on weight discrimination. In: Brownell KD, Puhl RM, Schwartz MB, et al., eds. Weight Bias: Nature, Consequences, and Remedies. New York: Guilford Press, 2005:195–211.

46. Puhl R, Latner J. Obesity, stigma, and the health of the nation's children. Psychol Bull 2007; 133(4):557–580.

47. Neumark-Sztainer D, Falkner N, Story M, et al. Weight-teasing among adolescents: correlations with weight status and disordered eating behaviors. Int J Obes 2002; 26: 123–131.

48. Griffiths LJ, Wolke D, Page AS, et al. Obesity and bullying: different effects for boys and girls. Arch Dis Child 2006; 91:121–125.

49. Janssen I, Craig WM, Boyce WF, et al. Associations between overweight and obesity with bullying behaviors in school-aged children. Pediatrics 2004; 113:1187–1194.

50. Hayden-Wade HA, Stein RI, Ghaderi A, et al. Prevalence, characteristics, and correlates of teasing experiences among overweight children vs. non-overweight peers. Obes Res 2005; 13:1381–1392.

51. Cramer P, Steinwert T. Thin is good, fat is bad: how early does it begin? J Appl Dev Psychol 1998; 19:429–451.

52. Brylinskey JA, Moore JC. The identification of body build stereotypes in young children. J Res Pers 1994; 28: 170–181.

53. Wardle J, Volz C, Golding C. Social variation in attitudes to obesity in children. Int J Obes Relat Metab Disord 1995; 19:562–569.

54. Neumark-Sztainer D, Story M, Faibisch L. Perceived stigmatization among overweight African-American and Caucasian adolescent girls. J Adolesc Health 1998; 23:264–270.

55. Neumark-Sztainer D, Story M, Harris T. Beliefs and attitudes about obesity among teachers and school health care providers working with adolescents. J Nutr Educ 1999; 31:3–9.

56. Price JH, Desmond SM, Krol RA, et al. Family practice physicians' beliefs, attitudes, and practices regarding obe-sity. Am J Prev Med 1987; 3:339–345.

57. Greenleaf C, Weiller K. Perceptions of youth obesity among physical educators. Soc Psychol Edu 2005; 8:407–423.

58. O'Brien KS, Hunter JA, Banks M. Implicit anti-fat bias in physical educators: physical attributes, ideology, and socialisation. Int J Obes Relat Metab Disord 2006; 31:308–314.

59. Weiler K, Helms LB. Responsibilities of nursing educa-tion: the lessons of Russell v Salve Regina. J Prof Nurs 1993; 9:131–138.

60. Canning H, Mayer J. Obesity: its possible effect on college acceptance. New Engl J Med 1966; 275:1172–1174.

61. Friedman KE, Reichmann SK, Costanzo PR, et al. Weight stigmatization and ideological beliefs: relation to psycho-logical functioning in obese adults. Obes Res 2005; 13:907–916.

62. Myers A, Rosen JC. Obesity stigmatization and coping: relation to mental health symptoms, body image, and self-esteem. Int J Obes Relat Metab Disord 1999; 23:221–230.

63. Davison KK, Birch LL. Processes linking weight status and self-concept among girls from ages 5 to 7 years. Dev Psychol 2002; 38:735–748.

64. Eisenberg ME, Neumark-Sztainer D, Story M. Associations of weight-based teasing and emotional well-being among adolescents. Arch Pediatr Adolesc Med 2003; 157:733–738.

65. Keery H, Boutelle K, van den Berg P, et al. The impact of appearance-related teasing by family members. J Adolesc Health 2005; 37:120–127.

66. Thompson JK, Coovert MD, Richards KJ, et al. Development of body image, eating disturbance, and general psychological functioning in female adolescents: covariance structure modeling and longitudinal investigations. Int J Eat Disord 1995; 18:221–236.

67. Grilo CM, Wilfley DE, Brownell KD, et al. Teasing, body image, and self-esteem in a clinical sample of obese women. Addict Behav 1994; 19:443–450.

68. Lunner K, Werthem E, Thompson JK, et al. A cross-cultural examination of weight-related teasing, body image, and eating disturbance in Swedish and Australian samples. Int J Eat Disord 2000; 28:430–435.

69. Puhl R, Henderson KE, Brownell KD. Social consequences of obesity. In: Kopelman P, Caterson I, Dietz W, eds. Clinical Obesity and Related Metabolic Disease in Adults and Children. London: Blackwell Publishing Ltd, 2005: 29–45.

70. Strauss CC, Smith K, Frame C, et al. Personal and interpersonal characteristics associated with childhood obesity. J Pediatr Psychol 1985; 10:337–343.

71. Strauss RS, Pollack HA. Social marginalization of overweight children. Arch Pediatr Adolesc Med 2003; 157: 746–752.

72. Falkner NH, Neumark-Sztainer D, Story M, et al. Social, educational, and psychological correlates of weight status in adolescents. Obes Res 2001; 9:32–42.

73. Harris MB, Walters LC, Waschull S. Gender and ethnic differences in obesity-related behaviors and attitudes in a college sample. J Appl Soc Psychol 1991; 21:1545–1566.

74. Miller CT, Rothblum ED, Barbour L, et al. Social interactions of obese and nonobese women. J Pers 1990; 58:365–380.

75. Snyder M, Haugen JA. Why does behavioral confirmation occur? A functional perspective on the role of the perceiver. J Exp Soc Psychol 1994; 30:218–246.

76. Snyder M, Haugen JA. Why does behavioral confirmation occur? A functional perspective on the role of the target. Pers Soc Psychol Bull 1995; 21:963–974.

77. Haines J, Neumark-Sztainer D, Eisenberg ME, et al. Weight teasing and disordered eating behaviors in adolescents: longitudinal findings from Project EAT (Eating Among Teens). Pediatrics 2006; 117:209–215.

78. Puhl R, Moss-Racusin C, Schwartz MB. Internalization of weight bias: implications for binge eating and emotional wellbeing. Obesity 2007; 15:19–23.

79. Storch EA, Milsom VA, DeBraganza N, et al. Peer victimization, psychosocial adjustment, and physical activity in overweight and at-risk-for-overweight youth. J Pediatr Psychol 2007; 32(1):80–89.

80. Faith MS, Leone MA, Ayers TS, et al. Weight criticism during physical activity, coping skills, and reported physical activity in children. Pediatrics 2002; 110:e23.

81. Vartanian LR, Shaprow JG. Effects of weight stigma on exercise motivation and behavior: a preliminary investigation among college-aged females. J Health Psychol 2008; 13(1):131–138.

82. Matthews KA, Salomon K, Kenyon K, et al. Unfair treatment, discrimination, and ambulatory blood pressure in black and white adolescents. Health Psychol 2005; 24: 258–265.

83. Bell SK, Morgan SB. Children's attitudes and behavioral intentions toward a peer presented as obese: does a medical explanation for the obesity make a difference? J Pediatr Psychol 2000; 25:137–145.

84. Sigelman CK. The effect of causal information on peer perceptions of children with physical problems. J Appl Dev Psychol 1991; 12:237–253.

85. Anesbury T, Tiggermann M. An attempt to reduce negative stereotyping of obesity in children by changing controllability beliefs. Health Educ Res 2000; 15:145–152.

86. DeJong W. Obesity as a characterological stigma: the issue of responsibility and judgments of task performance. Psychol Rep 1993; 73:963–970.

87. DeJong W. The stigma of obesity: the consequences of naïve assumptions concerning the causes of physical deviance. J Health Soc Behav 1980; 21:75–87.

88. Teachman BA, Gapinski KD, Brownell KD, et al. Demonstrations of implicit anti-fat bias: the impact of providing causal information and evoking empathy. Health Psychol 2003; 22:68–78.

89. Crandall CS. Prejudice against fat people: ideology and self-interest. J Pers Soc Psychol 1994; 66:882–894.

90. Puhl R, Schwartz MB, Brownell KD. Impact of perceived consensus on stereotypes about obese people: new avenues for bias reduction. Health Psychol 2005; 24:517–525.

91. Gapinski KD, Schwartz MB, Brownell KD. Can television change anti-fat attitudes and behavior? J Appl Biobehav Res 2006; 11:1–28.

92. Wiese HJ, Wilson JF, Jones RA, et al. Obesity stigma reduction in medical students. Int J Obes Relat Metab Disord 1992; 16:859–868.

93. Hague AL, White AA. Web-based intervention for changing attitudes of obesity among current and future teachers. J Nutr Educ Behav 2005; 37:58–66.

6

Impact of Voluntary Weight Loss on Morbidity and Mortality

EDWARD W. GREGG

Division of Diabetes Translation, National Center for Chronic Disease Prevention and Health Promotion, Centers for Disease Control and Prevention, Atlanta, Georgia, U.S.A.

RATIONALE FOR WEIGHT LOSS AS A PUBLIC HEALTH INTERVENTION

While the health of the U.S. population, based on mortality and crude morbidity indicators, has improved to unprecedented levels, obesity has emerged as one of the most prominent threats to continued advances in health status. Prevalence of obesity has increased from 15% to 31% between 1976 and 2004, with the greatest relative increase observed in the very obese categories (1–4). During this period the prevalence of class III obesity has tripled, now comprising 5% of adults. These trends have affected both genders, virtually all ethnic groups and all age ranges, including children (1,3).

An increasing prevalence of obesity is of concern because it is associated with so many adverse health conditions, including diabetes, cardiovascular diseases (CVDs), renal disease, arthritis and disability, depression, sleep apnea, certain cancers, and ultimately worsened quality of life (5–10). The most tangible population level impact on the trends in health of the public is seen in diabetes, disability, and in health care expenditures (11–13). For example, the prevalence of diabetes has tripled during the last 40 years and doubled during the past 25 years, with virtually all of this increase in diabetes prevalence contributed by people who are overweight and obese and one-fourth of cases coming from those with

class III obesity (14). Some of the greatest concern surrounds obesity, fueling speculation that the new cohort of youth with an unprecedented obesity prevalence will ultimately have a health outlook worse than that of their parents (15,16). Although medical and public health systems have reduced some risk factors among obese persons, this has come at a large cost and is unlikely to compensate for the wide-ranging impacts of obesity (12,17–20).

In the absence of major progress in the prevention of obesity, voluntary weight loss is considered central to the clinical and public health response to prevent overweight and obesity-related conditions. Yet ironically, recommendations of weight loss as a clinical and public health intervention remain controversial for several reasons. First, weight loss is perceived as being relatively ineffective due to the large proportion of persons who regain weight, raising questions of whether the short-term benefits are likely to influence long-term health outcomes. This concern is compounded by the lack of long-term intervention trials examining the effects of weight loss on major causes of morbidity and mortality. Second, weight loss remains controversial because of epidemiological literature associating weight loss with increased mortality. This latter concern may have been spuriously affected by weaknesses in the methodology of observational epidemiology. Finally, weight loss is controversial because its ramifications are so broad. Weight loss is one of the most common health-related interventions undertaken by adults in the United States, as more than a third of all adults and more than two-thirds of obese adults are trying to lose weight at any given time (21). The fact that overweight and obesity affect most Americans at some point in their life means that clinical and public health interventions have a huge potential to positively affect health or, alternatively, waste resources if interventions are either ineffective or contribute to adverse health outcomes.

In this chapter, we review the evidence that voluntary weight loss is associated with long-term benefits in major health outcomes, ranging from diabetes to disability to mortality.

TYPES OF VOLUNTARY WEIGHT LOSS

In the examination of the effectiveness of weight loss as a clinical and public health intervention, we view voluntary weight loss from two general perspectives: (*i*) intentional weight loss as determined in observational studies and (*ii*) weight loss as obtained from structured clinical and community interventions designed to achieve a high efficacy of weight loss. The fundamental difference between the two perspectives is that the first assesses the effects of weight loss as it is performed in the population by those who choose to perform it, whereas the second perspective specifically examines the impact of interventions that are given or imposed on a segment of the population.

Observational studies capture the impact of weight loss in all of its diversity, from brief, fleeting, ineffective methods undertaken by individuals to state-of-the-art intensive interventions. Overall, 29% of men and 44% of women report trying to lose weight (Fig. 1).

Prevalence of trying to lose weight is consistently higher among women, peaks in middle age, and is somewhat higher among persons of higher education. Among men, about a third of overweight men and almost two-thirds of obese men report trying to lose weight. Notably, more than a fourth of normal weight women and almost three-fourths of obese women report trying to lose weight. Of those trying to lose weight, most have a weight loss goal of <10 kg, but about one-fourth would like to lose 15 kg or more (21). The methods of reported weight loss are diverse. While the vast majority report dieting and physical activity, only one-fifth report the recommended combination of eating fewer calories and exercising >150 min/wk (21). At the same time, many use other methods, including skipping meals (17%), attending special programs (7%), eating special products (22%), taking supplements or diet pills

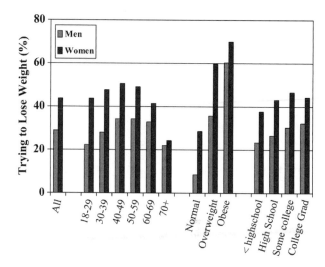

Figure 1 Prevalence of U.S. population reporting intentional weight loss by sex, age group, education, and body mass index, Behavior Risk Factor Surveillance System. *Source*: Adapted from Ref. 21.

(14%), fasting, or purging (3%), which may have varied success (22). Many attempts are short-lived using fairly innocuous, if ineffective, changes in lifestyle, carried out without professional or clinical assistance. Other attempts are carried out with professional or clinical help using largely healthy improvements in lifestyle. Other attempts are carried out using extreme, potentially deleterious or dubious methods (22,23). Observational studies typically evaluate weight change and intent to lose weight using simple self-report questions at one point in time, which is followed by a period of outcome ascertainment. The advantage to this perspective is that it examines the "average" impact of weight loss attempts as it truly exists in the real world. A disadvantage is that the benefits of highly efficacious methods may be counterbalanced or obscured by the nonbenefits or risks of ineffective methods.

For these reasons, observational studies should generally not be used to guide clinical and public health intervention strategies but rather to gauge the impact in the general population and to prioritize the types of intervention and subpopulations to be tested using controlled intervention trials.

The second main category of voluntary weight loss, structured weight loss programs, has the advantage of providing stronger evidence about the cause and effect, dose response, and clinical utility of weight loss interventions. Thus, they are more valuable in prioritizing the types of clinical and public health interventions likely to be most effective in overweight and obese people at risk of disease. An inherent limitation of structured weight loss programs is that they frequently test interventions that are either not practical in the real world and/or do not reflect the real ways that people in the community go about weight loss. Thus, they tell us about the potential efficacy of the approach but not the net effect in the population. A key challenge in interpreting intervention studies is determining whether intervention's health effects will be different when translated into the real world.

SUMMARY OF SHORT-TERM EFFECTS OF WEIGHT LOSS

Weight loss leads to several short-term physiological changes that could affect long-term disease incidence and mortality (Fig. 2). Weight loss has some of its most direct and important effects on insulin sensitivity, glucose tolerance, blood pressure, lipid parameters, and inflammatory factors. Meta-analyses suggest that 12-month weight loss programs on average achieve a 4- to 5-kg weight loss at one year and reductions of 4 mmHg systolic blood pressure, 3 mmHg of diastolic blood pressure, 5 to 8 mg/dL of total and low-density lipoprotein (LDL) cholesterol and about 18 mg/dL of triglyceride (24). Weight loss reduces left ventricular hypertrophy and resting heart rate, increases stroke volume and cardiac output, improves coagulation and fibrinolytic factors, reduces angina symptoms, and consistently improves functional status and cardiorespiratory capacity (25,26). Meta-analyses of data from patients with diabetes show that lifestyle and behavioral weight loss interventions led to a net 0.3% reduction in HbA1c (27,28). This effect tended to parallel the magnitude of weight loss but ranged across studies, from 1%

gain to 2.6% decline in A1c. Recent studies suggest that levels of inflammatory markers are also improved with short-term weight loss. A recent two-year lifestyle intervention conducted in obese middle-aged women achieved a 10% weight loss and resulted in approximate 25% reductions in interleukin-6, interleukin-18, and C-reactive protein and 50% increase in adiponectin levels (29,30). Finally, underlying these overt effects in humans is a broad set of tissue-specific effects of dietary restriction that have been demonstrated in a range of animal models, with several studies suggesting that dietary restriction results in a lengthening of mean and maximum life span (31,32).

Despite the short-term benefits of weight loss, there are several reasons to question whether losing weight in the short term will influence long-term disease outcomes. First, most people who try to lose weight regain weight; on average, one-third of peak weight loss is regained in the year following weight loss (33). Second, even in the cases of successful weight loss it is unclear whether the physiological benefits are maintained over a long-enough period of time to reverse preexisting pathology and thus influence long-term health outcomes.

Finally, while most physiological adaptations to moderate weight loss are positive, weight loss is associated with increased bone loss, decreased lean muscle mass, gallstone development, and perhaps, decreased immunity associated with multiple weight loss attempts (34–37,38). The reduction in bone loss may be offset by increased physical activity, but the implications of bone loss for subsequent osteoporotic fracture risk and disability remain a concern of weight loss in older populations. It has also been suggested that weight loss leads to a release of toxins from the mobilization of fat that ultimately increase risk for cancer (39).

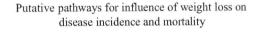

Putative pathways for influence of weight loss on disease incidence and mortality

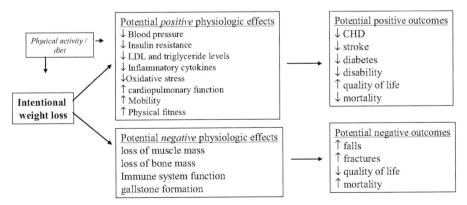

Figure 2 Putative pathways for the influence of weight loss on disease incidence and mortality. *Source*: Adapted from Ref. 39.

IMPACT OF WEIGHT LOSS INTERVENTIONS ON MORBIDITY

Hypertension

The strong association of weight loss with improved blood pressure levels led to a series of trials to test whether clinically defined hypertension could be prevented or altered using multidisciplinary lifestyle interventions. In the Trials of Hypertension Prevention I and II, overweight persons aged 30 to 54 years with high normal blood pressure assigned to a weight loss condition had a 2% to 4% weight loss over 1.5 to 4 years and achieved a 21% to 34% decreased hypertension incidence (40,41). The magnitude of risk reduction was related to the magnitude of weight loss, as persons who maintained a 5% weight loss over three years had a 65% reduced hypertension incidence, whereas those who had similar initial weight loss and regained half of their weight back had a 25% reduced hypertension incidence (42).

A subsequent lifestyle intervention conducted among adults aged 60 to 80 years (the Trial of Nonpharmacologic Interventions in the Elderly, TONE) achieved an average of 4% weight loss over 2.5 years and found a 30% reduction in combined hypertension and CVD outcomes. Thirty-nine percent of intervention participants remained free of medications and did not have a hypertensive or CVD event, compared to 26% remaining event-free in the control group (43). In addition, a recent major lifestyle-based trial tested the impact of a multicomponent behavioral intervention over an 18-month period among 810 middle-aged adults with either prehypertension or mild hypertension (44). The trial compared three conditions: brief advice; "established" (i.e., standard) behavioral intervention with an approximate 7% weight loss goal to the established intervention; and the specific Dietary Approaches to Stop Hypertension (DASH) diet, a diet high in fruits and vegetables and low-fat dairy products and low in saturated fat, total fat, and cholesterol. The trial was conducted over an 18-month period, achieved roughly 2.5% weight loss and 20% lower probability of hypertension for persons randomized to the intervention condition.

Each of the hypertension prevention and management studies described above used multidisciplinary behavior–based weight loss approaches to achieve modest weight losses through reduced fat and total intake, increased intake of complex carbohydrates, and physical activity. The magnitude of effects on hypertension was modest in comparison to what medical management may achieve, but the trials nonetheless justified lifestyle-based weight loss approaches as a viable supplement to medical management and as a means of reducing the need for anti-hypertensive medication. In addition, the lifestyle-based antihypertensive trials also established the feasibility of multiyear, multidisciplinary weight loss programs, serving as precursors for trials in diabetes prevention.

Type 2 Diabetes

Type 2 diabetes provides one of the strongest cases for the benefits of intentional weight loss. A series of multiyear prevention studies have shown that weight loss achieved through combined dietary intervention and physical activity with strong behavioral support can significantly reduce the incidence of diabetes in overweight persons with impaired glucose tolerance (IGT) (45–50). The first published lifestyle intervention trials were conducted in Sweden and China (48,51–53). In a nonrandomized intervention study of 260 Swedish men aged 47 to 49 years with IGT, those assigned to a diet and exercise condition maintained a modest (2.3%) weight loss over six years and had a 63% lower diabetes incidence (48,51). A study conducted in the oil city of Da Qing in northern China from 1986 to 1992 assigned clinics of high-risk adults to a diet, exercise, or combined diet and exercise condition. Interventions were achieved using a combination of dietary counseling, exercise counseling, and structured sessions. A reduction in diabetes incidence of 29% to 32% was achieved in all the three interventions among both lean and overweight persons in spite of negligible change in weight loss at the six-year point of the study (51).

The next major diabetes prevention trial was conducted in Finland among overweight persons with IGT (47). Five hundred twenty-two overweight men and women, again with IGT, were randomized to either a normal care or a lifestyle intervention. The lifestyle intervention group received tailored advice to lose weight, reduce saturated and total fat, increase fiber intake, and increase physical activity levels. The intervention achieved a net 3.4% weight loss after one year and 2.7% weight loss after two years, and ultimately, a 58% reduced diabetes incidence after a median four years of follow-up.

The next year, results from the U.S. Diabetes Prevention Program (DPP) were reported (45,54), demonstrating an overall effect on diabetes incidence identical to that of the Finnish study. Overweight men and women with IGT assigned to the intervention condition achieved a 7% weight loss after one year, 4.5% weight loss after three years, and ultimately a 58% reduced incidence of diabetes that were mediated by both improved insulin sensitivity and reduced insulin secretion. Findings were similar across genders, race/ethnicity, and age groups. Participants randomized to a metformin arm had a 2% weight loss and a 31% reduced diabetes incidence. In 2004–2005, a randomized controlled trial comparing the effects of lifestyle modification, metformin, and both among

502 Asian Indians found significant, equivalent reductions in diabetes incidence of 38%, 35%, and 37%, respectively over a three-year period (49).

The effects of these lifestyle and weight loss–based diabetes prevention trials along with seven additional smaller studies were also recently quantified in a meta-analysis by Gillies et al. (55). The meta-analysis notes that virtually all studies were conducted among overweight, middle-aged (40s and 50s) populations at a high baseline risk of diabetes, often defined by presence of IGT. The pooled effect was a 49% (95% CI, 41–60%) reduced diabetes incidence, with strong consistency across studies. Five-year pooled diabetes incidence in control conditions was 37%, compared with an incidence of about 20% among person receiving lifestyle intervention. There was no interaction between underlying baseline risk and the effectiveness of interventions. In other words, lifestyle interventions had similar levels of effectiveness in studies with somewhat lower risk populations (46,56,57) as studies with noted high-risk populations (45,48,49).

Figure 3 summarizes the differences in yearly diabetes incidence between the intervention and control conditions in six major diabetes prevention trials. The magnitude of difference in incidence between intervention and control groups was remarkably similar (four to six events per year difference) across the lifestyle-based studies, despite the fact that the absolute level of body mass index (BMI) and country of location varied considerably. The level of incidence and corresponding difference between control and intervention conditions were lower in the Swedish Obese Subjects (SOS) study presumably because it is the one study that did not have IGT as inclusion criteria. Thus,

baseline risk in SOS was lower than other studies in spite of the high level of obesity. Taken as a whole, these diabetes prevention studies have provided a consistent case for the role of intentional weight loss to delay diabetes in high-risk individuals and has provided the basis and hope for new strategies to prevent type 2 diabetes.

Questions remain unanswered about the degree to which reductions in type 2 diabetes incidence are due principally to weight loss or to the behaviors that lead to the weight loss. The DPP, for example, achieved a 7.2% weight loss at year 1, but also an increase in seven to eight metabolic equivalent task hours of physical activity, and 7% reduction in fat intake (45,58). However, post hoc analyses showed that weight change was the dominant factor, as physical activity and fat intake were not significant predictors of diabetes risk in multivariate analyses, and each kilogram of weight loss was associated with a 16% reduced risk. Compared with participants who met none of the three major goals (7% weight loss, 150 minutes walking per week, <30% of fat in the diet), relative risk of diabetes was reduced by 89% among people who met all the three goals. However, participants who met the weight change goal without meeting the exercise or fat goal also had an 80% reduced risk of diabetes (58). In the Finnish Diabetes Prevention Study, achievement of the weight loss goal also appeared to drive the main study findings. In multivariate analyses, achievement of the 5% weight loss goal was associated with a 57% reduced diabetes incidence, adjusting for attainment of goals related to fat intake, saturated fat intake, fiber, and physical activity (50,57).

Weight change was less associated with diabetes prevention in the two Asian studies (48,49), as each study found reduced diabetes incidence in lifestyle intervention arms that achieved no weight loss. It is conceivable that these interventions reduced visceral adiposity in combination with a modest increase in lean mass, leading to a potent reduction in diabetes risk, without materially influencing BMI. This raises the question of whether the behaviors contributing to weight loss, increases in physical activity levels, or specific factors related to dietary change (e.g., reduced saturated fat intake, reduced refined carbohydrate intake) ultimately play a greater role in diabetes prevention than the weight loss per se. This notion is supported by a large body of observational studies but has not been tested in the form of large randomized controlled trials (59). Nevertheless, the effectiveness of lifestyle behaviors to influence diabetes risk above and beyond weight loss has important implications for the ways that public health messages and community interventions are delivered.

The most dramatic effects of weight loss on type 2 diabetes risk have been observed in nonrandomized studies of obesity surgery (60,61). In the SOS bariatric surgery among over 800 very obese men and women had an

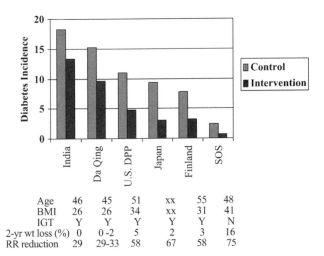

	India	Da Qing	U.S. DPP	Japan	Finland	SOS
Age	46	45	51	xx	55	48
BMI	26	26	34	xx	31	41
IGT	Y	Y	Y	Y	Y	N
2-yr wt loss (%)	0	0 -2	5	2	3	16
RR reduction	29	29-33	58	67	58	75

Figure 3 Differences in incidence (y-axis) of diabetes between control and intervention groups according to baseline body mass index (x-axis) from major diabetes prevention trials. *Source:* Adapted from Ref. 47.

average net weight loss of 23% two years after surgery and 14% 10 years after surgery. The surgery group had net reductions in fasting glucose of 18 to 20 mg/dL compared with the control group. Incidence of diabetes among the surgery condition was 7% versus 24% among control participants, corresponding to a 75% reduced odds of diabetes. There were also substantial improvements in levels of fasting insulin, uric acid, triglycerides, and high-density lipoprotein (HDL) cholesterol that were diminished somewhat but still maintained after 10 years. There were essentially no differences in total cholesterol, but this was compensated and explained by large increases in HDL cholesterol among the intervention groups (60).

Several key questions remain related to weight loss and diabetes prevention. First, it is unclear whether less intense, community-driven approaches can achieve suitable efficacy. In a review of community-based studies, Satterfield et al. identified several community-based diabetes prevention studies that have successfully improved knowledge and preventive behaviors, but the ultimate impact of these interventions on diabetes and related clinical outcomes was unclear (62). Second, it is unknown whether effectiveness will be sufficient among people in lower-risk states to expand recommendations beyond persons with IGT. In the Multiple Risk Factor Intervention Trial (MRFIT), men with CVD risk factors assigned to a six-year, multidisciplinary, risk factor reduction intervention had a significant 18% reduced diabetes incidence, but this benefit was limited to nonsmokers (63). Most prevention trials were limited to persons with IGT, and in some cases, additional risk factors. To alter trends in prevalence in the population as a whole, it may be necessary to intervene earlier in the pathophysiological process. In other words, once someone has IGT, it may be too late to do more than delay diabetes. Finally, it is unclear whether interventions will have sustained effects on type 2 diabetes beyond the life of the study and whether the benefits of lifestyle interventions also extend beyond type 2 diabetes to also influence microvascular and macrovascular complications of disease (63).

Cardiovascular Disease

In theory, the reliable improvements in glucose tolerance, blood pressure, lipid profiles, inflammatory markers, and cardiorespiratory fitness caused by intentional weight loss should all combine to reduce cardiovascular incidence. Despite this potential, the long-term effects of weight loss on incidence and survival of CVD is surprisingly unstudied. This is, in part, due to the practical limitations of conducting weight loss intervention over a long enough period of time to accrue CVD outcomes.

In the 1990s, the Lifestyle Heart Trial examined the effects of intensive weight loss and cardioprotective dietary interventions. The studies recruited 48 people with heart disease and randomized half of them to an aggressive low-fat, high-fiber diet achieving an 8% weight loss over one year, with the other group randomized to a usual-care control condition (64,65). The study observed significant reductions in coronary stenosis, angina symptoms, and cardiac events over five years. Similarly, a small study examining a 12-month diet and exercise intervention program among patients with coronary artery disease demonstrated a 5% reduction in body weight and significant reductions in myocardial ischemia as well as coronary artery stenosis relative to patients in a usual care condition. In the Stanford Coronary Risk Intervention Project (SCRIP), a multifactorial risk factor reduction consisting of intensive total and saturated fat reduction, increases in physical activity, and a 4% weight loss resulted in about a 40% reduced probability of cardiac events and a slower rate of coronary artery stenosis (66).

One observational study found a beneficial effect of weight loss among a cohort of high-risk patients aged 50 to 75 years. Persons who successfully dieted and lost weight during the first six months of the intervention had a 30% reduced odds of a coronary heart disease (CHD) event over a three-year period (67). Cumulative CHD incidence was 18% among patients who gained weight, 14% among those who lost <2 kg or gained weight, 14% among those with 2- to 7-kg weight loss, and only 8% among those with at least 7-kg weight loss. However, it was unclear whether follow-up time was equivalent between groups. A greater follow-up among those with less weight loss would permit more time for a CHD event to occur and thus overestimate the benefit of weight loss. The study did not report how many patients initiated lipid-lowering therapy or whether this varied according to quintile of weight loss.

Despite the encouraging findings related to multifactorial risk factor reduction and CVD-related outcomes, interpreting the effect of weight loss on these studies is difficult. Although each study observed greater weight loss in the intervention groups, it is likely that treatment with lipid-lowering medications and the reduction in saturated fat intake were major factors driving the study results, and these effects may have occurred independent of changes in body weight. Furthermore, there have been no studies examining whether intentional weight loss prevents CVD in the first place. Two studies underway should provide answers to whether weight loss prevents CVD. The Diabetes Prevention Program Outcomes Study is underway to examine whether the successful effects of lifestyle intervention on diabetes prevention also extend to reduction of CVD incidence and other diabetes-related complications. The Look AHEAD (Action for Health in Diabetes) study, currently underway, is the largest study to examine the impact of intentional weight loss on long-term health outcomes. The study includes a four-year intensive weight loss intervention period, employing dietary reduction including portion-controlled diets, regular physical activity, and behavioral support, using a multidisciplinary intervention team. Release of first-year findings of the study showed that persons assigned to multidisciplinary lifestyle intervention lost 8% of their initial weight (net of control) and had substantial increases in fitness (15% net improvement), declines in mean A1c (0.6% vs. −0.1%), fasting glucose levels (−21 mg/dL), blood pressure (−6.8/3 mmHg), triglycerides (−30 mg/dL), and had declines in the proportion of taking diabetes medications or lipid-lowering drugs (68). The study is designed to last 11.5 years and ultimately determines whether the established risk factor reductions are maintained long enough to influence incidence of CVD and related outcomes.

Disability and Musculoskeletal Morbidity

Physical disability has emerged as one of the most consistent consequences of obesity in the population and possibly, one of the outcomes likely to persist into the future due to declining mortality rates (12,69–72). The link between obesity and disability is probably multifactorial, with diabetes, arthritis, CHD and heart failure, stroke and depression all being potential disease-related mediators (69–71). Additional nondisease consequences include inflammation, lean muscle loss, gait abnormalities, and impaired cardiorespiratory fitness. Although this constellation of potential mediators points to weight loss as a potentially effective intervention, few studies have specifically examined its effectiveness on disability related outcomes.

Observational studies examining the association of weight loss with disability have given mixed conclusions. Some previous studies have suggested that weight loss in older populations may be associated with functional decline and disability (72). Among adults aged 70 to 79 years in the Health, Aging, and Body Composition (Health ABC) Study, incidence of mobility limitation was strongly associated with BMI, with lowest incidence (about 10% per year) observed among persons with BMI <25 and 25 to 30, about 18% per year incidence among moderately obese persons (BMI 30–34.9), and over 40% incidence among very obese persons (BMI > 35) (73). Persons reporting intentional weight loss had a higher incidence of mobility limitations than stable weight, but this appeared to be explained by persons who lost weight being more obese at baseline. In analyses stratified by BMI category, intentional weight loss was associated with a 59% increased risk of mobility limitation among overweight adults but not significantly associated with either

an increase or decrease in risk in all other BMI categories. Unintentional weight loss and weight fluctuation were each associated with increased incidence of mobility limitation.

While mobility and functioning may be improved in some high-risk subgroups, an increased risk of osteoporotic fractures may occur in others. A report by Ensrud and colleagues (74) found that older women who had a 10% unintentional weight loss had a significant 80% increased risk of osteoporotic fracture, but those who lost weight intentionally did not have an increased fracture risk. However, both intentional and unintentional weight loss were associated with slight but statistically significant (relative risk = 1.16–1.18) increased risks of falling (35,36,72,74). An analysis of Nurses' Health Study data, however, demonstrated an association between weight loss and improved physical functioning and vitality (75). Interpretation of observational weight loss studies in the elderly population remains difficult because of the possibility for reverse causality, with frailty and aging-related illness leading to weight loss at the same time as increased weight loss (76).

The benefits of weight loss appear more clear for arthritis-mediated functional impairment. An observational study in 1992 suggested that weight loss of about 5 kg over 10 years was associated with a 59% reduced incidence of arthritis (77). More recently, a series of randomized controlled trials have suggested that structured weight loss programs with exercise for overweight older adults with osteoarthritis can reduce osteoarthritis symptoms and improve functional status. The Arthritis, Diet, and Activity Promotion Trial (ADAPT) randomized 316 older adults (aged >60 years) with BMI >28 and knee pain and disability to a control condition, diet, exercise, or diet plus exercise weight loss interventions, wherein the intervention conditions achieved a 5% to 6% weight loss over 18 months (78). The diet- and exercise-based weight loss group had the most substantial improvements of the groups, with significant improvements in lower extremity and physical functioning, six-minute walking distance, and knee pain.

Mortality

Most observational studies of the effects of weight loss on mortality over the years have suggested that weight loss is actually associated with increased mortality rather than decreased mortality (79,80). However, interpretation of this literature is difficult because people who lose weight are a mixture of healthy people losing weight using positive lifestyle changes and others who have lost weight because of either overt or underlying illnesses that increase their risk of death. Allison et al. demonstrated, for example, a separation of mortality effects depending upon whether the weight change was primarily attributed to fat or lean mass, as loss of fat mass was associated with reduced mortality whereas loss of lean mass was associated with increased mortality (81). Most studies have relied on assessment of weight loss without measurement of the characteristics or the weight change or without finding out whether the weight change was intentional. This limitation of observational studies led to a series of observational studies attempting to assess the effect of "intentional" weight loss on mortality, which only partially resolved the controversy related to weight loss and mortality (79,80).

In a 13-year follow-up of over 43,000 middle-aged (40–64 years) women in the Cancer Prevention Study, women with obesity-related conditions and a modest (0–9 kg) weight loss over time was associated with a 20% decrease in all-cause mortality, 40% to 50% decrease in cancer-related mortality and a 30% to 40% reduction in diabetes mortality but no difference in CVD mortality (82). However, there was no association between weight loss and mortality among healthy women. Among men, there was no association of weight loss with all-cause, CVD, or cancer mortality, but there was a 33% reduced mortality among those with preexisting disease (83). In a supplemental analysis of over 5000 diabetic men and women from the Cancer Prevention Study, self-reported intentional weight loss was associated with a 25% to 28% reduced all-cause, CVD, and diabetes-related mortality (84). The greatest reduction in mortality (33%) was associated with a 10% to 15% (20–29 lb) weight loss.

A nine-year mortality follow-up of the National Health Interview Survey showed that among overweight and obese U.S. adults aged >35 years, persons reporting intentional weight loss had a 24% lower mortality rate than persons reporting no weight change and not trying to lose weight (85). Unexpectedly, however, mortality rates were 20% lower among persons reporting trying to lose weight but no weight change during the previous year. Thus, reporting trying to lose weight appeared as important as weight loss itself. Unintentional weight loss, on the other hand, was associated with a 31% increased mortality rate. Results were similar among diabetic adults in the United States. Compared with persons reporting no weight loss and no weight loss attempt, those who lost weight over the previous year had a nonsignificant 17% decrease in those with modest intentional weight loss (86). Unexpectedly, persons who reported trying to lose weight but reported no weight change over the previous year had a 23% lower mortality rate than those not trying to lose weight at all. Those reporting unintentional weight loss had a significant 58% increased mortality risk. This could be attributed to health benefits associated with weight loss attempts or, alternatively, an indication that people who report trying to lose weight engage in other healthier behavior (Fig. 4).

An analysis by Wannamethee et al. provided yet another insight into the potential role of intentional weight loss (87). Among about 5000 British men aged 56 to 75 years, intentional weight loss was associated with a 41% reduced risk of all-cause mortality and a 64% reduced risk of non-CVD-related mortality if the weight loss was as a result of personal choice. However, intentional weight loss that was attributed primarily to ill health or a physician's advice was associated with a 37% increased mortality risk. There was no association of intentional weight loss and

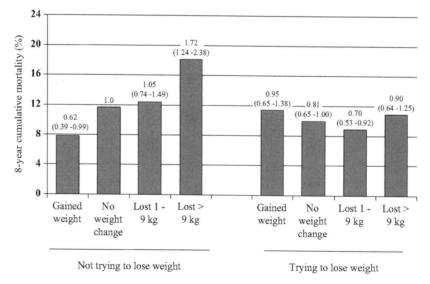

Figure 4 Eight-year cumulative mortality rates and hazard rates according to amount of intentional and unintentional weight loss. *Source*: Adapted from Ref. 85.

CVD-related mortality. This study served as a reminder of the diversity of intentional weight loss and the association of this diversity with health outcomes.

Other observational studies have been less encouraging about the benefits of intentional weight loss on mortality. A study of about 26,000 women aged 55 to 69 years in the Iowa Women's Health Study found no association between intentional weight loss and mortality (88). Similarly, a cohort study of adults aged 65 years and older found no association of weight loss (89) with mortality.

One observational study even makes a case that intentional weight loss increases mortality risk (90). In an 18-year follow-up of the Finnish Twin Study, persons reporting intentional weight loss over a six-year period had an 87% greater risk of all-cause mortality than persons with stable weight who were not trying to lose weight. Weight gain was associated with a 58% increased mortality rate. Lowest mortality rates were observed in persons who either had stable weight without trying to lose weight or persons who reported trying to lose weight but had no weight change. Excess mortality was somewhat greater among persons who reported trying to lose weight principally by dieting than among those who used exercise. On the whole, the study by Sorensen had stronger methods than previous observational studies, as all body weights were measured (as opposed to self-report) and assessment of intentionality was assessed at baseline (as opposed to retrospectively). The study also had thorough assessment of comorbid conditions and found no confounding or effect modification. The study could not explain why intentional weight loss was associated with excess mortality, but the authors speculated that the loss of fat-free mass associated with weight loss may be a key factor.

No randomized controlled trials have been adequately powered to examine the association of weight loss with mortality. However, at least two nonrandomized intervention studies have conducted extended follow-ups of individuals who had undergone weight loss interventions. A 12-year follow-up of the Malmo Prevention Study observed a 50% reduced mortality due to ischemic heart disease and all-causes, effectively negating the excess mortality risk associated with IGT (91). However, the control group had lower blood pressure values at baseline by about 6 mmHg, making it difficult to distinguish the effects of the intervention from an underlying variation in risk factor status.

In the SOS Study, 2010 bariatric surgery patients were compared with 2037 control subjects over a 10-year period (60,61). Average age of the participants was 46 years at baseline and average BMI was 42. The study population ranged in age from 37 to 60 years at baseline (average 46 years for intervention, 47 years for control) and had minimum BMIs of 34 for men and 37 for women. Average weight loss after 10 years was 32% for gastric

bypass, 26% for vertical-banded gastroplasty, and 20% for banding. Surgery patients had a 27% reduced mortality risk (relative risk = 0.73, 95% CI, 0.56–0.95). The difference in mortality rate between surgery and control patients appeared to be driven by the lower number of deaths due to myocardial infarction and cancers. These findings corroborated earlier smaller studies of bariatric surgery that lacked matched control groups.

In a study of bariatric surgery patients in Utah and BMI-matched controls, mortality was 40% lower among 9000 surgery patients than among control patients who were matched for age and BMI (92). The reduced mortality was observed for both CVD and cancer deaths as well as diabetes-related deaths, which were reduced by a dramatic 92%. Of note, however, surgery patients had a significant 58% increased risk of mortality due to "non-disease" causes, including accidents, poisonings, and suicide. Despite the powerful effect sizes observed in the surgery studies, the lack of randomization leaves open some possibility for selection biases, wherein surgery patients somehow have better health status, socioeconomic status, or health behaviors that make them more favorable surgery candidates, also reducing their mortality risk. However, there was no overt evidence of this in the SOS study, wherein baseline prevalences of comorbid conditions were similar between groups.

Finally, one fascinating ecological study explored the impact of population-wide weight change on health trends (Fig. 5A, B). Franco et al. (93) examined trends in energy intake, physical activity, weight loss, and mortality during the extended economic crisis in Cuba following the fall of the Soviet Union. Between 1988 and 1993, average per capita daily energy intake decreased over 1000 calories, a doubling of the proportion of citizens considered physically active doubled, obesity prevalence declined from 14% to 7%, and the prevalence of overweight remained relatively stable. During the same period, mortality due to diabetes, CHD mortality, and all-cause mortality, declined by 51%, 35%, and 18%, respectively, while there was no change in cancer mortality rates. By 2000, the economic crisis had subsided and energy intake and obesity levels returned to precrisis periods. Declines in mortality due to diabetes, CHD, and all-causes ceased declining around 2002.

SUMMARY AND CONCLUSIONS

We draw several conclusions from this summary of the impact of voluntary weight loss on long-term morbidity and mortality:

1. *Strong and consistent evidence relates intentional weight loss to reduced incidence of diabetes among high-risk individuals.* These findings appear strongest

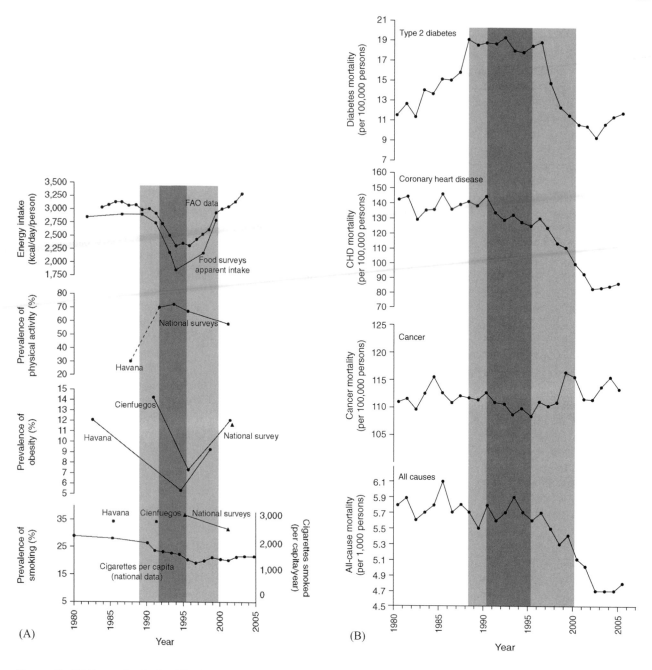

Figure 5 (**A**) Energy intake (kcal/day/person), prevalences (%) of physical activity, obesity, and smoking, and per capita cigarette use (per year) in Cuba, 1980–2005. Shaded zones illustrate period of economic crisis (1989–2000), including the most severe years of the crisis (1991–1995). (**B**) Incidence of mortality due to diabetes, coronary heart disease, cancer, and all-causes in Cuba, 1980–2005. Shaded zones illustrate period of economic crisis (1989–2000), including the most severe years of the crisis (1991–1995). *Source:* Adapted from Ref. 93.

for obese persons with IGT, among whom multidisciplinary lifestyle intervention that achieves modest weight loss can reduce incidence by 40% to 60%. These benefits have made lifestyle intervention a first-line intervention for persons at risk of diabetes. Key remaining questions include whether similar benefits also exist for the broader segment of the population at slightly lower risk, whether less intensive, community-based approaches will be similarly effective, and whether the interventions will have sustained effects on diabetes beyond the life of the study.

2. *Intentional weight loss has been consistently associated with reduced incidence of hypertension and improved control of blood pressure.* The magnitude of effect on hypertension-related outcomes is weaker than the effects on diabetes risk and may be outweighed by pharmacological interventions. Nevertheless, modest weight loss remains a key aspect of hypertension prevention and management.

3. *Weight loss may reduce disability and improve mobility and functioning in daily living among older populations.* However, this evidence has been limited to selected populations such as older persons with arthritis. Furthermore, these benefits may be offset somewhat by an increased fracture risk in frail or osteopenic or osteoporotic older adults. More research on the impact of weight loss on disability in other segments of the older and middle-aged population is needed. Notably, an equal or stronger body of literature supports the effectiveness of exercise to reduce disability irrespective of weight loss.

4. *Increasing evidence suggests that intentional weight loss reduces overall mortality and possibly CVD incidence among persons of high risk.* However, this evidence base is limited to studies of weight loss surgeries and a few observational studies of intentional weight loss. Each of these types of studies has caveats that prevent translation directly into public health policy. Specifically, the proportion of the population that is eligible and appropriate for weight loss surgery remains unclear. Observational studies of weight loss are limited because they do not actually test the impact of interventions per se. On the whole, these studies do, however, suggest that intentional weight loss is not harmful and that previous associations of weight loss with increased mortality appear to be explained by confounding of health status and the lack of assessment of weight loss intent.

Two fundamental dilemmas remain in the application of weight loss into effective public health policy. First, the relative value of a high-risk strategy versus population strategy to weight loss in the population remains unresolved. A high-risk strategy would target people at high risk for conditions wherein clear established intervention efficacy exists. For example, health systems and communities would attempt to identify overweight people with IGT and refer them to intensive weight loss programs conducted by trained personnel. A population strategy would attempt to reduce weight of the population more broadly through health promotion approaches, health policies affecting food availability, and environmental changes to influence physical activity and dietary patterns. The high-risk strategy has the advantage of being more evidence based whereas the population strategy may be more sustainable and perhaps more likely to influence trends in disease of the population over the long term. The choice between these strategies will ultimately depend on future research to examine the long-term effects of weight loss on CVD, quality of life, and disability, new approaches to efficiently target high-risk populations, and economic studies to assist in the prioritization of effective interventions.

REFERENCES

1. Wang Y, Beydoun MA. The obesity epidemic in the United States—gender, age, socioeconomic, racial/ethnic, and geographic characteristics: a systematic review and meta-regression analysis. Epidemiol Rev 2007; 29:6–28.

2. Flegal KM, Carroll MD, Ogden CL, et al. Prevalence and trends in obesity among US adults, 1999–2000. JAMA 2002; 288(14):1723–1727.

3. Ogden CL, Carroll MD, Curtin LR, et al. Prevalence of overweight and obesity in the United States, 1999–2004. JAMA 2006; 295(13):1549–1555.

4. Sturm R. Increases in clinically severe obesity in the United States, 1986–2000. Arch Intern Med 2003; 163(18):2146–2148.

5. Anandacoomarasamy A, Caterson I, Sambrook P, et al. The impact of obesity on the musculoskeletal system. Int J Obes (Lond) 2008; 32(2):211–222.

6. Must A, Spadano J, Coakley EH, et al. The disease burden associated with overweight and obesity. JAMA 1999; 282(16):1523–1529.

7. Wilson PW, D'Agostino RB, Sullivan L, et al. Overweight and obesity as determinants of cardiovascular risk: the Framingham experience. Arch Intern Med 2002; 162(16):1867–1872.

8. Wilson PW, Meigs JB, Sullivan L, et al. Prediction of incident diabetes mellitus in middle-aged adults: the Framingham Offspring Study. Arch Intern Med 2007; 167(10): 1068–1074.

9. Visscher TL, Seidell JC. The public health impact of obesity. Annu Rev Public Health 2001; 22:355–375.

10. Kasen S, Cohen P, Chen H, et al. Obesity and psychopathology in women: a three decade prospective study. Int J Obes (Lond) 2007 (Epub ahead of print).

11. Alley DE, Chang VW. The changing relationship of obesity and disability, 1988–2004. JAMA 2007; 298(17): 2020–2027.

12. Gregg EW, Guralnik JM. Is disability obesity's price of longevity? JAMA 2007; 298(17):2066–2067.

13. Leveille SG, Wee CC, Iezzoni LI. Trends in obesity and arthritis among baby boomers and their predecessors, 1971–2002. Am J Public Health 2005; 95(9):1607–1613.

14. Gregg EW, Cheng YJ, Narayan KM, et al. The relative contributions of different levels of overweight and obesity to the increased prevalence of diabetes in the United States: 1976–2004. Prev Med 2007; 45(5):348–352.

15. Speiser PW, Rudolf MC, Anhalt H, et al. Childhood obesity. J Clin Endocrinol Metab 2005; 90(3):1871–1887.

16. Olshansky SJ, Passaro DJ, Hershow RC, et al. A potential decline in life expectancy in the United States in the 21st century. N Engl J Med 2005; 352(11):1138–1145.

17. Gregg EW, Cheng YJ, Cadwell BL, et al. Secular trends in cardiovascular disease risk factors according to body mass index in US adults. JAMA 2005; 293(15):1868–1874.

18. Thorpe KE, Florence CS, Howard DH, et al. The rising prevalence of treated disease: effects on private health insurance spending. Health Aff (Millwood) 2005; Suppl Web Exclusives:W5-317–W5-325.

19. Thorpe KE. Factors accounting for the rise in health-care spending in the United States: the role of rising disease prevalence and treatment intensity. Public Health 2006; 120(11):1002–1007.

20. Truesdale KP, Stevens J, Cai J. Nine-year changes in cardiovascular disease risk factors with weight maintenance in the atherosclerosis risk in communities cohort. Am J Epidemiol 2007; 165(8):890–900.

21. Serdula MK, Mokdad AH, Williamson DF, et al. Prevalence of attempting weight loss and strategies for controlling weight. JAMA 1999; 282(14):1353–1358.

22. Weiss EC, Galuska DA, Kettel Khan L, et al. Weight-control practices among U.S. adults 2001–2002. Am J Prev Med 2006; 31:18–24.

23. Dwyer JT, Allison DB, Coates PM. Dietary supplements in weight reduction. J Am Diet Assoc 2005; 105(5 suppl 1): S80–S86.

24. Avenell A, Broom J, Brown TJ, et al. Systematic review of the long-term effects and economic consequences of treatments for obesity and implications for health improvement. Health Technol Assess 2004; 8(21):iii–iv, 1–182.

25. Hankey CR, Lean ME, Lowe GD, et al. Effects of moderate weight loss on anginal symptoms and indices of coagulation and fibrinolysis in overweight patients with angina pectoris. Eur J Clin Nutr 2002; 56(10):1039–1045.

26. Poirier P, Giles TD, Bray GA, et al. Obesity and cardiovascular disease: pathophysiology, evaluation, and effect of weight loss: an update of the 1997 American Heart Association Scientific Statement on Obesity and Heart Disease from the Obesity Committee of the Council on Nutrition, Physical Activity, and Metabolism. Circulation 2006; 113(6):898–918.

27. Aucott L, Poobalan A, Smith WC, et al. Effects of weight loss in overweight/obese individuals and long-term hypertension outcomes: a systematic review. Hypertension 2005; 45(6):1035–1041.

28. Norris SL, Zhang X, Avenell A, et al. Long-term effectiveness of lifestyle and behavioral weight loss interventions in adults with type 2 diabetes: a meta-analysis. Am J Med 2004; 117(10):762–774.

29. Esposito K, Pontillo A, Di PC, et al. Effect of weight loss and lifestyle changes on vascular inflammatory markers in obese women: a randomized trial. JAMA 2003; 289(14): 1799–1804.

30. Ryan AS, Nicklas BJ. Reductions in plasma cytokine levels with weight loss improve insulin sensitivity in overweight and obese postmenopausal women. Diabetes Care 2004; 27(7):1699–1705.

31. Bishop NA, Guarente L. Genetic links between diet and lifespan: shared mechanisms from yeast to humans. Nat Rev Genet 2007; 8(11):835–844.

32. Vasselli JR, Weindruch R, Heymsfield SB, et al. Intentional weight loss reduces mortality rate in a rodent model of dietary obesity. Obes Res 2005; 13(4):693–702.

33. Fitzwater SL, Weinsier RL, Wooldridge NH, et al. Evaluation of long-term weight changes after a multidisciplinary weight control program. J Am Diet Assoc 1991; 91(4): 421–426, 429.

34. Shade ED, Ulrich CM, Wener MH, et al. Frequent intentional weight loss is associated with lower natural killer cell cytotoxicity in postmenopausal women: possible long-term immune effects. J Am Diet Assoc 2004; 104(6):903–912.

35. Ensrud KE, Ewing SK, Stone KL, et al. Intentional and unintentional weight loss increase bone loss and hip fracture risk in older women. J Am Geriatr Soc 2003; 51(12):1740–1747.

36. Ensrud KE, Fullman RL, Barrett-Connor E, et al. Voluntary weight reduction in older men increases hip bone loss: the osteoporotic fractures in men study. J Clin Endocrinol Metab 2005; 90(4):1998–2004.

37. Ryan AS, Nicklas BJ, Dennis KE. Aerobic exercise maintains regional bone mineral density during weight loss in postmenopausal women. J Appl Physiol 1998; 84(4): 1305–1310.

38. Syngal S, Coakley EH, Willett WC, et al. Long-term weight patterns and risk for cholecystectomy in women. Ann Intern Med 1999; 130(6):471–477.

39. Gregg EW, Williamson DF. The relationship of intentional weight loss to disease incidence and mortality. In: Wadden TA, Stunkard RJ, eds. Handbook of Obesity Treatment. New York, NY: Guilford Press.

40. No author listed. The effects of nonpharmacologic interventions on blood pressure of persons with high normal levels. Results of the Trials of Hypertension Prevention, Phase I. JAMA 1992; 267(9):1213–1220.

41. The Trials of Hypertension Prevention Collaborative Research Group. Effects of weight loss and sodium reduction intervention on blood pressure and hypertension incidence in overweight people with high-normal blood pressure. The Trials of Hypertension Prevention, phase II. Arch Intern Med 1997; 157(6):657–667.

42. Stevens VJ, Obarzanek E, Cook NR, et al. Long-term weight loss and changes in blood pressure: results of the Trials of Hypertension Prevention, phase II. Ann Intern Med 2001; 134(1):1–11.

43. Whelton PK, Appel LJ, Espeland MA, et al. Sodium reduction and weight loss in the treatment of hypertension in older persons: a randomized controlled trial of nonpharmacologic interventions in the elderly (TONE). TONE Collaborative Research Group. JAMA 1998; 279(11): 839–846.

44. Elmer PJ, Obarzanek E, Vollmer WM, et al. Effects of comprehensive lifestyle modification on diet, weight, physical fitness, and blood pressure control: 18-month results of a randomized trial. Ann Intern Med 2006; 144(7): 485–495.

45. Knowler WC, Barrett-Connor E, Fowler SE, et al. Reduction in the incidence of type 2 diabetes with lifestyle intervention or metformin. N Engl J Med 2002; 346(6):393–403.

46. Kosaka K, Noda M, Kuzuya T. Prevention of type 2 diabetes by lifestyle intervention: a Japanese trial in IGT males. Diabetes Res Clin Pract 2005; 67(2):152–162.

47. Lindstrom J, Ilanne-Parikka P, Peltonen M, et al. Sustained reduction in the incidence of type 2 diabetes by lifestyle intervention: follow-up of the Finnish Diabetes Prevention Study. Lancet 2006; 368(9548):1673–1679.

48. Pan XR, Li GW, Hu YH, et al. Effects of diet and exercise in preventing NIDDM in people with impaired glucose tolerance. The Da Qing IGT and Diabetes Study. Diabetes Care 1997; 20(4):537–544.

49. Ramachandran A, Snehalatha C, Mary S, et al. The Indian Diabetes Prevention Programme shows that lifestyle modification and metformin prevent type 2 diabetes in Asian Indian subjects with impaired glucose tolerance (IDPP-1). Diabetologia 2006; 49(2):289–297.

50. Tuomilehto J, Lindstrom J, Eriksson JG, et al. Prevention of type 2 diabetes mellitus by changes in lifestyle among subjects with impaired glucose tolerance. N Engl J Med 2001; 344(18):1343–1350.

51. Li G, Hu Y, Yang W, et al. Effects of insulin resistance and insulin secretion on the efficacy of interventions to retard development of type 2 diabetes mellitus: the DA Qing IGT and Diabetes Study. Diabetes Res Clin Pract 2002; 58(3):193–200.

52. Eriksson KF, Lindgarde F. Prevention of type 2 (non-insulin-dependent) diabetes mellitus by diet and physical exercise. The 6-year Malmo feasibility study. Diabetologia 1991; 34(12):891–898.

53. Eriksson KF, Lindgarde F. No excess 12-year mortality in men with impaired glucose tolerance who participated in the Malmo Preventive Trial with diet and exercise. Diabetologia 1998; 41(9):1010–1016.

54. Kitabchi AE, Temprosa M, Knowler WC, et al. Role of insulin secretion and sensitivity in the evolution of type 2 diabetes in the diabetes prevention program: effects of lifestyle intervention and metformin. Diabetes 2005; 54(8):2404–2414.

55. Gillies CL, Abrams KR, Lambert PC, et al. Pharmacological and lifestyle interventions to prevent or delay type 2 diabetes in people with impaired glucose tolerance: systematic review and meta-analysis. BMJ 2007; 334 (7588):299.

56. Liao D, Asberry PJ, Shofer JB, et al. Improvement of BMI, body composition, and body fat distribution with lifestyle modification in Japanese Americans with impaired glucose tolerance. Diabetes Care 2002; 25(9):1504–1510.

57. Lindstrom J, Eriksson JG, Valle TT, et al. Prevention of diabetes mellitus in subjects with impaired glucose tolerance in the Finnish Diabetes Prevention Study: results from a randomized clinical trial. J Am Soc Nephrol 2003; 14(7 suppl 2):S108–S113.

58. Hamman RF, Wing RR, Edelstein SL, et al. Effect of weight loss with lifestyle intervention on risk of diabetes. Diabetes Care 2006; 29(9):2102–2107.

59. Hu FB, van Dam RM, Liu S. Diet and risk of Type II diabetes: the role of types of fat and carbohydrate. Diabetologia 2001; 44(7):805–817.

60. Sjostrom L, Lindroos AK, Peltonen M, et al. Lifestyle, diabetes, and cardiovascular risk factors 10 years after bariatric surgery. N Engl J Med 2004; 351(26):2683–2693.

61. Sjostrom L, Narbro K, Sjostrom CD, et al. Effects of bariatric surgery on mortality in Swedish obese subjects. N Engl J Med 2007; 357(8):741–752.

62. Satterfield DW, Volansky M, Caspersen CJ, et al. Community-based lifestyle interventions to prevent type 2 diabetes. Diabetes Care 2003; 26(9):2643–2652.

63. Davey SG, Bracha Y, Svendsen KH, et al. Incidence of type 2 diabetes in the randomized multiple risk factor intervention trial. Ann Intern Med 2005; 142(5):313–322.

64. Ornish D. Can lifestyle changes reverse coronary heart disease? World Rev Nutr Diet 1993; 72:38–48.

65. Ornish D, Scherwitz LW, Billings JH, et al. Intensive lifestyle changes for reversal of coronary heart disease. JAMA 1998; 280(23):2001–2007.

66. Haskell WL, Alderman EL, Fair JM, et al. Effects of intensive multiple risk factor reduction on coronary atherosclerosis and clinical cardiac events in men and women with coronary artery disease. The Stanford Coronary Risk Intervention Project (SCRIP). Circulation 1994; 89(3):975–990.

67. Eilat-Adar S, Eldar M, Goldbourt U. Association of intentional changes in body weight with coronary heart disease event rates in overweight subjects who have an additional coronary risk factor. Am J Epidemiol 2005; 161(4):352–358.

68. Pi-Sunyer X, Blackburn G, Brancati FL, et al. Reduction in weight and cardiovascular disease risk factors in individuals with type 2 diabetes: one-year results of the look AHEAD trial. Diabetes Care 2007; 30(6):1374–1383.

69. Al SS, Ottenbacher KJ, Markides KS, et al. The effect of obesity on disability vs. mortality in older Americans. Arch Intern Med 2007; 167(8):774–780.

70. Alley D, Chang VW. Obesity's changing impact on disability: 1988–2004. JAMA 2007; 298(17):2020–2027.

71. Boult C, Altmann M, Gilbertson D, et al. Decreasing disability in the 21st century: the future effects of controlling six fatal and nonfatal conditions. Am J Public Health 1996; 86(10):1388–1393.

72. Launer LJ, Harris T, Rumpel C, et al. Body mass index, weight change, and risk of mobility disability in middle-aged and older women. The epidemiologic follow-up study of NHANES I. JAMA 1994; 271(14):1093–1098.

73. Lee JS, Kritchevsky SB, Tylavsky F et al. Weight change, weight change intention, and the incidence of mobility limitation in well-functioning community-dwelling older adults. J Gerontol A Biol Sci Med Sci 2005; 60(8):1007–1012.

74. Ensrud KE, Cauley J, Lipschutz R, et al. Weight change and fractures in older women. Study of Osteoporotic Fractures Research Group. Arch Intern Med 1997; 157(8):857–863.

75. Fine JT, Colditz GA, Coakley EH, et al. A prospective study of weight change and health-related quality of life in women. JAMA 1999; 282(22):2136–2142.

76. Heiat A, Vaccarino V, Krumholz HM. An evidence-based assessment of federal guidelines for overweight and obesity

as they apply to elderly persons. Arch Intern Med 2001; 161(9):1194–1203.

77. Felson DT, Zhang Y, Anthony JM, et al. Weight loss reduces the risk for symptomatic knee osteoarthritis in women. The Framingham Study. Ann Intern Med 1992; 116(7):535–539.

78. Messier SP, Loeser RF, Miller GD, et al. Exercise and dietary weight loss in overweight and obese older adults with knee osteoarthritis: the Arthritis, Diet, and Activity Promotion Trial. Arthritis Rheum 2004; 50(5): 1501–1510.

79. Williamson DF. Intentional weight loss: patterns in the general population and its association with morbidity and mortality. Int J Obes Relat Metab Disord 1997; 21 (suppl 1):S14–S19.

80. Williamson DF. Weight loss and mortality in persons with type-2 diabetes mellitus: a review of the epidemiological evidence. Exp Clin Endocrinol Diabetes 1998; 106(suppl 2): 14–21.

81. Allison DB, Zhu SK, Plankey M, et al. Differential associations of body mass index and adiposity with all-cause mortality among men in the first and second National Health and Nutrition Examination Surveys (NHANES I and NHANES II) follow-up studies. Int J Obes Relat Metab Disord 2002; 26(3):410–416.

82. Williamson DF, Pamuk E, Thun M, et al. Prospective study of intentional weight loss and mortality in never-smoking overweight US white women aged 40–64 years. Am J Epidemiol 1995; 141(12):1128–1141.

83. Williamson DF, Pamuk E, Thun M, et al. Prospective study of intentional weight loss and mortality in overweight white men aged 40–64 years. Am J Epidemiol 1999; 149(6):491–503.

84. Williamson DF, Thompson TJ, Thun M, et al. Intentional weight loss and mortality among overweight individuals with diabetes. Diabetes Care 2000; 23(10):1499–1504.

85. Gregg EW, Gerzoff RB, Thompson TJ, et al. Intentional weight loss and death in overweight and obese U.S. adults 35 years of age and older. Ann Intern Med 2003; 138(5): 383–389.

86. Gregg EW, Gerzoff RB, Thompson TJ, et al. Trying to lose weight, losing weight, and 9-year mortality in overweight U.S. adults with diabetes. Diabetes Care 2004; 27(3): 657–662.

87. Wannamethee SG, Shaper AG, Lennon L. Reasons for intentional weight loss, unintentional weight loss, and mortality in older men. Arch Intern Med 2005; 165(9): 1035–1040.

88. French SA, Folsom AR, Jeffery RW, et al. Prospective study of intentionality of weight loss and mortality in older women: the Iowa Women's Health Study. Am J Epidemiol 1999; 149(6):504–514.

89. Diehr P, Bild DE, Harris TB, et al. Body mass index and mortality in nonsmoking older adults: the Cardiovascular Health Study. Am J Public Health 1998; 88(4):623–629.

90. Sorensen TI, Rissanen A, Korkeila M, et al. Intention to lose weight, weight changes, and 18-y mortality in overweight individuals without co-morbidities. PLoS Med 2005; 2(6):e171.

91. Eriksson KF, Lindgarde F. Prevention of type 2 (non-insulin-dependent) diabetes mellitus by diet and physical exercise. The 6-year Malmo feasibility study. Diabetologia 1991; 34(12):891–898.

92. Adams TD, Gress RE, Smith SC, et al. Long-term mortality after gastric bypass surgery. N Engl J Med 2007; 357(8): 753–761.

93. Franco M, Ordunez P, Caballero B et al. Impact of energy intake, physical activity, and population-wide weight loss on cardiovascular disease and diabetes mortality in Cuba, 1980–2005. Am J Epidemiol 2007; 166(12): 1374–1380.

7

Weight Cycling as an Instance of False Hope

JANET POLIVY
Department of Psychology, University of Toronto at Mississauga, Mississauga, Ontario, Canada

C. PETER HERMAN
Department of Psychology, University of Toronto, Toronto, Ontario, Canada

INTRODUCTION

The research literature documents various medical and psychological consequences of weight cycling. In the present chapter, we will attempt to identify why people engage in "yo-yo dieting" with its repeated cycles of weight loss and regain (i.e., weight cycling), and in particular, why they keep trying to lose weight despite previous repeated failures. This pattern of failure followed by renewed effort is reminiscent of the false-hope syndrome that appears to characterize many self-change efforts. We will explore the role of false hope of self-change in the phenomenon of repeated weight cycling.

THE FALSE-HOPE MODEL OF SELF-CHANGE

Most people occasionally make resolutions to change themselves for the better; many do so every New Year's Eve (1). Whether the resolutions involve trying to lose weight, quit smoking, or spend less money, a large proportion of them end in failure (1,2). Despite their often lengthy histories of failed attempts at self-change, individuals nevertheless persist in making new resolutions. Each fresh attempt begins with renewed hope of quick,

easy, and extremely rewarding success, but all too frequently the outcome is failure accompanied by feelings of discouragement and self-denigration. Polivy and Herman (3) have named this cycle of failure and renewed hope the "false-hope syndrome" (Fig. 1).

Resolutions to lose weight are among the most prevalent self-change efforts (3). That is, many individuals resolve to lose weight, and the same individuals tend to renew their resolutions repeatedly. In many ways, weight-loss resolutions epitomize the false-hope syndrome characterizing self-change efforts. People have high hopes that they will succeed at losing weight, and beyond the success of weight loss itself there lies the prospect that weight loss will improve various aspects of their lives. People do tend to succeed in the early stages of weight-loss attempts, and so most dieters have at least some early success to spur them on. When weight loss slows or stops, however, people tend to become vulnerable to elements that interfere with further weight loss. Many succumb to temptations, overeat, and give up on the current diet or weight-loss program. The weight-loss attempt is judged to have failed. Over time, however, most people experience a renewed desire to lose weight, and begin a new weight-loss program or effort. This subsequent effort usually follows the same pattern (initial small success, ultimate

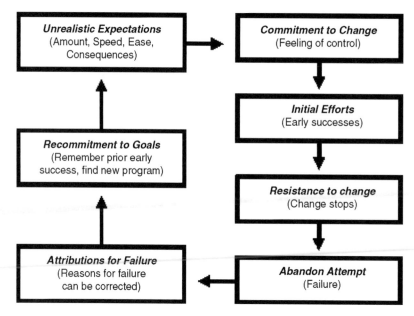

Figure 1 The false-hope model.

failure, and the regain of whatever weight was lost) (3–5). These repeated dieting attempts then eventuate in cycles of weight loss and regain, or what is called yo-yo dieting, in which the individual loses weight (sometimes a substantial amount of weight) only to regain the lost weight, often regaining more weight than was lost. This cycle often occurs in a relatively short period of time. In this chapter, we will explore such weight cycling, and discuss how the false-hope syndrome contributes to both the repeated failures and to the renewed efforts that usually produce further failures.

Contributions of Unrealistic Expectations to Self-Change Failure

The false-hope cycle begins with individuals setting unrealistic goals for themselves as they approach a difficult self-change task such as weight-loss dieting. The goals for change are often based for the most part on a set of self-change expectations that are themselves highly unrealistic. We have identified four kinds of unrealistic expectations that frequently characterize self-change attempts; and because they are so unrealistic, these expectations almost inevitably lead to failure. These unrealistic expectations pertain to the amount, speed, and ease of the self-change attempt, as well as the expected rewards attendant on success (3–5). For example, individuals embarking on a weight-loss diet often believe that they will lose more weight than is realistically feasible, that they will lose the weight more rapidly and more easily than is likely, and

that when they succeed at losing weight, their lives will improve dramatically in many or all respects. Given these unrealistically high expectations, failure is more likely than is success (3–5) if only because success is defined in terms of the benchmarks set by the expectations, which themselves are unrealistic.

The typical dieter provides a good illustration of the negative effects of these inflated expectancies. A young woman who is dissatisfied with her weight (and her life) sees an advertisement for a new diet program that promises she will lose 25 lb in four weeks, with little or no effort on her part, and that many aspects of her life will improve as and after she loses the weight. This hypothetical advertised diet is typical of how self-change programs promise everything the prospective self-changer wants to hear, raising her expectations to an unrealistic level. Still, is there not an advantage to embarking on an ambitious program? Do we not accomplish more if our reach exceeds our grasp? Are these high expectations not motivating? What exactly is the problem with such elevated expectations?

We propose that the expectations themselves make success less attainable. For one thing, unrealistic expectations increase the probability of failure by making smaller successes seem inadequate. Thus, the dieter who is promised that she will lose 25 lb in four weeks is disappointed if she loses "only" 3 lb a week, because that means that in four weeks she has lost a mere 12 lb, not the 25 that she was promised. She may therefore abandon her diet, feeling that it is "not working." Thus, inflated expectations may cause dieters who are actually succeeding at losing weight to reject the successful effort as "not successful enough" (3). In fact, weight-loss programs do find that clients losing significant amounts of weight still report themselves as disappointed that the weight loss was not greater (6). If inflated expectations disappoint those who are experiencing some reasonable degree of success, how disheartened will those be who are not even reaching a minimal level of weight loss?

Why would people believe these inflated promises about weight loss, especially in light of the hard-won experience of their own previous failed attempts to diet? Most importantly, these promises are exactly what people want to hear or already believe. Their prior experience notwithstanding, people believe that weight is easy to change (7). (Below we will examine this disjunction between people's beliefs and their own experiences.) Moreover, people want to lose weight—indeed, they are often desperate to lose weight—and they want to believe that they can do so easily and quickly, that they can lose huge amounts of excess poundage, and that their wildest dreams will be fulfilled if they do succeed. The attractiveness of these promises makes them more believable (7), for it is a basic feature of human nature to believe what we want to believe. The unrealistic promises made by unscrupulous weight-loss programs are thus designed to pander to people's desires. From a psychological standpoint, these promises of success are also reinforcing in and of themselves. If change is thought to be both achievable and likely to generate sizeable benefits, then committing to such a change brings these desirable outcomes under one's own control, which is in itself reinforcing (4). Believing that we have the power to accomplish our goals makes us feel good about ourselves, and optimistic.

Attributions for Previous Failures

Self-change efforts are generally difficult, the enthusiastic promises of many programs notwithstanding. When people abandon these efforts, they may recognize, at least temporarily, the strenuous effort required to achieve the desired goal, and they may acknowledge that they were inadequate to the task (8). But over time, people appear to change how they view their previous (failed) weight-loss attempt(s). Instead of continuing to blame their lack of ability or willpower to effect and maintain the change, and/or the inadequate programs that do not produce lasting weight loss, and/or the inherent difficulty of the task, as people move further away from an earlier failure they begin to listen again to the siren call of weight-loss as the means to solve all of their problems. As the desire to lose weight reawakens, people begin to reattribute their previous failures away from unchangeable features of the endeavor such

as its inherent difficulty or their own limited willpower, and instead they explain away their past failures, "concluding that what caused them to fail is something that can be corrected on the next attempt" (3, p. 682). In other words, people reattribute their previous failure away from intrinsic, unalterable aspects of the task to more extrinsic, unstable factors than can be "improved" in a new effort. This time they will really try, or their lives will be more in control and will not interfere with their efforts, or the new program is a better one that will really work. (Whether the rekindled attractiveness of weight loss produces the reattribution or whether the reattribution makes it possible to reconsider the lures of weight loss is a research question that has not yet been answered. For present purposes, however, it matters little whether reattribution precedes or follows the rekindled desire to lose weight. In either case, the cycle is ready to begin anew.)

Renewed Efforts to Lose Weight

Numerous mechanisms have been proposed to explain the apparently irrational behavior of perseverance at self-change attempts such as dieting despite a prior history of failure (often repeated failures). We have just described the subtle change in attributions for previous failures that allows people to believe that the next attempt may well have a different and more positive outcome. Reattribution is only one of the mechanisms that encourage such perseverance. Expectations of reinforcement, such as the rewards thought to be associated with being thin, and the same elevated expectations of success as in previous efforts provide motivation to try again (9). That is, it is not only the explaining away of past failure that is motivating; the original positive rewards of success retain their allure. Also, the mere commitment to change in and of itself, before any actual change has been accomplished, produces feelings of control and enthusiasm (as well as overconfidence), and is thus reinforcing (3,4,10). This aspect of the process is particularly insidious: simply making a commitment to change makes the individual feel efficacious and even accomplished, and is therefore quite seductive.

In addition, repeated self-change attempts despite failure may be encouraged by a superior memory for the initial success of the effort rather than for the subsequent failure (3,4). Given that most self-change attempts involve an initial period of success before they ultimately fail, differential recall of this initial success may contribute to self-changers' renewed attempts to change. Because most dieters lose weight early in the diet episode and only later fail at their weight-loss attempt, regaining the lost weight, insofar as the initial success is better remembered and subsequently retrieved more easily, in retrospect it may overshadow the failure outcome, encouraging future diet attempts. And insofar as the anticipated rewards of self-change act as motivators, remembering the quick and easy successes from the earliest stages of previous self-change attempts may allow or even encourage one to maintain unrealistic expectations about how quickly and easily one will be able to change during a new attempt. In fact, our data indicate that the behavior of repeat dieters may be explained at least in part by their tendency to remember the successful aspects of previous dieting attempts better than the unsuccessful aspects (11). Moreover, early success not only influences subsequent memories of the attempt, but also makes people feel better about themselves (than does failing immediately), and also makes people remember having been more successful than they actually were (11). Thus, a sequence that at least begins successfully has less of a negative impact on mood and self-esteem than does one that begins with failure (12). This primacy effect of memory might further contribute to the willingness of failed self-changers to initiate another change attempt.

Repeated Failure

The repeated failures characteristic of the false-hope syndrome reflect the negative effects of overconfidence. In dieters, this overconfidence reflects the belief that they will lose a lot of weight in a short period of time with minimal effort, and that this weight loss will produce substantial benefits in every aspect of their lives (3–5,7,9). Overconfidence is at least partially a product of the inflated promises made by diet programs and devices, but the individual contributes as well. Baumeister et al. (10) noted that when people commit to a specific goal, "their positive illusions or overconfidence should create a tendency to set goals too high for themselves, with the result that their likelihood of eventual failure increases" (p. 142). Positive illusions about the likelihood of succeeding at (12) or of quickly completing tasks (13) abound. False hopes and overconfidence about an outcome desired as strongly as weight loss are thus only to be expected.

When people do not learn that they must modify their expectations and be more realistic about changing, the odds are high that they will continue to fail at these attempts. But as we have indicated, the circumstances surrounding most weight-loss attempts maintain the unrealistic expectations and positive illusions that set the stage for failure. Moreover, resolving to achieve a future goal such as weight loss is much easier than is resisting an immediate reward such as a favorite, fattening food (14,15); as a result, we often encounter scenarios in which commitments to dieting are immediately followed by dietary lapses.

What happens when people fail at their self-change efforts? They appear to blame themselves for lacking sufficient willpower (16) and feel disappointed and describe themselves as failures and as not meeting their expectations (8,9). It is worth noting at this point that self-blame is not the only possible outcome; one could just as easily blame the difficulty of the goal or the inadequacies of the particular diet strategy that was used. These alternatives are rarely invoked, however. For one thing, dieters are all aware—and if they are not, then the diet promoters will quickly make them aware—of the "numerous" inspirational cases of success that often form a central part of the advertising for the diet program. Secondly, the diet program, by focusing on testimonials endorsing the program, leaves dieters with the impression that the program has been proven to be successful, so if they fail, they are hardly in a position to blame the program; the fault must lie in themselves. Eventually, dieters about to embark on a new diet face a choice: either rededicate themselves to the program that failed before or try a new program. Dieters who choose the former implicitly (and probably even explicitly) acknowledge that the previous failure was due not to the inadequacies of the program but to their own inadequacies (especially insufficient effort). The new attempt will feature more dedication, more effort, and more perseverance. This strategy is particularly ill-advised, inasmuch as it not only places all the blame on the self, but sets things up so that future success depends on dieters displaying a degree of effort and commitment that they have not shown in the past and are therefore unlikely to be able to summon up in the future. It represents a profound misunderstanding of the consistency of behavior and personality over time and occasions.

Deciding instead to lay the blame for prior failure on the program rather than on the self has obvious advantages. It does not require a personality transformation whereby a weakling suddenly becomes strong; in that respect, it is more realistic. The difficulty arises, though, when the individual is required to regard as inadequate what was initially presented as a proven weight-loss technique. What about those testimonials and the case histories brimming with success? The dieter who is about to switch diet programs is required to redirect attention away from those positive (if bogus) features of the old diet and to focus on the positive (if bogus) features trumpeted by the new diet. Most notably, the new diet is likely to include a brief discussion of why all previous diets are inadequate (the testimonials and case histories attendant upon those old diets notwithstanding). Typically, the new diet involves a newly discovered, quasi-magical nutritional principle of which previous diet-mongers were unaware. The new diet offers hope because it exploits this new principle, which, if adhered to, will make dieting easy, fast, and effective. And so we return to the starting point of the cycle.

To summarize, the false-hope syndrome begins with a decision to change based on unrealistic expectations about how fast, easy, successful, and rewarding the change process will be. The resolution to change is accompanied by positive feelings associated with hope, the sense of being in control of oneself, and the expected rewards of self-change. These positive feelings are reinforced by early successes, because most self-change attempts succeed at least initially; but the long-term vicissitudes of self-change soon make change difficult to maintain and relapse-inducing temptations increasingly difficult to resist. Moreover, as the anticipated successes do not accumulate or reach the unrealistic level anticipated by the changer, disappointment and discouragement set in. Ultimately, the effort is abandoned as unsuccessful, and dieters blame themselves. But as time passes, a new self-change program appears and/or dieters experience a rekindled desire for the perceived benefits of changing. Memories of the previous attempt focus differentially on the early successes and initial good feelings (at the expense of the eventual failure), so the dieters try again, resuming the cycle (3–5).

WEIGHT CYCLING: AN INSTANCE OF FALSE HOPE?

How well does weight cycling or yo-yo dieting fit the model of the false-hope syndrome? We will examine the pattern of weight loss and regain and associated psychological features that characterize weight cycling to determine whether they resemble what has been described as the false-hope syndrome.

Initial Success Followed by Weight Regain

According to the false-hope model, false hope occurs when initial success at self-change is not maintained, so the effort ultimately fails and initial gains are followed by reversion to pre-change levels (3–5). Weight cyclers are people who have succeeded at losing weight (often as much as 10–15% of initial body weight), but who then regained the weight, usually going through this cycle more than once. Thus, all weight cyclers have successfully lost weight, usually more than once, although the number of cycles varies considerably and is not always specified. Weight cycling is generally defined as intentional weight loss of some amount, usually 5 kg or greater (17,18) or at least 5% of initial body weight (19) followed by unintentional weight (re)gain. There is, however, no universally accepted definition of weight cycling (20). What is universal in studies of weight cycling is that initial weight loss (of whatever degree) occurs, but is followed by regain of most or all of the lost weight. This loss-gain cycle

occurs at least once and often three or more times for a given individual. Thus, yo-yo dieters meet the first criterion of the false-hope syndrome: They tried to change (lose weight) and did initially meet with some success, which was then followed by failure (weight regain).

Psychological Reactions to Weight Loss and Regain

According to the false-hope model, the early stage of a self-change effort, when some success is being achieved, is generally a time of improved mood and well-being for the person attempting to change (3–5). In fact, during the initial weight-loss phase of weight cycling, yo-yo dieters exhibit enhanced positive feelings about themselves (21), consistent with the false-hope syndrome. These enhanced pleasant feelings revert to baseline levels when weight is regained (21), just as in the false-hope syndrome when disappointment replaces initial optimism (3). Similarly, moderately obese women engaged in a weight-loss diet showed the pattern of mood effects predicted by the false-hope model; after three months of dieting, their mood had improved; in particular, they were more confident and calmer (22). By eight months, though, their mood had deteriorated, and this deterioration was evident at the two-year follow-up assessment. Moreover, those participants whose motivation to diet at the beginning of the study was higher exhibited larger decreases in mental well-being at the end of the study. Furthermore, compared to successful weight losers who maintain their weight loss for at least one year, dieters who lose weight but regain it within the year report that they had not achieved their weight goals and felt dissatisfied with the weight loss that they did achieve (23).

More generally, although there are some minor inconsistencies in the literature, yo-yo dieters' reactions to the weight-regain phase of weight cycling resemble the psychological effects postulated by the false-hope model. Like the false-hope syndrome, weight cycling results in negative feelings that seem to be directly associated with the self-change effort. Psychological correlates of weight cycling are measured, for the most part, before, during, and following a weight-loss program, so short-term changes may escape observation. Despite this shortcoming of the literature, the overall long-term effects of weight cycling do seem to correspond to what the false-hope model would predict. Weight cyclers report a variety of negative responses, including frustration, shame, and disappointment (24); feelings of perceived deprivation (25); dietary helplessness; pessimism about losing weight (26); feeling less physically healthy (27); binge eating (27,28); covert hostility (29); declines in self-esteem, eating self-efficacy, and life satisfaction

(30,31); and increased body dissatisfaction (31). The consensus is that weight cycling, like the false-hope syndrome, is related to dysphoric feelings—in the case of weight cycling, those feelings focus on eating, dieting, and the body—and more general dissatisfaction, but is not usually associated with diagnosable psychopathology (24,27,32,33). There is some evidence that the actual extent of weight cycling is less closely related to these negative indices of psychological functioning than is one's self-perception as a weight cycler, which is only partially correlated with one's history of cycling (31). That is, seeing oneself as a weight cycler is a stronger predictor of adverse psychological states than are some objective measures of weight cycling. We may conclude, then, that as with other instances of the false-hope syndrome, cycles of successful and then failed dieting can elevate the risk for dysphoria and psychological problems but do not produce actual psychological pathology.

Repeated Weight Loss and Regain— Prevalence of Weight Cycling

The false-hope syndrome is posited to occur in those individuals who attempt difficult changes, achieve some initial success but ultimately fail in their attempt, and some time later try again (3–5). Attempted weight loss has frequently been cited as an example of the sort of self-change effort likely to entail false hope (3–5,9). How prevalent, then, is this sort of cycling between successful weight loss and failure/weight regain? The two or three dozen studies that focus on weight cycling examine the physical and/or psychological effects of repeated fluctuations, but only one specifically focused on the prevalence of these cycles of weight loss and regain. Lahti-Koski and colleagues (18) randomly sampled Finnish adults in order to determine the prevalence of weight cycling in this population. Among 3320 men and 3540 women aged 25 to 64 years, 66% of the men and 56% of the women were nonobese nondieters, whose weight had not changed in 10 years. Mild weight cycling was defined as intentionally losing and regaining 5 kg or more one or two times; 11% of the men and 19% of the women met this criterion and were identified as mild cyclers. The criterion for severe weight cycling was intentionally losing and regaining 5 kg or more on three or more occasions; 7% of men and 10% of women were classified as severe cyclers.

The Finnish population studied by Lahti-Koski and colleagues (18) may not be fully representative of Western weight cyclers, especially because the proportion of the population classified as normal weight is so much higher than is found in North America, where overweight and obesity have become increasingly prevalent (19,34) and

where we would expect more weight-loss motivation. Although we were unable to find any other studies directed at determining the prevalence of weight cycling in adults, several of the studies looking at other aspects of weight cycling provide data indicating what percentage of participants were weight cyclers. For example, a large-scale study (8) tracking weight changes over two years in 18,000 middle-aged men and women found that fewer than 60% of them maintained a stable weight over this time. Carmody and colleagues (26,29) followed healthy adults participating in the RENO Diet-Heart Study (RDHS) over several years. Of 385 adults studied initially (26), 41.55% were self-reported weight cyclers; among the obese participants, the proportions were much higher (65% of obese women and 55% of obese men reported cycling, whereas only 38% of nonobese women and 15% of nonobese men reported these weight changes). Looking at their actual weights after five years of study, 48.05% did not maintain their weights within 2.4 kg (5 lb) of their baseline weight on every six-month weigh-in over the five years. Only 18.96% of participants truly maintained their weights this consistently for five years. A later study of 331 of these adults (29) found that 37.16% were self-reported weight cyclers; it is unclear whether the degree of cycling declined a bit over time, or the missing participants in the later study were more likely to have been weight cyclers. Similar rates of self-reported cycling were reported by Foreyt et al. (30), who studied 475 volunteers, of whom 43.16% were self-described as yo-yo dieters.

Simkin-Silverman et al. (33) also divided their 429 female participants from the Healthy Woman Study into normal ($n = 232$) and overweight ($n = 197$) groups; 38% of normals and 75% of the obese women reported at least one weight cycle, with 14.66% of the normals and 52.80% of the obese reporting two or more cycles. Venditti et al. (27) also found that approximately 75% of their obese female participants reported weight cycling.

Field et al. (35) mailed questionnaires asking about weight to over 46,000 female nurses in 1989, 1991, 1993, and 1995. During the four years of the study, 78.2% of the women intentionally lost at least 2 to 4 kg (5–10 lb) one or more times; 16.5% did this only once, 41% did this twice or more. In addition, approximately 19% lost up to 4.5 kg (10 lb) three or more times plus 1.5% lost 9 kg (20 lb) or more three or more times, and another 5% lost 23 kg (50 lb) once or twice. Thus, even in this very large population, who are themselves involved in health care, over 40% exhibited weight cycling. When groups are not divided by weight into normal versus obese, the percentage of women who exhibit cycles of weight loss and gain seems fairly consistent at about 40%.

One study (19) that did examine the prevalence of large weight gains and losses within a year found fewer weight cyclers among 1200 healthy men and women aged 20 to

45 years than were found in the other studies summarized above, with only 24.3% fluctuating by 5% in one year. These participants were, however, enrolled in a three-year study to prevent weight gain over time and were thus neither a general population nor obese dieters. (On average, the group as a whole did gain a small amount of weight—about 2 kg—over the three-year course of the study.)

It seems, then, that among the general population, whether measured by degree of self-reported weight cycling or weight stability over time, there is consistent evidence that weight cycling occurs with some regularity (and the frequency is similar regardless of the method of measuring it). Females and overweight or obese individuals are more likely to report weight cycling and to exhibit such cycles in prospective studies of weight over time than are males and normal-weight people in general. The false hope associated with weight-loss dieting seems to be widespread.

Weight Regain—Why Success Turns to Failure

The false-hope syndrome reflects the adverse results of self-change attempts that are based on unrealistic, unattainable goals (3–5). Thus, dieters' initial efforts often meet with some success, but inflated expectations about how much (and how quickly, and how easily) weight will be lost make even successful weight losses seem disappointingly small (6). When the goal is not met, even what a dispassionate observer might regard as successful weight-loss efforts may be abandoned. There is no mention in the weight-cycling literature of whether yo-yo dieters achieve their initial weight loss goals when they lose weight and then regain the lost weight. Even studies of "successful dieters" (36) define their populations by the degree of weight lost (e.g., 15% of initial weight) and length of time the loss is maintained (e.g., 1 year), rather than by whether or not the dieter has reached the goal weight. We do know, however, from studies such as that by Foster et al. (6), that a loss as great as 15 kg may be seen as a "disappointed weight" by obese dieters, suggesting that the degree of "success" involved in the initial weight loss by yo-yo dieters may not represent true success at reaching one's personal weight goal. Thus, part of the problem may be that the goals set by weight cyclers are unrealistically ambitious, as is posited by the false-hope model. When weight loss slows or stops, and continued losses become difficult or impossible to achieve, the dieter expecting a larger loss is likely to become discouraged (3,4,9). Indeed, research on those who have lost weight and then either maintained the loss or regained the weight (37) indicates that those who regained their lost weight reported that they had failed

to reach their weight-loss goals and felt dissatisfied with the amount of weight they had managed to lose. Moreover, of obese patients seeking weight-loss treatment, more than half discontinue their weight-loss attempt in less than one year (38). Those who left the weight-loss program had initially reported lower goal weights and had higher expected weight losses. In fact, the risk of dropping out of treatment at 12 months was directly related to degree of expected one-year BMI decrease. Many weight cyclers may therefore be people who did not believe that they had succeeded at losing enough weight and gave up their efforts because they were discouraged by their perceived failure.

In addition, continued efforts to lose weight require resisting the temptations of attractive, fattening foods, temptations that increase in intensity as weight loss proceeds. Resisting temptation requires self-control, which takes energy—energy that may be a finite resource (39). The difficulty of resisting temptations may be due at least in part to the fact that both temptations and actual dietary lapses are associated with feeling sad, deprived, stressed, and out of control (40), feelings that are probably draining or fatiguing.

The lure of temptations reminds us that, in fact, weight loss is really only one of a set of conflicting goals; that is, although on the one hand dieters want to lose weight, on the other hand, they also want to eat the high-calorie foods that they enjoy, and eat larger quantities of all of their preferred foods (41). Moreover, the perception that one has lost or been denied something increases desire more than does a perceived gain (42), making temptations that must be resisted more attractive than goals that are slowly being attained. Therefore, resisting attractive foods becomes more difficult because the tempting foods become more desirable the more they are resisted, whereas losing weight does not increase in attractiveness while one is engaged in attempting to achieve the weight-loss goal.

It seems, then, that the various factors that contribute to failure according to the false-hope model operate for weight cyclers. Elevated expectations that cause weight losers to be dissatisfied with their losses lead to discouragement and disappointment, making the dieter even more depleted in resources/willpower. The inevitable temptations posed by attractive foods that are ubiquitous in our culture then become increasingly difficult to resist, until the diet is overwhelmed and abandoned, and the lost weight is regained. It is clear that weight-loss maintenance and the avoidance of weight regain require continuing vigilance and sacrifice. Because commensurate enhancements in self-image and quality of life do not often immediately accompany weight loss (thus providing the necessary reinforcement for the sacrifices made to achieve the weight loss), sustained weight loss is rare (43).

Factors Contributing to Repeated Attempts/Weight Cycling

Given the difficulties inherent in weight-loss attempts, and the rarity of successfully maintaining losses, one has to wonder why people weight cycle, losing and regaining weight repeatedly. After an episode of weight loss followed by regain, weight cyclers eventually make another attempt, often succeeding temporarily yet again. The false-hope model posits that these sorts of repeated attempts at self-change occur for several reasons. We will examine here the degree to which these reasons for trying anew characterize weight cycling, bearing in mind that the weight-cycling literature does not directly address the parallel with false hope.

According to the false-hope model, the first reason for trying again is that starting a self-change effort feels good (3–5). One study (24) examined weight-cycling women entering a weight-control program. The authors expected these women to report negative feelings; the absence of such negative feelings among weight cyclers was attributed by the authors as a reflection of the positive mood that weight cyclers experience when embarking on a new weight-loss program.

Another factor that contributes to repeated self-change attempts is the tendency to differentially remember previous early successes at changing (3–5). When one experiences success before ultimately failing, information associated with that early success is remembered better than is information associated with the subsequent failure (11). The individual remembers these good feelings and forgets the disappointment and discouragement that followed when failure ultimately set in. There is ample evidence that, as posited by the false-hope syndrome, initial weight loss (i.e., early success at self-change) is associated with increased feelings of well-being, at least early on while weight is still decreasing (21–23,44).

In addition, dieters who did manage to reach their weight-loss goals (mostly through larger initial losses) succeeded at maintaining greater long-term losses than did those who failed to reach their goals (45), although by 30 months there was no relation between psychological well-being and initial degree of weight loss or initial goal level. Moreover, when both self-reported weight cycling and history of weight losses and gains were used to determine the relation of weight cycling to psychological well-being, it was self-reported or perceived weight cycling (rather than history of weight changes) that predicted the presence of psychological problems (31). This suggests that even the memory of cycling may be inflated as compared to the actual history of cycling, further heightening dysphoria. Although there is no clear evidence that weight cyclers actually are displaying disproportionately heightened (i.e., inaccurate) recall for their previous weight

losses, their self-perception as weight cyclers could represent, at least in part, inflated memories of amounts of weight change. Moreover, the pattern of early weight loss leading to elevated mood and more positive feelings about the self that occurs in weight cycling seems to correspond to the sort of early elevations in mood and self-image postulated by the false-hope model.

Finally, the false-hope model postulates that as their desire for the anticipated benefits of the self-change reemerges (some time after the last failure), people find a new program promising them success at changing—this time, for sure—and begin the false-hope cycle again. Some studies of weight cycling (24,32,37,38,46) use patients currently in weight-loss treatment as participants. Weight cyclers who are in weight-loss treatment appear to have found a new program in order to try again.

In summary, although there are limited data on some of the factors postulated to lead to repeated efforts to change, it seems that weight cyclers exhibit many of the posited characteristics normally associated with the false-hope syndrome.

CONCLUSIONS—WEIGHT CYCLING AND FALSE HOPE

Despite the absence of studies directed at testing the propositions of the false-hope model as they might apply to weight cycling, the evidence does suggest that weight cyclers exhibit many if not all of the features of the false-hope syndrome. What does this mean for the average yo-yo dieter?

Weight Cycling as an Instance of False Hope

The false-hope syndrome begins with unrealistic expectations about self-change. Weight cyclers seem often to have been unable either to meet their weight-loss goals or to persist in their diets when these goals are not met. In fact, female dieters experience negative affect when their diet goals appear difficult to attain (47), suggesting that it is important to identify and pursue goals that are personally "achievable."

Despite the positive feelings associated with starting a weight-loss effort (24), and despite early successes in their weight loss endeavors (with their attendant positive self-evaluations and emotions) (21), weight cyclers do not end up feeling any better, especially when the weight is regained (22). One study (48) found that over time "there was no significant association between weight loss and psychological well-being among obese women" (48, p. 181) (mainly because the losses are not maintained, so neither are the positive feelings), and concluded that maintenance of stable weight is more likely to contribute to psychological well-being in women than is weight loss (if weight loss is followed by weight gain). When resistance to change begins and the weight-loss attempt is abandoned as a failure, weight cyclers regain their lost weight and feel even worse about themselves than they felt before they began the attempt (22).

In fact, the process of giving up on the weight-loss attempt is associated with negative feelings about the self. Feeling tempted and lapsing from one's diet are each associated with believing that one is deficient in willpower; giving in to temptation is also associated with feeling sad, and stressed, and less confident in one's ability to resist temptations, maintain a diet, or control one's eating now or in the future (40).

Part of the false-hope syndrome is the tendency to remember the positive aspects of earlier self-change efforts (3–5). Although memory for positive events can serve as a protective factor promoting psychological well-being in some instances (49), in terms of dieting/weight loss, memory for fleeting successes may actually be counter-productive, contributing to repeated futile attempts to change by preserving memories of short-lived success. These memories, even if accurate as far as they go, do not accurately reflect the entire diet (loss-and-gain) experience, and therefore seduce the cycler into an experience that is on balance negative, even if part of it is positive.

For the most part, the effects of the false-hope syndrome consist of psychological discomfort and negative feelings about the self. For weight cyclers, repeated weight-loss attempts not only adversely influence their psychological well-being, but may have physical and health ramifications as well.

Physical Effects of Weight Cycling

Previous discussions of the false-hope syndrome have not mentioned any physical consequences of repeated self-change failures. Yo-yo dieting or weight cycling has been as widely investigated as it has largely because of its presumed medical/physical ramifications; however, the evidence regarding the health risks of weight cycling is mixed. For example, body composition and function, along with corresponding ease of subsequent weight loss are presumed to alter as a result of repeated episodes of dieting-induced weight loss and subsequent weight regain (19,46,50). Weight cycling may have metabolic effects that make subsequent weight loss efforts more difficult (46) and contribute to subsequent obesity (19) (both of which do seem to be associated with weight cycling), but it does not appear to do this by affecting lean body mass (50), and it is not yet clear how weight cycling actually contributes to increased overweight.

Serious health outcomes such as coronary artery disease have been linked to body weight variability in the Framingham population (51), though a selected sample of obese participants (selected for not having weight-related complications) did not exhibit cardiovascular problems in a cross-sectional study (52). Reviews of the literature find mixed data; the National Task Force on the Prevention and Treatment of Obesity (53) noted a correlation between weight cycling and increases in morbidity and mortality, but concluded that this association was not compelling enough to warrant abandoning weight-loss efforts. Muls et al. (54) concluded that despite disagreements between studies, there is evidence that weight cycling is related to excess mortality (not to mention disordered eating, impaired glucose tolerance, and preference for dietary fat). Some recent studies (35,55) conclude that weight/BMI is responsible for any associations noted between weight cycling and such health problems as hypertension and type 2 diabetes. Given that weight cycling appears to increase the risk of overweight/obesity, however, it seems likely that weight cycling may contribute to these problems through its ultimately elevating effect on body weight. Weight cycling thus appears to entail at least some risk, if only from the ratcheting upward of weight that seems to result from cycles of success and failure at weight loss.

What Causes Weight Cycling?

In reviewing the literature on weight cycling, we were unable to find any speculation concerning the causes of weight cycling. As we have mentioned, many studies have investigated the physical or psychological effects of weight cycling, but this research seems to be focused exclusively on effects rather than causes of weight cycling. The false-hope model offers some possible insights into why weight cycling occurs. As we have shown, weight cyclers exhibit most of the characteristics of the false-hope syndrome. Starting a self-change attempt with unrealistically elevated expectations makes eventual failure more likely. Then the combination of reattributing the weight-loss failure to factors that can be changed (such as lack of effort or the specifics of a particular diet program), remembering the initial successful weight loss in preference to the eventual weight regain, and finding a new diet program all lead to further (unsuccessful) attempts to lose weight. Weight cycling thus reflects attempts to change in inappropriate and unrealistic ways. False hope is probably only one route to weight cycling, but at this point, it is the only one proposed. Put differently, weight cycling would appear to be a classic instance of the false-hope syndrome. If it is true that weight cycling has certain adverse consequences, research exploring and bemoaning those adverse consequences may have some value. Rather than focus exclusively on the consequences of weight cycling, however, it might be of benefit if researchers devoted some attention to attempting to learn more about weight cycling's causes. Knowing that weight cycling poses problems for the dieter is probably not enough to dissuade dieters from pursuing their dreams. Exploring the mechanisms that seduce dieters into unrealistic weight-loss efforts that are likely to fail would appear to be a better approach to getting dieters to behave more sensibly.

REFERENCES

1. Norcross JC, Mrykalo MS, Blagys MD. Success predictors, change processes, and self-reported outcomes of New Year's resolvers and nonresolvers. J Clin Psychol 2002; 58:397–405.
2. Prochaska JO, DiClemente CC, Norcross JC. In search for how people change: applications to addictive behaviors. Am Psychol 1992; 47:1102–1114.
3. Polivy J, Herman CP. If at first you don't succeed: false hopes of self-change. Am Psychol 2002; 57:677–689.
4. Polivy J, Herman CP. The false hope syndrome: unfulfilled expectations of self-change. Curr Direcs Psychol Sci 2000; 9:128–131.
5. Polivy J. Why is it so hard to change? False hope of self-change. Can Clin Psychol 2005; 16:8–9.
6. Foster GD, Wadden TA, Vogt RA, et al. What is a reasonable weight loss? Patients' expectations and evaluations of obesity treatment outcomes. J Consult Clin Psychol 1997; 65:79–85.
7. Brownell K. Personal responsibility and control over our bodies: when expectation exceeds reality. Health Psychol 1991; 10:303–310.
8. Polivy J, Herman CP. The effects of resolving to diet on restrained and unrestrained eaters: the "False Hope Syndrome." Int J Eat Disord 1999; 26:434–447.
9. Trottier K, Polivy J, Herman CP. Effects of exposure to unrealistic promises of dieting: are unrealistic expectations of dieting inspirational? Int J Eat Disord 2005; 37:142–149.
10. Baumeister RF, Heatherton TF, Tice DM. When ego threats lead to self-regulation failure: negative consequences of high self-esteem. J Pers Soc Psychol 1993; 64: 141–156.
11. Hargreaves D, Polivy J, Herman CP, et al. False hope: understanding the cycle of repeated, unsuccessful self-change. Manuscript under review, 2007.
12. Taylor SE. Asymmetrical effects of positive and negative events: the mobilization-minimization hypothesis. Psych Bull 1991; 110:67–85.
13. Buehler R, Griffin D, Ross M. Exploring the "planning fallacy": why people underestimate their task completion times. J Pers Soc Psychol 1994; 67:366–381.
14. Loewenstein G, Angner E. Predicting and indulging changing preferences. In: Loewenstein G, Read D, Baumeister R, eds. Time and Decision: Economic and Psychological Perspectives on Intertemporal Choice. New York: Russell Sage Foundation, 2003:351–191.
15. Trope Y, Liberman N. Temporal construal and time-dependent changes in preference. J Pers Soc Psychol 2000; 79:876–889.
16. Heatherton TF, Nichols PA. Personal accounts of successful versus failed attempts at life change. Perspect Soc Psych Bull 1994; 20:664–675.
17. Kroke A, Liese AD, Schulz M, et al. Recent weight changes and weight cycling as predictors of subsequent two year weight change in a middle-aged cohort. Int J Obes Relat Metab Disord 2002; 26:403–409.
18. Lahti-Koski M, Mannisto S, Pietinen P, et al. Prevalence of weight cycling and its relation to health indicators in Finland. Obes Res 2005; 13:333–341.
19. Jeffery R, McGuire M, French S. Prevalence and correlates of large weight gains and losses. Int J Obes Relat Metab Disord 2002; 26:969–972.
20. Blackburn GL, Borrazzo ECL. Weight cycling. JAMA 1995; 273:998.
21. Wilson GT. The controversy over dieting. In: Fairburn CG, Brownell KD, eds. Eating Disorders and Obesity: A Comprehensive Handbook. New York: Guilford Press, 2002: 93–97.
22. Karlsson J, Hallgren P, Kral J, et al. Predictors and effects of long-term dieting on mental well-being and weight loss in obese women. Appetite 1994; 23:15–26.
23. Byrne S, Cooper Z, Fairburn CC. Weight maintenance and relapse in obesity: a qualitative study. Int J Obes Relat Metab Disord 2003; 27:955–962.
24. Bartlett SJ, Wadden TA, Vogt RA. Psychosocial consequences of weight cycling. J Consult Clin Psychol 1996; 64:587–592.
25. Timmerman GM, Gregg EK. Dieting, perceived deprivation, and preoccupation with food. West J Nurs Res 2003; 25:405–418.
26. Carmody TP, Brunner RL, St Jeor ST. Dietary helplessness and disinhibition in weight cyclers and maintainers. Int J Eat Disord 1995; 18:247–256.
27. Venditti EM, Wing RR, Jakicic JM, et al. Weight cycling, psychological health, and binge eating in obese women. J Consult Clin Psychol 1996; 64:400–405.
28. Marchesini G, Cuaaolaro M, Mannucci E, et al. Weight cycling in treatment-seeking obese persons: data from the QUOVADIS study. Int J Obes Relat Metab Disord 2004; 28:1456–1462.
29. Carmody T, Brunner R, St Jeor ST. Hostility, dieting, and nutrition attitudes in overweight and weight-cycling men and women. Int J Eat Disord 1999; 26:37–42.
30. Foreyt JP, Brunner RL, Goodrick GK, et al. Psychological correlates of weight fluctuation. Int J Eat Disord 1995; 17:263–275.
31. Friedman MA, Schwartz MB, Brownell KD. Differential relation of psychological functioning with the history and experience of weight cycling. J Consult Clin Psychol 1998; 66:646–650.
32. Foster GD, Wadden TA, Kendall PC, et al. Psychological effects of weight loss and regain: a prospective evaluation. J Consult Clin Psychol 1996; 64:752–757.

33. Simkin-Silverman LR, Wing RR, Plantinga P, et al. Lifetime weight cycling and psychological health in normal-weight and overweight women. Int J Eat Disord 1998; 24:175–183.

34. Wadden TA, Brownell KD, Foster GD. Obesity: responding to the global epidemic. J Consult Clin Psychol 2002; 70:510–525.

35. Field A, Byers T, Hunter D, et al. Weight cycling, weight gain, and risk of hypertension in women. Am J Epidemiol 1999; 150:573–579.

36. Ferguson KJ, Spitzer RL. Binge eating disorder in a community-based sample of successful and unsuccessful dieters. Int J Eat Disord 1995; 18:167–172.

37. Byrne S, Cooper Z, Fairburn CC. Weight maintenance and relapse in obesity: a qualitative study. Int J Obes Relat Metab Disord 2003; 27:955–962.

38. Dalle Grave R, Calugi S, Molinari E, et al. Weight loss expectations in obese patients and treatment attrition: an observational multicenter study. Obes Res 2005; 13: 1961–1969.

39. Muraven M, Baumeister RF. Self-regulation and depletion of limited resources: does self-control resemble a muscle? Psych Bull 2000; 126:247–259.

40. Carels RA, Hoffman J, Collins A, et al. Ecological momentary assessment of temptation and lapse in dieting. Eat Behav 2001; 2:307–321.

41. Baumeister RF, Heatherton TF. Self-regulation failure: an overview. Psychol Inquir 1996; 7:1–15.

42. Faber R, Vohs KD. To buy or not to buy: self-control and self-regulatory failure in purchase behavior. In: Baumeister RF, Vohs KD, eds. Handbook of Self-Regulation: Research, Theory and Applications. New York: Guilford Press, 2004:509–524.

43. Sarlio-Lahteenkorva S. Weight loss and quality of life among obese people. Soc Indic Res 2001; 54:329–354.

44. Wadden TA, Mason G, Foster GD, et al. Effects of a very low calorie diet on weight, thyroid hormones and mood. Int J Obes 1990; 14:249–258.

45. Jeffery RW, Wing RR, Mayer RR. Are smaller-weight losses or more achievable weight loss goals better in the long term for obese patients? J Consult Clin Psychol 1998; 66:641–645.

46. Blackburn GL, Wilson GT, Kanders BS, et al. Weight cycling: the experience of human dieters. Am J Clin Nutr 1989; 49:1105–1109.

47. Roncolato WG, Huon GF. Subjective well-being and dieting. Brit J Health Psych 1998; 3:375–386.

48. Rumpel C, Ingram DD, Harris TB, et al. The association between weight change and psychological well-being in women. Int J Obes Relat Metab Disord 1994; 18:179–183.

49. Taylor SE, Brown JD. Illusion and well-being: a social psychological perspective on mental health. Psych Bull 1988; 103:193–210.

50. Prentice A, Jebb S, Goldberg G, et al. Effects of weight cycling on body composition. Am J Clin Nutr 1992; 56:209S–216S.

51. Lissner L, Odell PM, D'Agostino RB, et al. Variability of body weight and health outcomes in the Framingham population. New Eng J Med 1991; 324:1839–1844.

52. Jeffery RW, Wing RR, French S. Weight cycling and cardiovascular risk factors in obese men and women. Am J Clin Nutr 1992; 55:641–644.

53. National Task Force on the Prevention and Treatment of Obesity. Weight cycling. J Am Med Assoc 1994; 272: 1196–1202.

54. Muls E, Kempen K. Vansant G, et al. Is weight cycling detrimental to health? A review of the literature in humans. Int J Obes Relat Metab Disord 1995; 19:S46–S50.

55. Field A, Manson J, Laird N, et al. Weight cycling and the risk of developing type 2 diabetes among adult women in United States. Obes Res 2004; 12:267–274.

8

Obesity and the Primary Care Physician

ROBERT F. KUSHNER

Feinberg School of Medicine, Northwestern University, Chicago, Illinois, U.S.A.

LOUIS J. ARONNE

Department of Medicine, Weill Medical College of Cornell University, New York, New York, U.S.A.

INTRODUCTION

With nearly two-thirds of U.S. adults currently categorized as overweight or obese, this condition represents one of the most common chronic medical problems seen by the primary care physician (1). Since obesity is associated with an increased risk of multiple health problems, these patients are also more likely to present with silent diseases, e.g., hypertension, dyslipidemia, type 2 diabetes, metabolic syndrome, or with a variety of complaints requiring further medical attention. For this reason, the U.S. Preventive Services Task Force (2) along with multiple other societies and organizations (3–11) has endorsed periodic measurement of height and weight for all patients. Additionally, the new U.S. Department of Health and Human Services Agency for Healthcare Research and Quality (AHRQ) checklist for health recommends that all men and women have their body mass index (BMI) calculated to screen for obesity (12). In practice, however, obesity is underrecognized and undertreated in the primary care setting. Survey studies conducted among patients (13–20) and physicians (21–27) uniformly demonstrate that physicians are failing to adequately identify the overweight and mildly obese patient, although there is greater recognition for the moderately to severely obese patient, particularly when accompanied by comorbid conditions. In general, less than half of obese adults are being advised to lose weight by health care professionals. The low rates of identification and treatment of obesity are thought to be due to multiple factors including lack of reimbursement, limited time during office visits, lack of training in counseling, competing demands, or low confidence in ability to treat and change patient behaviors (28–31).

This chapter is divided into two parts. The first provides an overview of the general issues and concerns related to treating overweight and obese patients in the primary care setting and the second provides a practical review of the obesity evaluation and treatment process that should be incorporated into the care of all patients.

OFFICE-BASED OBESITY CARE

The Practice Setting and Office-Based Systems

In addition to the multiple practice barriers noted above, one of the most significant obstacles to obesity care during a routine office visit is the current health care system that is geared to treating acute care problems rather than chronic conditions (32). Whereas the former system emphasizes short appointments, brief patient education, rendering a rapid diagnosis, and dispensing a prescription, the chronic care model focuses on relationship-centered communication and creating informed, active patients with improved self-management skills (33). Obesity must be recognized as a chronic condition (34). Accordingly, successful treatment for obesity will require two factors: systematic organization of office-based processes and functions, and physician training in obesity care. The focus on the system comes from organizational theories that promote change by altering the system of care. The emphasis is not on the "bad apple" (i.e., the doctor that does not practice obesity care) but on the "bad system" (i.e., a practice environment that does not assist in provision of obesity care) (35). The second factor, physician training in obesity care, can be achieved from multiple interventions including medical school curricular development, seminars, conferences, workshops, primers, and journal articles.

Care of the obese patient would be greatly facilitated by incorporating efficient and effective office-based systems. Put Prevention Into Practice (PPIP), a national campaign by the Agency for Health Care Policy and Research (AHCPR) to improve the delivery of clinical preventive services such as counseling for health behavior change, provides a useful framework for analyzing the office systems designed to deliver patient care (36). PPIP identifies key components that can either expedite or hinder the care of patients in the office. They include organizational commitment, clinicians' attitudes, staff support, establishing policies and protocols, using simple office tools, and delegating tasks, among others.

A second useful framework is Improving Chronic Illness Care (ICIC), a national program of the Robert Wood Johnson Foundation (37,38). Perhaps not surprisingly, the essential elements for improving the care of people with chronic illness overlap with the components described by PPIP and include the need for assisting with self-management, decision support based on guidelines, development of clinical information systems, using well-designed delivery systems that meet the needs of patients, adapting a unified organizational philosophy of health care, and involvement of community resources. ICIC provides several useful tools including a step-by-step manual for improving clinical practice, a care model checklist, and a self-assessment of chronic illness care (38). These tools are excellent resources for initiating and conducting ongoing quality improvement initiatives regarding obesity care. The ICIC recommends that the system undergo a "PDSA" cycle of evaluation: Plan-Do-Study-Act. By planning it, trying it, observing the results, and acting on what is learned, a systematic method is used for improving the care of the overweight and obese patient population.

Although currently there are only limited evidence-based interventions shown to specifically improve health professionals' management of obesity (39–43), the following sections review the office-based systems that should be

Table 1 Office-Based Obesity Care

The physical environment	Accessibility and comfort: stairs, doorways, hallways, restrooms, waiting room chairs and space, reading materials and other educational materials
Equipment	Large adult and thigh blood pressure cuffs, large gowns, step stools, weight and height scales, tape measure
Materials	Educational and behavior promoting handouts on diet, exercise, medications surgery, BMI, obesity-associated diseases
Tools	Previsit questionnaires, BMI stamps, food and activity diaries, pedometers
Protocols	Patient care treatment protocols for return visit schedule, medications, referrals to dietitians and psychologists
Staffing	Team approach to include office nurse, physician assistant, nurse practitioner, health advocate

considered when caring for the obese patient (Table 1). Collectively, they address a need for heightened sensitivity and thoroughness throughout all office systems.

The Physical Environment

Accessibility to the office is critical for the obese patient. Facility limitations include difficult access from the parking lot or stairs, narrow doors and hallways, and cramped restrooms. These are the same problems that face other patients with disabilities and are covered under the regulations of the Americans with Disabilities Act of 1990. One of the first concerns obese patients have upon entering the waiting room is where they can safely sit. Office chairs of standard width and side arm rests will not comfortably accommodate moderately to severely obese patients. Ideal chairs have no arms so that patients do not have to squeeze themselves into predefined "normal" dimensions. Although often thought insignificant, hanging artwork and magazines in the waiting and examination rooms can convey misinterpreted messages to patients. Magazines, newspapers, television, movies, and billboards constantly remind overweight individuals of society's beauty ideals. Magazines, newsletters, and artwork can be chosen that don't contribute to these unattainable images.

Equipment

Measurement of an accurate height and weight is paramount to treating patients with obesity. All too often, the physician's office has a scale that does not measure above

350 lb, or the foot platform is too narrow to securely balance the overweight individual. Although a wall-mounted sliding statiometer is the most accurate instrument, a sturdy height meter attached to the scale will suffice. The weight scale should preferably have a wide base with a nearby handlebar for support if necessary. Depending on the patient population, it is reasonable to select a scale that measures in excess of 350 lb. To protect privacy, the scale should be located in a private area of the office to avoid unnecessary embarrassment.

Examination rooms should have large gowns available to wear as well as a step stool to mount the examination tables. Each room should be equipped with large adult and thigh blood pressure cuffs for measurement of blood pressure. A bladder cuff that is not the appropriate width for the patient's arm circumference will cause a systematic error in blood pressure measurement. The error in blood pressure measurement is larger when the cuff is too small relative to the patient's arm circumference than when it is too large—a situation commonly encountered among the obese. It has been demonstrated that the most frequent error in measuring blood pressure is "miscuffing" with undercuffing large arms accounting for 84% of the miscuffings (44). According to an updated American Heart Association Scientific Statement on blood pressure measurement, the "ideal" cuff should have a bladder length that is 80% and a width that is at least 40% of arm circumference (a length-to-width ratio of 2:1) (45). Therefore, a large adult cuff (16 × 36 cm) should be chosen for patients with mild to moderate obesity (or arm circumference 14 to 17 inches) while an adult thigh cuff (16 × 42 cm) will need to be used for patients whose arm circumferences are greater than 17 inches. In patients who have very large circumferences with short upper arm length, blood pressure can be measured from a cuff placed on the forearm and listening for sounds over the radial artery (although this may overestimate systolic blood pressure). Lastly, a cloth or metal tape should be available for measurement of waist circumference as per the National Heart, Lung, and Blood Institute (NHLBI) Practical Guide for Obesity Classification (3).

Using an Integrated Team Approach

How practices operate on a day-to-day basis is extremely important for the provision of effective obesity care. Several key office-based strategies have been shown to improve practice performance in relation to goals for primary care. Two of the most successful features are use of a multidisciplinary or interdisciplinary team and incorporation of protocols and procedures (46). Current therapies for obesity may be best provided using an integrative team approach (47,48). Because of limited time, physicians are generally unable to provide all of the care necessary for treatment. Moreover, other personnel are often better qualified to deliver the dietary, physical activity, and behavioral counseling. Accordingly, there is an opportunity for other office staff to play a greater role in the care of obese patients. A sense of "groupness," defined as the degree to which the group practice identifies itself and functions as a team, will enhance the quality and efficiency of care (49).

The optimal team composition and management structure will vary among practices. However, as an example of an integrative model, receptionists can provide useful information about the program including general philosophy, staffing fee schedules, and other written materials; registered nurses can obtain vital measurements including height and weight (for BMI) and waist circumference, instruction and review of food and activity journals and other educational materials; and physician assistants can monitor the progress of treatment and assume many of the other responsibilities of care. A new position of health advocate, whose role is to serve as a resource to the physician and to patients by providing additional information and assisting in arranging recommended follow-up, may be particularly useful (50). Regardless of how the workload is delegated, the power of the physician's voice should not be underestimated. The physician should be perceived as the team leader and source of common philosophy of care (51).

Protocols and Procedures

A significant portion of the time spent in the evaluation and treatment of the obese patient can be expedited by use of protocols and procedures. A self-administered medical history questionnaire can be either mailed to the patient prior to the initial visit or completed in the waiting room (52). In addition to standard questions, sections of the form should inquire about past obesity treatment programs, a body weight history, current diet and physical activity levels, social support, and goals and expectations. The review-of-systems section can include medical prompts that are more commonly seen among the obese, such as snoring, morning headaches and day time sleepiness (for obstructive sleep apnea), urinary incontinence, intertrigo and sexual dysfunction among others. An example of a patient history questionnaire can be obtained from the American Medical Association's Assessment and Management of Adult Obesity: A Primer for Physicians (53).

Identifying BMI as a fifth vital sign may also increase physician awareness and prompt counseling. This method was successfully used in a recent study where a smoking status stamp was placed on the patient chart, alongside blood pressure, pulse temperature, and respiratory rate (54).

Use of prompts alerts, or other reminders has been shown to significantly increase physician performance of other health maintenance activities as well (46,55). Once the patient is identified as overweight or obese, printed food and activity diaries and patient information sheets on a variety of topics such as the food guide pyramid, deciphering food labels, healthy snacking, dietary fiber, aerobic exercise and resistance training, and dealing with stress can be used to support behavior change and facilitate patient education. Ready-to-copy materials can be obtained from a variety of sources free of charge such as those found in the Practical Guide, on www.mypyramid.gov., or for a minimal fee from other public sites and commercial companies.

On the basis of the health promotion literature, use of written materials and counseling protocols should lead to more effective and efficient obesity care. In a study of community-based family medicine physicians, Kreuter et al. (56) showed that patients were more likely to reduce smoking, increase physical activity, and limit dairy fat consumption when physician advice is supported by health education materials. In another randomized intervention study by Swinburn et al. (57) a written goal-oriented exercise prescription, in addition to verbal advice, was more effective than verbal advice alone in increasing the physical activity level of sedentary individuals over a six-week period. Several exercise assessment and counseling protocols have been developed that can be easily incorporated into obesity care. These include Project PACE (Provider-Based Assessment and Counseling for Exercise) (58), ACT (the Activity Counseling Trial) (59), and STEP (the Step Test Exercise Prescription) (60). Finally, protocols and procedures for various treatment pathways can be established for obtaining periodic laboratory monitoring and referral to allied health professionals, such as registered dietitians, exercise specialists, and clinical psychologists.

The Patient-Physician Encounter

Although all of the office-based systems reviewed above are important, the cornerstone of effective treatment for obesity is grounded in skillful and empathetic physician-patient communication. This vital interaction is affirmed by Balint's assertion that "the most frequently used drug in medical practice is the doctor himself" (61). From the patient's perspective, a caring physician is compassionate, supportive, trustworthy, open-minded, and nonjudgmental. He or she takes into account the patient's needs, values, beliefs, goals, personality traits, and fears (62). In a review of the literature, Stewart found that the quality of communication between the physician and patient directly influenced patient health outcomes (63). A large body of literature has described key elements of communication that foster behavior change. Since the primary

aim of obesity counseling is to influence what the patient does *outside* the office, the time spent *in* the office needs to be structured and effective.

Effective counseling begins with establishing rapport and soliciting the patient's agenda. Attentively listening to the patient to understand his or her goals and expectations is the first essential step. Asking the patient, "How do you hope that I can help you?" is an information-gathering open-ended question that directly addresses his or her concerns. Among 28 identified elements of care that were inquired about with patients before the office visit, Kravitz found that "discussion of own ideas about how to manage condition" was ranked as the highest previsit physician expectation (64). Interestingly, this is not always done in the primary care office. In a survey of 264 patient-physician interviews, patients completed their statement of concern only 28% of the time, being interrupted by the physician after an average duration of 23 seconds (65). Physicians were found to redirect the patient and focus the clinical interviews before giving patients the opportunity to complete their statement of concern. Obesity interviewing and counseling should be patient centered, allowing the patient to be an active participant in setting the agenda and having his or her concerns heard. This requires skillful management by the physician to structure the interview within the time allocated.

The style of communication used by the physician refers to the approach taken when interacting with and counseling patients. Emanuel and Emanuel (66) describe four models of the physician-patient relationship: paternalistic—the physician acts as the patient's guardian, articulating and implementing what is best for the patient; informative—the physician is a purveyor of technical expertise, providing the patient with the means to exercise control; interpretive—the physician is a counselor, supplying relevant information and engaging the patient in a joint process of understanding; and deliberative—the physician acts as a teacher or friend, engaging the patient in dialogue on what course of action would be best.

Roter et al. (67) define four similar prototypes of doctor-patient relationships using a "power" balance sheet. In this model, power relates to who sets the agenda, whether the patient's values are expressed and considered, and what role the physician assumes. As illustrated in Table 2, high physician and high patient power (upper left) depicts a

Table 2 Patient-Physician Communication Relationships

Patient power	Physician power	
	High	Low
High	Mutuality	Consumerism
Low	Paternalism	Dysfunctional

Source: From Ref. 67.

relationship of mutuality, balance, and shared decision making. High physician and low patient power (lower left) is consistent with Emanuel's paternalistic model where the doctor sets the agenda and prescribes the treatment. In the low physician and high patient power relationship (upper right), the patient sets the agenda and takes sole responsibility for decision making. Roter et al. (67) call this interaction consumerism. Lastly, in a low physician and low patient power relationship (lower right), the role of the doctor and patient is unclear and undefined. This is a dysfunctional relationship. According to Roter et al., the optimal relationship is that of mutuality or what they call "relationship-centered medicine." In the course of providing obesity care, it is likely that more than one of these relationships is used among patients. The important point is that the encounter should be functional, informative, respectful, and supportive.

Depending on the patient's course of treatment and response, various strategies and techniques are used during the visit. The traditional therapeutic role of the physician is to address concerns, build trust, give advice, and be supportive (68). Novack (69) describes four therapeutic interventions that support patient behavior change. Each of the therapeutic strategies listed in Table 3 is directed toward keeping the patient motivated and providing a sense of control. Among the components of effective counseling, empathy is perhaps the most important. The feeling of being understood is intrinsically therapeutic. Patients with obesity typically provide emotionally laden testimony about the frustration, anger, and shame of losing (and gaining) weight, the discrimination they feel

Table 3 Therapeutic Aspects of the Clinical Encounter

Strategy	Characteristic
Cognitive	Negotiation of priorities
	Giving an explanation
	Suggestion
	Patient education
	Giving a prognosis
Affective	Empathy
	Encouragement of emotional expression
	Encouragement
	Offering hope
	Touch
	Reassurance
Behavioral	Emphasizing patient's active role
	Praising desired behaviors
	Suggesting alternative behaviors
	Attending to compliance
Social	Use of family and social supports
	Use of community agencies and other health care providers

Source: From Ref. 69.

in the workplace and society for being overweight, and the ridicule they may have experienced with other health care providers. Recognizing and acknowledging the patient's concerns and experiences is an extremely important element in communication (70). In sum, it is important for patients to have the opportunity to tell the story of their weight journey in their own words and for the physician to validate the patients' experience.

Regardless of whether a good therapeutic and supportive relationship is established, many patients will not achieve their behavioral and weight loss goals. In this case, it is extremely important not to label these patients as noncompliant. The word "compliance" suggests that a submissive patient should obey the authoritative physicians' instructions. "Noncompliance" then denotes failure or refusal to cooperate. This description is consistent with the paternalistic physician-patient relationship model discussed above. Some authors have suggested that the word "adherence" is a better alternative to compliance, emphasizing the patient's role as an active decision making (71,72). Still others have abandoned both terms because they exaggerate the importance of the clinician and do not aid in helping the patient overcome behavioral obstacles (73). Simply asking the patient what is hard about a particular behavioral change is more productive in problem solving than giving them purposeless labels.

This brief review of the office environment and office systems that facilitate provision of obesity care is intended to provide a backdrop for the section that follows in this chapter. Herein we review the process of assessment, classification, and treatment of the overweight and obese adult patient in the primary care setting. Other chapters in the book address each of these processes in detail. Our focus is on the practical implementation of obesity care, highlighting the key elements of each step and the associated decision making that occurs in the process.

ASSESSMENT, CLASSIFICATION, AND TREATMENT

The clinical approach to the patient follows three steps used in the care of any patient with a multifactorial, chronic disease: assessment, classification, and treatment (3). Assessment includes determining the degree of obesity using BMI and waist circumference, and evaluating the overall health status of the patient. Information collected during the assessment is then used to classify the severity of obesity and related health problems. Decisions about treatment can be made based on the results of the assessment and classification. Treatment includes not only acute treatment of obesity but maintenance of weight loss as well as management of comorbid conditions. An obesity-specific approach is outlined in Table 4.

Table 4 Assessment and Management of the Overweight and Obese Patient

---

Measure height and weight; estimate BMI.

Measure waist circumference.

Review the patient's medical condition; assess comorbidities:
  How many are present, and how severe are they?
  Do they need to be treated in addition to the effort at weight loss?

Look for causes of obesity including the use of medications known to cause weight gain.

Assess the risk of this patient's obesity using Table 7.

Is the patient ready and motivated to lose weight?

If the patient is not ready to lose weight, urge weight maintenance and manage the complications.

If the patient is ready, agree with the patient on reasonable weight and activity goals and write them down.

Use the information you have gathered to develop a treatment plan based on Table 8.

Involve other professionals, if necessary.

Don't forget that a supportive, empathetic approach is necessary throughout treatment.

Source: From Ref. 74.

Assessment

History and Physical Examination

The history is important for evaluating risk and deciding upon treatment. Questions should address age of onset of obesity, minimum weight as an adult, events associated with weight gain, recent weight loss attempts, and previous weight loss modalities used successfully and unsuccessfully and their complications. For example, loss of weight to below a patient's minimum weight as an adult is unusual, and an earlier age of onset of obesity often, but not always predicts a less successful outcome. A treatment modality that was previously unsuccessful or during which the patient experienced adverse complications should generally be avoided. A history of eating disorders, bingeing, and purging by vomiting or laxative abuse are relative contraindications to treatment, and referral to a specialist in these areas should be considered. Alcohol and substance abuse require specific treatment that should take precedence over obesity treatment. Cigarette smoking can complicate treatment history because weight is often gained upon stopping smoking. While smoking cessation is of paramount importance, implementing a diet and exercise program on or before stopping can minimize weight gain.

The patient's current level of physical activity is important to determine the starting point for exercise recommendations. Some individuals may be completely sedentary while others are vigorously active. Providing the same recommendation to both patients would be inappropriate. Similarly, the patient's level of understanding of nutrition will determine whether a basic or more sophisticated level of nutrition education should be taught. This is crucial toward helping the patient get the most out of each session. Material that is too advanced won't be retained, and material that is too basic will be boring to the patient.

Diseases that may affect weight, such as polycystic ovarian syndrome (PCOS) and hypothyroidism, require specific treatment even though that treatment alone may not result in weight loss. In addition, patients may also exhibit substantial weight gain in the months or years before developing overt type 2 diabetes.

The clinician should search for complications of obesity, such as hypertension, type 2 diabetes, hyperlipidemia, coronary heart disease, osteoarthritis of the lower extremities, gallbladder disease, gout, and some forms of cancer. In men, obesity is associated with colorectal and prostate cancer; in women, it is associated with endometrial, gallbladder, cervical, ovarian, and breast cancer. Signs and symptoms of these disorders, such as vaginal or rectal bleeding, may have been overlooked by the patient and should be carefully reviewed by the physician.

Obstructive sleep apnea is a disorder often overlooked in obese patients. Symptoms and signs include very loud snoring, cessation of breathing during sleep followed by a loud clearing breath, nighttime awakening, daytime fatigue with episodes of sleepiness at inappropriate times, and morning headaches. Associated findings on examination may include hypertension, narrowing of the upper airway, scleral injection, and leg edema. Laboratory studies may show polycythemia. If signs of sleep apnea are recent, the patient should have a diagnostic sleep study performed. The onset of sleep apnea is sometimes associated with further weight gain, and management of sleep apnea may assist with weight loss by preventing the physiologic sequelae of sleep deprivation.

A number of medications are known to cause weight gain in some patients (Table 5). These include antidepressants, antiepileptics, phenothiazines, lithium, glucocorticoids, progestational hormones, antihistamines, sulfonylureas, insulin, thiazolidinediones, and β-blockers, among others (75). If possible, medications should be changed to those that do not cause weight gain or may even induce weight loss. The use of medications that may interact with planned treatment, such as monoamine oxidase (MAO) inhibitors and other antidepressants should be reviewed. In addition, some patients take over-the-counter weight control products and cold remedies that may cause side effects and interactions with medications that may be prescribed. Examples include pseudoephedrine, which may be found in cold remedies and over-the-counter diet products, and synephrine a nonspecific beta agonist found in diet products. Both are contraindicated if prescribing a sympathomimetic appetite suppressant.

Table 5 Drugs That May Promote Weight Gain
and Alternatives

Category	Drugs that may promote weight gain	Alternatives
Psychiatric/ neurologic	Lithium	
	Phenothiazines	
	Antidepressants, SSRI	Buproprion, Nefazadone, Short-term fluoxetine, sertraline
	Antipsychotics	Ziprasidone, Aripiprazole
	Antiepileptics	Topiramate, Zonisamide, Lamotrigine
Steroid hormones	Hormonal contraceptives	Barrier methods of contraception
	Corticosteroids	Nonsteroidal anti-inflammatory drugs
	Progestational steroids	Weight loss for menometrorrhagia
Diabetes treatments	Insulin	Metformin, acarbose, miglitol
	Sulfonylureas	Exenatide, pramlintide
	Thiazolidinediones	Orlistat, sibutramine, rimonabant
Antihistamines	Diphenhydramine, others	Decongestants, inhaled steroids
β-Adrenergic blockers	Propranolol, others	ACE inhibitors, Ca-channel blockers

Source: Modified from Ref. 75.

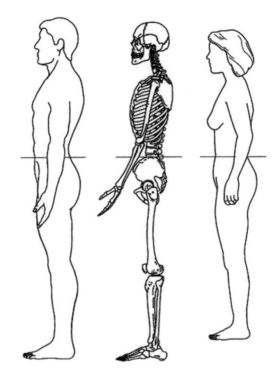

Figure 1 Measuring waist circumference. To measure waist circumference, locate the upper hip bone and the top of the right iliac crest. Place a measuring tape in a horizontal plane around the abdomen at the level of the iliac crest. Before reading the tape measure, ensure that the tape is snug, but does not compress the skin and is parallel to the floor. The measurement is made at the end of a normal expiration. Men with a waist circumferences >40 in (>102 cm) and women with a waist circumferences >35 in (>88 cm) are at higher risk because of excess abdominal fat and should be considered one risk category above that defined by their BMI. *Source*: From Ref. 3.

Clinical manifestations of the causes and complications of obesity should be particularly sought during the physical exam. Height and weight should be measured and the BMI calculated in order to categorize the severity and risk of obesity. Waist circumference should be assessed using a tape measure (Fig. 1). Blood pressure should be checked with an appropriately sized cuff. Other key features include examining the thyroid and looking for manifestations of hypothyroidism; looking for skin tags and acanthosis nigricans around the neck and axilla, which suggest hyperinsulinemia; and identifying leg edema, cellulitis, and intertriginous rashes with signs of skin breakdown. Leg edema may be secondary to right heart failure or direct compression by an abdominal pannus in the very obese patient.

The physician should look for the common disorders seen in the obese: type 2 diabetes, hyperlipidemia, coronary heart disease, osteoarthritis of the lower extremities, gallbladder disease, gout, colorectal and prostate cancer in men, and endometrial, gallbladder, cervical, ovarian, and breast cancer in women. Type 2 diabetes, gout, hyperlipidemia, and hepatic steatosis are the disorders most often discovered by laboratory evaluation (Table 6). Other labs may indicate disorders that may be involved in the induction of obesity and require specific treatment, such as hypothyroidism and hyperinsulinemia. Complete laboratory evaluation might include blood glucose, uric acid, BUN, creatinine, uric acid, ALT, AST, total and direct bilirubin, alkaline phosphatase, total cholesterol, HDL, LDL, triglycerides, complete blood count, TSH, and urinalysis. In some cases, a two-hour postprandial insulin level is of value in diagnosing hyperinsulinemia. Measurements of body composition utilizing methods such as bioelectrical impedance, while motivating to some patients, are not necessary for treating the average patient.

Table 6 Laboratory and Diagnostic Evaluation of the Obese Patient Based on Presentation of Symptoms, Risk Factors, and Index of Suspicion

If there is a suspicion of ...	Consider ...
Alveolar hypoventilation (Pickwickian) syndrome (hypersomnolence, possible right-sided heart failure)	CBC (to rule out polycythemia); pulmonary function tests (reduced lung volume), blood gases (pCO_2 often elevated); ECG (to rule out right heart strain)
Cushing's syndrome	Screen with 24-hr urine for free cortisol (>150 µg/24 hr considered abnormal) and overnight dexamathasone suppression test: 1 mg at 11 PM. At precisely 8 AM next morning, draw serum cortisol (<5 is normal suppression; axis intact). Failure of suppression indicates dysregulation, possibly Cushing's syndrome
Gallstones	Ultrasonography of gallbladder
Hepatomegaly/nonalcoholic steatohepatitis	Liver function tests, hepatic CT scan or MRI
Hypothyroidism	Serum TSH (normal generally < 5 µU/mL)
Insulinoma	Elevated levels of insulin and C-peptide in absence of sulfonylurea in plasma, especially during hypoglycemic episode
Sleep apnea	Polysomnography for oxygen desaturation apneic and hypopneic events; ENT examination for upper airway obstruction
Polycystic ovarian syndrome (PCOS) (oligomenorrhea, hirsutism, probable obesity, enlarged ovaries may be palpable, impaired glucose tolerance, persistent acne, and androgenic alopecia)	AM blood draw for total testosterone, free and weakly testosterone, DHEAS, prolactin, TSH and early morning 17-hydroxyprogesterone level. Testing should be OFF of oral contraceptives

Abbreviations: CBC, complete blood count; ECG, electrocardiogram; TSH, thyroid-stimulating hormone; ENT, ear, nose, and throat.
Source: From Ref. 76.

Before beginning treatment, results of the physical examination and laboratory tests should be shared with the patient. Emphasis should be placed on any new findings, particularly those associated with obesity that would be expected to improve with weight loss. The patient should focus on improvements in these health parameters, rather than focus on achieving an ideal or "dream" body weight or a similarly large weight loss that may not be attainable. Improvements in health complications should be discussed on an ongoing basis, because

they are achievable with the 5% to 10% weight loss frequently seen in clinical practice. Many patients find this a helpful motivator because, at some point, weight is likely to stabilize at a level above their own "ideal" weight. By focusing patients on the medical rather than the cosmetic benefits of weight loss, they may be more satisfied and better able to attain their goals and succeed long term.

The relative risk associated with a given degree of overweight and obesity can be estimated from Table 7.

Table 7 Classification of Overweight and Obesity by BMI, Waist Circumference, and Associated Disease Risk[a]

	BMI (kg/m^2)	Obesity class	Disease risk[a] (relative to normal weight and waist circumference)	
			Men $\leq$ 40 in. ($\leq$102 cm) and Women $\leq$ 35 in. ($\leq$88 cm)	Men $>$ 40 in. ($>$102 cm) and Women $>$ 35 in. ($>$88 cm)
Underweight	<18.5		–	–
Normal[b]	18.5–24.9		–	–
Overweight	25.0–29.9		Increased	High
Obesity	30.0–34.9	I	High	Very high
	35.0–39.9	II	Very high	Very high
Extreme obesity	$\geq$40	III	Extremely high	Extremely high

[a]Disease risk for type 2 diabetes mellitus, hypertension, and CVD.
[b]Increased waist circumference can also be a marker for increased risk even in persons of normal weight.
Source: From Ref. 3.

Contraindications to Treatment

Obesity treatment is contraindicated in patients who are pregnant, have anorexia nervosa, or have terminal illness. Medical or psychiatric illnesses such as cardiovascular disease, depression, and anxiety should be stable before weight reduction begins and may influence the choice of pharmacotherapy, if used. Furthermore, patients with cholelithiasis and osteoporosis should be warned that these conditions might be aggravated by weight loss.

Considering the Patient's Readiness to Lose Weight

The decision to attempt weight-loss treatment should consider the patient's readiness to make lifestyle changes. Evaluation of readiness should include the following: (1) reasons and motivation for weight loss; (2) previous attempts at weight loss; (3) support expected from family and friends; (4) an understanding of risks and benefits; (5) attitudes toward physical activity; (6) time availability; and (7) potential barriers, including financial limitations.

For the patient to succeed, he or she must be ready to make the effort to lose weight. An unwilling patient rarely if ever succeeds, frustrating both the patient and the practitioner. If the patient does not wish to lose weight and is not at high risk, weight maintenance should be encouraged. If the patient is at high risk as a result of obesity, the clinician should make an effort to motivate the patient by discussing the medical consequences related to the patient's case. However, negative and pejorative statements should be avoided since they are of no therapeutic value and tend to be demoralizing.

Classification and Treatment

While healthy eating and an increase in activity should be encouraged in every patient, the primary targets for treatment should be those individuals at health risk because of increased weight. This includes overweight patients with a BMI ≥ 25, and obese patients with a BMI ≥ 30,

especially if complications are present. Table 8 outlines a guide to selecting the appropriate treatment based on BMI. Individuals at lesser risk should be counseled about effective lifestyle changes. Goals of therapy are to reduce body weight and maintain a lower body weight for the long term; the prevention of further weight gain is the minimum goal. An initial weight loss of 10% of body weight achieved over six months is a recommended target. Even more modest weight loss can reduce visceral fat and improve comorbid conditions. The rate of weight loss should be 1 to 2 lb each week but will vary from patient to patient. Greater rates of weight loss have not been shown to achieve better long-term results. Weight maintenance, achieved through the combined changes in diet, physical activity, and behavior, should be the priority after the first six months of weight loss.

Given our current state of knowledge and the treatments currently available, the goal of obesity treatment should be the lowest weight the patient can comfortably maintain, which in the average patient is about 5% to 10% of total body weight or 2 BMI units. Attaining ideal body weight, or a loss of 20% to 30% or more of total body weight, is not possible for the vast majority of overweight and obese people. Loss of 5% to 10% of body weight can significantly improve cardiovascular and other risk factors associated with obesity (77,78) even though many patients may be disappointed with not reaching their "dream weight." Counseling about achievable goals and alternative goals such as an improvement in lipids or glucose, improved mobility, reduced waist circumference, or simply compliance with the regimen are worthy alternative goals.

Patients on a weight loss regimen should be seen in the office within approximately two to four weeks of starting treatment in order to monitor both the treatment's effectiveness and its side effects. Visits every four weeks are adequate during the first three months if the patient has a favorable weight loss and few side effects. More frequent visits may be required based on clinical judgment, particularly if the patient has comorbid conditions. The patient should be weighed each visit, with waist circumference

Table 8 A Guide to Selecting Treatment

	BMI category				
Treatment	25–26.9	27–29.9	30–34.9	35–39.9	≥40
Diet, exercise, behavior therapy	With comorbidities	With comorbidities	+	+	+
Pharmacotherapy		With comorbidities	+	+	+
Surgery				With comorbidities	+

Prevention of weight gain with lifestyle therapy is indicated in any patient with a BMI > 25, even without comorbidities, while weight loss is not necessarily recommended for those with a BMI of 25 to 29.9 kg/m^2 or a high waist circumference, unless they have two or more comorbidities. Combined intervention with a low-calorie diet, increased physical activity, and behavior therapy provide the most successful therapy for weight loss and weight maintenance.
Source: From Refs. 3,74.

measured less often. Blood pressure and pulse should be monitored if the patient is taking an appetite suppressant such as sibutramine or phentermine. The visit should be used to monitor compliance with the program, provide encouragement, and set new goals. This can be accomplished by reviewing food and exercise records, discussing progress or lack therefore, and solving problems which the patient has encountered. Less frequent follow-up is required after the first six months.

Available Treatments

Treatment

There are a number of available treatments that can be used for obesity. The backbone of conventional therapy includes behavior and lifestyle change, exercise, and diet. These are discussed in detail in the Practical Guide from National Institutes of Health/North American Association for the Study of Obesity (NIH/NAASO) (74) and in chapters 53 to 55. Medications can also be used as an adjunct to treatment programs using lifestyle change, diet, and exercise. Orlistat, noradrenergic drugs including sibutramine, newer drugs such as rimonabant, and thermogenic drugs are discussed in chapters 14 through 18. Finally, surgical treatments may be considered for individuals with a BMI ≥ 40 kg/m^2 or BMI ≥ 35 kg/m^2 if they have comorbidities. Further details on this therapy are available in chapter 18.

Resources Available to Health Care Practitioner

Referral to health care providers with an interest in obesity treatment including dietitians, psychologists, nurses, and nurse practitioners is an efficient way to manage the obese patient. For example, while many physicians feel uncomfortable prescribing a diet, community or hospital-based dietitians are available in most communities to assist with patient education and support. For the clinician interested in treating obesity in the office, important educational information including sample diets and other patient material may be found in the NIH publication, the Practical Guide: Identification, Evaluation, and Treatment of Overweight and Obesity in Adults (74) or on the NIH/NHLBI Web site (79). A comprehensive program for patient education can be found in the LEARN manual (80). Clinical practice guidelines on pharmacologic and surgical management of obesity in the primary care setting have been published by the American College of Physicians (81). Several recent review articles may also be helpful to the practitioner in crafting an approach to the overweight and obese patient (82–84). In some cases patients may choose to utilize commercial weight loss programs such as Weight Watchers, TOPS (Take Off Pounds Sensibly), or groups such as Overeaters

Anonymous for support in addition to the efforts made by the health care provider. These groups can be helpful addition to the support mechanism required for long-term success. Internet-based support may also be of value as an adjunct for some individuals. Information from the Practical Guide is available through the NIH Web site (85). For patients who have serious problems that are beyond the scope of what can be comfortably managed in the primary care office, referral to an obesity specialist or endocrinologist with an interest in obesity would be appropriate. NAASO, The Obesity Society lists its members on its Web site (86).

SUMMARY

Care of the obese patient can be improved by reevaluation of the processes and functions of office-based systems. PPIP and ICIC provide two frameworks for analyzing the office systems designed to deliver efficient and effective patient care. Key components to address include the physical environment, equipment, using an integrated team approach, protocols and procedures, and the patient-physician encounter. Clinical guidelines developed by the NHLBI can be used to provide an organized approach to the assessment, classification, and treatment of the overweight and obese patient.

REFERENCES

1. Ogden CL, Carroll MD, Curtin LR, et al. Prevalence of overweight and obesity in the United States, 1999–2004. JAMA 2006; 295:1549–1555.
2. US Preventive Services Task Force. Screening for obesity in adults: recommendations and rationale. Ann Intern Med 2003; 139:930–932.
3. U.S. Department of Health and Human Services, Public Health Service, National Institutes of Health, National Heart, Lung, and Blood Institute, NIH Publications No. 98-4083, September 1998.
4. Pearson TA, Blair SN, Daniels SR, et al. AHA guidelines for primary prevention of cardiovascular disease and stroke: 2002 update. Consensus panel guide to comprehensive risk reduction for adult patients without coronary or other atherosclerotic vascular diseases. Circulation 2002; 106:388–391.
5. Smith SC, Allen J, Blair SN, et al. AHA/ACC guidelines for secondary prevention for patients with coronary and other atherosclerotic vascular disease: 2006 update. Circulation 2006; 113:2363–2372.
6. Guzman SE and the American Academy of Family Physicians Panel on Obesity. Practical advice for family physicians to help overweight patients. An American Family Physician Monograph. AAFP, Leawood, KS, 2003. Available at: http://www.aafp.org/obesitymonograph.xml. Accessed March 21, 2005.

7. Nawaz, H, Katz DL. American College of Preventive Medicine practice policy statement. Weight management counseling of overweight adults. Am J Prev Med 2001; 21:73–78.

8. Lyznicki JM, Young DC, Riggs JA, et al. Obesity: assessment and management in primary care. Am Fam Physician 2001; 63:2185–2196.

9. Cummings S, Parham ES, Strain GW. Position of the American Dietetic Association: weight management. J Am Diet Assoc 2002; 102:1145–1155.

10. National Task Force on the Prevention and Treatment of Obesity. Medical care for obese patients: advice for health professionals. Am Fam Physician 2002; 65:81–88.

11. Eyre H, Kahn R, Robertson RM. Preventing cancer, cardiovascular disease, and diabetes. A common agenda for the American Cancer Society, the American Diabetes Association, and the American Heart Association. Circulation 2004; 109:3244–3255.

12. US Department of Health Services Agency for Healthcare Research and Quality (AHRQ). Available at: www.ahrq/ppip/healthymen.html.

13. Galuska DA, Will JC, Serdula MK, et al. Are health care professionals advising obese patients to lose weight? JAMA 1999; 282:1576–1578.

14. Nawaz H, Adams ML, Katz DL. Weight loss counseling by health care providers. Am J Public Health 1999; 89: 764–767.

15. Sciamanna CN, Tate DF, Lang W, et al. Who reports receiving advice to lose weight? Results from a multistate survey. Arch Intern Med 2000; 160:2334–2339.

16. Jackson JE, Doescher MP, Saver BG, et al. Trends in professional advice to lose weight among obese adults, 1994–2000. J Gen Intern Med 2005; 20:814–818.

17. Loureiro ML, Nayga RM. Obesity, weight loss, and physician's advice. Soc Sci Med 2006; 62:2458–2468.

18. Potter MB, Vu JD, Groughan-Minhane M. Weight management: what patients want from their primary care physicians. J Fam Pract 2001; 50:513–518.

19. Mehrotra C, Naimi TS, Serdula M, et al. Arthritis, body mass index, and professional advice to lose weight. Implications for clinical medicine and public health. Am J Prev Med 2004; 27:16–21.

20. Huang J, Yu H, Martin E, et al. Physicians' weight loss counseling in two public hospital primary care clinics. Acad Med 2004; 79:156–161.

21. Bramlage P, Wittchen HU, Pittrow D, et al. Recognition and management of overweight and obesity in primary care in Germany. Int J Obes Relat Metab Disord 2004; 28: 1299–1308.

22. Simkin-Silverman LR, Gleason KA, King WC, et al. Predictors of weight control advice in primary care practices: patient health and psychosocial characteristics. Prev Med 2005; 40:71–82.

23. Kristeller JL, Hoerr RA. Physician attitudes toward managing obesity: differences among six specialty groups. Prev Med 1997; 26:542–549.

24. Stafford RS, Farhat JH, Misra B, et al. National patterns of physician activities to obesity management. Arch Fam Med 2000; 9:631–638.

25. Bertakis KD, Azari R. The impact of obesity on primary care visits. Obesity Res 2005; 13:1615–1623.

26. Davis NJ, Emerenini A, Wylie-Rosett J. Obesity management: physician practice patterns and patient preference. Diabetes Educ 2006; 32:557–561.

27. Dilley KL, Martin LA, Sullivan C, et al. Identification of overweight status is associated with higher rates of screening for comorbidities of overweight in pediatric primary care practice. Pediatrics 2007; 119:148–155.

28. Kushner RF. Barriers to providing nutrition counseling by physicians: a survey of primary care practitioners. Prev Med 1995; 24:546–552.

29. Foster GD, Wadden TA, Makris AP, et al. Primary care physicians' attitudes about obesity and its treatment. Obes Res 2003; 11:1168–1177.

30. Block JP, DeSalvo KB, Fisher WP. Are physicians equipped to address the obesity epidemic? Knowledge and attitudes of internal medicine residents. Prev Med 2003; 36:669–675.

31. Forman-Hoffman V, Little A, Wahls T. Barriers to obesity management: a pilot study of primary care clinicians. BMC Fam Pract 2006; 7:35.

32. Kane RL, Priester R, Totten AM, eds. Meeting the Challenge of Chronic Illness. Baltimore: Johns Hopkins University Press, 2005.

33. Casalino LP. Disease management and the organization of physician practice. JAMA 2005; 293:485–488.

34. Serdula MK, Khan L, Dietz WH. Weight loss counseling revisited. JAMA 2003; 289:1747–1750.

35. Gross PA, Greenfield S, Cretin S, et al. Optimal methods for guideline implementation. Conclusions from Leeds Castle meeting. Med Care 2001; 8(suppl 2):II85–II92.

36. 10 Steps: Implementation Guide. Put prevention into practice. Adapted from the Clinicians' Handbook of Preventive Services. 2nd ed. Publication No. 98-0025, Rockville, MD: Agency for Healthcare Research and Quality, 1998. Available at: http://www.ahrq.gov/ppip/impseteps.htm.

37. Bodenheimer T, Wagner EH, Grumbach K. Improving primary care for patients with chronic illness. JAMA 2002; 288:1775–1779.

38. Improving chronic illness care. Available at: http://improvingchroniccare.org/. Accessed August 2007.

39. Harvey EL, Glenny AM, Kirk SFL, et al. A systematic review of interventions to improve health professionals' management of obesity. Int J Obes 1999; 23:1213.

40. Harvey EL, Glenny AM, Kirk SFL, et al. Improving health professionals' management and the organization of care for overweight and obese people. Cochrane Database Syst Rev 2001; (2):CD000984.

41. McQuigg M, Brown J, Broom J, et al. Empowering primary care to tackle the obesity epidemic: the Counterweight Programme. Eur J Clin Nutr 2005; 59(suppl 1): S93–S100.

42. Moore H, Summerbell CD, Greenwood DC, et al. Improving management of obesity in primary care: cluster randomized trial. BMJ 2005; 327:1085–1089.

43. Davis Martin P, Rhode PC, Dutton GR, et al. A primary care weight management intervention for low-income African-American women. Obesity 2006; 14:1412–1420.

44. Manning DM, Kuchirka C, Kaminski J. Miscuffing: inappropriate blood pressure cuff application. Circulation 1983; 68:763.

45. Pickering TG, Hall JE, Appel LJ, et al. Recommendations for blood pressure measurement in humans and experimental animals: part 1: blood pressure measurement in humans: a statement for professionals from the Subcommittee of Professional and Public Education of the American Heart Association Council on High Blood Pressure Research. Circulation 2005; 111(5):697–716.

46. Yano EM, Fink A, Hirsch SH, et al. Helping practices reach primary care goals. Lessons from the literature. Arch Intern Med 1995; 155:1146–1156.

47. Kushner R, Pendarvis L. An integrated approach to obesity care. Nutr Clin Care 1999; 2:285–291.

48. Frank A. A multidisciplinary approach to obesity management: the physician's role and team care alternatives. J Am Diet Assoc 1998; 98(supp 2):S44–S48.

49. Crabtree BF, Miller WL, Aita VA, et al. Primary care practice organization and preventive services delivery: a qualitative analysis. J Fam Pract 1998; 46:404–409.

50. Scholle SH, Agatisa PK, Krohn MA, et al. Locating a health advocate in a private obstetrics/gynecology office increases patient's receipt of preventive recommendations. J Women Health Gen-B 2000; 9:161–165.

51. Dickey L, Frame P, Rafferty M, et al. Providing more- and better-preventive care. Patient Care 1999; 15:189–210.

52. Hornberger J, Thom D, MaCurdy T. Effects of a self-administered previsit questionnaire to enhance awareness of patients' concerns in primary care. J Gen Intern Med 1997; 12:597–606.

53. Kushner RF. Roadmaps for Clinical Practice: Case Studies in Disease Prevention and Health Promotion—Assessment and Management of Adult Obesity: A Primer for Physicians. Chicago, IL: American Medical Association, 2003. Available at: www.ama-assn.org/ama/pub/category/10931. html. Accessed August 2007.

54. Ahluwalia JS, Gibson CA, Kenny E, et al. Smoking status as a vital sign. J Gen Intern Med 1999; 14:402–408.

55. Balas EA, Weingarten S, Grab CT, et al. Improving preventive care by prompting physicians. Arch Intern Med 2000; 160:301–308.

56. Kreuter MW, Chheda SG, Bull FC. How does physician advice influence patient behavior? Evidence for a priming effect. Arch Fam Med 2000; 9:426–433.

57. Swinburn BA, Walter LG, Arroll B, et al. The green prescription study: a randomized controlled trial of written advice provided by general practitioners. Am J Public Health 1998; 88:288–291.

58. Calfas KJ, Long BJ, Sallis JF, et al. A controlled trial of physician counseling to promote the adoption of physical activity. Prev Med 1996; 25:225–233.

59. Albright CL, Cohen S, Gibbons L, et al. Incorporating physical activity advice into primary care. Physician-delivered advice within the activity counseling trial. Am J Prev Med 2000; 18:225–234.

60. Petrella RJ, Wight D. An office-based instrument for exercise counseling and prescription in primary care. The Step Test Exercise Prescription (STEP). Arch Fam Prac 2000; 9:339–344.

61. Balint M. The Doctor, his Patient, and the Illness. New York: International University Press, 1972.

62. Groopman JE, Kunkel EJ, Platt FW, et al. Sharing decision making with patients. Patient Care 2001; 15:21–35.

63. Stewart MA. Effective physician–patient communication and health outcomes: a review. Can Med Assoc J 1995; 152:1423–1433.

64. Kravitz RL. Measuring patients' expectations and requests. Ann Intern Med 2001; 134:881–888.

65. Marvel MK, Epstein RM, Flowers K, et al. Soliciting the patient's agenda. Have we improved? JAMA 1999; 281:283–287.

66. Emanuel EJ, Emanuel LL. Four models of the physician–patient relationship. JAMA 1992; 267:2221–2226.

67. Roter D. The enduring and evolving nature of the patient-physician relationship. Patient Educ Couns 2000; 39:5–15.

68. Branch WT, Malik TK. Using 'windows' of opportunities' in brief interviews to understand patients' concerns. JAMA 1993; 269:1667–1668.

69. Novack DH. Therapeutic aspects of the clinical encounter. J Gen Intern Med 1987; 2:346–355.

70. Suchman AL, Markakis K, Beckman HB, et al. A model of empathic communication in the medical interview. JAMA 1997; 277:678–682.

71. Luftey KE, Wishner WJ. Beyond "compliance" is "adherence." Improving the prospect of diabetes care. Diabetes Care 1999; 22:635–639.

72. Jaret P. 10 ways to improve patient compliance. Hippocrates 2001, (Feb/Mar), 22–28.

73. Steiner JF, Earnest MA. The language of medication-taking. Ann Intern Med 2000; 132:926–930.

74. National Heart, Lung, and Blood Institute (NHLBI) and North American Association for the Study of Obesity (NAASO). Practical guide on the identification, evaluation, and treatment of overweight and obesity in adults. Bethesda, MD: National Institutes of Health, 2000. NIH Publication number 00-4084, Oct. 2000.

75. World Health Organization. Obesity: Preventing and Managing the Global Epidemic. Report of the WHO Consultation of Obesity. Geneva: WHO, 1997:926.

76. Kushner RF, Weinsier RL. Evaluation of the obese patient. Practical considerations. Med Clin North Am 2000; 84: 387–399.

77. Poirier P, Giles TD, George A, et al. Obesity and cardiovascular disease: pathophysiology, evaluation, and effect of weight loss. Circulation 2006; 113:898–918.

78. Blackburn G. Effect of degree of weight loss on health benefit. Obes Res 1995; 3:211S–216S.

79. National Institutes of Health/National Heart, Blood, and Lung Institute. Clinical Guide: Identification, Evaluation, and Treatment of Overweight and Obesity in Adults. Available at: http://www.nhlbi.nih.gov/guidelines/obesity/ ob_home.htm.

80. Brownell KD, Wadden TA. The LEARN Program for Weight Control. Dallas: American Health Publishing Company, 1998.

81. Snow V, Barry P, Fitterman N. Clinical practice guidelines on pharmacologic and surgical management of obesity in the primary care setting have been published by the American College of Physicians. Ann Intern Med 2005; 142:525–531.

82. Kushner RF, Roth JL. Assessment of the obese patient. Endocrinol Metab Clin North Am 2003; 32(4):915–933.

83. Kushner RF, Jackson Blatner D. Risk assessment of the overweight and obese patient. J Am Diet Assoc 2005; 105(suppl 1):S53–S62.

84. Anderson DA, Wadden TA. Treating the obese patient. Suggestions for primary care practice. Arch Fam Med 1999; 8:156–167.

85. National Institutes of Health. Aim for a Healthy Weight. Available at: http://www.nhlbi.nih.gov/health/public/heart/obesity/lose_wt/index.htm.

86. NAASO. The Obesity Society. Available at: http://www.naaso.org.

9

The Prevention of Obesity in Childhood and Adolescence

TIM LOBSTEIN

*Child Obesity Research Program, International Association for the Study of Obesity, London, U.K.,
and SPRU–Science and Technology Policy Research, University of Sussex, Brighton, U.K.*

OVERVIEW

Prevention of obesity is a priority for the simple reason that it is far easier in the modern food-rich environment to gain excess weight than it is to lose it. A specific focus on child obesity is considered important for two reasons: first, lifestyle patterns are learned at an early age, and unhealthy patterns can lead to a lifetime of increased risk of ill-health; and second, the pathological effects of obesity are in many cases a product of the time the individual has been obese as well as the severity of the obesity. Interventions that can maintain or improve health behavior from an early age and that prevent long-term obesity are likely to be far more cost-effective over the longer period than managing and treating obesity and obesity-related diseases after they have developed.

Evidence for the effects of different approaches to preventing child and adolescent obesity and for developing dietary and physical activity patterns is growing rapidly, and this chapter includes a summary of recent literature reviews and the recommendations of expert consultations and a summary table of recent systematic reviews relating to child obesity prevention and healthy weight promotion.

In summary, the evidence suggests that multiple actions—such as those that form a whole school approach to health (including meals, classroom activities, vending machines, sports and play activities)—are more likely to

have a sustainable beneficial impact than single actions alone. This perhaps is not surprising; it might be assumed that the more that an environment is consistently able to promote healthy behavior, the greater the likelihood that such behavior will occur.

There are, however, some important caveats. Interventions in free-living populations are hard to assess: the nonintervention group may be affected by some of the factors designed to influence the intervention group, and both groups may be influenced by external events that reduce the size of the effect of the intervention. The most common settings for controlled interventions are in schools, where specific inputs can be measured and the experimental designs can ensure a degree of scientific validity to the results, but this focus on the school creates a strong "settings bias" in the scientific evidence. The settings bias has limited the information available to policy-makers, and has led to concerns that "evidence-based policy" is too narrow in its focus and other types of evidence should be utilized, including modeling, observational studies, and expert opinion.

Three WHO expert consultations have made recommendations on measures to prevent overweight and obesity, and all have indicated the need to consider population-based interventions and to tackle the determinants of food choices and physical activity levels. Regulatory approaches—such as controls on marketing to children or mandatory clear nutritional food labeling—need to be included as policy options despite an absence of extensive evidence that such measures would have an effect on obesity levels.

Several tools have been developed to assist the development of obesity prevention policies and practices, such as the Angelo analysis grid and cost-effectiveness modeling, and these are discussed in the chapter. Obesity prevention, like other health promotion strategies, can be described using an investment paradigm, in which prevention initiatives are considered speculative ventures. An investment portfolio should carry a mixture of "safe" low-return initiatives and "risky" potentially high-return initiatives. Researchers should report information on the costs of intervention, and policy-makers need to attend to the social and environmental contexts in which children's health behavior occurs.

OBESITY PREVENTION IN YOUNG PEOPLE

Obesity and its prevention have risen rapidly up the policy-making agenda in the last decade. Although prevention strategies targeting adults may provide economic value in the short-term (1), policy-makers accept that in the longer term, there are reasons to prevent obesity occurring in childhood or as a result of behaviors learned in childhood. Policy-makers are also sensitive to prevention of obesity in children because children are generally not held responsible for their own health behavior, their behavior is assumed to be more open to influence than that of adults, and they can be more readily targeted than adults, for example, in school settings. Perhaps as a result of this perceived set of advantages, funding for research into childhood obesity prevention tends to be more easily obtained and the evidence base has consequently grown more rapidly.

Obesity prevalence among school-age children is rising in virtually all countries of the world for which data are available (2). An obese child faces a lifetime of increased risk of various diseases, including cardiovascular disease, diabetes, liver disease, and certain forms of cancer (3). A child is also likely to experience excess bodyweight as a cause of psychological distress.

At present, pediatric services have few treatment options available. Once a child is substantially overweight, successful weight loss is difficult to achieve, as it is for adults, and requires intensive health care resources. Prevention of obesity is to be preferred for the child's sake as much as for the social and economic costs that otherwise ensue.

In this chapter, we consider obesity prevention in its primary form: the prevention of obesity among children in the general population. We do not consider targeted programs for already-overweight children or the treatment of obese children to prevent them from becoming obese adults or developing obesity-related comorbidities.

Prevention: Who, Where, and How?

There is an accumulated body of evidence that examines the causes of weight gain in childhood (3–5) and has demonstrated the influence of parental BMI, maternal smoking and diabetes status, infant feeding patterns, dietary energy density and meal patterns, and sedentary behavior patterns, such as TV watching, on the risk of developing obesity. Some of these determinants are open to manipulation and can be utilized in health promotion initiatives.

The classical framework for the development of health promotion strategies is one that describes interventions in terms of "target groups" ("who," e.g., children, adolescents, pregnant women, minority ethnic groups, or those on low incomes), "settings" ("where," e.g., homes, clinics, kindergartens, schools, youth clubs), and "approaches" ("how," e.g., antenatal educational leaflets, kindergarten food service standards, school physical activity programs).

Following the model given in the WHO Global Strategy on Diet, Physical Activity and Health (6), target groups can be specified through reference to the life course: this starts with maternal health and prenatal nutrition and proceeds through pregnancy outcomes, infant nutrition, preschool and school-age children, adolescents, adults of reproductive age, and older people (with these last two categories able to exert a strong influence on the health behavior of the next generation). Crosscutting this sequence are gender and socioeconomic groupings, including racial and ethnic groups, migrant status, income and educational levels. The choice of target group will influence the nature of the approach used and the setting where the intervention takes place.

However, a limitation to the use of this analysis for identifying target groups is that it can be interpreted to mean that interventions should only act upon the group whose health is in question, e.g., those for whom an improvement in diet or physical activity would be beneficial. This may be considered too narrow a target for tackling obesity, as it does not consider how to tackle the determinants of individual behavior, namely the environmental, economic, and cultural influences, which may need to be changed so that healthy behavior changes are easier to make. In this respect, the definition of target groups may need to be widened to include the providers of the determinants of health, such as the providers of health information—the health services, schools, the media, commercial producers—and widened still further to include those who set the policies that shape access to healthy lifestyles through, for example, pricing, distribution, and marketing. In this sense, target groups may include shareholders in companies, members of learned societies, policy makers, and other public opinion leaders, including politicians and celebrities.

Similarly, the classical settings for interventions in health promotion, such as family health services, preschool and school settings, may be considered too restricted given the range of environments that shape health behavior, such as those provided by commercial operators (e.g., shops, restaurants) and by planners and designers (e.g., roads, parks, buildings).

Settings and approaches are interlinked. Economic interventions, such as those commonly made by commercial operators to increase sales, are in need of greater research attention, especially as much useful information on the manipulation of dietary preferences and food choices is kept commercially confidential. Short-term effects have been noted by French in a series of studies on changes to food services and vending machines in labeling and pricing of goods, which have indicated a significant effect—especially for pricing—on food selection, but this effect remains significant only while the intervention occurs (7).

Further work is needed to determine how manufacturers and retailers could support health promotion strategies though changes in production, pricing, marketing, and labeling of foods. The catering sector has an important role to play, with the growing tendency for people to eat their meals outside of the home. Food labeling and menu labeling opportunities that highlight healthy options have been considered a useful adjunct to consumer information in health promotion campaigns, although their long-term effectiveness on food intake has not been well documented. Reduced energy density and reduced portion sizes may also have an effect on reducing caloric intake (8,9).

Interventions set in the context of the built environment have also been poorly researched in terms of their health-promoting potential. The provision of cycle routes, walkways, sports, and leisure facilities may be assumed to be beneficial for the local population's body weight, fitness, and cardiovascular health, but there is a need for better evidence to show that this is the case, and to identify the variables which play the most significant role. Neighborhood safety or perceived safety may be more important in determining the use of recreational facilities than the distance or price, for example.

In its widest sense, a health promotion setting is any place in which it is possible to influence policies and practices toward improved health. In this wider sense, a setting could be a parliamentary hearing, a corporate shareholder meeting, or a transport authority board meeting.

Equally, the various approaches used for health promotion include mass media, written materials, skills training and counseling, but might be extended to include community development and advocacy. While several of these approaches are oriented directly toward the intended beneficiaries (e.g., educational materials, health messages through the mass media, community development) others may be oriented indirectly, for example, skills training may involve training health professionals and others to develop their ability to undertake health promotion work, or indeed to become advocates. Advocacy is primarily an indirect approach, attempting to influence the decisions made by policy-makers and program managers. Advocates for public health may be supported by professionals (e.g., in the health professions), patients' organizations, and other consumer groups. Advocacy organizations acting on behalf of public interests (such as consumer and environmental groups) tend to be trusted by the public at large to a greater extent than are commercial lobbying organizations or political parties (10).

It should be noted that healthy behavior patterns may require financial resources (e.g., to purchase healthier foods or to use sports facilities) and education and skills (e.g., to understand food labels or create healthy recipes). Some interventions may inadvertently increase health inequalities in society (11), especially if they rely on individual capacity to respond to health messages. Thus, individualized or family-based health promotion combined with an emphasis on personal responsibility or "making healthy choices" (12) may widen the health gap between rich and poor unless the strategy is supported by public interventions to ensure that healthier choices are fairly and widely available and their selection is easy and likely to be made by default.

Furthermore, strategies that rely on individual approaches effectively pass the responsibility for disease prevention onto those at risk. This begs a number of questions about the ability of the target groups to make and maintain the necessary behavior changes and the nature of the forces ranged against them. If the necessary support measures are not in place, the potential for the individual to fail is high. Individuals who experience failure, in the context of individuals being held responsible for their own health, are likely to suffer loss of self-esteem and a loss of further motivation. Adults can find this hard enough to deal with, children surely more so.

Examples of Preventive Interventions

Adipose tissue expansion occurs when food energy intake exceeds bodily energy expenditure. Some interventions are designed to change dietary patterns (e.g., to reduce caloric intake, increase fruit and vegetable consumption or, for infants, an increase in the opportunities for breast-feeding, as this appears to have a protective role against infant and young child obesity) and some are designed to increase physical activity, or decrease sedentary behavior, in order to increase energy expenditure. Many interventions are designed to tackle both energy intake and energy expenditure in a combined program.

By way of illustration, Table 1 lists some examples of recent or current programs in a variety of different social

Table 1   Examples of Controlled, Evaluated Obesity Prevention Trials

Source (reference)	Setting	Conclusion
13	*Australia (Perth)*. School-home program to enrich the opportunities for physical activity, for 11-yr-old urban children.	Significant improvements in fitness levels in boys and girls during the enrichment program, but no significant difference in physical activity at the end of the intervention.
14	*United States*. Native Americans. School-based series of interventions on nutrition and physical activity.	Improved awareness and self-reported improved nutrition, but not validated by observed food intake. No effects on activity levels and no improvements in adiposity.
15	*China (Taiwan)*. Health promotion counseling for overweight adolescent students at nursing college.	Counseling enabled subjects to adopt healthier lifestyles, showing reduced weight and improved CVHD indicators.
16	*U.S. Mexico* border. Elementary school-based cardiovascular health program for low-income Spanish speakers	Overweight increased, but less in participating than control schools. Research team recommended more community participation in forming and evaluating the program.
17	*Austria* "PRESTO" multiprofessional school educational intervention with children aged 10–12 yr (pilot study).	Improved nutritional knowledge, especially in higher attainment students. No change in BMI measures.
18	*Israel*. Clinical dietary-behavioral-exercise intervention with children and adolescents.	A combined, structured multidisciplinary intervention for childhood obesity resulted in decreased body weight, decreased BMI, and improved fitness, especially if the parents are not overweight.
19	*United States*. Family dietary changes for overweight parents: impact on child diets.	Increasing the intake of healthy food (fruit and vegetable) by overweight parents can improve nutrient intake for children. Decreasing the amount of unhealthy foods was less effective.
20	*United States*. Head Start schemes school beginners. Parent-child-teacher program.	Meal-time behavior may be significant in affecting child nutrient intake. Teachers need training to promote children's early nutrition socialization.
21	*Germany*. "StEP TWO" school-based intervention with children aged 7–9 yr	Reduced rate of increase in BMI, reduced systolic blood pressure.
22	*China*. Kindergarten interventions targeting obese children by training parents and care workers.	Child care workers, parents, and child health care doctors using a range of interventions reduced obesity prevalence and improved child nutrition and activity in care and at home.
23	*U.S. school students*. Systematic review of physical activity opportunities.	Physical activity can be increased during school break periods. Extracurricular, school-based interventions had problems with low attendance, which might be removed if delivered through existing community organizations. Active travel to school offers potential, but is impaired by traffic congestion and parental fears for child safety.
24	*United Kingdom*. School-based intervention focusing on reduced soft drink consumption, with children aged 7–11 yr.	Reduced consumption of soft drinks. Reduced prevalence of overweight compared to controls.
25	*Chile*. 6-mo nutrition education and physical activity intervention for primary school children. Included education for parents.	Increased physical activity observed for both genders. Reduced adiposity for boys only.
26	*Japan*. Support for parent and child weight loss.	Children of overweight parents who became non-overweight also lost weight and improved CV risk factors. Children of parents who remained overweight did not improve.
27	*Australian* aboriginals. Family and school programs, targeting cooking skills, school breakfasts, school snacks, parent education, shopping skills, breast-feeding promotion.	Project ongoing. More schools and teacher involvement being planned.
28,29	*Crete*. School-based health education prospective study for children aged 6 yr (through to age 12 yr).	BMI improvements in intervention group compared with the control group, although BMI and overweight in both groups rose during the period.

(Continued)

Source (reference)	Setting	Conclusion
30	*Thailand.* School-based weight control program.	Adiposity increased significantly less among children in the program compared with controls.
31	*Thailand.* Exercise program for kindergarten children, duration 30 wk.	Both the exercise and control groups decreased adiposity. Girls in the exercise group had a lower likelihood of having an increasing BMI slope than the control girls did.
32	*Germany* Kiel Obesity Prevention Study "KOPS." 8-yr duration school-based intervention, children initially aged 5–7 yr.	Improved nutrition knowledge and physical activity, reduced television viewing. Reduced adiposity indices (skinfold, % fat mass) vs. controls.
33	*Denmark.* Family counseling, shopping, and meal planning.	21 out of 25 children lost weight over a 2-yr intervention.
34	*Australia (New South Wales).* Group education program for families with overweight children.	After 6 mo, half of overweight/obese children stabilized or reduced their BMI for age, and obese parents also lost weight. Program could transfer from clinic to school as part of curriculum for all children.
35	*Singapore.* Clinic-based session with preschool children (age 3–6 yr). Dietetic interventions for the most overweight, and nurse-led counseling for moderate overweight.	After 1 yr 40% of the children improved their obesity status and 20% reached normal status.
36	*United Kingdom.* "MAGIC" Preschool (3- to 4-yr-olds) 12-wk program to increase physical activity (pilot study).	Aimed to increase physical activity. Results showed increases up to 40%. Unknown changes in adiposity.
37,38	*United Kingdom.* "APPLES" School-based intervention with children aged 7–11 yr	Some improvements in dietary patterns. No change in physical activity. No change in BMI.
39	*China (Zhejiang Province).* Three primary and three secondary health promoting schools. Used school-based working groups, nutrition training for staff, nutrition education for students, school-wide health promotion efforts and outreach to families and communities	Improvements in students' nutrition knowledge, attitudes, and behavior. Improvements to school facilities and school health services. Improved school policies and a positive school climate.
40	*France.* School and nonschool physical activity program for adolescents	Improved participation in activities compared with controls, especially for girls. Reduced sedentary behavior. Little impact on proportion overweight in 6 mo
41,42	*Singapore.* School-based nutrition and physical activity interventions. Teacher training and Ministry of Education input.	Decrease in the prevalence of obesity (from around 16% to 14% over an 8-yr period). Not been fully evaluated or peer reviewed.
43	*United Kingdom.* "Be Smart" 5- to 7-yr-olds, school and family intervention.	Increase in nutrition knowledge and fruit and vegetable intake. No significant change in overweight prevalence.
44	*Australia (Victoria)* small town, after-school activity program, healthier take away food (hot chips) formulation, community newsletter.	Ongoing project. Has benefited from strong community participation.
45	*New Zealand (South Auckland).* School-based awareness-raising for adolescent students, involved food, activity, and body-size perceptions.	Ongoing project. Draws in many cultural groups: Samoan, Cook Islands, Tongan, Maori, and New Zealand European.
46	*Tonga.* Awareness raising meetings. Focus on secondary school children in village setting. Assessing role of food supplies.	Ongoing project. Concern over imported high-fat meat products, protected by trade agreements.
47	*China (Taiwan).* Screening for overweight among elementary school children. Involvement of parents and caregivers.	Screening indicated that severely obese children using inappropriate methods to lose weight. Children staying in foster families or with grandparents, or from families of low socioeconomic status, had poorest weight-control behavior. Parents and foster families with low-income need support.
48	*Japan.* Screening and treatment for overweight among elementary school children.	Older children and those most overweight showed reduced adiposity in both control and intervention groups, but intervention group showed greater degree of improvement.

and economic contexts, which have been designed to tackle obesity or to encourage healthy body weight in child populations and which include control groups and have received some degree of scientific evaluation of their effectiveness. The construction of interventions with control groups is difficult to achieve in communities with open borders, and researchers frequently opt for settings that offer the least risk of contamination between control and intervention groups, usually in the school, home, or clinic.

In addition to these examples of structured, evaluated programs, a remarkable number of initiatives have been launched that are likely to have an impact on obesity levels even if obesity prevalence was not a measured outcome variable. Some are being evaluated, though not necessarily for their impact on obesity prevalence; examples include the Brazilian program "Agito São Paulo" (49), the Danish "Six-a-day" fruit and vegetable promotion program (50), the extensive network of Health Promoting Schools (51), the Baby Friendly Hospitals program, which includes breast-feeding promotion (52), programs promoting drinking water in schools (53) and active transport, such as "Walking Buses" that take children to and from school (54). Further examples of these types of initiatives are shown in Table 2.

Several features need to be noted concerning these interventions. These types of activity are introduced without strong evidence of effectiveness but on the assumption that they would be better than doing nothing and that the potential benefits outweigh the likely costs. Many of these initiatives grew out of local community action and were supported politically after rather than before they were launched. Thus, many came about largely as a result of public pressure being put on the relevant sections of the legislature or through voluntary action on the part of school authorities, local businesses, or community groups. As a result, many of these initiatives were introduced in a piecemeal way, and few of the actions have been or will be rigorously evaluated for their effectiveness in preventing adiposity.

THE EVIDENCE BASE

This section examines the reviews of evidence concerning interventions to prevent overweight and obesity and to promote healthy bodyweights. As indicated earlier, scientific investigations are most easily undertaken where interventions can be controlled so that comparable groups of subjects can receive different levels of treatment. The most common settings for controlled trials are in schools where specific inputs (e.g., classroom education, food services, physical activity sessions) can be measured and the experimental designs can ensure a degree of scientific validity to the results.

Table 2 Examples of Community and Population Initiatives That May Affect Child Obesity Rates

Action	Location(s)
Long maternity leave to encourage breast-feeding	Norway, Sweden
Heart-healthy meals in kindergartens	Manitoba, Canada
Healthy Heart Awards for kindergartens	New Zealand
Sport Waikato "Teddy Bear" project for fitness in under fives	New Zealand
Vending machines banned in schools	Taiwan, Japan
Nutrition standards for school food shops	Greece, Brazil
School teaching: the mobile Food Museum	Mexico
Fruit and vegetable eating will help get school swimming pool	United Kingdom
15-min workout for school staff and pupils every morning	Cyprus
Subsidized use of sports centers for local schools	Hong Kong
Liverpool School milk bar replaces vending machines	United Kingdom
Nutrition standards for school canteens	Japan, United Kingdom, Malaysia, Crete
"Ever Active" school sports program	Alberta, Canada
Breakfast for Learning, nutrition in schools project	Ontario, Canada
Collectif Action Alternative en Obésité	Quebec, Canada
Nutrition and Activity Awards, $2000 to Healthy School Zones	Pennsylvania, United States
Project LEAN for schools, with "Bright Ideas" suggestions zone	California, United States
Supermarkets provide activity areas while parents shop	Sweden, Cambodia
Companies give advice to employees regarding their child's overweight	Switzerland
Eat More Live, resource kit for primary school teachers	New Zealand
Children leaving schools in cars must stay back 10 min	Wales (United Kingdom)
Reduce the use of coloring additives in energy dense foods	Cambodia, Latvia
Tax on adverts for soft drinks	France
Controls on TV advertising to children	Sweden, Quebec, United Kingdom
Sales tax on sweet or fatty food (proposed)	Switzerland
Community programs for mass physical activity	Brazil, Kazakhstan

Source: Adapted from Ref. 55

However, even with evaluated trials such as these, there are serious problems with sustainability (few trials report on long-term effects), transferability, and resource requirements. Furthermore, as noted earlier, this settings bias restricts the types of intervention that can be reliably evaluated and has inevitably led to concerns that evidence-based policy will be far too narrow in its focus (56,57). These issues are considered further in the sections below.

Systematic Reviews

A listing of systematic reviews is given in Table 3. It includes those that conform to the Cochrane criteria and are listed in the Cochrane Library, along with other reviews undertaken in a systematic format. A summary of their conclusions is given in this chapter.

It should be noted that, for most interventions, long-term follow-up was not undertaken, making it difficult to evaluate the efficacy of these interventions for population wide effects on obesity prevalence. In their favor, most of the studies were able to show improvements in eating and/or exercise habits, and the large trials used for school-based interventions indicate that such programs are feasible.

We are not aware of any systematic reviews of interventions to prevent child obesity in commercial settings, although various researchers have looked at the effects of food prices, labeling, and marketing on food choices (7,118,119).

Breast-feeding Promotion

Four types of interventions have been shown to be useful in promoting breast-feeding:

- *Peer support given in the ante- and postnatal periods*: This can increase breast-feeding initiation and duration rates among women on low incomes. Peer-support programs should be targeted at women on low incomes who have expressed a wish to breast-feed.
- *Small-group health education sessions during the antenatal period*: These have been shown to be effective in increasing initiation and duration among women of all income groups and women from minority ethnic groups.
- *One-to-one health education*: This can be effective at increasing initiation rates among women on low incomes. It may be more effective than group sessions in increasing initiation among women who have made a prior decision to bottle-feed.
- *Maternity ward practices*: Programs to promote mother-infant contact and autonomy, such as "rooming in" and breast-feeding support, can increase the initiation and duration of breast-feeding.

In addition, initiation and duration of breast-feeding may be undermined by the physical hospital environment and by hospital routines, e.g., feeding at set times, separation of mother and baby, use of infant formula,

and by the attitudes and expectations of the health professionals who are involved. A beneficial effect on both initiation and duration of breast-feeding has been found in studies of the Baby Friendly Hospital initiative promoted by UNICEF, at least in European settings (Table 3).

Family-Based and Preschool Interventions

The effectiveness of interventions targeted at two- to five-year-olds and their families and caregivers, in terms of helping children maintain a healthy weight or prevent overweight or obesity, is equivocal (111). Three studies showed positive significant intervention effects, but a further two studies failed to show significant improvements. The studies suggest that small changes may be possible and that interventions are more likely to be effective if they are specifically focused on preventing obesity (rather than changing diet and physical activity behaviors), are intensive (e.g., include several behavior change techniques taught to both parents and children), fully resourced (primarily a function of the intensity), targeted, and tailored to individual needs.

A review of the effectiveness of interventions specifically designed to promote healthy eating in preschool settings showed most interventions improved nutrition knowledge, but the effect on eating behavior was less frequently assessed and the results were inconsistent (63). There was no assessment of long-term effectiveness on knowledge or behavior. There is some justification to assume that early establishment of good nutritional habits are valuable for both parents and children (92).

In the United States, assessors of the Women, Infants and Children (WIC) program noted the barriers faced by health professionals when counseling parents of overweight children (120). It found that mothers were focused on surviving their daily life stresses, used food to cope with these stresses and as a tool in parenting, had difficulty setting limits with their children around food, lacked knowledge about normal child development and eating behavior, were not committed to sustained behavioral change, and in many cases did not believe their overweight children were overweight.

The effectiveness of family interventions targeted at older children, in terms of helping children maintain a healthy weight or prevent overweight or obesity, is also equivocal. Studies of family-based treatment for overweight have indicated the need to consider the role of parents in the treatment process. One study indicated that treating the mother and child separately appeared to be significantly more effective than treating them together or treating the child alone, while in another study there was no significant difference in effect on weight outcomes between treating the parent and child together or separately (87).

(*text continues on page 147*)

Table 3 Reviews of Interventions to Prevent Obesity and Promote Healthy Weights in Infants and Children, 1996–2007

Review	Notes
Guidelines for School Health Programs to Promote Lifelong Healthy Eating. CDC, 1996 (58)	Recommendations for action at school and community level: • Review of policies that would be useful in supporting physical education and health education in schools. • Establishment of safe and pleasant environments and opportunities for physical activity. • Promote development of knowledge, attitudes, skills, and confidence to maintain physically active lifestyle. • Implement health education curricula to support. • Provide activities to meet needs/interests of all students. • Include parents in instruction and encourage support of physical activity. • Training for school and community personnel to promote lifelong physical activity. • Assess, counsel, refer, and advocate for health promoting physical activity. • Provide a range of sports and recreation programs. • Monitor and evaluate community and school physical activity programs and facilities.
The prevention and treatment of obesity. NHS-CRD, 1997 (59)	Progression of obesity in high-risk children may be prevented by family therapy. Interventions to reduce sedentary behavior can reduce overweight in children.
School-based cardiovascular disease prevention studies: review and synthesis. Resnicow and Robinson, 1997 (60)	The majority of school-based studies reported significant effects on health knowledge, attitudes, and behavioral outcomes. The diet and physical activity changes reported in some studies were modest in magnitude, although from a population perspective they could translate into potentially sizable reductions in population-attributable CVD risk. The results of school-based intervention research showed only modest change in physiological indicators including serum cholesterol, blood pressure, and measures of adiposity.
Effects of physical activity interventions in youth. Review and synthesis. Stone et al., 1998 (61)	Studies showing the best results used randomized designs, valid and reliable measurements, and more extensive interventions. Some follow-up results showed physical activity was sustained after interventions ended. Special attention is needed for girls, middle schools, and community settings for all youth. More objective assessments are needed for measuring physical activity outside of school and in younger children, since they cannot provide reliable self-report.
Effectiveness of interventions to promote healthy feeding in infants under one year of age: a review. Tedstone et al., 1998 (62)	Individual educational sessions were more successful than group sessions when they were aimed at promoting initial breast-feeding with women who had already made a decision to bottle-feed. Breast-feeding promotions delivered in the period both before and after birth were most likely to have a positive effect on breast-feeding. These interventions were intensive, involving multiple contacts with a professional promoter or peer counselor. Weaker evidence shows that including partners, providing incentives and changing the content of commercial hospital packs given to women upon discharge from hospital may aid promotion. The least successful interventions were those where breast-feeding promotion was only one part of the focus of multiple health promotion programs and involved special visits to the hospital/clinic or took place by telephone.
Effectiveness of interventions to promote healthy eating in preschool children aged 1 to 5 years. Tedstone et al., 1998 (63)	Most studies show an effect on nutrition knowledge, but few assessed the effect on eating behavior. There were no data to evaluate long-term effects on knowledge or behavior. Involvement of parents strengthened effects. Repeated exposure to initially novel foods combined with taste trials enhanced acceptance. Reward schemes not consistently effective. Pressing need for better quality research.
School-based approaches for preventing and treating obesity. Story, 1999 (64)	School-based treatment showed positive, though modest short-term results. Relatively few primary prevention studies have been conducted and therefore efficacy has not been established. Both primary and secondary obesity interventions have a role in schools. A model, building upon the comprehensive school health program model, consists of eight interacting components: health instruction, health services, school environment, food service, school-site health promotion for faculty and staff, social support services, physical education classes, and integrated and linked family and community health promotion efforts.

Role of physical activity in the prevention of obesity in children. Goran et al., 1999 (65)	The beneficial effect of physical activity in children is supported by controlled exercise intervention programs. The successful prevention of childhood obesity through physical activity promotion will involve theory-based, culturally appropriate school, family, and community interventions. Policy changes, environmental planning, and educational efforts in schools and communities provide increased opportunities and encouragement for physical activity.
Interventions to prevent weight gain, a systematic review of psychological models and behavior change methods. Hardeman et al., 2000 (66)	Effects on weight were mixed but follow-up was generally short. Smaller effects on weight gain were found among low-income participants, students, and smokers. Study dropout was higher among thinner and lower-income subjects. Interventions to prevent weight gain exhibited various degrees of effectiveness. Definite statements about the elements of the interventions that were associated with increased effect size cannot be made as only one of the five studies that involved an randomized controlled trial design reported a significant effect on weight. This intervention involved a correspondence program and a mix of behavior change methods including goal setting, self-monitoring, and contingencies.
Consolidation and updating the evidence base for the promotion of breast-feeding. Stockley, 2000 (67)	• Interventions should be long term, intensive, span both the antenatal and postnatal periods, and involve multiple contacts. Professionals need to be consistent in the advice and support they provide. Hospital practices should reflect current knowledge. • Information provision alone is not effective, and may exacerbate inequalities. Peer support programs are particularly promising. • Different approaches are needed for women who originally intended to bottle-feed. There is a negative impact of returning to full-time work on duration of breast-feeding. • Fathers have an important role in the initiation and establishment of breast-feeding. This is more likely to be positive if they are included in breast-feeding during pregnancy. • Workplace initiatives can address the barriers that currently exist, including negative attitudes and lack of facilities. • More coordinated and consistent education about breast-feeding is needed in schools for both girls and boys.
Toward Public Health Nutrition Strategies in the European Union to implement Food Based Dietary Guidelines and to enhance healthier lifestyles. Sjöström and Stockley, 2000 (68)	There are wide variations in rates of breast-feeding initiation and continuation in the member states of the European Union. Hospital practices and the support of community health services are important influences in this. Systematic reviews of the literature show that opportunities and barriers to good nutritional health in infants are associated with the physical hospital environment and routines, e.g., feeding at set times, separation of mother and baby, use of infant formula, but also importantly by the attitudes and expectations of the health professionals who are involved.
A systematic review to evaluate the effectiveness of interventions to promote the initiation of breast-feeding. Fairbank et al., 2000 (69)	• There is some evidence that breast-feeding literature alone is not effective in promoting breast-feeding among women of different income and ethnic groups. • Group health education can be effective among women from different ethnic and low-income groups. • One-to-one educational programs were more effective for women who planned to bottle-feed, whereas group programs were more effective for women who planned to breast-feed. Paying participants to attend has been shown to be effective at increasing participation rates for group. • The provision of additional health education from community staff through face-to-face and telephone contacts in the antenatal and postnatal periods had no significant effect. • In Sweden, advice, leaflets, and routine health education plus intensive staff training had significant effects on initiation rates.
School-based interventions for primary prevention of cardiovascular disease: evidence of effects for minority populations. Meininger, 2000 (70)	There were no consistent effects of school-based interventions on blood pressure, lipid profiles, or measures of body mass and obesity. There was evidence that changes in knowledge and health behaviors occurred. Findings are interpreted within the context of population-wide approaches to prevention, and recommendations for future research directions are discussed.

(Continued)

Table 3 Reviews of Interventions to Prevent Obesity and Promote Healthy Weights in Infants and Children, 1996–2007 (*Continued*)

Review	Notes
Preventing obesity in children and adolescents. Dietz and Gortmaker, 2001 (71)	Families and schools represent the most important foci for preventive efforts in children and adolescents. An examination of factors that affect energy balance can identify more proximal influences on those factors. For example, television viewing affects both energy intake and energy expenditure, and therefore represents a logical target for interventions. Guidance by pediatricians may help to change parental attitudes and practices regarding television viewing. School-based interventions can be directed at changes in food choices and sedentary behavior.
The importance of physical activity in the prevention of overweight and obesity in childhood: a review and an opinion. Steinbeck, 2001 (72)	The role of physical activity in the prevention of obesity (primary and secondary prevention) is not clear. However, a number of school-based interventions directed at either increasing physical activity and/or decreasing sedentary behaviors have shown encouraging results. On balance, increasing physical activity in children is an attractive and nonrestrictive approach to obesity prevention. To adopt this approach requires the support and involvement of many community sectors other than health.
The effectiveness of school-based interventions in promoting physical activity and fitness among children and youth, a systematic review. Dobbins et al., 2001 (73)	There was moderate improvement in physical activity among children and adolescent girls exposed to promotional campaigns, but with little measurable effect on BMI, blood pressure, or heart rate. The most effective initiatives involved children through the whole school day, including lunch and recesses as well as class time and physical education lessons. Adults who had participated in school-based physical activities as children were more likely to be active in adulthood than those that had not. • Interventions should be multifaceted including classroom instruction and changes in school environment. • Interventions should be behaviorally focused. • Longer-lasting interventions and/or frequent booster sessions improve effectiveness. • Age, gender, and ethnicity may affect outcomes and require further study.
Interventions for preventing obesity in childhood: a systematic review. Campbell et al, 2001 (74)	Two long-term studies resulted in a reduction in the prevalence on obesity, but a third found no effect. Of four short-term studies, two resulted in a reduction in the prevalence of obesity in intervention groups compared with control groups, another study found a nonsignificant reduction, and a fourth study found no effect on obesity but a reduction in fat intake. Overall, there is only limited quality data on the effectiveness of obesity prevention programs and no generalizable conclusions can be drawn.
Formula milk versus term human milk for feeding preterm or low birth weight infants. Henderson et al., Cochrane Library, 2001[a]	*Cochrane Review:* In preterm and low birth weight infants, feeding with formula milk, compared with unfortified term human milk, leads to a greater rate of growth in the short term. The limited data available do not allow definite conclusions on whether adverse outcomes occur in the longer term, and there are no data from randomized trials on the comparison of feeding with formula milk versus nutrient-fortified breast milk.
Extending breast-feeding duration through primary care: a systematic review of prenatal and postnatal interventions. de Oliveira et al., 2001 (75)	Interventions that were most effective in extending the duration of breast-feeding generally combined information and support and were long term and intensive. During prenatal care, group education was the only effective strategy reported. Home visits used to identify mothers' concerns with breast-feeding, assist with problem solving, and involve family members in breast-feeding support were effective during the postnatal period or both periods. Individual education sessions were also effective in these periods, as was the combination of 2 or 3 of these strategies in interventions involving both periods. Strategies that had no effect were characterized by no face-to-face interaction, practices contradicting messages, or small-scale interventions.
Environmental influences on eating and physical activity. French et al., 2001 (76)	Recent trends in food supply, eating out, physical activity, and inactivity are reviewed, as are the effects of advertising, promotion, and pricing on eating and physical activity. Public health interventions, opportunities, and potential strategies to combat the obesity epidemic by promoting an environment that supports healthy eating and physical activity are recommended.

The prevention and treatment of childhood obesity. Centre for Reviews and Dissemination, 2002 (77)

There is some evidence that school-based programs that promote physical activity, the modification of dietary intake and the targeting of sedentary behaviors may help reduce obesity in children, particularly girls. Family-based programs that involve parents, increase physical activity, provide dietary education, and target reductions in sedentary behavior may help reduce childhood obesity. Future research must be of good methodological quality, involve large numbers of participants, and be of longer duration and intensity.

Achieving physiological change in school-based intervention trials: what makes a preventive intervention successful? Lytle et al., 2002 (78)

A commentary on school-based interventions, noting that only a few interventions have had significant effect on physiological measures. Improved success rates may result from an adequate length of intervention and a reduction in dropout rates. Participants from diverse cultural backgrounds are rarely catered for in the experimental designs where "one size fits all," and this may compromise the ability to show significant effects.

Recommendations to increase physical activity in communities. Task Force on Community Preventive Services, 2002 (79)

- School-based physical education: strongly recommended.
- Classroom-based health education focused on information provision: insufficient evidence.
- Classroom-based health education focused on reducing television viewing and video game playing: insufficient evidence.
- Family-based social support: insufficient evidence.
- Individually adapted health behavior change programs: strongly recommended.
- Enhanced access to places for physical activity plus informational outreach activities: strongly recommended.

The effectiveness of interventions to increase physical activity, a systematic review. Kahn et al., 2002 (80)

Changes in physical activity behavior and aerobic capacity were used to assess outcome. Two informational interventions ("point-of-decision" prompts to encourage stair use and community-wide campaigns) were effective, as were three behavioral and social interventions (school-based physical education, social support in community settings, and individually adapted health behavior change) and one environmental and policy intervention (creation of or enhanced access to places for physical activity combined with informational outreach activities). Evidence is insufficient to assess classroom-based health education, family-based social support, mass media campaigns, college-based health education and physical education, or classroom-based health education focused on reducing television viewing and video game playing.

The effectiveness of school-based strategies for the primary prevention of obesity and/or for promoting physical activity and/or nutrition, the major modifiable risk factors for type 2 diabetes: A review of reviews. Micucci et al., 2002 (81)

A "review of reviews" on interventions to prevent chronic disease concluded that the most effective interventions should be based on a whole school approach, including cafeterias, PE classes, lunch and recess activities, and classroom teaching, and also include links to home and the community. The longer the intervention, the greater the change in outcome measures. Different age groups, ethnic groups, and genders needed different approaches.

Obesity, diagnosis, prevention, and treatment, evidence based answers to common questions. Reilly et al., 2002 (82)

"There is some doubt as to whether obesity is preventable in school-age children, using currently available intervention strategies. . . . Further research is indicated, though more recent evidence, published after the present literature review had been completed, is not promising."

Prevention of obesity. Schmitz and Jeffrey, 2002 (83)

- Environmental changes, such as alterations in school physical education or television viewing time, are at least as important as classroom-based educational interventions.
- Most of the studies were able to show improvements in eating and/or exercise habits of children and the large trials indicate the feasibility of implementing school wide changes for the purpose of obesity prevention. The absence of long-term treatment effects makes it difficult to evaluate the efficacy of interventions on obesity prevalence.
- A 5-yr school-based nutrition education program showed significantly raised awareness of nutritional knowledge, but no difference in energy or macronutrient intake.
- Future studies need to evaluate the cost-effectiveness of school and/or community-based obesity prevention interventions in youth, including long-term follow-up of obesity prevalence and incidence.

(Continued)

Table 3 Reviews of Interventions to Prevent Obesity and Promote Healthy Weights in Infants and Children, 1996–2007 (*Continued*)

Review	Notes
Obesity—problems and interventions. Swedish Council on Technology Assessment in Health Care, 2002 (84)	Most population-based preventive programs that have been scientifically assessed have not demonstrated any favorable effects on the prevalence of obesity. However, there are examples of successful programs for both adults and children. New outreach strategies need to be developed.
Physical activity interventions in the prevention and treatment of pediatric obesity: systematic review and critical appraisal. Reilly and McDowell, 2003 (36)	The evidence on childhood obesity prevention is not encouraging, although a promising focus for prevention is reduction in sedentary behavior. There is stronger evidence that targeting activity and/or inactivity might be effective in pediatric obesity treatment, but there are doubts as to the generalizability of existing interventions, and the clinical relevance of the interventions is unclear.
Prevention of obesity—is it possible? Muller et al., 2003 (85)	Programs can reduce cardiovascular risk factors but not affect mean BMI of the target populations. Selective prevention directed at high-risk individuals (e.g., at children with obese parents) exhibited various degrees of effectiveness. Health promotion, counseling, better school education and social support are promising strategies.
Management of obesity and overweight: Evidence briefing. Mulvihill and Quigley, 2003 (86)	The use of multifaceted school-based interventions can reduce obesity and overweight in schoolchildren, particularly girls. These interventions included nutrition education, physical activity promotion, reduction in sedentary behavior, behavioral therapy, teacher training, curricular material, and modification of school meals and tuck shops. There is limited evidence to support school-based health promotion (classroom curriculum to reduce television, videotape and video game use). Family-based behavior modification programs (family therapy in addition to diet education, regular visits to a pediatrician, and encouragement to exercise) can impede weight gain in obese children. There is a lack of evidence for school-based physical activity programs led by specialist staff or classroom teachers for the prevention of obesity and overweight in children. There is a lack of evidence to show that family-based health promotion interventions impact on obesity and overweight, even though these interventions focused on dietary and general health education and increased activity, with sustained contact with children and parents.
Family involvement in weight control, weight maintenance, and weight-loss interventions: a systematic review of randomized trials. McLean et al., 2003 (87)	Parental involvement is associated with weight loss in children, and the use of a greater range of behavior change techniques improves weight outcomes for both parents and children. Adolescents achieved greater weight loss when treated alone. Future interventions should pay attention to which family members are targeted and how they are involved in setting goals for behavior change.
The effectiveness of public health interventions to promote the initiation of breast-feeding: Evidence briefing Protheroe et al., 2003 (88)	Breast-feeding literature alone is not effective in promoting breast-feeding among women of different income and ethnic groups in the United Kingdom, Republic of Ireland, and United States. Group health education can be effective among women from different ethnic and low-income groups in westernized countries. Advice, leaflets, and routine health education plus intensive staff training had significant effects on initiation rates. Breast-feeding promotions delivered over both the ante- and postnatal period were most likely to have a positive effect on breast-feeding. The interventions involved were intensive, involving multiple contacts with a professional promoter or peer counselor. The confidence and commitment to breast-feed successfully are best achieved by exposure to breast-feeding rather than talking or reading about it.
Increasing activity to reduce obesity in adolescent girls: a research review. Clemmens and Hayman, 2004 (89)	Five out of six effective multifaceted interventions included a media campaign in combination with health education programs, training of health professionals, and/or changes in government and hospital policies. Four included a peer support program in combination with health education programs, media programs, and/or legislative and structural changes to the health care sector. Physical activity interventions with adolescent girls give inconsistent results, but school-based, multicomponent interventions that were also designed to decrease sedentary behavior were effective in increasing physical activity. Future research should focus on determinants of long-term adherence and the duration and intensity of interventions necessary to prevent obesity in adolescent girls.

Exercise prescription for the prevention of obesity in adolescents. Carrel and Bernhardt, 2004 (90)	School personnel report lack of training in intervention and health providers report ineffective clinic-based intervention strategies. Coordination of interventions in the school and clinic can improve child obesity prevention and treatment, although the evidence base is insufficient to provide specific guidelines for assessment and treatment. General recommendations are made.
Addressing childhood obesity: the evidence for action. Casey and Crumley, 2004 (91)	A review of systematic reviews identified the following: • Long-term follow-up is critical to determine the relationship between physical activity interventions and life-long patterns of activity and should be included as a measure of efficacy of the intervention. • Interventions to increase physical activity in schools should include measures of both in-school and out-of-school physical activity to determine the effect of these interventions on total activity levels. • Comparative studies on dietary interventions should be conducted specifically in populations of overweight children to determine the characteristics associated with improved dietary habits. • Age at intervention should be evaluated to assist in targeting available resources. • Research should be systematically reviewed to determine appropriate strategies for minority populations.
Review of children's healthy eating interventions. Worsley and Crawford, 2004 (92)	Good evidence that interventions to promote healthy eating in most settings can be effective in primary and secondary school populations in the short term. Poor definitions of healthy eating, confused outcome measurements and a lack of theoretical bases marked many studies. There is a paucity of studies of under fives and adolescents. Few studies of community-wide programs.
Noncurricular approaches for increasing physical activity in youth: a review. Jago and Baranowski, 2004 (23)	Time available for school physical education has declined. Children are active during school break periods and inexpensive interventions further increased activity during these times. Active travel to school offered potential, but its effectiveness was impaired by traffic congestion and parental fears for child safety. Extracurricular, school-based interventions had problems with low attendance, which might be removed if delivered through existing community organizations. Summer day camps offered potential for increasing activity of youth, but research is required to determine how best to convert camp activity into increased post-camp habitual activity.
Cardiovascular health promotion in the schools. Hayman et al., 2004 (93)	Across well-controlled and well-conducted studies, differential results in physiological outcome indicators point to the need for researchers to pay more attention to developmental age, gender, culture, and sociodemographic factors. The results indicate that the modification of risk factors for CVD in "real-world" school settings must be reinforced and complemented at multiple levels of intervention. Broader public health interventions are warranted, requiring partnerships between healthcare and educational professionals, policymakers, and community leaders.
Interventions for preventing obesity in children. Summerbell et al., Cochrane Library, 2005[a]	The majority of studies were short term. Studies that focused on combining dietary and physical activity approaches did not significantly improve BMI, although nearly all studies resulted in some improvement in diet or physical activity. There is not enough evidence from trials to prove that any one particular program can prevent obesity in children, although comprehensive strategies that address diet and physical activity with psychosocial support and environmental change may help. Future research should look at environments such as food availability and playing area facilities. Most interventions lasted less than 1 yr. More details are needed on costs as well as effectiveness.
Public health strategies for preventing and controlling overweight and obesity in school and worksite settings. Katz et al., 2005 (94)	The Task Force found insufficient evidence to determine the effectiveness of combined nutrition and physical activity interventions to prevent or reduce overweight and obesity in school settings because of the limited number of qualifying studies and their noncomparable outcomes.
Physical activity and obesity prevention: a review of the current evidence. Wareham et al., 2005 (95)	Low levels of activity are only weakly associated with future weight gain and the direction of causality is uncertain as individuals who are overweight are less likely to stay active. The review found eleven trials with children published since 2000, with no clear conclusion on whether increasing activity could prevent obesity.
Prevention of childhood obesity. Ells et al., 2005 (96)	Preventative interventions that encourage physical activity and a healthy diet, restrict sedentary activities, and offer behavioral support should involve not only the child but the whole family, school, and community. Large-scale, well-designed prevention studies are required, particularly within settings outside of the United States, in order to expand the evidence base for formulating clinical recommendations and public health approaches.

(Continued)

Table 3 Reviews of Interventions to Prevent Obesity and Promote Healthy Weights in Infants and Children, 1996–2007 (*Continued*)

Review	Notes
Preventing Childhood Obesity: Health in the Balance. Koplan et al., 2005 (97)	There is limited experimental evidence and other forms of available evidence—across different categories of information and types of study design—need to be included in policy-making. Actions should be based on the best available evidence, as opposed to waiting for the best possible evidence. There is an obligation to accumulate appropriate evidence not only to justify a course of action but to assess whether it has made a difference. Therefore, evaluation should be a critical component of any implemented intervention or change.
Screening and interventions for childhood overweight: a summary of evidence and recommendations statement. U.S. Preventive Services Task Force, 2005 (98,99)	Interventions to treat overweight adolescents in clinical settings have not been shown to have clinically significant benefits, and they are not widely available. The Task Force found insufficient evidence for the effectiveness of behavioral counseling or other preventive interventions with overweight children and adolescents that can be conducted in primary care settings.
Do baby-friendly hospitals influence breast-feeding duration on a national level? Merten et al., 2005 (100)	Two studies have evaluated the UNICEF BFH program in Europe. The most recent finds that children in Switzerland born in a baby-friendly health facility are more likely to be breast-fed for a longer duration, and this is particularly marked in those hospitals showing the greatest compliance with the UNICEF BHF guidelines. A second study, in Italy (101), found that an increase in the number of baby-friendly staff practices was related to a large rise in breast-feeding initiation and duration. Similar findings have been noted in Brazil (102) and in Asia and Africa (103).
Effectiveness of school programs in preventing childhood obesity: a multilevel comparison. Veugelers and Fitzgerald, 2005 (104)	Students from schools participating in a coordinated program that incorporated recommendations for school-based healthy eating programs exhibited significantly lower rates of overweight and obesity, had healthier diets, and reported more physical activities than students from schools without nutrition programs.
Interventions for promoting the initiation of breast-feeding. Dyson et al., Cochrane Library, 2005[a]	Five trials involving women on low incomes in the United States showed breast-feeding education increased initiation rates by 50% compared with routine care.
School- and family-based interventions to prevent overweight in children. Muller et al., 2005 (105)	The few controlled studies available differ in relation to strategy, setting, duration, focus, variables of outcome, and statistical power, and therefore do not allow general conclusions to be made about the value of preventive measures. All school-based interventions aimed at the prevention of overweight and obesity show some improvement of health knowledge and health-related behaviors. Short-term effects on nutritional state seem to be more pronounced in girls than in boys. School-based interventions can reduce the incidence of overweight. There is evidence that families of intermediate and high socioeconomic status as well as intact families benefit more from treatment than families sharing other characteristics. Selected prevention in obese children is most successful when children are treated together with their parents, but there are social barriers limiting the success of family-based interventions. Although some positive effects have been reported, simple interventions in a single area (e.g., a school health education program) are unlikely to work on their own. The development of effective preventive interventions probably requires strategies that affect multiple settings simultaneously. National campaigns and action plans on childhood overweight and obesity may increase the value of localized approaches (e.g., in schools and families).
Interventions for increasing fruit and vegetable consumption in preschool children.	There is currently no evidence-based guidance on effective methodologies for conducting 5-a-day type programs in preschool children. This information is important particularly when resources including time and money are limited.
Obesity Prevention in Schools. French and Story, 2006 (106)	School-based interventions targeting eating and physical activity behaviors, including those specifically aimed at obesity prevention, have generally shown positive effects, although they have been less successful at altering body weight or fatness. Emerging innovative interventions need to be developed and evaluated.

Reducing obesity and related chronic disease risk in children and youth: a synthesis of evidence with "best practice" recommendations. Flynn et al., 2006 (107)

- Some interventions show short-term improvements in outcomes relating to obesity and chronic disease prevention with no adverse effects noted.
- Engagement in physical activity is a critical component of successful interventions.
- Programs require sustained long-term resources to facilitate comprehensive evaluation.
- There is a need for consistent indicators to compare program outcomes.
- Few programs address the needs of subgroups, e.g., immigrants new to developed countries.
- Children 0–6 yr of age and males were underrepresented.
- There were few interventions in home and community settings, and very few population-based interventions.

The prevention of overweight and obesity in children and adolescents: a review of interventions and programs. Doak et al., 2006 (108)

This review was limited to school-based studies with quantitative evaluations. Seventeen of the 25 interventions were "effective" based on a statistically significant reduction in BMI or skinfolds for the intervention group. Four interventions were effective by BMI as well as skinfold measures, of which two reduced television viewing and two used a physical education program combined with nutrition education. One intervention was effective in reducing childhood overweight but increased underweight prevalence. The review recommends giving more attention to preventing adverse outcomes such as underweight.

An integrative research review: effective school-based childhood overweight interventions. Cole et al., 2006 (109)

A review of theoretical characteristics of effective school-based interventions found that Social Cognitive Theory was the stated or implied theory in 8 of the 10 studies. Healthy lifestyle education was initiated in nine studies, dietary habits in four, and physical activity in eight. Four of the 10 studies used a combination of all 3 interventions; 3 used a combination of 2 interventions; and 3 used only 1 intervention.

Interventions to prevent obesity in children and adolescents: a systematic literature review. Flodmark et al., 2006 (110)

A review of recent controlled studies with follow-up of at least 12 mo and results measured as BMI, skinfold thickness or the percentage of overweight/obesity found 24 studies of which 8 had a positive effect on obesity and 16 reported neutral results. This indicates that it is possible to prevent obesity in children and adolescents through school-based programs that combine the promotion of healthy dietary habits and physical activity, with little risk of negative effects.

Obesity prevention: evidence statements and reviews. NICE, 2006 (111)

Two systematic reviews: one preschool and family-based and one school-based (sections 8 and 9, and appendices 6 and 7, respectively). Preschool interventions can show small effects on weight gain and favorable changes in diet and physical activity levels. School-based interventions equivocal with some studies showing effects on weight but most showing effects only on diet and activity. Lack of large-scale and longer-term studies. Some evidence supporting a multicomponent or "whole-of-school" approach. Some evidence that environment—e.g., pricing and availability of different foods—can influence children's food choices.

The Role of Schools in Obesity Prevention. Story et al., 2006 (112)

USA: Evaluations of a small number of school-based controlled interventions have shown success at reducing weight gain among children. These interventions typically involve components that teach children about nutrition, promote reductions in television viewing, and engage children in physical activity. Many also involve parents to promote more healthful eating and greater physical activity when children are not in school. These studies indicate that school-based programs, policies, and environments can make a difference in childhood obesity.

The role of child care settings in obesity prevention. Story et al., 2006 (113)

United States: Little evidence is available, but existing research suggests that the nutritional quality of meals and snacks may be poor and activity levels may be inadequate. With a large share of young children attending child care and preschool programs, policymakers should place a high priority on understanding what policies and practices in these settings can prevent childhood obesity.

(Continued)

Table 3 Reviews of Interventions to Prevent Obesity and Promote Healthy Weights in Infants and Children, 1996–2007 (*Continued*)

Review	Notes
The role of parents in preventing childhood obesity. Lindsay et al., 2006 (114)	United States: There is insufficient high-quality evidence on the effectiveness of obesity-prevention programs that center on parental involvement. The authors also review research evaluating school-based interventions that include components targeted at parents and conclude that intervention programs and policies need to be multifaceted and community wide. Research shows that successful intervention must involve and work directly with parents from the very early stages of child development and growth to make healthful changes in the home and to reinforce and support healthful eating and regular physical activity.
School-based interventions for childhood and adolescent obesity. Sharma, 2006 (115)	Most of the 11 U.K. and U.S. interventions analyzed were focused on individual behavior change approaches, and observed modest short-term changes in behaviors and mixed results with indicators of obesity. TV watching seemed the most modifiable behavior, followed by physical activity and nutrition behaviors. Outcome measures such as lowered BMI, triceps skinfold thickness, and waist circumference were not measured in all studies.
International school-based interventions for preventing obesity in children. Sharma, 2007 (116)	Of the 21 non-U.S. interventions analyzed, 9 targeted nutrition behaviors and 7 aimed to modify both physical activity and nutrition behaviors. Only five were based on any explicit behavioral theory. All interventions that documented parental involvement successfully influenced obesity indices. Most interventions (16) focused on individual-level behavior change approaches and most used experimental designs with at least 1-yr follow-up.
Strategies for the prevention and control of obesity in the school setting: systematic review and meta-analysis. Katz et al., 2007 (117)	Nutrition and physical activity interventions resulted in significant reductions in body weight compared to controls. Parental or family involvement seemed to modify the effects of nutrition and physical activity interventions on weight reduction: the magnitude of weight reduction was larger when the analysis was limited to studies where parental or family involvement was incorporated in the intervention curriculum.

[a]Cochrane Library services are available at http://www.cochrane.org/index.htm.

Abbreviations: CVD, cardiovascular disease; UNICEF, United Nations Children's Fund; BFH, Baby Friendly Hospital; BMI, body mass index.

Interventions that link school and home activities appear to influence knowledge but not necessarily behavior (121). Family-based interventions tend to be more expensive than school-based interventions. Furthermore, family-based interventions may be least effective when trying to prevent obesity in adolescents.

School-Based Interventions

There is now a fairly large body of evidence on school-based interventions, which in summary shows that gains in understanding of children's nutrition, increases in physical activity, and alterations in diet are possible, but that only a small number of interventions appear able to demonstrate a significant effect on indicators of adiposity. Furthermore, very few studies last longer than a year, and in those that have followed children over a longer period there is evidence that the initial advantages gained by the intervention may be reduced over time (122).

Most of the formal reviews have identified the need to combine multiple approaches to obesity prevention—including education, food services, and physical activity—as a means of increasing the likelihood of achieving change. Effectiveness may be increased by linking the school-based program to out-of-school action through the family and community. Increases in school physical activity opportunities and reduced television viewing time in school hours and at home appear to be at least as important as classroom health education.

Further points identified in the reviews include the following:

- Approaches need to be tailored to age groups, ethnic groups, and gender of the target population.
- Effective initiatives to increase physical activity are those which involve children through the whole school day, including lunch and breaks/recesses, as well as class time and physical education lessons.
- Physical exercise should include not only the traditional sports and gymnastic activities but also others that appeal to children, such as dance clubs, self-defense lessons and skills training, and interventions that aim to reduce screen-watching behavior (television, computer, and video game use).
- Although schemes to encourage walking and cycling to school may be beneficial to health, there is no good evidence available on which to base a recommendation.
- Dietary change appears most likely if the intervention focuses on promoting one aspect of a healthy diet, such as increasing fruit and vegetable intake. Restricting the choices of food available to children is associated with healthier eating.
- Introducing nutrition standards for school foods needs to be supported by measures to ensure the healthy

options are selected, including price, availability (queues), and eating environment. A comprehensive school food service policy should include snacks brought to school, vending machines, snack bars, and access to local shops during breaks.
- Children will choose healthier options from vending machines, such as mineral water, pure fruit juice, and skimmed milk, even when healthy drinks vending machines are set alongside the school's usual vending machine. The key to successful healthy drinks vending is pupil involvement, appropriate location of the vending machine close to the dining area, product pricing, and ensuring continuity of provision (that the machine is full and in working order).
- Breakfast clubs (food provided when children arrive early at school) can have a beneficial effect on behavior, dietary intake, health, social interaction, concentration and learning, attendance and punctuality. The clubs can reach lower income families and so address inequalities.

Lytle et al. reviewed the evidence base for school interventions and suggested several factors that may improve success rates, notably ensuring an adequate length of intervention and ensuring the involvement of all participants to prevent dropout (78). The authors also noted that heterogeneity, i.e., the involvement of participants from diverse cultural backgrounds, is rarely catered for in the experimental designs where "one size fits all," and this may compromise the ability to show significant effects. The authors recommend programs that are more flexible and responsive to the social and cultural environments in which they occur, perhaps inviting the active participation of community members during the design of the intervention.

Richter et al. reviewed health promotion schemes among children and youth and concluded that such interventions are more likely to be successful if they occur in the context of health-promoting environments rather than being introduced in isolation (123). This raises the wider context for health promotion and the need to consider interventions that change the social, cultural, and economic environments. Few controlled scientific studies are able to undertake the degree of community intervention necessary to provide rigorous evidence of the effects of changing cultural or social aspects of the environment, although there is some evidence on altering economic aspects: French and Story have undertaken a series of interventions to examine the impact of pricing on food choices by children and have shown dramatic changes in behavior induced by alterations in relative price (106). That there are so few studies of the influence on a child of his or her surrounding environment is a significant evidence gap which is only gradually being filled (124).

Expert Recommendations

Besides the evidence reviews, policies are informed by the assessments made by expert consultations. Such assessments are able to consider target groups, settings, and approaches that are not amenable to controlled trials but that, on the basis of other forms of evidence, are likely to be important in controlling the obesity epidemic at a population level.

Most expert consultations have reflected on the systematic reviews of the sort summarized in Table 3 and have concluded that the intervention successes have been small compared with the public health change required and that a wider range of policy options will need to be considered to tackle obesity. Three World Health Organization expert consultations have reached conclusions similar to those already summarized here, and for reasons of space we have focused below on the additional recommendations they have made in relation to obesity prevention among children and youth.

WHO Consultation on Obesity 1997 (3)

This consultation described strategies for implementing obesity prevention and treatment in different health service systems. The report urges national governments to develop their commitment to obesity control and to implement food-based dietary guidelines. Actions require shared responsibilities between government, commercial operators, consumers, and the media, all of whom have roles to play in obesity prevention. The report suggests that successful public health campaigns need

- to be sustained over time, allowing 10 years or more to show signs of success;
- to be introduced in stages to support a transition from awareness through motivation and experimentation and resulting in behavior change;
- to be supported by legislation as well as education, as was the case with cigarette sales to minors and car seat belt use;
- the educational elements to be consistent across different media, including health and education professionals, industry promotional messages and mass media; and
- full use to be made of the support available from advocacy organization and experts and role models who can drive public attitudes and influence politicians.

WHO/FAO Expert Consultation on Diet, Nutrition and the Prevention of Chronic Diseases, 2002 (125)

This consultation made recommendations for diet and nutrition in prevention of chronic diseases including obesity.

Specifically for the prevention of child obesity, it recommended the following:

- Promotion of exclusive breast-feeding for infants, avoiding the use of sugars and starches in feeding formula, allowing infants to self-regulate their energy intake
- Promotion of active lifestyles, limited television viewing, promotion of plentiful fruit and vegetable consumption, restricted consumption of energy-dense, micronutrient-poor foods (e.g., snacks, soft drinks) for older children
- Limiting the exposure of young children to heavy marketing practices for energy-dense, micronutrient-poor foods
- Special attention, in some communities, to avoid overfeeding of stunted individuals (e.g., infants of low weight for age but normal weight for height)
- Protection and promotion of traditional diets that promote health (e.g., diets with a high level of fruits and vegetables)
- Education for parents with experience of food insecurity should stress that adiposity in children does not represent good health
- Measures for modification of the environment in order to enhance physical activity

WHO Expert Meeting on Childhood Obesity, 2005 (126)

An expert meeting on child obesity issues made a number of recommendations concerning the most appropriate forms of intervention at school and community level and the types of intervention that are needed at national and international levels to ensure that community-level interventions are supported. The meeting endorsed the WHO Global Strategy on Diet, Physical Activity and Health (6) and in addition recommended:

Maternity and early year services need greater attention.

Health service staff should be routinely monitoring and advising women, even before reproductive age.

Parents should be encouraged to interact with their children, and especially infants in their earliest years, to promote active play and developmental growth.

Nurseries and kindergartens should ensure that they do not unnecessarily restrict physical activity during the growing years.

Interventions to ensure adequate growth should avoid excess weight gain.

Schools are important for access to children and can set an example in their community. Multidisciplinary and "whole-of-school" approaches are desirable and may benefit the wider community.

Schools need to be fully funded so that they do not need to raise funds from commercial interests, especially those with potentially conflicting eating messages.

Schools should set high standards to ensure a health promoting food environment.

Daily exercise periods should be provided in all grades, with the programs appealing to children.

Health care facilities need to offer preventive services and health promoting activities, in cooperation with schools and community services. Health care staffs have a role in monitoring children's growth to recognize early signs of malnourishment, including stunting and overweight, and provide appropriate responses.

Governments need to consider cross-departmental, cross-sectoral policies that should be implemented through a responsible lead department. The policies and programs should be monitored by a separate agency, such as a parliamentary scrutiny committee or an "obesity observatory." In addition, governments can

help build capacity at national and at local levels to support public health initiatives;

ensure that research support and fiscal incentives given to food and agricultural enterprises include health criteria;

ensure that political donations from food companies are restricted or banned;

improve access to and affordability of fruits and vegetables, especially for low income and disadvantaged population groups; and

support moves to ensure that all UN agencies have policies that are consistent with the WHO Global Strategy.

Commercial enterprises should ensure that the promotion of food products should be consistent with a healthy diet.

Enterprises should implement the WHO-UNICEF Code of Marketing of Breast Milk Substitutes in all countries and support the development of an International Code of Marketing of Food to Children.

The meeting also noted that, in some cultures, high levels of obesity are acceptable, or even considered desirable, while in other cultures there is strong prejudice against overweight people, which many children are clearly aware of. Measures to reduce the prevalence of obesity need to be introduced that emphasize healthy behaviors and activities rather than idealized weight or appearance.

Furthermore, although there appears to be little evidence suggesting that treatments of obesity can lead to eating disorders, there is a theoretical risk that preventive programs that focus on dietary restrictions may induce anxiety and disrupted eating patterns in vulnerable children, which may in turn trigger a disorder.

Some children are resistant to participation in sports activities for various reasons, and schools may need to help staff promote and provide physical activities that children are attracted to, and to recognize and prevent discriminatory behavior.

RESEARCH AND POLICY GAPS

The WHO Kobe meeting described above (126) made several recommendations on research needs, including the following:

- All interventions should provide resource and cost estimates. Evaluation should include process evaluation measures and can include impact on other parties, such as parents and siblings.
- Interventions using control groups should be explicit about what the control group experiences. Phrases like "normal care" or "normal curriculum" or "standard school PE classes" are not helpful, especially if normal practices have been changing over the years.
- There is a need for more interventions looking into the needs of specific subpopulations, including immigrant groups, low income groups, and specific ethnic and cultural groups.
- New approaches to interventions, including prospective meta-analyses, should be considered.
- There is a need for an international agency to encourage networking of community-based interventions, support methods of evaluation, and assist in the analysis of the cost-effectiveness of initiatives.
- Research reviews should not be funded by commercial interests. There is a need to evaluate the impact of programs funded by industry and other sources of potential bias in order to examine their contribution to the evidence base.

A Wider Scope for the Evidence Base

Such suggestions for improving the evidence base are welcome, but may not be sufficient to meet the needs of policy-makers. While evidence-based public health should incorporate the same rigor and attention to internal validity as clinical trials, it should also maintain contextual and policy relevance, have a realistic chance of implementation, and show potential sustainability (56). Evidence of effectiveness is not sufficient by itself to guide appropriate decision-making, and true evidence-based policy-making is probably quite rare (127). Asking policy-makers to set out the forms of evidence they may need can help move from the classical "evidence-based practice" approach toward a model using "practice-based evidence" more closely linked to the prevailing economic and political processes that shape the policy context.

Evidence in its widest sense is information providing a level of certainty about the truth of a proposition (128). In relation to obesity prevention, Swinburn has grouped evidence into observational, experimental, extrapolated, and experience-based sources of evidence and information (56). In practice, there is considerable variation in the quantity and quality of information available in respect of different settings, approaches, and target groups for interventions to prevent obesity. There is virtually no evidence concerning the potential effects on obesity of altering social and economic policies, such as agricultural production, trade, or food-pricing policies, even though these are certain determinants of food availability and powerful influences on dietary intake. Much more evidence is available on localized attempts to influence the consumer through various means: education, exhortation, school training, parental training, and similar approaches that target the individual.

It is clear from the recent economically based analyses for the U.K. Treasury (129) that interventions relating to smoking, obesity, and physical inactivity require economic modeling in order to compare cost-benefit or cost-effectiveness ratios.

In a review of the determinants of dietary trends, Haddad (130) notes the need to consider several macroeconomic factors, including income growth, urbanization, and the relative prices of foods and their availability, which are affected by mass production technology and commodity costs, along with retail distribution chains and catering outlets. Similarly, more evidence is needed on the impact of investment strategies, such as foreign direct investment in sectors affecting food supplies—agriculture, food manufacturing, retailing, and catering (e.g., fast-food catering)—for their potential effects on the recipient population's diet and health, mediated through food prices and availability. Routine economic planning approaches have not been applied sufficiently for analyses of options for social policy change. The evidence required to show how policy changes in these areas might affect consumption patterns, and subsequent chronic disease rates have received too little attention.

In all the above suggestions, similar analyses could be undertaken relating to the products that affect physical environment and influence physical activity, or which encourage sedentary behavior. The commercial and upstream production and marketing of products relating to physical activity—such as television program consumption, video game playing, passive music playing, use of cars for short journeys, street design, building design, safety of outdoor play areas and parks—are all in need of better research understanding to demonstrate to policy-makers that interventions can be a worthwhile investment.

Evidence for Prevention as an Investment

In the last decade there has been increasing interest in the suggestion that health promotion should be described in the language of investment, with obesity prevention policy seen as an investment portfolio (131). Portfolios should carry a mixture of safe low-return reliable savings schemes and risky potentially high-return gambles, so investments in preventing obesity can carry a mixture of low-risk, low-cost approaches and high-risk, high-cost initiatives. A return on investment can be measured in terms of expected health gains and other desired outcomes. The risk can be measured in terms of the consistency of the impact of an intervention and indications of its likely effectiveness (56,132). Thus, intensive interventions within small groups or individuals might be low risk, as they consistently result in changes in behavior and other outcomes. However, the overall return may only be small to moderate as the effect of the intervention may result in only a slight impact on the health status of the community as a whole.

An important observation here is that investments require different types of information including costs, likely effectiveness, likely depth and reach of impact, sustainability and acceptability. Furthermore, when making investment decisions, attention needs to be paid to the contextual influences that can affect investment potential—the social, economic, and physical environments that can inhibit or enhance the chance of success.

Evidence of Costs and Cost Benefits

Although of primary concern to policy-makers and managers in public health, a remarkable feature of the evaluations and systematic reviews of interventions is that they rarely mention the costs of the various programs they examine, and make no estimates of cost effectiveness. A recent review of workplace and community interventions noted that only two studies that met the criteria for inclusion provided cost-effectiveness analyses of worksite interventions to prevent and control overweight and obesity (94). These indicated that costs of less than $1 per employee per year could engage 1% of the population at risk in onsite programs for weight loss.

For child obesity prevention, we have identified only one study that examined in detail the costs of an intervention program (the U.S. Planet Health Program) (133). This study estimated the intervention to have cost some $34,000 (or $14 per student per year), and that the program would prevent an estimated 1.9% of the female students from becoming overweight adults. As a result, society could expect to save an estimated $16,000 in medical care costs and $25,000 in loss of productivity, indicating a net saving

Table 4 Benefits and Costs of Different Child Obesity Interventions

Type of intervention	Reduction per child participant	Reduction for population	Gross cost per DALY[a]
Curbs on TV advertising	<0.02 DALY	37,000 DALYs	Under $8
Targeted multifaceted school-based program	0.08 DALY	360 DALYs	Over $1,000
Curbs on soft drink consumption	0.01 DALY	5,300 DALYs	Over $1,000
Curbs on TV viewing	0.03 DALY	8,600 DALYs	Over $1,500
Targeted family-based program	0.9–1.4 DALYs	2,700 DALYs	Over $3,000
Multifaceted school-based program including active PE	<0.08 DALY	8,000 DALYs	Over $5,000
Multifaceted school-based program without active PE	<0.02 DALY	1,600 DALYs	Over $6,000
Orlistat therapy	0.5–0.8 DALY	450 DALYs	Over $8,000
Laparoscopic adjustable gastric banding	2.7–3.3 DALYs	12,000 DALYs	Over $9,000
Targeted GP program	<0.06 DALY	510 DALYs	Over $15,000
Active After School Communities	<0.01 DALY	450 DALYs	Over $50,000
Walking School Bus	<0.01 DALY	30 DALYs	Over $120,000

[a]Australian dollars (Aus$1 = US$0.78)
Abbreviation: DALY, disability-adjusted life year.
Sources: From Ref. 135 and 136.

of around $7000 to society. It is not clear if the costs of such a program would be favorable in other economic contexts, where the intervention, productivity, and medical costs may be different. Planet Health's estimated cost-effectiveness ratio gives a value of $4305 per quality-adjusted life year, which compares favorably with interventions such as the treatment of hypertension, low-cholesterol diet therapies, some diabetes screening programs and treatments, and adult exercise programs (134).

A study undertaken in Australia by the government of Victoria (135,136) has calculated the likely health gains (in terms of reduced disability-adjusted life years) for a range of obesity interventions based on Australian data and estimated for Australian child demographics. This suggests that, although some policies have only small effects in reducing an individual child's risk, when adjusted for likely reach across population groups and penetration within population groups, the results can be illuminating for policy-makers (Table 4).

The cost element of an intervention is clearly a highly significant factor in the appraisal of interventions, and yet these details are rarely included in the published scientific reports on interventions. Details about costs should be collected prospectively and reported explicitly, and instruments need to be developed for obtaining cost data (both direct costs for materials and personnel, and indirect costs such as those for travel time or time lost from school or lost by parents in employment). At the very least, intervention trials should report their budgets for the intervention and provide details of the resources required for running the intervention.

Policy-makers make judgments on alternative options to tackle obesity on several dimensions, including cost, public support and political acceptability, proportionality and transferability, as well as scientific validity (57,137), and obesity researchers need to provide evidence on all these dimensions whenever and wherever they can.

REFERENCES

1. Seidell JC, Nooyens AJ, Visscher TL. Cost-effective measures to prevent obesity: epidemiological basis and appropriate target groups. Proc Nutr Soc 2005; 64(1):1–5.
2. Wang Y, Lobstein T. Worldwide trends in childhood overweight and obesity. Int J Ped Obesity 2006; 1(1):11–25.
3. World Health Organization. Obesity, preventing and managing the global epidemic. Report of a WHO Consultation. Technical Report Series 894. Geneva: World Health Organization, 2000.
4. Lobstein T, Baur L, Uauy R, IASO International Obesity TaskForce. Obesity in children and young people: a crisis in public health. Obes Rev 2004; 5(suppl 1):4–104.
5. Parsons TJ, Power C, Logan S, et al. Childhood predictors of adult obesity: a systematic review. Int J Obes Relat Metab Disord 1999; 23(suppl 8):1–107.
6. World Health Organization. Global Strategy on Diet, Physical Activity and Health. Geneva: World Health Organization, 2004.
7. French SA. Public health strategies for dietary change: schools and workplaces. J Nutr 2005; 135(4):910–912.
8. Ledikwe JH, Ello-Martin JA, Rolls BJ. Portion sizes and the obesity epidemic. J Nutr 2005; 135(4):905–909.
9. Drewnowski A, Rolls BJ. How to modify the food environment. J Nutr 2005; 135(4):898–899.
10. Eurobarometer. European Union citizens and sources of information about health. Eurobarometer special report 58.0. Brussels: European Commission DG Sanco, 2003.

Available at: http://europa.eu.int/comm/public_opinion/archives/ebs/ebs_179_en.pdf. Accessed August 2007.

11. Cockerham WC, Rütten A, Abel T. Conceptualizing contemporary health lifestyles. Moving beyond Weber. Sociol Q 1997; 38(2):321–342.

12. Department of Health. Choosing Health: Making Healthy Choices Easier. London: The Stationery Office, 2004.

13. Burke V, Milligan RA, Thompson C, et al. A controlled trial of health promotion programs in 11-year-olds using physical activity "enrichment" for higher risk children. J Pediatr 1998; 132(5):840–848.

14. Caballero B, Clay T, Davis SM, et al. Pathways: a school-based, randomized controlled trial for the prevention of obesity in American Indian schoolchildren. Am J Clin Nutr 2003; 78(5):1030–1038.

15. Chen MY, Huang LH, Wang EK, et al. The effectiveness of health promotion counseling for overweight adolescent nursing students in Taiwan. Public Health Nurs 2001; 18(5):350–356.

16. Coleman KJ, Tiller CL, Sanchez J, et al. Prevention of the epidemic increase in child risk of overweight in low-income schools: the El Paso coordinated approach to child health. Arch Pediatr Adolesc Med 2005; 159(3): 217–224

17. Damon S, Dietrich S, Widhalm K. PRESTO—Prevention study of obesity: a project to prevent obesity during childhood and adolescence. Acta Paediatr Suppl 2005; 94(448):47–48.

18. Eliakim A, Kaven G, Berger I, et al. The effect of a combined intervention on body mass index and fitness in obese children and adolescents—a clinical experience. Eur J Pediatr 2002; 161(8):449–454.

19. Epstein LH, Gordy CC, Raynor HA, et al. Increasing fruit and vegetable intake and decreasing fat and sugar intake in families at risk for childhood obesity. Obes Res 2001; 9(3):171–178.

20. Gable S, Lutz S. Nutrition socialization experiences of children in the Head Start program. J Am Diet Assoc 2001; 101(5):572–577.

21. Graf C, Rost SV, Koch B, et al. Data from the StEP TWO program showing the effect on blood pressure and different parameters for obesity in overweight and obese primary school children. Cardiol Young 2005; 15:291–298.

22. He YF, Wang WY, Fu P, et al. Effects of a comprehensive intervention program on simple obesity of children in kindergarten. Zhonghua Er Ke Za Zhi 2004; 42(5): 333–336.

23. Jago R, Baranowski T. Non-curricular approaches for increasing physical activity in youth: a review. Prev Med 2004; 39(1):157–163.

24. James J, Kerr D. Prevention of childhood obesity by reducing soft drinks. Int J Obes 2005; 29(suppl 2):54–57.

25. Kain J, Uauy R, Albala C, et al. School-based obesity prevention in Chilean primary school children: methodology and evaluation of a controlled study. Int J Obes 2004; 28(4):483–493.

26. Kanda A, Kamiyama Y, Kawaguchi T. Association of reduction in parental overweight with reduction in children's overweight with a 3-year follow-up. Prev Med 2004; 39(2):369–372.

27. Gill T, King L, Webb K. Best Options for Promoting Healthy Weight and Preventing Weight Gain in NSW. Sydney: University of Sydney, 2005. Available at: http://www.cphn.mmb.usyd.edu.au/resources/FinalHealthy-Weightreport160305.pdf. Accessed August 2007.

28. Mamalakis G, Kafatos A, Manios Y, et al. Obesity indices in a cohort of primary school children in Crete: a six year prospective study. Int J Obes 2000; 24(6):765–771.

29. Manios Y, Moschandreas J, Hatzis C, et al. Health and nutrition education in primary schools of Crete: changes in chronic disease risk factors following a 6-year intervention program. Br J Nutr 2002; 88(3):315–324.

30. Mo-suwan L, Junjana C, Puetpaiboon A. Increasing obesity in school children in a transitional society and the effect of the weight control program. Southeast Asian J Trop Med Public Health 1993; 24(3):590–594 [erratum in Southeast Asian J Trop Med Public Health 1994; 25 (1):224].

31. Mo-suwan L, Pongprapai S, Junjana C, et al. Effects of a controlled trial of a school-based exercise program on the obesity indexes of preschool children. Am J Clin Nutr 1998; 68(5):1006–1011.

32. Muller MJ, Asbeck I, Mast M, et al. Prevention of obesity—more than an intention. Concept and first results of Kiel Obesity Prevention Study (KOPS). Int J Obes 2001; 25(suppl 1):66–74.

33. Nielsen J, Gerlow J. Evalution of a Project for Families with Overweight Children [original report in Danish: Evaluering af projekt for familier med overvaegtige born]. Copenhagen: Udviklings- og Formidlingscenter for Born og Unge, 2004.

34. New South Wales Nutrition Project Register, 2001. Reported in Gill T, King L, Webb K. Best Options for Promoting Healthy Weight and Preventing Weight Gain in NSW. Sydney: University of Sydney, 2005. Available at: http://www.cphn.mmb.usyd.edu.au/resources/FinalHealthy-Weightreport160305.pdf. Accessed August 2007.

35. Ray R, Lim LH, Ling SL. Obesity in preschool children: an intervention program in primary health care in Singapore. Ann Acad Med Singapore 1994; 23(3):335–341.

36. Reilly JJ, McDowell ZC. Physical activity interventions in the prevention and treatment of pediatric obesity: systematic review and critical appraisal. Proc Nutr Soc 2003; 62(3):611–619.

37. Sahota P, Rudolf MCJ, Dixey R, et al. Evaluation of implementation and effect of primary school based intervention to reduce risk factors for obesity. BMJ 2001; 323:1027–1029.

38. Sahota P, Rudolf MCJ, Dixey R, et al. Randomised controlled trial of primary school based intervention to reduce risk factors for obesity. BMJ 2001; 323:1029–1032.

39. Shi-Chang X, Xin-Wei Z, Shui-Yang X, et al. Creating health-promoting schools in China with a focus on nutrition. Health Promot Int 2004; 19(4):409–418.

40. Simon C, Wagner A, DiVita C, et al. Intervention centred on adolescents' physical activity and sedentary behavior (ICAPS): concept and 6-month results. Int J Obes 2004; 28(suppl 3):96–103.

41. Singapore Ministry of Health. The State of Health 2001. The Report of the Director of Medical Services. Singapore: Ministry of Health, 2002.

42. Toh CM, Cutter J, Chew SK. School based intervention has reduced obesity in Singapore. BMJ 2002; 324:427.

43. Warren JM, Henry CJ, Lightowler HJ, et al. Evaluation of a pilot school program aimed at the prevention of obesity in children. Health Promot Int 2003; 18(4):287–296.

44. WHO Collaborating Centre for Obesity Prevention. Sentinel Site for Obesity Project: Be Active Eat Well. Available at: http://www.deakin.edu.au/hmnbs/who-obesity/downloads/reports/baew-2005pr.php. Accessed August 2007.

45. WHO Collaborating Centre for Obesity Prevention. OPIC Mangere project. Available at: http://www.deakin.edu.au/hmnbs/who-obesity/downloads/reports/mangere-2004pr.php. Accessed August 2007.

46. WHO Collaborating Centre for Obesity Prevention. OPIC Ma'alahi program. Available at: http://www.deakin.edu.au/hmnbs/who-obesity/downloads/reports/maalahi-2004pr.php. Accessed August 2007.

47. Wu FL, Yu S, Wei IL, et al. Weight-control behavior among obese children: association with family-related factors. J Nurs Res 2003; 11(1):19–30.

48. Yoshinaga M, Sameshima K, Miyata K, et al. Prevention of mildly overweight children from development of more overweight condition. Prev Med 2004; 38(2):172–174

49. Matsudo V, Matsudo S, Andrade D, et al. Promotion of physical activity in a developing country: the Agita Sao Paulo experience. Public Health Nutr 2002; 5(1A):253–261.

50. World Health Organization Fruit and Vegetable Promotion Initiative. A Meeting Report, August 24–27, 2003 (Document WHO/NMH/NPH/NNP/0308). Geneva: World Health Organization, 2003.

51. Aimbetova G. A health boost for school children. In: Network News—The European Network of Health Promoting Schools, 2002. Available at: http://www.euro.who.int/document/enhps/ENHPSnews072002.pdf. Accessed August 2007.

52. UNICEF. The Baby Friendly Hospital Initiative, 2007. Available at: http://www.unicef.org/program/breastfeeding/baby.htm. Accessed August 2007.

53. Carr S. Water in school is cool! Health News for Schools. 2004; 16:2. Available at: http://www.beh.nhs.uk/healthwise/pdf/Schlnews16.pdf. Accessed August 2007.

54. http://www.walkingbus.com/. Accessed August 2007.

55. International Obesity TaskForce (IOTF). Collected sources held in the International Obesity TaskForce archives (IOTF), International Association for the Study of Obesity, 231 North Gower Street, London. Available at: http://www.iotf.org. Accessed December 2005.

56. Swinburn B, Gill T, Kumanyika S. Obesity prevention: a proposed framework for translating evidence into action. Obes Rev 2005; 6(1):23–33.

57. Lobstein T. Comment: preventing child obesity—an art and a science. Obes Rev 2006; 7(suppl 1):1–5.

58. Centers for Disease Control and Prevention (CDC). Guidelines for school health programs to promote lifelong healthy eating. MMWR 1996; 45(RR-9):1–33.

59. NHS Centre for Reviews and Dissemination (NHS-CRD). The prevention and treatment of obesity. Effective Health Care 1997; 3(2):1–12. Available at: http://www.york.ac.uk/inst/crd/ehc32.pdf. Accessed August 2007.

60. Resnicow K, Robinson TN. School-based cardiovascular disease prevention studies: review and synthesis. Ann Epidemiol 1997; 7(suppl), S14–S31.

61. Stone EJ, McKenzie TL, Welk GJ, et al. Effects of physical activity interventions in youth. Review and synthesis. Am J Prev Med 1998; 15(4):298–315.

62. Tedstone A, Dunce N, Aviles M, et al. Effectiveness of Interventions to Promote Healthy Feeding in Infants Under One Year of Age: A Review. London: Health Education Authority, 1998.

63. Tedstone A, Aviles M, Shetty PS et al. Effectiveness of Interventions to Promote Healthy Eating in Preschool Children Aged 1 to 5 Years. London: Health Education Authority, 1998.

64. Story M. School-based approaches for preventing and treating obesity. Int J Obes 1999; 23(suppl 2):S43–S51.

65. Goran M, Reynolds KD, Lindquist CH. Role of physical activity in the prevention of obesity in children. Int J Obes 1999; 23(suppl 3):S18–S33.

66. Hardeman W, Griffin S, Johnston M, et al. Interventions to prevent weight gain, a systematic review of psychological models and behavior change methods. Int J Obes 2000; 24(2):131–143.

67. Stockley L. Consolidation and Updating the Evidence Base for the Promotion of Breastfeeding. Cardiff: National Assembly for Wales, 2001. Available at: http://www.wales.nhs.uk/publications/bfeedingevidence-base.pdf. Accessed August 2007.

68. Sjostrom M, Sockley L. Toward Public Health Nutrition Strategies in the European Union to Implement Food Based Dietary Guidelines and to Enhance Healthier Lifestyles. Working Party 3: EURODIET Final report. Heraklion: University of Crete. 2000. Available at: http://eurodiet.med.uoc.gr/. Accessed August 2007.

69. Fairbank L, O'Meara S, Renfrew MJ, et al. A systematic review to evaluate the effectiveness of interventions to promote the initiation of breastfeeding. Health Technol Assess 2000; 4(25):1–169. Available at: http://www.hta.ac.uk/project/1084.asp. Accessed August 2007.

70. Meininger JC. School-based interventions for primary prevention of cardiovascular disease: evidence of effects for minority populations. Annu Rev Nurs Res 2000; 18:219–244.

71. Dietz W, Gortmaker S. Preventing obesity in children and adolescents. Annu Rev Publ Health 2001; 22:337–353.

72. Steinbeck K. The importance of physical activity in the prevention of overweight and obesity in childhood: a review and an opinion. Obes Rev 2001; 2(2):117–130.

73. Dobbins M, Lockett D, Michel I, et al. The Effectiveness of School-based Interventions in Promoting Physical Activity and Fitness Among Children and Youth, A Systematic Review. Final Report. Effective Public Health Practice Project. Hamilton, Ontario: Public Health Branch, Ministry of Health and Long Term Care,

2001. Available at: http://www.nhsru.com/documents/Physical-Activity-Review.pdf. Accessed August 2007.

74. Campbell K, Waters E, O'Meara S, et al. Interventions for preventing obesity in childhood: A systematic review. Obes Rev 2001; 2(3):149–157.

75. de Oliveira MI, Camacho LA, Tedstone AE. Extending breastfeeding duration through primary care: a systematic review of prenatal and postnatal interventions. J Hum Lact 2001; 17(4):326–343.

76. French S, Story M, Jeffery RW. Environmental influences on eating and physical activity. Annu Rev Publ Health 2001; 22:309–335.

77. NHS Centre for Reviews and Dissemination (NHS-CRD) The prevention and treatment of childhood obesity. Effective Health Care Bull 2002; 7(6):1–12. Available at: http://www.york.ac.uk/inst/crd/ehc76.pdf. Accessed August 2007.

78. Lytle LA, Jacobs DR, Perry CL, et al. Achieving physiological change in school-based intervention trials: what makes a preventive intervention successful? Brit J Nutr 2002; 88(3):219–221.

79. Task Force on Community Preventive Services. Recommendations to increase physical activity in communities. Am J Prev Med 2002; 22(suppl 4):67–72.

80. Kahn EB, Ramsey LT, Brownson RC, et al. The effectiveness of interventions to increase physical activity, a systematic review. Am J Prev Med 2002; 22(suppl 4):73–107.

81. Micucci S, Thomas H, Vohra J. The Effectiveness of School-Based Strategies for the Primary Prevention of Obesity and for Promoting Physical Activity and Nutrition, the Major Modifiable Risk Factors for Type 2 Diabetes: Review of Reviews. Hamilton: City of Hamilton Public Health Research, Education and Development Program, 2002.

82. Reilly JJ, Wilson ML, Summerbell CD, et al. Obesity, diagnosis, prevention, and treatment, evidence based answers to common questions. Arch Dis Child 2002; 86(6):392–394.

83. Schmitz KH, Jeffrey RW. Prevention of obesity. In: Wadden TA, Stunkard AJ, eds. Handbook of Obesity Treatment New York: Guilford Press, 2002:556–593.

84. Swedish Council on Technology Assessment in Health Care. Obesity—problems and interventions. Report No. 160. Stockholm: The Swedish Council on Technology Assessment in Health Care, 2002. Available at: http://www.sbu.se/Filer/Content0/publikationer/1/obesity_2002/obsesityslut.pdf. Accessed August 2007.

85. Muller MJ, Mast M, Asbeck I, et al. Prevention of obesity—is it possible? Obes Rev 2003; 2(1):15–28.

86. Mulvihill C, Quigley R. The Management of Obesity and Overweight: An Analysis of Reviews of Diet, Physical Activity and Behavioral Approaches. Evidence briefing. London: Health Development Agency, 2003. Available at: http://www.nepho.org. uk/view_file.php?c=1612. Accessed August 2007.

87. McLean N, Griffin S, Toney K, et al. Family involvement in weight control, weight maintenance and weight-loss interventions: a systematic review of randomised trials. Int J Obes 2003; 27(9):987–1005.

88. Protheroe L, Dyson L, Renfrew MJ, et al. The Effectiveness of Public Health Interventions to Promote the Initiation of Breastfeeding: Evidence Briefing. London: Health Development Agency, 2003. Available at: http://www.publichealth.nice.org.uk/download.aspx?o=502585. Accessed August 2007.

89. Clemmens D, Hayman LL. Increasing activity to reduce obesity in adolescent girls: a research review. J Obstet Gynecol Neonatal Nurs 2004; 33(6):801–808.

90. Carrel AL, Bernhardt DT. Exercise prescription for the prevention of obesity in adolescents. Curr Sports Med Rep 2004; 3(6):330–336.

91. Casey L, Crumley E. Addressing Childhood Obesity: The Evidence for Action. Ottawa: Canadian Association of Pediatric Health Centres, 2004. Available at: http://www.cihr-irsc.gc.ca/e/23293.html. Accessed August 2007.

92. Worsley A, Crawford D. Review of Children's Healthy Eating Interventions. Public Health Nutrition Evidence Based Health Promotion Research and Resource Project. Healthy Eating Programs for Children Ages 0–15 Years. Melbourne: Deakin University, 2004.

93. Hayman LL, Williams CL, Daniels SR, et al. Cardiovascular health promotion in the schools: a statement for health and education professionals and child health advocates from the Committee on Atherosclerosis, Hypertension, and Obesity in Youth (AHOY) of the Council on Cardiovascular Disease in the Young, American Heart Association. Circulation 2004; 110(15):2266–2275. Available at: http://www.circ.ahajournals.org/cgi/content/full/110/15/2266. Accessed August 2007.

94. Katz DL, O'Connell M, Yeh MC, et al. Public health strategies for preventing and controlling overweight and obesity in school and worksite settings: a report on recommendations of the Task Force on Community Preventive Services. MMWR 2005; 54(RR-10):1–12.

95. Wareham NJ, van Sluijs EM, Ekelund U. Physical activity and obesity prevention: a review of the current evidence. Proc Nutr Soc 2005; 64(2):229–247.

96. Ells LJ, Campbell K, Lidstone J, et al. Prevention of childhood obesity. Best Pract Res Clin Endocrinol Metab 2005; 19(3):441–454.

97. Koplan JP, Liverman CT, Kraak VA, eds. Preventing Childhood Obesity: Health in the Balance. Institute of Medicine Committee on Prevention of Obesity in Children and Youth. Washington DC: The National Academies Press, 2005.

98. Whitlock EP, Williams SB, Gold R, et al. Screening and interventions for childhood overweight: a summary of evidence for the US Preventive Services Task Force. Pediatrics 2005; 116(1):e125–e144.

99. US Preventive Services Task Force. Screening and interventions for overweight in children and adolescents: recommendation statement. Pediatrics 2005; 116(1):205–209.

100. Merten S, Dratva J, Ackermann-Liebrich U. Do baby-friendly hospitals influence breastfeeding duration on a national level? Pediatrics 2005; 116(5):e702–e708.

101. Cattaneo A, Buzzetti R and the Breastfeeding Research and Training Working Group. Effect on rates of breastfeeding

of training for the Baby Friendly Hospital Initiative. BMJ 2001; 323:1358–1362.

102. Caldeira AP, Goncalves E. Assessment of the impact of implementing the Baby Friendly Hospital Initiative. J Pediatr (Rio J) 2007; 83(2):127–132.

103. Perez-Escamilla R. Evidence based breast-feeding promotion: the baby-friendly hospital initiative. J Nutr 2007; 137(2):484–487.

104. Veugelers PJ, Fitzgerald AL. Effectiveness of school programs in preventing childhood obesity: a multilevel comparison. Am J Public Health 2005; 95(3):432–435.

105. Muller MJ, Danielzik S, Pust S. School- and family-based interventions to prevent overweight in children. Proc Nutr Soc 2005; 64(2):249–254.

106. French SA, Story M. Obesity prevention in schools. In: Goran MI, Sothern MS, eds. Handbook of Pediatric Obesity: Etiology, Pathophysiology and Prevention. Boca Raton: CRC Taylor & Francis, 2006:291–309.

107. Flynn MA, McNeil DA, Maloff B, et al. Reducing obesity and related chronic disease risk in children and youth: a synthesis of evidence with "best practice" recommendations. Obes Rev 2006; 7(suppl 1):7–66.

108. Doak CM, Visscher TLS, Renders CM, et al. The prevention of overweight and obesity in children and adolescents: a review of interventions and programs. Obes Rev 2006; 7(1):111–136.

109. Cole K, Waldrop J, D'Auria J, et al. An integrative research review: effective school-based childhood overweight interventions. J Spec Pediatr Nurs 2006; 11(3):166–177.

110. Flodmark CE, Marcus C, Britton M. Interventions to prevent obesity in children and adolescents: a systematic literature review. Int J Obes 2006; 30(4):579–589.

111. National Institute for Health and Clinical Excellence (NICE). CG43 Obesity: Full Guideline, Section 3. Prevention: Evidence Statements and Reviews. London: NICE, 2006. Available at: http://www.guidance.nice.org.uk/CG43/guidance/section3/word/English. Accessed August 2007.

112. Story M, Kaphingst KM, French S. The role of schools in obesity prevention. In: McLanahan S et al., eds. Childhood Obesity (special issue). Future Child 2006; 16(1):109–142.

113. Story M, Kaphingst KM, French S. The role of child care settings in obesity prevention. In: McLanahan S, et al., eds. Childhood Obesity (special issue). Future Child 2006; 16(1):143–168.

114. Lindsay AC, Sussner KM, Kim J, Gortmaker S. The role of parents in preventing childhood obesity. In: McLanahan S, et al., eds. Childhood Obesity (special issue). Future Child 2006; 16(1):169–186.

115. Sharma M. School-based interventions for childhood and adolescent obesity. Obes Rev 2006; 7(3):261–269.

116. Sharma M. International school-based interventions for preventing obesity in children. Obes Rev 2007; 8(2):155–167.

117. Katz DL, O'Connell M, Njike VY, et al. Strategies for the prevention and control of obesity in the school setting: systematic review and meta-analysis. Int J Obes 2007;

advance online publication 31 July 2007; doi: 10.1038/sj.ijo.0803684.

118. Hastings G, Stead M, McDermott L, et al. Review of research on the effects of food promotion to children. Final report. Prepared for the Food Standards Agency. London: FSA, 2003. Available at: http://www.ism.stir.ac.uk/projects_food.htm. Accessed August 2007.

119. McGinnis JM, Gootman JA, Kraak VI, eds. Food Marketing to Children and Youth: Threat or Opportunity? Washington: Institute of Medicine Committee on Food Marketing and the Diets of Children and Youth; Washington DC: The National Academies Press, 2006.

120. St Jeor ST, Perumean-Chaney S, Sigman-Grant M, et al. Family-based interventions for the treatment of childhood obesity. J Am Diet Assoc 2002; 102(5):640–644.

121. Hopper CA, Gruber MB, Munoz KD, et al. School-based cardiovascular exercise and nutrition programs with parent participation. J Health Edu 1996; 27(5):S32–S39.

122. Kafatos A, Manios Y, Moschandreas J, et al. Health and nutrition education in primary schools of Crete: follow-up changes in body mass index and overweight status. Eur J Clin Nutr 2005; 59(9):1090–1092.

123. Richter KP, Harris KJ, Paine-Andrews A, et al. Measuring the health environment for physical activity and nutrition among youth: a review of the literature and applications for community initiatives. Prev Med 2000; 31(suppl):S98–S111.

124. McLanahan S, Haskins R, Paxson C, et al., eds. Childhood Obesity (special issue). Future Child 2006; 16(1):3–224.

125. World Health Organization. Diet, Nutrition and the Prevention of Chronic Disease. Report of a Joint WHO/FAO Expert Consultation. WHO Technical Report Series 916. Geneva: World Health Organization, 2003.

126. World Health Organization. WHO Expert Meeting on Childhood Obesity, Held in Kobe, Japan, June 20–24, 2005. Geneva: World Health Organization (report in press).

127. Marmot MG. Evidence based policy or policy based evidence? BMJ 2004; 328:906–907.

128. Rychetnik L, Hawe P, Waters E, et al. A glossary for evidence based public health. J Epidemiol Community Health 2004; 58(7):538–545.

129. Wanless D. Securing Our Future Health: Taking a Long-Term View. Final report. London: HM Treasury, 2002.

130. Haddad L. Redirecting the diet transition: What can food policy do? Dev Policy Rev 2003; 21(5–6):599–614.

131. Hawe P, Shiell A. Preserving innovation under increasing accountability pressures: the health promotion investment portfolio approach. Health Prom Aust 1995; 5(2):4–9.

132. Swinburn B, Gill T. "Best investments" to Address Child Obesity: A Scoping Exercise. New South Wales: Centre for Public Health Nutrition; Melbourne: Deakin University, 2004.

133. Wang LY, Yang Q, Lowry R, et al. Economic analysis of a school-based obesity prevention program. Obes Res 2003; 11(11):1313–1324.

134. Ganz ML. Commentary: the economic evaluation of obesity interventions—its time has come. Obes Res 2003; 11(11):1275–1277.

135. Department of Human Services. ACE-Obesity: Assessing Cost-Effectiveness of Obesity Interventions in Children and Adults: Summary of Results. Melbourne: Victorian Government Department of Human Services, 2006. Available at: http://www.health.vic.gov.au/healthpromotion/downloads/ace_obesity.pdf. Accessed August 2007.

136. Haby MM, Vos T, Carter R, et al. A new approach to assessing the health benefit from obesity interventions in children and adolescents: the assessing cost-effectiveness in obesity project. Int J Obes 2006; 30(10):1463–1475.

137. Millstone E, Lobstein T. The PorGrow project: overall cross-national results, comparisons and implications. Obes Rev 2007; 8(suppl 2):29–36. Available at: http://www.sussex.ac.uk/spru/porgrow. Accessed August 2007.

10

Prevention of Obesity

W. PHILIP T. JAMES
International Obesity TaskForce, London, U.K.

TIMOTHY P. GILL
Institute of Obesity, Nutrition and Exercise, The University of Sydney, New South Wales, Australia

INTRODUCTION

Obesity is now accepted as a serious public health problem throughout most of the world and is firmly on the agenda of policy makers, health professionals, and the general public across the world. The rates of obesity throughout both the developed and developing world are increasing at a dramatic rate. Indeed, the pandemic of overweight and obesity is now so advanced and so widespread that few regions of the world (with the possible exception of parts of sub-Saharan Africa) appear to have escaped its effects. The effective prevention of obesity has been widely acknowledged as the only feasible solution to addressing the problem in the long term. However, assessments of past obesity prevention initiatives (1–3) have come to a common conclusion that their impact has been very limited. However, they all conceded that given the considerable health risks associated with obesity, the high rates of overweight and obesity in most countries, the cost implications, and the limited long-term success of current weight reduction methods, priority should be given to the prevention of obesity and weight maintenance in preference to weight loss interventions. Jeffery and French (4) have also argued that the behavior change required to prevent small increments in weight with age is likely to be easier to sustain than the behavior change required to achieve and maintain large weight losses. This makes sense not just in terms of the magnitude of effort needed but also because of the adaptive response in humero-hypothalamic mechanisms, which operate to maintain weight gain.

In the last decade, there has been a considerable increase in the focus on obesity prevention issues but little systematic research and evaluation of the most efficacious preventive measures. A brief survey of the scientific literature indicates the much larger body of information that exists around the epidemiology, physiology, and clinical management of obesity. Furthermore, very few countries have introduced a comprehensive prevention plan, which allows detailed analysis of the effectiveness and costs of different strategies.

The literature also reveals a disproportionate focus on programs to address childhood obesity through individual behavior change, despite the fact that overweight and obesity are much more prevalent and represent a much greater immediate threat to the health of adults. This chapter therefore confines itself to the importance of addressing obesity prevention in adults and takes account of the subsequent chapters' contribution on public policy and the need to reengineer the environment.

THE IMPORTANCE OF OBESITY PREVENTION IN ADULTS

An examination of global data on weight status shows that the prevalence of overweight and obesity usually rises gradually throughout life, reaching a peak in the sixth or even seventh decade. A number of recent analyses (5–7) have clearly noted that although there is significant tracking of obesity from childhood to adulthood, a very high proportion of those who develop obesity in adulthood did not have a weight problem in childhood. These data relate to a time when children's environments were very different from those to which children are exposed today, so we need to be very aware of possible powerful cohort and period effects (8). However, it remains clear that adulthood is a period where there are considerable gains in weight that are associated with significant weight-related morbidity. The previous chapter has made a very strong case for the value of addressing obesity as early as possible, which justifies vigorous intervention in children. However, there are several important reasons why the prevention of overweight and obesity in adulthood should not be neglected and why a narrow focus on childhood obesity prevention is imprudent. These include (9,10) (i) the sharpest increase in the incidence of obesity is in (early) adulthood; (ii) adults usually continue to gain weight during adulthood; (iii) adult weight gain is almost always fat gain except in athletes in training; (iv) the relative risks for many diseases associated with obesity decrease with age but the absolute and population-attributable risks for disease increase with age; (v) interventions in children and adolescents need to be maintained for many more years or decades to have a considerable effect on the number of new cases of type 2 diabetes mellitus and heart disease or cancer compared with interventions in older individuals; and (vi) adults who

are parents act as role models and have other responsibilities toward the diet and physical activity behaviors of children. Thus, the prevention of obesity in childhood is dependent on the successful engagement of parents.

These arguments about the particular importance of adult interventions have been reinforced by a new British government analysis, which models the potential gains that might occur if children or adult prevention are the primary focus of action. This is illustrated in Figure 1, which shows that if the emphasis of obesity prevention efforts are focused solely on children and further deterioration in obesity levels are halted, this would have an almost negligible impact on the disease burden over the next 40 years, while interventions that address adults have the potential for a much more profound effect. This analysis also suggests that preventing weight gain is likely to produce better returns than attempting to achieve population weight loss, with the gain achieved by preventing those who are overweight becoming obese only slightly less than that produced by a (unachievable) reduction of 4 body mass index (BMI) units in the population BMI. The modeling of illness and costs shows very clearly the benefits of identifying and focusing preventive efforts on those who are most at risk of developing chronic diseases and indicates that it is a major mistake to focus only on those younger than 50 years, as immediate benefit comes from addressing those older than 50 years as well (11).

SPECIAL ISSUES IN ADULT OBESITY

Rapid Weight Gain in Early Adulthood

A number of large-scale epidemiological studies (8,12,13) have shown that the period of early adulthood has now become the new age group that is gaining weight the fastest and thus has the greatest incidence of overweight

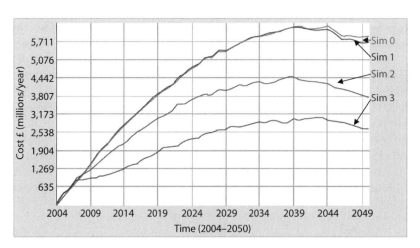

Figure 1 The increase in obesity attributable costs (above 2004 levels) within the United Kingdom under a variety of scenarios.

and obesity. In previous decades, the rate of weight gain began to rise slowly from the early 20s and peaked in the fifth or sixth decade of life. This meant that in past generations most adults attained excessive weight late in life only and thus limited the length of time that they were overweight and at increased risk of illness. The more rapid development of obesity in young adults has been associated with accelerated development of chronic diseases such as coronary atherosclerosis and cardiovascular disease (CVD) (14,15), diabetes (16), fertility problems (17), and quality of life (18). The decline in the age in onset of type 2 diabetes has been tied to early weight gain and development of obesity in early adulthood (19), and it has been predicted that the current generation may be the first not to outlive their parents (20). This means that the estimated benefit of interventions in different age groups as shown in Figure 1 will shift to earlier ages but the effect is likely to be relatively modest over the next 10 to 20 years.

Pregnancy and Weight Gain

The problem of mothers accumulating excess weight and developing obesity during pregnancy has been described for over 50 years (21) and is a common reason given by obese women for their weight problem. There is considerable variation in the amount of weight gained during gestation and this excess weight is often retained postpartum (22). Although the mean weight gain is quite small, some women experience extreme weight gains and others have cumulative increases in body weight after each pregnancy (23). Of equal concern is the potential impact on the adiposity of a child born to an obese woman. Although only recently identified as of concern, the propensity of obese women to produce large babies, whether or not they display their increased susceptibility to gestational diabetes, is now linked to a much greater likelihood of these children becoming obese during childhood (24).

Age-Related Changes in Body Weight, Body Composition, and Fat Distribution

Survey data from wealthier countries show that the level of overweight and obesity begins to climb rapidly in early adulthood and reaches its peak in the middle age. This is true for both males and females. These surveys also indicate that rates of overweight and obesity begin to decline from the seventh decade. This has sometimes been falsely interpreted as a decline in the weights of individuals as they get older. While there is some age-related weight loss as a result of sarcopenia, longitudinal studies indicate that this reduction in mean BMI is a bias created by the disproportionately higher early death rate in obese people and that survivors tend to continue to increase weight over time until late in life (25,26)

In addition, these increases in body weight are accompanied by changes in body composition that result in middle-aged and older adults having a higher level of body fatness for any level of BMI when compared with younger adults. Aging results in a loss of lean muscle tissue in both men and women and can decline by as much as 40% between the ages of 30 and 70 years (27). This decline in lean tissue is certainly influenced by a reduction in resistance exercise with age and a decline in the level of circulating anabolic hormones such as growth hormone and androgens. It may also be related to dietary changes.

Abdominal Obesity

Another detrimental consequence of aging on the development of obesity-related illness is the increase in central distribution of body fat that occurs in both men and women with age. Abdominal obesity has now been clearly linked to an enhanced risk of comorbidities and is a key feature of syndrome X or the metabolic syndrome (28,29). Although no clear-cut definition has yet been agreed on internationally, the syndrome includes a relative excess of abdominal fat, hypertension, insulin resistance with glucose intolerance or diabetes, dyslipidemia, and microproteinuria. In general, men have a higher proportion of body fat stored centrally than women, and the level of abdominal fat increases gradually with age. Women generally enter the middle years with a lower level of abdominal fat but it begins to accumulate rapidly within this period so that by the seventh decade of life men and women have a more equal distribution of body fat. Some studies have suggested that abdominal obesity does not really increase in women until after menopause (30) but other studies indicate that the increase among women is more related to age (31). The reasons for this increase in abdominal fat accumulation are similar to those that precipitate the decrease in lean muscle tissue and include changes in the level of sex hormones and lifestyle factors such as decreased physical activity and increased smoking, alcohol consumption, and positive energy balance (32).

Certain ethnic groups such as Asians, Mexican-Indians, and Australian Aborigines tend to have a higher level of abdominal fat for every level of body weight when compared with Caucasians and may preferentially deposit fat centrally (33). As a consequence, age-related increases in central adiposity may be exaggerated and occur at younger ages in these groups. This is commonly considered to have a genetic basis but it is increasingly evident that from a prevention point of view, the fetal and infantile provision of nutrients and the avoidance of deleterious

Table 1 NIH Classification of Overweight in Adults According to BMI, Waist Circumference, and Associated Disease Risk

	BMI (kg/m^2)	Obesity class	Disease risk[a] relative to normal weight and waist circumference	
			Men < 102 cm / Women < 88 cm	Men > 102 cm / Women > 88 cm
Underweight	<18.5		—	—
Normal[b]	18.5–24.9		—	—
Overweight	25.0–29.9		Increased	High
Obesity	30.0–34.9	1	High	Very high
	35.0–39.9	2	Very high	Very high
Extreme obesity	≥40.0	3	Extremely high	Extremely high

[a]Disease risk for type 2 diabetes, hypertension, and CVD.
[b]Increased waist can also be a marker for increased risk in normal-weight individuals.
Abbreviations: NIH, National Institutes of Health; BMI, body mass index; CVD, cardiovascular disease.
Source: From Ref. 36.

infections, mother's smoking, etc., are probably important because of the increasing evidence of epigenetic and other programming effects perhaps relating to the development and setting of the hypothalamic/pituitary/adrenal axis. Babies of low birth weight (taken as a crude index of in utero inadequate nutrition) tend to selectively put on weight abdominally. Abdominal obesity has also been linked in primate studies with the ingestion of trans fats that may have selective biochemical effects (34). This fact then emphasizes the importance of preventive measures, particularly in late adolescence and in the early adult lives of women of reproductive age, but the impact of any preventive measures are likely to be delayed by at least two if not five decades.

Recently, a Centers for Disease Control and Prevention (CDC)-based working group (35) reaffirmed the importance of addressing abdominal obesity, but the validity of identifying those with an elevated waist circumference as high-risk now needs to be set out in a more integrated way in obesity prevention and management strategies (Table 1).

WHO TO TARGET

No country, regardless of how wealthy it might be, has unlimited resources to apply to health care. Although the chapter on the economics of obesity indicates the potential savings from the effective prevention and management of obesity, finite health resources will always mean making decisions about where to target interventions. The report of the WHO Consultation on obesity (3) suggests that that there are three different but equally valid and complementary levels of obesity prevention. These levels are shown in Figure 2 with the inner circle representing the *targeted* prevention, which is aimed at those with an existing weight problem, while the second ring represents the selective approach directed at high-risk individuals and groups. The broad outside ring represents universal or

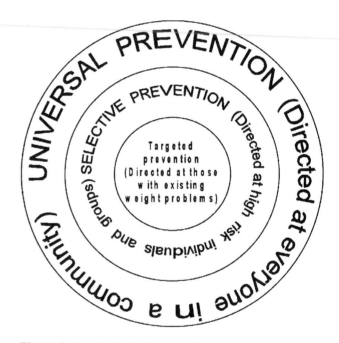

Figure 2 Levels of obesity prevention.

public health prevention approaches, which are directed at all members of the community.

Individuals or Populations?

The criteria chosen for the targeting of preventive strategies raise many issues. It might seem logical to consider identifying those who are on the borderline of obesity (i.e., adults with BMIs of perhaps 28 to 29 kg/m^2) and attempting to prevent them from gaining further weight and thus entering the obese category (i.e., a BMI ≥ 30 kg/m^2). Success would relate to maintaining a maximum BMI of 29 kg/m^2 for individual adults (37). This targeted approach has the advantage that individuals could be

Probability density

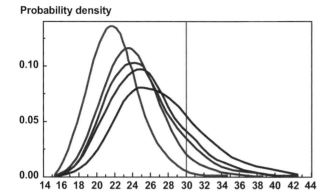

Figure 3 The shifting distributions of BMI of five population groups of men and women aged 20 to 59 years derived from 52 surveys in 32 countries. *Abbreviation*: BMI, body mass index.

selected and special efforts then be focused on these obesity-susceptible individuals. In medical terms, this would seem to provide substantial benefit and limit costs (see above) because a substantial part of the population would not have to be dealt with.

The effect of such a strategy in different societies is illustrated in Figure 3. It is taken from the quintile distribution curves found by Rose and his colleagues in the Intersalt Study, which was concerned with monitoring age and sex-related differences in blood pressure in 52 surveys in 32 societies throughout the world (38). This shows that in some countries, there would need to be a much bigger proportion of the population being targeted. In regions such as North America and Europe, with obesity rates of 20% to 30%, a substantial proportion of individuals would need to be identified if the aim is to not only prevent a further increase in obesity rates but also to ensure that the BMI of obese individuals reduces to below 30 kg/m² and that they are prevented from weight regain. Two flaws are evident in this approach. First, the shifting nature of the problem: the quintile distribution curves in Figure 2 reflect a dynamic process described as the global nutritional transition. As societies become more affluent, the BMI distribution shifts from quintile 1 toward quintile 5 so that more and more individuals will have to be targeted if the sole focus is on the prevention of individuals becoming obese. In the Scottish Intercollegiate Guidelines Network (SIGN) for the Primary Health Care approach to obesity management (39), it was estimated that a Scottish health center with 10,000 children and adults and five doctors would have to cope with about 80 additional obese patients per year because of the growing obesity epidemic. Similar conclusions can be drawn for most countries, and thus the effort of this approach has to be progressively expanded as the obesity epidemic gathers pace. Secondly,

Figure 2 also shows that the upper quintile curves simply reflect a shift in the whole societal pattern of body weights. Therefore, the logic is to target the whole population rather than a smaller group with BMIs of 28 to 29 kg/m². This is why obesity prevention has recently become very focused on population preventive strategies since both individuals and societies have to contend with the "obesogenic" environment.

Higher-Risk Groups

A range of higher-risk groups can be defined for special attention on the basis of their increased propensity to obesity or enhanced health hazards from obesity. Four key high-risk groups of adults include: those with abdominal obesity, Asians and other susceptible ethnic groups, families with a history of obesity and/or type 2 diabetes, and obese pregnant women. Their risks then are magnified as they grow older and have accentuated age-specific rates of developing disease.

Susceptible Ethnic Groups

A number of different ethnic groups have shown an increased propensity to develop obesity (particularly abdominal obesity) or to develop weight-related comorbidities at a lower BMI than Caucasians. For many years, it has been apparent that emigrants from the Indian subcontinent are particularly susceptible to coronary heart disease (CHD) whether they live in South Africa, the Caribbean, or Europe (40). This susceptibility was apparent in McKeigue's observations of the enhanced diabetes rates linked to unusual degrees of selective abdominal obesity with insulin resistance among migrants from the Indian subcontinent living in the United Kingdom (41). More recently, a WHO expert consultation meeting in Singapore in 2003 proposed that some populations may require lower or higher BMI cutoff points to define action in terms of overweight and obesity. These proposed cutoff points are set out in Figure 4.

Similarly, it has been noted that Australian Aborigines are also more likely to store fat abdominally and are more prone to diabetes, hypertension, and CHD at much lower levels of BMI than European-Australians (42). Aborigines who follow a more traditional way of life remain very lean and suffer very little chronic disease, but once they become acculturated to a Western lifestyle and begin to put on weight, their rates of comorbid illness increase rapidly (43). In the United States, Hispanics have disproportionately higher rates of obesity, diabetes, and hypertension when compared with non-Hispanic whites, although this does not translate into greater mortality from CHD (44). Mexican national studies also reveal the additional propensity to abdominal obesity and to excess

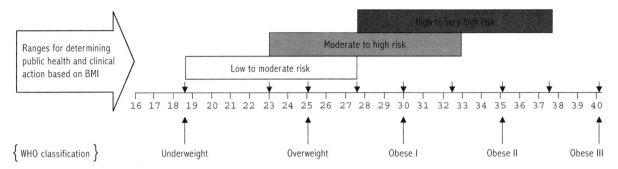

Figure 4 WHO proposed range of body mass index cutoff points for public health action.

diabetes and hypertension when compared with the U.S. non-Hispanic whites (45).

Some researchers have attempted to explain these differences in obesity-related comorbidity risk on the basis of variations in the levels of body fat at any given BMI, with Asians and particularly Indians having much higher levels of body fat at lower levels of BMI when compared with Europeans (46). However, other studies have shown that the relationship between body fat and BMI is more dependent on body proportions than on any genetic differences among ethnic groups (47,48).

Family History of Obesity and/or Diabetes

It has long been known that obesity runs in families, although the determinants of that heritability are not likely to be all genetic, with parental influence on dietary and physical activity patterns also playing a role (49,50). Whitaker and others (51) examined the influence and parental obesity on the development of childhood obesity and its persistence into adulthood. They found that having at least one obese parent greatly increased one's risk of becoming obese as an adult. However, the risks of adult obesity were magnified in subjects who had an obese parent and were also obese as children. In younger children, this effect was small or nonexistent (OR = 1.3 for children aged 1–2 years) but was very pronounced in older children (OR = 17.5 in 15- to 17-year-olds). Thus, it would appear that identifying children with obese parents and intervening early to prevent unhealthy weight gain may prevent the progression to adult obesity.

It has also been well recognized for sometime that the children of parents with type 2 diabetes are particularly susceptible to type 2 diabetes should they gain weight. Recent studies have found that this susceptibility is much stronger in children whose mothers, rather than fathers, had type 2 diabetes and have attributed this problem to the diabetic intrauterine environment (52). Therefore, preventive measures should properly be focused on the children of obese adults with or without a family history of diabetes and pregnant women with a history of type 2 diabetes.

Lower Socioeconomic Status Groups

A number of reviews have assessed the relationship between markers of socioeconomic status and levels of obesity and found a firm, if inconsistent, connection between low status and weight. This relationship is dependent on the level of economic development as obesity is still more prevalent in higher social classes in the poorest countries but this inverse relationship in less developed countries is beginning to become less pronounced (53,54). Many analyses have found that social status is a much better predictor of obesity in women than in men and children, and a recent study indicated that this association was much stronger in older adults (55), suggesting that extended periods of disadvantage may contribute to worsening weight gain.

Those with Existing Obesity or Weight-Related Comorbidities

Prevention of weight gain is an important strategy in people with existing obesity as a means of avoiding or delaying the onset of associated illness. It is also an important management strategy for those with existing weight-related comorbidities. However, perhaps the greatest impact of weight gain prevention can be achieved in those groups who are at high risk of comorbid illness. Those with existing impaired glucose tolerance have been shown to have less progression to full diabetes if they are able to maintain their weight when compared with those who continue to gain weight with age (see sect. "Sweetened Drinks").

APPROPRIATE GOALS FOR OBESITY PREVENTION IN ADULTS

Setting appropriate and achievable goals is an important component of the planning of any health promotion intervention. Past obesity prevention programs have been criticized for failing to adequately define a successful outcome (2). Jeffrey (56) considers that a failure to set specific weight-related goals was a contributing factor to the ineffectiveness of community CHD programs to prevent increases in the mean BMI of participants over time. Clear goals for obesity prevention not only provide outcome measures against which preventive programs can be evaluated but they also guide the nature and the content of preventive efforts. Setting inappropriate goals, such as unattainable reductions in the prevalence of obesity in the community or reductions in the mean population BMI, are in practice counterproductive and dangerous. Failure to achieve them will be taken as a measure of the weakness of an intervention and can often lead to the premature curtailment of potentially useful obesity prevention initiatives. The perspectives provided by the modeling of disease in terms of different preventive initiatives (Figs. 1–3) need to take this into account—thus, expecting a 4- to 8-unit drop in BMI is generally considered unobtainable without dramatic and unrealistic changes on the whole environment affecting both intake and physical activity.

A Focus on Weight Gain Prevention in Adults

In recent years, there has been considerable discussion as to whether all individuals or populations who are classified as overweight or obese using the existing WHO BMI cutoff points are actually at greater risk of ill health (57,58). Much of this discussion has been driven by the reevaluation of the CDC estimates of obesity-related mortality by Flegal and others (59), which indicated that there was a decreased mortality risk associated with a BMI in the overweight range in contrast to previous studies, which indicated an increased risk. Although there has been some debate about the methodology of this study (60,61), these findings have also been reported in a number of other assessments including a recent meta-analysis (62). In addition, the appropriateness of current BMI cutoff points to define health risks in different ethnic groups has also been raised by a number of researchers (63,64). In contrast, the relationship between increasing BMI (in contrast to absolute cutoff points) and morbidity appears to be strong and continuous regardless of the population group assessed (16,65,66).

Research suggests that a large weight gain in a lean individual may carry equivalent risk to maintaining a stable but slightly elevated BMI in an overweight individual. In addition, the risk of developing many chronic diseases begins to increase quite rapidly from a BMI of around 21 kg/m^2 and may reach substantial levels within the "healthy" BMI range. Recent analysis has shown that weight gain per se is one of the principal factors relating to increased health risk, and this risk is independent of the actual level of BMI. In 1989, a 40-year retrospective study of Danish draftees showed that hypertension was highest in those men who entered the army with a high BMI, but at any BMI level (in both normal and overweight subjects), the level of hypertension was higher in people who had gained weight in adulthood to reach that BMI (67). Similar interactions between absolute BMI and weight gain in adulthood have been found in the relationship between weight and the development of diabetes in cohort studies in both men (66) and women (16). In both these studies, larger weight gains led to increased risk of diabetes at each level of BMI. The relationship was extremely strong. An assessment of women in the Nurses Health study found that those who entered adulthood overweight and put on more than 20 kg over the 18-year follow-up were 70 times more likely to develop diabetes than those who entered adulthood lean and maintained their weight over time (65). Similar relationships have been found between weight gain and CHD, hypertension, and gallbladder disease (65), with the risk of each of these conditions being greater with larger increases in weight. There are a number of other important reasons why a focus on weight gain prevention should be central to all strategies to tackle the obesity problem. Although the process of weight gain is still poorly understood, it is widely recognized that once a person has entered a phase of weight gain, the longer the period, the more difficult it becomes to slow or reverse. Almost all weight gain in adulthood is fat gain and is usually associated with a disproportionate increase in abdominal fat stores. As a consequence, the relationship between BMI and risk varies with age and there appear to be similar variations between absolute BMI and the level of health risk between different ethnic groups. These issues are redundant at a population level if the major focus is weight gain and not absolute BMI.

Criteria have not been specifically set for obesity prevention, but it would seem appropriate to ensure that individuals avoid weight gain, which has the potential to impact appreciably on their "well-being" and capacity to live a full life. However, this general definition leads to a plethora of issues because in affluent western societies, women in particular are striving to prevent even modest weight increases often when they are within the normal BMI range. The concept of well-being, therefore, involves recognition that the quality of life of children and adults is in part determined by their cultural setting and not just by whether or not they have symptoms relating to physical comorbidities. Prevention strategies could be defined for simplicity as strategies which (*i*) allow individuals to remain within the normal BMI range and restrict adult weight gain to less than 5 kg, (*ii*) prevent further weight gain in existing

Table 2 Reasons for Focusing on Weight Gain Prevention in Adults

Weight gain in adulthood carries an independent risk of ill health

- Risk for chronic disease begins to increase from low BMI levels and significant weight gain can occur within normal limits.
- Extended periods of weight gain are difficult to reverse.
- Weight gain in adulthood is mostly fat gain.
- A focus on weight gain prevention avoids exacerbation of inappropriate dieting behaviors.
- The message is equally relevant to all sections of the adult population.
- It avoids further stigmatization of people with an existing weight problem.
- It avoids reference to poorly understood terms such as "healthy weight".

overweight and obese individuals, and (*iii*) successfully prevent weight regain in overweight and obese patients who have lost a reasonable amount of weight (e.g., >5%). In the SIGN guidelines, weight maintenance was defined as the weight regain of less than 3 kg in the long term (i.e., >2 years) (39). These three categories of successful prevention are chosen arbitrarily but demand very similar strategies.

In addition, weight maintenance can also serve as an appropriate goal of weight control programs in individuals with an existing weight problem (68). Shifting the focus away from weight loss to weight maintenance also avoids exacerbating inappropriate dieting behaviors, which have been reported in some young adults (Table 2).

Defining Appropriate Objectives That Focus on Energy Balance

Despite the difficulty in achieving weight stability and a reduction in the level of overweight and obesity in the community, it is important that objectives of any program or intervention addressing this problem be clearly related to achieving energy balance and preventing weight gain. This does not mean that there should be an excessive focus on weight and weight loss but rather that an intervention be planned to achieve sufficient impact on dietary intake and/or energy expenditure to influence energy balance and weight status. Imprecise objectives relating to healthy eating or active living are not an accurate reflection of the changes sought. Weight gain prevention is not achieved by merely putting together a range of interventions focusing on nutrition and physical activity into a healthy weight program.

ACHIEVING ENERGY BALANCE

Obesity develops from a sustained period of energy excess leading to weight gain. There remains much speculation as to the true size of the energy imbalance that is required to drive weight gain and contribute to the current rates of obesity. Most short-term studies of weight gain and loss have utilized a relatively large energy surplus or deficits of around 500 kcal to achieve significant shifts in weight status within a matter of weeks or months. However, most cohort studies that have studied weight gain over time have found that the average weight gain over one year is well below 1 kg even after excluding weight losers and those who were weight stable. It has been estimated that this level of weight gain could result from very small, persistent excesses of intake over expenditure of approximately 0.3% of the daily calorie consumption (around 50–100 kcal) (69). It is difficult to measure and detect these levels of energy imbalance even with tightly controlled laboratory conditions and translate this into everyday behaviors that individuals could consciously change (70). In addition, it is understood that daily energy intake and expenditure vary greatly within individuals (71) and that small deviations from energy balance can be attenuated or removed by variations in the activity of uncoupling proteins or other thermogenic processes (72,73). Therefore, the true energy imbalance associated with weight gain may be higher than the calculated figure but is likely to still be relatively small. It is therefore perplexing that so few efforts to prevent weight gain at an individual or community level have achieved success.

Evidence from Past Obesity Prevention Trials

A range of systematic and selective reviews have examined the evidence in relation to obesity prevention in adults and highlighted the paucity of trials addressing this issue. While the number of intervention trials in adults that had an index of adiposity as a specific outcome has increased in the last decade, the number of studies that have targeted weight gain prevention as a primary endpoint remains very low.

A recent systematic review undertaken by the Swedish Council on Technology Assessment in Health Care (SBU) (74) identified over 30 acceptable (although not high quality) studies addressing obesity prevention in adults while other reviews by Reeder and Katzmarzyk (75) and Gill and others (76) contained fewer studies. An assessment of the efficacy of these studies in the SBU review found that around half of the studies produced a positive impact on weight status in the intervention compared with control groups, half had no effect while a small number (three studies) resulted in worsening weight status in the intervention population. Many of the studies in this review focused on preventing weight in groups at greater risk of weight gain, such as women during and after pregnancy, around menopause, or couples starting to live together. Most of the studies that addressed the population as a whole were interventions to reduce the risk of chronic diseases such as CHD, and the largest group of studies dealt with programs addressing people at high risk of CVD. The majority of the studies had durations of one to two years and many were implemented within the workplace. Worksite interventions can be useful as they improve access to obese individuals but the CDC systematic review (77) emphasizes the need for nonfamily social support if interventions are to be effective in preventing weight gain.

The review by Reeder and Katzmarzyk (75) also found that communitywide weight gain prevention initiatives had been restricted to broader CVD prevention programs. However, a wider range of strategies had been employed to address weight gain prevention in individuals and small groups. Individual and small-group counseling produced some benefit, particularly in those at higher risk of weight gain such as menopausal women (78,79). However, the use of mail and telephone support did not appear to yield any benefit in terms of improved prevention of weight gain (80). There was generally good evidence that more intensive individual or small-group counseling on dietary change produced reasonable results (79,81,82) but there is also some evidence to support the inclusion of intensive aerobic exercise (83) and strength training (84).

Mass media campaigns, sometimes developed at considerable expense, have generally been shown to have little impact on indices of weight status, although very few have specifically targeted obesity (77). The only study to assess the impact of the use of mass media over a reasonable time frame, e.g., three years (85) showed no significant effect on weight. In 1999, the British Broadcasting Corporation (BBC) ran a large-scale health education program to encourage people to eat a more healthy diet and to become more active with the explicit aim of helping them to control their weight. The "Fighting Fat, Fighting Fit" campaign ran for seven weeks of peak and daytime programming across BBC television and radio. The campaign consisted of a series of programs and advertisements, with accompanying book, literature, and video (86). The community was encouraged to register for an additional support program, which involved returning three registration cards that charted their progress in weight loss, eating, and exercise behavior change over a six-month period. An evaluation of the progress of 6000 people randomly selected from the 33,474 campaign registrants found significant self-reported reductions in weight and improvements in dietary and exercise behaviors (87). Although the authors of the evaluation point out

the limitations of such a study and of mass media campaigns in general, they believed that such an approach could make a significant contribution to the management of population weight when combined with other strategies.

Evidence from Community Chronic Disease Prevention Programs

Conducting large-scale community-wide trials to address the prevention of obesity is a very expensive and difficult process, and as a consequence evidence of this nature is very limited. However, there have been a number of large CVD and diabetes prevention trials, which have included weight as an intermediary outcome. Such trials have demonstrated that it may be possible to prevent weight gain, if not reduce weight, at a population level and thus can provide useful information about effective strategies to address obesity.

The results of the early large-scale community-wide CVD prevention trials, such as the Stanford Three Community (88) and Five Community studies (89), as well as the Minnesota Heart Health Program (56), had limited impact on weight status and reinforced the difficulty of preventing weight gain in the community. However, later programs, such as the Pawtucket Heart Health Program (90), were able to make a modest impact on weight gain in the intervention community. These programs demonstrated the large time lag (5–10 years) that can be expected between the implementation of a truly community-wide program and the extent of behavior change likely to be required to impact on the weight status of the community. An analysis of the trials by Jeffery (56) suggests that unless weight is the primary outcome of the intervention, it is unlikely that sufficient focus will be placed on achieving the level of change required to impact on energy balance and community weight status.

Recent large community-based trials examining the progression to diabetes in persons identified as glucose-intolerant have become a major focus of adult preventive interventions using weight reduction as a specific intermediate goal. Table 3 shows that significant reductions in diabetes rates can be induced by attention to exercise and diet, with small, but significant, weight losses of around 3 to 4 kg on average.

Clearly, there are marked reductions in risk but this varies depending on the trial. There is a suggestion that Asians with higher risk have a lower response, as shown by the Chinese and Indian studies, but the Japanese study shows the most benefit. In this surprising study, the control group was asked to keep their BMI <24 kg/m^2 and the intervention group had detailed instructions on changing their lifestyle every three to four months and was provided with a goal of maintaining their BMIs

Table 3 Results from Recent Type 2 Diabetes Prevention Trials

Country (reference)	Sweden 1991 (91)	China 1997 (92)	Finland 2001 (93)	United States 2002 (94)	Japan 2005 (95)	India 2005 (96)
Weight loss						
Control	+1.7%	+0.3 kg	−0.8 kg	−0.1	0.39	+
Intervention	−3.7%	−1.8 kg	−3.5 kg	2.1 kg	−2.18	NS
				−5.6 kg		
Percentage reduction in diabetes	50%	42%	58%	31% (Drugs)	67%	29%
				58% (Lifestyle)		

<22 kg/m^2. This suggests that the remarkably modest average weight losses were of benefit (95).

It is noteworthy that there were several specific features, which may prove important in inducing effective changes. These include the fact that the individuals were selected on the basis that they were found to have a definite risk of a disease, i.e., glucose intolerance with the risk of diabetes. This disease is well known to the public so the intervention then may well be seen to have much more general validity than simply appealing to the general concept of gaining a hypothetical benefit. Furthermore, the Diabetes Prevention Program (DPP) study showed very clearly that it was participants older than 60 years who had the greatest benefit with more than 78% of the likely diabetes being prevented. Thus, on this basis one should now be able to advocate a much more vigorous approach to the identification of high-risk individuals.

Further, evidence that the benefits of specific interventions in clinical and everyday practice come from the follow-up to the Malmo study in Sweden, which showed that even 12 years after the intervention those who had glucose intolerance and had lifestyle advice to induce the very modest weight losses shown in Table 4, nevertheless, not only benefited from lower risks of diabetes but over a 12-year period had a death rate which was the same as that of individuals with normal glucose tolerance. Compared with those who had glucose intolerance and no intervention, the intervention reduced the mortality risk by more than 50% (91). These data therefore seem to highlight the importance of adult interventions, particularly in those older than 40 years with glucose intolerance. The challenge then is how to predict the likelihood of adults having glucose intolerance.

Interventions Addressing Diet and Physical Activity Behaviors

Several reviews have identified a number of promising interventions that have the potential to positively influence physical activity and dietary behaviors to a sufficient level to impact energy balance and assist with the prevention of weight gain. The most successful of these interventions involved targeting high-risk groups or small groups, were based on theory, and included goal setting. Also, interventions were more likely to succeed if they were part of an integrated program of actions, rather than an isolated intervention. Interventions to increase incidental activity through modification of the physical environment, improvement of facilities, and policy reform offer the strongest promise for improving the level of physical activity in the community.

Although workplace settings remain the most common settings for interventions to address physical activity and dietary behaviors in adults, reviews have indicated that supermarkets and other points of sale and mass media interventions also offer promise, when included as part of a larger program of action.

Table 4 Matrix for Determining the "Promise" of an Intervention

	Potential population impact (return)		
Certainty of effectiveness	Low	Moderate	High
Risk			
Quite low	Least promising	Less promising	Promising
Medium	Less promising	Promising	Very promising
Quite high	Promising	Very promising	Most promising

Source: Adapted from Ref. 97.

BEST OPTIONS TO ACHIEVE ENERGY BALANCE IN ADULTS

Many other chapters in this handbook have highlighted the complex, multifactorial nature of the etiology of obesity. Some of these factors are nonchangeable such as genetics, gender, and age, and others, such as physiological disturbances in hormonal regulatory systems, can only be dealt with at an individual level (if at all). However, this still leaves a large number of potential influences over energy intake or energy expenditure and thus body weight regulation, which could be the focus of interventions to prevent obesity. Unfortunately, we have gained few insights into the most effective obesity prevention strategies from the limited number of programs that have attempted to address this issue in the past (see sect. "Achieving Energy Balance"). Thus, it is necessary to speculate on what are the key behaviors to address that are most likely to support the attainment and maintenance of energy balance at both an individual and population level.

To facilitate this process, Gill and others (97,98) have proposed a system that allows the integration of the available information from the literature together with other forms of evidence including experience from past public health and health promotion action to identify the target groups and settings most likely to produce effective action on obesity. This is achieved by producing a classification system, which is based on potential for change rather than demonstrated effectiveness. To achieve this, interventions are selected and assessed in terms of how promising they may be in addressing population weight gain, using a health gain/risk framework. This allows the selection of interventions to be based on the best available evidence, while not excluding untried but promising strategies (Table 4). The return or health gain can be defined in terms of demonstrated or modeled efficacy (from previous studies), potential population reach, and likely uptake (estimated). Uncertainty or risk can be defined in terms of the level of information or evidence to support the effectiveness of the intervention.

Using the "promise" approach enables the development of a comprehensive and coherent program of action through the selection of a portfolio of action that provides the best mix of interventions to effectively address community weight issues. Although the initial selection of programs for a portfolio will be based on the evidence of efficacy together with potential impact, a range of secondary issues associated with local implementation—such as community acceptability, resource needs, workforce capacity, sustainability, and likely cost-effectiveness—will influence the final selection of a portfolio.

Increasing Energy Expenditure to Achieve Energy Balance

Although it is difficult to accurately measure changes in physical activity, there can be little doubt that energy expenditure from activity has decreased substantially over the last 50 years. James (99) compared food intake data with population weight gain to estimate that it is likely that the average, adult energy expenditure in the United Kingdom decreased by around 800 kcal between 1970 and 1990. The fact that this reduction in energy expenditure occurred in a period where surveys suggested that participation in leisure time physical activity was increasing in the same countries (100–102) supports the contention that the greatest contribution to this reduction in physical activity comes from the enormous changes in occupational and incidental activity. Prentice and Jebb (103) demonstrated the close association between increasing rates of obesity in the United Kingdom and two key indicators of inactivity (hours per week of television viewing and numbers of cars per household). Although there are few data to support the nature of this association, the extent of mechanization, computerization, and control systems imposed in the workplace and the shifting employment patterns away from manual to more sedentary occupations has markedly reduced the need for energy expenditure at work. In addition, the rapid increase in use of mechanized transport and labor-saving devices, such as elevators, has reduced the need to expend energy going about our daily lives.

There is widespread support for the promotion of physical activity in the prevention of weight gain, although it is not clear from current studies whether increased physical activity actually prevents or reverses age-related weight gain at the population level (104). Cohort studies in both Finland and the United States have shown that weight gain is less in those who are more active (105–107), and similar findings have emerged from assessments of a register of people who have been successful in losing and maintaining weight (108,109). However, reviews of the literature have shown mixed success of program aimed at improving physical activity in adults. Fogelholm and others (110) identified only five studies that utilized physical activity to prevent obesity and found no effect on improved weight status. This of course does not mean, as highlighted above, that one of the complications of obesity, namely diabetes, cannot be prevented by physical activity even if the weight loss is modest. A more recent review by Reeder and Katzmarzyk (75) identified further six studies of mixed quality, which used exercise alone as a strategy for preventing weight gain. Results were disappointing but two intensive exercise programs targeted at middle-aged women, one using endurance exercise (84) and the other using strength training (85), produced positive changes in weight or body composition.

It is also proving difficult to predict how much physical activity is required to prevent weight gain, with Schoeller and others (111) estimating that an additional 80 minutes of moderate activity or 35 minutes of vigorous activity may be needed to be added to our usual sedentary lifestyle to prevent weight regain in subjects who have previously been obese. However, there are numerous health benefits to be gained from a regular exercise regardless of the impact of physical activity on weight gain prevention (112,113). Bauman and others (114) believe that a focus solely on leisure time physical activity is inappropriate and may explain the lack of efficacy of physical activity programs in the prevention of weight gain. They argue that leisure time physical activity actually accounts for only a minor component of total physical activity and that the more dramatic decline in occupational and incidental physical activity should be addressed by weight gain prevention programs. Their modeling shows the difficulty in achieving sufficient leisure time physical activity to achieve the estimated required level of energy expenditure necessary to prevent weight gain (3) in a person employed in a sedentary occupation. In contrast, the inclusion of active commuting and more active housework into a daily routine has greater capacity to achieve energy balance.

Decreasing Sedentary Behaviors

Technological advances have allowed a reduction in hours spent at work and in undertaking household chores, leading to a substantial increase in leisure time while at the same time spawning the development of numerous entertainment options to fill this time. Almost all of these new entertainment options, such as television, video games, and computers, are sedentary activities, requiring little energy expenditure. In recent times, these activities, which initially were used to complement existing forms of leisure activity, are occupying more hours in the day and displacing more active pursuits and games. This has raised concerns for both adults and children, and a number of studies have found association between the number of hours spent watching television and increased levels of BMI in children (115–117). These associations, although small, have been relatively consistent but have not been demonstrated for other sedentary behaviors.

It is important to make a distinction between sedentary behavior and lack of physical activity, as the mechanism for their impact on body weight may be different, and a high level of sedentary behavior can coexist with a high level of physical activity. In the study of Andersen and others (117), most of the children reported relatively high frequency of activity, and although there was a strong association between TV watching and weight status, the association between physical activity and fatness was weak. Robinson indicates that the mechanisms by which sedentary behavior influences body fatness are still to be elucidated. He suggests that a reduction in energy expenditure from a displacement of physical activity seems logical (although not clearly found) but television viewing may also be associated with an increased dietary intake, potentially driven by food advertising (118). It is interesting to note that studies of the treatment of overweight children have found that reinforcing decreased sedentary behavior leads to a greater weight loss than promoting increased physical activity (119).

Decreasing Energy Intake to Achieve Energy Balance

Jeffrey has argued that while both diet and physical activity could plausibly contribute to the development of weight gain and obesity, interventions involving dietary change are likely to be more efficacious than those involving change in physical activity alone (120). He argues that as physical activity only contributes 15% to 25% of energy expenditure while food intake contributes 100% of energy intake, it would be much easier to achieve appropriate reduction in energy intake through diet than through physical activity. There have been very few trials on the prevention of weight gain in adults, which have only included a diet component but those that have included diet as well as physical activity have consistently shown better outcomes in terms of weight status. One very large study of 50,000 postmenopausal women with a high dietary fat intake, who were given individual dietary counseling, resulted in a small but significant reduction in BMI that was maintained at a 7.5-year follow-up (121). Individual or group counseling on both diet and exercise behaviors has been used in a number of studies addressing weight gain identified in systematic reviews (74,75). This approach has also been a feature of the successful diabetes prevention trials. The most promising dietary behaviors to influence weight gain include reducing sweetened drinks (especially in young adults), reducing intake of high fat/energy snack foods, and reducing foods eaten away from home.

Reducing Intake of High-Fat, High-Energy-Dense Foods

The role of a high-fat diet in inducing weight gain was highlighted by the WHO Consultation on obesity (3) and gained general acceptance as an appropriate strategy for the prevention of obesity until questioned by some authors who expressed doubts about the efficacy and safety of this approach (122–124). Their skepticism was based on the association of increasing levels of obesity with decreasing proportion of dietary energy from fat in the U.S. national diet, a belief that high-carbohydrate diets resulted in increased CHD risk, and the variable and inconsistent outcome of trials of low-fat diets. However, a review of the U.S. dietary patterns over the period 1970–1994 by the U.S. Department of Agriculture (125) revealed that while there was a decrease in the percentage of energy from fat (42–38%), the absolute amount of fat in grams available for consumption actually increased by 3%. This apparent paradox is possible because over the same time period, the energy available per capita increased by 15% (3300–3800 kcal). Astrup and others (126) have undertaken a meta-analysis of trials involving low-fat diets and shown that the lower the fat intake, the greater the weight loss, with this loss being more marked in the more overweight subjects. In addition, recent detailed assessments on the matter (127–129) have all concluded that the balance of evidence supports an important role for dietary fat in the genesis of obesity and support the potential for weight gain prevention of reducing fat in the diet. This does not mean however that the other dietary components do not have an important role to play in the prevention of weight gain. There is some evidence, which suggests that the source of dietary carbohydrate and the glycemic index may influence cardiovascular risk factors (130) and has the potential to amplify the risk of the metabolic syndrome in those who gain weight (131).

Food Eaten Away from Home

One of the most profound changes to affect the food supply in almost all developed and many developing countries has been the rapid increase in the proportion of food prepared away from home. The proportion of household budget spent on food eaten away from the home is as high as 40% in the United States (125) and around 25% to 30% in many other countries, such as Australia and the United Kingdom (132,133). The spread of fast-food outlets across the world is responsible for the biggest proportion of food eaten away from home with the number of outlets increasing from 30,000 to 140,000 in the United States between the period 1970–1980 and fast-food sales increasing 300% in the same period (134). Some analyses have linked the increase in fast-food consumption to increasing rates of obesity (135). French and others (136) have found that fast-food use was associated with increased energy and fat intake as well as higher body weight in females (but not males) in the subjects who participated in the "Pound of Prevention" study. The portion size of fast-food items has also been increasing rapidly in recent times and has been identified as a key issue in the consumption of dietary energy in excess of need (134). Evidence suggests that as portion size increases, the ability of consumers to estimate accurately

their intake deteriorates (137). The sheer volume of sales achieved by fast-food outlets and the association with increased fat and energy intake make them a useful target for obesity prevention efforts.

Sweetened Drinks

Evidence is accumulating from a range of sources that energy consumed as sweetened drinks is less compensated for than when consumed as solid food (138,139). A recent longitudinal study has shown that children who consumed more soft drinks at baseline were more likely to become obese and that every one-serving increase in soft drink consumption resulted in a 1.6 times increase in the risk of obesity (140). Special trials in adult volunteers allowing plentiful soft drinks, with either sugars or sweeteners for 10 weeks in double-blind trials, also show progressive weight gain only in the sugar drink-consuming group (141). Market research data suggest that soft drink consumption is increasing worldwide at a rate faster than any other food group (142) and is replacing water and milk as the most popular drinks among children. The widespread availability of soft drinks from vending machines could be contributing to this trend (134).

Social and Physical Environments

Physical, social, political, and economic environments have a profound effect on the way people live and behave. Each day, people interact with a wide range of services, systems, and pressures in settings such as schools, workplace, home, and commercial settings. In turn, these settings are influenced by laws, policies, economic imperatives, and attitudes of governments, industry, and society as a whole. Each of the features of this complex system has the capacity to inhibit or encourage appropriate dietary and physical activity patterns. A range of environmental factors such as the availability of open space, access to public transport, design of suburbs, access to buildings, the perceived level of safety, provision of lighting, and many other factors that influence our capacity and desire to be more physically active in our daily lives. Similarly, advertising pressures, access to appropriate food choices, school food policies, nutrition information, and labeling all potentially influence food selection. In society today, there is also a large commercial drive to promote products that contribute to obesogenic behaviors (cars and food are the two most advertised products on television). The economic imperative (i.e., profits) behind these promotions creates a challenge for policies and attitudes to turn the tide on the obesity epidemic.

Recent analyses of the obesity problem have focused discussion on moving beyond strategies that focus solely on changing personal or community behaviors to tackling some of the underlying structural and environmental determinants, which shape these behaviors (143–146).

The Long-Term Prevention of Weight Regain

Recent studies with a liquid diet and meal replacement scheme have produced a better initial weight loss in obese patients than a standard energy restricted regimen. In addition, persisting with the replacement of a single meal together with an energy-restricted diet after a three-month weight loss period allowed patients to both amplify their weight loss for a time and then maintain the reduced weight at three months for a further four years (147). Although this trial involved supervision, another five-year trial with the same meal and snack replacement scheme but self-administered by obese patients achieved and maintained a 6% weight loss, whereas their rural counterparts in Wisconsin, United States, gained about 7% (148). After the initial three-month weight-loss phase, the subjects were only seen twice a year. So, it would appear that this dietary device was capable of allowing adjustments in intake to be maintained despite the lack of supervision and without the explicit advice and help to take more exercise, which has been a crucial part of maintaining longer-term weight loss in other programs.

Beneficial Effects of Dietary and Physical Activity Interventions That Aim to Lower Weight but also Have Selective Effects on Obesity Comorbidities

Note has already been made of the very substantial benefits of dietary change or increased physical activity even when the weight loss induced is modest or not significant. It is clear that the potential benefit in terms of diabetes prevention is considerable, and it could be argued that the enhanced insulin sensitivity induced by physical activity together with the reduction in dietary fat with its specific effects on insulin resistance are two very reasonable explanations for the benefits of lifestyle interventions, which by itself would not be capable of inducing significant weight loss. In addition, there is increasing evidence that the elimination of trans fats from the diet may not only help to reduce the tendency to accumulate abdominal fat but may also have a selective effect on insulin resistance (149)—a feature which was recognized many years ago when the effects of unusual *cis*- and *trans*-fatty acids were shown to inhibit the insulin-induced process of desaturation and elongation of the essential polyunsaturated fatty acids. Now other mechanisms can also be invoked.

It is well recognized that even modest weight loss is effective in achieving significant and meaningful reductions in blood pressure (150). Other studies have produced additional evidence that a fall in the fat intake together with an increase in vegetable and fruit consumption can have a marked selective blood pressure–lowering effect even when there is no weight change (151). The longer-term benefits of these interventions were recognized many years ago by Stamler and his colleagues, who showed over a 10-year period in those patients with what they termed prehypertension that it was possible with dietary change as well as modest weight losses to induce a marked reduction in the development of hypertension (152).

CONCLUSIONS

Weight gain prevention is important in adults, and more effort should be applied to find successful intervention to achieve this outcome. Current obesity prevention efforts in adults have been limited and may have been inhibited by a number of factors including a lack of acceptance of the importance of obesity as a serious health problem, the setting of inappropriate or unachievable goals, a lack of focus on weight gain prevention as the main outcome, a poor understanding of effective prevention strategies, underfunding of public health and obesity prevention research, problems identifying and targeting at risk individuals and groups, and inadequate public health and practical prevention skills within the health workforce. Determining the most effective strategies for the prevention of obesity at the community level must be seen as a priority.

REFERENCES

1. Glenny AM, O'Meara S, Melville A, et al. The treatment and prevention of obesity: a systematic review of the literature. Int J Obes 1997; 21(9):715–737.
2. Reeder BA, Katzmarzyk PT. Prevention of overweight and obesity. Canadian Clinical Practice Guidelines on the Management and Prevention of Obesity. CMAJ 2007; 176(8): 92–94 (online).
3. World Health Organization (WHO). Obesity: Preventing and Managing the Global Epidemic. Report of a WHO Consultation: WHO Technical Report Series 894. Geneva: World Health Organization, 2000.
4. Jeffery RW, French SA. Preventing weight gain in adults: design, methods and one year results from the Pound of Prevention study. Int J Obes 1997; 21(6):457–464.
5. Venn AJ, Thomson RJ, Schmidt MD, et al. Overweight and obesity from childhood to adulthood: a follow-up of participants in the 1985 Australian Schools Health and Fitness Survey. Med J Aust 2007; 186:458–460.
6. Power C, Lake JK, Cole TJ. Body mass index and height from childhood to adulthood in the 1958 British born cohort. Am J Clin Nutr 1997; 66:1094–1101.

7. Freedman DS, Khan LK, Serdula MK, et al. The relation of childhood BMI to adult adiposity: the Bogalusa Heart Study. Pediatrics 2005; 115:22–27.

8. Allman-Farinelli MA, Chet T, Bauman AE, et al. Age, period and birth cohort effects on prevalence of over-weight and obesity in Australian adults from 1990 to 2000. Eur J Clin Nutr 2007 (Epub ahead of print).

9. Seidell JC, Nooyens AJ, Visscher TLS. Cost-effective measures to prevent obesity: epidemiological basis and appropriate target groups. Proc Nutr Soc 2005; 64(1):1–5.

10. Gill T. The importance of preventing weight gain in adulthood. Asia Pacific J Clin Nutr 2002; 11:S632–S636.

11. Butland B, Jebb S, Kopelman P, et al. Foresight. Tackling Obesities: Future Choices—Project Report. London: Government Office for Science, 2007.

12. McTigue KM, Harris R, Hemphill B, et al. Screening and interventions for obesity in adults: summary of the evidence for the U.S. Preventive Services Task Force. Ann Intern Med 2003; 139(11):933–949.

13. Lewis CE, Jacobs DR Jr., McCreath H, et al. Weight gain continues in the 1990s: 10-year trends in weight and overweight from the CARDIA study. Coronary Artery Risk Development in Young Adults. Am J Epidemiol 2000; 151:1172–1181.

14. McGill HC Jr., McMahan CA, Herderick EE, et al. Obesity accelerates the progression of coronary atherosclerosis in young men. Circulation. 2002; 105:2712–2718.

15. McMahan CA, Gidding SS, Fayad ZA, et al. Risk scores predict atherosclerotic lesions in young people. Arch Intern Med 2005; 165:883–890.

16. Colditz GA, Willett WC, Rotnitzky A, et al. Weight gain as a risk factor for clinical diabetes mellitus in women. Ann Intern Med 1995; 122:481–486.

17. Gunderson EP, Murtaugh MA, Lewis CE, et al. Excess gains in weight and waist circumference associated with childbearing: The Coronary Artery Risk Development in Young Adults Study (CARDIA). Int J Obes Relat Metab Disord 2004; 28:525–535.

18. Daviglus ML, Liu K, Yan LL, et al. Body mass index in middle age and health-related quality of life in older age: the Chicago heart association detection project in industry study. Arch Intern Med 2003; 163:2448–2455.

19. Alberti G, Zimmet P, Shaw J, et al. The International Diabetes Federation Consensus Workshop. Type 2 diabetes in the young: the evolving epidemic. Diabetes Care 2004; 27:1798–1811.

20. Adams KF, Schatzkin A, Harris TB, et al. Overweight, obesity, and mortality in a large prospective cohort of persons 50 to 71 years old. N Engl J Med 2006; 355: 763–778.

21. Sheldon JH. Maternal obesity. Lancet 1949; 2:869–873.

22. Ohlin A, Rossner S. Maternal body weight development after pregnancy. Int J Obes 1990; 14:159–173.

23. Rossner S. Long term intervention strategies in obesity treatment. Int J Obes 1995; 19:S29–S33.

24. Eriksson KF, Lindgårde E. Prevention of type2 (non-insulin-dependent) diabetes mellitus by diet and physical exercise: the 6-year Malmö feasibility study. Diabetologia 1991; 34:891–898.

25. Manson JE, Willey WC, Stampfer MJ, et al. Body weight and mortality among women. N Engl J Med 1995; 333:677–685.

26. Lee IM, Manson JE, Hennekens CH, et al. Body weight and mortality: a 27-year follow-up of middle-aged men. JAMA 1993; 270:2823–2828.

27. Evans WJ. What is sarcopenia? J Gerontol 1995; 50A: 5–8.

28. Després JP. The insulin resistance-dyslipidemic syndrome of visceral obesity: effect on patients' risk. Obes Res 1998; (suppl 1):8S–17S.

29. Kopelman PG, Albon L. Obesity, non-insulin-dependent diabetes and the metabolic syndrome. British Med Bull 1997; 53(2):322–340.

30. Svendsen OL, Hassager C, Christiansen C. Age and menopause-associated variations in body composition and fat distribution in healthy women as measured by dual-energy X-ray absorptiometry. Metabolism 1995; 44:369–373.

31. Wang Q, Hassager C, Raven P, et al. Total and regional body composition changes in early post-menopausal women: age-related or menopause-related? Am J Clin Nutr 1994; 60:843–848.

32. Seidell JC, Bouchard C. Visceral fat in relation to health: is it a major culprit or simply an innocent bystander? Int J Obes 1997; 21(8):626–631.

33. WHO Expert Consultation. Appropriate body-mass index for Asian populations and its implications for policy and intervention strategies. Lancet 2004; 363(9403):157–163.

34. Kavanagh K, Jones KL, Sawyer J, et al. Trans fat diet induces abdominal obesity and changes in insulin sensitivity in monkeys. Obesity 2007; 15(7):1675–1684.

35. Seidell JC, Kahn HS, Williamson DF, et al. Report from a Centers for Disease Control and Prevention Workshop on use of adult anthropometry for public health and primary health care. Am J Clin Nutr 2001; 73(1):123–126.

36. National Institutes of Health. Clinical Guidelines on the Identification, Evaluation, and Treatment of Overweight and Obesity in Adults: The Evidence Report. Washington, D.C.: U.S. Department of Health and Human Services, 1998.

37. Cole TJ, Bellizzi MC, Flegal KM, et al. Establishing a standard definition for child overweight and obesity worldwide: international survey. BMJ 2000; 320: 1240–1243.

38. Rose G. Population distributions of risk and disease. Nutr Metab Cardiovasc Dis 1991; 1:37–40.

39. Scottish Intercollegiate Guidelines Network (SIGN). Obesity in Scotland. Integrating Prevention and Weight Management. Edinburgh: SIGN, 1996.

40. McKeigue PM, Miller GJ, Marmot MG. Coronary heart disease in south Asians overseas: a review. J Clin Epidemiol 1989; 42:597–609.

41. McKeigue PM, Shah B, Marmot MG. Relation of central obesity and insulin resistance with high diabetes prevalence and cardiovascular risk in South Asians Lancet 1991; 337:382–386.

42. O'Dea K, Patel M, Kubisch D, et al. Obesity, diabetes, and hyperlipidemia in a central Australian aboriginal

community with a long history of acculturation. Diabetes Care 1993; 16(7):1004–1010.

43. Rowley KG, Best JD, McDermott R, et al. Insulin resistance syndrome in Australian aboriginal people. Clin Exp Pharmacol Physiol 1997; 24(9–10):776–781.

44. Stern MP, Patterson JK, Mitchell BD, et al. Overweight and mortality in Mexican Americans. Int J Obes 1990; 14(7):623–629.

45. Sánchez-Castillo CP, Velásquez-Monroy O, Lara-Esqueda A, et al. Diabetes and hypertension increases in a society with abdominal obesity: results of the Mexican National Health Survey 2000. Public Health Nutr 2005; 8:53–60.

46. Deurenberg P, Yap M, Van Staveren WA. Body mass index and percent body fat: a meta analysis among different ethnic groups. Int J Obesity 1998; 22:1164–1171.

47. Norgan NG. Interpretation of low body mass indices: Australian Aborigines. Am J Physical Anthropol 1994; 94:229–237.

48. Deurenberg P, Deurenberg-Yap M, Wang J, et al. The impact of body build on the relationship between body mass index and body fat percent. Int J Obes Relat Metab Disord 1999; 23:537–542.

49. Bouchard C. Can obesity be prevented? Nutr Rev 1996; 54(4):S125–S130.

50. Fogelholm M, Nuutinen O, Pasanen M, et al. Parent-child relationship of physical activity patterns and obesity. Int J Obes Relat Metab Disord 1999; 23(12):1262–1268.

51. Whitaker RC, Wright JA, Pepe MS, et al. Predicting obesity in young adulthood from childhood and parental obesity. N Engl J Med 1997; 337:869–873.

52. Dabelea D, Pettitt DJ. Intrauterine diabetic environment confers risks for type 2 diabetes mellitus and obesity in the offspring, in addition to genetic susceptibility. J Pediatr Endocrinol Metab 2001; 14(8):1085–1091.

53. McClaren L. Socio-economic status and obesity. Epidemiol Rev 2007; 29(1):29–48.

54. Monteiro CA, Moura EC, Conde WL, et al. Socioeconomic status and obesity in adult populations of developing countries: a review. Bull World Health Organ 2004; 82(12):940–946.

55. Regidor E, Gutiérrez-Fisac JL, Banegas JR, et al. Obesity and socioeconomic position measured at three stages of the life course in the elderly. Eur J Clin Nutr 2004; 58(3):488–494.

56. Jeffery RW. Community programs for obesity prevention: the Minnesota Heart Health Program. Obes Res 1995; 3:283s–288s.

57. Campos P, Saguy A, Ernsberger P, et al. The epidemiology of overweight and obesity: public health crisis or moral panic? Int J Epidemiol 2006; 35(1):55–60.

58. Oliver JE, Lee T. Public opinion and the politics of obesity in America. J Health Polit Policy Law 2005; 30: 923–954.

59. Flegal KM, Graubard BI, Williamson DF, et al. Excess deaths associated with underweight, overweight, and obesity. JAMA 2005; 293:1861–1867.

60. Hu FB. Overweight and increased cardiovascular mortality: no French paradox. Hypertension 2005; 46:1–2.

61. Willett WC, Hu FB, Colditz GA, et al. Excess deaths associated with underweight, overweight, and obesity (Letter). JAMA 2005; 294:551.

62. McGee D. Body mass index and mortality: a meta-analysis based on person-level data from twenty-six observational studies. Ann Epidemiol 2005; 15(2):87–97.

63. James WPT. Assessing obesity: are ethnic differences in body mass index and waist classification criteria justified? Obes Rev 2005; 6:179–181.

64. Pan WH, Flegal KM, Chang HY, et al. Body mass index and obesity-related metabolic disorders in Taiwanese and US whites and blacks: implications for definitions of overweight and obesity for Asians. Am J Clin Nutr 2004; 79:31–39.

65. Willett WC, Dietz WH, Colditz GA. Guidelines for healthy weight. N Engl J Med 1999; 341(6):427–434.

66. Chan JM, Rimm EB, Colditz GA, et al. Obesity, fat distribution, and weight gain as risk factors for clinical diabetes in men. Diabetes Care 1994; 17:961–969.

67. Sonne-Holm S, Sorensen TIA, Jensen G, et al. Independent effects of weight change and attained body weight on prevalence of arterial hypertension in obese and non-obese men. BMJ 1989; 299:767–770.

68. Rossner S. Long term intervention strategies in obesity treatment. Int J Obes Relat Metab Disord 1995; 19: S29–S33.

69. Hill JO, Wyatt HR, Reed GW, et al. Obesity and the environment: where do we go from here? Science 2003; 299:853–855.

70. Ravussin E, Lillioja S, Anderson TE, et al. Determinants of 24-hour energy expenditure in man. J Clin Invest 1986; 78(6):1568–1578.

71. Schulz LO, Schoeller DA. A compilation of total daily energy expenditures and body weights in healthy adults. Am J Clin Nutr 1994; 60:676–681.

72. Levine JA, Eberhardt NL, Jensen MD. Role of nonexercise activity thermogenesis in resistance to fat gain in humans. Science 1999; 283:212–214.

73. Garvey WT. Uncoupling protein 3 and human metabolism. J Clin Endocrinol Metab 2006; 91(4):1520–1525.

74. The Swedish Council on Technology Assessment in Health Care (SBU). Interventions to prevent obesity: a systematic review. An update of the chapter on preventing obesity in the SBU Report "Treating and Preventing Obesity—An Evidence Based Review." Stockholm: SBU, 2005.

75. Reeder BA, Katzmarzyk PT, and Canadian Task Force on Preventive Health Care. Prevention of Weight Gain and Obesity in Adults: a Systematic Review. London, Ontario: Canadian Task Force on Preventive Health Care, 2007.

76. Gill T, Bauman A, Rychetnik L, et al. Detailed review of intervention studies: how do we best address the issues of overweight, obesity and cardiovascular disease? National Heart Foundation of Australia, 2004. Available at: http://www.heartfoundation.org.au/document/NHF/OO_Detailed Review_InterventionStudies_2003.pdf.

77. Centers for Disease Control and Prevention. Increasing physical activity: a report on recommendations of the Task

Force on Community Preventive Services. MMWR Recomm Rep 2001; 50(RR-18):1–16.

78. Simkin-Silverman LR, Wing RR, Boraz MA, et al. Lifestyle intervention can prevent weight gain during menopause: results from a 5-year randomized clinical trial. Ann Behav Med 2003; 26:212–220.

79. Henderson MM, Kushi LH, Thompson DJ, et al. Feasibility of a randomized trial of a low-fat diet for the prevention of breast cancer: dietary compliance in the women's health trial Vanguard study. Prev Med 1990; 19:115–133.

80. Jeffery RW, Sherwood NE, Brelje K, et al. Mail and phone interventions for weight loss in a managed-care setting: weigh-to-be one-year outcomes. Int J Obes Relat Metab Disord 2003; 27:1584–1592.

81. Williams PT, Krauss RM, Vranizan KM, et al. Changes in lipoprotein subfractions during diet-induced and exercise-induced weight loss in moderately overweight men. Circulation 1990; 81:1293–1304.

82. Kristal AR, Curry SJ, Shattuck AL, et al. A randomized trial of tailored, self-help dietary intervention: the Puget Sound eating disorders study. Prev Med 2000; 31: 380–389.

83. Slentz CA, Duscha BD, Johnson JL, et al. Effects of the amount of exercise on body weight, body composition, and measures of central obesity: STRRIDE-a randomized controlled study. Arch Intern Med 2004; 164:31–39.

84. Schmitz KH, Jensen MD, Kugler KC, et al. Strength training for obesity prevention in midlife women. Int J Obes Relat Metab Disord 2003; 27:326–333.

85. Meyer AJ, Nash JD, McAlister AL, et al. Skills training in a cardiovascular health education campaign. J Consult Clin Psychol 1980; 48(2):129–142.

86. Wardle J, Rapoport L, Miles A, et al. Mass education for obesity prevention: the penetration of the BBC's "Fighting Fat, Fighting Fit" campaign. Health Educ Res 2001; 16(3):343–355.

87. Miles A, Rapoport L, Wardle J, et al. Using the mass-media to target obesity: an analysis of the characteristics and reported behavior change of participants in the BBC's "Fighting Fat, Fighting Fit" campaign. Health Educ Res 2001; 16(3):357–372.

88. Fortmann SP, Williams PT, Hulley SB, et al. Effect of health education on dietary behaviors: the Stanford Three Community Study. Am J Clin Nutr 1981; 34:2030–2038.

89. Farquhar JW, Fortmann SP, Flora JA, et al. Effects of community-wide education on cardiovascular disease risk factors: the Stanford Five City Project. JAMA 1990; 264:359–365.

90. Lefebvre RC, Lasater TN, Carleton RA, et al. Theory and delivery of health programming in the community: The Pawtuckett Heart Health Program. Preventive Med 1987; 16:80–95.

91. Pan X-R, LI G-W Hu Y-U, et al. Effects of diet and exercise in preventing NIDDM in people with impaired glucose tolerance. Diabetes Care 1997; 20(4):537–544.

92. Eriksson KF, Lindgärde F. No excess 12-year mortality in men with impaired glucose tolerance who participated in the Malmö Preventive Trial with diet and exercise. Diabetologia 1998; 41(9):1010–1016.

93. Tuomilehto J, Lindstrom J, Eriksson JG, et al. Prevention of Type 2 diabetes mellitus by changes in lifestyle among subjects with impaired glucose tolerance. N Engl J Med 2001; 344(18):1343–1350.

94. Knowler WC, Barrett-Connor E, Fowler SE, et al. Reduction in the incidence of type 2 diabetes with lifestyle intervention or metformin. N Engl J Med 2002; 346: 393–403.

95. Kosaka K, Noda M, Kuzuya T. Prevention of type 2 diabetes by lifestyle intervention: a Japanese trial in IGT males. Diab Res Clin Pract 2005; 67:152–162.

96. Ramachandran A, Snehalatha C, Mary S, et al. The Indian Diabetes Prevention Programme shows that lifestyle modification and metformin prevent type 2 diabetes in Asian Indian subjects with impaired glucose tolerance (IDPP-1). Diabetologia 2006; 49(2):289–297.

97. Gill T, King L, Webb K. Best Options for the Promoting Healthy Weight and Preventing Weight Gain in NSW. Sydney: NSW Centre for Public Health Nutrition and NSW Department of Health 2005.

98. Swinburn B, Gill T, Kumanyika S. Obesity prevention: a proposed framework for translating evidence into action. Obesity Rev 2005; 6:23–33.

99. James WP. A public health approach to the problem of obesity. Int J Obes 1995; 19(suppl 3):S37–S45.

100. Cox BD. Changes in body measurements. In: Cox BD, Huppert FA, Whitchelow MA, eds. The Health and Lifestyle Survey, Seven Years On. Aldershot, U.K.: Dartmouth Publishing, 1993:103–117.

101. Barengo NC, Nissinen A, Pekkarinen H, et al. Twenty-five-year trends in lifestyle and socioeconomic characteristics in Eastern Finland. Scand J Public Health 2006; 34:437–444.

102. Craig CL, Russell SJ, Cameron C, et al. Twenty-year trends in physical activity among Canadian adults. Can J Public Health 2004; 95(1):59–63.

103. Prentice AM, Jebb SA. Obesity in Britain: gluttony or sloth? BMJ 1995; 311(7002):437–479.

104. DiPietro L. Physical activity in the prevention of obesity: current evidence and research issues. Med Sci Sports Exerc 1999; 31(suppl 11):S542–S546.

105. Rissanen AM, Heliovaara M, Knekt P, et al. Determinants of weight gain and overweight in adult Finns. Eur J Clin Nutr 1991; 45(9):419–430.

106. Haapanen N, Miilunpalo S, Pasanen M, et al. Association between leisure time physical activity and 10-year body mass change among working-aged men and women. Int J Obes Relat Metab Disord 1997; 21(4):288–296.

107. Williamson DF, Madans J, Anda RF, et al. Recreational physical activity and ten-year weight change in a US national cohort. Int J Obes Relat Metab Disord 1993; 17(5):279–286.

108. Sherwood NE, Jeffery RW, French SA, et al. Predictors of weight gain in the Pound of Prevention study. Int J Obes Relat Metab Disord 2000; 24(4):395–403.

109. Klem ML, Wing RR, McGuire MT, et al. A descriptive study of individuals successful at long-term maintenance

of substantial weight loss. Am J Clin Nutr 1997; 66(2): 239–246.

110. Fogelholm M, Kukkonen-Harjula K. Does physical activity prevent weight gain–a systematic review. Obes Rev 2000; 1:95–111.

111. Schoeller DA, Shay K, Kushner RF. How much physical activity is needed to minimize weight gain in previously obese women? Am J Clin Nutr 1997; 66(3):551–556.

112. Blair SN, Kohl HW, Barlow CE, et al. Changes in physical fitness and all-cause mortality. A prospective study of healthy and unhealthy men. JAMA 1995; 273(14): 1093–1098.

113. Pate RR, Pratt M, Blair SN, et al. Physical activity and public health. A recommendation from the Centers for Disease Control and Prevention and the American College of Sports Medicine. JAMA 1995; 273(5):402–407.

114. Bauman A, Allman-Farinelli M, Huxley R, et al. Leisure time physical activity alone may not be a sufficient public health approach to prevent obesity—a focus on China. Obesity Rev 2008; 9(suppl 1):119–126.

115. Dietz WH, Gortmaker SL. Do we fatten our children at the television set? Obesity and television viewing in children and adolescents. Pediatrics 1985; 75(5):807–812.

116. Gortmaker SL, Must A, Sobol AM, et al. Television viewing as a cause of increasing obesity among children in the United States, 1986–1990. Arch Pediatr Adolesc Med 1996; 150(4):356–362.

117. Andersen RE, Crespo CJ, Bartlett SJ, et al. Relationship of physical activity and television watching with body weight and level of fatness among children: results from the Third National Health and Nutrition Examination Survey. JAMA 1998; 279(12):938–942.

118. Robinson TN. Does television cause childhood obesity? JAMA 1998; 279(12):959–960.

119. Epstein LH, Paluch RA, Gordy CC, et al. Decreasing sedentary behaviors in treating pediatric obesity. Arch Pediatr Adolesc Med 2000; 154(3):220–226.

120. Jeffrey RW, Linde J. Evolving environmental factors in the obesity epidemic. In: Jeffrey RW, Crawford D, eds. Obesity Prevention and Public Health. New York: Oxford University Press, 2005.

121. Howard BV, Manson JE, Stefanick ML, et al. Low-fat dietary pattern and weight change over 7 years: the Women's Health Initiative Dietary Modification Trial. JAMA 2006; 295(1):39–49.

122. Katan MB, Grundy SM, Willett WC. Should a low-fat, high-carbohydrate diet be recommended for everyone? Beyond low-fat diets. N Engl J Med 1997; 337(8):563–566.

123. Willett WC. Dietary fat and obesity: an unconvincing relation. Am J Clin Nutr 1998; 68(6):1149–1150.

124. Taubes G. Nutrition. The soft science of dietary fat. Science 2001; 291:2536–2545.

125. Frazao E, ed. America's Eating Habits: Changes and Consequences. Washington, D.C.: USDA Economic Research Services, 1999.

126. Astrup A, Grunwald GK, Melanson EL, et al. The role of low-fat diets in body weight control: a meta-analysis of ad libitum dietary intervention studies. Int J Obes Relat Metab Disord 2000; 24(12):1545–1552.

127. Bray GA, Popkin BM. Dietary fat intake does affect obesity? Am J Clin Nutr 1998; 68:1157–1173.

128. Astrup A, Toubro S, Raben A, et al. The role of low fats diets and fat substitutes in body weight management: what have we learned from clinical studies? J Am Diet Assoc 1997; 97:82S–87S.

129. Shick SM, Wing RR, Klem ML, et al. Persons successful at long-term weight loss and maintenance continue to consume a low-energy, low-fat diet. J Am Diet Assoc 1998; 98:408–413.

130. Frost G, Leeds AA, Dore CJ, et al. Glycemic index as a determinant of serum HDL-cholesterol concentration. Lancet 1999; 353:1045–1048.

131. Liu S, Willett WC, Stampfer MJ, et al. A prospective study of dietary glycemic load, carbohydrate intake, and risk of coronary heart disease in US women. Am J Clin Nutr 2000; 71(6):1455–1461.

132. Lester IH. Australia's Food and Nutrition. Canberra, Australia: Australian Government Publishing Service, 1994.

133. Kearney JM, Hulshof KF, Gibney MJ. Eating patterns—temporal distribution, converging and diverging foods, meals eaten inside and outside of the home–implications for developing FBDG. Public Health Nutr 2001; 4(2B):693–698.

134. French SA, Story M, Jeffery RW. Environmental influences on eating and physical activity. Ann Rev Public Health 2001; 22:309–335.

135. Binkley JK, Eales J, Jekanowski M. The relation between dietary change and rising US obesity. Int J Obes Relat Metab Disord 2000; 24(8):1032–1039.

136. French SA, Harnack L, Jeffery RW. Fast food restaurant use among women in the Pound of Prevention study: dietary, behavioral and demographic correlates. Int J Obes Relat Metab Disord 2000; 24(10):1353–1359.

137. Young LR, Nestle MS. Portion sizes in dietary assessment: issues and policy implications. Nutr Rev 1995; 53:149–158.

138. Mattes R. Dietary compensation by humans for supplemental energy provided as ethanol or carbohydrate in fluids. Physiol Behav 1996; 59:179–187.

139. De Castro JM. The effects of the spontaneous ingestion of particular foods or beverages on the meal pattern and overall nutrient intake of humans. Physiol Behav 1993; 53:1133–1144.

140. Ludwig DS, Peterson KE, Gortmaker SL. Relation between consumption of sugar-sweetened drinks and childhood obesity: a prospective, observational analysis. Lancet 2001; 357:505–508.

141. Raben A, Møller AC, Vasilaras TH, et al. A randomised 10-week trial of sucrose vs. artificial sweeteners on body weight and blood pressure after 10 weeks. Obes Res 2001; 9(suppl 3):86S.

142. Beverage Marketing Corporation of New York. The Global Multiple Beverage Marketplace. New York: Beverage Marketing Corporation, December 2000.

143. Kumanyika SK. Minisymposium on obesity: overview and some strategic considerations. Annu Rev Public Health 2001; 22:293–308.

144. James WP. A public health approach to the problem of obesity. Int J Obes Relat Metab Disord 1995; 19(suppl 3): S37–S45.

145. Egger G, Swinburn B. An "ecological" approach to the obesity pandemic. BMJ 1997; 315(7106):477–480.

146. Nestle M, Jacobson MF. Halting the obesity epidemic: a public health policy approach. Public Health Rep 2000; 115:12–24.

147. Flechtner-Mors M, Ditschuneit HH, Johnson TD, et al. Metabolic and weight loss effects of long-term dietary intervention in obese patients: four-year results. Obes Res 2000; 8:399–402.

148. Rothacker DQ. Five-year self-management of weight using meal replacements: comparison with matched controls in rural Wisconsin. Nutrition 2000; 16:344–348.

149. Kavanagh K, Jones KL, Sawyer J, et al. Trans fat diet induces abdominal obesity and changes in insulin sensitivity in monkeys. Obesity 2007; 15(7):1675–1684.

150. Stevens VJ, Obarzanek E, Cook NR. Long-term weight loss and changes in blood pressure: results of the Trials of Hypertension Prevention, phase II. Ann Intern Med 2001; 134(1):72–74.

151. Sacks FM, Svetkey LP, Vollmer WM, et al. Effects on blood pressure of reduced dietary sodium and the Dietary Approaches to Stop Hypertension (DASH) diet. N Engl J Med 2001; 344(1):3–10.

152. Stamler J, Farinaro E, Mojonnier LM, et al. Prevention and control of hypertension by nutritional-hygienic means. Long-term experience of the Chicago Coronary Prevention Evaluation Program. JAMA 1980; 243(18):1819–1823.

11

Analyzing and Influencing Obesogenic Environments

BOYD SWINBURN

School of Exercise and Nutrition Sciences, Deakin University, Melbourne, Victoria, Australia

GARRY EGGER

School of Health and Applied Sciences, Southern Cross University, Lismore, Australia, and Centre for Health Promotion and Research, Sydney, Australia

INDIVIDUAL VS. POPULATION PERSPECTIVE OF OBESITY

Introduction

Obesity is now at pandemic levels. Its prevalence is increasing in almost all countries—developed and developing (1). To curtail and eventually reverse the rise in obesity prevalence rates, a broad population-based approach will be needed (1,2). The majority of the current global efforts on obesity, however, are centered on establishing biological mechanisms related to energy imbalance and finding appropriate methods of treatment for individuals with obesity. The move to tackle whole populations with obesity requires conceptual shifts at many levels.

Individual and Population Examples

Consider the following two examples of obesity. The first example is of Penny who is 45-years old and, apart from a few years around the time of her wedding, she has always been quite chubby. Over the last 15 years she has gained a lot more weight and now has a body mass index (BMI) of 34 kg/m^2. Her husband, on the other hand, has a BMI of about 25 kg/m^2, and this virtually has not changed since

he left school. The second example is of England, where the prevalence of obesity (BMI > 30 kg/m^2) in 2002 was 24% (3), having increased from 7% in 1980 (4). England's neighbor just across the English Channel is the Netherlands, where the prevalence of obesity in 2004 was only 11%, up from about 5% in 1981 (5).

These two examples illustrate the different perspectives needed for dealing with individuals or populations. The etiologies and management strategies will be quite different for Penny's obesity compared with England's obesity (Table 1).

The etiology of Penny's obesity will tend to be ascribed to genetic and behavioral factors and perhaps socioeconomic status (SES), whereas for England it will be ascribed to economic, environmental, sociocultural, and behavioral factors. For example, the transport environment in England will stand out as "obesogenic" (obesity promoting) because of its car-dependence compared with the relatively "leptogenic" (leanness promoting—leptos is Greek for thin) transport environment in the Netherlands with its strong emphasis on bicycle and public transport travel.

The management strategies for obesity at the individual and population levels are also quite different (Table 1). The volume of studies and information about weight loss is

Table 1 Differences Between the Individual-Based and Population-Based Approaches to Obesity

Approaches to obesity	Individual-based approach	Population-based approach
Key measures	Body weight, waist, BMI, comorbidities	Prevalence of overweight and obesity, mean BMI, and waist
Key etiology question	Why is this particular person obese (or gaining weight)?	Why does this particular population have a high (or rising) prevalence of obesity?
Main etiological mechanisms	Genetic, behavioral, socioeconomic	Economic, environmental, cultural, behavioral
Key management question	What are the best long-term strategies for reducing the person's body fat?	What are the best long-term strategies for reducing the population's mean BMI?
Main management actions	Patient education, behavioral modification, drugs, surgery	Improving food and physical activity environments, policies, programs, social marketing
Volume of information on etiology and management	Vast	Minimal
Driving forces for research and action	Immediate and powerful	Distant and weak
Potential for long-term benefit to individuals	Modest	Modest
Potential for long-term benefit to populations	Modest	Significant

Abbreviation: BMI, body mass index.

huge compared with the amount available on population-based prevention. For example, the 150-page report of the British Nutrition Foundation Task Force on Obesity dedicated 51 pages to treatment of individuals and only one page to population prevention strategies (6). This is in part because the driving forces for research and action are quite different. For individual treatment, the forces are powerful and immediate and include the clinical imperative to help people with obesity, the pressure from individuals to lose weight, and the huge potential profits for pharmaceutical companies from weight loss medications. Contrast this with the relatively weak and distant driving forces for population-based prevention research and action. These are funded largely from government sources, and the lack of political will due to a short-term political focus and limited public pressure for change remain major obstacles. As discussed later, the driving forces for the obesity epidemic are linked to much broader sectors such as transport, the food industry, education, urban planning, building design, and local government, and this adds to the sense of impotence among health authorities about obesity prevention.

As a general rule, individual-directed interventions bring about significant benefits to those individuals being treated but have little impact on the population rates of disease or condition in question and vice versa for population-based interventions, which generally bring little benefit to each individual but have the potential to influence the prevalence or incidence of the condition (7). With obesity, this discrepancy is even more exaggerated (compared with, say, hypertension or hypercholesterolemia) because available

individual interventions, apart from surgery, have modest long-term effects for the individuals under treatment (8,9). The efforts on population-based interventions related to obesity are much needed but are still in their infancy (1,10,11).

The potential for population-wide effects is particularly strong for high-volume foods or physical activities. For example, a survey of fast-food outlets in New Zealand showed that the mean fat content of french fries was 11.5% by weight (12). There was an enormous range across the country from 5% to 20% and in many instances the deep frying practices were very poor. It should be possible to reduce the mean fat content to 10% through a national training program for fast-food outlet operators or regulatory approaches. If this could be achieved, the consumption of french fries is such that the reduction in fat intake would be about 0.5 kg/capita. This is not insubstantial compared with the increase in weight of the New Zealand adult population of about 0.33 kg/person/yr (13). In other words, such an intervention would reduce about a year's worth of increase in mean weight.

Linking the Individual and Population Approaches

There are synergies to be achieved by bringing the individual and population approaches together. This can be seen most clearly at the general practice/primary care level. For example, a general practitioner will have a greater chance of helping Penny to lose weight and keep it off if her obesogenic environments are acknowledged and, where possible, acted upon. Part of Penny's weight gain response to her obesogenic environment may be genetically determined, and recognition of this also helps to remove moral judgments about her obesity and places her individual behaviors into a wider context. The more limited behavior-based perspective can be judged too easily (by her and others) in "sloth-and-gluttony" terms. Penny may even be able to take action to make her own environments more leptogenic, such as changing the types of food available at home or on offer at the work cafeteria.

On the flip side, it makes sense to use the high contact that primary health care has with the public on a regular basis to further the population health goals for obesity. Educating and upskilling large numbers of patients increases the dissemination of knowledge through the community and promotes advocacy to make health choices easier.

MODELS OF OBESITY THAT INCORPORATE THE INDIVIDUAL AND POPULATION PERSPECTIVES

There are a large number of models of intervention in common usage in health promotion and clinical care (14). The value of any particular model is that it helps to explain the problem and to provide a framework for action, and in the obesity area, it should ideally incorporate both treatment and prevention aspects as these should be considered on a continuum. We have found two models of particular value: one is an "ecological model" based on the energy balance equation. The other is the epidemiological triad, which has been successfully applied in other epidemics.

Ecological Model of Obesity

The energy balance equation is a logical place to start trying to understand obesity at the individual and population level. The most accurate version of the energy balance equation is the "dynamic, physiological" version (15), which incorporates "rates of change" (16) and an interconversion between energy balance and fat balance (17,18).

$$\text{Rate of change of energy (fat) stores} = \text{rate of energy (fat) intake} - \text{rate of enery (fat) expenditure}$$

While this equation has served reasonably well as a model for understanding weight gain and obesity at an individual level, it is not helpful in incorporating the broader influences on weight gain and obesity, especially the environmental influences. We have expanded the energy/fat balance equation into an ecological model (2)

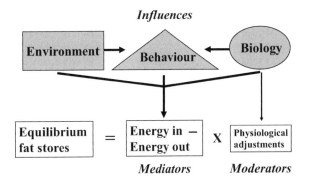

Figure 1 An ecological model of obesity.

to help visualize the interplay between the broad influences on energy balance (Fig. 1) and used this in a planning approach to diagnose obesogenic environments (19).

Ecological models help to conceptualize the interdependence of people, their health, and their environments in the broadest sense (20). The model regards an individual's or population's level of obesity at any one time as being at an equilibrium or a "settling point"—the net result of multiple influences, which impact on fat mass by acting through the mediators of energy intake (especially through high-fat, energy-dense food and large portion sizes) (21) and/or energy expenditure (especially through the impact of machines on reducing physical activity). The concept of a single fixed "set point" to explain why people tend to return toward their original body weight following a period of weight loss (22) does not fit with the metabolic evidence (23), and it is an unhelpful term because it is clearly not "set." Most individuals increase their body fat levels over a lifetime, and most populations are getting fatter over time.

The influences are broadly defined as biological, behavioral, and environmental. Biological influences include the effects of genes, hormones, age, gender, ethnicity, and drugs on one or more of the myriad pathways that influence energy balance. The behavioral influences typically attributed to obesity are sloth and gluttony, which imply a willful control over the forces affecting body weight. However, this is simplistic and judgmental because all behaviors are the net result of complex individual factors (including habits, knowledge, emotions, cognitions, attitudes, and beliefs) interacting with environmental influences (see later).

Biological differences also explain the heterogeneous physiological adjustments that the body makes in response to weight loss or gain. A period of energy imbalance is moderated by a somewhat "exaggerated" counterresponse in such things as hunger, metabolic rate, nutrient partitioning, and the energy costs of physical activity (23,24). These all serve to moderate the impact of energy imbalance on changes in fat mass.

Epidemiological Triad

Another way to visualize these influences is using the classic epidemiological triad (Fig. 2), which has proved to be a robust model with epidemics such as infectious diseases, smoking, coronary heart disease, and injuries (25–27).

The Host encompasses the biological and behavioral influences and the physiological moderators of weight change from the ecological model. The Agent is defined as energy imbalance and its Vectors are energy-dense food, large portion sizes, time- or energy-saving machines (e.g., cars) and time-using machines (e.g., television). These are analogous to the mediators. The Environment is the same in both models. The strategies for intervention are different for each corner of the triad (Fig. 2); however, the main lesson learned from other epidemics is that all three corners need to be addressed together. For the host, the intervention strategies encompass both prevention and treatment and range from education (awareness raising to intensive counseling) through behavioral modification to medical strategies such as drugs and surgery. A diagnostic approach to analyze the diet, activity, and related behaviors of individuals has recently been developed (28). For the vectors, the strategies are often technology based, such as food technology approaches to reduce the fat content of food. Unfortunately, many technological advances appear to be the vectors for inactivity (especially cars, television, and computers) with only a few (such as exercise equipment) being vectors for physical activity. The underlying drivers creating the obesogenic environments are mainly commercial (29). The food, car, and electronic entertainment industries are among the biggest in the world and it is hard to see these forces abating in the near future. The best hope for reversing the obesogenic environments lies

with public policies promoting healthier environments in concert with social demands for healthier choices. At a clinical level, the model also is helpful in showing that the individual is part of a wider system, including influential environments.

OBESOGENIC AND LEPTOGENIC ENVIRONMENTS

A central concept to emerge from considering these models is that while environments are external to the person, they have a powerful influence on the person's behaviors and thus energy balance and obesity. Genetic variation remains an important cause of individual body size variation, but as George Bray memorably stated, "genetics load the gun, but the environment pulls the trigger" (30). The term "obesogenic environments" can be defined as "the sum of influences that the surroundings, opportunities, or conditions of life have on promoting obesity in individuals or populations" (19). By contrast, leptogenic environments would promote healthy food choices and encourage regular physical activity. The obesogenic environment is synonymous with other terms, which have been coined, such as the "toxic environment" (31) or "pathoenvironment" (15), but a term for the other end of the spectrum (i.e., the "leptogenic environment") may also be of value in defining the direction of desired environmental change.

We have defined environments in a broad sense to include more than just the visible, tangible aspects of the physical environment. They include costs, laws, policies, social and cultural attitudes, and values, and indeed any external factors that might affect an individual's behavior. From this perspective, the increasingly obesogenic environments are a fundamental driving force for the global obesity epidemic (32).

WHY THE FOCUS ON ENVIRONMENTS?

A broad approach is required for reducing obesity at a population level. Biological research will continue to map the metabolic and molecular pathways involved in the development of obesity and will therefore help to explain some of the differences in obesity risk among individuals. Identifying key molecules in the pathways may lead to the development of effective drugs to treat obesity, but unless costly, mass medication is undertaken for a large proportion of the population, there will be little impact on the population burden of obesity.

One of the primary weight loss interventions aimed at the host is education (including awareness raising, public education, and individual counseling and skills training). The expectation is that new knowledge will be turned into

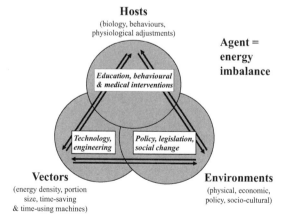

Figure 2 Epidemiological triad as it applies to obesity. The circles refer to the predominant strategies to address each corner of the triad.

sustained behavior changes. This may be true for some individuals and appears to be a moderately successful approach for obese men (33). However, for most obese people and for population-based prevention, just knowing about what the healthy choices are is a relatively weak force for sustained behavior change (8,9). Education about healthy choices, therefore, appears *necessary but not sufficient* to reverse obesity.

The key role of environmental change is "to make the healthy choices the easy choices." Unfortunately, the environments in relation to obesity have received little attention to date. Compare the vast human and financial efforts to sequence the human genome with the minor and nascent efforts to sequence the human environment. Yet, environmental change can have an important and lasting impact on behaviors (34), especially if it is a "passive" intervention that does not require an active decision by the individual, such as car-free central business districts or lower-fat french fries (see sect. "Individual and Population Examples") or potato chips (see below) (35). An intervention for another purpose that has increased physical activity or healthier eating as a side effect has been called a "stealth intervention" (36). It is possible that the issue of reversing climate change will become a major driver of population behavior change and therefore interventions such as personal carbon trading may become important stealth interventions for increasing physical activity (37). Table 2 lists some of the key strengths of an environmental/systems-based approach underpinning the obesity prevention efforts.

Obesity, like diabetes and coronary heart disease, has higher prevalence rates among the lower SES populations in developed countries. Low income and educational attainment bring with them reduced options for low SES groups and a lower uptake of health messages about behavioral changes for a healthy future. One of the key strengths of an environmental focus is its potential impact among lower SES groups. By influencing the default choices in key environments, there is a much greater potential to affect overall diet and physical activity patterns in lower SES groups than by education strategies alone. Education-based campaigns are complementary to

Table 2 Strengths of an Environmental/Systems-Based Approach to Underpin Obesity Prevention Efforts

Strength	Examples
Addresses underlying determinants (i.e., potential for true prevention)	Parental fears for children's safety as the major reason for driving children to school—addressing the substance and perceptions related to the fears is likely to result in more active transport to school
Becomes structural/systemic	Changing the physical environment for recreation, agricultural subsidies, local government transport policies, etc., embeds the changes into the system
Becomes the accepted norm	Regular availability of reduced fat milk, salad options, vegetable-based dishes, etc., makes them normative choices, just as legislation quickly made smoke-free indoor environments the norm
Likely to be sustained	Systemic changes such as safe, attractive cycle networks, or healthy school food, which are backed by strong policies and traditions are more likely to sustain behaviors over the long term than, say, media campaigns
Influences the hard to reach	Disadvantaged populations such as those with low income or low educational attainment tend not to respond to health messages but they can still benefit from the fast-food outlet which cooks lower-fat french fries
Less language dependent	Health messages and information are often aimed at a narrow population segment and are often not transmitted in the native tongue of ethnic minorities, but all ethnic groups can take advantage of public transport
Can address inequities	Environmental interventions can not only reach populations with poor health outcomes but they can also be differentially targeted to them, such as improving bus services, school food programs, and active recreation amenities
Usually cost-effective	Environmental interventions (especially policy-based initiatives) are relatively inexpensive compared with individual-based approaches and media-based public education campaigns and even the expensive ones (e.g., improving public transport) are often cost-effective in the long term
Changes default behavior	Some food choices are highly influenced by price, labeling, and availability, and changing these factors shifts the "default" food choices
Minimizes message distortion	Education messages related to obesity (or foods which might promote weight loss) may be misconstrued or misapplied and this risk is minimized by a greater emphasis on providing the choices rather then preaching the choices

the environmental approach but the priority needs to be on ensuring that the healthy choices are available first, before embarking on such campaigns to educate people about taking up those choices. The dictum "legislate and regulate where you can, educate and motivate where you can't" provides health promotion with a wide broom for making healthy choices the easy choices (37).

One of the principles of environmental intervention on the energy intake side is to affect small changes in high-volume foods. Take potato chips (potato crisps) as an example, where, say, 90% of the sales are in the regular higher-fat chips (35% fat) and 10% of sales are in the lower-fat chips (25%). There are three main options for reducing the population's dietary fat burden from potato chips by 10%. The first is to reduce the total consumption of chips by 10%, which would probably require a major, sustained public education campaign by health authorities to eat fewer chips, no doubt in the face of stiff opposition from the potato chips manufacturers. The second is to expand the proportion of the sales of lower-fat chips to 44% of the market share. Food companies are already heavily marketing the healthier options to the high-income, high-education consumers in an effort to expand that market share. Such healthier options often come at a premium price and are marketed to the healthiest section of the community, making this a relatively ineffective option for reducing the fat intake of low-income people who are at higher risk of obesity. The sales growth in low- or no-energy drinks in recent years is another example of the food and beverage industry successfully marketing higher-profit products to health-conscious customers. The third option is to reduce the fat content of higher-fat crisps from 35% to 31%. This is technologically feasible, would not be detectable by the consumer, and impacts on a large section of the community including low-income groups. The barriers to reducing the fat content of the high-volume potato chips are perhaps some increases in cost of production (changing plant and adding fans to blow off the fat after cooking) and the lack of a marketing angle to make it appear worthwhile to the manufacturers.

DISSECTING OBESOGENIC ENVIRONMENTS

The ANGELO Framework

The development and execution of health promotion programs, including environmental interventions, require the following steps: (i) analysis, (ii) problem identification, (iii) strategy development, (iv) intervention, and (v) evaluation (38). Major barriers to progressing through these steps for environmental programs include the lack of suitable paradigms and tools for understanding and measuring the environment (39). We have previously described the development and use of the ANGELO

(Analysis Grid for Elements Linked to Obesity) framework for steps (i) and (ii) above (19). This has proved to be a valuable conceptual and practical framework for dissecting the rather nebulous concept of the environment and identifying concrete elements within it, which are amenable to measurement and interventions (40–42). The model has since been used and expanded on to examine the environmental correlates of dietary behaviors (43) and physical activity (44) in youth and in different settings (45).

The first step in using the model is to dissect eating and physical activity behaviors into the settings in which they occur and then link those settings to the wider sectors that influence them. An example of this analysis is shown in Table 3. The interactions among all these levels can be expanded into a full "causal web" such as the one developed by the International Obesity Task Force (46).

The ANGELO framework is a grid, which is comprised of two sizes of environment on one axis and four types of environments on the other (Fig. 3) and is used to scan the environments in question (19). Individuals interact with the environment in multiple (local) microenvironments or settings, including schools, workplaces, homes, and neighborhoods. Microenvironmental settings, in turn, are influenced by the broader macroenvironments or sectors (such as the education and health systems, all levels of government, the food industry, and society's attitudes and beliefs), and these tend to be less amenable to the influence of individuals.

Within these settings or sectors, there are different types of environments. We have categorized these as physical, economic, policy, or sociocultural. Put in simple terms, one can scan the four types of environments by asking the four respective questions: What is or is not available? What are the financial factors? What are the rules? What are the attitudes, perceptions, values, and beliefs? Both food and physical activity (the two mediators) then become subcategories within these cells and it is either (or both) of these that mediate the effects of the broader environments on body fat levels.

The Physical Environment

The physical environment ("what is or is not available?") includes not only the visible world (food and physical activity choices) but also less tangible factors such as the availability of educational training opportunities, nutrition and exercise expertise, technological innovations, information, and food labels. Some factors such as the weather or terrain may be important determinants of behavior but because they are not amenable to influence there is little value in including them in the ANGELO scan, which is selecting factors for potential interventions.

Table 3 Dissection of Some Important Environments That Influence the Mediators of Energy Balance: Energy Intake and Energy Expenditure

Mediator = Energy intake (Energy density, portion size)		
Behaviors	Settings	Sectors
Home food	Home	Food industry, media/marketing
Food prepared outside the home	Fast-food outlets	Food industry, media/marketing
	Cafes/restaurants	Food industry
	Institutions	Food industry
	Cafeterias	Food industry
School food	Schools (+home)	Education sector, food industry, media/marketing

Mediator = Energy expenditure (Physical activity)		
Behaviors	Settings	Sectors
School PE/sports/transport	Schools/transport network	Education sector, local government
Active recreation	Neighborhood (streets, recreation spaces and facilities)	Local government, sports/exercise industry
Passive recreation	Home	Television networks, home entertainment industry, media
Active transport	Transport network (for walking, cycling, public transport)	Local/central government
Car transport	Transport network (for cars, including parking spaces)	Local/central government, media/marketing
Incidental activity	Home Workplace	Local/central government

Abbreviation: PE, physical education.

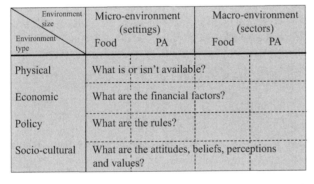

Figure 3 The ANGELO framework. *Abbreviation*: ANGELO, analysis grid for elements linked to obesity.

The Economic Environment

The economic environment ("what are the financial factors?") refers to both the costs related to food and physical activity and the income available to pay for them. These are very important at a household level because of the strong relationship between low incomes and high rates of obesity (47). However, at a macro level, it is the drive to maximize profits of industries, particularly transnational corporations, which dominate in a free market society. In the United States alone, the food and soft drink industries are amongst the largest spenders on mass media (48) accounting for over 14% (about $14 billion) of the top 100 advertisers in 2006 (49). Among the biggest spenders are McDonalds Corporation ($1.7 billion) and PepsiCo ($1.3 billion). The budget allocations of local and central governments are tangible indicators of the importance placed on, say, active transport versus car transport or nutrition and physical activity monitoring.

The Policy Environment

The policy environment ("what are the rules?") refers to laws, regulations, policies (formal or informal), and institutional rules (including in the home) that impact on physical activity and eating behaviors. These rules can have profound effects on the behavior of individuals and organizations. Some examples include home rules on television watching (50,51), school food policies (52), regulations (or lack of them) on fast-food advertising on children's television (53), food labeling laws (54), traffic-zoning bylaws (55), building codes (limiting stair access), and urban planning regulations (56).

The Sociocultural Environment

The sociocultural environment ("what are the attitudes, perceptions, values, and beliefs?") establishes the context for what is considered normative behaviors within a particular societal group. At a micro or setting level, these sociocultural influences combine to give what is variously described as the culture, ethos, or climate of a school, home, workplace, or neighborhood. In schools, for example, the school ethos is considered a central component of a health-promoting school (52). It is influenced by, among other things, the relationships among staff and students, the value a school places on participation in sports and physical education, the degree to which the teachers serve as healthy role models for the students, and how much good nutrition features in the philosophy of the school food service.

Some cultural values or attitudes such as hospitality expectations on hosts to provide and guests to consume large amounts of food could promote overconsumption of food (57). Also, some cultures consider that it is inappropriate for its members to be physically active, thus promoting inactivity (57,58). One could therefore consider individuals to be culturally predisposed to (or protected from) obesity, depending on their cultural affiliations in the same way that they would be considered genetically predisposed or protected according to their genotypes.

At the macroenvironmental level, the mass media are an important sector influencing the sociocultural aspects of food and physical activity (59–61). They directly and indirectly influence society's attitudes, beliefs, and values because they not only reflect and reinforce the common culture but also shape it, particularly through the effects of advertising and marketing (62,63).

PRIORITIZING ENVIRONMENTAL FACTORS FOR INTERVENTION

Using the ANGELO framework with a group of stakeholders usually identifies a large number of potential environmental influences that may affect eating and physical activity patterns. The major challenge then is to hone them down to a few high-priority areas for further action. There are many potential criteria which could be used for prioritizing, including effectiveness, cost, feasibility, sustainability, effects on equity, strength of evidence, and so on. At a practical level with communities, it may be easier to consolidate these as two key criteria: changeability (is the environmental factor amenable to change?) and importance (how big a problem is the environmental factor in our area and will changing it influence behaviors?). Getting stakeholders to score each element along these criteria quickly sorts out the high-priority environmental factors. Action

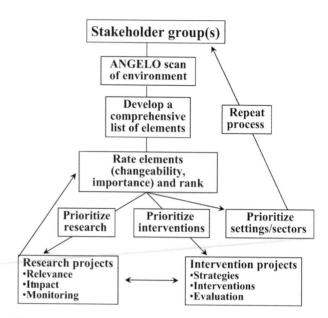

Figure 4 A proposed process for applying the ANGELO framework to prioritize interventions and research. *Abbreviation*: ANGELO, analysis grid for elements linked to obesity.

usually takes the form of interventions ("we know enough now to strengthen existing interventions or begin new ones"), research ("we need more hard data before we can proceed to intervention"), or further consultation ("we need more stakeholder consultation before we can prioritize"). This prioritizing process (as shown in a flow diagram in Fig. 4) has been found to be valuable in a variety of settings (19,43,44), although in real life such processes rarely proceed along such a linear path.

MEASURING ENVIRONMENTAL INDICATORS

The development of indicators of obesogenic environments (and related behaviors) is a fundamental requirement of an environment or systems-based approach to obesity (64). The indicators are needed primarily to monitor progress over time but they also allow comparisons among neighborhoods/cities/regions/countries and provide the basis for testing the impact of environmental change and behavior change.

Curtailing and reversing the obesity epidemic will not occur without the underlying environmental driving forces becoming more leptogenic. To positively and systematically influence the environments requires a robust set of indicators. The attributes of an ideal indicator are listed in Table 4, although, as with most measurements in science, all criteria are rarely met. The assessment of the impact of particular environmental factors on a behavior of interest is often problematic. Cross-sectional and ecological studies have inherent limitations in assessing the nature and

Table 4 Criteria for Ideal Indicators of Obesogenic Environments

Criterion	Comments
Impact	The environmental factor it reflects should have a significant impact on behaviors, e.g., TV advertising on food choices.
Validity	It should faithfully reflect the environmental factor in question, e.g., local government budgets for public transport support and cycleways versus major road works as a true reflection of the public investment in active transport versus car transport.
Responsiveness	It should be able to detect small changes in the environmental factor, e.g., a yes/no question about the presence of a school food policy may not be sensitive enough to detect differences in effectiveness of policies
Reliability	The intra and inter observer error and random error should be minimal, e.g., questionnaire-based indicators often need test-retest reliability assessments, whereas, the number of cars per household from census data would be considered reliable.
Easy to measure	Ideally it would use data, which are already collected for other purposes, e.g., food sales from supermarkets by category.
Inexpensive to measure	Questionnaire-based indicators, e.g., sociocultural indicators will be relatively expensive to measure.
Easily understood	Indicators that have complex derivations and are highly adjusted are less likely to be well understood, e.g., access to recreational facilities that is measured using distance-decay formulae and adjusted for attractiveness of the facility and the type of facility.

strength of associations (65) and even intervention studies are either multidimensional or have design weaknesses (such as no-comparison group) that make interpretation difficult (66).

INFLUENCING OBESOGENIC ENVIRONMENTS—GENERAL STRATEGIES

Using the ANGELO framework with stakeholders across various environments generates dozens, even hundreds, of potential aspects of the environments that might be amenable to leptogenic changes. Several authors have also outlined lists of potential environmental interventions for obesity prevention (19,41–44,67–69). The key difficulty in converting good ideas into action is narrowing down the many "could do" activities into a few "can do" ones and gaining the community and political commitment to then make them "must do" actions. This has not been achieved in a coherent way for any population, but on the basis of the experience of other epidemics and the obesity epidemic to date, a few general principles can be extracted.

Keeping Obesity Prevention Firmly Environment Based

One of the risks of developing a momentum for environment-led obesity prevention is that obesity as an issue gets combined with diabetes and cardiovascular diseases and then most of the funding and efforts are channeled into clinical interventions and/or mass media strategies. While the rationale for such clumping is readily defendable, and these strategies are important, a primary focus on improving the environments for healthy food and physical activity choices is needed if population-based prevention is to be a priority.

Keeping the Interventions Achievable and Sustainable

The vastness of the task of preventing obesity is a classic barrier to action. To build the political and community case for action, the interventions need to be doable. Expanding existing programs that have shown some success (50,70,71), limiting the geographical reach of interventions in the first instance (i.e., establishing demonstration or sentinel sites), or focusing on a small number of settings are all strategies that can overcome the "inertia of enormity."

Priority on Children

Perhaps the strongest cases for priority environments to influence are those related to children and adolescents. Nowhere does the ounce of prevention versus the pound of treatment apply more appropriately than with obesity because of the difficulty of losing excess fat once it has been gained. Also the range of achievable environmental interventions for children is greater than for adults (see later).

Broad-Based Community and Political Commitment

Most of the environments that influence eating and activity patterns lie outside the jurisdiction of health and therefore need the engagement of a range of stakeholders.

The strong backing from the community, the setting stakeholders, and the politicians is vital to securing the momentum and funding for interventions.

High-Quality Programs

A high-quality program to reduce obesity would have a long duration, be sufficiently well funded to achieve a high dose of the intervention(s) and a wide reach to priority populations, and have robust evaluations. One of the temptations for governments with a low commitment to long-term solutions for obesity is to establish one or two short-term, low-dose, high-profile interventions. Another temptation is to shift the responsibility onto individuals (to make the healthy choices), private industry (to use market forces to create healthy environments), or the nongovernment health organizations (to fund the programs). High-dose programs over long periods are needed and this inevitably means government vision and funding. Evaluation is needed at every step: early formative inquiry, process evaluation (including the implementation and roll out phases), outcome analysis, and ongoing monitoring (72). Highly controlled, one-off interventions provide useful information about efficacy (or lack of efficacy) (11,73), but what is probably much more valuable are long-term evaluation studies (often less well controlled) of the real-world effectiveness of ongoing programs (72).

INFLUENCING OBESOGENIC ENVIRONMENTS— PRIORITY SETTINGS

Schools and Other Educational Settings

Rationale and Evidence of Impact

Schools are a natural setting for influencing the food and physical activity environments for several reasons (74): children are a high-priority population, they are almost all captive in the school environment, they spend a large proportion of their waking hours at school, they eat and do sport and activities at school, there are links to the curriculum, and schools provide some access to the home environment. In a review of environment-based interventions to reduce energy intake or energy density (66), 24 of the 75 identified studies were school based. There was a wide variety of interventions including changes to the school lunch menus and food choices, award certificates for school canteens, curriculum changes, healthy choice information to students and parents, and changing the price of food items. Overall, the evaluation designs were of mixed quality, but most showed a positive impact on nutrient intake and dietary patterns (70,75,76), nutrition knowledge (77), and food sales (71,78).

Stone et al. (79) reviewed the impact of 14 school-based interventions on physical activity knowledge and behavior. Most of the outcome variables showed significant improvements for the intervention schools or groups. One interdisciplinary intervention program (mainly curriculum based) aimed at influencing the eating patterns, television viewing, and activity levels among six- to eight-year-old children resulted in a reduction in obesity prevalence among the girls but not the boys (50).

In addition to the areas targeted for intervention in the published studies, there are other areas of growing concern in relation to schools. One is the increasing proportion of children who are being driven to school because of parental fears for the children's safety (from injury from cars) and security (from abduction) (80). In the United Kingdom, the proportion of seven- to eight-year-old children who traveled to school on their own plummeted from 80% in 1971 to only 9% in 1990 (80). Another area of concern is the increasing pressure from soft drink companies on schools to place soft drink vending machines in the schools with contracts for a required volume of sales (34). Also, low participation rates in sports and physical education, particularly among adolescent girls, may set the pattern for activity patterns in adulthood (81).

Despite the crowded curriculum and the pressure on schools and teachers to take on a variety of health programs, there is a strong imperative for schools to be a major setting for obesity prevention. In fact, efforts to prevent obesity could hardly be deemed serious without schools being a central component.

Potential Interventions

There are many different models of school food programs, depending on the school food services offered (66). Interventions may be in the form of new programs or enhanced existing programs, stand-alone programs, or part of a wider health-promoting schools concept (52). Whatever form they take, they need to be funded to achieve a high-enough dose of intervention and achieve a wide-enough reach, particularly to schools in disadvantaged areas. The major elements of a school-based program are (*i*) a school food and nutrition policy (including the types of foods and drinks available and promoted at school through the school food service or vending machines), (*ii*) training and resources for teachers and food service staff, (*iii*) guidelines for offering healthy food and drink choices, (*iv*) encouraging healthy options in food brought from home, and (*v*) curriculum content on food and nutrition.

Substantial increases in sports participation and/or physical education time can be successful at reducing adiposity but the programs need to have policy support both at the school and the education sector levels (82).

Home Environment

Rationale and Evidence of Impact

The home environment is undoubtedly the most important setting in relation to shaping children's eating and physical activity behaviors, but, surprisingly, we know very little about what those specific home influences are (102). As a setting, however, it is difficult to influence because of the sheer numbers and heterogeneity of homes and the limited options for access (with television being the most effective but very expensive access option). Potential areas to target in terms of the home food environment would be the food available and served in the home, the parents as role models for healthy eating, and the eating ethos of the household (is a meal simply fuel eaten on the run or in front of television or is it a focus for family communion?). For physical activity/inactivity, the home environment provides rules for television, the Internet, and video game use (103) and establishes the activity ethos of the family, again with parents as critical role models, and whether there are television sets in children's bedrooms. Of all these aspects of the home environment, television viewing has been the most researched (50,104). It appears that gains can be made in obesity prevention through restricting television viewing, although it seems that reduced eating in front of television is at least as important as decreasing inactivity or increasing activity (103).

Potential Interventions

Apart from the studies aimed at reducing television viewing, some of which used a locking device on the television (103), there are no major studies to guide potential interventions aimed at influencing the home environment (66,101). The medium for any interventions on the home environment for children and adolescents will have to depend heavily on educating parents. While the use of mass media might achieve the desired reach, it is expensive, and other access points such as through school or preschool or early-childhood health systems might be more sustainable alternatives.

Indicators of Change

Surveys of time spent in front of television, videos, and computer screens are conducted regularly in some countries and are good indicators of inactive recreation. More specific indicators to capture the home environment in terms of television sets in children's bedrooms, family rules on food and television viewing, and parental role model behavior would require more extensive household survey questionnaires.

Other Potentially Changeable Obesogenic Environments

A variety of other environments warrant consideration for interventions. A few short-term studies have shown that a simple sign on stairs or elevators can increase stair walking (105,106). What is now needed is an implementation program to widely deploy such signs as well as advocacy to influence building codes and architectural designs so that stairs are an attractive easy option for everyday use rather than being hidden and dingy and intended for emergency use only.

The design and development of built environments that are conducive and attractive for physical activity is a major challenge. It will be a long process involving urban planners, architects, engineers, government infrastructure departments, as well as end users, but it is in sympathy with current drive to make environment and infrastructure decisions more environmentally and socially sound.

Restaurants (66,107), workplaces (66,108,109), supermarkets (66,110), sports venues (111), and whole communities (34,68,112) have been studied as settings for influencing dietary intake and physical activity patterns. The impacts have ranged from none to modest and many of the interventions have been of relatively short duration. Nevertheless, modest changes adopted by a high proportion of the population are undoubtedly going to be the manner in which the obesity epidemic is to be curtailed. The magnitude of changes seen in individual-based trials cannot expect to be found in population-based interventions.

CONCLUSIONS

Increasingly obesogenic environments (mainly economic) are the predominant driving forces behind the escalating obesity pandemic. It is therefore surprising that little attention has been paid to this area by way of academic analysis, etiological research, and intervention studies. We have proposed a framework for dissecting and analyzing obesogenic environments that we have found to be a useful and robust scanning tool to identify environmental elements worthy of intervention. However, this is only the first stage and prioritizing the elements or settings to invest in for obesity prevention is difficult in the absence of much evidence to guide decisions. Priorities will vary according to local, regional, and national circumstances, and building intervention efforts onto existing activities will probably be a more successful approach than creating de novo intervention programs. Some of the strategies for reducing obesogenic environments such as banning the marketing of obesogenic foods to children will be met by substantial opposition. One only has to revisit the lessons from the tobacco epidemic to see that the efforts of government, society, and science can overcome such powerful vested interests if they are synergistic and sustained.

We have suggested that the priority population for obesity prevention should be children and adolescents because of the difficulty of reversing obesity in adults once it is established. We have also suggested that the key settings for interventions could be schools and other education settings, neighborhoods, transport networks, fast-food outlets, and home environments. In general, the studies to date have been short to medium term in duration, the study designs have been of mixed quality and the results have ranged from no effect to modest effects. However, the strength of an environmental approach is that even modest impacts can have positive population benefits if there is a high volume of people exposed to that environment. "Small changes times large volumes" is the nature of both the ascending and descending trajectories of the noncommunicable disease epidemics.

The challenge ahead of us is to identify obesogenic environments and influence them so that the healthier choices are more available, easier to access, and widely promoted to a large proportion of the community. This will require a paradigm shift within the health sector to see obesogenic environments as the drivers and the nonhealth sectors as essential allies in tackling the obesity epidemic. Similarly, for the nonhealth sectors such as local governments, schools, and the food industry, a paradigm shift is needed for them to see their contributions toward reversing the obesity epidemic.

REFERENCES

1. Obesity: Preventing and Managing the Global Epidemic, . Report of a WHO Consultation. WHO Technical Report Series 894. Geneva: World Health Organization, 1998: 157–162.
2. Egger G, Swinburn BA. An "ecological" approach to the obesity pandemic. BMJ 1997; 315:477–480.
3. Rennie KL, Jebb SA. Prevalence of obesity Great Britain. Obesity Rev 2005; 6:11–12.
4. Knight I. The Heights and Weights of Adults in Great Britain. London: HMSO, 1984.
5. Schokker DF, Visscher TLS, Nooyens ACJ, et al. Prevalence of overweight and obesity in the Netherlands. Obes Rev 2006; 8:101–107.
6. Obesity. The Report of the British Nutrition Foundation Task Force. Oxford: Blackwell Science, 1999.
7. Rose G. The Strategy of Preventive Medicine. London: Oxford University Press, 1993.
8. Swinburn BA, Metcalf PA, Ley SJ. Long term (5 year) effects of a reduced fat diet in individuals with glucose intolerance. Diabetes Care 2001; 24(4):617–624.

9. Brownell K. Relapse and the treatment of obesity. In: Wadden TA, VanItallie TB, eds. Treatment of the Seriously Obese Patient. New York: The Guilford Press, 1992:437–455.
10. Doak CM, Visscher TL, Renders CM, et al. The prevention of overweight and obesity in children and adolescents: a review of interventions and programmes. Obes Rev 2006; 7(1):111–136.
11. Summerbell C, Waters E, Edmunds L, et al. Interventions for preventing obesity in children. Cochrane Database Syst Rev 2005; (3):CD001871.
12. Morley JJ, Swinburn BA, Metcalf PA, et al. Fat content of chips, quality of frying fat and deep-frying practices in New Zealand fast food outlets. Aust N Z J Public Health 2002; 26(2):101–107.
13. Wilson BD, Wilson NC, Russell DG. Obesity and body fat distribution in the New Zealand population. N Z Med J 2001; 114:127–131.
14. Nutbeam D, Harris E. Theory in a Nutshell: A Practical Guide to Health Promotion Theories. Sydney: McGraw-Hill, 2004.
15. Swinburn BA, Ravussin E. Energy and macronutrient metabolism. In: Caterson ID, ed. Baillière's Clinical Endocrinology and Metabolism: Obesity. Vol. 8(3). London: Baillière Tindall, 1994:527–548.
16. Alpert S. Growth, thermogenesis, and hyperphagia. Am J Clin Nutr 1990; 48:240–247.
17. Abbott WGH, Howard BV, Christin L, et al. Short term energy balance: relationship with protein, carbohydrate, and fat balances. Am J Physiol 1988; 255:E332–E337.
18. Swinburn BA, Ravussin E. Energy balance or fat balance? Am J Clin Nutr 1992; 57(suppl):766S–771S.
19. Swinburn BA, Egger GJ, Raza F. Dissecting obesogenic environments: the development and application of a framework for identifying and prioritising environmental interventions for obesity. Prev Med 1999; 29:563–570.
20. Sallis JF, Owen N. Ecological models. In: Glanz K, Lewis FM, Rimer BK, eds. Health Behavior and Health Education: Theory, Research and Practice. San Francisco: Jossey-Bass, 1996:403–424.
21. Rolls BJ, Roe LS, Meengs JS. Reductions in portion size and energy density of foods are additive and lead to sustained decreases in energy intake. Am J Clin Nutr 2006; 83(1):11–17.
22. Keesey RE. The body weight set-point. What can you tell your patients? Postgrad Med 1988; 83:114–127.
23. Ravussin E, Swinburn BA. Metabolic predictors of obesity: cross-sectional versus longitudinal data. Int J Obes 1994; 17(suppl 3):S28–S31.
24. Leibel RL, Rosenbaum M, Hirsch J. Changes in energy expenditure from altered body weight. N Engl J Med 1995; 332:621–628.
25. Teris M. Epidemiology and the public health movement. J Publ Health Policy 1987; 8(3):315–329.
26. Haddon W. Advances in the epidemiology of injuries as a basis for public policy. Public Health Rep 1980a; 95(5): 411–420.
27. Chapman S. Unwrapping gossamer with boxing gloves. BMJ 1993; 307:429–432.

28. Egger G, Pearson S, Pal S, et al. Dissecting obesogenic behaviours: the development and application of a test battery for targeting prescription for weight loss. Obes Rev 2007; 8:481–486. Available at www.professortrim.com/DAB-Q.

29. Moodie R, Swinburn B, Richardson J, et al. Childhood obesity—a sign of commercial success but market failure. Int J Ped Obesity 2006; 1(3):133–138.

30. Bray G. Leptin and leptinomania. Lancet 1996; 348: 140–141.

31. Battle EK, Brownell KD. Confronting the rising tide of eating disorders and obesity: treatment versus prevention and policy. Addict Behav 1996; 21:755–765.

32. Hill JO, Peters JC. Environmental contributions to the obesity epidemic. Science 1998; 280:1371–1374.

33. Egger G, Bolton A, O'Neill M, et al. Effectiveness of an abdominal obesity reduction programme in men: The GutBusters 'waist loss' programme. Int J Obes 1996; 20: 227–231.

34. French SA, Story M, Jeffrey RW. Environmental influences on eating and physical activity. Ann Rev Public Health 2001; 22:309–335.

35. King AC. Community and public health approaches to the promotion of physical activity. Med Sci Sports Exerc 1994; 26:1405–1412.

36. Robinson TN, Sirad JR. Preventing childhood obesity: a solution oriented research paradigm. Am J Prev Med 2005; 28(suppl 2):194–201.

37. Egger G. Personal carbon trading: a potential "stealth intervention" for obesity reduction? Med J Aust 2007; 187(3):185–187.

38. Egger G, Spark R, Donovan R. Health Promotion: Strategies and Methods. 2nd ed. Sydney: McGraw Hill, 1999:113–122.

39. Nutbeam D. Creating health-promoting environments: overcoming barriers to action. Aust N Z J Public Health 1997; 21(4):355–359.

40. Egger G, Fisher G, Piers S, et al. Abdominal obesity reduction in indigenous men. Int J Obes 1999; 23: 564–569.

41. Acting on Australia's Weight. National Medical and Health Research Council. Canberra: Commonwealth of Australia, 1997.

42. Balancing Policies for Healthy Weight: Preparing an Action Plan for the Prevention and Management of Overweight and Obesity. London: International Obesity Task Force, 2000:32–36.

43. van der Horst K, Oenema A, Ferreira I, et al. A systematic review of environmental correlates of obesity-related dietary behaviors in youth. Health Ed Res 2007; 22(20): 203–226.

44. Ferreira I, van der Horst K, Wendel-Vos W, et al. Environmental correlates of physical activity in youth—a review and update. Obes Rev 2007; 8(2):129–154.

45. Schultz, Utter J, Mathews L, et al. Action plans and interventions—The Pacific OPIC Project (Obesity Prevention in Communities). Pac Health Dialog (in press).

46. Kumanyika SK. Mini symposium on obesity: overview and some strategic considerations. Ann Rev Public Health 2001; 22:293–308.

47. Aguirre P. Socioanthropological aspects of obesity in poverty. In: Pena M, Bacallo J, eds. Obesity and Poverty. A New Public Health Challenge. Scientific Publication No 576. Washington, D.C.: Pan-American Health Organization, 2000.

48. Gallo AE. Food advertising in the United States. In: Frazao E, ed. America's Eating Habits: Changes and Consequences. Washington DC: USDA/Econ Res Serv 1999:173–180.

49. Advertising Age. 2007. 2007 Marketer Profiles Yearbook. 100 Leading National Advertisers. Available at: http://adage.com/datacenter/.

50. Gortmaker SL, Peterson K, Wiecha J, et al. Reducing obesity via a school-based interdisciplinary intervention among youth: planet health. Arch Pediatr Adolesc Med 1999; 153:409–418.

51. Epstein LH, Valoski A, Wing RR, et al. Ten-year outcomes of behavioural family-based treatment for childhood obesity. Health Psychol 1994; 13:373–383.

52. Booth ML, Samdal O. Health-promoting schools in Australia: models and measurements. Aust N Z J Public Health 1997; 21(4):365–370.

53. Dibb S, Castwell A. Easy to Swallow, Hard to Stomach: The Results of a Survey of Food Advertising on Television. London: The National Food Alliance, 1995.

54. Glanz K, Mullis RM. Environmental interventions to promote healthy eating: a review of models, programs, and evidence. Health Ed Quart 1988; 15:395–415.

55. Crawford JH. Carfree Cities. Utrecht: International Books, 2000.

56. Cervero R, Gorham R. Commuting in transit versus automobile neighborhoods. J Am Plan Assoc 1995; 61:210–225.

57. Packard DP, McWilliams M. Cultural foods heritage of Middle Eastern immigrants. Nutr Today 1993; 28:6–13.

58. Stahl T, Rutten A, Nutbeam D, et al. The importance of the social environment for physically active lifestyle—results from an international study. Soc Sci Med 2001; 52:1–10.

59. MacLaren T. Messages for the masses: food and nutrition issues on television. J Am Diet Assoc 1997; 97(7): 733–738.

60. Hertzler AA, Grun I. Potential nutrition messages in magazines read by college students. Adolescence 1990; 25(99):717–723.

61. Strasburger VC. Adolescents and the Media: Medical and Psychological Impact. California: Sage, 1995.

62. Billington R, Strawbridge S, Greensides L, et al. Culture and Society. London: MacMillan Education, 1991:156–171.

63. Serwer AE. McDonald's conquers the world. Fortune 1994; 130(8):103–107.

64. Cheadle A, Kristal A, Wagner E, et al. Environmental indicators: a tool for evaluating community-based health promotion programs. Am J Prev Med 1992; 8:345–350.

65. Beaglehole R, Bonita R, Kjellstrom T. Basic Epidemiology. Geneva, World Health Organization 1993:31–53.

66. Hider P. Environmental interventions to reduce energy intake or density. A critical appraisal of the literature. NZHTA Report 2001 4(2). Christchurch: New Zealand Health Technology Assessment, 2001.

67. Nestle M, Jacobson MF. Halting the obesity epidemic: a public health policy approach. Public Health Rep 2000; 115:1–13.

68. Sallis JF, Bauman A, Pratt M. Environmental and policy interventions to promote physical activity. Am J Prev Med 1998; 15:379–397.

69. King AC, Jeffrey RW, Fridinger F, et al. Environmental and policy approaches to cardiovascular disease prevention through physical activity: issues and opportunities. Health Ed Quart 1995; 22(4):499–511.

70. Flynn MAT, McNeill DA, Maloff B, et al. Reducing obesity and related chronic disease risk in children and youth: a synthesis of evidence with 'best practice' recommendations. Obes Rev 2007; 7(suppl 7):7–66.

71. Taylor RW, McAuley KA, Barbezat W, et al. APPLE Project: 2-y findings of a community-based obesity prevention program in primary school-age children. Am J Clin Nutr 2007; 86:735–742.

72. Swinburn BA, Bell AC, King L, et al. Obesity prevention programs demand high quality evaluations. Aust N Z J Public Health 2007; 31:305–307.

73. Caballero B, Clay T, Davis SM, et al. Pathways: a school-based, randomized controlled trial for the prevention of obesity in American Indian schoolchildren. Am J Clin Nutr 2003; 78(5):1030–1038.

74. Resnicow K, Robinson TN. School-based cardiovascular disease prevention studies: review and synthesis. Ann Epidemiol 1997; S7:S14–S31.

75. Synder P, Anliker J, Cunningham-Sabo L, et al. The pathways study: a model for lowering the fat in school menus. Am J Clin Nutr 1999; 69(suppl 4):810S–815S.

76. Snyder P, Story M, Trenkner L. Reducing fat and sodium in school lunch programs: the Lunchpower intervention study. J Am Diet Assoc 1992; 92:1087–1091.

77. Dollahite J, Hosig K, White K, et al. Impact of a school-based community intervention program on nutrition knowledge and food choices in elementary school children in the rural Arkansas Delta. J Nutr Ed 1998; 30:289–301.

78. Meiselman H, Hedderley D, Staddon S, et al. Effect of effort on meal selection and acceptability in a student cafeteria. Appetite 1994; 23:43–55.

79. Stone EJ, McKenzie TL, Welk GJ, et al. Effects of physical activity interventions in youth. A review and synthesis. Am J Prev Med 1998; 15:298–315.

80. Frank LD, Engelke P. How land use and transportation systems impact public health: a literature review of the relationship between physical activity and the built form. Report to the Centers for Disease Control and Prevention. Georgia Institute of Technology, 2001.

81. Booth M, Maskill P, McClelland L, et al. NSW Schools Fitness and Physical Activity Survey. Sydney: NSW Department of School Education, 1997.

82. Dwyer T, Coonan WE, Leitch DR, et al. An investigation of the effects of daily physical activity on the health of primary school students in South Australia. Int J Epidemiol 1983; 12(3):308–313.

83. Sallis JF, Hovell MF, Hofstetter CR, et al. Distance between homes and exercise facilities related to frequency of exercise in San Diego residents. Public Health Rep 1990; 105(2):179–185.

84. Bauman A, Smith B, Stoker L, et al. Geographical influences upon physical activity participation: evidence of a 'coastal effect'. Aust N Z J Public Health 1999; 23(3):322–324.

85. Wright C, MacDougall C, Atkinson R, et al. Exercise in daily life: supportive environments. National Heart Foundation of Australia Report. Adelaide: Commonwealth of Australia, 1996.

86. Rutten A, Abel T, Kannas L, et al. Self reported physical activity, public health and perceived environment: results from a comparative European study. J Epidemiol Community Health 2001; 55(2):139–146.

87. Corti B, Donovan RJ, D'Arcy C, et al. Factors influencing the use of physical activity facilities: results from qualitative research. Health Prom J Aust 1996; 6(1):16–21.

88. Housmann RA, Brown DR, Jackson-Thompson J, et al. Promoting physical activity in rural counties—walking trails access, use and effects. Am J Prev Med 2000; 18:235–241.

89. Lancaster RA, ed. Recreation, Park and Open Space Standards and Guidelines. Virginia: National Recreation and Park Association, 1983.

90. Llewelyn-Davies. Sustainable Residential Quality—New Approaches to Urban Living. London: London Planning Advisory Committee, 1997.

91. Dora C. A different route to health: implications of transport policies. BMJ 1999; 318:1686–1689.

92. Kitamura R, Mokhtarian PL, Laidet L. A micro-analysis of land use and travel in five neighborhoods in the San Francisco Bay area. Transportation 1997; 24:125–158.

93. TravelSmart (Transport). Available at: www.travelsmart.transport.wa.gov.au.

94. Bachels M, Newman P, Kenworthy J. Indicators of Urban Transport Efficiency in New Zealand's Main Cities: An International City Comparison of Transport, Land Use and Economic Indicators. Perth: Institute for Science and Technology Policy, Murdoch University, 1999.

95. Jeffrey RW, French SA. Epidemic obesity in the United States: are fast foods and television viewing contributing? Am J Public Health 1998; 88:277–280.

96. Wilson N, Quigley R, Mansoor O. Food advertisements on TV: a health hazard for children. Aust N Z J Public Health 1999; 23(6):647–650.

97. Hill JM, Radimer KL. A content analysis of food advertisements in television for Australian children. Aust N Z J Public Health 1997; 54(4):174–181.

98. Guthrie JF, Kox JJ, Cleveland LE, et al. Who uses nutrition labeling and what effects does label use have on diet quality? J Nutr Ed 1995; 27:163–172.

99. Young L, Swinburn B. The impact of the Pick the Tick food information program on salt content of food in New Zealand. Health Prom Int 2002; 17(1):13–19.

100. Institute of Medicine. Food Marketing to Children and Youth. Threat or opportunity? Washington: National Academy of Sciences, 2006.

101. The Sydney Principles, International Obesity Taskforce. Available at: www.iotf.org/sydneyprinciples.

102. Campbell K, Crawford D. Family food environments as determinants of preschool-aged children's eating behaviours: implications for obesity prevention policy. A review. Aust J Nutr Diet 2001; 58(1):19–25.

103. American Academy of Pediatrics Committee on Communications, . Children, adolescents and television. Pediatrics 1995; 96(4):786–787.

104. Dietz WH, Gortmaker SL. Preventing obesity in children and adolescents. Annu Rev Public Health 2001; 22:337–353.

105. Russell WD, Dzewaltowski DA, Ryan GJ. The effectiveness of a point-of-decision prompt in deterring sedentary behavior. Am J Health Prom 1999; 13(5):257–259.

106. Brownell KD, Stunkard AJ, Albaum JM. Evaluation and modification of exercise patterns in the natural environment. Am J Psych 1980; 137:1540–1545.

107. Colby J, Elder J, Peterson G, et al. Promoting the selection of health food through menu item description in a family style restaurant. Am J Prev Med 1987; 3:171–177.

108. Chu C, Driscoll T, Dwyer S. The health-promoting workplace: an integrative perspective. Aust N Z J Public Health 1997; 21(4):377–384.

109. Schmitz M, Fielding J. Point-of-choice nutrition labeling—evaluation in a worksite cafeteria. J Nutr Ed 1986; 18(suppl 1):S65–S68.

110. Winett R, Wagner J, Moore J, et al. An experimental evaluation of a prototype public access nutrition information system for supermarkets. Health Psychol 1991; 10:75–78.

111. Corti B, Holman CDJ. Warning: attending a sport, racing or arts venue may be beneficial to your health. Aust N Z J Public Health 1997; 21(4):371–376.

112. Bell AC, Swinburn BA, Amosa H, et al K. A nutrition and exercise intervention program for controlling weight in Samoan communities in New Zealand. Int J Obes 2001; 25:920–927.

12

Reengineering the Built Environment: Schools, Worksites, Neighborhoods, and Parks

DEBORAH A. COHEN

Rand Corporation, Santa Monica, California, U.S.A.

WHAT IS THE BUILT ENVIRONMENT?

The term "built environment" refers to man-made surroundings that provide the setting for human activity, from the largest-scale civic structures to the smallest personal places (1). The built environment consists of four different structures: physical structures; social structures; specific products like consumer items, including their accessibility and availability; and the media environment (2).

Physical structures are fixed in the environment or are characteristics of products. They influence behavior by creating or inhibiting opportunities for behavior (e.g., gun-safety locks, abandoned houses, sidewalks), sending messages about rules of behavior (e.g., blighted housing), and facilitating or constraining social interactions (e.g., porches, fences).

Social structures include laws, policies, and social rules that regulate individual and interpersonal behavior, and organizations in society that influence behavior indirectly. They influence behavior by directly constraining or promoting behaviors, communicating norms of behavior, encouraging or discouraging social interactions, or providing people with a purpose, social niche, or status. Examples of social structures include indoor smoking bans, mandatory seat belt laws, and schools, jobs, and recreation programs.

Accessibility of consumer products affects health in that limited availability reduces use and widespread availability encourages greater use. Accessibility includes quantity, prominence, and price. Examples of relevant products include tobacco, alcohol, guns, condoms, needles, drugs, and healthy and unhealthy foods.

Messages in the mass media include television, radio, magazines, newspapers, and the Internet. They influence behavior by communicating behavioral norms and values, creating a new reality (framing events), and increasing consumption. Examples include violence on television (which has been shown to cause aggressive behavior among those who watch) and food advertising, associated with greater consumption of advertised foods.

All of these structures are engineered by people, and their distribution across geographic space is determined by them. Therefore, reengineering these structures is also feasible.

Behavioral Settings

The built environment forms what has been termed "behavioral settings" based on the idea that behavioral cues are produced by the places we visit or inhabit (3). As people go about their daily routines, moving from home to school or work or to other destinations outside the home, each of the settings influences their behavior, including physical activity (PA) and diet, depending on the design of the location, its accessibility, the presence or absence of food, and the messages and cues regarding food and PA.

Food environments include any place where food is available, such as restaurants, markets, vending machines, and kitchens. Increasingly, food is available at more and more places, including sites that in previous decades never had food. Food is available now at car washes, hardware stores, bookstores, pharmacies, department stores, and gas stations. Typically, these sites only provide highly processed foods that are relatively nonperishable, energy-dense, and with low nutrient value. Moreover, such sites are generally not regulated by health departments that otherwise license and inspect outlets that sell fresh and perishable food items. The inspection and licensing process from the level of the United States Department of Agriculture (USDA) to the local health department has contributed to the control of food-borne diseases, and is a social structure that influences how food is prepared (4).

Environments also determine the level of PA people engage in: sedentary, moderately active, or vigorously active. Typically, most indoor settings (except for gyms, dance floors, health clubs, and swimming pools) are considered inappropriate for vigorous activity, since the structural features of the environment (walls, furniture, small spaces) are incompatible with vigorous exercise like running and are most conducive to sedentary behavior. Outdoor settings are the venues where people move from one site to another. Sidewalks, streets, paths, as well as parks are the places where moderate-to-vigorous PA is the most appropriate.

Why is the Environment Important?

The traditional medical approach to health views individuals and individual behavior and physiology as the source of disease. The belief that people are rational and act in their own interest if they have the appropriate information is the basis for the myriad educational and informational programs that are intended to change people's behaviors. The traditional approach suggests that individuals can act contrary to cues in their environment if they are armed with appropriate knowledge and skills.

However, even when people have knowledge about behaviors that are beneficial and have the relevant behavioral skills, this can be trumped by behavioral settings that dictate how people should behave. It is very difficult for a person to act in a way that is inconsistent with the behavioral setting. A large part of the reason why behavioral settings exert such a powerful influence has to do with human neurophysiology and how the environment governs our behaviors.

Although it seems obvious that physical structures can be barriers or facilitators of PA, there are other reasons and pathways through which the built environment influences human behaviors. If people really wanted to, they could jog in place, use treadmills indoors, and exercise in front of a television in their living room. The reality is that much home exercise equipment is unused and most people do not engage in vigorous exercise at home. Homes imply sedentary behaviors and relaxation—a respite from the outside world. We respond to the settings and cues in our environment automatically. If we want to behave in a manner that is contrary to all the cues in our environment, we need to purposefully change and reorient our behaviors. While this is not impossible, it is extremely difficult to maintain over the long term for one simple reason: human beings have limited cognitive capacities that fatigue over time.

The part of our brains that constitute our conscious awareness has the ability to process about 40 to 60 bits/sec, equivalent to a short sentence. Fortunately, we do not rely solely on our conscious awareness to function. Our entire processing capacity also includes our sight, other senses, and the unconscious thinking, and is estimated to have a much larger capacity, about 11 million bits/sec (5). Therefore, unconscious thinking and processes beyond conscious awareness play an inordinately large role in our decisions and behaviors. Given the wealth of stimuli and the millions of bits of information in our environment and the fact that people cannot concentrate on two things simultaneously, much of our daily behavior occurs without the involvement of our conscious awareness.

Since the beginning of the social and behavioral sciences, researchers have explored why people make the decisions they do. Decades ago researchers realized that the analysis of situations and appraisals of the environment occur at unconscious levels, to which individuals *cannot* bring conscious awareness (6–8). There are many instances in which people are unaware of a particular stimulus that causes a behavior or judgment and instances where people are unaware of their response. Even if they are aware of the stimulus and the response, they may be unaware that the stimulus was the cause of the responses (9). After an extensive review of the studies on insight into mental processes, Nisbett and Wilson concluded that people only have insight into their decisions when the potential causes are few in number, are salient, seem plausible given cultural norms, and when causes have been observed to be associated with the outcome in the past (9). The wealth of randomized controlled intervention trials in which people's behaviors are influenced without their awareness and the documented lack of insight provide a foundation that could explain why many people often do not recognize the cues that lead them to eat, nor the cues that lead them to be sedentary, and therefore, may not easily control their responses to these cues (10–14).

Evidence of how the environment influences our diet without our awareness comes from a myriad of studies on eating behaviors. The mere sight of food can stimulate people to eat. For example, Wansink showed that secretaries ate 3.1 more chocolate "kisses" (75 kcal) when they were present on their desks in transparent jars than when they were in opaque jars (15). In an experiment, investigating whether visual cues influence quantity consumed, two groups of individuals were asked to sample soup. One group had bowls that automatically refilled, while the other group had normal bowls. The group with the self-refilling bowls consumed 73% more soup, yet did not realize they did so, nor did they report feeling more full than the group that ate less. In fact, both groups estimated they consumed less soup than they actually did (16). Wansink's work demonstrates repeatedly that environmental cues influence the frequency and quantity of what we eat and people do not typically recognize these cues.

Food portion sizes in particular appear to be very important; people served larger portions simply eat more food, regardless of their age, gender, race, body weight, or personality characteristics (17–21). For example, people served a baked pasta dish at a restaurant that was 50% larger than the normal portion, increased their caloric consumption by 159 kcal (17). People given 175 g instead of 25 g bags of potato chips tripled the amount of chips they ate, consuming an extra 311 kcal (20). The temptation to eat food at hand is so strong that humans eat more even if the food tastes bad: people going to the movies given large boxes of stale, 14-day-old popcorn ate one third more popcorn than those given medium-sized boxes (22).

Beyond portion size, one principle is that the amount of food consumed increases as the effort to eat it decreases, even if the differences in effort are small. For example, during a workday, secretaries who had chocolate "kisses" within reach on their desks ate an average of 5.6 more candies (amounting to 136 kcal) a day compared to secretaries who had to walk 6 ft across the room (23).

The context in which eating takes place can also greatly influence consumption. The longer the meal, the more people eat (24). The amount of food people eat is associated with the number of people at the table with food consumption increasing by 33% when one other person is present and increasing steadily to 96% when the number of companions is seven or more (25). Eating with other people introduces "mimicry" effects, in which we automatically and unconsciously copy another person's behaviors and expressions. In one study, an interviewer and a participant were each given two bowls, one of goldfish crackers and one of animal crackers. If the interviewer snacked on only goldfish while talking about

an unrelated subject, the participant was more likely to eat goldfish, and if the interviewer ate animal crackers, the participant ate more animal crackers. The participants had no awareness that they were copying the interviewer. Moreover, they subsequently reported that they preferred the snacks the interviewer had eaten, without recognizing that their preference was influenced by the interviewer's choice (12).

Another important determinant of how humans respond to any feature of their environment is simply its salience, that is, how much it attracts their attention. For example, marketing researchers have shown that in grocery stores when the amount of shelf space for a consumer item is doubled, sales increase by about 40% (26,27). This effect is seen regardless of whether the item is generally popular or unpopular. Sales also increase with special displays or end-aisle displays, or if items are placed at eye level (27,28). Grocery chains aware of this principle maximize their revenue by arranging large, prominent displays of high-profit items. Prices are also important. Several studies have shown that price reductions can lead people to purchase lower-fat food products and more nutritious foods (29–31).

People, however, do not recognize that they are not actively making decisions about their behavior. In fact we resist the notion that we are not in complete control. Typically, after we behave in a certain way, we rationalize why we did it and fabricate a plausible reason to explain why we behaved as we did (9). In some cases, the reason may be correct, but when it comes to understanding why we eat too much and exercise too little, our insight is quite poor.

REENGINEERING BUILT ENVIRONMENTS AND BEHAVIOR SETTINGS

A fundamental principle of public health is to address the conditions in which people live. Targeting common environments that reach large numbers of people is more efficient than targeting individual, unique environments. The environments of the greatest interest for targeting PA and dietary outcomes include schools, worksites, and neighborhood and community settings. Within community settings, reengineering venues like markets, restaurants, any kind of food outlet, parks and facilities that support PA, and the design of our cities, streets, and thoroughfares have a great deal of promise in the control of the obesity epidemic.

School Environments

Several behavioral settings occur before, during, and after school that influence diet and PA. These include (*i*) getting to school and school location, (*ii*) being in school (in classes vs. moving between classes), (*iii*) recess, (*iv*) school size, (*v*) indoor versus outdoor facilities and after school activities, and (*vi*) cafeteria food options, vending machines, school stores, and school policies.

Getting to School and School Location

There are many studies measuring the activity gained from commuting to school showing increased PA among active commuters (32–37). Walking and biking to school are more common in denser neighborhoods with smaller schools (38). An evaluation of the "safe routes to school" program, which funded the transformation of streets and sidewalks to make them pedestrian friendly, suggests that these changes increased the percentage of youth walking to school past these improvements by 12% compared with youth who did not pass by these areas (39). Distance to school was negatively related to PA in 6th grade girls (40).

Being in School

While one might intuitively think that most PA in school would come from being in physical education (PE) classes, in a study of PA of 6th grade students wearing pedometers during school, most steps were accumulated at lunchtime (more than in PE class and during recess) (41). Many studies of PE classes indicate that youth are active less than 50% of the time during PE because of teaching techniques that result in many students watching and waiting and that solutions may be as simple as having more equipment (a ball for each student) or promoting exercise and sports that allow all the students to be active simultaneously (42,43). Studies have tried to promote more vigorous PA during PE, and the most positive effects have been among boys (44). Supervision during recess and the presence of outdoor equipment was strongly associated with PA during recess in middle schools (45). One study in elementary school settings found that simply painting playgrounds using multicolored paints resulted in increased minutes of PA, with the largest effects seen among children who initially were the most sedentary (46).

Building size has been associated with PA: students in schools with larger footprints had more activity than students in smaller schools (47). On the other hand, students who attend larger schools serving more students are less likely to participate in sports and after-school activities (48). PA during school hours was increased when schools had more outdoor physical amenities, although when accounting for weather, the association was not significant (47).

After School

Opportunities for increasing PA can be provided after school, yet several studies that have tried to promote these activities have difficulty in recruiting and sustaining participation (49,50). Barriers to participation in after-school sports and PA programs include transportation, lack of funding, and the increased emphasis on academic achievement. In addition, a study of the accessibility of schoolyards and school facilities on weekends indicates that in many localities a large proportion of schools lock their gates. An analysis of the data showed a correlation between girls' body mass indices (BMIs) and weekend schoolyard accessibility such that girls who lived in neighborhoods with more locked schoolyards had higher BMIs (51). Descriptive studies of after-school PA programs show that large schools may offer more programs, but typically have lower rates of participation considering the size of the student body (52). In addition, schools that serve lower-income populations tend to have fewer after-school opportunities for PA (53).

Food at School

Over the past decade schools have installed vending machines and have begun to sell fast food in their cafeterias (54). Given the increased concern about obesity among youth, some states are passing laws that prohibit the sales of sugar-sweetened beverages in schools and control the quality of the food that can be sold in cafeterias and in vending machines. Efforts are also being directed to have schools develop wellness policies and adopt practices that limit the types of foods that can be served in classrooms, to eliminate using food and candy as a reward for academic or other school performance, and to eliminate sales of candy, cookies, or other food items from school fund-raisers. The ability to consistently implement these changes and whether these changes will have an impact on youth diet and weight gain is still unknown.

Future Directions

The recent trend to build larger size schools on large areas of land on the outskirts of town reduces the ability of youth to walk or bike to school and to stay for after-school programs. Therefore, if the goal is to increase PA, in the future, schools should be built in closer proximity to residences, be smaller, and serve fewer students. The extra PA gleaned from a larger school footprint is likely to be smaller than the potential PA that could be gained from walking to and from school. Furthermore, if schools did require daily PE for students that include at least 50% of the time involvement in moderate-to-vigorous physical activity (MVPA), the PA deficit could be solved for a large portion of students. The restriction or elimination of energy-dense, low-nutrient foods and beverages at school will likely reduce the consumption of these products at school over time and may address some of the issues of overweight and obesity among youth. It remains to be seen whether youth will compensate by eating more when they leave school.

Work Environments

The worksite is a potentially promising environment for promoting healthy behaviors because of the huge percentage of the population that could potentially be reached. The total U.S. civilian labor force is 153 million. At the end of 2006, about 96% (145 million) of Americans able to work were employed; of these, 22.5 million of nonfarm jobs are considered "goods producing" ("blue collar" employees), while another 113.8 million are "service providing" ("white collar" employees) (55).

Obesity is associated with higher rates of chronic medical conditions and with health-related quality of life worse than that resulting from a lifetime of smoking, problem drinking, or poverty (56). From a societal perspective, the health care costs associated with obesity exceed the short-term costs of smoking or problem drinking, and the health-related quality of life from obesity has been compared with that associated with aging by 20 years (57). Several studies have assessed the costs to employers of employee obesity. Burton and colleagues (58) studied 3266 employees at Bank One and found that sick days and medical claims increased with obesity. Employees with a BMI above 27.8 kg/m^2 for women and 27.3 kg/m^2 for men averaged considerably higher health care costs than those below these levels. Female employees older than 45 years with a high BMI spent an average of $3610/yr in health costs, while those with low BMI spend just over half that ($2064/yr); men with high BMI spent $2666 versus $1599 spent by those with low BMI. A study that measured worker productivity among customer service employees using objective computer-generated data on variables such as total calls answered, talk time, transfer hold time, and total unavailable time found that obesity was associated with failure to meet productivity standards (59). These findings provide a strong rationale for employers to invest in obesity prevention, especially if it means only small changes in the worksite environment at a relatively little cost.

Hill et al. estimate that as little as 100 cal/day make a difference as to whether people gain, lose, or maintain their weight. Small changes in behavior, such as walking an additional 2000 steps/day, or substituting a low energy-dense snack for higher energy-dense snack might make a significant difference, without being uncomfortable or very noticeable (60).

The CDC and many states have developed guidelines and recommendations for promoting health in worksite settings (61). Specific worksite conditions that have been shown to affect health include clean air laws and other smoking restrictions (62,63) and safety regulations controlling exposures to toxins (64). Many policies that govern worksite conditions are the consequence of federal, state, and local laws and regulations; other conditions are unique to the worksite and reflect preferences of company leadership and demands of the specific duties and goals of the business. However, the fact that a company has a worksite practice or condition does not mean that all employees are equally exposed. Their job duties and location in the worksite may affect their access to a particular food or PA environment.

Worksites can address sedentary behavior. Many of them voluntarily promote active transport to work and some state and local regulations require employers to offer incentives. For example, Ordinance 1604 in Santa Monica, California, requires local employers with 10 or more employees to help reduce employee commute trips (65). Employers with 10 to 49 employees must give each employee information about ride sharing, and educate employees about air quality issues and alternatives to driving alone to work everyday. Employers of 50 or more employees must further motivate employees to reduce individual commuting trips by implementing a variety of incentives. California's Parking Cash Out Program (AB2109) requires employers of 50 or more employees who lease their parking and subsidize any part of their employee parking to offer their employees the opportunity to relinquish their parking space and find an alternative means to work. The employer gives the cost of the parking space to employees who accept the offer (65). The primary rationale for these regulations is geared to reduce air pollution from motor vehicle emissions; however, they could also promote more walking and biking.

Currently, only eight states require breaks during the workday (66). Most of these states require a minimum of 10 minutes break for every four hours worked. Rest breaks are also often negotiated by labor unions or are voluntarily provided by employers. If employees are sedentary all day, as increasingly U.S. workers are, it makes more sense to give employees an exercise break, rather than a resting break. Developing walking programs could address this easily without any particular investment in exercise equipment or gymnasiums. Constraints due to weather may be a problem, and small offices may not have hall space or stairwell that is conducive to walking. However, more than 50% of the labor force works for companies that employ over 500 persons (67), so even if only large employers followed this, it could make a substantial difference in PA among workers.

Building Design/Stairwells

Building design and the placement of features such as stairwells whose use requires additional energy expenditure also contributes to PA. While the Task Force on Community Preventive Services reviewed a variety of interventions promoting PA and identified signage promoting stairwell use as effective in increasing PA (68), it is critical that stairs be made accessible. A recent study of stairwell features that reviewed both spatial and aesthetic qualities found that the spatial components were the most important in determining stair use. Stairs that were highly visible and in the main pathway of use were used more than stairs that may have been more attractive, leading the researchers to conclude that "a well-placed stair is more important than a well-dressed stair" (69).

Oldenburg et al. (70) developed a "Checklist of Health Promotion Environments at Worksites (CHEW)" to assess environmental characteristics of worksites that could promote healthy behaviors including PA and better nutrition and found that visible stairs were relatively uncommon. Many states and localities have also developed unique worksite assessment tools, but to date, none of the instruments have been validated with respect to how well worksite features actually do predict health outcomes. Workers typically do not stay in one employment setting their whole lives and each worker may interact uniquely with the worksite environment depending upon his or her job. However, as jobs are increasingly sedentary, altering physical environmental features like the length of hallways or the location of stairs alone may be insufficient to increase PA.

Worksites can also address the over consumption of energy-dense food with low nutrient values. Just as youth in schools are exposed to fast food and sugar-sweetened beverages, most office buildings also have vending machines that sell such beverages and a wide variety of energy-dense beverage and snack foods. Worksites could restrict these machines or eliminate them altogether. Worksite cafeterias are no different than restaurants and food outlets (discussed below), but employers have a vested interest in taking steps to control the quality and quantity of food that is made available to employees. Cafeteria interventions that have subsidized lower-fat and lower-calorie items have shown increased levels of purchases of these foods, but no long-term studies documenting whether this translates eventually to weight control have been completed (31,71). Worksites could make efforts to control the portion sizes of meals served, to control the quality of foods that are served at meetings, such as substituting fruits and vegetable for pastries and cookies, or substituting water for sugar-sweetened beverages. Even regulations that restrict eating at one's desk might be useful, similar to restriction of the use of tobacco in smoke-free buildings and alcohol at work. To date, most worksites have implemented wellness programs that focus more on education than on environmental changes.

No systematic evaluations of the cues to eat during work have been made.

Future interventions and research in this area should focus on factors such as building design, policies related to PA and nutrition, and structuring PA into the workday.

Neighborhood Environments

Elements related to PA and nutrition include: (*i*) street network design, street connectivity, and sprawl; (*ii*) proximity to and accessibility of parks and recreational facilities, (*iii*) traffic safety/sidewalks, (*iv*) bike paths and trails, (*v*) land use/zoning and population density, and (*vi*) food availability.

Street Networks, Street Connectivity, and Sprawl

Many studies that have examined street design in relationship to PA among adults show that adults walk more in neighborhoods with more intersections and that are more densely populated (72,73). Frank et al. developed an index of walkable neighborhoods strongly based on land use and found that a 1 standard deviation difference in walkability could increase PA by more than 8% (72). The association between street connectivity and children appears to be mixed. In one study, no association with street design was found (40), in another, more PA was observed in boys (74), while in another, the association with PA in youth was opposite to that of adults (more PA in streets with lower connectivity) (75).

Sprawl is defined as an urbanized area with separated residential, shopping, and business areas, limited street connections, and lower population density, with dependence on automobiles for transportation. While empirical evidence to support the popular assumption that suburban sprawl is bad for one's health remains limited, plausible pathways exist through which suburban sprawl can affect health (72,76,77). Pathways that have been documented include: increased traffic fatalities, increased air pollution from motor vehicles, decreased walking trips, and a higher BMI (78–80). A movement dubbed the New Urbanism advocates building dense, mixed-use residential commercial neighborhoods and transforming low-density areas into ones that are more pedestrian friendly, allowing people to accomplish the majority of their daily errands on foot. An empirical test of some of the principles advocated by the New Urbanism approach confirms that having a wide variety of destinations and businesses is associated with increased walking; however, the residential densities associated with increased walking are much higher than those currently proposed (81). Changing urban design is a long-term approach to promote PA and most applicable for the construction of new communities.

Proximity to Parks and Recreational Facilities

Recreation professionals and governments are becoming increasingly aware of the importance of both accessibility of PA venues and policies that support these venues. In the spring of 2004, the National Association of Counties (NACo), Center for Sustainable Communities, and the International City/County Management Association (ICMA) jointly designed a survey to understand how local government leaders view their role in enabling active living in communities. Local leaders consider it an important public duty to provide opportunities for PA in their communities. When asked which departments should take a leading, supportive, minor, or no role in developing active living communities, the majority said that Parks and Recreation departments (89%) should have a leading role in developing a community conducive to active living, followed by Planning (71%), Health (50%), and other departments (50%) (82).

Parks provide places for PA, recreation, and relaxation (83,84). One study that investigated the relationship between perceived environmental variables and PA found that convenient facilities, including public parks, were correlated with vigorous exercise (85). Although the authors note that much of the association was mediated by socioeconomic status, this study provides evidence supporting a linkage between parks and PA and highlights the need for a more-focused research. Reviews of environmental interventions to promote PA cited additional studies that support convenient exercise facilities as a correlate of PA (86,87). Other studies have shown associations between children's activity levels and the number of play spaces near their homes (44,88). The authors conclude that interventions to increase PA by providing opportunities and removing barriers are likely to be effective.

Neighborhood parks are the most common parks in the United States and form the basic unit of the park system (89). They serve as the recreational and social focus of the neighborhood and provide settings for structured activities (e.g., sports) as well as informal active and passive recreations. Neighborhood parks are typically 5 to 10 acres in size, serve residents within an area ¼ to ½ mile in radius, are centrally located within a service area, and are uninterrupted by nonresidential roads and other physical barriers. Neighborhood parks are larger than mini- or pocket parks, and usually contain several recreational areas, including playgrounds, multipurpose fields, areas for sitting or picnicking, and basketball courts (89).

Parks are extensively supported with infrastructure throughout the United States and are critical venues already being used in interventions to promote PA. According to the National Recreation and Parks Association (NRPA), approximately 75% of all Americans live within two miles of a park (82). The National Heart, Lung, and Blood Institute (NHLBI) has recognized the potential for parks to play an important role in cardiovascular health and obesity prevention. NHLBI funded "Hearts N' Parks," a national, community-based program that aims to reduce the growing trend of obesity and risk of coronary heart disease in the United States by encouraging Americans of all ages to aim for a healthy weight, follow a heart-healthy eating plan, and engage in regular PA (90). Hearts N' Parks, however, was conceived primarily as an educational intervention, with 25 participants per class, and a curriculum that teaches about healthy eating, PA, obesity and overweight, high blood pressure, and high blood cholesterol. The program has developed a wide variety of materials for parks and a mobilization packet to distribute; yet at present its goals for outreach are exceedingly modest. After being in more than 48 Hearts N' Parks sites (magnet centers) across the country, the program has reached only 2800 individuals, only 25 to 50 participants per park. Parks have a considerably greater capacity than that, as they are designed to serve tens of thousands of people. If each park served an average of 25,000 people, reaching only 10% of them per park could have an enormous impact. Rather than limiting resources to serve few people, funders and policy-makers should be broadening the vision to develop routine opportunities that reach millions of people.

Several studies indicate that proximity of parks and recreational facilities is associated with increased PA among youth (91–94). Supervision and organized activities appear to be key to utilization of neighborhood public parks (95). We also found that, in parks with walking paths, a greater percentage of the park users were engaged in moderate-to-vigorous activity than in parks without designated paths (96).

Traffic and safety concerns are barriers to PA (97–99), although in one study, those who walk more perceive greater barriers than those who walk less (100), and in another study, perceptions of safety do not seem to matter (101). Perceptions of lack of safety however have also been associated with obesity (102), while objective measures of crime have not been associated with obesity (103).

Land use refers to the mix of types of building and facilities and spaces that are in a particular area. The most common terms to describe land use include residential, commercial, industrial, and open and green space. Additional uses have been dividing the commercial uses to retail and service-related functions. Many studies of walkability have focused on neighborhoods with multiple land uses, so that people who live nearby can walk to engage in their daily routines and run errands. Most of these studies indicate that mixed land use neighborhoods are associated with higher levels of PA (81). Some also point to a relationship between land use and BMI (73,79,80,104), while others do not (105). Studies on "walkable communities" with greater mixed land use and increased population density show associations with more PA among youth (77,105). There are few studies of changing the environment with children's PA as the outcome. Studies of the impact of engineering changes of roads to make them more pedestrian friendly on PA are mixed (106,107).

Bike Paths and Walking Trails

The idea, "build it and they will come," has been an inspiration for the creation of new bike paths and trails, yet evaluations of many of these projects have been disappointing. A recent review of alterations in bike paths noted three relevant studies, one with a 3% increase in biking after three years, the other two resulting in bicycling declines (107), while similar mixed results were found for walking trails (108,109). For new facilities to be used, people have to be aware that the facilities exist. As well, the facilities need to be convenient and accessible (110). Although new bike paths and roadways are frequently being built in the United States, there are few studies using objective measures that prospectively document increases in PA in response to environmental changes (111,112). A recent evaluation of a new bike path built along a transit way in the San Fernando Valley of Los Angeles showed a significant increase in use, mainly among adult males during weekday commuting hours (Fig. 1) (113).

Food Promotion and Availability

The most promising strategies for controlling food consumption include regulating the availability of food to influencing consumption at the point of purchase. Most

food purchases are impulsive, they occur in direct response to the appeal of the item at the moment (114). One strategy is to restrict the number and type of outlets where food can be sold. Since food itself stimulates consumption, removing snacks and the nonperishable items from outlets where food is not the primary business may reduce impulsive eating. Removing energy-dense food items like candy bars and chips from car washes, gas stations, bookstores, and other nonfood establishments should be considered.

Another strategy being implemented in the United Kingdom is the use of traffic light signal labeling. Items with large amounts of unhealthy ingredients are labeled red, amber signifies a medium amount of unhealthy ingredients, and green signifies a low amount of unhealthy ingredients but a large amount of healthy ingredients. The interpretation is that one should respond to the food similar to traffic signals: avoid red, be cautious with yellow, and go ahead with green (115). Although this system is new and the impact yet unknown, the direction of the intervention provides a simple heuristic, and is likely to help moderate people's choices of foods.

The Potential to Expand Restaurant Inspections and Food Preparation Guidelines to Cover the Risk of Chronic Diseases

All localities have a system whereby they regulate and inspect outlets that serve fresh foods to help prevent food-borne diseases. Los Angeles County initiated a unique restaurant rating system that focused on the prevention of food-borne diseases in 1998, in which they posted the results of kitchen inspections outside of restaurants within 5 ft of an entrance. Within one year of program initiation, inspection scores increased from about 25% having "A" to over 50% performing at an A level (score 90–100). Improved scores were generally maintained on subsequent inspections. Higher risk establishments were inspected more frequently than were lower risk establishments. Over 30,000 food handlers were certified. The rate of outlet closures also decreased (116). In the year after the introduction of grade posting, the number of patients admitted to the hospital for food-related illnesses dropped by 13% (4). The quality of restaurants in the entire county became more equitable, with the average score going in areas below the median county income becoming equal to those in areas above the median county income. Consumer demand was affected and restaurants with A increased their sales and restaurants with "C" lost revenue (117,118).

This model of restaurant inspections is currently limited to safety issues with respect to infectious diseases and could be expanded to cover reduction of the risk of chronic diseases. Standards that dictate appropriate

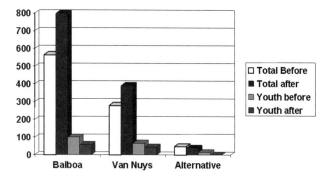

Figure 1 Numbers of bike path users before and after construction of a bike path between Balboa and Van Nuys transit stops. *Source*: From Ref. 113.

ingredients, like eliminating the use of trans fats, are already being regulated by health departments like the New York City Department of Health and are being considered by a number of others. Standards could include how items are labeled and presented on menus, on portion sizes, on availability of low-fat or sugar-free items, fresh fruits, and vegetables, and could make it easier and more likely for customers to obtain healthier, lower-calorie meals. Menu items could be rated for health using simple symbols rather than a complex description of ingredients, such as grams of nutrients and calories, thereby allowing people to make decisions based on of easily understood information at their fingertips.

Controlling the Available Portion Sizes

Given that portions sizes are closely tied to overconsumption, serious consideration should be made for controlling them. There is some precedent for controlling portion sizes in the field of alcohol control; however, the regulations that define alcohol servings as 12 oz for beer, 5 oz for wine, and 1 oz for spirits were initially designed to prevent people from being cheated by being served watered-down drinks. Regulatory authorities could define appropriate serving sizes for meal items on the basis of calories. If people wanted to purchase more, they could simply order additional portions. Since individuals are unable to judge appropriate portion sizes by looking, having these specified quantities defined and served by an establishment could go a long way in helping people avoid overeating.

SUMMARY AND CONCLUSION

The principal barrier to controlling the obesity epidemic is the firmly held belief that it is just a matter of willpower for people to control their own dietary and exercise behaviors, regardless of the environmental cues around them. Because of the illusion we have that individuals can consistently resist the environment that promotes overeating and sedentary behaviors, there is little-to-no political will to regulate the marketing and availability of food products nor to invest in the infrastructure and programming that could ensure that the average person meets minimum PA guidelines. In contrast, when we believe that the consequence of toxic exposures are beyond individual control, like exposures to air pollution or contaminated water, as a society we have enacted regulations that limit pollution and we have invested in extensive sanitary systems to ensure that people can have clean water. Yet the toxic environment also includes the marketplace that promotes unhealthy foods and provides excessive calories as well as school and worksite environments that demand sedentary behaviors. These settings remain inadequately regulated because we believe that the chain of events from perception to behavior is easily interruptible by any person who is concerned with his or her health.

Future interventions to promote PA and a nutritious, calorie-appropriate diet should target venues and products that are most likely to reach the majority of the population. Therefore, settings of schools to reach youth and worksites to reach adults are the most appropriate. Others who are not in school or are unemployed can be reached through neighborhood settings by having easy accessibility to recreational facilities and increasing the odds of utilitarian PA by creating communities where active transport can be a part of daily life. Community-level interventions may have relatively small impacts at the individual level, but at the community level an increase in PA of only 3% to 5% among an entire population could potentially have significant results (119). PA is contextually dependent, and therefore tends to be venue based. Investments in public services and spaces, establishing standards for school and work settings, and regulations of the food environment are the most promising for controlling the obesity epidemic and facilitating a minimum amount of PA among all.

REFERENCES

1. Wikipedia. Built environment. Available at: http://en.wikipedia.org/wiki/Built_environment; 2006. Accessed April 2007.
2. Cohen D, Scribner R, Farley T. A structural model of health behavior: A pragmatic approach to explain and influence health behaviors at the population level. Prev Med 2000; 30:146–154.
3. Barker R. Ecological Psychology: Concepts and Methods for Studying the Environment of Human Behavior. Stanford, California: Stanford University Press, 1968.
4. Simon PA, Leslie P, Run G, et al. Impact of restaurant hygiene grade cards on foodborne-disease hospitalizations in Los Angeles County. J Environ Health 2005; 67:32–36, 56.
5. Dijksterhuis A. Think different: The merits of unconscious thought in preference development and decision making. J Pers Soc Psychol 2004; 87:586–598.
6. Wilson TD, Nisbett RE. The accuracy of verbal reports about the effects of stimuli on evaluations and behavior. Soc Psychol 1978; 41:118–131.
7. Vallacher RR, Wegner DM. What do people think they're doing? Action identification and human behavior. Psychol Rev 1987; 94:3–15.
8. Neisser U. Cognitive Psychology. East Norwalk, CT; Appleton-Century-Crofts, 1967.
9. Nisbett RE, Wilson TD. Telling more than we can know: Verbal reports on mental processes. Psychol Rev 1977; 84:231–259.
10. Bargh JA, Chartrand TL. The unbearable automaticity of being. Am Psychol 1999; 54:462–479.

11. Bargh JA. Losing consciousness: Automatic influences on consumer judgment, behavior, and motivation. J Consum Res 2002; 29:280–285.

12. Chartrand T. The role of conscious awareness in consumer behavior. J Consum Psychol 2005; 15:203–210.

13. Dijksterhuis A, Smith P, van Baaren R, et al. The unconscious consumer: Effects of environment on consumer behavior. J Consum Psychol 2005; 15:193–202.

14. Dijksterhuis A, Smith PK. What do we do unconsciously? And how? J Consum Psychol 2005; 15:225–229.

15. Wansink B, Painter JE, Lee YK. The office candy dish: proximity's influence on estimated and actual consumption. Int J Obes (Lond) 2006; 30:871–875.

16. Wansink B, Painter JE, North J. Bottomless bowls: why visual cues of portion size may influence intake. Obes Res 2005; 13:93–100.

17. Diliberti N, Bordi PL, Conklin MT, et al. Increased portion size leads to increased energy intake in a restaurant meal. Obes Res 2004; 12:562–568.

18. Levitsky DA, Youn T. The more food young adults are served, the more they overeat. J Nutr 2004; 134: 2546–2549.

19. Rolls BJ, Morris EL, Roe LS. Portion size of food affects energy intake in normal-weight and overweight men and women. Am J Clin Nutr 2002; 76:1207–1213.

20. Rolls BJ, Roe LS, Kral TV, et al. Increasing the portion size of a packaged snack increases energy intake in men and women. Appetite 2004; 42:63–69.

21. Rolls BJ, Roe LS, Meengs JS. Larger portion sizes lead to a sustained increase in energy intake over 2 days. J Am Diet Assoc 2006; 106:543–549.

22. Wansink B, Kim J. Bad popcorn in big buckets: portion size can influence intake as much as taste. J Nutr Educ Behav 2005; 37:242–245.

23. Painter JE, Wansink B, Hieggelke JB. How visibility and convenience influence candy consumption. Appetite 2002; 38:237–238.

24. Feunekes GI, de Graaf C, van Staveren WA. Social facilitation of food intake is mediated by meal duration. Physiol Behav 1995; 58:551–558.

25. de Castro JM, Brewer EM. The amount eaten in meals by humans is a power function of the number of people present. Physiol Behav 1992; 51:121–125.

26. Curhan RC. The effects of merchandising and temporary promotional activities on the sales of fresh fruits and vegetables in supermarkets. J Mark Res 1974; 11:286–294.

27. Wilkinson JB, Mason JB, Paksoy CH. Assessing the impact of short-term supermarket strategy variables. J Mark Res 1982; 19:72–86.

28. Frank RE, Massey WF. Shelf position and space effects on sales. J Mark Res 1970; 7:59–66.

29. French SA. Pricing effects on food choices. J Nutr 2003; 133:841S–843S.

30. French SA, Jeffery RW, Story M, et al. Pricing and promotion effects on low-fat vending snack purchases: the CHIPS Study. Am J Public Health 2001; 91:112–117.

31. French SA, Jeffery RW, Story M, et al. A pricing strategy to promote low-fat snack choices through vending machines. Am J Public Health 1997; 87:849–851.

32. Tudor-Locke C, Ainsworth BE, Adair LS, et al. Objective physical activity of Filipino youth stratified for commuting mode to school. Med Sci Sports Exerc 2003; 35: 465–471.

33. Cooper AR, Andersen LB, Wedderkopp N, et al. Physical activity levels of children who walk, cycle, or are driven to school. Am J Prev Med 2005; 29:179–184.

34. Rosenberg DE, Sallis JF, Conway TL, et al. Active transportation to school over 2 years in relation to weight status and physical activity. Obesity (Silver Spring) 2006; 14:1771–1776.

35. Saksvig BI, Catellier DJ, Pfeiffer K, et al. Travel by walking before and after school and physical activity among adolescent girls. Arch Pediatr Adolesc Med 2007; 161:153–158.

36. Cooper AR, Wedderkopp N, Wang H, et al. Active travel to school and cardiovascular fitness in Danish children and adolescents. Med Sci Sports Exerc 2006; 38: 1724–1731.

37. Sirard JR, Riner WF Jr., McIver KL, et al. Physical activity and active commuting to elementary school. Med Sci Sports Exerc 2005; 37:2062–2069.

38. Braza M, Shoemaker W, Seeley A. Neighborhood design and rates of walking and biking to elementary school in 34 California communities. Am J Health Prom 2004; 19: 128–136.

39. Boarnet MG, Anderson CL, Day K, et al. Evaluation of the California Safe Routes to School legislation: urban form changes and children's active transportation to school. Am J Prev Med 2005; 28(2 suppl 2):134–140.

40. Cohen D, Ashwood S, Scott M, et al. Proximity to school and physical activity among middle school girls: The trial of activity for adolescent girls study. J Phys Act Health 2006; 3:S129–S138.

41. Tudor-Locke C, Lee SM, Morgan CF, et al. Children's pedometer-determined physical activity during the segmented school day. Med Sci Sports Exerc 2006; 38: 1732–1738.

42. McKenzie TL, Sallis JF, Nader PR. SOFIT: System for observing fitness instruction time. J Teach Phys Educ 1991; 11:195–205.

43. McKenzie TL, Catellier DJ, Conway T, L, et al. Girls' activity levels and lesson contexts in middle school PE: TAAG baseline. Med Sci Sports Exerc 2006; 38: 1229–1235.

44. Sallis JF, McKenzie TL, Alcaraz JE, et al. The effects of a 2-year physical education program (SPARK) on physical activity and fitness in elementary school students. Sports, play and active recreation for Kids. Am J Public Health 1997; 87:1328–1334.

45. Sallis JF, Conway TL, Prochaska JJ, et al. The association of school environments with youth physical activity. Am J Public Health 2001; 91:618–620.

46. Stratton G, Mullan E. The effect of multicolor playground markings on children's physical activity level during recess. Prev Med 2005; 41:828–833.

47. Cohen D, Scott M, Wang Z, et al. School design and physical activity among middle school girls. J Phys Act Health (in press).

48. Barker RG, Gump PV. Big School, Small School: High School Size and Student Behavior. Stanford, CA: Stanford University Press, 1964.

49. Pate RR, Saunders RP, Ward DS, et al. Evaluation of a community-based intervention to promote physical activity in youth: lessons from active winners. Am J Health Prom 2003; 17:171–182.

50. Urban After-School Programs: Evaluations and Recommendations. ERIC/CUE Digest, Number 140. 071 Information Analyses—ERIC IAPs. New York, NY: ERIC Clearinghouse on Urban Education, 1998 12-00. Report No.: EDO-UD-98-0.

51. Scott MM, Cohen DA, Evenson KR, et al. Weekend schoolyard accessibility, physical activity, and obesity: 3 The Trial of Activity in Adolescent Girls (TAAG) study. Scott, Prev Med 2007; 44(5):398–403.

52. McNeal RB Jr. Participation in high school extracurricular activities: Investigating school effects. Soc Sci Q 1999; 80:291–309.

53. Cohen DA, Taylor S, Zonta M, et al. Availability of high school extra-curricular sports programs. J School Health 2007; 77:80–86.

54. Nestle M. Soft drink "pouring rights": marketing empty calories to children. Public Health Rep 2000; 115:308–319.

55. Bureau of Labor Statistics. The employment situation, January 2007, US Dept of Labor. Available at: http://www.bls.gov/news.release/empsit.nr0.htm.

56. Sturm R, Wells KB. Does obesity contribute as much to morbidity as poverty or smoking? Public Health 2001; 115:229–235.

57. Sturm R. The effects of obesity, smoking, and drinking on medical problems and costs. Obesity outranks both smoking and drinking in its deleterious effects on health and health costs. Health Aff (Project Hope) 2002; 21:245–253.

58. Burton WN, Chen CY, Schultz AB, et al. The costs of body mass index levels in an employed population. Stat Bull Metropol Life Insur Co 1999; 80:8–14.

59. Burton WN, Conti DJ, Chen CY, et al. The role of health risk factors and disease on worker productivity. J Occup Envir Med 1999; 41:863–877.

60. Hill JO, Wyatt HR, Reed GW, et al. Obesity and the environment: where do we go from here? Science 2003; 299:853–855.

61. CDC. Healthier Worksite Initiative. Available at: http://www.cdc.gov/nccdphp/dnpa/hwi/index.htm. Accessed June 2007.

62. Kadowaki T, Kanda H, Watanabe M, et al. Are comprehensive environmental changes as effective as health education for smoking cessation? Tob Control 2006; 15:26–29.

63. Levy DT, Friend KB. The effects of clean indoor air laws: what do we know and what do we need to know? Health Educ Res 2003; 18:592–609.

64. Baggs J, Silverstein B, Foley M. Workplace health and safety regulations: Impact of enforcement and consultation on workers' compensation claims rates in Washington State. Am J Ind Med 2003; 43:483–494.

65. Santa Monica Transportation Management Office: Doing Business in Santa Monica. Available at: http://www.smgov.net/planning/transportation/abouttransmanagementtmo.html. Accessed June 2007.

66. Department of Labor. Minimum Paid Rest Period Requirements Under State Law for Adult Employees in Private Sector—January 1, 2007. Available at: http://www.dol.gov/esa/programs/whd/state/rest.htm. Accessed June 2007.

67. Hopkins J. Workforce shifts to big companies. In: USA Today, 2002. Available at: http://www.usatoday.com/money/general/2002/03/19/big-business.htm.

68. CDC. Increasing physical activity. A report on recommendations of the Task Force on Community Preventive Services. MMWR Recomm Rep 2001; 50:1–14.

69. Nicoll G. Spatial measures associated with stair use. Am J Health Promot 2007; 21(4 suppl):346–352.

70. Oldenburg B, Sallis JF, Harris D, et al. Checklist of Health Promotion Environments at Worksites (CHEW): development and measurement characteristics. Am J Health Promot 2002; 16:288–299.

71. Faith MS, Fontaine KR, Baskin ML, et al. Toward the reduction of population obesity: macrolevel environmental approaches to the problems of food, eating, and obesity. Psychol Bull 2007; 133:205–226.

72. Frank LD, Schmid TL, Sallis JF, et al. Linking objectively measured physical activity with objectively measured urban form: findings from SMARTRAQ. Am J Prev Med 2005; 28(2 suppl 2):117–125.

73. Frank LD, Andresen MA, Schmid TL. Obesity relationships with community design, physical activity, and time spent in cars. Am J Prev Med 2004; 27:87–96.

74. Roemmich JN, Epstein LH, Raja S, et al. The neighborhood and home environments: disparate relationships with physical activity and sedentary behaviors in youth. Ann Behav Med 2007; 33:29–38.

75. Norman GJ, Nutter SK, Ryan S, et al. Community Design and Access to Recreational Facilities as correlates of adolescent physical activity and body mass index. J Phys Act Health 2006; 3:S118–S128.

76. Handy SL, Boarnet MG, Ewing R, et al. How the built environment affects physical activity: views from urban planning. Am J Prev Med 2002; 23(2 suppl):64–73.

77. Frank L, Kerr J, Chapman J, et al. Urban form relationships with walk trip frequency and distance among youth. Am J Health Promot 2007; 21(4 suppl):305–311.

78. Brownson RC, Chang JJ, Eyler AA, et al. Measuring the environment for friendliness toward physical activity: a comparison of the reliability of 3 questionnaires. Am J Public Health 2004; 94:473–483.

79. Ewing R, Brownson RC, Berrigan D. Relationship between urban sprawl and weight of United States youth. Am J Prev Med 2006; 31:464–474.

80. Ewing R, Schmid T, Killingsworth R, et al. Relationship between urban sprawl and physical activity, obesity, and morbidity. Am J Health Promot 2003; 18:47–57.

81. Boer R, Zheng Y, Overton A, et al. Neighborhood design and walking trips in ten U.S. metropolitan areas. Am J Prev Med 2007; 32:298–304.

82. ICMA, NaCO. Active Living Approaches by Local Government. In: ICMA, 2006.

83. Godbey GC, Caldwell LL, Floyd M, et al. Contributions of leisure studies and recreation and park management research to the active living agenda. Am J Prev Med 2005; 28(2 suppl 2):150–158.

84. Bedimo-Rung AL, Mowen AJ, Cohen D. The significance of parks to physical activity and public health: A conceptual model. Am J Prev Med 2005; 28(2S2):159–168.

85. Sallis JF, Hovell MF, Hofstetter CR, et al. Distance between homes and exercise facilities related to frequency of exercise among San Diego residents. Public Health Rep 1990; 105:179–185.

86. Brownson RC, Baker EA, Housemann RA, et al. Environmental and policy determinants of physical activity in the United States. Am J Public Health 2001; 91: 1995–2003.

87. Sallis JF, Bauman MP. Environmental and policy interventions to promote physical activity. Am J Prev Med 1998; 15(4):379–397.

88. Sallis JF, Bauman A, Pratt M. Environmental and policy interventions to promote physical activity. Am J Prev Med 1998; 15:379–397.

89. Mertes J, Hall J. Park, Recreation, Open Space and Greenway Guidelines. Ashburn, VA: National Recreation and Park Association, 1996.

90. NHLBI. Hearts N' Parks. Available at: http://www.nhlbi.nih.gov/health/prof/heart/obesity/hrt_n_pk/index.htm. Accessed May 2006.

91. Babey SH, Brown ER, Hastert TA. Access to safe parks helps increase physical activity among teenagers. Policy brief (UCLA Center for Health Policy Research) (Policy Brief UCLA Cent Health Policy Res) 2005 Dec(PB2005-10):1–6.

92. Cohen D, Ashwood J, Scott M, et al. Public parks and physical activity among adolescent girls. Pediatrics 2006; 118:e1381–e1389.

93. Nelson MC, Gordon-Larsen P, Song Y, et al. Built and social environments associations with adolescent overweight and activity. Am J Prev Med 2006; 31: 109–117.

94. Gordon-Larsen P, Nelson MC, Page P, et al. Inequality in the built environment underlies key health disparities in physical activity and obesity. Pediatrics 2006; 117: 417–424.

95. Cohen DA, McKenzie TL, Sehgal A, et al. Contribution of public parks to physical activity. Am J Public Health 2007; 97:509–514.

96. Cohen D, Sehgal A, Williamson S, et al. Park Use and Physical Activity in a Sample of Public Parks in the City of Los Angeles. Santa Monica: RAND, 2006.

97. Gómez JE, Johnson BA, Selva M, et al. Violent crime and outdoor physical activity among inner-city youth. Prev Med 2004; 39:876–881.

98. Molnar BE, Gortmaker SL, Bull FC, et al. Unsafe to play? Neighborhood disorder and lack of safety predict reduced physical activity among urban children and adolescents. Am J Health Promot 2004; 18:378–386.

99. CDC, Neighborhood safety and the prevalence of physical inactivity–selected states, 1996. MMWR Morb Mortal Wkly Rep 1999; 48:143–146.

100. Alton D, Adab P, Roberts L, et al. Relationship between walking levels and perceptions of the local neighbourhood environment. Arch Dis Child 2007; 92:29–33.

101. Burdette HL, Whitaker RC. A national study of neighborhood safety, outdoor play, television viewing, and obesity in preschool children. Pediatrics 2005; 116: 657–662.

102. Burdette HL, Wadden TA, Whitaker RC. Neighborhood safety, collective efficacy, and obesity in women with young children. Obesity (Silver Spring) 2006; 14: 518–525.

103. Burdette HL, Whitaker RC. Neighborhood playgrounds, fast food restaurants, and crime: relationships to overweight in low-income preschool children. Prev Med 2004; 38:57–63.

104. Rutt CD, Coleman KJ. Examining the relationships among built environment, physical activity, and body mass index in El Paso, TX. Prev Med 2005; 40:831–841.

105. Kligerman M, Sallis JF, Ryan S, et al. Association of neighborhood design and recreation environment variables with physical activity and body mass index in adolescents. Am J Health Promot 2007; 21:274–277.

106. Morrison DS, Thomson H, Petticrew M. Evaluation of the health effects of a neighbourhood traffic calming scheme. J Epidemiol Community Health 2004; 58:837–840.

107. Ogilvie D, Mitchell R, Mutrie N, et al. Evaluating health effects of transport interventions methodologic case study. Am J Prev Med 2006; 31:118–126.

108. Evenson KR, Herring AH, Huston SL. Evaluating change in physical activity with the building of a multi-use trail. Am J Prev Med 2005; 28(2 suppl 2):177–185.

109. Merom D, Bauman A, Vita P, et al. An environmental intervention to promote walking and cycling—the impact of a newly constructed Rail Trail in Western Sydney. Prev Med 2003; 36:235–242.

110. King WC, Brach JS, Belle S, et al. The relationship between convenience of destinations and walking levels in older women. Am J Health Promot 2003; 18:74–82.

111. Morrison DS, Thomson H, Petticrew M. Evaluation of the health effects of a neighborhood traffic calming scheme. J Epidemiol Community Health 2004; 58: 837–840.

112. Killoran A, Doyle N, Waller S, et al. Transport interventions promoting safe cycling and walking: Evidence briefing. Available at: http://www.nice.org.uk/page.aspx?o=346196. Accessed July 2007.

113. Cohen D, Sehgal A, Williamson S, et al. Impact of a new bicycle path on physical activity. Prev Med 2007; Available online July 26, 2007.

114. Hausman A. A multi-method investigation of consumer motivations in impulse buying behavior. J Consum Mark. 2000; 17:403–419.

115. Food Standards Agency. Traffic light labelling. Available at: http://www.eatwell.gov.uk/foodlabels/trafficlights/. Accessed April 2007.

116. Fielding JE, Aguirre A, Spear MC, et al. Making the grade: changing the incentives in retail food establishment inspection. Am J Prev Med 1999; 17:243–247.

117. Jin G, Leslie P. The case in support of restaurant hygiene grade cards. choices 2005; 20:97–102.

118. Jin G, Leslie P. The effect of information on product quality: Evidence from restaurant hygiene grade cards. Q J Econ 2003; 118:409–451.

119. Rose G. The Strategy of Preventive Medicine. New York: Oxford University Press, Inc., 1992.

13

Agriculture and the Food Industry's Role in America's Weight Pandemic

JAMES E. TILLOTSON

Friedman School of Nutrition Science and Policy, Tufts University, Boston, Massachusetts, U.S.A.

INTRODUCTION

Universally today the world's industrial and developing industrial nations suffer from rapid increases in number of their citizens—young and older—becoming overweight and obese. In the United States—arguably the world's most industrialized nation—this pandemic is the most severe.

This raises the health issue of the potential relationship between a nation's industrialization process, with its many food ramifications, and the universal occurrence of high-levels of population-wide overweight and obesity in these countries.

Industrialization markedly changes the relationship of a nation's population to its food supply. Germane to this change with industrialization is the extensive commercialization of the food supply that occurs. Harvey Levenstein, the noted food historian, has labeled this transformation as nothing less than a *revolution at the table* in the United States (1).

During recent decades, this transformation of the American food supply has gathered speed, while during this same time frame, overweight and obesity have markedly increased among Americans. This raises the obvious question of the degree of association between these two events.

As the United States industrialized, continuous changes occurred in its food supply. With this, there has occurred an increased delegation to its commercial sector of production, processing, and delivery of food to its population. As a result, a large, powerful, varied commercial food sector—reaching from the farm and ranch to the final consumer—has developed to feed Americans.

Over the last century this commercial sector has become increasingly dominant to Americans' food, often being the sole food source for the majority of Americans. As a result, Americans have become increasingly dependent on the commercial sector for their daily food. Through this process the agricultural and food-processing sector collectively has come to exert ever greater environmental influence on Americans' food consumption simply by nature and matter of its commercial food and beverage offerings. Today the commercial food supply is American's food.

This increased commercial dominance in supplying food leads to an additional question beyond its more general role in the societal industrialization process: namely, what specific role does the food industry play in the nation's pandemic? Is the commercial food sector merely a passive feeder of Americans with ravenous, unchecked appetites, or is it a compelling commercial force stimulating them to eat ever larger amounts of unneeded food, or more likely, a mixture of both roles?

When considering the causes of overweight and obesity, the relative importance of different factors are commonly stressed depending on whether these conditions are being considered at the individual or population level. At the individual level the importance of diet, food habits, and lifestyles (physical activity) are commonly thought to be more significant. At the population level, greater attention is attributed to environmental conditions (cultural, economic, education, industrialization, ethnic, etc.). This results in differing opinions on dealing with this pandemic.

In spite of differing but valid viewpoints in understanding the causes of overweight and obesity, there is wide agreement on the primary importance of *one demand-side* factor, whether on an individual or on a population basis: the *personal responsibility* of the individual for his or her diet, eating behavior, and physical activity determining whether the individual becomes overweight or obese.

A major controversy, still unresolved, revolves around the contribution of personal responsibility versus other factors—environmental factors such as the food industry—in the etiology of obesity. Hard evidence is lacking. However, personal responsibility does *not* occur in a social vacuum. It occurs under diverse environmental conditions (social, political economic, and technological) having potentially significant influence on the individual's ultimate eating behavior and, in turn, the individual's weight.

The modern commercial food sector, with its varied and ubiquitous food offerings, coupled with its aggressive marketing methods, is a leading environmental condition presently being questioned as a major factor in the marked increase of overweight and obesity in recent decades among Americans.

Guiding the U.S. agricultural and food-processing activities—between *consumer demand* and *supply conditions*—is a framework of *public policies* (agricultural, economic, and industrial as well as public health) shaping the population's behavior between supply and demand, influencing their diet and, in turn, their weight.

The purpose of this chapter is to examine the role of the commercial food supply chain in the present pandemic, starting with agriculture through processing to delivery to the ultimate consumer. While people's organoleptic desires and their purchase of food are important factors in shaping the commercial food supply chain, the food industry and the government with its institutions are also key factors in determining the nature of the U.S. consumer-food supply interface. Therefore, the following also examines the role of our nation's agricultural, economic, industrial, food, and public health policies in shaping the commercial food supply chain and its citizens' food choices.

The chapter is written from the viewpoint that the American food system, while not a direct causal agent (such as an individual's diet, physical activity, or eating behavior), yet the commercial sector gives evidence of being an ever more powerful environmental force contributing to Americans' overeating, resulting in the nation's growing overweight and obesity problems (2).

While this chapter deals specifically with the American problem, this nation's weight problem is instructive for other nations, as the U.S. problem is the most severe today, and the industrial transformation of its diet the most extensive, globally, of any industrialized country.

As a case study, the United States is also instructive for other nations in demonstrating the degree to which its current public policies have been successful or unsuccessful in curbing this pandemic. A further aspect to consider is that a number of major American food companies that are commercially active in the United States are also globally active in commerce, and, as they have played a part in the industrial transformation of the American diet, they are playing or may play a important role in the industrial transformation of other nations' diets (3).

The reader should be aware that the following analysis rests heavily on anecdotal and observational information (partly based on the author's 50 years of observing the commercial food sector from within the industry and, more recently, as an academic, studying the food sector). Realizing there are many views but unfortunately little hard evidence, it is meant more to raise questions rather than to provide definitive answers to the commercial food sector's role in our nationwide overweight and obesity problems.

INDUSTRIALIZATION OF THE FOOD SUPPLY CHAIN

Industrialization of the food supply is a relatively recent event in humankind's long food history, occurring mainly during the last century. With industrialization, centuries-old fear of starvation and hunger disappear; food becomes plentiful and dependable; food takes on new social roles beyond solely survival (4).

During the 20th century, food supply industrialization in this country put an end to many of the earlier food security concerns. Commercially prepared food became ever more available, ample, and affordable to practically all Americans (5).

Industrialization of the food supply was, and is, driven by strong market factors. Using agricultural products that are readily available (and plentiful), processors developed, produced, and aggressively marketed food products desired by the fast-growing population that previously the population had prepared (even grown) the food for their own subsistence. This changed the dynamics of Americans' relationship to their food supply.

As a result of the industrialization (particularly during the latter half century), Americans were faced with great changes in their food supply—and at the same time—became increasingly dependent on the new industrial system. With this rise in commercial activities between producers and consumers, the food sector had ever stronger economic incentives to keep increasing Americans' food consumption. As Americans would become increasingly overweight and obese, the food seller's commercial interests and the buyer's health interests would become increasingly divergent (6).

Industrialization also resulted in widespread laborsaving technologies that, in turn, reduced the actual amount of daily food required by Americans—a seemingly never-ending process. At the same time, food becomes ever more plentiful, economical, readily available, and enticing to eat.

Industrialization results, therefore, in a paradox; food becomes ever more available, while the individual's caloric requirement lessens. While the industrialization of a nation's food supply shields its population from the historical dangers of hunger and starvation, it increases their risk of overnutrition with overweight and obesity.

Industrialization also gave rise to labor *differentiation* as well as a rise in the population's income. Fewer and fewer workers are required for food production, while others are increasingly employed in other types of labor, enabling them to purchase ever larger amounts of commercially processed foods with their increasing wages. Along with these social and economic changes, food is no longer gathered, produced, exchanged, or bartered, but *sold*.

During much of this industrialization era in the 20th century, governmental policies were mainly concerned with economic issues rather than nutritional issues. The public's choice of food from this industrialization process was dictated by traditional market factors (taste, price, and convenience); nutritional issues were not a defining factor beyond subsistence.

Industrialization itself has also proven to be a powerful environmental condition *favoring overconsumption*. With industrialization, there have come new health problems related to excesses and unbalances in Americans' food consumption (nutrition-related noncommunicable diseases).

At a societal level, Americans' present widespread overweight condition can be seen as a lack of successful acculturation by Americans to these markedly changed food conditions brought about by industrialization. At a policy level, pandemic obesity can be considered to be a symptom of the inability of people to self-adjust their food intake in this new era-of-plenty from commercial foods and their reduced caloric requirement as a result of currently active governmental health policies. To date,

our present public health policies have unfortunately met with mixed success in resolving this diet dilemma.

This raises still other policy issues: the social responsibilities, rights and duties of those responsible for food availability on the *supply side* (agriculture and the food industry) versus people's responsibilities, rights and duties of consumers on the *demand side*. What are the appropriate public policies—health, agricultural, and economic—to pursue in achieving appropriate balance among these interests? The accelerating rate of obesity—among the young as well as adults—gives new urgency to resolve the conflict between our current economic and public health policies.

U.S. FOOD POLICY HISTORY

Widespread obesity in the United States is a new concern in our long history of food concerns. Public health concerns through much of this history have been *undernutrition*, not *overnutrition*.

In America, obesity has become a significant population-wide problem only in very recent decades; throughout much of our country's development, food and public health concerns have been mainly for food security for its citizens (during the Great Depression of the 1930s) and proper subsistence for all (feeding programs for needy women and children).

Historical timing has apparently played a role in the unforeseen and unintentional weight dilemma we find ourselves in today. During the last century, two major events occurred that have had greatly influenced our obesity problem in the 21st century: industrialization of the U.S. economy (including the food supply system) and increasing knowledge of the role of diet in human health.

Significantly, these important food events have occurred at *different times* in our country's history: the basic industrialization of the food supply was largely completed and entrenched *prior* to much of the discovery of the present knowledge concerning the relationship between diet and chronic diseases, particularly overnutrition, and certainly, prior to the high levels of overweight and obesity occurring today among Americans—young and adult.

We must also recognize that the majority of present food policies—agricultural, economic, and industrial—affecting our food supply were developed in the past with valid objectives far different from those that might be applied if these policies were being developed today. It is probable that our present obesity genesis is partially rooted in the public policies and policy decisions of the past that were so instrumental in forming and shaping our dynamic and powerful commercial food sector of today.

In the past, one of the primary challenges of these public policies at their inception was to assure adequate and affordable food for all Americans and to economically support the agricultural sector. This occurred at a time when an increasing number of our population were leaving the agricultural life to enter a new industrial lifestyle, dependent on ever fewer and fewer of their fellow citizens to feed them.

Today our policy challenges are far different (and more difficult); we suffer not from a lack of food, but rather an oversupply of food. However, the policy legacies of the past and the resulting food supply they created are still with us today, successfully and aggressively functioning. These earlier public policies apparently act as an impediment to the creation of an environment that can maximize the opportunity for the individual to control his or her own weight. Unfortunately, we do not yet have the necessary research to confirm such beliefs, and in the absence of hard research, we have to rely heavily on anecdotal impressions (always a risky basis for public policy development).

NUTRITIONAL POLICIES AND OBESITY

The 20th century (particularly the latter half) saw nutritional science making monumental progress in its understanding of the relationship between diet and long-term human health. The government attempted to implement public health policies as this new knowledge became available (Fig. 1).

Newly discovered nutritional knowledge offers those following a prudent diet hope in reducing the risks of many types of disabling and deadly chronic diseases. This startling new dietary knowledge with its potential for improving human health became well known to the public through wide media coverage; nutrition became a subject of general public interest and discussion. Because of these happenings, the 1990s have been often referred to as the *nutrition decade*.

In spite of the government's attempts to put this new knowledge to broad use by Americans (assisted by the public's intellectual interest in nutrition), the latter part of the century saw the rapid rise of a serious nutrition-related problem: widespread and increasing overweight and obesity throughout the United States.

Policy makers were faced with a discouraging paradox: during a period in which there were large increases in nutritional information (as well as wider public understanding of its meaning for human health), there occurred one of this country's most serious nutritional crises—upward of two-thirds of adult Americans became overweight or obese by the start of the 21st century.

Looking back at the start of the 21st century, it is obvious that our governmental health agencies were slow to react to the fast-rising pandemic, only acknowledging by the 1990s the increasing numbers of Americans—both adults and children—were becoming dangerously overweight and obese. The reason(s) for the government's slow reaction remains an open question. Today—even in government circles where there is much rhetoric about Americans' overweight and obesity problems—no formal nationwide program to deal with the pandemic has yet emerged.

As we attempt to craft new public health policies to control overweight and obesity, we need to better

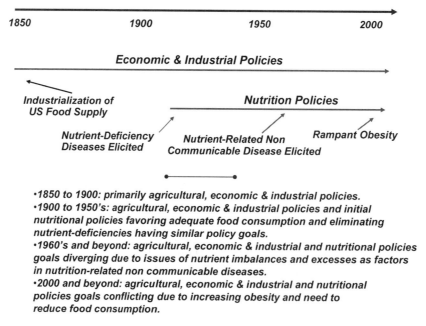

Figure 1 Economic and industrial policies. *Source*: From Ref. 2.

understand why past nutritional policies have not been effective in dealing with these new nutritional problems. Many reasons have been advanced for the inability of these policies to check rampant overweight and obesity at the end of the 20th century. The following have been advanced as likely (but not proven) causes.

During the last century, as there occurred a dramatic increase in the understanding of nutrition and its relation to health, government policy makers, scattered throughout different federal agencies [the US Departments of Health and Human Services (HHS), United States Department of Agriculture (USDA), Federal Food and Drug Administration (FDA), and the Federal Trade Commission (FTC)] operating under different—and sometimes conflicting—laws and legal mandates, attempted to incorporate this new knowledge into America's health policies. Policy makers were challenged by new, but changing, knowledge available to them, requiring ongoing changes in public health responses (Fig. 1).

In the period from the 1900s to the 1950s, many nutrient-deficiency diseases were discovered. This was soon followed by government-initiated nutritional policies aimed at *adequate food consumption*, to eliminate nutrient-deficiency diseases, particularly in low-income households.

In the period from the 1950s to the 1980s, great advances were made in the understanding of nutrient-related noncommunicable diseases (for example, diabetes and cardiovascular diseases), which policy makers quickly incorporated into nutrition policies aimed at eliminating imbalances and excesses of certain nutrients (fats, oils, and saturated fatty acids) in the American diet associated with such diseases.

It was during this time period that the Senate Select Committee on Nutrition and Human Needs released the first Dietary Goals for Americans. This was followed soon after by the Dietary Guidelines for Americans in 1980. Consumption of the appropriate diet rather than weight control was the core message of these policy documents.

In the current period, nutritional science emphasis and policies are shifting again to obesity-related issues, now stressing *reduced* food consumption or energy imbalance.

Accordingly, during the 20th century, government policy makers and their policies—due to new and different emerging science—have had to deal with constantly changing policy objectives. The result has been *unintended and unforeseen* conflicting government directives to Americans on food consumption over the 20th century, which no doubt diluted the effectiveness of any nutritional advice given to the public (7).

Agricultural and other food policies involving the commercial food sector did not suffer this policy vacillation; as outlined below they stayed the same during the 20th century through today. Their singular, unwavering objective was continuously increasing selective food pro-

duction (government-subsidized commodities) and consumption, resulting in a food environment very favorable to overconsumption of high-caloric foods by Americans.

While an analysis of 20th century public health diet initiatives is not the purpose here, nevertheless, the constantly changing thrust of these policies is potentially one of the significant factors in explaining why agricultural and industrial policies were so successful, while diet and health policies were *not*, especially in relation to Americans' weight problems.

Another important factor to consider was the different financial resources employed to accomplish the mission of these differing governmental policies—nutrition and related activities received a *few million* dollars annually while agricultural and food sector programs were funded in many *billions* of dollars annually.

The government's organizational structure may also have been a contributing factor. Government nutritional initiatives have been historically scattered throughout various agencies. As a result, their overall effectiveness may have been diminished by not being centralized in one government agency, with a strong primary nutritional mandate and authority.

Another factor to be considered is the traditional approach of the U.S. government agencies to advising its citizens on issues concerning their nutritional health. Up to the present time, the predominant government nutritional philosophy has been for government agencies to serve in an *advisory role* to its citizens in matters of diet and health (food pyramids, guidelines, food labels), believing it is the responsibility of the *individual* to use this advice to maintain his or her nutritional health (weight). Nutritional advice to Americans was long on what they should eat but short on how they might do this living on an increasingly enticing commercially supplied food and drink diet.

Obviously, this laissez-faire nutritional philosophy has not prevented nationwide overweight and obesity. (As we shall see below, agricultural and other food policies relating to the commercial sector were far from laissez-faire.) Unfortunately, with the scanty evidence available, it is not clear whether other ideological approaches would have fared better in the prevention of our nation's overweight and obesity.

Further, during the latter part of the 20th century, an overall analysis of government nutritional initiatives with regard to the rising obesity problem could identify the government responses (labeling, guidelines, food pyramids, etc.) as *tactical* in nature rather than *strategic* (coordinated policies and programs to reach health objectives). This, no doubt, also hampered overall effectiveness.

In addition, compounding the government's organizational, philosophical, and strategic problems, the agricultural and food industrial sector was generally resistant to the application of new nutritional science to their governmental policies, being concerned about the potentially negative influence on the businesses of the commercial food sector.

To summarize, the 20th century saw both the greatest advances in diet and health knowledge and the greatest changes in the Americans' eating behavior (not always for the best of nutritional health). However, public health policies arising from new nutritional knowledge apparently had only a limited influence on the long-established, successful agricultural, economic, and industrial public policies focusing on ever-increasing American food consumption. This *disjunction between supply-side and demand-side public policies* has apparently been a major contributing factor to the rise in overweight and obesity, and it warrants further study.

THE PARADOX OF U.S. FOOD POLICIES AND OBESITY

America's overweight problems present a paradox in public policies affecting our food supply: on one hand great success and on the other great failure. Our policies supporting the commercial food sector have worked, and those aimed at controlling the public's weight have failed.

The abundance of food and its wide availability, low cost, high quality, and great palatability to Americans attest to the great success of our agricultural, industrial, and economic policies and of the governmental programs supporting these policies. That two out of three adult Americans are now either overweight or obese confirms a serious failing of our current health policy programs. Resolving this policy paradox is one of our great health challenges of the 21st century.

Yet, there is far from universal agreement on the relationship between the successes and failures in our public policies and the causes in recent years of the steady onslaught of overweight and obesity among Americans, young and old. However, concern over the health risks (and their potential medical costs) associated with America's skyrocketing overweight problem is motivating new interest and thinking in examining all possible causal and environmental factors.

Beyond the influence of demand-side factors (eating behavior), there is growing recognition of the importance of supply-side factors (amount, nature, and cost of commercial food) in this pandemic: the role of social, economic, technological, and political environmental conditions that assist or deter the individual in maintaining his or her desirable weight.

Confirming the need to better understand the supply-side influence is the conclusion reached by the 2005 report of the U. S. Dietary Guidelines Advisory Committee, "In conducting the research on which this report is based, the Committee was struck by the critical and likely predom-

inant role of the environment in determining whether or not individuals consume excess calories, eat a healthful diet, and are physically active." (7). Further, the Committee added the observation that environmental influences tend to be *beyond individual control*, implicitly recognizing the supply-side factors role in the pandemic.

One of our future public policy challenges is to determine what those *supply-side policies* might, or should, be and the role of our government in developing the environmental conditions for citizens to attain and maintain optimum weight. These yet unresolved issues promise to be an area of nutrition and policy requiring future research (challenging and difficult), and also an area of great potential public controversy, due to the lack of evidence-based research on agriculture and food industry's role in our weight pandemic.

AMERICAN AGRICULTURE AND OBESITY

A necessary environmental condition for overweight and obesity to occur in the individual is the availability of ample food. For population-wide occurrence, this basic environmental condition is the wide availability of ample, affordable, liked food. U.S. agriculture, with its abundant commodities' production is the *starting point* in making such a food environment possible for Americans.

America's food supply chain starts with farms and ranches of unparalleled agricultural commodity productivity. This agricultural productivity is a key supply input in the ability of our food and restaurant industries to supply Americans with ubiquitous, inexpensive, plentiful, commercial food.

Our food availability and its economics are greatly dependent on our agricultural sector's commodity productivity. This agricultural supply condition affords our food-processing industries low-cost, high-quality, reliable, basic agricultural commodities (grains, oilseeds, dairy and livestock) to process into highly desired and economical consumer food products.

Furthermore, in the United States today, consumers' food costs require, on average, only 10% of their disposable income, resulting in Americans presently having one of the world's most economical, varied, and consumer-enjoyed food supplies. This inexpensive food largesse is largely based on high-caloric density food ingredients (corn-derived sweeteners, vegetable oils, dairy, and meat ingredients) derived from our government-subsidized agricultural commodities.

As a result, Americans can enjoy among other diets, if they wish, those that include superlarge food portions, fast-food dollar deals, and all-you-can-eat restaurants plus gigantic packaged soft drinks and sweet treats, as well as supermarkets offering more than 40,000 great-tasting foods at minimum costs. Food and food practices are based largely on our major agricultural-subsidized commodities. Foods and food practices are questioned now as being implicated in our present overweight and obesity problems.

Americans' lifestyles are shaped by this plentiful, inexpensive food. Today, food is everywhere in our daily lives: at home, in our social lives, and at work. This makes for an American lifestyle that is extremely food oriented, resulting in ubiquitous opportunities for Americans to overeat. The temptation to eat is everywhere today, 24×7. Our agricultural prowess is the starting supply-side condition making such food-based American lifestyle possible.

While ample and economical agricultural commodities by themselves are not a direct causal factor of our pandemic, U.S. agriculture—with its supportive governmental policies—does create a commodity supply making possible more than ample food (processed and supplied by the food industry as food products) that allow Americans to overconsume, if they wish, which many have.

The U.S. agriculture and its governmental policies have only recently been questioned concerning their negative influence on Americans' health and weight. Our agricultural policies are commonly recognized as pivotal to our great agricultural abundance, but have been often overlooked when analyzing environmental factors that could contribute to our pandemic (2).

U.S. AGRICULTURE

The United States is one of the world's leading industrial nations, but agriculture remains a large, vital part of the U.S. economy. Agriculture is, in fact, one of the largest businesses of this country and most successful when all elements are included.

The American agricultural system includes much more than farmers and ranchers alone, it includes also the many industries that supply the agricultural sector the necessary inputs and services (agricultural chemicals, equipment, and assorted financial services) as well as the industries that collect, handle, distribute, and process the agricultural commodities the agricultural sector produces. American agriculture, beyond its importance in feeding us, has great economic importance to our nation. Its economic welfare has been, and continues to be, a primary concern of our government.

American agriculture supplies the world's largest consumer food market, which will reach some one trillion in retail food sales in 2007. Our consumer food industry is the world's largest and most diverse in food processing, benefiting from the availability of an array of low-cost major commodities produced by the agricultural sector. Further, the United States is one of the world's largest exporters of agricultural commodities (estimated $62 billion in export

sales in 2004). Agriculture, including its related industries, is of great economic significance to our nation.

Americans, in general, enjoy and desire a diet that is greatly dependent on the major agricultural commodities (grain, oilseeds, dairy, and livestock). Agriculture's role in supplying the necessary building-block commodities to make our food abundance possible is widely recognized and supported by Americans. Americans overwhelmingly favor government policies supporting major agricultural commodity programs and have been willing to fund the government's great involvement in agriculture through their taxes for decades. As a result, agriculture and its production-oriented government policies for major commodities have had, and continue to have, wide political support.

Our agricultural system, with its many related industries, creates strong economic and political pressures for its continuous increase in production and utilization of the commodities it produces. Further, our agricultural system and its related government policies and programs operate on the implicit assumption that our domestic commodities demand will continue to increase.

The long-term economic viability of our agricultural system is currently based on this assumption: ever greater production, ever greater consumption. From a public health perspective, this is of minimum concern in a nation with a rapidly growing population to be fed as in our past. However, presently, with the U.S. population growth rate of approximately only 1% and most Americans already consuming too much food (calories) for their good health, this continuous growth production and consumption strategy—supported by present governmental agricultural policies—becomes more questionable.

Today in the United States, as an increasing number of our population becomes overweight and obese, we are facing a growing public policy debate over present policies aimed at ever-increasing consumption of favored agricultural commodities versus public health policies aimed at moderating our overconsumption of these same agricultural commodities as consumer foods.

AGRICULTURAL PUBLIC POLICIES

To fully understand any potential relationship between America's current obesity problem and its agricultural policies, it is necessary to understand the development of agriculture and agricultural policies, their objectives, accomplishments, and support over the last 150 years.

Strong political support for agriculture has its foundation in America's history. At our nation's founding, America was prominently an *agricultural nation* with 90% of its people directly depending on agriculture for their livelihoods. Its founders, many having their own agricultural holdings, greatly valued agriculture and its way of life. Many of these men hoped our nation would remain an agricultural nation.

This agrarian orthodoxy would fuel agricultural growth and prosperity up to the present. It has given rise to our strong, enduring agricultural tradition (the family farm). These agrarian sentiments that are still widely held by many Americans today serve as a powerful reservoir of political support for agricultural interests.

Americans also recognize the uniqueness of agriculture as compared with other types of businesses. Farming requires the favorable interaction of a unique and complex set of environmental conditions (weather, temperature, etc.) with varying degrees of unpredictability. As a result, agriculture is commonly recognized as a high-risk undertaking.

This environmental uncertainty, coupled with the economic variability of commodity markets, and the resulting risks to its farmers are further reasons for which agriculture has long been highly favored by American public policies to provide economic stability to the farm sector. Government policies are, and have been, practically favorable to the economic viability of a number of our major subsidized agricultural commodities. Fruits and vegetable crops have not been so favored.

U.S. agricultural productivity is also greatly assisted by its unparalleled *comparative advantage* of resources (land, climate, and water). Much of our agricultural land, climate, and environmental conditions are highly favorable for the production of grains, oilseeds, dairy and cattle, which become low-cost, building-block ingredients of a potentially high-caloric diet for Americans.

However, American agriculture supply-side achievements are the result of more than natural resources, they are also due to a favorable combination of governmental policies, the U.S. agricultural education and research system, abundant technology and, not to be forgotten, its industrious and innovative farmers and livestock producers.

AGRICULTURE AND GOVERNMENT

Strong, politically backed, long-active government policies have played a key role in shaping American agricultural productivity. Since the Civil War, the U.S. government has been involved in agriculture. The U.S. Congress created the Department of Agriculture in 1862. In this same period, it also enacted the Morrill Land-Grant College Act, commonly considered the most important piece of agricultural legislation in American history, which provided for the appropriation of public land for the establishment of agricultural and industrial colleges in each state.

In 1887, the Hatch Act, in combination with the previous act, established the country's land-grant universities and their agricultural experimental stations. This sequence of congressional legislation resulted in the establishment of the country's agricultural education and research system, commonly acknowledged to be the world's leading national agricultural research system. By the creation of this government-sponsored system, American agriculture would be supplied with a constant stream of world-class, cutting-edge technologies, allowing it to become ever more efficient and productive in agriculture.

These scientific resources have favored and been predominantly applied to the crops that our nation was historically most proficient at production (grains, oilseed, dairy, and livestock) and enjoyed a broad market demand (both domestically and internationally), which has resulted in continuous cycle of increased productivity, efficiency, and economic improvement for production of these agricultural commodities. Through no fault of American agriculture, our dominant agriculture system and its commodities favor a supply of economical, high-quality, consumer-liked, high caloric-density foods; an unintended, unplanned outcome of historically agricultural production policies.

American agriculture continues to be favored by government policies, right up to the present. During the period of 1902 to the present, the U.S. Congress passed some 70 or more major federal acts, which were highly beneficial to production agriculture. These congressional actions have, over time, created a favored agricultural economy within the broader U.S. economy, strongly supported and financed by federal government programs.

As recently outlined:

> As a result, US agriculture developed its own agricultural regime of market institutes and public investment and finance—subsidies, marketing assistance programs, special taxation, a farm credit system, market regulations, commodity programs and trade policies. All of these were highly favorable to US agriculture. It also included a nationally supported rural infrastructure encompassing country roads, drainage systems, flood controls, postal service, as well as technical assistance in the form of market information sources, extension education and assistance, and federally funded world-class production agricultural research (2).

This powerful regime has, as its overarching objective, constantly increasing agricultural productivity, efficiency, and production of our major commodities (grains, oilseeds, livestock, and dairy). Historically, public policies aimed at furthering these objectives had great social utility for a nation that was rapidly industrializing, accelerating in population growth, and desiring food security at reduced cost and processed foods favored by Americans.

American agricultural policies have been phenomenally successful in meeting these production objectives through the agricultural commodities they have championed. These policies should be highly regarded for their accomplishments.

Only now, as we face the grim reality of America's pandemic obesity, is there any need to question them from a public health perspective: its agricultural regime, its political power, and continuing production goals. However, given the scope of the present pandemic, *all factors* in our food environment need to be questioned. Whether a less-productive agriculture resulting from past, and present, agricultural policies would have made us less prone to overweight and obesity is an open question.

AGRICULTURE'S POLITICAL POWER

During the 20th century, U.S. agriculture's congressional political power has played a significant role in the growth of American production agriculture. No other business sector has equaled the agricultural interests' ongoing *bipartisan* political power in the U.S. Congress. Its power centers are the agricultural committees in both houses of Congress. These powerful committees, staffed and controlled by congressional members from predominantly agricultural states, are historically where U.S. food policy is formed, and then implemented by the U.S. Congress' control of the public purse. What senator or congressman from an agriculture-oriented state can be anything but supportive of agricultural production policies?

The political system by which this comes about has been described in the following manner:

> A "structural" view of farmers' political power focuses on a "gold triangle" of members of the committees that authorize legislation and appropriate funds, the executive branch department that administers the programs (USDA) and the lobbyists representing farm interests (8).

As a result, the U.S. Congress and its agriculture committees have strongly favored, funded, and protected production agriculture. In this mission, the U.S. Congress has been backed by American voters' support, the acceptance of the *special business* status of farming, and the agricultural sector's electoral power in predominantly farm states.

Under this American agricultural regime, agricultural interests have dominated and directed much of this policy to its production objectives—ever greater commodity yields of favored crops and livestock and increased consumer utilization of these commodities.

The ultimate success of these policies can be judged by the results: per capita U.S. food *utilization* has increased from 1800 lb/yr in the early 1980s to 2000 lb/capita at present. This increase in food utilization is mirrored by an increase in per capita caloric consumption; during the period 1971–2000 the average American man added 168 calories to his daily fare, while the average woman added 335 calories a day. This has occurred while the country's never-ending process of the application of new laborsaving technologies continues, resulting in an ongoing reduction in people's general food requirement (calories).

At this point, projections are that the agricultural production policies will continue, as in the past, to be successful and Americans will continue consuming ever greater amounts of agricultural commodities in their diets.

In summary, overproduction, and the consequently inexpensive foods, is now being increasingly questioned as one of the potential environmental factors favoring the occurrence of overweight and obesity. Today, ever more productive U.S. agriculture in a number of high-calorie-yielding commodities supported by unceasing technological innovation, generous governmental crop subsidies, and public policies favoring production agriculture as well as the country's comparative advantage in natural resources are all contributing elements in varying degrees in creating an environment that favor the occurrence of America's obesity problem—*excess food commodity production*. However, confirming current agricultural policies as a significant environmental factor in overweight and obesity is not yet supported by evidence-based studies.

THE DEVELOPMENT OF THE AMERICAN FOOD INDUSTRY

In the 19th century a food supply revolution began in America. Throughout the 19th and 20th centuries a fast growing commercial food sector would grow and evolve to answer Americans' ever-changing needs and desires in food. As this supply revolution has progressed to the present day, Americans would become increasingly dependent on the commercial sector to feed themselves ever more completely (even with ready-prepared, ready-to-eat foods) (9).

This food-oriented revolution was first triggered by increasing number of people leaving the farm to work in the new, rising industrial cities; these workers would require food, now having wages to pay others to feed them. America needed a commercial food supply to nourish a nation undergoing rapid industrialization.

A commercial-based processing and distribution system arose—massive in size and diversity of products—to answer Americans' growing food requirements. This nascent industry would respond by supplying the food required and desired by the country's growing nonagrarian population.

Aided by the fast-growing food demand, abundant agricultural commodities, new food-processing technologies, an expanding transportation network (railroads, later trucking) and a new diverse communication system (telegraph, newspapers and magazines), the food industry developed and prospered, becoming one of our nation's largest industries.

The industry's growth was further aided by growing numbers of retail stores and chains, new business methods (marketing, branding, and advertising), eager entrepreneurs (sensing great economic opportunities backed by ample venture capital) and, most importantly, very favorable governmental economic policies.

The industry prospered by supplying large volumes of low-cost, processed food, which Americans were eager for and very willing to buy. The commercial sector development would be further shaped and expanded by changing American social trends, evolving consumer food needs, and importantly, the nation's almost continuous economic expansion, generating consumer purchasing power for commercial food. As with our agricultural sector's commodities, the food sector's strategy assumed a continuously increasing market for its processed foods, which Americans would endorse by their ever-increasing purchases of the industry's food and beverages.

Through the 19th and 20th centuries the commercial food supply would have ever-increasing influence on Americans' diet through their products and their promotional and distribution methods (6).

THE FOOD INDUSTRY, ITS ECONOMIC ORIENTATION, AND AMERICA'S PANDEMIC

Over the last half century, the food industry—with its enticing food and beverage products coupled with its aggressive promotional practices—has become widely acknowledged as an environmental factor in determining what, where, and how much Americans eat. With its *present* size, resources, products, and new business methods, the industry is today without question a powerful, if not the most powerful, environmental force determining Americans' diet.

The role that the industry serves in the American diet is best understood through considering our nation's economic orientation. The United States is one of the world's most capitalistic-oriented nations, being so since its founding. Its capitalism is based on the principle of open markets regulated by market conditions rather than governmental regulation, resulting in an economic system that promotes economic growth as its overriding (if not sole) business objective. The food industry has thrived under American capitalism, resulting in the industry becoming collectively the world's leading food marketing juggernaut.

Key to this phenomenal growth was, and is, the industry's great ability to sell food and beverages that Americans like and that answers their eating choices and provides affordable, widely distributed products that respond to Americans' ever-changing lifestyles and food needs. The industry's success depended on satisfying Americans' immediate food wants, not what government health policies might recommend.

During its development the food sector—along with the overall industrialization of the nation—was widely accepted as a necessary part of our nation's industrial growth, which it was. The food industry's economic importance and well-being are to this day a major factor in all public policy consideration affecting the sector. Our government's economic and industrial policies have been highly supportive of the industry's economic growth while having little or no concern over possible health-related problems (overweight) occurring among Americans from such economically oriented public policies.

The remarkable industrialization of our food supply over its 150 years of development is largely attributable to its economic orientation under our American capitalistic system. Under this national economic agenda, the food-processing sectors have attracted great financial investment, on the basis of the expectation of continuing growth and profitability, which the industry has generally achieved through most of its history. Economic return—through market growth—rather than social objectives has been the paramount objective of the industry from its founding to the present.

During much of its development era, the industry's food and beverage products and their consumption were also greatly influenced by consumer demand. Granted that the industry's advertising and promotion methods have stimulated consumer demand for its products, yet in the final analysis we must also acknowledge that the consumers' inherent food desires—particularly for sugars and fat- and oil-based foods and beverages rather than fruits and vegetables—have also served as a motivating condition in determining the industry's structure and commercial offerings. The food industry thrives by selling food products that consumers organoleptically wanted and were willing to purchase, not by what government health policies recommend.

Of late, governmental health policy makers—previously fixated on personal behavior as *the* causal factor—have come to recognize that the food industry, under the nation's economic and agricultural policies, strongly sets *the American table* with its attractive commercial offering for the weight pandemic to occur; many Americans—following both their inherent unhealthy eating behavior and a physically less-demanding modern sedentary lifestyles—have made the pandemic occur. Both supply- and demand-side factors contribute to the cause of the pandemic (2).

THE FOOD INDUSTRY'S IMPACT ON AMERICANS' DIET

In analyzing the impact the food industry has on the American diet and, in turn, the role the industry plays in America's pandemic, it is common to attribute its effect to a few of its products (soft drinks, fast food) or its marketing methods (advertising and product promotion) as well as its political power and financial resources (Table 1).

While these are important factors in themselves in explaining the industry's influence on Americans' diet, the following will attempt to show that to fully comprehend the *overwhelming power* of the food industry on today's diet, it is necessary to understand industry's *business strategies* and the nature of *their food products* as well as the changing industrial *structure* for implanting these factors. Rather than attributing the dietary influence to one, or even several, environmental factors in attempting to explain our pandemic, a broader approach—structural in nature—is warranted.

Further, over the last few decades as outlined below, the food industry evolved from selling largely food ingredients to prepare our own daily food into an industry that increasingly fed us completely with ready-prepared, ready-to-eat food and beverages. The industry moved from supplying us to feeding us. This trend markedly increased the environmental influence of the industry in determining what many Americans ate and, no doubt, how much many Americans ate. This change in commercial food products has helped to create an American eating environment—especially in recent decades—that is highly conducive to overeating, which apparently two of three Americans have done (2).

The major influence of the food industry on many Americans' diet rests in its composite structure, products and marketing methods. (Table 2) The food industry's power in defining Americans' diet is believed to arise initially in the following manner: Michael Porter, the well-respected Harvard economist, who has extensively studied the basis for various nations' world prominence in various industries, including the American food-processing industry, proposes a growth model based on a few diverse broad environmental conditions that favor the growth of world-leading companies in any industrial nation.

Table 1 Factors Commonly Attributed as the Source of the Marketing Power of American Food Companies

Advertising and promotional activities
Brands and products
Financial resources
Political power

Source: From JE Tillotson.

Table 2 Major Strategic Objectives of the American Food Industry

Great innovation in products, processing, distribution, and marketing
Organoleptic quality of products
Consumer convenience of products
Better product economics
Improving product distribution
Market growth and development of large market share for products

Source: From JE Tillotson.

Determinants of National Advantage

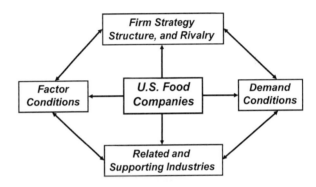

Figure 2 Determinants of national advantage. *Source*: From JE Tillotson.

To explain this industrial prominence—both domestically and globally in any industry—Porter has identified, through his extensive research, four broad, nationwide, environmental conditions (Fig. 2). In the case of American food industry, these environmental conditions are the following (11).

Factor Conditions

This refers to the necessary factors of production such as labor, arable land, natural resources, capital and infrastructure (road and transportation), which America has in abundance to support its agriculture and commercial food production.

Related and Supporting Industry Conditions

These are the necessary industries and companies that supply the food industry with equipment, supplies, and services (financial, marketing, etc.) as well as the education system, which train employees and serve as a source of intellectual capital for the industry. The United States exceeds at these industrial inputs.

Demand Conditions

The United States is a large, highly competitive market for processed food and a market that is highly receptive to new food products. Market conditions motivate the American food companies to be highly innovative and to continuously seek a competitive advantage versus their competitors through new products and services. It is through this dynamic and intense market competition that food companies become ever more competent in answering consumers' changing food desires.

Firm Strategy, Structure, and Rivalry Conditions

The United States is recognized as being a nation that is highly encouraging of business activities (founding, expanding, and profitability of businesses) under the nation's capitalistic economy. Under America's positive business culture the food industry has grown and prospered.

These four domestic environmental conditions have nurtured a score of very large, highly successful American food companies operating in different major food sectors (foods, beverages, and restaurants), all highly successful both financially and in terms of their abilities to market their food products in great amounts to Americans.

During the last century and a half, all of these Porter economic conditions have been strongly present in the United States for the food-processing industry, arguably to a greater degree in the United States than in any other nation.

The food industry has thrived under these four economic environmental conditions in the United States, resulting in the industry becoming collectively the world's leading food-marketing juggernaut. For example, presently, among the world's 10 largest food companies, eight are founded and developed and continuing to operate in the United States, remembering that consumer acceptance—*consumption*—of a food company's production—*food products*—goes hand in hand with a company's capability for market dominance—*market share*.

A prime example of the above is Americans' increasing consumption in recent years of discretionary caloric foods and beverages in the form of snack foods—most of which are high-caloric, low-nutrient-density products. These much-enjoyed snacks have grown phenomenally in recent decades in consumption. In 1977–1978, an American's daily total calorie average was 1798 with 12% coming

from snack foods; in 1994–1996, total daily calories increased to 2003 with 21% coming from snacks; and a recent study reporting on 1999–2000 calculated that, on average, one-third of Americans' total daily calories— slightly less than 2700—now come from snack foods (25% from sweets and desserts, soft drinks, and alcoholic beverages) (12).

Concurrently with this change in consumer snack consumption, the market structure of companies marketing many of these snacks has changed: presently, eight large food companies (alone or with one of the other seven companies) market 50% to 70% of each major categories of snack foods (soft drinks, candy, cookies and crackers, salty snacks) to Americans. These large companies (six are among the 10 largest of all food companies and two among the 20 largest) have great marketing and promotional abilities, as well as the financial resources and distribution capabilities, to aggressively promote their consumer-popular branded snacks. Together these few snack food companies form a powerful marketing force in shaping Americans' daily eating behavior (12).

We have similar changes in recent years in consumption from fast-food restaurants and in the market concentration of retail outlets supplying often high-caloric meals to Americans. Industry data report that Americans currently eat restaurant-prepared food slightly more than 200 times a year on average (both in restaurants and taken out). Industry sources estimate that approximately 70% of all restaurant-source food originates from a fast-food type outlet.

Further, with fast-food restaurants we have the same concentrated market trend as with snack foods. The concentration of fast-food outlets is occurring in ever larger restaurant chains, with the six largest fast-food chains of United States reported as having a combined control over 49,198 American outlets in 2002. These six largest fast-food chains were estimated to be selling approximately 11.8% of all $426 billion of away-from-home prepared food purchases in 2002, while spending a combined $1.68 billion in that year in the advertising and promotion of their meals. Again, we have a food sector with a few very large companies with large business resources with great ability in shaping Americans' eating behavior (14).

Were it not for the serious long-term health implications, the development of our commercial food system and its resulting products would be seen as a model example of America's industrialization, aided by the country's development-favoring governmental policies. In fact, even today, much of public policy (agricultural, industrial, and economic) still greatly favors growth of the American processed-food industry rather than acknowledging the current industrial policy's serious negative health implications.

The role of our government can be seen in the growth of increasingly sophisticated food products marketed by the food industry that have required sustained industrial entrepreneurship and innovation. We see great governmental support of the food industry in its innovation.

History has demonstrated repeatedly that governments are notoriously ineffective as agents for industrial product-innovation; however (and most important for sustained industrial economic development), only governments can foster the necessary economic and social conditions to allow entrepreneurship to achieve beneficial innovation. The United States has been extraordinarily successful with its industrial and economic policies and the public services available for entrepreneurs to achieve innovation. The food industry has shared greatly in this favorable American entrepreneurial environment.

Beyond the general support of America's agricultural and economic policies, the food industry was further favored in its growth by specific policies to encourage innovation in the food sector (such as product and processing research at land grant universities and USDA laboratories) (8).

Agricultural interests and policies were also supportive of the food-processing sector because a growing food industry was necessary for greater utilization of America's subsidized agricultural commodities production. As the present size and diversity of food industry's products attest, American economic and development policies have been markedly successful in their objective of encouraging *great innovation* in the food sector.

Viewed from a historical prospective the industry's innovation was largely aimed at answering Americans' organoleptic convenience and food price objectives rather than health and wellness considerations. History also demonstrates that public showed enthusiasm for the industry's stream of innovations by constantly increasing their purchases (as they continue to do) of new processed foods that fulfill their current food needs and lifestyles requirements.

As happened in agriculture, without government-sponsored research it is doubtful that the food industry would have reached the current range and sophistication of its products or its present industrial structure. During the industry's development—under the nation's public policies—government institutions (state and federal) would supply the necessary food science and technology research while the industry would supply the required innovation, yielding a plethora of attractive new consumer products that defined the American commercially sourced diet (8).

In general, the food industry throughout its history has been highly dependent on government-sponsored research as the basis for its innovation (it still is). Food companies historically invest relatively less in research than most other major industrial sectors, spending, on average, the equivalent of only 0.5% to 1% of their sales on research and development.

The food industry's research efforts historically have been directed to applied product development plus quality control efforts rather than to new industry-reshaping technological innovations. The industry, in general, is basically not high-technology-driven, but uses technology as necessary to accommodate the American public's changing wants and desires in food. Academic and government research laboratories, as well as suppliers' research efforts (new processing methods, packaging, and ingredients), have supplied much of the new technology used by the food industry for product innovation, leading to its economic growth (8).

The industry's day-to-day research objectives are— *new products, processing, packaging, and distribution*— of food and beverages to encourage consumer purchase. While success of any new product from a single company can be problematic (and always will be), overall the industry-wide new-product efforts have been highly successful. Predominantly, during much of the food industry's development, Americans chose and bought their food mainly on *taste, convenience, and economic motivations* rather than for any health reasons (6).

While a detailed, full account of the commercial development of the industry during the 20th century is beyond the scope of this chapter, the following brief overview may be helpful in understanding the diet-determining power the industry gained through product innovation—*first commodity to packaged to ready-prepared, ready-to-eat foods*—to meet Americans' changing food needs. The introduction of waves of new products with ever-increasing consumer utility, in turn, gave the food industry ever greater influence over what Americans ate and will eat (6).

The development of the commercial diet in the United States can be divided into three historical industrial eras as outlined below (Figs. 3 and 4).

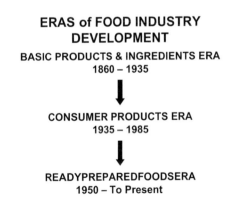

ERAS of FOOD INDUSTRY DEVELOPMENT

BASIC PRODUCTS & INGREDIENTS ERA
1860 – 1935

↓

CONSUMER PRODUCTS ERA
1935 – 1985

↓

READYPREPAREDFOODSERA
1950 – To Present

Figure 3 Eras of food industry development. *Source*: From JE Tillotson.

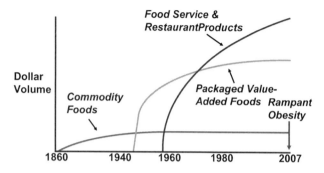

Figure 4 Industrialization eras of the U.S. food supply. *Source*: From Ref. 2.

RETAIL COMMODITY FOODS— 19TH CENTURY TO 1930s

This was the formative stage of the food industry in which the first food-processing plants producing basic food ingredients (flour, sugar, salt, fat and oils, dairy, meat, and other food staples, as well as vegetables and fruits) packaged in economic, convenient, and consumer-acceptable units were established in the industrial countries. The agricultural products chosen for processing by such technologies as canning, freezing, drying, milling, and other food-engineering unit operations were based on a balance between those suitable for processing and storage and those that people would purchase for consumption.

This era also saw the growth of long-distance distribution (railroads, trucking) and long-period storage of commercial food products (warehouses, frozen and chilled storage), as well as the first establishment of retail sales outlets (grocery stores). Product branding and salesmanship were introduced as aids in the sale and distribution of manufacturers' products. The manufacturing strategy was production of high volumes, produced at low unit costs, using investment in efficient processing plants to minimizing labor inputs.

As the public purchased and used the commodities in their meal preparation with time—in ever-increasing amounts—Americans became accustomed to these as ongoing components in their daily diet. This established the beginning elements of the American commercial, high-caloric diet that, from the first, was often high in sugar, salt, white flour, fat and oils, and animal-source ingredients and foods. This initial product stage began the food industry's environmental influence on the American diet. A trend that would increase as the food industry developed during the 20th century (2).

PACKAGED CONVENIENCE FOODS— 1930s TO 1980s

In this second era—while the earlier commodity type food products continue to be sold—aided by advances in food science and technology, increasing numbers of food companies successfully transformed themselves from processors and sellers of undifferentiated low-profitability commodity type foods to producers and marketers of branded, profitable, packaged convenience foods (TV dinners, cake and dessert mixes, frozen fully prepared items, crackers and snacks, and frozen and bottled beverages of all types).

The vast number and amounts of these new food products being produced by the industry found the growing new supermarket chains as a perfect distribution channel to the public that now lived increasingly in the suburbs with automobiles to shop at these large, consumer acceptable new retail outlets (6).

The germane strategy used by these companies was to develop new and unique, attractively packaged foods that met the fancy, needs, and budgets of consumers, based on taste, low cost, and convenience and then to build their products into a national brand, using skillful advertising and promotion, aided greatly by (then new) television. As the public grew to know and want the new branded product through compelling marketing programs, sales increased, yielding both profitability—and importantly—funds for additional market development.

Companies successful at using this strategy came to, and still do, dominate America's shopping carts. These products further acculturated Americans to commercial foods often with product characteristics of energy-dense/low-nutrient content, high fat and sugar, and high in animal-source content, and extended the consumer acceptance of commercial food products into their diet (15).

Industry economics, distribution, and marketing power favored increasing industry consolidation. Today the companies supplying us with retail consumer products are larger and fewer in number. This is an industry consolidation trend that has been occurring at increasing rate in the last decade through all food industry sectors. For example, by 2001 it was estimated that America's 10 largest food companies sold consumers 44% of all food at retail ($213 billion retail sales), and if this number is expanded to the 40 largest companies, their sales were 81% ($365 billion in sales). Today relatively few companies supply much of the food Americans purchase at retail. As a result these few consumer goods companies have a greater influence on Americans' diet than ever before (2).

READY-PREPARED, READY-TO-EAT FOODS— 1950s TO THE PRESENT

Starting in the 1950s with the founding of one of the first national fast-food chains—McDonalds—a new type of convenience food started rapidly entering the American market: ready-prepared foods that offered the public the ultimate in utility and convenience at very affordable prices—food requiring no preparation; food and beverages, both as handheld snacks or full meals that could be purchased in fast-food outlets or restaurants as well as in supermarkets and stores of all kinds. Food and beverages developed to be eaten at the site of purchase, in the home, or on the move. This trend would diminish the previous high growth rate of consumer-packaged food products that occurred in the 1930s–1980s era in favor of the rapid market growth of new ready-prepared, ready-to-eat foods.

The rapid and extensive growth plus the commercial origin of these modern ready-prepared foods were without parallel. *By the early 1990s Americans would be spending approximately half of their total food purchase dollars on ready-prepared, ready-to-eat foods and beverages* (Table 3).

Socioeconomic factors, in particular, were largely responsible for the success of these new ready-prepared convenience foods. Americans were experiencing unprecedented economic growth, affluence was molding their expectations, and ready-prepared foods and beverages became *affordable luxuries* for all.

A major factor in the growth of these foods was the increasing participation by women in the work force; overworked, time-constrained consumers, often in dual-income or single-parent households (particularly with children), not having the time, energy, or desire to cook, consumed these products in record amounts.

Ready-prepared foods were ideally suited, in both form and price, to newly developing eating pattern of consumers. At the forefront of the changing eating habits were the fast-food outlets, which increased from one outlet per 2000 Americans in 1990, to one per 1400 Americans in 2000, to presently one outlet for every 1000 Americans (2,13).

In addition, Americans' food from fast-food outlets became increasingly concentrated in ever larger chains. By 1998, the 20 largest fast-food chains would have 79,922 outlets in the United States, with annual sales of $56 billion, accounting for 22% of total restaurant sales (2).

From this century-long, three-stage industrial development outlined above has evolved a small number of leading food companies both consumer food products and ready-prepared, ready-to-eat foods (chain restaurants) with the following operating characteristics having, no doubt, great environmental influence on many Americans' diet (3,10).

- Producing commercial food products that the majority of the population find enjoyable to eat and use as a major source of their daily diet through repeated purchases, offered at convenient delivery sites.
- Products heavily oriented to those offering energy-dense/low-nutrient content foods and beverages, high added sugar and fat content foods and beverages, and products with high animal-source content.
- Producing increasing percentages of finished food products requiring no or very minimal further preparation, distributed ever more widely beyond traditional food channels.
- Producing attractive mass-produced branded food and beverages that are relatively inexpensive, accounting for decreasing percentage of consumers' rising disposable income.
- Marketing and distributing by ever larger food companies with continuously greater resources, competing in markets with markedly decreasing numbers of competing firms with often one to four brands dominating food product categories.
- Skilled marketing firms with single business strategies aimed at economic and volume growth based on continuously answering consumers' changing organoleptic and lifestyle needs through ongoing distribution and technical innovation.
- Firms that have continuously improved, through innovation of the marketing, promotional, and selling capabilities of their market-leading brands.

Table 3 U.S. Annual Expenditures for Food

	Preparation of food				
	Food at home		Food away from home[a]		Total
Year	Billions	Percent (%)	Billions	Percent (%)	Billions
1990	$304	55	$248	45	$552
1995	$349	53	$303	47	$652
2000	$422	52	$391	48	$813
2006	$553	51	$529	49	$1082

[a]Both meals and snacks.
Source: From U.S. Department of Agriculture.

- Food firms that, due to their great size, employment, resources, and their pivotal importance in the use and distribution of agricultural products, are favored by government and financial institutions.

In thinking of potentially successful public health policies, one must realize that the American type of processed food diet is the product of a food delivery system that, over the 20th century, has marshaled the strengths, resources, and abilities of the largest free-market capitalistic economy, aided by highly favorable agricultural, economic, and industrial governmental policies.

As a result, never in the long history of food has a nation's population faced such a powerful environmental force as Americans have during the last few decades than with its food industry and its promotional methods or as large and diverse number of highly capable food marketers.

Under the environmental commercial conditions that have existed in recent decades in the United States—*particularly associated with the food industry*—and the inherent organoleptic appeal of the American commercial diet—*coupled with the many Americans' excess eating behaviors and low physical activity levels*—any other population dietary outcome other than widespread overweight and obesity occurrence would have been highly unlikely.

THE FUTURE CHALLENGE

The prevalence of overweight and obesity in the United States today is motivating new thinking and questioning of present public health policies. Motivating this reevaluation are the predicted future staggering human suffering and economic costs that this pandemic may cause. Human suffering will be staggering and are unquantifiably large. Estimated financial costs to our nation are already in the range of $69 billion to $117 billion/yr. Lack of success to date in curbing this pandemic requires new thinking and the realization that the cause and solution can no longer be considered as solely the individual's problem, but rather as a broad population-wide problem requiring societal thinking.

With this new thinking, there is growing interest in the supply-side's role—*especially the commercial sector*—in creating an environment influencing the individual's eating behavior. Along with this general interest in environmental conditions, there is growing realization of the role that public policies—agricultural, economic, and industrial—serve in creating an *environment* that can assist or hinder the individual in maintaining proper body weight. While environmental conditions are not the cause of obesity, they can strongly influence individual eating behavior that, in turn, can lead to overweight and obesity.

Advances in the nutritional sciences have given us considerable understanding of the causes and potential control of obesity, at the *individual level*; however, at the societal level, we have only started our investigation of the causes and prevention of population-wide obesity. Therefore, before embarking on new policy initiatives aimed at solving the pandemic, we should ask to what extent we understand the environmental and structural conditions—*especially the commercial sector*—as a contributing factor to today's overweight population.

Therefore, in spite of the looming problem of population-wide overweight and the specter of its future human and economic costs, we need to be cautious. There is much we do not know about the influence of environmental and structural conditions—especially the commercial sector; our knowledge base is minimal.

Recent public policy history demonstrates how difficult it is to develop effective nutrition-based policies. As an example, it might be worthwhile to reconsider the high hopes that the nation shared for Americans' future diet and health upon the passage of the *Nutrition Labeling and Education Act in 1990*, with its required nutritional labeling of almost all packaged foods. Only recently we discovered, in people's everyday life, a low level of effective label use; on the contrary, there was an extensive change in their daily diets to non-nutritional-labeled, ready-prepared, ready-to-eat foods.

This, among other recent public health initiatives (the health significance of total-fat-dietary-intake initiatives) should give us pause—*to evaluate our understanding of the environmental forces contributing to the pandemic*—before rushing into new public policies without fully anticipating the dynamics of any proposed new public policies.

Presently, concerned health experts and citizen advocates are calling for immediate societal responses to curb obesity, with *tactics* such as targeting foods high in fat and sugar for new taxes, rigid controls of commercial communications to children, eliminations of certain foods from educational institutions, and increased interventions in matters of diet and physical activity.

As attractive as such tactics seem, we need to question if we have any firm evidence that such environmental tactics *alone* will work to control obesity? While such tactics may well be *part* of any eventual solution, we need to question the success of any such *limited tactical initiatives*—given that the present powerful promotional abilities of the commercial sector with Americans, both adult and young, outlined above are still in effect—as opposed to broader *strategic and structural approaches*.

A further issue to consider is the public's current opinion on overweight and obesity. According to recent public opinion studies, the American public is not yet overly concerned about obesity, showing a low level of support for obesity-targeted public policies aimed at the food industry. They apparently view obesity as resulting mainly from individual behavior rather than being any responsibility of industry (some public opinion polls have reported up to 90% of those questioned attributing obesity to individual behavior alone). The introduction of new policies aimed at environmental factors must first overcome the public's present indifference to environmental factors (*the food industry*) involvement with overweight and obesity.

Assuming that future research demonstrates that the commercial sector and its agricultural, economic, and industrial policies do, in fact, lead to negative environmental conditions in the individual's quest for maintaining proper body weight, what action do we then take?

New public policies and initiatives are, therefore, likely to be required to contain and solve this ubiquitous American health problem. If so, which policies and public health initiatives (supply side, demand side, or both) will be successful, considering that overweight and obesity are the result of widely varying types of *both* individual behavior and environmental forces? Which of various current agricultural, industrial, and developmental public policies are significant factors? All this is still further complicated by a complex set of interacting, and often conflicting social, economic, and political factors.

Could more progress be made in solving the obesity problem, prior to deciding on specific remedial actions, by framing the issue as the conflicting objectives of long-established agricultural, industrial, and economic policies versus necessary, new health policies requiring resolution at a societal level? There is the need to determine if Americans are willing to place national health goals (including often needed, difficult personal dietary changes) *before* traditional food sector economic goals (and their own current eating behavior)? We need to remember that all industrial nations are facing the same pandemic—with no present solution.

Designing successful public policies for addressing pandemic obesity at a national level presents daunting new challenges to policy makers: first, devising population-wide policy strategies (presently far from obvious) to control Americans' large appetites in a society highly food-oriented; second, convincing a skeptical public that obesity initiatives are the appropriate role for governmental action (recent public opinion polls show antipathy to this action); and finally, successfully implementing these policies in the daily lives of Americans, whose diverse-lifestyle popula-

tion is now reaching 300 millions! Further, any proposed policies, to be seriously considered, need to be acceptable to the majority of Americans culturally, economically, legally and—most difficult of all—*practically.*

REFERENCES

1. Levenstein H. Revolution at the Table—The Transformation of the American Diet. Berkeley, CA: University of California Press, 2003.
2. Tillotson JE. America's Obesity: conflicting public policies, industrial economic development, and unintended consequences. Annu Rev Nutr 2004; 24:617–643.
3. Tillotson, JE. Multinational Food Companies and Developing Nations' Diets, Food Policy Options: Preventing and Controlling Nutrition-Related Non-communicable Diseases. Washington, D.C.: WHO/World Bank, 2003.
4. Femández-Amesto F. Near a Thousand Tables—a History of Food. New York: Free Press, 2002.
5. Levenstein H. Paradox of Plenty—A Social History of Eating in Modern America. Berkeley, CA: University of California Press, 2003.
6. Tillotson J. Convenience Foods, Encyclopedia of Food Sciences and Nutrition, 2nd ed. London: Academic Press, 2003.
7. U. S. Department of Health and Human Services and the Department of Agriculture. The report of the Dietary Guidelines Advisory Committee on Dietary Guidelines for Americans. Washington, D.C., 2005.
8. Gardner BL. American Agriculture in the Twentieth Century: How it Flourished and What it Cost. Cambridge, MA: Harvard University Press, 2002.
9. Morison SE, Commager HS, Leuchtenburg W. The Growth of the American Republic. Vol. 2, 11th ed. New York: Oxford University Press, 1980.
10. Tillotson JE. 10 Things congress needs to know about obesity. Nutr Today 2005; 40(3):126–129.
11. Porter ME. The Competitive Advantage of Nations. New York: The Free Press, 1990.
12. Tillotson JE. Who's filling your grocery bag? (Part 1 and 2) Nutr Today 2004; 39(4,5). 176–179 and 217–219.
13. Sloan AE. What, when, and where Americans eat. Food Technol 2003; 57(8):48–66.
14. Tillotson JE. Our ready-prepared ready-to-eat nation. Nutr Today 2002; 37(1):36–38.
15. Tillotson JE. The mega-brands that rule our diet (Part 1 and 2). Nutr Today 2005; 40(6):257–260 and Nutr Today 2006; 41(1):17–21.

14

Behavioral Approaches to the Treatment of Obesity

RENA R. WING

Department of Psychiatry and Human Behavior, Brown Medical School, The Miriam Hospital,
Weight Control and Diabetes Research Center, Providence, Rhode Island, U.S.A.

THE BEHAVIORAL APPROACH TO OBESITY: A THEORETICAL OVERVIEW

The behavioral approach to obesity grew out of the Learning Theory (1,2) and was first applied to the treatment of obesity between 1960 and 1970 (3,4). The primary assumptions of the behavioral approach are that (*i*) eating and exercise behaviors affect body weight; by changing eating and exercise behaviors, it is possible to change body weight; (*ii*) eating and exercise patterns are learned behaviors and, like other learned behaviors, can be modified; and (*iii*) in order to modify these behaviors long term, it is necessary to change the environment that influences them.

The behavioral approach does not deny the fact that an individual's genetic background may have a strong influence on his or her body weight. However, despite a predisposition to be of a certain weight, changes in energy balance (i.e., decreases in energy intake and/or increases in energy expenditure) will produce weight loss.

Likewise, the behavioral approach recognizes the importance of an individual's past history. The individual's family and cultural background influence body weight by determining food preferences, food choices, and the preferred level of physical activity. However, while accepting the importance of historical antecedents, the focus of a behavioral approach is on current behaviors and the environmental factors controlling these current behaviors.

The essence of the behavioral approach to obesity is the functional analysis of behavior, delineating the association between eating and exercise behaviors and environmental events, such as time of day, presence of other people, mood, and other activities (5,6). Patients are asked to self-monitor their eating and exercise behaviors to determine specific problem areas that should be targeted in treatment. The environment controlling these behaviors is then restructured to modify these problem behaviors.

A key technique in behavioral approaches is self-monitoring (7), which involves writing down exactly what is eaten and what type of physical activity is performed. This record allows the patient and the therapist to identify problem behaviors that might be changed. For example, the self-monitoring record may reveal that a large percentage of an individual's caloric intake is consumed in the form of desserts, which between-meal eating constitutes a major problem, or that an individual's portion size is unusually large. Alternatively, the individual may consume relatively few calories but lead a very sedentary lifestyle. These different behavior patterns would lead to different targets for the behavior change intervention.

Often in changing overall behavior, it is necessary to break the target behavior into several components, and

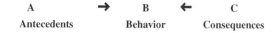

A → B ← C
Antecedents   Behavior   Consequences

Figure 1 A-B-C model of the behavioral approach to the treatment of obesity.

then to work on each part in turn (i.e., "shape" the behavior). For example, to lower calorie intake in an overweight individual, a therapist might work first on reducing calories consumed at breakfast and later move to lunch and dinner, or focus initially on decreasing the quantity of food consumed (i.e., portion sizes) and later work on changing the quality of the diet.

After defining the behavior to be changed, the next step is to change the environment that controls the behavior. The behavioral approach assumes that behavior is controlled by *antecedents*, or cues in the environment that set the stage for the behavior, and by *consequences*, or reinforcers, that come after the behavior and lead to its recurrence (8). This A-B-C model is shown schematically in Figure 1. For example, the sight of food on a buffet table may lead a person to overeat, or the cue of seeing someone else eating may arouse feelings of hunger.

Likewise, the positive consequences that come from the good taste of food or from reduction in feelings of hunger may lead to continued selection of these food items.

In the behavioral approach to weight control, patients are taught to restructure their home environment so that it will elicit the desired behaviors. These techniques are called stimulus-control strategies (3,4). For example, patients are encouraged to refrain from purchasing high-calorie desserts and to store all high-calorie foods in difficult to reach places; simultaneously, they are taught to buy more fruits and vegetables and to keep them readily accessible. Patients are also taught strategies for changing thoughts and emotions, which can serve as powerful cues for overeating and strategies for dealing with social cues and social pressure to overeat.

Patients in weight control programs often observe that they do not have the necessary "willpower" to avoid unhealthy foods. The behavioral approach is designed to restructure the environment to minimize the need for willpower. For example, if a patient opens the refrigerator and finds only low-calorie food items available, the chances are good that the patient will select a low-calorie item (even if the person lacks willpower). Likewise, if the patient plans ahead to meet a friend at the park for a walk after work, the chances are increased that the patient will actually take a walk. Planning ahead and developing a structure at a point in time when willpower is not required increase the likelihood that the desirable behavior will occur.

Finally, since environmental consequences are believed to play an important role in influencing behavior, behavioral programs attempt to develop new reinforcement contingencies. Behavior therapists use reinforcers, such as praise and positive feedback to encourage patients to adopt new healthier eating and exercise behaviors and teach patients to reinforce themselves for appropriate behavior change. Some behavioral programs also include more formal reinforcement systems, such as contingency procedures where patients deposit money with the therapist and earn back portions of their money contingent on behavior change (9,10).

HISTORY OF BEHAVIORAL APPROACHES TO OBESITY

The Development of Treatments from 1970 to 1990

The earliest report of a behavioral treatment program for obesity was by Stuart, who successfully treated eight overweight women (4). These women experienced an average weight loss of 17 kg over a 12-month period, ranging from a weight loss of 12 to 21 kg. It should be noted that Stuart (an eminent behavior therapist) conducted the treatment program himself, selecting each patient individually and tailoring the program to fit the needs of the individual patient. At the start of therapy, the treatment sessions were scheduled frequently (several times per week), and then gradually less frequently. Eating and exercise behaviors were targeted, and patients weighed themselves four times each day. The program included cognitive interventions, as patients were taught to deal with their weight-related fears, and the patients were helped to develop new hobbies as alternative sources of reinforcement.

Stuart's successful report led to a flood of behavioral research studies. These studies in the early 1970s typically involved 10 weeks of group treatment with mildly overweight subjects and were often conducted as part of a student's doctoral dissertation (5,11). Thus, in many ways these studies represented an abrupt departure from Stuart's landmark treatment. The emphasis in these programs was on changing eating patterns (where and when foods were eaten), but the nutritional aspects of the diet (number of calories, macronutrient distribution) were ignored, in part to distinguish behavioral treatment from traditional dieting interventions. These early studies showed that behavior modification was more effective than nutrition education (12) or psychotherapy (13). On average, participants lost 3.8 kg over an 8.4-week treatment interval (5). When followed up an average of 15.5 weeks later, participants had maintained a weight loss of 4.0 kg.

The evolution of behavioral treatments from 1974 to 1990 is shown clearly in Table 1, a summary table reprinted from (14). As seen in this table, behavioral treatments gradually evolved over this period (1974–1990) to include

Table 1 Summary Analysis of Selected Studies from 1974 to 1990 Providing Treatment by Behavior Therapy and Conventional Reducing Diet

	1974	1978	1984	1985–1987	1988–1990
No. of studies included	15	17	15	13	5
Sample size	53.1	54.0	71.3	71.6	21.2
Initial weight (kg)	73.4	87.3	88.7	87.2	91.9
Initial % overweight	49.4	48.6	48.1	56.2	59.8
Length of treatment (weeks)	8.4	10.5	13.2	15.6	21.3
Weight loss (kg)	3.8	4.2	6.9	8.4	8.5
Loss per week (kg)	0.5	0.4	0.5	0.5	0.4
Attrition (%)	11.4	12.9	10.6	13.8	21.8
Length of follow-up (weeks)	15.5	30.3	58.4	48.3	53
Loss at follow-up	4.0	4.1	4.4	5.3	5.6

Source: Ref. 14.

heavier participants (from 73 to 92 kg at entry), longer treatment intervals (from 8.4 to 21.3 weeks in length) and longer follow-up durations (increasing to a yearlong follow-up). The program itself changed as well, placing far greater emphasis on nutrition (14). Patients in behavioral programs were given calorie goals (usually 1200–1500 kcal/day) and self-monitored not only the events surrounding eating but also exactly what they ate (8,15). Calorie goals for exercise were also prescribed. Cognitive behavioral strategies were given greater emphasis (2), and financial incentives were often utilized. Thus, behavioral programs evolved from teaching strictly behavioral strategies to focusing equally on diet, exercise, and behavior modification. With this longer, more inclusive intervention, average weight losses increased to 8.5 kg in 1990. At the one-year follow-up, subjects had maintained an average weight loss of 5.6 kg (66% of their initial weight loss).

Refining Treatments (1990–2000)

Research during the period of 1990–2000 was designed to evaluate new strategies that might increase the magnitude of weight loss achieved in behavioral programs. Interestingly, years 1990–1995 focused mainly on diet, whereas 1996–2000 stressed physical activity. Each of these areas will be described in detail in later sections of this chapter.

Estimating the magnitude of weight loss that can be achieved with current behavioral weight loss programs is difficult, because a variety of different approaches have often been tried within a single study. Therefore, rather than tabulating results of all treatment studies and all intervention groups, Table 2 presents a highly selected listing of 12 of the largest and longest studies. Two of these 12 studies compared very low calorie diets (VLCD) with low-calorie diets (LCD) (16,17); results from the low-calorie conditions are included in the table to provide a more accurate appraisal of the usual outcome in behav-

ioral programs. Similarly, treatment conditions that include diet plus exercise were selected (aerobic exercise was selected if several types of exercise), since this is the recommended approach to behavioral treatment. Finally, if a study included several treatment groups that were prescribed diet plus exercise, results from the most effective intervention were used to determine what can be achieved in current intervention studies.

Table 3 averages across the treatment groups listed in Table 2. Comparing Table 3 with Table 1, it appears that there has been continued improvement in treatment outcomes. While in 1988–1990, the average patient lost 8.5 kg over 21 weeks, in 1990–2000, the average patient lost 10.4 kg over five months. Some of this improvement may be due to the fact that not all treatment groups were tabulated for 1990–2000; as noted above, the most effective LCD plus exercise intervention in each trial has been selected. However, much of the improvement appears to be the result of stronger behavioral techniques. These stronger behavioral techniques will be discussed in subsequent sections of this chapter.

Follow-up also appears to be improving. When reexamined at approximately 18 months (i.e., a year later), patients in studies conducted from 1900 to 2000 maintained a weight loss of 8.1 kg, or 82% of their initial weight loss. Again, this compares very favorably with the 5.6-kg loss at follow-up reported in 1988–1990.

Figure 2 presents the data from the 1990–2000 studies in graphical form showing the pattern of weight changes over time and the consistency of results across the 12 studies. There is a tight clustering of results at six months, suggesting that initial weight losses are produced quite consistently across different studies, different investigators, and different treatment populations (the only two outliers are the two studies that had three- and four-month treatments). Weight losses at 12 months (mean = 10.35 kg) are comparable to those seen at 6 months (mean = 10.37 kg). Studies with 18-month data (N = 7 studies) showed an average weight

Table 2 Results of Selected Behavioral Weight Loss Trials, 1990–2000

First author (reference)	Treatment format	Weight loss (kg)				
		Initial weight	Month 6	Month 12	Month 18	Month 24
Wadden (16)	Weekly for 12 mo Biweekly mo 12–18 Low-calorie diet	106	11.9	14.4	12.2	
Wing (17)	Weekly for 12 mo No Tx after 12 mo Low-calorie diet	106	13.5	10.5		5.7
Viegener (50)	Weekly for 6 mo Biweekly 6–12 mo Low-calorie diet	96	10.2	9.0		
Jeffery (52)	Weekly for 6 mo Monthly 6–18 mo SBT + food provision	90	10.0	9.1	6.4	
Wing (54)	Weekly for 6 mo Varied for next 12 mo SBT + food provision or menus	86	12.0		6.9	
Wadden (55)	Weekly for 6 mo Biweekly 6–12 mo Aerobic exercise 2–3 times perwk	96	16.2	13.7		8.5
Jeffery (67)	Weekly BT for 6 mo Monthly 6–18 mo Exercise on own	86	8.3		7.6	
Jakicic (64)	Weekly for 6 mo Biweekly 7–12 mo Monthly 12–18 mo Long-bout exercise	90	~7.5		5.8	
Perri (63)	Weekly for 6 mo Biweekly 6–12 mo Lifestyle exercise	88	10.6	12.4	11.9[a]	
Andersen (62)	Weekly 4 mo Lifestyle exercise	89	7.9[b]		7.1[c]	
Leermakers (60)	Weekly 6 mo Biweekly 6–12 mo Weight-focused maintenance	85	8.7	8.5	7.9	
Foreyt (59)	Weekly for 3 mo Biweekly/monthly for 3–12 mo Diet + exercise	97	6.9[d]	8.1		

[a]15 months
[b]4 months
[c]16 months
[d]3 months

Table 3 Summary of Results of Selected Behavioral Weight Loss Trials, 1990–2000

Number of treatment trials	12
Initial treatment	
Duration	5.6 mo
Weight loss	10.4 kg
Final follow-up	
Duration	17.6 mo
Weight loss	8.1 kg
Percent of weight loss retained	82%

loss of 8.2 kg. Thus weight regain appears to occur during the 12- to 18-month window. Only two studies provided 24-month data. In these studies, the average weight loss was 7.1 kg at 24 month, quite comparable to the results for studies with 18-month data. Since the two studies with 24-month follow-up included a full 12 months of treatment, the 24-month point actually reflects results one year after the end of weekly treatment, perhaps explaining the similarity between the 18-month and 24-month results. No studies were found that included 30-month, 36-month, or longer follow-up.

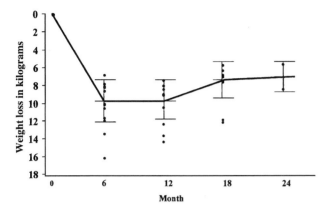

Figure 2 Weight loss outcome in behavioral treatments from 1990 to 2000.

Thus, results of behavioral programs appear to be continuing to improve, albeit only slightly. The strongest behavioral programs now produce weight losses of 10.4 kg, with maintenance of an 8.1-kg weight loss one year later.

Evidence that Modest Weight Losses Have Important Health Benefits (2000–2005)

One of the important achievements during 2000–2005 has been the demonstration that the magnitude of weight loss produced by behavioral weight control interventions is sufficient to produce marked improvements in health. The Diabetes Prevention Program (DPP), for example, demonstrated that a lifestyle intervention could significantly reduce the risk of developing type 2 diabetes (18). DPP was a randomized clinical trial in over 3000 individuals with impaired glucose tolerance who were randomly assigned to a lifestyle intervention, to metformin (a medication used to treat diabetes), or to placebo. The goals of the lifestyle intervention were a 7% weight loss and at least 150 minutes of physical activity per week. These goals were achieved through a behavioral lifestyle intervention, including frequent individual sessions; a low-calorie, low-fat diet; and home-based physical activity focused on brisk walking. On average, participants in the lifestyle intervention lost 6.8 kg at six months and maintained a weight loss of 4.1 kg at three years. The lifestyle intervention reduced the risk of developing diabetes over three years by 58%, whereas metformin reduced the risk by 31% relative to placebo. Both interventions had significant effects, but lifestyle was twice as effective as medication and worked in all age, weight, gender, and ethnic subgroups.

A further analysis of the lifestyle intervention (19) sought to determine whether the benefits of lifestyle resulted from the weight loss or the physical activity. Weight loss was clearly the major factor, with each kilogram of weight loss associated with a 16% reduction in risk. Although changes in dietary fat intake and physical activity were related to weight loss and weight loss maintenance, it was the weight loss per se that was related to reduced diabetes risk.

Weight loss not only helps reduce the risk of developing diabetes, it also improves glycemic control and cardiovascular risk factors in individuals who already have diabetes. Look AHEAD (Action for Health in Diabetes) is a randomized trial with over 5000 overweight individuals with diabetes who are assigned to a lifestyle intervention or control. Again, the lifestyle intervention is based on the behavioral approaches described in this chapter. The intervention includes a combination of group plus individual sessions, a structured low-calorie, low-fat diet that includes use of meal-replacement products, and a 200-min/wk physical activity goal. Results at one year showed that the lifestyle intervention was effective at producing a weight loss of 8.7 kg (8.6%) (20). Excellent weight losses were achieved both in individuals using insulin (7.1%) and in those not using insulin (8.1%). Moreover, these weight losses were associated with significant improvements in glycemic control. Glycosylated hemoglobin decreased from 7.25% at baseline to 6.61% at one year in the lifestyle intervention group, whereas the control group levels were 7.29% and 7.15%, respectively. At baseline, 11% of the lifestyle group and 10% of the control group met all three American Diabetes Association (ADA) goals for glycemic control, blood pressure, and lipids. At one year, this had increased to 24% in lifestyle and 16% in control. The Look AHEAD study will continue to year 2012 to examine the effects of this weight loss on cardiovascular morbidity and mortality.

DESCRIPTION OF CURRENT BEHAVIORAL TREATMENT PROGRAMS

Over time, behavioral programs have become fairly standardized. Therefore, it is possible to describe a "typical" program. These current programs discussed above differ quite markedly from both Stuart's early intervention and from the theoretical description of a behavioral program provided in the overview at the start of this chapter.

Currently, almost all behavioral programs are delivered in groups of 10 to 20 patients (8,14). With this many patients in a group, it is difficult to conduct an individualized functional analysis of behavior. The program is offered as a series of lessons, and the entire group of participants receives lesson 1 on week 1, lesson 2 on week 2, etc. There is no assessment of whether the lessons relate to the individual participant's problem areas or whether the participant has mastered the skill before moving on to the next skill. However, individualization of treatment occurs through lessons on problem solving, allowing participants the opportunity to focus on their specific problem areas. Therapists for behavioral programs are likewise quite different. Some programs use one therapist throughout, but many use a team of therapists (including a behavior therapist, an exercise physiologist, and a nutritionist) and rotate therapists by the topic. Treatment usually involves weekly meetings for 16 to 24 weeks (with some programs now using yearlong programs) and then less frequent contact.

Key strategies in current behavioral program include the following:

Self-Monitoring

Patients in behavioral programs are taught to write down everything they eat and the calories in these foods. In addition, many programs have begun to teach patients to self-monitor the grams of fat in each food. After a few weeks in the program, self-monitoring of physical activity is added (with activity monitored either in minutes or in calories expended). Self-monitoring is prescribed daily throughout the initial 20- to 24-week program and periodically (or daily) during maintenance. Self-monitoring is often considered the sine qua non of behavioral programs, and continued adherence to self-monitoring predicts long-term maintenance of weight loss (21,22).

Goal Setting

The goal in behavioral programs is to achieve a weight loss of 1 to 2 lb/wk (0.5–1 kg). To accomplish this, patients are given goals for total calories (usually 1000–1500 kcal/day), for grams of fat (usually given in grams of fat per day and set at a level to achieve a 20–30% fat diet), and for physical activity (gradually increased from 250 kcal/wk to 1000 kcal/wk). Patients may also set specific behavioral goals to achieve during various weeks of the project. Short-term goals that the participant can reasonably be expected to achieve are emphasized (23).

Nutrition

The nutritional aspects of weight loss are now given far more attention in behavioral weight loss programs (8,15). Virtually all programs ask participants to record what they are eating and the calorie and/or fat content of those foods. Lessons on healthy eating, which emphasize increasing intake of complex carbohydrates and fiber and decreasing dietary fat, are usually included. Moreover, the specific skills required to be able to consume a low-fat diet are taught during the course of the program, with lessons on topics such as recipe modification, label reading, restaurant eating, and demonstration of special cooking skills

such as stir-fry cooking. Thus, nutrition is taught both through educational classes designed to increase knowledge of what should be consumed and through demonstrations of how to accomplish the complex task of going from a high-calorie, high-fat diet to a lower-calorie, lower-fat regimen.

Exercise

Exercise is given a great deal of attention in behavioral weight loss programs because exercise is the single best predictor of long-term weight maintenance (24). Correlational studies comparing successful and unsuccessful weight losers consistently show that successful weight losers are best distinguished by their self-reported exercise behavior (25–27). The association between exercise and long-term weight loss has been observed in men, women, children, and adolescents, and is seen in programs involving LCDs and VLCDs (24). In addition, randomized controlled trials, in which diet alone, exercise alone, and diet plus exercise are compared, consistently show that the combination of diet plus exercise produces the best results (28–30).

To increase exercise, participants in behavioral programs are given goals for exercise, and these goals are gradually increased over time to shape an exercise routine. Most programs encourage patients to gradually work up to 1000 calories/wk of exercise, which can be accomplished by walking 10 miles/wk (2 miles on 5 days each week).

Behavioral treatment programs often distinguish between *lifestyle exercise,* such as using stairs instead of elevators or parking further from the store, and *programmed exercise,* in which a specific time is set aside for the purpose of exercise. Both types of exercise are strongly encouraged in behavioral treatment programs. Moreover, based on Epstein et al.'s findings that decreasing sedentary activities such as TV watching is very effective in promoting weight loss (31), many programs now include lessons on this topic as well.

Again, as in discussing nutrition, behavioral programs help patients learn the specific skills required to become more active, such as learning to monitor their heart rate to determine the intensity of exercise, learning how to dress for exercise in cold or hot weather, and learning how to deal with barriers that make exercise difficult. Some behavioral programs include supervised exercise sessions to model these skills and help provide participants with social support for exercise (32).

Stimulus Control

Stimulus control techniques remain the hallmark of behavioral treatment programs (3,4). Based on the assumption that behaviors are controlled by environmental antecedents, participants in weight control programs are taught to change their environments, so that there are an increased number of cues for appropriate diet and exercise behaviors and fewer cues for inappropriate behaviors. Specifically, participants in behavioral weight control programs are taught to increase their purchase of fruits and vegetables, to wash and prepare these foods for easy eating, and to place these foods prominently in the refrigerator. In contrast, high-fat/high-calorie products are to be decreased. If it is necessary to purchase these foods at all, they are to be stored in opaque containers or high cupboards, since "out of sight is out of mind." Some programs also encourage participants to select a designated eating place and to restrict all eating to that place, and to separate eating from other activities (such as watching television or reading). In this way, behavioral programs seek to limit the cues associated with eating.

Problem Solving

The problem-solving approach of D'Zurilla and Goldfried (33) is taught to participants in weight control programs. Participants learn to identify situations that pose a problem for their eating and exercise behaviors, to use brainstorming to generate possible solutions to the problem, to select one solution to try, and then to evaluate the success of their attempt. Through training in problem solving, behavioral programs are able to individualize the group-based weight control program and to teach patients strategies for dealing with their own personal problem areas.

Cognitive Restructuring

The cues for overeating and underexercising include not only physical cues such as the sight and smell of food but also cognitive cues. A person's thoughts, such as the thought, "I've had a bad day. I deserve a treat. I'll go for some ice cream," can lead to inappropriate behavior. Dividing the world into good and bad foods, developing excuses or rationalizations for inappropriate behavior, and making comparisons with others can all serve as negative thoughts. Behavioral programs teach participants to recognize that they are having these negative thoughts, to understand the function these thoughts serve for the participant, and then to counter these negative thoughts with more positive self-statements (34,35).

Relapse Prevention

On the basis of Marlatt and Gordon's theory of the relapse process (36,37), behavioral weight control programs now emphasize that lapses (or slips) are a natural part of the weight loss process. Patients are taught to anticipate the types of situations that might cause them to lapse and to plan strategies for coping with these situations. The goal is to keep lapses from becoming relapses.

EFFORTS TO IMPROVE TREATMENT OUTCOME

In an effort to improve treatment outcome, behavioral research from 1990 to 2000 has focused on strengthening the dietary component of the weight loss program, strengthening the exercise component, and/or strengthening the manner in which the behavioral strategies are implemented. Each of these areas of research will be discussed in turn.

Strengthening the Dietary Component

Combining Behavior Modification and VLCD

One approach to improving weight loss in behavioral treatment programs is to improve initial weight loss by using stricter dietary approaches, such as VLCDs. VLCDs are diets of <800 kcal/day, usually consumed as liquid formula or as lean meat, fish, and fowl (38). These diets have been shown to produce excellent weight losses (9 kg in 12 weeks) (38,39) and appear to be safe when used with carefully selected patients and appropriate medical monitoring (38). By using VLCDs to produce large initial weight losses and behavioral training to improve maintenance, it was hoped that a more successful treatment approach could be developed.

In one of the earliest studies of the combination of behavior modification and a VLCD (Table 4), Wadden and colleagues (40) randomly assigned 59 overweight subjects to one of three conditions: an 8-week VLCD administered in a physician's office with no behavioral counseling (VLCD alone), a 20-week group behavioral weight loss program that used behavior therapy (BT) and a balanced LCD throughout (BT + LCD), or a 20-week group behavioral program that included an 8-week period of VLCD (BT + VLCD). Subjects in the VLCD-alone group lost 14.1 kg during the 8-week diet, but then rapidly regained their weight, maintaining a weight loss of 4.1 kg at the one-year follow-up (i.e., maintaining only 29% of their initial weight loss). Better results were obtained in the BT + VLCD condition that lost 19.3 kg initially and maintained a weight loss of 12.9 kg at one year. However, while the initial weight losses in the BT + VLCD condition were better than those in the BT + LCD (19.3 vs. 14.3 kg, respectively), at the one-year follow-up, weight losses were no longer significantly different (12. 9 vs. 9.5 kg in BT + VLCD vs. BT + LCD conditions, respectively). Thus, the greater initial weight losses in the VLCD were not successful in producing significantly better long-term results.

Table 4 Weight Loss in Long-Term Studies of Behavioral Interventions with VLCD Vs. LCD

Trial (reference)	Short-term results			Long-term results		
	Duration (wk)	Weight loss		Duration (wk)	Weight loss	
		LCD (kg)	VLCD (kg)		LCD (kg)	VLCD (kg)
Wadden (40)	20	14.3	19.3[a]	52	9.5	12.9
Wing (41)	20	10.1	18.6[a]	72	6.8	8.6
Wadden (16)	52	14.4	17.3	78	12.2	10.9
Wing (17)	50	10.5	14.2[a]	102	5.7	7.2

[a]Difference in weight loss between LCD and VLCD significant at $p < 0.05$.
Abbreviations: VLCD, very low calorie diets; LCD, low-calorie diets.

A similar finding occurred in the Wing et al. study (41) with a sample of 36 obese patients with type 2 diabetes. At the end of a 20-week behavioral program that included an 8-week period of VLCD, weight losses averaged 18.6 kg and were significantly greater than those obtained when a 1000 to 1500 kcal LCD was used throughout (10.1 kg). At the one-year follow-up, subjects in the BT + VLCD condition had regained 54% of their initial weight loss, compared with only 33% in the BT + LCD group; consequently, the overall weight losses (8.6 for BT + VLCD vs. 6.8 kg for BT + LCD) no longer differed significantly between the two treatment groups.

These studies of VLCDs were indeed successful in improving initial weight loss, as researchers had anticipated; however, increasing initial weight loss did not improve long-term outcome; rather, it simply increased the magnitude of weight regained. To try to maintain these larger initial weight losses better, several investigators have used VLCDs in combination with yearlong behavioral programs. Wadden and colleagues (16) randomly assigned 49 overweight women to a behavioral treatment program that involved 52 weekly meetings and either used a balanced LCD throughout (1200 kcal/day) or included 16 weeks of VLCD. All subjects were then seen biweekly from week 52 to week 72. The BT + VLCD condition achieved their maximum weight loss at six months (21.1 kg) and then gradually regained (17.3 kg at 12 months and 10.9 kg at 18 months). The BT + LCD group lost significantly less weight initially (11.86 kg at 26 weeks), but then continued to lose weight between 26 and 52 weeks (14.4 kg at 52 weeks). Consequently, by week 52, differences between the VLCD and LCD condition were no longer significant. After week 52, subjects in the BT + LCD group regained weight despite continued contact, achieving a final weight loss of 12.2 kg at 18 months. Subjects in the LCD condition regained much less than the VLCD subjects, so that at the end of the study, overall weight loss in the BT + LCD condition exceeded but did not differ significantly from that of the BT + VLCD condition (12.2 kg vs. 10.9 kg).

Wing and colleagues (17) also examined the possibility of using the VLCD in the context of a yearlong behavioral treatment program. These investigators studied 93 patients with type 2 diabetes and randomly assigned them to either a balanced LCD (1000–1200 kcal) throughout the 52 weeks or to a program that included two 12-week periods of VLCD. Subjects in the BT + VLCD condition consumed 400 kcal/day for weeks 1 to 12 and 24 to 36 and then gradually increased their intake after these periods until they were eating 1000 to 1200 kcal/day. After 24 weeks of treatment, subjects in the BT + VLCD condition had lost 16.4 kg, while those in the BT + LCD condition had lost only 12.3 kg. Despite continued weekly contact and the use of a second 12-week interval of the VLCD, both groups regained approximately 2 kg over the next 6 months. At the end of the yearlong program, the BT + VLCD group had lost 14.2 kg versus 10.5 kg in the BT + LCD conditions. This difference approached statistical significance ($p = 0.057$), but is of questionable clinical significance. Treatment was then terminated and subjects were recontacted one year later. At that time, the VLCD group maintained a weight loss of 7.2 kg versus 5.7 kg in the LCD group.

VLCDs pose an interesting dilemma for behavior therapists. These regimens have been successful in accomplishing what they are designed to accomplish namely, increasing the magnitude of initial weight loss. The diets are well tolerated by patients, and most patients find them easier to follow than balanced LCDs. They have also improved glycemic control (42). Moreover, it appears that VLCDs of 800 kcal/day are just as effective for weight loss as those with 400 to 600 kcal and reduce the risks and the need for medical monitoring (43). However, to date it has not been possible to develop approaches that are effective in maintaining the large initial weight losses obtained with VLCDs. Creative approaches to using VLCDs that allow these regimens to be used over longer intervals may be helpful. For example, Williams et al (44) tested the efficacy of using intermittent VLCDs for individuals with type 2 diabetes. These investigators suggested that periodic VLCDs might improve both weight loss and glycemic control in patients with diabetes. One group of participants received a standard 20-week behavioral program with a 1500- to 1800-kcal diet throughout. A second group used a VLCD one day each week and a third group used the VLCD for five consecutive days every five weeks. Weight loss for the standard group averaged 5.4 kg over 20 weeks, compared to 9.6 kg in the 1 day/wk group and 10.4 kg in the 5 day/wk group. The 5 day/wk regimen also increased the percent of participants losing more than 5 kg (93% vs. 50–69%) and the percent who normalized glycemic control [47% vs. 8% in standard behavioral therapy (SBT)]. It remains unclear whether this intermittent regimen also improves long-term weight loss. Further research with novel approaches to using VLCDs is clearly warranted.

Low-Fat Diets

Another approach to improving weight loss in behavioral treatment programs has been to emphasize decreasing dietary fat intake, instead of or in addition to decreasing total calories. This approach is based on studies suggesting that subjects who are allowed to consume as much low fat, high carbohydrate food as they desire will decrease their calorie intake and lose weight (45,46).

Several behavioral studies have addressed the effects of restricting fat intake (Table 5). Jeffery and colleagues (47) compared the effectiveness of the usual behavioral approach of restricting calorie intake, with a program based on restricting only the intake of dietary fat. Moderately overweight women ($N = 122$) were recruited; half of the women were given a fat goal (20 g of fat per day), but no calorie goal; the other half were given a calorie goal (1000–1200 kcal/day), but no dietary fat goal. Both groups were seen weekly for 6 weeks, biweekly for 20 weeks and then monthly through 18 months. Weight losses at the end of six months were comparable in two conditions: 4.6 kg for fat restriction and 3.7 kg for calorie

restriction. Likewise no differences between conditions were seen at 12 or 18 months. By 18 months, both treatment groups had returned to their baseline levels. The weight losses of the calorie restriction condition are modest compared to most behavioral weight control studies, a finding that is not readily explained but may have been due to the fact that only six weekly meetings were held before turning to biweekly sessions.

Another group of investigators compared a low-fat, unrestricted-carbohydrate diet to the combination of calorie plus fat restriction. Schlundt et al. (48), randomly assigned 60 overweight subjects to a low-fat dietary intervention (20 g of fat) with either ad libitum carbohydrate intake or with calories restricted to 1200 kcal/day for women and 1500 for men. Forty-nine of the 60 subjects completed the 20-week treatment program. At the end of the 20 weeks, subjects in the low-fat, ad libitum carbohydrate condition had lost less weight than those who had both calorie and fat restriction (4.6 kg vs. 8.8 kg). Follow-up occurred after 9 to 12 months but included only 58% of the initial cohort. In these participants, follow-up weight losses averaged 2.6 kg for the ad libitum carbohydrate diet and 5.5 kg for the calorie-restricted subjects.

A calorie plus fat restriction condition similar to that used by Schlundt et al. (48) was also used by Pascale and colleagues (49), but compared in this study to the standard behavior approach of calorie restriction. Ninety subjects, half with type 2 diabetes and half with a family history of diabetes, were studied. Subjects in the calorie restriction condition were instructed to consume 1000 to 1500 kcal/day, depending on initial body weight, and monitor the calories in each food they consumed. Those in the calorie plus fat restriction group were given a similar calorie goal, but in addition were also given a fat gram goal corresponding to a fat intake of ≤20% of calories. These individuals recorded the calories and the grams of fat in each food they consumed. In the participants with type 2 diabetes, significant differences were seen between the two diet interventions, with greater weight loss in the

Table 5 Weight Loss in Long-Term Studies of Behavioral Interventions with Low-Fat Vs. Low-Calorie Diets

| | | Short-term results | | | | Long-term results | | |
| | | Weight loss | | | | Weight loss | | |
Trial (reference)	Duration (wk)	Low cal (kg)	Low fat (kg)	Low cal/ Low fat (kg)	Duration (wk)	Low cal (kg)	Low fat (kg)	Low cal/Low fat (kg)
Jeffery (47)	24	3.7	4.6	—	78	+1.8	+0.4	—
Schlundt (48)	20	—	4.6	8.8[a]	36–52	—	2.6	5.5[a]
Pascale (49)								
Type 2 diabetes	16	4.6	—	7.7[a]	52	1.0	—	5.2[a]
FH+	16	6.9	—	7.5	52	3.2	—	3.1
Viegener (50)	24	8.9	10.2	—	52	9.0	9.0	—

[a]Differences in weight loss between LCD and VLCD significant at p < 0.05.

calorie plus fat restriction condition both at the end of the 16 week treatment program (7.7 kg vs. 4.6 kg) and at the one-year follow-up (5.2 kg vs. 1.0 kg). There were no significant differences between the diet groups in the cohort of individuals at risk for diabetes. Weight losses in the calorie restriction alone condition in the diabetic patients were poorer than would be expected based on other similar studies.

The best overall results in a dietary comparison study were reported by Viegener et al. (50). Eighty-five obese women were randomly assigned to either follow a 1200 kcal/day diet throughout or to alternate between an 800 kcal/day low-fat diet used 4 days/wk and the 1200 kcal regimen. In this alternating condition, subjects were taught to restrict their fat intake to <25% of total calories on the 1200 kcal days and to <15% on the 800 kcal days. The goal of achieving "fat-free" days was also introduced during this program and subjects were gradually encouraged to develop 4 fat-free days/wk. The dropout rate from this study was quite high (26%), but in the subjects who completed the six-month behavioral program, there was a tendency toward greater weight losses in the alternating low-fat diet condition at months one to four of the program. At the end of the six-month treatment, weight losses were comparable (8.9 kg in standard low calorie and 10.2 kg in alternating low fat). Subjects were then offered a chance to participate in a maintenance program with meetings held every two weeks for six months. Weight losses at the end of this six-month maintenance program remained excellent in both groups (9.0 kg in both standard and alternating low fat).

Thus, taken as a whole, these studies suggest some potential benefit to a low-calorie, low-fat regimen versus the traditional calorie-focused approach. However, the differences are not very substantial. Moreover, the fact that several of the studies had a significant dropout rate makes conclusions from these studies more difficult.

Additional evidence suggesting the importance of reducing dietary fat in behavioral weight control studies comes from a correlational analysis by Harris and colleagues (51) of predictors of weight loss over an 18-month program in 82 men and 75 women. Changes in body mass index (BMI) were more strongly associated with changes in dietary fat intake than with changes in total calories. Moreover, decreases in consumption of certain specific foods—beef, hot dogs, and sweets—were associated with weight losses, as were increases in consumption of vegetables and increases in physical activity.

Providing More Structure Regarding Dietary Intake

As noted in the overview of the behavioral approach to obesity, teaching patients to rearrange their home environment is a key behavioral treatment strategy. Typically participants in behavioral weight control programs are encouraged to remove the high-calorie, high-fat foods from their home and to replace these items with healthier alternatives. Jeffery and colleagues (52) argued that better weight losses might be obtained if therapists intervened more directly on the home environment, by actually providing patients with the food they should eat in appropriate portion sizes. To test this hypothesis, these investigators recruited 202 overweight patients (half at the University of Minnesota and half at the University of Pittsburgh) and randomly assigned these participants to one of five groups. Group 1 was a no-treatment control group that received no weight control intervention and was simply followed over time. Group 2 received a standard behavioral treatment program (SBT) with weekly meetings for 20 weeks and then monthly meetings and weekly weigh-ins through an 18-month treatment program. These participants were given a daily calorie goal of 1000 or 1500 kcal (depending on their initial weight) and encouraged to restrict their intake of dietary fat. In group 3, the standard behavioral program was supplemented by actual food provision. The calorie goals remained at 1000 to 1500 kcal/day, but subjects in group 3 were given a box of food each week that contained exactly what should be eaten for five breakfasts and five dinners each week. Patients selected their own lunches and all three meals on the other two days each week. Group 4 was designed to test their hypothesis that more direct reinforcement for weight loss might improve treatment outcome. The subjects in this group received the SBT, and in addition, could earn up to $25 each week for losing weight and maintaining their weight loss. Group 5 included SBT, food provision, and payment for weight loss.

The main finding in this study (Fig. 3) was that food provision significantly increased weight loss. Weight losses with SBT averaged 7.7, 4.5, and 4.1 kg at 6, 12, and 18 months, compared to 10.1, 9.1, and 6.4 with addition of food. Provision of incentives had no effect on weight loss.

After the 18-month program, all intervention was terminated and subjects were recontacted at 30 months to assess weight maintenance (53). Unfortunately subjects in all four of the active treatment groups maintained weight losses of only 1.4 to 2.2 kg. These weight losses at 30 months were better than in the no-treatment control group, but did not differ among the four active treatment groups.

Since the use of food provision improved weight losses during the initial treatment program, actually doubling the results at month 12, a subsequent study was designed to determine which component of food provision was responsible for its success (54). Food provision includes actual food, which was provided free to subjects and a meal plan specifying which foods should be eaten at which times. To determine which of these components is necessary, a cohort

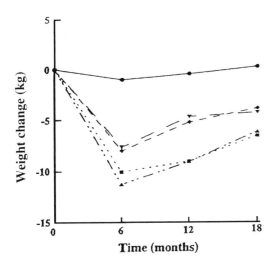

Figure 3 Weight change at 6, 12, and 18 months by treatment group. ●, Control; ▼, SBT; ◆, SBT + incentives; ■, SBT + food; ▲, SBT + food + incentives. SBT, standard behavioral treatment. (From Ref. 19.)

of 163 overweight women was recruited, and the women were randomly assigned to SBT-only, SBT plus meal plans and grocery lists, SBT plus meal plans plus food provided on a cost-sharing basis, or SBT plus meal plans plus food provided free. Results at the end of the six-month study showed that subjects in the SBT-only condition had lost 8.0 kg. Weight losses in the other three conditions, which were given meal plans or meal plans plus food, were all significantly better than those achieved by the SBT condition, and did not differ from each other (12.0, 11.7, and 11.4 kg, for groups 2–4, respectively). From these results, it appears that the most important component of food provision is the provision of structured meal plans and grocery lists; no further benefit was seen by actually giving food to the patients.

The meal plan and grocery lists appear to improve weight loss by changing the foods available in the home and creating a more regular meal pattern. Interestingly, the meal plans and grocery lists exerted as much of an effect on these variables as actual food provision. Subjects in the treatment groups that were given either meal plans or actual food reported an increase in the number of days per week that they ate breakfast, an increase in the number of days that they ate lunch, and a decrease in the frequency of snacks. Likewise, when asked to survey their homes and to indicate what foods were currently stored in their home, subjects given meal plans and those who were given the food reported greater increases than subjects in the SBT-only condition in the number of fruits and vegetables, low-fat meats, medium-fat meats, breads and cereals, and low-calorie frozen entrees. Subjects in these conditions also reported less difficulty having appropriate foods available, estimating portion sizes, finding time to

plan meals, and controlling eating when not hungry. On all these measures, the patients who were given the meal plans and grocery lists reported changes that were comparable to those in subjects who were actually given the food.

Several other studies have achieved excellent weight losses using portion-controlled diets in which some or all of the participants' food is provided to them. These diets often involve a combination of liquid formula and regular food and are designed for calorie levels of approximately 1000 kcal/day. Wadden and colleagues (55) used a 900- to 925-kcal/day diet that included four servings of liquid formula diet (at 150 kcal per serving) and a prepackaged entrée plus salad for dinner. After 18 weeks on this regimen, conventional foods were gradually reintroduced and calories increased to 1500 kcal/day. Average weight loss was 16.5 kg at 24 weeks. Participants continued to attend treatment meeting for a full year, and at week 48 had maintained a weight loss of 15.1 kg.

A portion-controlled diet using Slim-Fast has also been shown to improve short- and long-term weight losses (56). Participants ($N = 100$) were asked to consume a 1200- to 1500-kcal/day diet, but were randomly assigned to use either a self-selected diet of conventional foods or a daily regimen of two Slim-Fast meal replacements and two Slim-Fast snack bars plus a healthy dinner. At the end of three months, the conventional diet group had lost 1.3 kg versus 7.1 kg in the Slim-Fast group. Subsequently, both groups of participants were instructed to consume one Slim-Fast meal and one Slim-Fast snack bar each day for the next 24 months. At month 27, mean weight losses were 7.7 kg for the conventional food group and 10.4 kg for the Slim-Fast group. Four-year follow-up data (57) were available for 75% of the original 100 participants (Fig. 4). Those in the Slim-Fast group maintained a weight loss of 9.5 kg at four years, whereas the conventional group's weight loss was 4.1 kg. The excellent results from these portion-controlled diets suggest that it is the structure rather than the calorie levels of VLCDs that makes these regimens effective. By using diets of 1000 to 1500 kcal/day rather than 400- to 800-kcal VCLDs and having patients continue to consume regular food in addition to liquid formula, it appears possible to achieve large weight losses without the subsequent marked weight regain.

The Look AHEAD study described above (20) used structured diets and meal-replacement products as part of the lifestyle intervention. This highly structured approach to the dietary intervention may have helped achieve the excellent weight losses reported in this trial.

Strengthening the Exercise Component

As noted above, exercise is a key component of behavioral weight loss program and has been strongly associated with

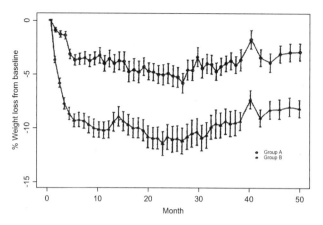

Figure 4 Mean (± SEM) percentage change from initial body weight in patients during 51 months of treatment with an energy-restricted diet (1200–1500 kcal/d). Data were analyzed on an available case basis. Patients received either a conventional energy-restricted diet (control group A, O) or a diet with two meals and snack replacements (group B, △) for 3 months. During the remaining 4 years, all patients received one meal and snack replacement daily. (From Ref. 60.)

the long-term maintenance of weight loss. Prior to 1990, there were a number of behavioral treatment studies showing that the combination of diet plus exercise was more effective for long-term weight control than diet or exercise alone (28,29,58). Foreyt and colleagues (59) replicated this finding in a study of 165 mildly overweight adults who were randomly assigned to an exercise only, diet only, diet plus exercise or waiting list control group. Each group attended 12 weekly meetings, followed by three biweekly meetings and eight monthly meetings. The goal for the exercise groups was to complete three to five aerobic exercise sessions per week with each session lasting 45 minutes. The diet program focused on reducing fat to <30% of calories and utilized the Help Your Heart Eating Plan. At the end of 12 weeks, the two diet groups had lost significantly more weight (7.1 kg for diet only and 6.9 kg for diet plus exercise) than the exercise alone condition (0.32 kg) or the waiting list control (0.98 kg). Approximately 75% of participants completed the one-

year study. At that time, the diet plus exercise group maintained a weight loss of 8.1 kg, which was significantly greater than the exercise alone condition (2.7 kg), but not different from diet alone (6.3 kg).

Leermakers et al. (60) examined the effect of focusing on exercise during the maintenance phase. All participants (N = 67) received the same initial six-month weight loss program and were then randomly assigned to an exercise-focused maintenance program or a weight-focused maintenance program. Both maintenance programs involved six months of biweekly treatment contact. The exercise-focused program included supervised walking sessions, contingencies for exercise, and relapse prevention strategies focused on maintaining physical activity. The weight-focused program involved general problem solving of weight-related problems. At month 12, the weight-focused group maintained a weight loss of 7.9 kg versus 5.2 kg (p < 0.05) in the exercise-focused intervention. Perhaps with the extensive focus on exercise, participants neglected to maintain their dietary change.

Rather than simply addressing the issue of whether exercise is important to include in the behavioral treatment or maintenance component of obesity programs, investigators have begun to ask what type of exercise is best to prescribe (i.e., what type of exercise will produce the greatest adherence and best long-term weight loss?) and how best to prescribe exercise to promote adherence.

Home-Based Vs. Supervised Exercise

Physical activity researchers have shown that it is possible to increase fitness using either supervised exercise or home-based physical activity (61). In weight loss programs, however, home-based programs appear to produce better maintenance of weight loss (Table 6). Andersen and colleagues (62) randomly assigned overweight participants to weight loss programs that involved either three supervised sessions of aerobic dance each week for 16 weeks or home-based activity (goal of 30 minutes of moderate to vigorous activity most days in the week). Weight losses in the two groups were similar at week 16 (8.3 kg for aerobics and 7.9 kg for lifestyle), but the aerobic dance group regained 1.6 kg from week 16 to

Table 6 Effects of Supervised Vs. Home-Based Exercise Programs for Long-Term Weight Loss

| | | Short-term results | | | Long-term results | |
| | | Weight loss | | | Weight loss | |
Trial (reference)	Duration (wk)	Supervised (kg)	Home based (kg)	Duration (wk)	Supervised (kg)	Home based (kg)
Andersen (62)	16	8.3	7.9	68	6.7	7.8[a]
Perri (63)	26	9.3	10.4	64	7.0	11.6[a]

[a]p < 0.5 for difference in weight regain.

1-year follow-up whereas the lifestyle group regained only 0.08 kg ($p = 0.06$). Perri and colleagues (63) also found evidence of similar initial weight losses in home-based and supervised programs, but better maintenance of weight loss in the home-based program. Forty-nine obese women participated in a yearlong behavioral weight loss program. All participants were instructed to complete a moderate-intensity walking program (30 min/day on 5 days/wk) but half completed this activity on their own, at home, whereas the other half attended three supervised group-exercise sessions per week for 26 weeks and then two supervised group-exercise sessions per week. Weight losses at six months were 10.4 kg for home based and 9.3 kg for group based. At month 15, the home-based program had an average weight loss of 11.6 kg versus 7.0 kg in the supervised program. Thus, home-based exercise appears most effective for long-term weight loss maintenance.

Short Bouts Vs. Long Bouts

Home-based and supervised exercise prescriptions differ in many ways, including the location used for exercise (and the convenience of access to this location), whether the activity is done alone or with others, and the flexibility regarding when the exercise is performed. Since lack of time is the most commonly reported barrier to physical activity, another important difference may be in the duration of each episode of activity. In supervised exercise programs, participants typically complete an hour of exercise three times per week. In home-based programs, the emphasis is on accumulating activity, with a goal of being active for 30 minutes each day. Jakicic et al. (64,65) have conducted two weight loss studies examining the effect of prescribing exercise in long bouts (40-minute sessions) versus several shorter bouts (four 10-minute sessions). In the first study (65), the use of short bouts led to better exercise adherence and somewhat greater weight losses at six months. The second study, which involved a larger number of participants ($N = 148$) and continued for 18 months, suggested that both long and short bouts can be equally effective for exercise adherence, weight loss, and long-term changes in fitness (64). At 18 months, weight losses averaged 5.8 kg for the long-bout group and 3.7 kg for the short-bout group, a nonsignificant difference. Thus, short bouts of exercise may be helpful as participants are beginning to increase their physical activity and represent a useful option for long-term participation in activity.

Providing Home Exercise Equipment

Another way to maximize adherence to physical activity may be to provide participants with home exercise equipment. Jakicic and colleagues observed a significant correlation between the number of pieces of exercise

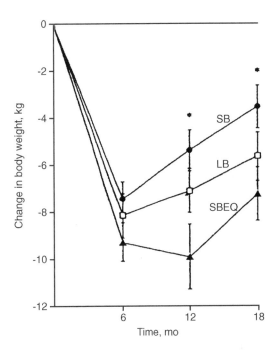

Figure 5 Changes in weight loss among treatment groups across 18 months of treatment (mean [SEM]). Asterisk indicates that data for the short-bout exercise (SB) group and multiple short-bout exercises plus home exercise equipment (SBEQ) group were significantly different ($P < .05$) at the same time period. LB indicates long-bout exercise. Error bars indicate standard error of the mean. (From Ref. 23.)

equipment in one's home and activity level (66). Although the direction of causation cannot be determined from these correlational data, it is possible that providing home equipment to participants would increase physical activity since the equipment may serve as a cue for activity and reduce some of the barriers to exercise. The benefit of providing home exercise equipment was examined in the study of long and short bouts of exercise described above (64). Participants were randomly assigned to long exercise bouts (40-minute bouts 5 days/wk), short bouts (four 10-minute bouts 5 days/wk) or short bouts with provision of a home treadmill. The group given the treadmill had higher physical activity levels from 13 to 18 months and better maintenance of weight loss over the 18-month study (Fig. 5). At month 18, the group given the treadmill had an average weight loss of 7.4 kg compared to 3.7 kg in the short-bout group without treadmills.

Personal Trainers and Financial Incentives

As described above, the behavioral approach suggests that by changing antecedents and consequence, it is possible to change behavior. Jeffery and colleagues (67) applied this model to increasing physical activity in participants in a weight loss program. They recruited 193 participants and randomly assigned them to one of five conditions. Group 1 received a standard behavioral program, with home-based exercise and a goal of expending 1000 kcal/wk in physical activity. Group 2 received the same behavioral program and same exercise goal, but these participants were asked to attend 3 supervised exercise sessions (walking at a track) each week for 18 months. Group 3 had the same interventions as group 2, except that they were provided a personal trainer or coach who called them regularly to encourage them to exercise and met them at the exercise facility and walked with them. This strategy was designed to increase the cues for exercise. Group 4 had the same intervention as group 2, but they could earn small financial incentives for attending the supervised exercise sessions ($1–$3 per session), thus increasing the positive consequence of exercising. Group 5 had the combination of the personal trainers or coaches and incentives.

The personal coaches and the incentives both significantly increased the number of supervised activity sessions attended by participants (Table 7). Group 2 attended 35 scheduled exercise sessions on average; the use of coaches increased this to an average of 80 walks, and the use of incentives increased this to 66 walks (thus each approach approximately doubled attendance at exercise sessions). When both approaches were combined (group 5), there was an additive effect and participants attended an average of 103 sessions. However, increased attendance at exercise sessions did not result in increased overall physical activity (all groups exceeded the 1000 kcal/wk goal) nor improved weight loss. Group 1 which had home-based exercise, actually maintained the largest weight loss (7.6 kg), confirming findings from the Perri (63) and Andersen (62) studies described above.

Table 7 Effects of Supervised Walks, Exercise Coaches, and Financial Incentives on Attendance, Activity Level, and Weight Loss

Group	Number of walks attended[a]	Self-reported activity at 18 mo (kcal/wk)	Weight loss at 18 mo (kg)
SBT	—	1119	7.6[b]
SBT + supervised walks	35	1063	3.8
SBT + walks + coach	80[b]	1294	2.9
SBT + walks + $	66[b]	1426	4.5
SBT + walks + coach + $	103[b]	1272	5.1

[a]Out of 222 total possible
[b]Difference between conditions is significant at $p < 0.05$.
Abbreviation: SBT, standard behavioral therapy.
Source: Adapted from Ref. 67.

Average weight losses at 18 months were 3.8, 2.9, 4.5, and 5.1 kg for groups 2 to 5, respectively. Hence, the cues and incentives increased the targeted behavior (attendance at exercise sessions), but this behavior did not increase overall physical activity (participants appeared to substitute the supervised activity for other approaches to activity) or long-term weight losses.

Resistance Vs. Aerobic Exercise

Typically behavioral weight loss programs stress aerobic exercise, such as walking or bicycling. Since resistance exercises may increase lean muscle mass, such changes may offset the decrease in metabolic rate that occurs with weight reduction. However, studies comparing aerobic and resistance exercise have typically reported no differences in long-term weight loss (68). For example, Wadden and colleagues (55) randomly assigned 128 obese women to diet alone, diet plus aerobic training, diet plus strength training or diet plus the combination of aerobic plus strength training. All participants received the same 48-week behavioral program and were prescribed the same portion-controlled diet (discussed above). Those in the exercise conditions attended supervised sessions three times per week for the first 28 weeks of the program and then two times per week through week 48. There were no significant differences in weight loss for the four conditions at week 24 or week 48 (14.4, 13.7, 17.2, and 15.2 kg for the four conditions at week 48, respectively). Participants in all four conditions regained 35% to 55% of their weight loss over the subsequent year of follow-up; at week 100, there was again no significant difference among conditions (overall weight loss of 13.7–17.2 kg). The excellent weight loss in all four conditions supports the use of the portion-controlled diet, but there is no evidence from this study of any differences due to the type of exercise prescribed.

Increasing Physical Activity Vs. Decreasing Sedentary Behavior

Epstein and colleagues reported the results of a treatment program for overweight children that focused on increasing physical activity versus a program that focused on decreasing sedentary activities or the combination (31). In the decreased sedentary activity condition, the amount of time that the children could spend watching television or playing computer games was gradually reduced. At the one-year follow-up, the group that was taught to decrease sedentary activities had greater decreases in percent overweight than the group that was taught to increase aerobic exercise or the combination group. All groups increased in fitness, suggesting that the decreased sedentary activity group had used their extra time for more physical activities. In addition, children in the decreased sedentary activity group increased their liking of high-intensity physical activities more than the exercise conditions. These results suggest an interesting new approach that could be used to change activity level in overweight adults.

Increasing the Amount of Physical Activity That Is Prescribed

Behavioral weight loss programs traditionally prescribe gradual increases in activity to a goal of 1000 kcal/wk. The rationale for selecting this goal is unclear, and several studies suggest that higher levels of activity may be associated with better weight loss maintenance. For example, in the National Weight Control Registry (69), successful weight loss maintainers are asked to complete the Paffenbarger Activity Questionnaire, indicating their current level of activity. Table 8 shows on average these individuals report expending 2800 kcal/wk. Similar levels of physical activity were reported by the highest quartile of exercisers in the Jeffery et al. study (67), described above, who also had the best long-term weight loss. Jakicic et al. (64) found that participants who reported at least 200 minutes of activity per week had better weight losses at 18 months than those reporting 150 minutes or less. Unpublished data from these participants who exercised 200 minutes or more showed exercise levels of approximately 2500 kcal/wk.

On the basis of these data, Jeffery et al. (70) conducted a randomized controlled trial comparing SBT programs which incorporated either the usual exercise goal of 1000 kcal/wk or a higher exercise goal of 2500 kcal/wk. To help participants in the high-exercise group achieve these levels, these participants were encouraged to recruit one to three exercise partners into the study and were given personal exercise coaching and small monetary incentives.

Table 8 Exercise Habits (kcal/wk) Reported by Successful Weight Loss Maintainers

	Energy expenditure (kcal/wk) of successful weight maintainers in NWCR[a]	Subjects in top quartile of energy expenditure in TRIM study[b]
Walking	1093	1125
Stair climbing	188	259
Sports		
Light	211	167
Medium	526	390
Heavy	798	608
Total	2829	2559

[a]From Ref. 69.
[b]From Ref. 67.
Abbreviation: NWCR, National Weight Control Registry.

The high physical activity group was able to achieve higher levels of activity than the standard group at 6, 12, and 18 months (e.g., 2317 kcal/wk vs. 1629 kcal/wk for high vs. standard exercise group at 18 months), and greater weight losses at 12 and 18 months. Weight losses in the high-exercise condition averaged 9.0, 8.5, and 6.7 kg at 6, 12, and 18 months, which were significantly greater than those of the standard group at the latter two time points (8.1, 6.1 and 4.1 kg at 6, 12, and 18 months).

At the 30-month follow-up, however, the high physical activity group did not differ in activity levels from the standard group (1696 kcal vs. 1390 kcal), and both groups had regained most of their weight (mean weight loss 0–30 months of 0.9 kg in SBT and 2.86 kg in high physical activity) (71). However, participants who maintained an activity level of >2500 kcal/wk at month 30 maintained a weight loss of 12 kg versus 0.8 kg for all other participants. Thus, these studies suggest the benefit of high exercise for weight loss and maintenance, but highlight the difficulty of producing sustained energy expenditures of this magnitude.

Strengthening the Behavioral Component

The studies by Jeffery (52), Wing (54), and Jakicic (64) described above are designed to strengthen the behavioral component of weight loss programs by more directly modifying the home environment. Other approaches to improving behavioral programs have included lengthening the program, increasing social support and motivation for weight loss, and increasing the target audience. Each of these approaches will be discussed below.

Lengthening Treatment

Over the period of 1970–1990, behavioral weight loss programs gradually succeeded in producing larger initial weight losses. Part of this improvement appeared to be due to lengthening of the treatment program. Whereas in 1974, the average treatment lasted eight weeks and weight loss averaged 3.8 kg (0.5-kg weight loss per week), by 1990, the program had been increased to 21 weeks, and the weight loss had increased to 8.5 kg (0.4-kg weight loss per week).

To investigate more systematically the effect of treatment length on outcome, Perri and colleagues compared a standard 20-week program to a 40-week program (72). The material presented was identical in the two conditions, but the 40-week program covered the lessons more gradually. At week 20, weight losses were comparable (8.9 kg in the standard 20-week program and 10.1 kg in the extended program). However, when treatment was terminated, subjects in the 20-week program began to regain weight, whereas those in extended treatment (who continued to participate in weekly therapy) increased their weight loss, thus producing significant differences between conditions at week 40 (6.4 kg in standard program vs. 13.6 kg in extended). Between weeks 40 and 72, both groups regained weight, but at week 72, the extended condition maintained a significantly greater weight loss (9.8 kg vs. 4.6 kg).

While these data clearly show that lengthening treatment improves weight loss, it has been suggested that such continued contact merely delays the point at which weight regain occurs. The standard condition regained 28% of their initial weight loss in the 20-weeks following cessation of therapy; the extended condition regained the identical percent of their weight loss in the 32 weeks following the end of their treatment. Although it would thus appear that extended treatment is not helping participants learn the behavioral skills to a greater extent, the fact that relapse can be delayed is an important step forward—especially if by continuing to lengthen programs, relapse can be pushed further and further back in time.

On the basis of these findings, several treatment studies have evaluated yearlong behavioral programs (16,17,73). Subjects in the Wadden et al. study (16), continued to lose weight over time, with weight losses averaging 11.9 kg at 26 weeks and 14.4 kg at 1 year. Wing et al. (17) found that the weight losses were best at six months (12.3 kg), and then subjects regained weight, maintaining a weight loss of 10.5 kg at one year. The changes between weeks 24 and 48 varied by treatment condition in the Andersen et al. study (73). From these results, it would appear that lengthening treatments to one year might be warranted. However, as noted by several of these investigators, attendance declines tremendously over time, and the cost-benefit ratio of extending treatment from 24 to 52 weeks is questionable.

Continuing regular contact with patients after the initial treatment program has also been shown to be beneficial for long-term maintenance of weight loss. Perri and colleagues (74) treated 123 women in a standard 20-week behavioral weight loss program, followed by different types of maintenance interventions over the subsequent year. One group of women received no further treatment contact over the year of follow-up; the others received 26 biweekly treatment contacts focusing on problem solving, problem solving plus aerobic exercise, problem solving plus social support or problem solving plus aerobic exercise and social support. All four of the groups that received continued contact maintained their weight losses better than the no-contact condition, with no significant differences between the four conditions. Other studies have shown benefit from phone contact during the maintenance period (75,76). Thus, providing some form of ongoing contact with participants appears to improve long-term outcome.

Increasing Social Support and Motivation for Weight Loss

Another approach to providing ongoing support for the participant is to involve significant others in the treatment program. For example, spouses have been involved in a variety of behavioral weight loss programs; a meta-analysis of this literature found a small positive effect on weight loss through two to three months of follow-up but not thereafter (77). Wing and Jeffery (78) examined the effect of natural and experimentally created social support. Participants enrolled in the weight loss program either alone or with three friends or family members (thus this aspect of the study was not randomized). These individuals or small groups were then randomly assigned to a standard behavioral program or to a program with enhanced social-support strategies (intragroup cooperation and intergroup competition activities). Participants recruited with friends had better weight losses at the end of the 4-month treatment and at the 10-month follow-up than participants recruited alone. Both recruitment strategy and the social support intervention affected maintenance of weight loss from month 4 to 10. Among participants recruited alone and given the standard behavioral treatment (representing the typical approach to recruitment and intervention), only 24% maintained their weight loss in full from month 4 to 10. In contrast, 66% of those recruited with friends and given the social support intervention maintained their weight loss in full.

Attention should also be given to a report evaluating the Trevose behavioral modification program (79). This program is lay-led and charges no fees. Standard behavioral strategies are presented at each weekly group meeting. There are two unique aspects of this program: First, it is indefinite in length; and second, attendance and achieving weight loss goals are strictly enforced for continued participation. At entry, participants set a weight loss goal that must be within the normal weight range and represent a weight loss of 20 to 100 lb. During the first five weeks (an initial trial period), attendance is required, and participants must achieve a weight loss of 15% of their weight loss goal. Subsequently, absences may be excused but failure to attend or meet the cumulative weight loss goals (22% of the total goal at two months, 30% at three months, and so forth until 90% of the goal is achieved) results in dismissal from the program. Attendance requirements are gradually decreased after achieving the weight loss goal.

Latner et al. (79) described the outcome of all applicants to the Trevose program from 1992 to 93. Of the 329 who applied, 286 were invited to join, 202 entered week 1 of the program, and 171 (52%) completed the five-week trial. Thereafter, 105 of these 171 entrants completed year 1, 54 completed year 3, and 37 completed year 5. The 37 who completed year 5 maintained a weight loss of

15.7 kg at five years. While this represents only 11% of the original applicant pool, it is still unusual to obtain a 15.7-kg weight loss at five years for even 10% of the patient population. Moreover, five-year weight loss data were collected by self-report from 77 of the 171 participants who completed the five-week trial period but were no longer in the program. Their average weight loss was 11.44 kg. Thus, the approach used in this program clearly deserves further empirical investigation. By requiring attendance and success at achieving realistic weight loss goals, this approach may help identify those participants who are most motivated to succeed.

Increasing the Audience Through Internet and Media-Based Treatments

In an effort to increase the audience served by behavioral weight loss programs, investigators have studied various media-based interventions. Although most of these programs have not achieved weight losses comparable to face-to-face programs, they may prove useful in reducing the cost of delivering treatments, expanding the number of individuals who are willing to participate, and providing a way to maintain long-term contact with participants.

Telephone calls have been used primarily as a way to maintain contact with participants during the maintenance phase of treatment. Wing and colleagues (80) suggested that an important effect of such calls was to prompt participants to continue to self-monitor their diet, exercise, and body weight. Consequently, after successful completion of a six-month weight loss program (weight loss of > 4 kg), participants were randomly assigned to either a no-contact control group or to receive weekly calls from a research assistant who collected data from the participant's self-monitoring record. Call completion and self-reported adherence to self-monitoring were significantly related to weight regain over the yearlong intervention, but average weight regain in the phone maintenance condition did not differ significantly from the control condition (3.9 kg. vs. 5.6 kg.). Similarly use of telephone calls as the primary mode of intervention (after two initial group meetings) did not increase weight loss relative to a no-contact condition (81).

Several studies here suggested that television might be a useful way to provide weight loss programming. In one study, an eight-week cable TV weight loss program produced weight losses equivalent to a face-to-face program (82). Harvey-Berino (83) used an interactive television technology, where participants can see and hear the therapists and the other participants. Weight losses were again comparable for those assigned to receive the 12-week program via interactive TV (−7.6 kg.) and those who participated in a face-to-face program (−7.9 kg.).

Computer technology has also been applied to weight loss, with most studies investigating the effects of hand-held computers for self-monitoring and reinforcement (84,85). More recently, Tate and colleagues (86) used the Internet and e-mail to deliver a more complete behavioral-therapy program. Ninety-one participants were randomly assigned to a six-month weight loss program of either Internet education or Internet behavior therapy. The Internet education condition was given access to a Web site that provided an organized directory of Internet weight loss resources related to self-monitoring, diet and nutrition, and physical activity. The Internet behavior-therapy program included, in addition, 24 weekly behavioral lessons sent via e-mail, weekly online submission of self-monitoring diaries, individualized therapist feedback via e-mail, and an online bulletin board. The Internet behavior-therapy group lost significantly more weight than the education group over the six-month program (4.1 kg vs. 1.6 kg), and more participants achieved the 5% weight loss goal (45% vs. 22%). Log-in frequency was significantly correlated with weight loss.

In the next of her programmatic studies using the Internet, Tate specifically addressed the impact of e-mail feedback (86). A total of 92 overweight individuals who were at increased risk of developing type 2 diabetes were randomly assigned to a basic Internet program or to an Internet program with weekly behavioral e-mail counseling. The latter group had significantly greater weight loss (5.3 kg vs. 2.3 kg, among completers, $p = 0.03$), showing the importance of the e-mail counseling.

The concern raised by these findings is that if a human is needed to provide individualized feedback to each participant, then Internet approach will remain expensive to implement. Therefore Tate and colleagues sought to determine whether the human counselor could be replaced by providing computer-automated tailored counseling (87). A total of 192 overweight adults participated in a six month Internet behavioral weight loss program that included the following arms: (*i*) no counseling, (*ii*) computer-automated counseling, or (*iii*) human counseling. All participants used Slim-Fast as part of their diet regimen. The feedback for the computer-generated group was based on weekly information submitted by the participant and compared the participant's self-reported intake, exercise, and weight loss to prespecified goals and then provided either positive reinforcement or suggestions for reducing barriers and achieving these goals. At three months, weight losses of completers in the computer-automated counseling were comparable to those in the human counseling group, and both were significantly greater than no counseling (5.3, 6.1, and 2.8 kg, respectively). At six months, weight losses were greater in the human counseling group (7.3 kg) than in either computer generated (4.9 kg) or no counseling (2.6 kg). This study suggests that there is tremendous potential in the use of computer-generated feedback. For three months, a first-generation computer-automated counseling system was as effective as a human counselor! Further research to extend this approach is clearly warranted.

Several other studies also attest to the efficacy of Internet-based weight loss programs. In a study of over 2800 overweight or obese members of Kaiser-Permanente (88), those randomly assigned to a Web site that provided just information about weight control lost 1.2% of their body weight over six months, compared to a 3% weight loss in members who had access to a Web site that provided a full six-week self-help program, including a tailored action plan.

Harvey-Berino and colleagues have been studying an Internet program (VTrim) that simulates all of the components of a face-to-face behavioral weight control intervention. During the first six months, participants attend weekly online chats and submit their self-reported weights, homework assignments, and diaries each week. This information is reviewed by a therapist and e-mail feedback is provided. During months 6 to 12, chats and e-mail contact are reduced to every other week. With this intensive Internet intervention, weight losses are similar to those achieved with a face-to-face program. Participants randomly assigned to VTrim lost 7.8 kg at 12 months, whereas those who were assigned to a commercial and online weight loss program (eDiets.com) lost only 3.4 kg (89). Supplementing this intensive Internet behavior program with occasional face-to-face meetings did not further increase weight loss (90). These studies show the tremendous potential of Internet approaches for increasing the audience that can be served by behavioral weight control programs.

Improving the Maintenance of Weight Loss

At this point in time, we are relatively effective in producing initial weight losses. As noted above, on average, participants in behavioral programs lose about 7% to 10% of their body weight and achieve significant health improvements. However, despite our best efforts, these weight losses are gradually regained. Consequently, there is increasing attention to approaches to improving maintenance of weight loss. Such approaches are described in detail in chapter 15.

In an effort to understand the behaviors of those who have achieved long-term maintenance of weight loss, Wing and Hill established the National Weight Control Registry (NWCR). To be eligible for the registry, individuals must have lost at least 30 lb (13.6 kg) and kept it off at least one year. The 5000-plus members of the registry far exceed these minimum criteria—having lost an average of 73 lb (33.2 kg) and kept it off 5.7 years. When asked to report their current behaviors, these registry members are quite consistent in reporting that they continue to consume a low-calorie, low-fat diet, and do high levels of physical activity. On average, they report consuming 1400 kcal/day with 24% to 29% from fat and expending about 2800 kcal/wk in physical activity (91).

Several other behaviors have been reported consistently by registry members. They report consuming breakfast on 6.3 of the 7 days in the week, with 78% reporting eating breakfast daily (92). This meal may help prevent hunger later in the day or may just be a marker of a low-calorie, low-fat eating style. Registry members also report consuming a diet with little variety (93). Since dietary variety has been associated with increased intake, the consumption of a limited diet may help these individuals restrict their intake. Although these individuals continue to eat out in restaurants, they eat in fast-food establishments less than once per week. Whereas Americans on average watch over four hours of television each day (28 hours/wk), only 10% of registry members watch this level of TV. Over 60% watch 10 hours or less of TV per week, with over 36% watching less than five hours (94).

Of particular note is the high degree of dietary restraint reported by NWCR members. Although they lost their weight almost six years ago, registry members report levels of dietary restraint that are typically observed at the end of a 24-week behavioral program (95). A key component of this restraint is their use of regular self-weighing. Thirty-six percent of Registry members weigh themselves at least once a day, and an additional 42% weigh at least weekly (69).

Further evidence of the importance of daily weighing for maintenance of weight loss comes from a recent trial by Wing et al. (96). This trial was unique in that it recruited participants after they had lost weight and focused entirely on maintenance of weight loss. Individuals who had recently lost weight ($N = 314$, mean $= 19.3$ kg) were randomly assigned to a control group that received quarterly newsletters, or to groups that received a self-regulation intervention via face-to-face meetings or through the Internet. The intervention focused on teaching participants to weigh themselves daily and to use the information from the scale to self-regulate their eating and exercise behavior. The intervention delivered face-to-face was effective in reducing the magnitude of weight gain over the 18-month follow-up, and both the face-to-face and Internet program reduced the proportion of participants who regained 5 lb or more over 18 months (72.4% in control, 54.8% in Internet, and 45.7% in face-to-face). An important component of the intervention was daily self-weighing which increased in both intervention groups and reduced the risk of regaining 5 lb or more by 82%.

These studies highlight the key behaviors associated with long-term weight loss maintenance, including continued consumption of a low-calorie, low-fat diet, increased physical activity, and vigilance about one's weight and weight-related behaviors.

CONCLUSION

Behavioral treatment programs focus on teaching participants to change their diet (calories and percent of fat consumed) and their exercise behaviors. It appears that there has been a fair amount of standardization in the way in which participants are helped to make these lifestyle changes. Currently, strong behavioral programs produce weight losses of 10.4 kg at the end of six months. When followed-up approximately one year later, participants maintain a weight loss of 8.1 kg. Thus, there appears to have been a gradual improvement in treatment outcome results over the past 10 years.

Efforts to improve weight loss results have focused on strengthening the diet and exercise components in weight loss programs. VLCDs have been shown to improve initial weight losses, but it has been difficult to maintain these weight losses long term. Better long-term results are seen with dietary approaches such as food provision, structured meal plans and grocery lists, or meal-replacement products that provide a high degree of structure for patients but use calorie intake goals of 1000 to 1500 kcal.

Research in the area of physical activity has shown benefits to home-based rather than supervised exercise. Related to this emphasis on lifestyle activity, there have been several studies indicating that exercise can be effective when divided into multiple short bouts and that providing home exercise equipment to participants increases their long-term adherence. Although participants in behavioral weight control programs are encouraged to gradually increase their physical activity to 1000 kcal/wk, there is increasing evidence that successful long-term weight losers may expend approximately 2500 kcal/wk in physical activity.

Behavioral researchers have also examined several other approaches to improving outcome, including lengthening the intervention program and increasing social support and motivation. Telephone calls have been shown to be a useful approach to extending treatment contact. Most recently, the Internet has been used to deliver a behavioral weight loss program. Further research using the Internet to increase the audience for behavioral weight loss programs is clearly warranted.

ACKNOWLEDGMENT

Preparation of this chapter was supported by NIH grants DK57413, DK56992, and DK66787.

REFERENCES

1. Skinner BF. The Behavior of Organisms: An Experimental Analysis. New York: Appleton-Century-Crofts, 1938.
2. Bandura A. Social Learning Theory. Englewood Cliffs, NJ: Prentice-Hall, 1977.
3. Ferster CB, Nurnberger JI, Levitt EB. The control of eating. J Math 1962; 1:87–109.
4. Stuart RB. Behavioral control of overeating. Behav Ther 1967; 5:357–365.
5. Brownell KD, Wadden TA. Behavior therapy for obesity: Modern approaches and better results. In: Brownell KD, Foreyt JP, eds. The Handbook of Eating Disorders: The Physiology, Psychology, and Treatment of Obesity, Bulimia, and Anorexia. New York Basic Books, 1986:180–190.
6. Wadden TA, Bell ST. Obesity. In: Kazdin AE, Hersen M, Bellack AS, eds. International Handbook of Behavior Modification and Therapy. New York: Plenum Publishing Corporation, 1990:449–473.
7. Kazdin AE. Self-monitoring and behavior change. In: Mahoney MJ, Thoresen CF, eds. Self-control: Power to the Person. Monterey, CA Brooks/Cole, 1974.
8. Wing RR. Behavioral strategies for weight reduction in obese type II diabetic patients. Diabetes Care 1989; 12: 139–144.
9. Jeffery RW, Thompson PD, Wing RR. Effects on weight reduction of strong monetary contracts for calorie restriction or weight loss. Behav Res Ther 1978; 16:363–369.
10. Jeffery RW, Gerber WM, Rosenthal BS, et al. Monetary contracts in weight control: effectiveness of group and individual contracts of varying size. J Consult Clin Psychol 1983; 51(2):242–248.
11. Jeffery RW, Wing RR, Stunkard AJ. Behavioral treatment of obesity: the state of the art. Behav Ther 1978; 9: 189–199.
12. McReynolds WT, Lutz RN, Paulsen BK, et al. Weight loss resulting from two behavior modification procedures with nutritionists as therapists. Behav Ther 1976; 7:283–291.
13. Penick SB, Filion R, Fox S, et al. Behavior modification in the treatment of obesity. Psychosom Med 1971; 33:49–55.
14. Wadden TA. The treatment of obesity: an overview. In: Stunkard AJ, Wadden TA, eds. Obesity: Theory and Therapy. New York: Raven Press, 1993:197–218.
15. Brownell KD. The LEARN Program for Weight Control. Dallas, TX American Health Publishing Company, 1991.
16. Wadden TA, Foster GD, Letizia KA. One-year behavioral treatment of obesity: comparison of moderate and severe caloric restriction and the effects of weight maintenance therapy. J Consult Clin Psychol 1994; 62:165–171.
17. Wing R, Blair E, Marcus MD. Year-long weight loss treatment for obese patients with type II diabetes: does inclusion of intermittent very low calorie diet improve outcome? Am J Med 1994; 97:354–362.

18. Diabetes Prevention Program Research Group. Reduction in the incidence of type 2 diabetes with lifestyle intervention or metformin. N Engl J Med 2002; 346:393–403.

19. Hamman RF, Wing RR, Edelstein SL, et al. Effect of weight loss with lifestyle intervention on risk of diabetes. Diabetes Care 2006; 29(9):2102–2107.

20. Look AHEAD Research Group. Reduction in weight and cardiovascular disease risk factors in individuals with type 2 diabetes: one year results of the Look AHEAD trial. Diabetes Care 2007; 30(6):1374–1383.

21. Wadden TA, Letizia KA. Predictors of attrition and weight loss in patients treated by moderate and severe caloric restriction. In: Wadden TA, VanItallie TB, eds. Treatment of the Seriously Obese Patient. New York: Guilford Press, 1992:383–410.

22. Guare JC, Wing RR, Marcus MD, et al. Analysis of changes in eating behavior and weight loss in type II diabetic patients. Diabetes Care 1989; 12:500–503.

23. Bandura A, Simon KM. The role of proximal intentions in self-regulation of refractory behavior. Cognit Ther Res 1977; 1:177–193.

24. Pronk NP, Wing RR. Physical activity and long-term maintenance of weight loss. Obes Res 1994; 2(6):587–599.

25. Kayman S, Bruvold W, Stern JS. Maintenance and relapse after weight loss in women: behavioral aspects. Am J Clin Nutr 1990; 52:800–807.

26. Jeffery RW, Bjornson-Benson WM, Rosenthal BS, et al. Correlates of weight loss and its maintenance over two years of follow-up among middle aged men. Prev Med 1984; 13:155–168.

27. Colvin RH, Olson SB. Winners Revisited: an 18-month follow-up of our successful weight losers. Addict Behav 1984; 9:305–306.

28. Dahlkoetter J, Callahan EJ, Linton J. Obesity and the unbalanced energy equation: exercise versus eating habit change. J Consult Clin Psychol 1979; 47:898–905.

29. Stalonas PM, Johnson WG, Christ M. Behavior modification for obesity: the evaluation of exercise, contingency management, and program adherence. J Consult Clin Psychol 1978; 46:463–469.

30. Wing RR, Epstein LH, Paternostro-Bayles M, et al. Exercise in a behavioural weight control programme for obese patients with type 2 (non-insulin-dependent) diabetes. Diabetologia 1988; 31:902–909.

31. Epstein LH, Valoski AM, Vara LS, et al. Effects of decreasing sedentary behavior and increasing activity on weight change in obese children. Health Psychol 1995; 14:109–115.

32. Craighead LW, Blum MD. Supervised exercise in behavioral treatment for moderate obesity. Behav Ther 1989; 20: 49–59.

33. D'Zurilla TJ, Goldfried MR Problem solving and behavior modification. J Abnorm Psychol 1971; 78:107–126.

34. Beck AT. Cognitive Therapy and the Emotional Disorders. New York International Universities Press, 1976.

35. Mahoney MJ, Mahoney K. Permanent Weight Control: A Total Solution to the Dieters Dilemma. New York: W. Norton, 1976.

36. Marlatt GA, Gordon JR. Determinants of relapse: implications for the maintenance of behavior change. In: Davidson PO, Davidson SM, eds. Behavioral Medicine: Changing Health Lifestyles. New York: Brunner/Mazel, 1979:410–452.

37. Marlatt GA, Gordon JR. Relapse Prevention: Maintenance Strategies in Addictive Behavior Change. New York: Guilford Press, 1985.

38. National Task Force on the Prevention and Treatment of Obesity. Very low-calorie diets. JAMA 1993; 270(8): 967–974.

39. Wadden TA, Stunkard AJ, Brownell KD. Very low calorie diets: their efficacy, safety, and future. Ann Intern Med 1983; 99:675–684.

40. Wadden TA, Stunkard AJ. Controlled trial of very low calorie diet, behavior therapy, and their combination in the treatment of obesity. J Consult Clin Psychol 1986; 54: 482–488.

41. Wing RR, Marcus MD, Salata R, et al. Effects of a very-low-calorie diet on long-term glycemic control in obese type 2 diabetic subjects. Arch Intern Med 1991; 151:1334–1340.

42. Wing RR, Blair EH, Bononi P, et al. Caloric restriction per se is a significant factor in improvements in glycemic control and insulin sensitivity during weight loss in obese type 2 diabetes patients. Diabetes Care 1994; 17:30–36.

43. Foster GD, Wadden TA, Peterson FJ, et al. A controlled comparison of three very-low-calorie diets: effects on weight, body composition, and symptoms. Am J Clin Nutr 1992; 55:811–817.

44. Williams KV, Mullen ML, Kelley DE, et al. The effect of short periods of caloric restriction on weight loss and glycemic control in type 2 diabetes. Diabetes Care 1998; 21(1):2–8.

45. Insull W, Henderson MM, Prentice RL, et al. Results of a randomized feasibility study of a low-fat diet. Arch Intern Med 1990; 150:421–427.

46. Kendall A, Levitsky DA, Strupp BJ, et al. Weight loss on a low-fat diet: consequence of the imprecision of the control of food intake in humans. Am J Clin Nutr 1991; 53: 1124–1129.

47. Jeffery RW, Hellerstedt WL, French S, et al. A randomized trial of counseling for fat restriction versus calorie restriction in the treatment of obesity. Int J Obes 1995; 19: 132–137.

48. Schlundt DG, Hill JO, Pope-Cordle J, et al. Randomized evaluation of a low fat 'ad libitum' carbohydrate diet for weight reduction. Int J Obes 1993; 17:623–629.

49. Pascale RW, Wing RR, Butler BA, et al. Effects of a behavioral weight loss program stressing calorie restriction versus calorie plus fat restriction in obese individuals with Type 2 diabetes or a family history of diabetes. Diabetes Care 1995; 18(9):1241–1248.

50. Viegener BJ, Perri MG, Nezu AM, et al. Effect of an intermittent, low-fat, low-calorie diet in the behavioral treatment of obesity. Behav Ther 1990; 21:499–509.

51. Harris JK, French SA, Jeffery RW, et al. Dietary and physical activity correlates of long-term weight loss. Obes Res 1994; 2:307–313.

52. Jeffery RW, Wing RR, Thornson C, et al. Strengthening behavioral interventions for weight loss: a randomized trial of food provision and monetary incentives. J Consult Clin Psychol 1993; 61(6):1038–1045.

53. Jeffery RW. Long-term effects of interventions for weight loss using food provision and monetary incentives. J Consult Clin Psychol 1995; 63:793–796.

54. Wing RR, Jeffery RW, Burton LR, et al. Food provision vs. structured meal plans in the behavioral treatment of obesity. Int J Obes 1996; 20:56–62.

55. Wadden TA, Vogt RA, Andersen RE, et al. Exercise in the treatment of obesity: effects of four interventions on body composition, resting energy expenditure, appetite, and mood. J Consult Clin Psychol 1997; 65:269–277.

56. Ditschuneit HH, Flechtner-Mors M., Johnson TD, et al. Metabolic and weight-loss effects of a long-term dietary intervention in obese patients. Am J Clin Nutr 1999; 69: 198–204.

57. Flechtner-Mors M, Ditschuneit HH, Johnson TD, et al. Metabolic and weight loss effects of long-term dietary intervention in obese patients: four-year results. Obes Res 2000; 8(5):399–402.

58. Pavlou KN, Krey S, Steffee WP. Exercise as an adjunct to weight loss and maintenance in moderately obese subjects. Am J Clin Nutr 1989; 49:1115–1123.

59. Foreyt JP, Goodrick GK, Reeves RS, et al. Response of free-living adults to behavioral treatment of obesity: attrition and compliance to exercise. Behav Ther 1993; 24: 659–669.

60. Leermakers EA, Perri MG, Shigaki CL, et al. Effects of exercise-focused versus weight focused maintenance programs on the management of obesity. Addict Behav 1999; 24(2):219–227.

61. Dunn AL, Marcus BH, Kampert JB, et al. Comparison of lifestyle and structured interventions to increase physical activity and cardiorespiratory fitness: a randomized trial. JAMA 1999; 281:327–334.

62. Andersen R, Frankowiak S, Snyder J, et al. Effects of lifestyle activity vs. structured aerobic exercise in obese women: a randomized trial. JAMA 1998; 281(4): 335–340.

63. Perri MG, Martin AD, Leermakers EA, et al. Effects of group- versus home-based exercise in the treatment of obesity. J Consult Clin Psychol 1997; 65:278–285.

64. Jakicic J, Wing R, Winters C. Effects of intermittent exercise and use of home exercise equipment on adherence, weight loss, and fitness in overweight women. JAMA 1999; 282(16):1554–1560.

65. Jakicic JM, Wing RR, Butler BA, et al. Prescribing exercise in multiple short bouts versus one continuous bout: effects on adherence, cardiorespiratory fitness, and weight loss in overweight women. Int J Obes 1995; 19:893–901.

66. Jakicic JM, Wing RR, Butler BA, et al. The relationship between presence of exercise equipment in the home and physical activity level. Am J Health Promot 1997; 11: 363–365.

67. Jeffery RW, Wing RR, Thornson C, et al. Use of personal trainers and financial incentives to increase exercise in a behavioral weight-loss program. J Consult Clin Psychol 1998; 66(5):777–783.

68. Wing RR. Physical activity in the treatment of adulthood overweight and obesity: current evidence and research issues. Med Sci Sports Exerc 1999; 31(S11):S547–S552.

69. Klem ML, Wing RR, McGuire MT, et al. A descriptive study of individuals successful at long-term maintenance of substantial weight loss. Am J Clin Nutr 1997; 66:239–246.

70. Jeffery RW, Wing RR, Sherwood NE, et al. Physical activity and weight loss: does prescribing higher physical activity goals improve outcome? Am J Clin Nutr 2003; 78(4): 684–689.

71. Tate DF, Jeffery RW, Sherwood NE, et al. Long-term weight losses associated with prescription of higher physical activity goals. Are higher levels of physical activity protective against weight regain? Am J Clin Nutr 2007; 8(4): 954–959.

72. Perri MG, Nezu AM, Patti ET, et al. Effect of length of treatment on weight loss. J Consult Clin Psychol 1989; 57(3): 450–452.

73. Andersen RE, Wadden TA, Bartlett SJ, et al. Relation of weight loss to changes in serum lipids and lipoproteins in obese women. Am J Clin Nutr 1995; 62:350–357.

74. Perri MG, McAllister DA, Gange JJ, et al. Effects of four maintenance programs on the long-term management of obesity. J Consult Clin Psychol 1988; 56(4):529–534.

75. King AC, Frey-Hewitt B, Dreon DM, et al. The effects of minimal intervention strategies on long-term outcomes in men. Arch Intern Med 1989; 149:2741–2746.

76. Perri MG, Shapiro RM, Ludwig WW, et al. Maintenance strategies for the treatment of obesity: an evaluation of relapse prevention training and posttreatment contact by mail and telephone. J Consult Clin Psychol 1984; 52:404–413.

77. Black DR, Gleser LJ, Kooyers KJ. A meta-analytic evaluation of couples weight-loss programs. Health Psychol 1990; 9:330–347.

78. Wing RR, Jeffery RW. Benefits of recruiting participants with friends and increasing social support for weight loss and maintenance. J Consult Clin Psychol 1999; 67(1): 132–138.

79. Latner JS, Wilson AJ, Jackson GT, et al. Effective long-term treatment of obesity: a continuing care model. In J Obes 2000; 24:893–898.

80. Wing RR, Jeffery RW, Hellerstedt WL, et al. Effect of frequent phone contacts and optional food provision on maintenance of weight loss. Ann Behav Med 1996; 18: 172–176.

81. Hellerstedt W, Jeffery R. The effects of a telephone-based intervention on weight loss. Am J Health Promot 1997; 11: 177–182.

82. Meyers A, Graves T, Whelan J, et al. An evaulation of a television-delivered behavioral weight loss program: are the ratings acceptable? J Consult Clin Psychol 1996; 64: 172–178.

83. Harvey-Berino J. Changing health behavior via telecommunications technology: using interactive television to treat obesity. Behav Ther 1998; 29:505–519.

84. Burnett KF, Taylor CB, Agras WS. Ambulatory computer-assisted therapy for obesity: a new frontier for behavior therapy. J Consult Clin Psychol 1985; 53(5):698–703.

85. Taylor CB, Agras WS, Losch M, et al. Improving the effectiveness of computer-assisted weight loss. Behav Ther 1991; 22:229–236.

86. Tate DF, Wing RR, Winett RA. Using internet technology to deliver a behavioral weight loss program. JAMA 2001; 285(9):1172–1177.

87. Tate DF, Jackvony EH, Wing RR. A randomized trial comparing human e-mail counseling, computer-automated tailored counseling, and no counseling in an Internet weight loss program. Arch Intern Med 2006; 166(15): 1620–1625.

88. Rothert K, Strecher VJ, Doyle LA, et al. Web-based weight management programs in an integrated health care setting: a randomized, controlled trial. Obesity 2006; 14(2):266–272.

89. Gold BC, Burke S, Pintauro S, et al. Weight loss on the web: a pilot study comparing a structured behavioral intervention to a commercial program. Obesity 2007; 15(1): 155–164.

90. Micco N, Gold B, Buzzell P, et al. Minimal in-person support as an adjunct to internet obesity treatment. Ann Behav Med 2007; 33:49–56.

91. Phelan S, Wyatt HR, Hill JO, et al. Are the eating and exercise habits of successful weight losers changing? Obesity 2006; 14:710–716.

92. Wyatt HR, Grunwald GK, Mosca CL, et al. Long-term weight loss and breakfast in subjects in the National Weight Control Registry. Obes Res 2002; 10(2):78–82.

93. Raynor HA, Jeffery RW, Phelan S, et al. Amount of food group variety consumed in the diet and long-term weight loss maintenance. Obes Res 2005; 13:883–890.

94. Raynor DA, Phelan S, Hill JO, et al. Television viewing and long-term weight maintenance: results from the National Weight Control Registry. Obesity 2006; 14: 1816–1824.

95. Klem ML, Wing RR, McGuire MT, et al. Psychological symptoms in individuals successful at long-term maintenance of weight loss. Health Psychol 1998; 17(4): 336–345.

96. Wing RR, Tate DF, Gorin AA, et al. A self-regulation program for maintenance of weight loss. N Engl J Med 2006; 355(15):1563–1571.

15

Preventing Weight Regain After Weight Loss

MICHAEL G. PERRI

Department of Clinical and Health Psychology, University of Florida, Gainesville, Florida, U.S.A.

JOHN P. FOREYT

Baylor College of Medicine, Houston, Texas, U.S.A.

STEPHEN D. ANTON

*Department of Aging and Geriatric Research and Department of Clinical and Health Psychology,
University of Florida, Gainesville, Florida, U.S.A.*

OVERVIEW

For most dieters, a regaining of lost weight is an all too common experience. Indeed, virtually all interventions for weight loss show limited or even poor long-term effectiveness. This sobering reality was reflected in a comprehensive review of nonsurgical treatments of obesity conducted by the Institute of Medicine (IOM). In its report, the IOM concluded, "those who complete weight-loss programs lose approximately 10 percent of their body weight, only to regain two thirds of it back within one year and almost all of it back within five years (1)."

In this chapter, we address the question of whether it is possible to prevent the regaining of weight that invariably seems to follow treatment-induced weight loss. We begin by reviewing the long-term outcomes of lifestyle interventions and by describing some of the physiological, environmental, and psychological factors that contribute to weight regain following weight loss. Next, we examine methods designed specifically to prevent regaining of lost weight, including strategies such as extended treatment, skills training,

portion-controlled diets, monetary incentives, social support, physical activity, and pharmacotherapy. We conclude the chapter by discussing future directions for the prevention of weight regain in the management of obesity.

LONG-TERM EFFECTS OF OBESITY TREATMENT

Numerous reviews have documented the effects of lifestyle interventions (2–6). Randomized trials conducted in the past decade show that lifestyle interventions, delivered in weekly group sessions over the course of four to six months, typically produce mean posttreatment weight reductions of 5 to 10 kg ($\sim$5–10% of initial body weight). Weight losses of this magnitude usually result in beneficial changes in blood pressure, blood glucose, lipid profiles, and psychological well-being (3,7). However, the clinical significance of 5% to 10% reductions in body weight is ultimately determined by long-term rather than short-term outcomes. If the weight reduction is not maintained, it is unlikely that the health benefits derived from that weight loss will be achieved or sustained.

Table 1 Behavioral Weight Loss Interventions with Follow-ups of Two or More Years

Study (yr)	(n)	Treatment length (wk)	Pre-tx wt (kg)	Initial loss (kg)	Follow-up (yr)	Net loss at follow-up (kg)	Initial loss maintained (%)
Behavioral treatments							
Blissmer et al. (2006)	104	24	90	5.6	2.0	2.7	48
Flechtner-Mors et al. (2000)	75	12[a]	93	4.2	4.0	6.8	122
Gotestam (1979)	11	16	87	9.4	3.0	2.1	22
Heshka et al. (2003)	148	52	94	4.3	2.0	2.9	67
Knowler et al. (2002)	1079	24	94	7.0	4.0	4.0	57
Kramer et al. (1989)	152	15	97	11.5	4–5	2.7	23
Lantz et al. (2003)	26	24	117	7.8	4.0	7.1	91
Latner et al. (2002)	30	52	86	15.5	5.0	15.6	100
Melin et al. (2006)	20	52	106.8	8.0	2.0	9.7	121
Riebe et al. (2005)	48	24	93.3	5.7	2.0	2.8	49
Simkin-Silverman (2003)	246	24	68	4.9	4.5	0.1	2
Stevens et al. (2001)	547	24	93.9	4.4	3.0	0.2	1
Stunkard and Penick (1979)	26	12	NA	8.0	5.0	4.4	55
Tuomilehto et al. (2001)	242	52	89	4.2	2.0	3.5	83
Villanova et al. (2006)	43	12	94	8.7	2.5	7.9	91
Wadden et al. (1988)	16	26	122	14.3	3.0	4.8	33
Wadden et al. (1989)	22	26	106	13.0	5.0	+2.7	None
Combined treatments (Behavioral therapy plus VLCD)							
Anderson et al. (1999)	112	22	108	29.7	5.0	6.8	23%
Kajaste et al. (2004)	29	24	136	19.1	3.0	6.6	35%
Lantz et al. (2003)	29	24	116	15.7	4.0	7.3	47
Lantz et al. (2003)	117	24	114	20.0	2.0	9.6	48
Melin et al. (2003)	32	52	96.6	11.5	2.0	7.7	67
Melin et al. (2006)	55	52	117	13.0	2.0	8.8	67
Wadden et al. (1988)	19	26	122	19.3	3.0	6.5	34
Wadden et al. (1989)	31	26	106	16.8	5.0	+0.8	None

[a]Included the use of meal replacements (1 meal and 1 snack per day) over four years of follow-up.

Table 1 summarizes the results of 21 studies (that included 25 behavioral intervention groups) with follow-ups of two or more years (8–28). Studies were only included if the initial treatment period was at least 12 weeks. The initial weight change for studies using behavioral treatments ranged from 4.2 to 15.5 kg with a mean loss of 8 kg (unadjusted for study n). In contrast, the initial weight change in studies that utilized combined interventions, behavior therapy plus very low calorie diets (VLCD), ranged from 11.5 to 29.1 kg with a mean loss of 18.1 kg (unadjusted for study n). Thus, studies that used VLCDs (i.e., daily energy intakes < 800 kcal) showed larger initial losses. The pretreatment weight of the samples and the length of initial treatment also appear to affect the magnitude of initial losses; studies with heavier subjects and longer initial treatments showed larger initial losses. Across all studies, final follow-up evaluations, conducted 2 to 12 years after initial treatment, showed mean weight changes that ranged from a gain of 2.7 kg to a net loss of 15.6 kg. For studies using standard behavioral treatment (with energy

intakes > 800 kcal/day), there was a mean long-term net loss of 4.4 kg (unadjusted for sample n); for studies testing combined interventions, there was a mean long-term net loss of 6.4 kg.

Modest weight reductions (i.e., 5–10% of initial body weight) result in significant health improvements in overweight individuals with known disease risk factors, such as elevated blood pressure or blood glucose levels (29). If we consider long-term maintenance of a 5-kg loss or a 5% reduction in body weight as reflecting a clinically significant outcome (1), then 5 of the 17 standard behavioral interventions showed successful long-term results, and seven of the eight combined interventions had successful long-term outcomes. However, if we raise the bar for successful weight loss maintenance to a 10-kg loss or a 10% reduction in body weight, then none of the standard behavioral interventions achieved successful long-term outcomes, and only one of the combined interventions would be considered successful. It is worth noting that the attrition rate for the one successful intervention was very high with only 44% of participants remaining in treatment at two years. Thus, studies to date indicate that few obese individuals succeed at sustaining weight losses of 10 kg or more over the long run. Moreover, many obese individuals may not view a 10-kg loss as a significant accomplishment, (30) and therefore, may not work to sustain such losses.

If we look at studies where participants achieved a 5% or greater reduction in body weight at two years, then results from studies conducted over the past seven years are encouraging. Prior to 2000, only two studies, both conducted in Europe, achieved a 5% or greater weight loss at two years (9,31). Both of these studies included intensive maintenance programs that incorporated ongoing therapist contacts and either the use of meal replacements (9) or occasional periods of VLCD for patients who relapsed (31). Since 2000, 8 of 15 additional studies have achieved long-term weight loss outcomes of 5% or greater at two years. The interventions used in these studies generally incorporated an intensive weight maintenance program that included continuous contact (e.g., monthly or bimonthly meetings) throughout the entire two years. An important caveat to these otherwise promising findings is that the attrition rate was high in studies that included follow-up assessments at two years (mean = 39%; range = 20–65%), and the follow-up rates were even lower in studies that extended beyond two years. These results may also be biased in a positive direction because individuals who have regained weight may be less likely to return for follow-up appointments (32,33). Taken as a whole, however, these findings suggest that interventions have improved over time and that extended treatment programs can assist individuals in maintaining modest but clinically significant weight losses (5–10 kg) for two years or longer.

In evaluating the significance of modest weight reductions, we must consider what would have happened had the individual's weight problem gone untreated (34). The natural course of obesity in untreated adults entails steady weight gain (35,36) with obese individuals gaining ∼0.6 kg/yr (36). Moreover, secular trend data suggest that weight tends to increase with age in young and middle-aged adults (35,37). Accordingly, a long-term finding of the maintenance of a small amount of weight loss may represent a relatively favorable outcome (38). Furthermore, simply examining mean weight changes may obscure the fact that some subsets of participants achieve clinically significant long-term outcomes (i.e., maintenance of losses of 5 kg or 5% of body weight). For example, in the Kramer et al. (13) study, the mean net weight loss at the 4.5-year follow-up was 2.7 kg; however, ∼20% of the participants maintained losses ≥5 kg for four or more years. Such findings suggest a significant percentage of participants in lifestyle treatments achieve successful long-term outcomes.

CONCEPTUALIZATION OF THE PROBLEM OF WEIGHT REGAIN

Factors That Promote Weight Regain

A complex interaction of physiological, environmental, and psychological factors makes the maintenance of lost weight difficult to achieve. Following a period of restrictive dieting, people often experience a heightened sensitivity to palatable food (39), including sweet and salty substances (40). Other evidence indicates that brain areas of obese individuals have greater sensitivity to the sensory processing of food intake (41), and self-reported sensitivity to the rewarding properties of taste and smell has been found to be related to overeating and preference for foods high in fat and sugar (42). Consequently, exposure to an environment rich in tasty high-fat, high-calorie foods virtually guarantees occasional lapses in dietary control (43–45). Many internal and external cues (in addition to hunger) may prompt an orientation toward certain foods and an increased desire to eat (46). Moreover, compared to lean individuals, overweight individuals have been reported to have a stronger preference for energy dense foods (46). This is of significance because over the long run even small changes in caloric intake may impact body weight (47). Consequently, some experts have recently argued that policy changes are needed to create environments that facilitate healthy eating and exercise behaviors (47,48).

Increased caloric intake during the post-dieting period may easily translate into weight regain. During the post-dieting period, a variety of physiological processes, including reduced metabolic rate (49–51); changes in catecholamine excretion and thyroid function (52); increases in grhelin, a gut peptide associated with the sensation of hunger (53); and increases in lipoprotein lipase activity (54–57) may facilitate the regaining of lost weight. Moreover, after a period of dieting, resting metabolic rate decreases beyond the level expected from the loss of body mass alone (51). Thus, even minor periods of positive energy balance may readily result in weight gain.

As a consequence of this unfriendly combination of factors, most individuals experience some regaining of weight during the post-dieting period. This weight gain often occurs at a time when there is less contact with a health care provider and fewer reinforcers to maintain adherence to changes in diet and activity. In addition, the most satisfying aspect of treatment, namely, weight loss, usually ceases with the completion of treatment. Consequently, the dieter sees a high behavioral "cost" of continued dietary control and little "benefit" in terms of weight loss. In line with this, a recent review of long-term (≥1 year) outcomes associated with calorie-reducing diets concluded that dieting alone does not lead to successful weight loss maintenance, and that one-third to two-thirds of individuals who initiate a diet regain more weight than they lost on the diet (58). Without professional assistance, a sense of hopelessness may ensue, and a small weight regain may lead to attributions of personal ineffectiveness, negative emotions, and an abandonment of the weight control endeavor (59–62).

Weight Loss Expectations

This problem is further compounded by unrealistic weight loss expectations, a minimization of the importance of "modest" weight losses, and a failure to achieve personal goals. Virtually, all obese clients begin weight loss therapy with unrealistically high expectations about the amount of weight loss they can achieve. For example, Foster et al. (63) found that obese persons commonly expect to lose 25% to 32% of their body weight; reductions of a magnitude that can only be reliably accomplished through surgery. Furthermore, Wadden and colleagues found that even informing participants about their expected weight loss had little effect on their unrealistically high weight loss expectations (64). Such unreasonable expectations may lead obese patients to discount the beneficial impact of modest weight losses such as the 5% to 10% reductions that are typically accomplished with lifestyle interventions. This mismatch between expected and actual weight changes may lead to demoralization and poor maintenance of the behavioral changes needed to sustain weight loss (65). Unrealistically high weight loss expectations may also lead to increased attrition rates in obesity prevention treatment programs (66). Nonetheless, some benefit may be associated with ambitious weight loss goals. One recent study observed that higher goals for weight loss were associated with greater weight reductions at 18 months, as well as the expectation that treatment would require more effort and produce larger rewards (67).

In addition to having unrealistic weight loss expectations, many obese persons expect that losing weight will help them to realize other personal goals, such as improving their physical attractiveness and gaining greater approval and affection from others (68). When these personal goals go unfulfilled, disappointment may follow and the motivation to continue with weight management may evaporate. Sustained weight loss, however, produces a number of important psychological benefits including increased satisfaction with physical appearance, fewer depressive symptoms, and improved health-related quality of life (66).

MAINTENANCE STRATEGIES

Long-term outcome in weight management may be improved by implementing strategies specifically designed to maintain the behavioral changes accomplished in initial treatment. The various maintenance methods that have been evaluated include extended treatments, skills training, provision of portion-controlled foods, social support, exercise/physical activity, monetary incentives for weight loss and exercise, multicomponent programs, and pharmacotherapy. In this section, we summarize the effectiveness of these strategies.

Extended Treatment/Professional Contact

Over the past two decades, the magnitude of weight reductions accomplished with behavioral lifestyle treatments has doubled: The increase in weight loss appears to be the result of increases in the length of treatment (i.e., from 10 to 12 weekly sessions in the 1980s up to current standard of 20 to 24 weekly sessions). The longer obese patients are in treatment, the longer they adhere to prescribed changes in eating and exercise behaviors. The effects of length of treatment on continued adherence and weight loss have been demonstrated experimentally. Perri and colleagues (69) investigated whether extending treatment would improve adherence and weight loss by comparing a standard 20-week program with an extended 40-week program. The results indicated that the extended treatment significantly improved outcome compared with the standard program. From week 20 to week 40, participants in extended treatment increased their weight losses by 35% while those in the standard length program regained a small amount of weight. Furthermore, the weight loss and adherence data showed that the longer participants were in treatment, the longer they adhered to the behaviors necessary for weight loss. Some recent studies suggest that the maintenance of long-term weight losses is often associated with treatment programs of indefinite duration (70), particularly those that incorporate a continuous care model with group support systems (71). Thus, extending the length of treatment may help patients to sustain the behavioral changes required to maintain lost weight.

Table 2 presents the results of 17 studies in which behavioral treatment was extended beyond six months through the use of weekly or biweekly treatment sessions (72–88). On average, the initial treatment was 24 weeks in these 17 studies, and the extended intervention included 18 sessions over the course of 31 weeks. Approximately one year after the initiation of treatment, those groups that received extended treatment maintained 95% of their initial weight losses. The inclusion of a control group (i.e., behavioral treatment without extended contact) in four of the studies allowed a rough comparison of behavioral treatment with and without extended contact. The groups without extended contact maintained about 61.5% of their initial weight reductions. Evaluating the impact of

Table 2 Behavioral/Lifestyle Interventions with Professional Contact Extended Beyond Six Months Through Weekly or Biweekly Sessions

Study (yr)	(n)	Initial treatment length (wk)	Mean initial weight loss (kg)	Type and number of extended contact sessions	Length of extended contact period (wk)	Net loss after extended contact (kg)	Initial loss maintained (%)	Additional follow-up without contact (wk)	Net loss at follow-up (kg)	Initial loss maintained (%)
Pi-Sunyer et al. (2007)	2570	26	NA	13 bw	26	8.6	NA	None	—	—
Jakicic et al. (1999)	148	26 Lb	8.2	13 bw	26	7.0	85	26	5.8	71
		26 Sb	7.5	13 bw	26	5.7	76	26	3.7[a]	49
		26 SbE	9.3	13 bw	26	10.0	108	26	7.4[b]	80
Jeffery et al. (2003)	74	26[c]	8.1	20 bw	52	4.1	51	None	—	—
	84	26	9.0	20 bw	52	6.7	74	None	—	—
Leermakers et al. (1999)	28	26	9.6	EF 13 bw	26	7.9	82	26	5.2	54[a]
	20	26	8.7	WF 13 bw	26	8.5	98	26	7.9	91[b]
Perri et al. (1987)	16	20	10.3	None	—	7.8[a]	76	48	3.1[a]	30
	27	20	10.7	15 bw	30	11.5[b]	107	48	6.4[b]	60
Perri et al. (1988)	16	20	10.8	None	—	5.7[a]	53	26	3.6[a]	33
	19	20	13.2	26 bw	52	12.9[b]	98	26	11.4[b]	86
Perri et al. (1989)	16	20	8.9	None	—	6.4[a]	71	32	4.6[a]	52
	16	20	10.1	20 wk	20	13.6[b]	135	32	9.9[b]	98
Perri et al. (1997)	24	26 H	10.4	13 bw	26	12.1[a]	116	13	11.7[a]	113
	25	26 G	9.4	13 bw	26	8.1[b]	86	13	7.01[b]	75
Perri et al. (2001)	15	20	9.5	None	—	4.1[a]	46	None	—	—
	20	20	8.4	RP 26 bw	52	5.9	70	None	—	—
	23	20	9.3	PST26 bw	52	10.8[b]	116	None	—	—
Viegener et al. (1990)	32	26	8.9	13 bw	26	9.0	101	None	—	—
Wadden et al. (1994)	16	26	11.9	26 wk + 13bw	52	12.2	103	None	—	—
Wadden et al. (1998)	17	20[d]	11.0	10 bw	20	12.4	113	None	—	—
Wadden et al. (1997,1998)	77	26[d]	17.4	22 wk	22	15.6	90	52	8.5	49
Wadden et al. (2005)	55	18[e]	6.7	10 bw	20	6.2	93	None	—	—
	60	18	12.1	12.1	100%					
Weinstock et al. (1998)	45	28[d]	13.8	10 bw	20	15.2	110	48	10.0	72
Wing et al. (1994)	41	26	13.5	26 wk	26	10.5	78	52	5.7	42
Wing et al. (1998)	37	26 D	9.1	13 bw	26	5.5	56	52	2.1	23
	40	26 DE	10.3	13 bw	26	7.4	72	52	2.5	24

[a,b] Means with differing superscripts indicate significant between-group differences ($p < 0.05$).

[c] Included high physical activity condition.

[d] Included short-term use of a low-calorie liquid diet (925 kcal/day).

[e] Included combination of lifestyle treatment and sibutramine condition.

Abbreviations: bw, biweekly; D, diet; E, exercise; EF, exercise focused; G, group-based exercise; H, home-based exercise; Lb, long-bout exercise; Sb, short-bout exercise; SbE, short-bout exercise; WF, weight focused; RP, relapse prevention; PST, problem-solving therapy.

Table 3   Randomized Trials of Maintenance Strategies Implemented or Continued After Initial Behavioral/Lifestyle Treatment

Study (yr)	Initial tx and length (wk)	(n)	Pre-tx weight (kg)	Mean initial weight loss (kg)	Maintenance strategies	Weeks of maintenance	Net loss after maintenance	Initial loss maintained (%)	Additional follow-up (wk)	Net loss at follow-up (kg)	Initial loss maintained (%)
Baum et al. (1991)	B	16	81.5	4.0	None	12	3.5	87	39	1.5^a	38
	B	16	81.5	3.9	C + R	12	5.4	138	39	3.6^b	92
	(26)										
Flechtner-Mors et al. (2000)	B	50	92.7	1.3^a	F 48 monthly mtgs	208	4.1^a	315	—	—	—
	B + F	50	92.6	7.1^b	F 48 monthly mtgs	208	9.5^b	134	—	—	—
	(12)										
Jakicic et al. (1999)	B + Lb	49	90	8.2	Lb 13 bw	26	7.0	85	26	5.8	71
	B + Sb	51	92	7.5	Sb 13 bw	26	5.7^a	76	26	3.7^a	49
	B + Sb + E	48	88.3	9.3	SbE 13 bw	26	10.0^b	108	26	7.4^b	80
	(26)										
Jeffery et al. (1993,1995)	B	40	89.4	7.5^a	C (monthly)	52	4.4	58.6	52	1.4	19
	B + I	41	92.3	7.9^a	C + I	52	3.8	48.1	52	1.6	20
	B + F	40	88.1	10.0^b	C + F	52	6.7^b	67.0	52	2.2	22
	B + I + F	41	91.1	10.2^b	C + I + F	52	6.2^b	60.8	52	1.6	16
Jeffery et al. (1998)	B	40	86	8.3	None	52	7.6^a	92	—	—	—
	B	41	87	6.0	Su. walks 3/wk	52	3.8^b	63	—	—	—
	B	42	85	5.6	PT walks 3/wk	52	2.9^b	52	—	—	—
	B	37	88	6.7	Su. walks + I	52	4.5^b	67	—	—	—
	B	36	86	7.9	PT walks + I	52	5.1^b	65	—	—	—
Leermakers et al. (1999)	B	28	94	9.6	EF 13 bw	26	7.9	82	26	5.2	54^a
	B	20	94	8.7	WF 13 bw	26	8.5	98	26	7.9	91^b
Perri, McAdoo et al. (1984)	B	17	90.9	5.6	None	65	2.1	38	26	0.4^a	7
	B	26	84.1	6.1	C: mail + phone	65	5.8^c	95	26	4.6^b	75
	(14) + peer mtg										
Perri, Shapiro et al. (1984)	B	21	88.6	7.5	None	26	7.6	98	26	6.3	84
	B + C	15	88.6	8.7	C: mail + phone	26	8.7	100	26	5.8	66
	B + R	15	88.6	8.5	None	26	4.9^a	58	26	3.0^a	35
	B + R + C	17	88.6	9.7	C: mail + phone	26	10.8^b	111	26	10.3^b	106
Perri et al. (1986)	B	16	92.1	7.5^a	None	52	0.3^a	4	26	0.7^a	9
	B	17	92.1	8.3^a	C: mail/phone	52	6.5^b	78	26	5.2^b	63
	B + A	16	92.1	10.3^b	None	52	5.2^b	50	26	3.1^b	30
	B + A	18	92.1	11.0^b	C: mail/phone + peer mtg	52	9.7^c	88	26	7.6^c	69

Study	Condition	n			Maintenance treatment						
Perri et al. (1987)	B	16	88.1	10.3	None	30	7.8[a]	76	48	3.1[a]	30
	B	32	94.2	10.9	Peer mtg	30	9.3[a]	85	48	6.5[b]	60
	B	27	89.8	10.7	C	30	11.5[b]	107	48	6.4[b]	60
Perri et al. (1988)	B	16	89.0	10.8	None	52	5.7[a]	52	26	3.6[a]	33
	B	19	97.4	13.2	C	52	12.9[b]	97	26	9.9[b]	98
	B	19	95.2	11.3	C + increased A	52	13.4[b]	117	26	8.4[b]	74
	B	18	96.9	13.1	C + S	52	13.0[b]	99	26	9.1[b]	70
	B	19	97.4	13.7	C + increased A + S	52	15.7[b]	114	26	13.5[b]	99
Perri et al. (2001)	B (20)	15	94.7	9.5	None	52	4.1[a]	46	—	—	—
	B	20	97.0	8.4	R 26 bw	52	5.9	70	—	—	—
	B	23	98.0	9.3	PS 26 bw	52	10.8[b]	116	—	—	—
Wadden et al. (1997,1998)	B	29	96.3	16.7	bw meetings	20	14.4	86	52	6.9	41
	B + A	31	98.7	16.2	aerobics 2/wk	20	13.7	85	52	8.5	52
	B + St	31	96.8	16.8	strength 2/wk	20	17.2	102	52	10.1	60
	B + A + St (26)	29	92.4	16.3	aerobics and strength 2/wk	20	15.2	93	52	8.6	53
Wing et al. (1996)	B	27	NA	14.2	None	52	8.6	60.6	—	—	—
	B	26		12.8	Phone prompts (wkly)	52	9.3	72.7	—	—	—
	B	22		13.4	None	52	9.2	68.7	—	—	—
	B (26)	26		13.2	Optional FP	52	9.0	68.2	—	—	—
Wing et al. (2006)	B	105	79	19.3	F 17 monthly mtgs	76	16.8	87	—	—	—
	B (In)	104	78	19.3	F 17 monthly mtgs	76	14.6	76	—	—	—

[a]Different superscripts denote significant between-group differences ($p < 0.05$).
[b]Different superscripts denote significant between-group differences ($p < 0.05$).
[c]Different superscripts denote significant between-group differences ($p < 0.05$).

Abbreviations: A, aerobic exercise; B, behavior therapy; C, therapist contact; E, exercise equipment; EF, exercise focused; FP, food provision; I, incentives; Lb, long-bout exercise; PS, problem-solving therapy; PT, personal trainer; R, relapse prevention training; S, social support; Sb, short-bout exercise; St, strength training; Su, supervised; WF, weight-focused; bw, biweekly sessions; In, Internet.

extended contact by comparison with the standard-length treatment suggests a beneficial impact for extended treatment (i.e., 95% vs. 61.5% maintenance of initial weight loss). Furthermore, the results of additional follow-ups conducted, on average, 21 months after the initiation of treatment showed that the extended treatment groups maintained 67% of their initial reductions. In contrast, the groups without extended contact maintained only 38.3% of their initial reductions.

Collectively, these findings suggest that extended treatment improves long-term outcome. However, following the conclusion of the extended contact periods, participants gradually begin to regain weight. Such findings may be interpreted as reflecting the futility of lifestyle interventions (88,89) or the necessity of a continuous care approach to the management of obesity (70,71,90).

Table 3 summarizes the long-term results of other strategies designed to improve long-term outcome in lifestyle interventions for weight loss. The findings are discussed in the following sections.

Telephone Prompts

Considerable professional time and effort is required to provide patients with extended treatment via additional face-to-face sessions. Thus, one might consider whether telephone contact might be employed as a more efficient method for continued contact. Wing et al. (91) studied the effects of weekly posttreatment phone calls intended to prompt self-monitoring of caloric intake and body weight. The phone calls were made by interviewers who were not the participants' therapists and who offered no counseling or guidance. Although participation in the telephone contact program was positively associated with better long-term outcome, the phone prompts did not improve the maintenance of lost weight compared to a no-contact control condition.

Some studies, however, have found beneficial effects for telephone contacts during the period following initial weight loss treatment. Perri et al. (76) found that patient-therapist contacts by telephone and mail significantly improved the maintenance of lost weight compared with a control condition without contact. In this study, the phone calls were made by the patients' therapists who provided counseling about ways to maintain behavioral changes in diet and exercise.

In a study that examined the effectiveness of delivering an entire intervention by phone or mail in a managed care setting, Sherwood and colleagues (92) found that neither mail nor phone-based interventions were more effective than a usual care group over a 24-month period. Because the phone and mail treatments were both used to induce initial weight losses, as well as to maintain those losses, their

potential effectiveness as maintenance strategies cannot be determined by this study. Moreover, the overall study participation rates were very low, just 56% in the phone condition and only 12% in mail group.

Internet and E-mail

In a recent review, Weinstein (93) found that internet-based weight loss programs produced significant weight loss in seven out of eight studies. Internet-based interventions, to date, have produced approximately half as much weight loss as traditional programs (94). Weight loss was enhanced, however, in internet interventions that included a behavioral therapy component (95).

The three studies that have tested use of the internet as a weight loss maintenance strategy have produced mixed results. Harvey-Berino et al. (96) found that a 22-week internet-based weight maintenance program was as effective as in-person therapist-led groups following a 15-week in-person behavioral weight loss program. Participants assigned to in-person counseling, however, had better attendance and greater satisfaction with their treatment than participants assigned to the internet program. Another study from this same group (97) found that a 12-month internet-based weight maintenance program consisting of biweekly online sessions was not as effective as a biweekly in-person support group. More recently, Harvey-Berino and colleagues (98) found that a 12-month internet-based weight maintenance program that included biweekly contacts was as effective as biweekly in-person support. In this study, participants in the internet-based condition had higher levels of peer contact and self-monitoring. Given these mixed findings, it is difficult to draw firm conclusions about the effectiveness of the internet in promoting weight loss maintenance at the present time. Nevertheless, the internet appears to have the potential to become an effective weight maintenance tool (99).

Skills Training

Can training in the skills needed to avoid or overcome lapses in dietary control enhance long-term outcome? Relapse prevention training (RPT) involves teaching participants how to avoid or cope with slips and relapses (100). Studies of the effectiveness of RPT on long-term weight management have revealed mixed results. Perri et al. (101) found that the inclusion of RPT during initial treatment was not effective, but that combining RPT with a posttreatment program of patient-therapist contacts by mail and telephone improved the maintenance of weight loss (102). Similarly, Baum et al. (100) showed that participants who received RPT combined with posttreatment therapist contacts maintained their end-of-treatment losses better than did participants in a minimal contact condition. In a recent study, Perri et al. (79) compared RPT and problem-solving therapy as yearlong extended treatments for weight management and found that only problem-solving therapy showed better long-term outcome than standard-length behavioral treatment. However, it should be noted that in this study, RPT was administered in a didactic fashion as a psychoeducational program. RPT may be more effective when implemented as an individualized therapy (103).

Food Provision

Jeffery and colleagues (104) examined whether long-term weight control could be improved through the use of portion-controlled meals and monetary incentives for weight loss. During initial treatment and the year following initial treatment, the researchers provided obese patients with prepackaged, portion-controlled meals (10 per week at no cost) or with monetary incentives for weight loss or with both. The monetary incentives had no significant impact on outcome. However, participants in the food provision groups showed significantly greater weight losses than those without food provision both during initial treatment and during the subsequent 12 months. The results of an additional 12-month follow-up, without food provision, revealed a significant weight regain (105). In a subsequent study (91), these researchers found that simply providing participants with the "opportunity" to purchase and use portion-controlled meals as a maintenance strategy was not effective, primarily because the participants elected not to purchase the portion-controlled meals.

The findings from a recent meta-analysis (106) showed that the use of partial meal replacements (PMRs) was associated with significant weight loss at one year in four of five studies reviewed. PMRs were effective in producing body weight reductions of 7% to 8%, and when pooled, weight loss in PMR conditions at both 3 months and 12 months exceeded that of reduced calorie diets (RCDs) by ~2.5 kg. Thus, in clinical trials, PMRs appear to promote greater weight loss and weight maintenance than RCDs. Although these results are encouraging, their external validity is questionable because the meal replacements were typically provided at no cost to the participants. As noted in a recent review (107), comparisons across studies are diffcult to make because the costs to participants associated with meal replacements varied across investigations. Nonetheless, it appears that the effectiveness of PMRs, as compared to RCDs, may be determined primarily by whether or not the meals are provided to participants at no cost.

To our knowledge, there have only been two studies that have evaluated the use of PMRs as a long-term (>1 year) weight loss maintenance strategy. Both of these were uncontrolled studies. Flechtner-Mors et al. (9) found excellent long-term maintenance of lost weight for participants who were provided with monthly clinician contacts and with no-cost portion-controlled meals and snacks (i.e., 7 meals and 7 snacks per week) over the course of a 48-month period. Quinn (108) observed that participants who received free meal replacement products ($n = 141$) maintained a 5-kg weight loss over five years, whereas individuals in a retrospectively matched control group ($n = 389$) gained 6.5 kg during the same time period. As noted above, these results may not be representative of the effect in the "real world" because in both studies the replacement meals were provided to the participants at no cost.

Monetary Incentives

Wall and colleagues (109) recently conducted a systematic review of randomized controlled trials examining the effectiveness of monetary incentives in modifying dietary behavior. Four trials (104,110–112) were identified that used monetary incentives as a central component of the intervention in a manner that could be separated from other intervention components. Of these, only two trials (104,110) reported the effects of monetary incentives on weight loss. Although both of these trials reported positive effects on weight loss at six months, the effects of monetary incentives may have been confounded with the beneficial effects associated with meal replacements in at least one of the trials (111). Similar to the provision of free meal replacements to participants, the external validity of these findings is questionable because most clinical treatment programs do not provide payment for weight loss.

To our knowledge, only one trial (110) has examined the effect of monetary incentives on weight loss greater than one year. This study found that participants in the monetary incentive condition maintained a weight loss of only 1.5 kg at 18 months, and no effect on weight loss maintenance was found one year after the intervention ended (i.e., 30 months). Thus, the limited research in this area suggests monetary incentives do not appear to be a promising maintenance strategy.

Peer Support

Can social support be utilized to improve long-term outcome? The benefits of a peer support maintenance program were investigated by Perri et al. (101). After completing standard behavioral treatment, participants were taught how to run their own peer group support meetings. A meeting place equipped with a scale was provided to the group, and biweekly meetings were scheduled over a seven-month period. Although attendance at the peer group meetings was high (67%), no advantage was observed in terms of adherence or weight change during the maintenance period compared with a control condition. The results of a long-term follow-up showed a trend toward better maintenance of lost weight in the peer support group compared with the control condition.

Wing and Jeffery (113) tested the effects of recruiting participants alone or with three friends or family members. The researchers used a partially randomized study in assigning participants (recruited alone vs. with friends) to receive either standard behavior therapy or behavior therapy with social support training. The results of a six-month follow-up showed that participants who were recruited with friends and were provided social support training maintained 66% of their initial weight losses. In contrast, the individuals who entered the study alone and received standard treatment maintained only 24% of their initial losses.

Milsom et al. (114) recently reviewed the literature to evaluate the long-term effects of guided group support on weight loss outcomes. In the 11 studies identified, lifestyle treatments with guided group support were found to produce greater weight loss over one year than interventions that did not include group contact during the follow-up period (7.3 kg vs. 5.3 kg). Moreover, a higher percentage of interventions with guided group support (85% vs. 55%) met the IOM (1995) (1) criterion (i.e., >5% reduction from baseline weight observed at follow-up of one year or more of initial treatment). Overall, these findings suggest that group support improves long-term weight loss outcomes. However, group support does not appear to completely prevent weight regain following treatment; participants in interventions with group support regained approximately one quarter of their posttreatment weight loss during the year following initial treatment.

Problematic attendance and ultimately program attrition are two problems that can significantly limit the effectiveness of extended group treatment. For example, Perri et al. (79) found that group session attendance rates decreased from 90% during initial treatment to 58% during the follow-up intervention and that the attrition rate was double that of initial treatment (32% vs. 15%, respectively). Other experts have reported that participants sometimes describe extended care sessions as "monotonous" or even "demoralizing" (115). These feelings typically occur at a point in time (i.e., after 6 months) when additional weight loss becomes increasingly more difficult. This may lead some participants to perceive the cons of attending group to outweigh the pros, which could ultimately lead to their discontinuing follow-up care (87).

One strategy that may increase the reward value of group sessions, and in turn increase participant retention, is short-term campaigns that focus on group cohesion and achievement of group goals. This strategy has been successfully used to promote physical activity in older adults (116) and is currently being used in a large-scale trial called Look AHEAD (Action for Health in Diabetes) (72). Participant retention may also be improved by varying the frequency or times of group sessions rather than maintaining a consistent interval meeting schedule; however, this approach has not been empirically tested. Future research should also attempt to identify the specific components of group treatment that influence long-term weight loss outcomes.

Dietary Composition

In a number of studies, low carbohydrate, high protein diets have been found to produce superior short-term (i.e., 6 month) weight loss as compared with conventional, low-fat diets (117–121). Only two studies have assessed the effects of low carbohydrate versus conventional, low-fat diets at one year. The first of these studies found no difference between conditions at one year (117). A more recent study, however, found the low-carbohydrate, high-protein diet (i.e., Atkins diet) produced greater weight loss than diets with higher carbohydrate content (i.e., LEARN, Ornish, and Zone) (121).

Long-term studies (i.e., ≥2 years) are needed to assess the potential effects of dietary composition on health and weight loss outcomes. Information regarding the effectiveness of diets differing in macronutrient content should be provided on the completion of the Preventing Overweight Using Novel Dietary Strategies (POUNDS) Lost trial, which is testing the effectiveness of four diets differing in fat and protein content for weight loss and weight maintenance over two years (see chap. 19).

Exercise/Physical Activity

The association between long-term weight loss and increased physical activity is a common finding in correlational studies (e.g., 122,123). Similarly, studies of obese persons who have achieved successful long-term weight losses (124) show that exercise is associated with the maintenance of lost weight. High levels of exercise (e.g., 200–300 min/wk or >2000 kcal/wk) appear to be necessary to improve long-term weight loss outcomes (74,125–127). Of importance, the evidence for the effectiveness of this dose comes from correlational analyses, and there is currently no prospective evidence regarding the effectiveness of this dose. Nevertheless, there is a growing body of literature that suggests that exercise can improve long-term weight loss outcomes, as long as it is performed at high levels (e.g., $\geq$60 min/day on most days). Noteworthy, this level of activity is greater than the amounts recommended to improve health outcomes (128).

In a review of controlled trials of exercise in obesity treatment, Wing (129) observed that only 2 of 13 studies showed significantly greater initial weight losses for the combination of diet plus exercise versus diet alone. Wing also noted that only two of six studies with follow-ups of one year or more showed significantly better maintenance of lost weight for diet plus exercise than for diet alone. However, in all the studies reviewed, the direction of the findings favored treatment that included exercise. The short duration of treatments and the relatively low levels of exercise prescribed in many of the studies may have accounted for the modest effects of exercise on weight loss. For example, Jakicic et al. (125) found that weight loss outcomes at one year were improved according to level of reported exercise participation; participants who exercised for < 150 min/wk had a mean weight loss of 4.7%, whereas participants who exercised for 150 min/wk or more had a mean weight loss of 9.5%, and participants who exercised for 200 min/wk or more had a mean weight loss of 13.6%. Similarly, Tate et al. (130) found that participants who sustained high levels of physical activity (>2500 kcal/wk) over 30 months lost significantly more weight (12 kg vs. 0.8 kg, respectively) than participants who reported lower levels of physical activity. Of importance, only a small number of individuals (13 of 141) were able to achieve and maintain this high level of physical activity. Another recent study evaluating the effects of a physical activity program on weight loss maintenance found that the probability of losing 5% to 10% of initial body weight increased by 20% for every 1000 steps/day ($\sim$10 min/day) (22).

The maintenance of treatment integrity often poses a significant problem in controlled trials of exercise. Participants assigned to exercise conditions often vary greatly in their adherence to their exercise prescriptions, and participants assigned to "diet only" conditions sometimes initiate exercise on their own. Poor adherence to assigned treatments can blunt or obscure the true effects of exercise interventions. For example, Wadden and colleagues (83) examined the effects of adding aerobic exercise, strength training, and their combination to a 48-week behavioral treatment program. None of the exercise additions improved weight loss or weight loss maintenance, compared to behavior therapy with diet only. In all four conditions, adherence to exercise assignments was highly variable, especially during follow-up. Nevertheless, the investigators observed a positive association between exercise and long-term weight loss. Participants who indicated that they "exercised regularly" had long-term

weight losses nearly twice as large as those who described themselves as "nonexercisers" (mean weight loss = 12.1 vs. 6.1 kg). Jakicic et al. (125) found a similar pattern of results in that there were no differences in weight loss outcomes at one year by intervention group (vigorous intensity/high duration, moderate intensity/high duration, moderate intensity/moderate duration, or vigorous intensity/moderate duration) with moderate duration based on 1000 kcal/wk estimated energy expenditure and high duration based on 2000 kcal/wk estimated energy expenditure. However, as noted above, weight loss outcomes for participants who reported exercising for $\geq$200 min/wk were almost three times that of participants who reported exercising for <150 min/wk (13.6% vs. 4.5% of initial body weight).

Given the potential benefits of exercise for long-term weight management, how can adherence to physical activity regimens be improved? The various strategies that have been examined include home-based exercise, the use of short bouts of exercise, the provision of home exercise equipment, monetary incentives for exercise, and post-treatment programs focused exclusively on exercise.

Home-Based Exercise

Although group-based exercise programs offer the opportunity for enhanced social support, over the long run, such benefits may be limited by potential barriers that one must overcome in meeting with others to exercise at a designated time and location. In contrast, home-based exercise offers a greater degree of flexibility and fewer obstacles. Perri et al. (78) investigated the use of home-based versus supervised group-based exercise programs in the treatment of obesity. After six months, both approaches resulted in significant improvements in exercise participation, cardiorespiratory fitness, eating patterns, and weight loss. However, over the next six months, participants in the home-based condition completed a significantly higher percentage of prescribed exercise sessions than subjects in the group program (83.3% vs. 62.1%, respectively). Moreover, at long-term follow-up, the participants in the home-based program displayed significantly better maintenance of lost weight than the subjects in the group-based program. Similarly, in a recent review, Ashworth et al. (131) concluded that home-based programs produced better long-term adherence to exercise than center-based programs in older adults ($\geq$50 years of age).

Personal Trainers/Financial Incentives

Jeffery and colleagues (132) studied the use of personal trainers and financial incentives as strategies to improve exercise adherence and long-term weight loss. The personal trainers exercised with participants and made phone calls reminding them to exercise. In addition, the participants could earn $1 to $3 per bout of walking. The use of personal trainers and financial incentives both increased attendance at supervised exercise sessions but neither improved weight loss. In fact, participants in the control condition, who received a home-based exercise regimen, showed superior maintenance of weight loss at follow-up compared with all other conditions. These results corroborated the findings of Perri et al. (78) regarding the benefits of home-based exercise in the management of obesity.

Short Bouts and Home Exercise Equipment

The benefits of home exercise may be enhanced by providing participants with exercise equipment and by allowing them to exercise in brief bouts. Jakicic et al. (73) tested the effects of intermittent exercise (i.e., four 10-min bouts per day vs. one 40-min bout per day) and the use of home exercise equipment on adherence and weight loss and fitness. The researchers provided half of the subjects in the short-bout condition with motorized treadmills for home use. The benefits from exercise in short or long bouts were equivalent. However, participants with the home exercise equipment maintained significantly higher levels of long-term exercise adherence and weight loss than participants without exercise equipment. Two recent studies found equivalent, and in some cases superior, health benefits for multiple bouts of exercise of 10- and 15-minutes duration as compared to a single 30-minute bout with adherence levels being similar across conditions (133,134). Overall, the literature suggests dividing exercise into multiple bouts produces similar health benefits as single bouts of equivalent duration, and it provides an option that may improve adherence for some individuals.

Exercise-Focused Maintenance Program

Leermakers and colleagues (75) examined whether a posttreatment program focused exclusively on exercise might improve long-term outcome in obesity treatment. These researchers compared the effects of exercise-focused and weight-focused posttreatment programs. The components of the exercise-focused program included supervised exercise, incentives for exercise completion, and RPT aimed at the maintenance of exercise. The weight-focused maintenance program included problem solving of barriers to weight loss progress. The results of a long-term follow-up study showed that participants in the weight-focused program had significantly greater decreases in fat intake and significantly better maintenance of lost weight compared with participants in the exercise-focused condition. These results highlight the necessity of focusing on dietary intake as well as exercise in the long-term management of obesity.

Multicomponent Posttreatment Programs

A number of investigations have studied the impact of posttreatment programs with multiple components. Perri et al. (101) tested the effects of a multicomponent program that included peer group meetings combined with ongoing client-therapist contacts by mail and telephone. The multicomponent program produced significantly better maintenance of weight loss compared with a control group that received behavioral treatment without a follow-up program. These findings were replicated in a later study (135) that employed a longer initial treatment (20 weeks vs. 14 weeks), included an aerobic exercise component, and achieved larger weight losses at posttreatment and at follow-ups.

Finally, Perri and colleagues (77) examined the effects of adding increased exercise (from 80 to 150 min/wk) and a social influence program (or both) to a posttreatment therapist contact program consisting of 26 biweekly group sessions. Compared to a control condition that received behavioral therapy without posttreatment contact, all four posttreatment programs produced significantly greater weight losses at an 18-month follow-up evaluation. The four maintenance groups succeeded in sustaining on average 83% of their initial weight losses, compared with 33% for the group without a posttreatment program. Although there were no significant between-group differences among the four maintenance conditions, only the group that received all three maintenance strategies (i.e., therapist contact + increased exercise + enhanced social support) demonstrated additional weight loss (4 kg) during the months following initial treatment.

Pharmacotherapy

Can pharmacotherapy prevent weight regain? At present there are only two FDA-approved weight loss medications for long-term use: orlistat and sibutramine. A recent meta-analysis (136) that evaluated the effectiveness of nine different weight loss medications showed that only sibutramine produced placebo-subtracted weight losses greater than 4.0 kg over one year (i.e., mean weight loss at 52 weeks = 4.5 kg) with average placebo-subtracted weight losses increasing from $\sim$2.8 kg at 3 months to 4.5 kg at 12 months. Orlistat was found to produce placebo-subtracted weight losses of 2.9 kg and total weight losses of 8.2 kg at one year.

The use of pharmacotherapy to prevent the almost inevitable weight regain that occurs following weight loss induced by a VLCD is a promising idea. Apfelbaum et al. (137) randomly assigned patients who had lost 6 kg or more during a four-week VLCD intervention to receive either sibutramine or placebo. From the four-week time of randomization to the one-year endpoint, patients who received sibutramine had an additional mean weight loss of 5.2 kg compared with a weight gain of 0.5 kg in those who received the placebo. A total of 75% of patients in the sibutramine group maintained at least 100% of the weight loss achieved with the VLCD, compared with 42% in the placebo group. Additionally, James and the STORM Study Group (138) randomly assigned 467 patients who lost more than 5% of their weight through a low-calorie diet to receive sibutramine or placebo for an additional 18 months. The dose was adjusted upward if weight gain occurred. Of the 204 patients who completed the study, 43% of those receiving sibutramine maintained at least 80% of the weight lost during the initial six months, compared to only 16% of patients who received the placebo. In a study similar in design to the STORM trial, obese patients who had lost at least 8% of their initial body weight during a six-month low-calorie diet lead-in were randomly assigned to receive placebo, 30 mg, 60 mg, or 120 mg of orlistat three times daily for one year. The patients treated with 120-mg orlistat regained a significantly smaller portion of their initial weight loss (32.8%) than those treated with placebo (58.7%) over the subsequent year (139).

The XENical in the prevention of Diabetes and Obese Subjects (XENDOS) trial is unique in that it was four years in duration. This double-blind prospective trial evaluated the effectiveness of orlistat in combination with lifestyle modification in 3305 obese, nondiabetic participants with both normal (79%) and impaired (21%) glucose tolerance (140). Participants receiving lifestyle changes plus orlistat lost significantly more weight than participants receiving lifestyle change with placebo at both one year (10.6 vs. 6.2 kg) and four years (5.8 kg vs. 3.0 kg). Retention rates over four years were relatively low (52% for orlistat and 34% for placebo) but were in line with previous drug trials of two years duration (e.g., 141).

Rimonabant, the first CB1 receptor blocker (142), is an antiobesity drug that may facilitate weight loss maintenance and is currently under consideration for FDA approval. In rodent models, rimonabant has been shown to produce a dose-dependent reduction in food intake (143,144), and it appears to have both central and peripheral effects. On the basis of one-year results from four double-blind, placebo-controlled trials, collectively known as the Rimonabant in Obesity (RIO) program (145–147), a 20-mg dose was effective in producing a 4.6-kg placebo-subtracted weight loss at one year (148). Similar to studies on orlistat and sibutramine (149), attrition rates at one year were high (i.e., 40–50%), so it is difficult to fully evaluate rimonabant's effectiveness. RIO–North America is the only trial to examine the effect of rimonabant for a two-year period. In this trial, participants who continued taking rimonabant during year two maintained almost the entire weight loss achieved in year one. In contrast, participants who received rimonabant during year one and were rerandomized to the placebo condition during year two regained almost all of their initial weight loss in year two (147).

Several studies have pointed to the significant advantage of combining pharmacotherapy with a strong lifestyle intervention. As compared with either pharmacotherapy or lifestyle interventions alone, most studies suggest that the combination of lifestyle treatment and pharmacotherapy leads to a greater decrease in total body weight (150). For example, in a one-year trial of the effectiveness of sibutramine alone compared with sibutramine plus lifestyle treatment (85), participants receiving the combination lost significantly more weight than participants in the sibutramine alone group (i.e., 12.1 kg vs. 5.0 kg).

Overall, it appears that certain pharmaceutical agents can help sustain lost weight. In particular, the data for orlistat, sibutramine, and rimonabant appear clear. In each case, these medications not only help participants lose weight, but they also help participants to sustain weight loss. However, conclusions regarding the effectiveness of weight loss medications need to be tempered by two notable limitations. First, follow-up rates in most pharmaceutical trials of one-year duration or longer have been relatively low (e.g., 40–60%), resulting in incomplete data regarding the true efficacy of these agents. Second, there is an absence of data regarding the effects and side effects of antiobesity agents beyond two years (151).

CONCLUSION

Regaining of Lost Weight

Long-term follow-ups of behavioral interventions show a reliable pattern of gradual regaining of lost weight. Four years after the completion of lifestyle treatment, a modest amount of weight loss remains evident in individuals who remain in treatment, ~4.5 kg or 53% of initial loss. This loss was increased to a mean of 7.1 kg or 35% of initial loss in two studies that tested the effect of behavior therapy combined with VLCD at four years. When viewed from the perspective of secular trends that show predictable weight gains for untreated obese adults, these results imply that behavioral treatment coupled with extended care may confer long-term benefit in weight management. Clinically significant, long-term losses of 5 kg or more may be sustained by as many as one in five participants in behavioral treatment. Moreover, many individuals who receive multicomponent treatment programs (behavior therapy plus VLCD) appear to achieve long-term losses of 5 kg or more. Such findings may be seen in a favorable light, particularly when one considers that a number of the intervention studies (listed in Table 1) did not provide participants with follow-up care or with strategies specifically designed to enhance the maintenance of lost weight.

Preventing the Regaining of Lost Weight

Our review of strategies designed to improve long-term outcome in obesity treatment reveals an interesting pattern of findings. RPT, peer group meetings, telephone prompts by nontherapists, monetary incentives for weight loss or exercise, supervised group exercise, the use of personal trainers, and the "availability" of portion-controlled meals do not appear effective in improving outcome. On the other hand, there is evidence suggesting that extending treatment beyond six months through the use of weekly or biweekly sessions and providing multi-component programs with ongoing patient-therapist contact, in person or via telephone and mail, may improve the maintenance of lost weight. In addition, supplying patients with no-cost portion-controlled meals, helping patients achieve high levels of physical activity through home-based exercise programs, and combining lifestyle treatment with pharmacotherapy may also contribute to improved long-term outcome. Although studies are limited, the Internet also appears to have promise in becoming a cost-effective weight maintenance tool.

Our review provides support for the proposition that extended treatment has a beneficial impact on the maintenance of lost weight. Follow-up assessments conducted on average 21 months after initiation of treatment showed that extended-treatment groups maintained mean net losses of 7.6 kg (67% of their initial reductions). Over the same time period, treatment groups without extended contacts showed mean net losses of 3.8 kg (38% of their initial reductions). Similarly, multicomponent approaches that combine ongoing client-therapist contacts (whether in person or by telephone and mail) with RPT or social support programs have demonstrated improved maintenance compared with behavioral treatment without such programs. Consistent with our findings, a recent review of multicomponent lifestyle interventions with follow-ups of at least two years concluded, "There is consistent and strong evidence that lifestyle interventions for obesity can produce modest but clinically significant reductions in weight with minimal risk (6)."

In those studies that directly tested behavior therapy with and without extended contact, greater maintenance of *behavior change* was observed in the groups with continuing contact than in those without it. Thus, continued adherence to prescribed eating and activity patterns is likely responsible for the better outcomes observed in extended treatments. Indeed, ongoing professional contact typically involves prompting of "appropriate" eating and exercise behaviors. Similarly, providing patients with no-cost meals or home-based exercise equipment and home-based activity regimens represent "environmental" manipulations that also prompt adherence to behaviors required for weight management. However, extended

contact with a treatment provider also allows opportunities for reinforcement of adherence and for problem solving of obstacles to continued maintenance (90).

Extended treatment is not a panacea for the problem of weight regain in the treatment of obesity. Several factors should be considered in evaluating the utility of extended treatment. Continuing therapy is labor-intensive and expensive. Yet these costs must be weighed against the alternative, namely, the seemingly inevitable weight gain that follows intervention without posttreatment care. A second issue concerns the changes in motivation of participants during extended care. As treatment duration approaches one year, session attendance becomes problematic, adherence begins to deteriorate, and participants often begin to regain weight. Furthermore, when weight loss plateaus during the course of long-term treatment, patients become disheartened and their participation in treatment flounders. Therefore, it becomes essential to address expectations about weight loss and personal goals and to have strategies available to address changes in motivation (152,153).

Clinical Directions

Several approaches to obesity treatment may improve the maintenance of lost weight, including a comprehensive initial assessment, using multiple indicators of success, focusing on the maintenance of behavior change, and adopting a continuous care approach to obesity management.

Comprehensive Assessment

The long-term treatment of obesity should be preceded by a comprehensive assessment of the effects of obesity on the individual's health and emotional well-being (154). The impact of obesity on risk factors for disease (e.g., hypertension, glucose tolerance, dyslipidemia) and quality of life (e.g., emotional state, body image, binge eating) should be assessed. As noted above, expectations regarding weight loss and personal goals should be assessed at this time. A careful individualized assessment will often reveal important behavioral and emotional targets for intervention, such as binge eating, body image disparagement, and anxiety or depression, problems that need to be addressed regardless of whether weight loss itself becomes an objective of treatment (90,155). For some obese individuals, self-acceptance independent of weight loss may be an important treatment objective (156).

Indicators of Success

Successful long-term outcome should not be viewed solely in terms of weight loss. Beneficial changes in risk factors for disease and improvements in quality of life

(157) represent important indicators of success in the care of the obese person. Improvements in the quality of diet should be a component of care independent of whether weight reduction is an identified objective of care (158). Reductions in amounts of dietary fats, particularly saturated fats, can improve health as well as assist in weight loss (159). Similarly, increased physical activity and a decrease in sedentary lifestyle can represent beneficial components of long-term care irrespective of the impact of exercise on weight loss (160).

Maintenance of Behavior Change

Because obese persons do not have direct control over how much weight they lose, goals for the posttreatment period should be framed in terms of behaviors that they can control, such as the quantity and quality of food they consume and the amounts and types of physical activity they perform. Moreover, obese persons should be informed that significant health benefits can be derived from even modest amounts of weight loss (161,162).

Continuous Care Approach

Finally, clinicians and patients alike must view obesity as a chronic condition requiring continuous care (90). Short-term interventions that strive to produce reductions to "ideal" weight are doomed to long-term failure. A continuous-care approach focused on the achievement of realistic long-term objectives appears more appropriate for most obese patients. Extended treatments have shown promise in promoting adherence to the behaviors required for the long-term maintenance of weight loss. Additionally, newer intervention methods, such as Internet-based programs, may offer the ability to intervene with large numbers of individuals at much lower costs than traditional treatments; thus, Internet-based interventions may be a cost-effective way to extend the reach of future treatments and maintenance programs.

SUMMARY

In this chapter, we addressed the question of whether it is possible to prevent the regaining of weight that invariably seems to follow treatment-induced weight loss. Our review of long-term follow-ups of lifestyle interventions for weight loss showed that moderate weight losses (5–10 kg) can be maintained for long periods of time (≥2 years). On average, individuals who remain involved with treatment maintain approximately half their initial weight loss (Mean, M = 4.4 kg for standard behavioral treatment and 6.4 kg for combined interventions) for up to two years; thus, more than 20% of participants may achieve clinically significant, long-term losses of 5 kg or

more. These numbers, however, may be positively biased as follow-up rates are relatively low in most long-term studies. If we assumed that everyone who did not return for their final clinic visit returned to their baseline weight, then the average weight loss in studies of at least two years duration would be lower (M = 2.7 kg for standard behavioral treatment and 4.2 kg for combined interventions). Thus, future studies should examine strategies to enhance long-term participation, as participant retention is critical to evaluate the effectiveness of weight loss maintenance programs.

The difficulty associated with maintaining lost weight appears to be the result of physiological, environmental, and psychological factors that combine to facilitate a regaining of lost weight and an abandonment of weight control efforts. A variety of methods to improve the long-term effects of treatment have been evaluated. RPT, peer group meetings, telephone prompts by nontherapists, monetary incentives for weight loss or exercise, supervised group exercise, the use of personal trainers, and the availability of portion-controlled meals do not appear effective in improving outcome. On the other hand, there is evidence suggesting that extending treatment beyond six months through the use of weekly or biweekly sessions and providing multicomponent programs with ongoing patient-therapist contact in person or via telephone and mail may improve the maintenance of lost weight. In addition, no-cost meal replacements, home-based exercise programs that assist patients in achieving high levels of physical activity, and the use of home exercise equipment and pharmacotherapy may enhance adherence as well as may contribute to improved long-term outcome. The most pressing challenge facing researchers is the improvement of programs for the long-term management of obesity. The greatest practical challenge is to convince health care professionals, obese individuals, and the general public that obesity is a complex, chronic condition that can be managed effectively through intensive programs of ongoing care.

ACKNOWLEDGMENTS

We would like to thank Joyce Corsica for her valuable assistance in the preparation of our previous version of this chapter.

REFERENCES

1. Thomas PR, Stern JSS. Weighing the Options: Criteria for Evaluating Weight-Management Programs. Washington: National Academy Press, 1995.
2. Jeffery RW, Drewnowski A, Epstein LH, et al. Long-term maintenance of weight loss: current status. Health Psychol 2000; 19(suppl 1):5–16.

3. National Heart, Lung and Blood Institute. Obesity education initiative expert panel on the identification, evaluation, and treatment of overweight and obesity in adults. Obes Res 1998; 6(suppl 2):51–209.

4. Perri MG. The maintenance of treatment effects in the long-term management of obesity. Clin Psychol Sci Pract 1998; 5:526–543.

5. Wadden TA, Brownell KD, Foster GD. Obesity: responding to the global epidemic. J Consult Clin Psychol 2002; 70:510–525.

6. Powell LH, Calvin JE, Calvin JE. Effective obesity treatments. Am Psychol 2007; 62:234–246.

7. Pi-Sunyer X, Blackburn G, Brancati FL, et al. Reduction in weight and cardiovascular disease risk factors in individuals with type 2 diabetes: one-year results of the look AHEAD trial. Diabetes Care, 30, 1374–1383.

8. Blissmer B, Riebe D, Dye G, et al. Health-related quality of life following a clinical weight loss intervention among overweight and obese adults: intervention and 24 month follow-up effects. Health Qual Life Outcomes 2006; 17:43–51.

9. Flechtner-Mors M, Ditschuneit HH, Johnson TD, et al. Metabolic and weight loss effects of long-term dietary intervention in obese patients: four-year results. Obes Res 2000; 8:399–402.

10. Gotestam KG. A three year follow-up of a behavioral treatment for obesity. Addict Behav 1979; 4:179–183.

11. Heshka S, Anderson JW, Atkinson RL, et al. Weight loss with self-help compared with a structured commercial program: a randomized trial. JAMA 2003; 289: 1792–1798.

12. Knowler WC, Barrett-Connor E, Fowler SE, et al. Diabetes Prevention Program Research Group. Reduction in the incidence of type 2 diabetes with lifestyle intervention or metformin. N Engl J Med 2002; 346:393–403.

13. Kramer FM, Jeffery RW, Forster JL, et al. Long-term follow-up of behavioral treatment for obesity: patterns of weight regain among men and women. Int J Obes 1989; 13:123–126.

14. Lantz H, Peltonen M, Agren L, et al. A dietary and behavioural programme for the treatment of obesity. A 4-year clinical trial and a long-term post-treatment follow-up. J Intern Med 2003; 254:272–279.

15. Latner JD, Wilson GT, Stunkard AJ, et al. Self-help and long-term behavior therapy for obesity. Behav Res Ther 2002; 40:805–812.

16. Melin I, Reynisdottir S, Berglund L, et al. Conservative treatment of obesity in an academic obesity unit. Long-term outcome and drop-out. Eat Weight Disord 2006; 11: 22–30.

17. Riebe D, Blissmer B, Greene G, et al. Long-term maintenance of exercise and healthy eating behaviors in overweight adults. Prev Med 2005; 40:769–778.

18. Simkin-Silverman LR, Wing RR, Boraz MA, et al. Lifestyle intervention can prevent weight gain during menopause: results from a 5-year randomized clinical trial. Ann Behav Med 2003; 26:212–220.

19. Stevens VJ, Obarzanek E, Cook NR, et al. Trials for the Hypertension Prevention Research Group. Long-term weight loss and changes in blood pressure: results of the trials of hypertension prevention, phase II. Ann Intern Med 2001; 134:1–11.

20. Stunkard AJ, Penick SB. Behavior modification in the treatment of obesity: the problem of maintaining weight loss. Arch Gen Psychiatry 1979; 36:801–806.

21. Tuomilehto J, Lindstrom J, Eriksson JG, et al. Prevention of type 2 diabetes mellitus by changes in lifestyle among subjects with impaired glucose tolerance. N Engl J Med 2001; 344(18):1343–1350.

22. Villanova N, Pasqui F, Burzacchini S, et al. A physical activity program to reinforce weight maintenance following a behavior program in overweight/obese subjects. Int J Obes (Lond) 2006; 30(4):697–703.

23. Wadden TA, Stunkard AJ, Liebschutz J. Three year follow-up of the treatment of obesity by very low calorie diet, behavior therapy, and their combination. J Consult Clin Psychol 1988; 56:925–928.

24. Wadden TA, Sternberg JA, Letizia KA, et al. Treatment of obesity by very low calorie diet, behavior therapy, and their combination: a five-year perspective. Int J Obes Relat Metab Disord 1989; 13(suppl 2):39–46.

25. Anderson JW, Vichitbandra S, Qian W, et al. Long-term weight maintenance after an intensive weight-loss program. J Am Coll Nutr 1999; 18(6):620–627.

26. Kajaste S, Brander PE, Telakivi T, et al. A cognitive-behavioral weight reduction program in the treatment of obstructive sleep apnea syndrome with or without initial nasal CPAP: a randomized study. Sleep Med 2004; 5(2):125–131.

27. Lantz H, Peltonen M, Agren L, et al. Intermittent versus on-demand use of a very low calorie diet: a randomized 2-year clinical trial. J Intern Med 2003; 253(4):463–471.

28. Melin I, Karlstrom B, Lappalainen R, et al. A programme of behaviour modification and nutrition counselling in the treatment of obesity: a randomised 2-y clinical trial. Int J Obes Relat Metab Disord 2003; 27(9):1127–1135.

29. Case CC, Jones PH, Nelson K, et al. Impact of weight loss on the metabolic syndrome. Diabetes Obes Metab 2002; 4(6):407–414.

30. Fabricatore AN, Wadden TA, Womble LG, et al. The role of patient's expectations and goals in the behavioral and pharmacological treatment of obesity. Int J Obes (Lond) 2007; 31:1739–1745

31. Bjorvell H, Rossner S. A ten year follow-up of weight change in severely obese subjects treated in a behavioural modification programme. Int J Obes Relat Metab Disord 1999; 16:623–625.

32. Grodstein F, Levine R, Troy L, et al. Three-year follow-up of participants in a commercial weight loss program. Can you keep it off? Arch Intern Med 1996; 156(12):1302–1306.

33. Hovell MF, Koch A, Hofstetter CR, et al. Long-term weight loss maintenance: assessment of a behavioral and supplemental fasting regimen. Am J Public Health 1988; 78(6):663–666.

34. Brownell KD, Jeffery RW. Improving long-term weight loss: pushing the limits of treatment. Behav Ther 1987; 18:353–374.

35. Lewis CE, Jacobs DR, McCreath H, et al. Weight gain continues in the 1990s: 10-year trends in weight and

overweight from the CARDIA study. Am J Epidemiol 2000; 151:1172–1181.

36. Shah M, Hannan PJ, Jeffery RW. Secular trends in body mass index in the adult population of three communities from the upper mid-western part of the USA: the Minnesota Heart Health Program. Int J Obes Relat Metab Disord 1991; 15:499–503.

37. Sternfeld B, Wang H, Quesenberry CP Jr., et al. Physical activity and changes in weight and waist circumference in midlife women: findings from the Study of Women's Health Across the Nation. Am J Epidemiol 2004; 160:912–922.

38. Norris SL, Zhang X, Avenell A, et al. Long-term effectiveness of weight-loss interventions in adults with pre-diabetes: a review. Am J Prev Med 2005; 28:126–139.

39. Rodin J, Schank D, Striegel-Moore R. Psychological features of obesity. Med Clin North Am 1989; 73:47–66.

40. Zverev YP. Effects of caloric deprivation and satiety on sensitivity of the gustatory system. BMC Neurosci 2004; 5:5.

41. Wang GJ, Volkow ND, Felder C, et al. Enhanced resting activity of the oral somatosensory cortex in obese subjects. Neuroreport 2002; 13:1151–1155.

42. Davis C, Patte K, Levitan R, et al. From motivation to behaviour: a model of reward sensitivity, overeating, and food preferences in the risk profile for obesity. Appetite 2007; 48(1):12–19.

43. Hill JO, Peters JC. Environmental contributors to the obesity epidemic. Science 1998; 280:1371–1374.

44. Poston WS, Foreyt JP. Obesity is an environmental issue. Atherosclerosis 1999; 146:201–209.

45. Hill JO, Wyatt HR, Reed GW, et al. Obesity and the environment: where do we go from here? Science 2003; 299:853–855.

46. Mela DJ. Determinants of food choice: relationships with obesity and weight control. Obes Res 2001; 9 (suppl 4): 249S–255S.

47. Hill JO. Understanding and addressing the epidemic of obesity: an energy balance perspective. Endocr Rev 2006; 27(7):750–761.

48. Hill JO, Peters JC, Wyatt HR. The role of public policy in treating the epidemic of global obesity. Clin Pharmacol Ther 2007; 81:772–775.

49. Dulloo AG, Jacquet J. Adaptive reduction in basal metabolic rate in response to food deprivation in humans: a role for feedback signals from fat stores. Am J Clin Nutr 1998; 68:599–606.

50. Ravussin E, Swinburn BA. Energy metabolism. In: Stunkard AJ, Wadden TA, eds. Obesity: Theory and Therapy. 2nd ed. New York: Raven, 1993:97–124.

51. Heilbronn LK, de Jonge L, Frisard MI, et al. Effect of 6-month calorie restriction on biomarkers of longevity, metabolic adaptation, and oxidative stress in overweight individuals: a randomized controlled trial. JAMA. 2006; 295(13):1539–1548 [erratum in JAMA 2006; 295(21): 2482].

52. Rosenbaum M, Hirsch J, Murphy E, et al. Effects of changes in body weight on carbohydrate metabolism, catecholamine excretion, and thyroid function. Am J Clin Nutr 2000; 71(6):1421–1432.

53. Cummings DE, Weigle DS, Frayo RS, et al. Plasma ghrelin levels after diet-induced weight loss or gastric bypass surgery. N Engl J Med 2002; 346:1623–1630.

54. Kern PA. Potential role of TNF alpha and lipoprotein lipase as candidate genes for obesity. J Nutr 1997; 127:1917S–1922S.

55. Kern PA, Ong JM, Saffari B, et al. The effects of weight loss on the activity and expression of adipose tissue lipoprotein lipase in very obese humans. N Engl J Med 1990; 322:1053–1059.

56. Ruge T, Svensson M, Eriksson JW, et al. Tissue-specific regulation of lipoprotein lipase in humans: effects of fasting. Eur J Clin Invest 2005; 35(3):194–200.

57. Nicklas BJ, Rogus EM, Berman DM, et al. Responses of adipose tissue lipoprotein lipase to weight loss affect lipid levels and weight regain in women. Am J Physiol Endocrinol Metab 2000; 279(5):E1012–E1019.

58. Mann T, Tomiyama AJ, Westling E, et al. Medicare's search for effective obesity treatments: diets are not the answer. Am Psychol 2007; 62(3):220–233.

59. Goodrick GK, Raynaud AS, Pace PW, et al. Outcome attribution in a very low calorie diet program. Int J Eat Disord 1992; 12:117–120.

60. Jeffery RW, French SA, Schmid TL. Attributions for dietary failures: problems reported by participants in the Hypertension Prevention Trial. Health Psychol 1990; 9:315–329.

61. Foster GD, Sarwer DB, Wadden TA. Psychological effects of weight cycling in obese persons: a review and research agenda. Obes Res 1997; 5(5):474–488.

62. Elfhag K, Rossner S. Who succeeds in maintaining weight loss? A conceptual review of factors associated with weight loss maintenance and weight regain. Obes Rev 2005; 6(1):67–85.

63. Foster GD, Wadden TA, Vogt RA, et al. What is a reasonable weight loss? Patients' expectations and evaluations of obesity treatment outcomes. J Consult Clin Psychol 1997; 65:79–85.

64. Wadden TA, Womble LG, Sarwer DB, et al. Great expectations: "I'm losing 25% of my weight no matter what you say." J Consult Clin Psychol 2003; 71(6): 1084–1089.

65. Polivy J. The false hope syndrome: unrealistic expectations of self-change. Int J Obes Relat Metab Disord 2001; 25(suppl 1):S80–S84.

66. Dixon JB, Anderson M, Cameron-Smith D, et al. Sustained weight loss in obese subjects has benefits that are independent of attained weight. Obes Res 2004; 12(11):1895–1902.

67. Linde JA, Jeffery RW, Finch EA, et al. Are unrealistic weight loss goals associated with outcomes for overweight women? Obes Res 2004; 12(3):569–576.

68. Cooper Z, Fairburn CG. A new cognitive-behavioural approach to the treatment of obesity. Behav Res Ther 2001; 39:499–511.

69. Perri MG, Nezu AM, Patti ET, et al. Effect of length of treatment on weight loss. J Consult Clin Psychol 1989; 57:450–452.

70. Latner JD, Stunkard AJ, Wilson GT, et al. Effective long-term treatment of obesity: a continuing care model. Int J Obes Relat Metab Disord 2000; 24(7):893–898.

71. Latner JD, Stunkard AJ, Wilson GT, et al. The perceived effectiveness of continuing care and group support in the long-term self-help treatment of obesity. Obesity (Silver Spring) 2006; 14(3):464–471.

72. Look AHEAD Research Group, Pi-Sunyer X, Blackburn G, Brancati FL, et al. Reduction in weight and cardiovascular disease risk factors in individuals with type 2 diabetes: one-year results of the look AHEAD trial. Diabetes Care 2007; 30(6):1374–1383.

73. Jakicic JM, Winters C, Lang W, et al. Effects of intermittent exercise and use of home exercise equipment on adherence, weight loss, and fitness in overweight women: a randomized trial. JAMA 1999; 282:1554–1560.

74. Jeffery RW, Wing RR, Sherwood NE, et al. Physical activity and weight loss: does prescribing higher physical activity goals improve outcome? Am J Clin Nutr 2003; 78(4):684–689.

75. Leermakers EA, Perri MG, Shigaki CL, et al. Effects of exercise-focused versus weight-focused maintenance programs on the management of obesity. Addict Behav 1999; 24:219–227.

76. Perri MG, McAdoo WG, McAllister DA, et al. Effects of peer support and therapist contact on long-term weight loss. J Consult Clin Psychol 1987; 55:615–617.

77. Perri MG, McAllister DA, Gange JJ, et al. Effects of four maintenance programs on the long-term management of obesity. J Consult Clin Psychol 1988; 56:529–534.

78. Perri MG, Martin AD, Leermakers EA, et al. Effects of group-versus home-based exercise in the treatment of obesity. J Consult Clin Psychol 1997; 65:278–285.

79. Perri MG, Nezu AM, McKelvey WF, et al. Relapse prevention training and problem solving therapy in the long-term management of obesity. J Consul Clin Psychol 2001; 69:722–726.

80. Viegener BJ, Renjilian DA, McKelvey WF, et al. Effects of an intermittent, low-fat, low-calorie diet in the behavioral treatment of obesity. Behav Ther 1990; 21:499–509.

81. Wadden TA, Foster GD, Letizia KA. One-year behavioral treatment of obesity: comparison of moderate and severe caloric restriction and the effects of weight maintenance therapy. J Consult Clin Psychol 1994; 62:165–171.

82. Wadden TA, Considine RV, Foster GD, et al. Short-and long-term changes in serum leptin in dieting obese women: effects of caloric restriction and weight loss. J Clin Endocrinol Metab 1998; 83:214–218.

83. Wadden TA, Vogt RA, Andersen RE, et al. Exercise in the treatment of obesity: effects of four interventions on body composition, resting energy expenditure, appetite, and mood. J Consult Clin Psychol 1997; 65:269–277.

84. Wadden TA, Vogt RA, Foster GD, et al. Exercise and the maintenance of weight loss: 1-year follow-up of a controlled clinical trial. J Consult Clin Psychol 1998; 66:429–433.

85. Wadden TA, Berkowitz RI, Womble LG, et al. Randomized trial of lifestyle modification and pharmacotherapy for obesity. N Engl J Med 2005; 353(20):2111–2120.

86. Weinstock RS, Dai H, Wadden TA. Diet and exercise in the treatment of obesity: effects of 3 interventions on insulin resistance. Arch Intern Med 1998; 158:2477–2483.

87. Wing RR, Blair E, Marcus M, et al. Year-long weight loss treatment for obese patients with type II diabetes: does including an intermittent very low-calorie diet improve outcome? Am J Med 1994; 97:354–362.

88. Wing RR, Vendetti E, Jakicic JM, et al. Lifestyle intervention in overweight individuals with a family history of diabetes. Diabetes Care 1998; 21:350–359.

89. Wilson GT. Behavioral treatment of obesity: thirty years and counting. Adv Behav Res Ther 1994; 16:31–75.

90. Perri MG, Nezu AM, Viegener BJ. Improving the Long-term Management of Obesity: Theory, Research, and Clinical Guidelines. New York: John Wiley & Sons, 1992.

91. Wing RR, Jeffery RW, Hellerstedt WL, et al. Effect of frequent phone contacts and optional food provision on maintenance of weight loss. Ann Behav Med 1996; 18:172–176.

92. Sherwood NE, Jeffery RW, Pronk NP, et al. Mail and phone interventions for weight loss in a managed-care setting: weigh-to-be 2-year outcomes. Int J Obes (Lond) 2006; 30(10):1565–1573.

93. Weinstein PK. A review of weight loss programs delivered via the internet. J Cardiovasc Nurs 2006; 21:251–258.

94. Wadden, TA, Butryn ML. Behavioral treatment of obesity. Endocrinol Metab Clin N 2003; 32:981–1003.

95. Tate DF, Wing RR, Winett RA. Using Internet technology to deliver a behavioral weight loss program. JAMA 2001; 285(9):1172–1177.

96. Harvey-Berino J, Pintauro SJ, Gold EC. The feasibility of using Internet support for the maintenance of weight loss. Behav Modif 2002; 26(1):103–116.

97. Harvey-Berino J, Pintauro S, Buzzell P, et al. Does using the Internet facilitate the maintenance of weight loss? Int J Obes Relat Metab Disord 2002; 26(9):1254–1260.

98. Harvey-Berino J, Pintauro S, Buzzell P, et al. Effect of internet support on the long-term maintenance of weight loss. Obes Res 2004; 12(2):320–329.

99. Wing RR, Tate DF, Gorin AA, et al. A self-regulation program for maintenance of weight loss. N Engl J Med 2006; 355:1563–1571.

100. Baum JG, Clark HB, Sandier J. Preventing relapse in obesity through post treatment maintenance systems: comparing the relative efficacy of two levels of therapist support. J Behav Med 1991; 14:287–302.

101. Perri MG, McAdoo WG, Spevak PA, et al. Effect of a multi-component maintenance program on long-term weight loss. J Consult Clin Psychol 1984; 52:480–481.

102. Perri MG, Shapiro RM, Ludwig WW, et al. Maintenance strategies for the treatment of obesity: an evaluation of relapse prevention training and posttreatment contact by mail and telephone. J Consult Clin Psychol 1984; 52:404–413.

103. Marlatt GA, George WH. Relapse prevention and the maintenance of optimal health. In: Shumaker SA, Schron EB, Ockene JK, et al., eds. The Handbook of Health Behavior Change. 2nd ed. New York: Springer, 1998:33–58.

104. Jeffery RW, Wing RR, Thorson C, et al. Strengthening behavioral interventions for weight loss: a randomized trial of food provision and monetary incentives. J Consult Clin Psychol 1993; 61:1038–1045.

105. Jeffery RW, Wing RR. Long-term effects of interventions for weight loss using food provision and monetary incentives. J Consult Clin Psychol 1995; 63:793–796.

106. Heymsfield SB, van Mierlo CA, van der Knaap HC, et al. Weight management using a meal replacement strategy: meta and pooling analysis from six studies. Int J Obes Relat Metab Disord 2003; 27(5):537–549.

107. Keogh JB, Clifton PM. The role of meal replacements in obesity treatment. Obes Rev 2005; 6(3):229–234.

108. Quinn, RD. Five-year self-management of weight using meal replacements: comparison with matched controls in rural Wisconsin. Nutrition 2000; 16:344–348.

109. Wall J, Mhurchu CN, Blakely T, et al. Effectiveness of monetary incentives in modifying dietary behavior: a review of randomized, controlled trials. Nutr Rev 2006; 64(12):518–531.

110. Wing RR, Jeffery RW, Burton LR, et al. Food provision vs structured meal plans in the behavioral treatment of obesity. Int J Obes Relat Metab Disord 1996; 20(1):56–62.

111. Anderson JV, Bybee DI, Brown RM, et al. 5 a day fruit and vegetable intervention improves consumption in a low income population. J Am Diet Assoc 2001; 101(2):195–202.

112. French SA, Jeffery RW, Story M, et al. Pricing and promotion effects on low-fat vending snack purchases: the CHIPS Study. Am J Public Health 2001; 91(1):112–117.

113. Wing RR, Jeffery RW. Benefits of recruiting participants with friends and increasing social support for weight loss and maintenance. J Consult Clin Psychol 1999; 67: 132–138.

114. Milsom VA, Perri MG, Rejeski WJ. Guided group support and the long-term management of obesity. In: Latner JD, Wilson GT, eds. Self-help for Obesity and Binge Eating. New York: Guilford Publications, Inc., 2006:205–222.

115. Wadden TA, Butryn ML, Byrne KJ. Efficacy of lifestyle modification for long-term weight control. Obes Res 2004; 12:151S–162S.

116. Rejeski WJ, Brawley LR, Ambrosius WT, et al. Older adults with chronic disease: the benefits of group mediated counseling in the promotion of physically active lifestyles. Health Psychol 2003; 22:414–423.

117. Foster GD, Wyat HR, Hill JO, et al. A randomized trial of a low-carbohydrate diet for obesity N Engl J Med 2003; 348:2082–2090.

118. Samaha FF, Iqbal N, Seshadri P, et al. A low-carbohydrate as compared with a low-fat diet in severe obesity. N Engl J Med 2003; 348:2074–2081.

119. Sondike SB, Copperman, N, Jacobson, MS. Effects of a low-carbohydrate diet on weight loss and cardiovascular risk factor in overweight adolescents J Pediatr. 2003; 142:253–258.

120. Brehm BJ, Seeley RJ, Daniels SR, et al. A randomized trial comparing a very low carbohydrate diet and a calorie-restricted low fat diet on body weight and cardiovascular risk factors in healthy women. J Clin Endocrinol Metab 2003; 88:1617–1623.

121. Gardner CD, Kiazand A, Alhassan S, et al. Comparison of the Atkins, Zone, Ornish, and LEARN diets for change in weight and related risk factors among overweight preme-nopausal women: the A to Z Weight Loss Study: a randomized trial. JAMA 2007; 297(9):969–977.

122. Harris JK, French SA, Jeffery RW, et al. Dietary and physical activity correlates of long-term weight loss. Obes Res 1994; 2:307–313.

123. Sherwood NE, Jeffery RW, French SA, et al. Predictors of weight gain in the Pound of Prevention study. Int J Obes 2000; 24:395–403.

124. McGuire M, Wing R, Klem M, et al. What predicts weight regain in a group of successful weight losers? J Consult Clin Psychol 1999; 67:177–185.

125. Jakicic JM, Marcus BH, Gallagher KI, et al. Effect of exercise duration and intensity on weight loss in overweight, sedentary women. A randomized trial. JAMA 2003; 290:1323–1330.

126. Hill JO, Wyatt HR. Role of physical activity in preventing and treating obesity. J Appl Physiol 2005; 99:765–770.

127. Schoeller DA, Shay K, Kushner RF. How much physical activity is needed to minimize weight gain in previously obese women. Am J Clin Nutr 1997; 66:551–556.

128. US Department of Health and Human Services. Physical activity and health: a report of the Surgeon General. Atlanta: US Department of Health and Human Services, Centers for Disease Control and Prevention, National Center for Chronic Disease Prevention and Health Promotion, 1996.

129. Wing RR. Physical activity in the treatment of the adulthood overweight and obesity: current evidence and research issues. Med Sci Sports Exerc 1999; 31:S547–S552.

130. Tate DF, Jeffery RW, Sherwood NE, et al. Long-term weight losses associated with prescription of higher physical activity goals. Are higher levels of physical activity protective against weight regain? Am J Clin Nutr 2007; 85(4):954–959.

131. Ashworth NL, Chad KE, Harrison EL, et al. Home versus center based physical activity programs in older adults. Cochrane Database Syst Rev 2005; 25(1):CD004017.

132. Jeffery RW, Wing RR, Thorson C, et al. Use of personal trainers and financial incentives to increase exercise in a behavioral weight-loss program. J Consult Clin Psychol 1998; 66:777–783.

133. Schmidt WD, Biwer CJ, Kalscheuer LK. Effects of long versus short bout exercise on fitness and weight loss in overweight females. J Am Coll Nutr. 2001; 20(5):494–501.

134. Quinn TJ, Klooster JR, Kenefick RW. Two short, daily activity bouts vs. one long bout: are health and fitness improvements similar over twelve and twenty-four weeks? J Strength Cond Res 2006; 20(1):130–135.

135. Perri MG, McAdoo WG, McAllister DA, et al. Enhancing the efficacy of behavior therapy for obesity: effects of aerobic exercise and a multicomponent maintenance program. J Consult Clin Psychol 1986; 54:670–675.

136. Li Z, Maglione M, Tu W, et al. Meta-analysis: pharmacologic treatment of obesity. Ann Intern Med. 2005; 142(7): 532–546.

137. Apfelbaum MD, Vague P, Ziegler O, et al. Long-term maintenance of weight loss after a very-low-calorie diet: a randomized blinded trial of the efficacy and tolerability of sibutramine. Am J Med 1999; 106:179–184.

138. James WPT, Astrup A, Finer N, et al. Effect of sibutramine on weight maintenance after weight loss: a randomized trial. Lancet 2000; 356:2119–2125.

139. Hill JO, Hauptman J, Anderson JW, et al. Orlistat, a lipase inhibitor, for weight maintenance after conventional dieting: a 1-year study. Am J Clin Nutr 1999; 69:1108–1116.

140. Torgerson JS, Hauptman J, Boldrin MN, et al. XENical in the prevention of diabetes in obese subjects (XENDOS) study: a randomized study of orlistat as an adjunct to lifestyle changes for the prevention of type 2 diabetes in obese patients. Diabetes Care 2004; 27(1):155–161.

141. Sjostrom L, Rissanen A, Andersen T, et al. Randomised placebo-controlled trial of orlistat for weight loss and prevention of weight regain in obese patients. European Multicentre Orlistat Study Group. Lancet 1998; 352 (9123):167–172.

142. Rinaldi-Carmona M, Barth F, Heaulme M, et al. Biochemical and pharmacological characterisation of SR141716A, the first potent and selective brain cannabinoid receptor antagonist. Life Sci 1995; 56(23–24):1941–1947.

143. Carai MAM, Colombo G, Gessa GL. Rimonabant: the first therapeutically relevant cannabinoid antagonist. Life Sci 2005; 77:2339–2350.

144. Boyd ST, Fremming BA. Rimonabant: a selective CB1 antagonist. Ann Pharmacother 2005; 39:684–690.

145. Despres JP, Golay A, Sjostrom L. Rimonabant in Obesity-Lipids Study Group. Effects of rimonabant on metabolic risk factors in overweight patients with dyslipidemia. N Engl J Med. 2005; 17353(20):2121–2134.

146. Van Gaal LF, Rissanen AM, Scheen AJ, et al. Effects of the cannabinoid-1 receptor blocker rimonabant on weight reduction and cardiovascular risk factors in overweight patients: 1-year experience from the RIO-Europe study. Lancet 2005; 365(9468):1389–1397.

147. Pi-Sunyer FX, Aronne LJ, Heshmati HM, et al. Effect of rimonabant, a cannabinoid-1 receptor blocker, on weight and cardiometabolic risk factors in overweight or obese patients: RIO-North America: a randomized controlled trial. JAMA 2006; 295(7):761–775.

148. Scheen AJ, Finer N, Hollander P, et al. Efficacy and tolerability of rimonabant in overweight or obese patients with type 2 diabetes: a randomized controlled study. Lancet 2006; 368(9548):1660–1672.

149. Padwal R, Li SK, Lau DCW. Long-term pharmacotherapy for overweight and obesity. Int J Obes Metab Disord 2003; 27:1437–1446.

150. Schnee DM, Zaiken K, McCloskey WW. An update on the pharmacological treatment of obesity. Curr Med Res Opin 2006; 22(8):1463–1474.

151. Simons-Morton DG, Obarzanek E, Cutler JA. Obesity research—limitations of methods, measurements, and medications. JAMA 2006; 295(7):826–828.

152. Miller WR, Rollnick S. Motivational Interviewing. New York: Guilford Press, 1991.

153. Smith DE, Heckmeyer CM, Kratt PP, et al. Motivational interviewing to improve adherence to a behavioral weight-control program for older obese women with NIDDM: a pilot study. Diabetes Care 1997; 20:52–54.

154. Beliard D, Kirschenbaum DS, Fitzgibbon ML. Evaluation of an intensive weight control program using a priori criteria to determine outcome. Int J Obes Relat Metab Disord 1992; 16:505–517.

155. Wadden TA, Foster GD. Behavioral assessment and treatment of markedly obese patients. In: Wadden TA, Van Itallie TB, eds. Treatment of the Seriously Obese Patient. New York: Guilford, 1992:290–330.

156. Wilson GT. Acceptance and change in the treatment of eating disorders and obesity. Behav Ther 1996; 27: 417–439.

157. Atkinson RL. Proposed standards for judging the success of the treatment of obesity. Ann Intern Med 1993; 119:677–680.

158. Hill JO, Drougas H, Peters JC. Obesity treatment: can diet composition play a role? Ann Intern Med 1993; 119: 694–697.

159. Insull W, Henderson M, Prentice R, et al. Results of a feasibility study of a low-fat diet. Arch Intern Med 1990; 150:421–427.

160. Paffenbarger RS, Lee IM. Physical activity and fitness for health and longevity. Res Q Exerc Sport 1996; 67:11–28.

161. Blackburn G. Effect of degree of weight loss on health benefits. Obes Res 1995; 3(suppl 2):211s–216s.

162. Wadden TA, Anderson DA, Foster GD. Two-year changes in lipids and lipoproteins associated with the maintenance of a 5% to 10% reduction in initial weight: some findings and some questions. Obes Res 1999; 7:170–178.

16

Diet Composition and Weight Loss

ANGELA P. MAKRIS and GARY D. FOSTER

Center for Obesity Research and Education, School of Medicine, Temple University, Philadelphia, Pennsylvania, U.S.A.

ARNE ASTRUP

Department of Human Nutrition, Faculty of Life Sciences, University of Copenhagen, Frederiksberg C, Denmark

INTRODUCTION

The perennial appearance of diet books on bestseller lists underscores the global perpetual search for the "best" weight loss diet. This search for novel approaches is driven in part by the limited long-term efficacy of the best clinic-based approaches to obesity treatment (1). It is also fueled by the public's perception that "experts can't make up their minds" when it comes to the best diet.

Currently, the best dietary strategy for tipping the energy balance equation in favor of weight loss is a matter of some debate among professionals and the public alike. During the last 20 years, there has been a focus on decreasing fat intake (2,3). This recommendation is guided by the high energy density of all dietary fat and the link between increased risk of chronic disease and saturated fat (4–6). Although low-calorie, low-fat approaches are effective in the short term, they have not proven to be sustainable for many living in an environment in which palatable, inexpensive, and high-fat foods are easily accessible (7). As such researchers have explored other means of reducing energy intake (e.g., manipulating the amount and/or type of carbohydrate and protein and altering the energy

density of the diet). Unfortunately, these approaches to weight loss have not proven to be any more sustainable than low-fat diets over the long term. While "energy in versus energy out" remains the cornerstone of obesity treatment, there is still controversy whether particular macronutrients or bioactive ingredients differentially affect satiety, thermogenesis, energy bioavailability, adherence, and other factors that would reduce energy intake, energy uptake, and energy expenditure, and shift energy balance. It is also unclear how diet affects the complex homeostatic systems that modulate appetite and energy balance.

This chapter reviews dietary approaches to obesity treatment, with an emphasis on the relative roles of fat, carbohydrate, and protein, as well as other nutrients with a putative role on energy balance. It begins with an overview of the general characteristics and functions of macronutrients. Then the relative effects of these macronutrients on hunger and satiety are discussed. In addition, the effects of unique characteristics of food, including glycemic index (GI) and energy density, on satiety and the regulation of energy balance are explored. Finally, the efficacy of various macronutrient- and micronutrient-based strategies for weight loss is examined.

GENERAL CHARACTERISTICS AND FUNCTIONS OF MACRONUTRIENTS

Dietary Fat

Dietary fat is a term used for a diverse group of water insoluble compounds (also referred to as lipids) that perform a variety of functions in the body as well as in food. Lipids deliver essential fatty acids that are vital for normal immune function and vision, carry fat soluble vitamins, comprise cell membranes, provide energy for immediate and long-term use, and contribute to satiety by delaying gastric emptying and by eliciting release of satiety hormones from the intestine. In addition, fats add flavor and texture to foods.

The most abundant type of fat in food (e.g., triglyceride) consists of a variety of fatty acids that differ in chain length and degree of saturation. Fatty acids are divided into two basic categories: saturated and unsaturated. Saturated fat is generally solid at room temperature and is most commonly found in animal sources (e.g., fat in whole milk, cheese, and butter). Monounsaturated and polyunsaturated fats are examples of unsaturated fats. Sources of monounsaturated fats include olive, canola (rapeseed), peanut oils, nuts, and avocados. Polyunsaturated fats can be found in corn, soybean, sunflower, safflower, and flaxseed oil, as well as fish.

Industrially produced *trans*-fatty acids are typically produced from vegetable oils by a hydrogenation process that makes them solid. The solid form makes the fat easier (and cheaper) to transport and store and has some functional advantages. Fats with high content of trans fat have therefore been used extensively by the food industry, and intakes have been up to 40 to 50 g/day in certain subsets of the population (8).

High saturated and trans fat intake can raise low-density cholesterol levels and increase the risk for cardiovascular disease (9,10). Due to increasing evidence that the industrially produced isomers may have adverse health effects, trans fats are gradually being eliminated from foods and are being replaced with healthier alternatives. Replacing saturated and trans fats with unsaturated fats, particularly monounsaturated fats, appears to lower cholesterol (i.e., low-density lipoprotein, LDL) and reduce the risk for cardiovascular disease (11). Two polyunsaturated fatty acids, linoleic acid and linolenic acid, are considered essential because the body cannot produce them. Thus, if not consumed in adequate amounts, symptoms of deficiency begin to appear. Consumption of approximately 4% of total energy intake from plant oils (e.g., about one tablespoon of oil) will prevent essential fatty acid deficiency (12).

Dietary fat can affect body weight regulation in a variety of ways. First, dietary fat (9 kcal/g) has more than double the energy of carbohydrate and protein (4 kcal/g each). Thus, reducing fat intake is an efficient way to reduce energy intake and create an energy deficit (13). This is the underlying concept behind low-fat diets, reduced-fat foods, and drugs that inhibit fat absorption.

Second, dietary fat is palatable. While good taste enhances the enjoyment of eating, it can undermine weight control. Flavor and taste are strong mediators of food intake (14). In one study, taste was rated as the most important determinant of food selection followed by cost, nutrition, convenience, and weight control (15). It has been demonstrated that intake of palatable high-fat foods can lead to overconsumption (16–20) without appropriate compensation (21,22). Moreover, high-fat preloads have been shown to increase the amount of fat consumed at a subsequent meal (23).

Protein

Protein is a unique macronutrient in that unlike fat or carbohydrate it provides the body with a usable form of nitrogen. Nitrogen is found in amino acids, the building blocks of protein. The amino acids that are consumed from food are used to synthesize a variety of proteins that have diverse functions in the body (i.e., enzymes, hormones, structural components, and antibodies).

As with some fatty acids, the body cannot produce certain amino acids; therefore, they are considered essential and must be obtained from the diet. Protein requirements vary as a function of one's age and health status. The goal for healthy adults is to maintain protein equilibrium. Assuming high-quality protein is consumed, protein equilibrium can be achieved on average by consuming 0.8 g of protein per kg of body weight per day (24). Requirements are generally greater for infants, children, adolescents, pregnant and lactating women, and athletes. The average American consumes approximately 1.2 g/kg/day (25).

Although protein appears to be an important promoter of satiety, excessive consumption can be associated with increased intake of saturated fat and cholesterol, if lean meat and meat products, low-fat dairy products, and vegetarian foods such as beans and lentils are not consumed. High protein intake also poses the risk of reduced consumption of carbohydrate-rich foods including whole grains, fruits, and vegetables, which are good sources of fiber, vitamins, and minerals (26). Reductions in potassium, calcium, and magnesium may have a negative effect on blood pressure (27,28), but increased calcium intake is normally achieved by a high-protein diet partly based on dairy products. Although there is no evidence that high-protein intake adversely affects kidney function in healthy adults, high-protein intake is contraindicated in those with mild renal insufficiency, renal disease, and diabetes, who are at risk of developing the condition (29).

Carbohydrate

Like fat, various forms of carbohydrate exist in food. Sugars (e.g., glucose, fructose, sucrose) are the simplest forms of carbohydrate. More complex carbohydrates are both digestible (i.e., multiple glucose units linked together like starch) and indigestible (i.e., fiber). Although simple sugars are readily consumed in the form of table sugar, soft drinks, and baked goods, they are also found in nutritionally rich foods such as fruits and milk. Fruits and vegetables also contain complex carbohydrates and dietary fiber. Whole grains and beans are also sources of dietary fiber. Most carbohydrates add flavor (e.g., sweetness) to food. Carbohydrates play an important role in inducing satiety. However, the primary function of dietary carbohydrate is to provide energy. Certain cells use glucose for energy exclusively (e.g., red blood cells and brain cells). As a survival mechanism during times of carbohydrate insufficiency, these cells (e.g., brain and heart cells) adapt to using ketones for energy, a condition referred to as ketosis. Consumption of 50 to 100 g of carbohydrate per day will prevent ketosis (30). Since protein, glycerol, and some organic acids can be converted to glucose, there is no absolute dietary requirement for carbohydrate (31). Like dietary fat, carbohydrate can positively and negatively affect weight regulation. Increased intake of fiber-rich foods can promote satiety; however, excess intake of digestible carbohydrate, like any other macronutrient, though the

in normal-weight women (33). Similarly, Holt et al. (34,35) found significant differences in energy consumption after individuals consumed six categories of foods varying in macronutrient content (e.g., fruits, bakery products, snack foods, carbohydrate-rich foods, protein-rich foods, breakfast cereals) but similar in energy content. Foods high in protein, fiber, and water content were more satiating than foods high in fat (34), and high-fat test foods were associated with higher daily fat and energy intakes than carbohydrate-rich test foods (35). The caloric content of the preloads was controlled and the weight of each preload was matched by adjusting water intake. However, other factors such as orosensory characteristics and visual cues were not controlled in these studies, which may have affected the results. To control for sensory characteristics (i.e., texture, taste) and cognitive factors (i.e., expectancy), Latner (36) and Rolls (16) utilized liquid and yogurt preloads, respectively, varying in macronutrient composition but similar in flavor. Intake and subjective ratings of hunger following the high-protein (72% protein) liquid meal was significantly less than intake after a high-carbohydrate (99% carbohydrate), but not the mixed macronutrient (36% protein, 55% carbohydrate), meal (36). In addition, high-carbohydrate yogurt preloads suppressed subsequent intake more than high-fat yogurt preloads (16). Considering dietary fat is energy dense, has weak effects on satiety, as well as has the greatest potential to trigger overeating, decreasing the proportion of fat in the diet is theoretically a logical strategy for managing appetite and caloric intake. These findings also suggest that increasing the proportion of protein in the diet may be one way to increase satiety and attenuate positive energy balance.

Gut Hormones

A variety of internal signals including neurotransmitters and central and peripheral neuropeptides are involved in appetite regulation and energy balance (37–40). These signals can be classified as short-acting satiation signals (e.g., neuropeptide Y, agouti-related peptide, ghrelin, cholecystokinin, melanocortins, glucagon-like peptide-1, peptide YY_{3-36}) and long-acting adiposity signals (e.g., insulin and leptin). Short-acting signals generally act rapidly to influence food intake while long-acting signals act more slowly to maintain the stability of fat stores. Peripheral signals may mediate the differences in satiation or satiety among macronutrients. Although the mechanisms are not well understood, there is some preliminary evidence suggesting that certain nutrients may produce a hormonal profile that favors positive energy balance.

Previous studies have reported that postprandial ghrelin secretion is differentially affected by macronutrient composition (41–46). One study compared the acute effects of different proteins (whey and casein) and carbohydrates (glucose and lactose) on appetite and appetite-regulatory hormones in 19 obese men (46). Four liquid preloads (1 MJ) containing whey (55 g), casein (55 g), lactose (56 g), or glucose (56 g) were consumed. Blood samples were taken at 15, 30, 45, 60, 90, 120, and 180 minutes after consumption of the preload. A buffet meal was served after the last blood sample. Bowen et al. reported that appetite and ad libitum energy intake were higher after consumption of the glucose-based liquid preload compared with the lactose- and protein (whey or casein)-based preloads. The glucose preload was also associated with an earlier return of ghrelin to fasting levels compared with the other preloads. These researchers suggest that the prolonged postprandial suppression of ghrelin of the protein preloads may explain in part the higher satiation associated with protein intake compared with glucose; however, some studies evaluating the effects of protein on ghrelin have reported increases or no change in ghrelin after protein intake (44,47–50). Differences in study design, macronutrient, and the physical state of the preload (i.e., liquid vs. solid) may reflect differences in findings.

Moran et al. compared the effects of isocaloric test meals differing in protein and fat on fasting and postprandial ghrelin in 57 overweight hyperinsulinemic adults before and after weight loss (49). Participants were randomly assigned an energy- (i.e., 6081 kJ/day) and carbohydrate-restricted (i.e., 37% of total energy), high-protein, low-fat (i.e., 34% protein, 29% fat) or low-protein, high-fat (i.e., 18% protein, 45% fat) diet, which they followed for 12 weeks. They consumed a diet with the same macronutrient composition for an additional four weeks but the caloric content was increased to achieve energy balance. At baseline and week 16, all participants completed a three-hour meal tolerance test. The test meal was the same macronutrient composition as the assigned diet. After 16 weeks, weight loss was similar with both groups. Fasting ghrelin increased and the postprandial ghrelin response improved with weight loss (i.e., the postprandial decrease in ghrelin was faster at week 16 compared with baseline and the decrease in ghrelin within the first 60 minutes was greater at week 16 compared with baseline). There were no significant differences in ghrelin concentrations as a function of diet; therefore, these data suggest that satiating effect of protein is not mediated by ghrelin.

Weigle et al. showed that compared with a two-week period of low-carbohydrate, moderate-fat (i.e., 45% of total energy as carbohydrate, 35% of total energy as fat) intake, plasma ghrelin levels were suppressed to a greater extent following a two-week period of a high-carbohydrate, low-fat diet (i.e., 65% of total energy as carbohydrate, 15% of total energy as fat) intake (41). Furthermore,

typical increases in plasma ghrelin during weight loss were not observed in individuals consuming a high-carbohydrate diet for 12 weeks (41). Similarly, greater reductions in ghrelin levels and hunger have been observed after an isocaloric high-carbohydrate breakfast compared with a high-fat breakfast (43). Given that glucose was the predominant carbohydrate in this study, these finding suggest that glucose and its effects on insulin may have suppressed ghrelin release. Teff et al. compared the effects of fructose and glucose on circulating levels of insulin, leptin, and ghrelin (51). In this study, participants consumed meals with either glucose- or fructose-containing beverages supplying 30% of total daily energy intake. This group found that ghrelin was less suppressed following consumption of a fructose beverage compared with a glucose beverage (51). Taken together, these findings suggest that altering the carbohydrate and fat composition of a diet, and more specifically, the type of carbohydrate consumed (i.e., glucose vs. fructose) may differentially affect ghrelin levels.

Studies have compared the effects of carbohydrate and fat on leptin secretion (41,52–54) but few have examined whether various types of carbohydrate differentially affect insulin, leptin concentrations, and food intake. It has been repeatedly demonstrated that high-fat diets reduce leptin sensitivity and 24-hour concentrations (41,52,53). In contrast, substitution of carbohydrate for fat has been shown to increase leptin sensitivity and increase both insulin secretion and leptin concentration over a 24-hour period (41,53). In addition to altering the amount of carbohydrate in the diet, others suggest that increasing protein from 15% to 30% of total energy increases leptin sensitivity (50). Teff et al. found that lower glucose and insulin responses as well as lower 24-hour circulating leptin concentrations were observed when fructose beverages were consumed with meals than when glucose beverages were consumed (51). Further research is needed to better understand the effects of macronutrients on internal signals that regulate appetite and energy balance.

Solids Vs. Liquids on Satiety

Interest in the relationship between intake of energy-yielding beverages and obesity has been increasing given observations from epidemiological and experimental studies, suggesting that intake of sweetened beverages and weight gain are linked (55–60). More specifically, these studies generally show inverse relationships with total sugar and body weight but positive associations between sugared soft drinks and body weight and obesity. It is hypothesized that beverages promote obesity not only by providing added calories but also by their poor ability to promote compensatory responses and satiety (61,62). It has been suggested that sugars in beverages may not possess the same satiating power as sugars in solid food (63,64). Drewnowski and Bellisle suggest that the latter belief rests on inconclusive evidence (65). There is also evidence to support that no differences in hunger ratings and/or subsequent energy intakes are observed following sugar-sweetened solid or liquid preloads (66).

Energy Density and Satiety

A concept that crosses all macronutrient categories is energy density. The energy density of a food is calculated simply by dividing energy content by amount. For example, the energy density of 80 g (i.e., ~½ cup) of grapes would be 0.75 kcal/g (i.e., 60 kcal/80 g). The energy density of the same portion of cheese would be 320 kcal/ 80 g or 4.0 kcal/g. Cheese is more energy-dense than grapes because it contains more energy for a similar weight of food. Given an equal amount of calories, an individual consuming a relatively low-energy-dense diet can eat a greater volume of food than an individual consuming a high-energy-dense diet. Figure 1 illustrates this point.

Reducing the energy density of a diet may be an effective weight management strategy considering individuals tend to eat a constant volume of food (67–69). Increasing the water and fiber content and reducing the fat of meals are two strategies for decreasing the energy content of a diet. Unfortunately, reducing the fat content also affects the flavor of food, so manufacturers often replace fat with significant amounts of carbohydrate in the form of sugar, often high-fructose corn syrup. Adding large amounts of carbohydrate will maintain or increase the energy density of a product. Some low-fat foods (e.g., melba toast, pretzels) can be as energy dense as high-fat foods (e.g., cheddar cheese) because of their low-moisture content (70). Thus, in terms of energy density, factors that affect the weight of food, including moisture and fiber

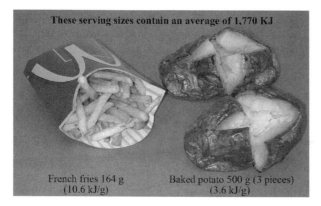

Figure 1 Differences in serving size as a function of energy density.

content, must be considered along with the caloric content. Otherwise, there is no benefit in eating certain low-fat foods because the end result will be the same— consumption of a significant amount of calories for a small weight of food.

In addition to macronutrient content and type, satiety appears to be influenced by energy density. There are a number of mechanisms by which energy density can affect satiety. One is through visual cues. Individuals make judgments regarding how full they will feel when they see a portion of food on a plate. A small portion may appear inadequate to some individuals, even if it is energy dense and packed with calories. This response is based on past eating experiences and learned behaviors. Another mechanism by which energy density can affect satiety is through volume and its effects on gastrointestinal distention and rate of gastric emptying. Mechanical (e.g., gastric stretch receptors) and chemical (e.g., peptides, hormones) signals from the gastrointestinal tract, in combination with dietary factors (e.g., caloric, macronutrient, fiber, and water content of food), can influence an individual's subjective evaluation of fullness, as well as physiological mechanisms that regulate food intake (71–73).

Several laboratory-based studies have evaluated the short-term effects of energy density on energy intake. These studies suggest that lowering the energy density, particularly by incorporating water into a food or recipe (as opposed to simply drinking water with a meal), is a more effective strategy for reducing food intake than altering the proportion of macronutrients in a meal (34,74–76). In a study in which macronutrient and energy content of a preload were held constant but energy density differed (by varying the water content), energy intake at a subsequent meal was significantly lower after consumption of a low-energy-dense preload compared with a high-energy-dense preload (74). Ratings of fullness corresponded with intake, and participants did not compensate for the reduced energy intake later in the day. Moreover, others have shown that energy intake increased with increasing energy density (68,76). Duncan et al. found that energy intake after consumption of energy-dense foods (e.g., meats, desserts) was twice as high as intake following low-energy-dense foods (e.g., fruit, vegetables, beans) (68). These findings suggest that individuals can feel satisfied eating fewer calories when they eat a standard weight of food.

DIETARY APPROACHES FOR THE TREATMENT OF OBESITY

The following section describes various dietary approaches to weight loss (i.e., low-, very low, and moderate-fat diets, low-carbohydrate diets, low-GI diets, high-protein diets, high-dairy diets). Descriptions of each approach are followed by a review of short- and long-term efficacy data. Studies prescribing macronutrient controlled ad libitum diets and macronutrient controlled energy-restricted diets are reviewed.

Lower-Fat Diets

Very Low Fat Diets

Some argue that a reduction in fat greater than 20% to 35% of calories is necessary for optimal health (77). Diets that provide <10% fat are defined as very low fat diets (78). Pritikin and Ornish diets are examples of very low fat diets. The Ornish diet is a plant-based diet and therefore encourages consumption of high complex carbohydrate, high-fiber foods (e.g., fruits, vegetables, whole grains), beans, soy, moderate amounts of reduced-fat dairy, eggs, and limited amounts of sugar and white flour (78). The Pritikin diet is similar. However, limited quantities of lean meats and fish are also allowed. The major difference between low- and very low fat diets is that the latter are more restrictive in terms of the types of foods permitted. Unlike low-fat plans that incorporate all foods, the very low fat diets strongly discourage consumption of foods containing high amounts of refined carbohydrate and/or fat such as sugar, high-fructose corn syrup, white flour, and rice.

The Lifestyle Heart Trial was a long-term randomized trial on 48 patients with coronary atherosclerosis that evaluated the effects of a very low fat diet and intensive lifestyle modification on the progression of this disease (79). Twenty participants were randomly assigned to an intervention group and 28 to a control group. The intervention group consumed a very low fat vegetarian diet and was prescribed a behavior modification program that included moderate aerobic activity, stress management, and smoking cessation. Those in the control group followed recommendations consistent with conventional guidelines for a healthy lifestyle (provided by their primary care physician).

Participants in the intervention group reduced their fat intake from 29.7% to 6.22% at one year. The decrease in the control group (30.5% to 28.8%) was less dramatic. Participants in the two groups lost 10.8 and 1.5 kg, respectively, at one year. Furthermore, there were significant differences in coronary artery outcomes. The average coronary artery percentage diameter stenosis in the intervention group decreased (i.e., 1.75 absolute percentage points) at one year, while it increased (i.e., 2.3 absolute percentage points) in the control group. These data suggest that a very low fat diet in combination with lifestyle change can result in regression of coronary atherosclerosis.

Low-Fat Diets

The *Dietary Guidelines for Americans* (along with My Pyramid) provides one example of a low-fat eating plan (80). The guidelines are based on the premise that a low-fat (20–30%), high-carbohydrate (55–60%) diet results in optimal health (81). By consuming a variety of foods and the recommended number of servings from each food group, individuals will meet their protein requirements, as well as their recommended daily allowances for vitamins and minerals, and consume adequate amounts of fiber. In addition, healthy limits on total fat, saturated fat, cholesterol, and sodium are encouraged. Other examples of a low-fat diet are the Dietary Approaches to Stop Hypertension (DASH) diet and those recommended by the American Diabetes Association (82), American Heart Association (83), and American Cancer Society (84), as well as commercial programs like Weight Watchers.

Low-fat diets are the best studied of all approaches to weight loss. It is generally recognized that a reduction of dietary fat content from 40% to 25% to 30% of energy intake under ad libitum conditions produces a 2- to 4-kg weight loss (85,86). Findings from the Women's Health Initiative trial (Table 1) comparing a low-fat diet with a control diet higher in fat suggest that an ad libitum reduced-fat (24–29% energy from fat) diet resulted in modest but greater weight loss during the first year of the trial and less weight gain over 7.5 years than the higher-fat (35–37% energy from fat) diet, despite the fact that neither group was instructed to lose weight (87). More specifically, the difference in weight between groups after the first year was 1.9 kg and after 7.5 years was 0.4 kg. Compliance to the low-fat diet was obviously poor during such a long period, but post hoc analysis of self-reported diet suggested that those who had reduced their fat intake had gained ~2 kg less than the control group after seven years. Similarly, three large multicenter randomized studies (i.e., the PREMIER trial, Diabetes Prevention Program, and the Finnish Diabetes Prevention study) have demonstrated that greater weight loss is achieved in groups consuming calorie-controlled low-fat diets compared with controls receiving standard lifestyle recommendations (88–90). Findings from these studies are summarized in Table 1.

The PREMIER trial investigated the effects of the DASH diet, a diet high in fruits and vegetables, fiber, and mineral content (such as calcium, magnesium, and potassium) and low in total and saturated fat and cholesterol and refined sugar. This diet was combined with recommendations known to individually lower blood pressure (i.e., sodium and alcohol restriction, exercise, and weight loss) and evaluated for reduction in weight loss and hypertension. Eight hundred and ten participants were randomly assigned to either a control group (single

Table 1 Summary of Findings from Low- and Moderate-Fat Studies

	PREMIER (88) (6-month data)	DPP (89) (6-month data)	Finnish Prevention (90) (12-month data)	McManus (99) (18-month data)	Women's Health Initiative (87) (7.5-year data)
Sample size (n)	810	3,234	522	101	48,835
Control	273	1,082	257	51	29,294
Intervention 1	268	1,079	265	50	19541
Intervention 2	269	1,073	N/A	N/A	N/A
Sex					
Male	310	1,043	172	10	N/A
Female	500	2,191	350	91	48,835
Age (yr)					
Control	49.5	50.3	55	44	62.3
Intervention 1	50.2	50.9	55	44	62.3
Intervention 2	50.2	50.6	N/A	N/A	N/A
Baseline BMI (kg/m^2)					
Control	32.9	34.2	31.0	33	29.1
Intervention 1	33.0	33.9	31.3	34	29.1
Intervention 2	33.3	33.9	N/A	N/A	N/A
Weight loss (kg)					
Control	−1.1	−0.1	−0.8	2.9	−0.1
Intervention 1	−4.9	−5.6	−4.2	−4.1	−0.8
Intervention 2	−5.8	−2.1	N/A	N/A	N/A

Premier: Intervention 1, established intervention; Intervention 2, established intervention plus DASH; Control, advice only
DPP: Intervention 1, intensive lifestyle group; Intervention 2, metformin; Control, placebo
Finnish PP: Intervention 1, detailed diet and exercise instruction in seven sessions during year 1; Control, diet and exercise information at baseline and annual visit
McManus: Intervention 1, moderate fat; Control, low fat
Women's Health Initiative: Intervention, group and individual sessions to promote decreases in fat and increases in fruits, vegetables, and whole grains; Control, diet-related education.
Abbreviations: DPP, Diabetes Prevention Program; BMI, body mass index.

advice-giving session for consuming a DASH diet) or one of two intervention groups. One intervention group instructed participants to reduce calories through the DASH diet (Established Intervention plus DASH) and exercise. The other group encouraged calorie restriction and exercise (Established Intervention) alone. Both intervention groups included behavior modification instruction.

There were significant differences in dietary intake and weight loss between the control and intervention groups at six months. The Established Intervention plus DASH group consumed more fruits and vegetables and dairy products than the other two groups. Significantly greater weight losses were observed in the Established Intervention and the Established Intervention plus DASH groups compared with the control group at six months (Table 1). There were no significant differences in weight loss between the Established Intervention and Established Intervention plus DASH groups.

The Diabetes Prevention Program was a 27-center randomized clinical trial that evaluated the effects of lifestyle intervention and pharmacotherapy on the incidence of type 2 diabetes in individuals with impaired glucose tolerance (89). In this study, 3234 overweight participants were randomly assigned to one of three

groups: (*i*) placebo plus standard lifestyle recommendations, (*ii*) metformin plus standard lifestyle recommendations, and (*iii*) intensive lifestyle intervention. Participants in the medication and placebo group were provided written information on the Food Guide Pyramid and the National Cholesterol Education Program Step 1 diet and were seen annually in individual sessions. Participants in the lifestyle intervention group were prescribed fat (i.e., less than 25% of calories) and calorie goals and were asked to monitor their intake daily. Calorie levels were based on initial body weight and were designed to produce a weight loss of 0.5 to 1.0 kg/wk.

Participants in the intensive lifestyle group lost significantly more weight than those in the metformin and placebo groups (Table 1). The intensive lifestyle group also had a significantly lower incidence of type 2 diabetes than the placebo or metformin groups at one year.

Similar to the Diabetes Prevention Program, the Finnish Diabetes Prevention study investigated the ability of lifestyle intervention to prevent or delay the onset of type 2 diabetes in 522 overweight participants with impaired glucose tolerance (90). Participants were randomly assigned either a control group, which received verbal and written diet and exercise information at baseline and at annual visits, or to an intervention group, which was provided detailed dietary and exercise instructions in seven sessions with a nutritionist during the first year and every three months after the first year. These latter participants were instructed to consume less than 30% of energy from fat (i.e., consuming low-fat dairy and meat products), less than 10% from saturated fat (i.e., increase consumption of vegetable oils rich in monounsaturated fat), 15 g/1000 kcal of fiber from whole grain products, vegetables, berries, and other fruits. They were also told to engage in moderate activity for 30 minutes or more per day.

Results showed that there was a significantly greater reduction in the incidence of type 2 diabetes and greater weight loss in the intervention group. Greater reductions in mean body weight were observed in the intervention group compared with the control group in the first year and remained significantly greater in the intervention group than after two years (Table 1). Subsequent post hoc analyses from both studies found that the best predictor of retained weight loss and diabetes protection was achieved by the reduction in dietary fat content (91).

Taken together, these findings suggest that consumption of a low-fat, low-calorie diet, in the context of intensive group and/or individual counseling and physical activity, is an effective strategy for weight management. In addition, low-fat diets are associated with health benefits, such as reduced incidence of diabetes and improved control of hypertension (92). Given these findings, should health professionals recommend low-fat diets over other diets for the long-term treatment of obesity? In their review of six randomized controlled trials comparing low-fat diets with other weight-reducing diets (i.e., low-carbohydrate, moderate-fat, energy-restricted diets), Pirozzo et al. reported that low-fat diets are no more efficacious than other diets in the long term (93). Swinburn et al. reported that weight loss in diabetics eating a low-fat diet after one year was 3.3 kg; however, when data were stratified according to compliance, more-compliant participants (defined as those who had better group attendance and completion of food records) lost 6 kg compared with less-compliant participants who lost 1 kg after one year (94). These findings clearly suggest that frequent contact with health professionals and self-monitoring improves outcome. The challenge that health professionals face is how to help individuals maintain behaviors that support low-fat eating over the long term when contact with health professionals is limited.

A major limitation of these studies is that the control and intervention groups did not receive the same number of treatment visits. Participant-clinician contact and instruction were greater in the intervention groups. It can also be argued that these studies do not simulate treatment in the "real" world because of their high intensity and frequency. While not effectiveness studies, these

well-designed efficacy studies show that low-calorie, low-fat, high-fiber diets have positive effects on weight control and, more importantly, on comorbid conditions.

Implementation of lower fat diets and safety considerations

If fat is reduced from 40% to 10% to 30% of energy intake and protein is held constant at 15%, the percentage of carbohydrate consumed increases from 45% to 55% to 75%. Given that fat may promote satiety by delaying gastric emptying, replacing fat with fiber-rich carbohydrates, also known to delay nutrient absorption, may be an effective strategy for managing appetite and promoting health. This can be achieved by increasing intake of whole grain bread and pasta, brown or wild rice, beans, and vegetables, and replacing highly refined carbohydrate-containing foods like sugary cereals, instant oatmeal, and low-fat/high-calorie baked goods with whole grain cereal, steel cut oatmeal, and fruit for dessert. Although the flavor and texture of foods may be compromised when fat is reduced, these characteristics are not necessarily lost when unrefined foods are consumed since they contain many unique flavors and textures of their own.

Dietary changes such as these may lead to reductions in total energy and body weight and improvements in lipid parameters. Few safety concerns emerge with low-fat diets; however, reducing fat intake below 4% of total energy intake may increase risk of essential fatty acid deficiency. Unless increased gradually, very high fiber diets may result in gastrointestinal distress. The efficacy of very low fat diets for long-term weight management remains uncertain however because adherence to these dietary and lifestyle recommendations outside of clinical trials is unknown.

Moderate-Fat Diets

While many argue that intake of 30% fat or less is the most favorable approach for treating obesity and preventing chronic disease, others note that many European countries with relatively high percentages of fat intake (e.g., France, Italy) have a low prevalence of obesity (95) and lower rates of cardiovascular disease (96,97) and mortality (98–100). Moreover, there is some evidence to suggest that individuals who follow a diet higher in fat may be better able to sustain weight losses over the long-term compared with those who adhere to a diet lower in fat (101).

Mediterranean diets are considered moderate-fat diets because they generally contain over 30% of total calories from fat (102,103), although the percentage of fat can range from 26% to 42% of total calories from fat. Mediterranean diets differ depending on the region of the Mediterranean from which they originate. Despite differences in the total percentage of fat, Mediterranean diets generally contain a higher proportion of monounsaturated fat and ω-3 fatty acids than Western diets. A traditional Mediterranean diet is rich in natural whole foods and relies heavily on foods from plant sources like fruits, vegetables (including wild types such as purslane), legumes, breads and grains, and nuts and seeds. These plant foods along with olive oil and low-to-moderate amounts of cheese, yogurt, and wine are consumed daily (104). Rather than red meat, fish, chicken, and eggs are consumed on a weekly basis. The diet is low in saturated and trans fat due to limited intakes of butter, red meat, and processed foods. Fresh or dried fruit with nuts (e.g., figs stuffed with walnuts) is viewed as a typical daily dessert rather than commercially baked foods.

Few studies have evaluated the effects of moderate-fat diets on weight (105). McManus et al. (101) examined the effects of a moderate-fat diet (35% of total energy) and a lower-fat control diet (20% of total energy) in 101 overweight men and women. Women were instructed to consume 1200 kcal/day while men were asked to consume 1500 kcal/day in both groups. All subjects participated in weekly behavior modification sessions. There were no differences between the moderate-fat and low-fat groups in weight loss at 6 and 12 months. However, at 18 months they were significantly different because participants in the intervention group maintained their weight loss while the low-fat group regained weight (Table 1). Furthermore, there were greater reductions in percentage body fat and waist circumference in the intervention group. No difference in body weight was observed after three months in another study comparing the effects of an ad libitum Mediterranean diet and ad libitum low-fat diet (106).

Due et al. (107) compared the effects of three ad libitum diets varying in the type of fat and carbohydrate in the prevention of weight gain. One hundred thirty-one nondiabetic overweight or obese adults followed an energy-restricted diet for eight weeks and then were randomized to one of three diets for six months: (*i*) monounsaturated fatty acids (MUFA) diet consisting of 40% energy from fat (20% monounsaturated fatty acids) and low-GI foods, (*ii*) low-fat diet consisting of 25% energy from fat and medium-GI foods, or (*iii*) control diet consisting of 35% fat and high-GI foods. An average weight loss of approximately 13 kg was observed after the eight-week energy restriction phase. Weight was regained after six months but there were no significant differences in regain among the three groups. These findings suggest that diets higher in fat are as effective as low-fat diets in preventing weight regain.

Implementation of moderate-fat diets and safety considerations

Moderate-fat and relatively low-fat Mediterranean diets are less studied for weight loss but have impressive risk-reducing effects on cardiovascular disease (i.e., decreasing markers of vascular inflammation and lipids) and type 2 diabetes (i.e., improving insulin sensitivity) and have been shown to decrease mortality from cardiovascular disease, coronary heart disease, and cancer (70,71,108,109). Shifting the focus from low fat to eating more nuts, fish, and unsaturated oils (so-called healthy fats) and focusing on portion control may be a more enjoyable and sustainable approach to weight management for some people. Additional studies comparing the effects of low-fat and moderate-fat diets on weight loss, satiety, and adherence would help clarify the amount of fat that is most effective for long-term weight control and health.

In summary, many studies have assessed the effects of fat intake on weight loss. Compared with very low-fat and moderate-fat diets, low-fat diets are the best studied. These diets have been shown to be effective in treating obesity and preventing disease. Although the low-fat diet is an effective weight loss strategy, there are questions concerning long-term adherence. The moderate-fat Mediterranean diet is less studied for weight loss and maintenance but has impressive effects on the prevention of disease (99).

HIGH-PROTEIN DIETS

There is no standard definition of a "high-protein diet"; however, intakes of 25% total energy or greater or of 1.6 g/kg/day can be considered high (110). The Zone diet (30% protein, 40% carbohydrate, and 30% fat) is an example of a high-protein diet. The most prominent difference between a high-protein diet such as the Zone and a low-carbohydrate diet like the Atkins New Diet Revolution is that a high-protein diet is typically low in fat.

A limited number of studies have investigated the effects of high-protein diets on weight loss. In one study, 50 overweight and obese [body mass index (BMI) of 25–35 kg/m^2] individuals were randomly assigned to an ad libitum low-protein diet (12% protein, 30% fat, 58% carbohydrate) or a high-protein regimen (25% protein, 30% fat, 45% carbohydrate) (111). During the first six months of the study, foods were provided to ensure that the prescribed diet was consumed. Between months 6 to 12, foods were no longer provided but participants were asked to maintain their dietary prescription and attend biweekly group behavior therapy sessions.

The high-protein group lost significantly more weight than the low-protein group after six months (−9.4 kg vs. −5.9 kg). Not surprisingly, the high-protein group had a greater decrease than the low-protein group in waist circumference, waist-to-hip ratio, and intra-abdominal adipose tissue (assessed by dual-energy X-ray absorptiometry). At the 24-month assessment, the former group continued to have a greater weight loss than the latter group (-6.4 kg vs. -3.2 kg) but this difference was not significant because a large number of participants were lost to follow-up.

These findings suggest that although participants in the high-protein group regained weight after six months, there was a trend toward better weight maintenance in these individuals. The authors speculated that the greater weight loss in the high-protein group may have been attributable to the satiating effect of protein, to smaller reductions in resting energy expenditure, or to greater diet-induced thermogenesis. In addition to weight loss, there was a greater reduction in waist circumference, waist-to-hip ratio, and intra-abdominal adipose tissue even after weight was regained, which is important because these measures are highly correlated with certain chronic conditions such as cardiovascular disease. Similarly, Skov et al. (112) and Parker et al. (113) reported greater total fat and intra-abdominal fat losses in individuals following high-protein ad libitum or energy-restricted diets for three to six months, while others reported no differences in total or intra-abdominal fat as a function of diet condition (114,115).

Other studies have also reported that high-protein diets are superior to high-carbohydrate diets in reducing hunger, body weight, preserving lean body mass, and promoting fat loss (112,116–119). In one study in which macronutrient composition was controlled but quantity was unrestricted, reductions in body weight (i.e., 8.7 kg vs. 5.0 kg) and intra-abdominal adipose tissue (33.0 cm^2 vs. 16.8 cm^2) were significantly greater in the high-protein group (i.e., 46% carbohydrate, 25% protein, and 29% fat) compared with the high-carbohydrate group (e.g., 59% carbohydrate, 12% protein, and 29% fat) at six months (112). The decrease in energy intake in the latter study was not associated with increased ratings of hunger. Another study showed that slightly overweight adults (BMI 26.2 $\pm$ 2.1 kg/m^2) reported decreases in hunger and increases in fullness, experienced spontaneous decreases in caloric intake of approximately 500 kcal/day, and had a weight loss of 4.9 $\pm$ 0.5 kg after consuming an ad libitum 30% protein diet for 12 weeks, despite the fact that this was not a weight-reduction study and participants were excluded if they expressed any interest in losing weight (120). Farnsworth et al. found that women who consumed a high-protein diet lost significantly less lean body mass after 16 weeks than women who ate a standard protein diet (116). The researchers stated that the high-protein diet provided women approximately 1.4 g protein/kg ideal body weight, a level sufficient to suppress proteolysis in women but not in men, as it only provided approximately 1.1 g protein/kg ideal body weight for men. Intakes of 1.5 g protein/kg ideal body weight have also been shown to prevent loss of lean body mass (118,121).

Westerterp-Plantenga and colleagues investigated whether addition of protein to a diet improves weight maintenance by preventing or limiting weight regain after weight loss (122). One hundred and forty-eight overweight (BMI 29.5 $\pm$ 2.5 kg/m^2) adults followed a very low-energy diet (2.1 MJ/day) for four weeks and were then randomized to a high-protein (18% energy from protein) or control group (15% energy from protein) for an additional 12 weeks. Body weight, body composition, and leptin concentrations were measured. Total body water (TBW) was measured using the deuterium dilution technique and fat-free mass was calculated by dividing the TBW by a hydration factor. Fat mass was obtained by subtracting fat-free mass from total body weight.

Significant differences in weight and body composition were observed between the high-and low-protein groups. Participants in the high-protein group regained less weight at three months than those in the low-protein group (i.e., 1 kg vs. 2 kg). Reductions in fat mass were significantly greater at three months in the high-protein group compared with the low-protein group while reductions in fat-free mass were significantly less in the high-protein group compared with the low-protein group, suggesting that a greater percentage of the weight regained in the high-protein group was fat-free mass compared with the low-protein group. Leptin concentrations were significantly lower in the high-protein group compared with the low-protein group at three months, which may reflect differences in fat mass between groups. These researchers conclude that higher protein intake during weight maintenance is more effective in limiting weight regain and regain of fat mass than lower protein intakes (122).

When studied under isocaloric conditions, high- and low-protein diets appear to be equally effective at reducing weight. Luscombe-Marsh et al. (123) compared the effects of a high-protein, low-fat (i.e., 34% protein, 29% fat, 37% carbohydrate) diet and a lower-protein, high-fat (i.e., 18% protein, 45% fat, 37% carbohydrate) diet on weight loss over 12 weeks of energy restriction (30% restriction of total energy) in 57 overweight and obese individuals. Weight loss was not significantly different between the high-protein (-9.7 ± 1.1 kg) and low-protein (-10.2 ± 1.4 kg) groups. Bone turnover and calcium excretion did not change significantly. Brinkworth et al. (124) compared a high-protein, low-fat diet (i.e., 30% protein, 30% fat, 40% carbohydrate) with a low-protein, low-fat diet (i.e., 15% protein, 30% fat, 55% carbohydrate) during 12 weeks of energy restriction ($\sim$6.5 MJ/day) in 58 obese hyperinsulinemic individuals. After 12 weeks, weight ($-9.1\% \pm 0.7\%$ in the low-protein group and $-8.7\% \pm 0.7\%$ in the high-protein group) and fat mass decreased by a similar amount in both groups. There was a significant regain in weight by week 68 but there were no differences between groups ($-2.9\% \pm 0.8\%$ in the low-protein group and $-4.1\% \pm 1.3\%$ in the high-protein group).

Taken together, these studies suggest that energy-restricted high- and low-protein diets are equally effective in producing weight loss in the short term; however, replacing some dietary carbohydrate with protein results in greater weight loss in the context of an ad libitum low-fat diet (125). Although further research is needed, findings from ad libitum studies suggest that it may be easier for individuals to consume fewer calories when following a high-protein, low-fat diet than a low-protein, low-fat diet because they feel more satiated during and between meals. If proven to be true, high-protein diets may be more efficacious than low-protein diets for long-term weight maintenance. There is also some evidence to suggest that diets higher in protein are better at preserving lean body mass and may facilitate regain of fat-free mass rather than fat mass, which is favorable because lean mass is more metabolically active than adipose tissue (116,118,121).

Implementation of a high protein diet and safety considerations

If protein is increased in the diet from standard recommended levels of 10% to 15% of total energy to 25% to 30%, respectively, and fat is held constant at 30% of total energy, the percentage of carbohydrate consumed is reduced to 40% to 45% of total energy. Given that carbohydrates rich in fiber contribute to satiety, replacing refined carbohydrate with protein would be preferable to replacing fiber-rich carbohydrate with protein. More specifically, the shift in the proportion of protein and carbohydrate in the diet could be achieved by replacing soft drinks containing refined sugar with high-protein beverages like milk and shifting the proportion of carbohydrate (i.e., smaller portions of white bread, rice, and pasta) and protein (i.e., larger portions of lean meat, fish, and beans) during meals (126). These dietary changes may lead to a spontaneous reduction in total energy consumed and body weight.

Unless lean protein sources are consumed and intake of unrefined carbohydrate is maintained, high protein intake may result in increases in intake of saturated fat and cholesterol and reduced consumption of fiber, vitamins, and minerals (i.e., potassium, calcium, and magnesium), which could negatively impact cardiovascular, bone, and kidney function. Although these are reasonable possibilities, many studies suggest that replacement of some carbohydrate by protein has a neutral or even positive influence on inflammation, risk factors for type 2 diabetes, cardiovascular disease, and osteoporosis (123,127). Beneficial effects on weight and LDL cholesterol have been observed even in diabetic patients without renal failure (113).

LOW-CARBOHYDRATE DIETS

Standard Low-Carbohydrate Diet

Many versions of the low-carbohydrate diet exist (e.g., Atkins New Diet Revolution, South Beach diet), each with a unique interpretation of optimal low-carbohydrate eating. Unlike low-fat diets, the FDA has not established a clear definition for "low carbohydrate." Much attention has focused on the high fat and protein content of the diet. However, the focus of low-carbohydrate diets, as the name implies, is on carbohydrate, not fat or protein. Low-carbohydrate approaches encourage consumption of controlled amounts of nutrient-dense carbohydrate-containing foods (i.e., low-GI vegetables, fruits, and whole grain products) and eliminate intake of carbohydrate-containing foods based on refined carbohydrate (i.e., white bread, rice, pasta, cookies, and chips). Although consumption of foods that do not contain carbohydrate (i.e., meats, poultry, fish, as well as butter and oil) is not restricted, the emphasis is on moderation and quality rather than quantity.

Six randomized studies conducted over 6 to 12 months have compared the effects of a low-carbohydrate diet and a calorie-controlled, low-fat diet on weight and body composition in obese adults (128–134). (Note that the Samaha and Stern papers refer to the same study but report 6- and 12-month data, respectively.) With the exception of one study that prescribed nutritional supplements including vitamins, minerals, essential oils, and chromium picolinate to the low-carbohydrate group but not the low-fat group (132), diet prescriptions in these studies were comparable (e.g., a low-carbohydrate diet containing 20–60 g of carbohydrate). BMI and ages ranged from 33 to 43 kg/m^2 and 43 to 54 years, respectively, in all studies. While there were many similarities in diet prescriptions and participant characteristics, a few differences emerged. The majority of the studies consisted of female participants (128,129,132–134) except for one (130,131). Comorbidities and amount of clinician contact also differed slightly among these studies. Three of the investigations evaluated effects in obese but otherwise healthy adults (128,129,133), three examined effects in adults with significant comorbidities such as diabetes, metabolic syndrome (129,130), hyperlipidemia (132), and other cardiovascular risk factors (133). Treatment occurred primarily in a self-help setting in one study (128) and in individual and/or group treatment in the others (129–133). Only four studies evaluated effects at one year (128,131,133,134). Findings of these studies are summarized in Table 2.

Participants who consumed a low-carbohydrate diet lost significantly more weight than those who consumed a low-fat diet during the first six months of treatment in

Table 2 Summary of Findings from Low-Carbohydrate Studies

	Brehm (129) (6-month data)	Yancy (132) (6-month data)	Stern (131) (12-month data)	Foster (128) (12-month data)	Dansinger (133) (12-month data)	Gardner (134) (12-month data)
Sample size (n)	53	119	132	63	80	156
LC	26	59	64	33	40	77
C	27	60	68	30	40	79
Sex						
Male	N/A	28 (15 LC/13C)	109 (51 LC/58C)	20 (12 LC/8 C)	36 (19 LC/17 C)	N/A
Female	53 (26 LC/27C)	91 (44 LC/47C)	23 (13 LC/10 C)	43 (21 LC/22C)	44 (21 LC/23C)	156 (77 LC/79C)
Age (yr)						
LC	44.2	44.2	53.0	44.0	47.0	42.0
C	43.1	45.6	54.0	44.2	49.0	40.0
Baseline BMI (kg/m^2)						
LC	33.2	34.6	42.9	33.9	35.0	32.0
C	34.0	34.0	42.9	34.4	35.0	31.0
Weight loss (% change)						
LC	−9.3	−12.9	−3.9	−7.3	−3.9	−5.5
C	−4.2	−6.7	−2.3	−4.5	−4.8	−2.9

Abbreviations: LC, low carbohydrate; C, conventional diet; BMI, body mass index.

four of the studies (128–130,132). Despite differences at six months, there were no differences in weight loss at one year (128,131,133,134) (Table 2). Two studies (128,133) observed weight regain in both groups after six months with a greater regain in the low-carbohydrate group. While participants in the low-carbohydrate group did not regain weight in the third one-year study, those in the low-fat group continued to lose weight after six months, resulting in similar weight losses at one year (131).

Data from the studies described above suggest that although participants in the low-carbohydrate group were not instructed to limit their energy intake, as were individuals in the conventional group, the low-carbohydrate group consumed fewer calories (129,132). Thus, at six months, subjects who were instructed to count carbohydrate consumed fewer calories than those who were instructed to count calories. The reason for this is unknown but may include greater satiety on a higher-protein, low-GI diet. In a small inpatient study examining the effects of a low-carbohydrate diet on body weight, energy intake, and expenditure in 10 obese diabetic patients, Boden et al. (135) reported that weight loss (i.e., −1.65 kg) was completely accounted for by a reduction in caloric intake. Mean energy intake in this two-week study decreased from 3111 kcal/day to 2164 kcal/day. Greater weight loss may also be the result of the increased structure (i.e., clear boundaries about what foods are allowed result in eating fewer calories). Structured approaches, including meal replacements and food provision, have been shown to increase the magnitude of weight loss (136–141).

Although few in number, it is interesting to note that findings are remarkably consistent despite differences across studies (e.g., gender, comorbid conditions, and clinician contact). These initial results are encouraging but very preliminary and do not signal a call for revised dietary guidelines. Limitations of these studies include small sample sizes, high attrition, and short duration of treatment and assessments limited to glycemic control and lipids. These preliminary data need to be replicated in larger and longer trials that include more comprehensive assessment of compliance (i.e., urinary nitrogen excretion), safety including measures of bone, renal, and endothelial function.

Implementation of a low carbohydrate diet and safety considerations

A principal concern about low-carbohydrate approaches is that the high-fat content of the diet may adversely affect serum lipids and increase the risk for cardiovascular disease. Preliminary findings challenge this argument. In studies that compared low-carbohydrate and low-fat diets over the course of 6 to 12 months there were no differences in total cholesterol or LDL cholesterol concentrations among groups (128–132). One study reported that the low-carbohydrate diet was less effective than the low-fat diet in reducing total cholesterol and LDL cholesterol at one year (133). Only one study reported a small transient increase in total cholesterol and LDL cholesterol during the third month of a one-year treatment (128). Furthermore, compared with the conventional group, those in the low-carbohydrate group experienced greater improvements in high-density lipoprotein (HDL) cholesterol (128,132) and triglycerides (128–130,132). Only one study reported decreases in HDL cholesterol in participants following a low-carbohydrate diet but the decrease was less than the decrease in the low-fat group (131). It is worth noting that in the Yancy et al. study, two subjects in the low-carbohydrate group withdrew because of high LDL levels while none did so in the low-calorie group. These small numbers are difficult to interpret, but they suggest that mean values may obscure important individual differences. A meta-analysis of these data suggests that while the low-carbohydrate diet produced more favorable changes in triglycerides and HDL cholesterol concentrations, the low-fat diet produced more favorable changes in total cholesterol and LDL cholesterol concentrations (142). As such, further research is needed to understand whether the improvements in triglycerides and HDL concentrations outweigh the relatively smaller effects low-carbohydrate diets have on total and LDL cholesterol as compared with low-fat diets. No significant differences in blood pressure were observed among groups in any of the studies.

Low-GI Diet

Carbohydrates vary in the degree to which they raise blood glucose and insulin levels. The term "glycemic index" refers to a property of carbohydrate-containing foods that affects the change in blood glucose following food consumption (143). GI is a value calculated by dividing the incremental area under the glucose response curve after consumption of a standard 50 g portion of a test food (during a two-hour period) by the area under the curve after consumption of an equal portion of a control substance (e.g., white bread or glucose) (143,144). Carbohydrate-containing foods are ranked in relation to glucose or white bread, which both have a GI of 100. Thus, foods with a GI between 0 and 55 are considered low-GI foods (e.g., apple, beans), those with a GI of 70 or greater are considered high-GI foods (e.g., corn flakes, potatoes), and those that fall between these two ranges are categorized as intermediate-GI foods (e.g., raisins, boiled long grain rice). A variety of factors such as carbohydrate type, amount and type of fiber, degree of processing, cooking, storage, acidity, food structure, and macronutrient content can all affect GI.

Glycemic load (GL) is another concept related to GI. Unlike GI, which predicts the impact of a standard amount of carbohydrate (i.e., 50 g portion) on blood glucose levels, GL predicts the impact of various types and amounts of carbohydrate-containing food on blood glucose levels. GL is calculated by multiplying the GI value of a food by the amount of carbohydrate in a normal serving size (as opposed to a standard serving size). The product is then divided by 100. It is important to understand the distinction and underlying principle behind these two concepts. The 50-g portion was selected to standardize the glycemic response to various foods since the glycemic response increases with increasing amounts of carbohydrate up to 50 g (145). However, since individuals do not usually consume the large portions of carbohydrate used in GI testing, GL was developed to understand better the differences in glycemic response following intake of more realistic servings of carbohydrate-containing foods. Although some feel that GL is a more accurate measure of glycemic response than GI, there is debate about its validity.

Some investigators believe that high-GI foods or meals disrupt homeostatic mechanisms and spawn undesirable endocrine and metabolic responses such as hyperinsulinemia, hypoglycemia, increased hunger, and hyperphagia (146). More specifically, the high insulin-glucagon ratio (caused by the rapid spike in glucose from a high-GI meal) causes metabolic processes to shift from oxidation toward nutrient storage and blood sugar levels to drop below normal physiological ranges. Together these effects are thought to increase hunger and result in weight gain. However, clinical trials comparing low- and high-GI diets have not provided convincing evidence of any clinically relevant advantage of low-GI diets for appetite and body weight control (147).

GI Methodology and GI of Mixed Meals

As consumption of carbohydrate has increased, more attention has been focused on the impact of high- and low-GI foods on food intake and obesity. The glycemic response to a certain food is influenced by numerous factors that make the prediction of the GI value of a meal from table values very complex, and according to some studies, unreliable. Since GI varies by shelf life, storage, preparatory methods, and finally by incorporation into mixed meals, even GI testing of individual products will not guarantee a valid prediction of the GI value. For example, a recent study measured GI of eight different potato varieties, all served freshly boiled, and demonstrated GI values ranging from 56 to 94, showing wide variations simply among varieties (148). On top of that come differences in methods in preparation and storing that further increase the variation of GI, as exemplified in a recent study demonstrating a 25% decrease in the GI of potatoes following cold storage (149). Finally, incorporation into a meal with protein and fat will make prediction of the glycemic response highly unreliable (150).

Effects of GI on Satiety and Weight Loss

It has been suggested that low-GI foods, (i.e., those foods that produce smaller changes in glucose and insulin response), are more desirable in part because they prolong satiety. The claim that low-GI foods have a positive effect on obesity is partly based on the assumption that reduction of postprandial glucose and insulin responses will decrease carbohydrate oxidation and fat storage and increase fat oxidation. Furthermore, lower and slower glucose and insulin responses are believed to promote satiety and suppress hunger, because large increases in blood glucose and insulin may subsequently induce hypoglycemia, which leads to increased hunger. However, experimental evidence has failed to substantiate that link (151,152).

Roberts reported that compared with low-GI meals, individuals consume approximately 29% more energy following high-GI meals (143). Ludwig et al. (153) compared the effects of three isocaloric breakfasts varying in GI on subsequent food intake and a variety of metabolic parameters including glycemic response. The area under the glycemic response curve of the high-GI meal was two times higher than the medium-GI meal and four times higher than the low-GI meal. Energy intake during a subsequent meal (lunch) was significantly higher after the high-GI meal compared with the medium- and low-GI meals. Furthermore, latency to the next meal request after lunch was significantly less after the high-GI lunch compared with the low-GI lunch. These findings suggest that low-GI diets may potentially be efficacious in reducing both energy intake and frequency of eating.

In contrast to these findings, Ball et al. (154) did not observe any significant differences in energy consumed following a high-GI meal replacement, low-GI meal replacement, or a low-GI whole food meal. The authors did observe a decreased latency between the test meal and the next request for food after the high-GI meal replacement. Another study evaluating the effects of high- and low-GI/GL meals, matched on macronutrient composition and palatability, on plasma glucose and insulin, appetite, and food intake in 39 healthy adults did not observe any significant differences in plasma glucose or insulin responses, appetite ratings, or food intake after consumption of ad libitum high- and low-GI/GL meals (152). These data do not support a positive association between plasma glucose or insulin and appetite and food intake.

Dumesnil et al. (155) compared an ad libitum low-GI, high-protein diet with a pair-fed or ad libitum American Heart Association (AHA) phase I diet (e.g., 55% carbohydrate, 15% protein, 30% fat) in 12 overweight men. Participants followed each dietary condition for six days with a washout period of two weeks between conditions. Compared with energy intake in the ad libitum AHA condition, energy intake was less in the ad libitum low-GI condition. Interestingly, participants did not report any changes in hunger or desire to eat during either ad libitum condition. However, increased hunger and desire to eat

were reported when participants consumed the pair-fed AHA diet. These findings suggest that isocaloric low-GI, high-protein and low-fat diets are both effective in producing weight loss but a low-GI, high-protein combination may be more satisfying. If poor compliance to a low-fat diet and weight regain are associated with hunger and discontent with food choice, a low-GI, high-protein diet may be a more appealing and sustainable strategy for weight management. Further research is needed before any conclusions can be made regarding the efficacy of low-GI diets for weight loss.

There is considerable discussion regarding whether clinicians should recommend low-GI diets to overweight and obese patients (156,157). Some suggest that low-GI diets produce greater decreases in weight and fat (158–160), and better preservation of lean body mass (161). Others argue that these findings are not consistently observed and that there is insufficient evidence to conclude that low-GI diets are more effective than high-GI, low-fat diets in reducing food intake and producing weight loss (157). The effects of low-GI diets on weight loss have not been extensively studied. Two studies have examined outcomes in obese but otherwise healthy children (158) and adolescents (159). Three small crossover studies have compared the effects of low- and high-GI diets in obese hyperinsulinemic women (162), patients with non-insulin-dependent diabetes (161), and overweight but healthy nondiabetic men (160). A small parallel design randomized 12-week controlled-feeding trial with a 24-week "free-living" follow-up phase, comparing the effects of a hypocaloric, reduced GI/GL diet with other hypocaloric diets (i.e., high-GI/GL and high-fat diets) on weight loss was conducted in obese men and women (163). One large multicenter randomized trial evaluated the effects of diets consisting of simple versus complex carbohydrates on body weight in obese adults (165). Although all studies evaluated the effects of increased intake of low-GI foods, these studies differed in study duration and dietary instruction and macronutrient composition, making it difficult to compare studies.

In a nonrandomized study, Speith et al. (158) compared the effects of an ad libitum low-GI diet (45–50% carbohydrate, 20–25% protein, 30–35% fat) with an energy-restricted low-fat diet (55–60% carbohydrate, 15–20% protein, 25–30% fat) in 107 children (mean age 10 years) attending an outpatient obesity program. Participants in the low-GI group were instructed to follow the low-GI pyramid and focus on food selection rather than energy restriction while those in the low-fat group were prescribed a calorie-controlled diet based on the Food Guide Pyramid. Children who consumed a low-GI diet had a significantly larger decrease in BMI (-1.53 kg/m^2) compared with children who followed a low-fat diet (-0.06 kg/m^2).

Ebbeling et al. (159) found similar effects on weight in a study comparing an ad libitum reduced-GL diet with an energy-restricted low-fat diet in 16 obese adolescents (aged 13–21 years). Macronutrient distributions were the same as those in the Speith study. Participants also received behavior therapy during treatment. The study consisted of a six-month intervention phase and a six-month follow-up. Significantly greater reductions in BMI (-1.3 kg/m^2 vs. 0.7 kg/m^2) and fat mass (-3.0 kg vs. 1.8 kg) were observed in the low-GI group at 12 months.

Taken together, these studies suggest that children who follow an ad libitum low-GI diet are more successful in losing weight than those who adhere to a standard low-fat diet. However, it is unclear whether these effects are due to differences between diets in GI or macronutrient composition.

Slabber et al. (164) compared the effects of low- and high-GI energy-restricted diets on weight loss and plasma insulin concentrations in 42 obese, hyperinsulinemic women during a 12-week period. Both diets were similar in macronutrient composition (50% carbohydrate, 20% protein, and 30% fat) and differed primarily in the types of carbohydrate-containing foods permitted (i.e., high-GI foods were excluded from the low-GI food plan). The Exchange List for Meal Planning was used in both groups to aid in meal selection. Participants in the low-GI group lost 9.3 kg while those in the high-GI group lost 7.4 kg after 12 weeks of treatment. Despite similar weight loss, fasting insulin concentrations dropped significantly more in the low-GI group than the high-GI group.

Similarly, Bouche et al. (160) examined whether differences in glucose and lipid metabolism, as well as in total fat mass would be observed in nondiabetic men adhering to low-GI diets or high-GI diets for five weeks. With the exception of the type of carbohydrate prescribed, total energy and macronutrient intakes of the experimental diets were similar to those of the regular diet for each participant. Participants in the low-GI group were instructed to consume foods with a GI <45% while those in the high-GI group were asked to consume foods with a GI >60%. Each participant was provided a substitution list allowing exchanges within food groups and a list of commonly consumed foods. No significant changes in body weight were observed during the five weeks in either group. However, participants who consumed a low-GI diet had lower postprandial plasma glucose and insulin profiles as well as lower postprandial cholesterol and triglycerides compared with those in the high-GI group. In another small six-week study that compared low- and high-GI diets, overall blood glucose and lipid control were improved in patients with type 2 diabetes following a low-GI diet. Similar amounts of weight were lost on both diets (i.e., 1.8 kg on the low-GI diet and 2.5 kg on the high-GI diet) (161). Similarly, Saris et al. (165) found that simply substituting simple carbohydrate for complex carbohydrate in the context of a low-fat diet does not result in significant differences in weight after six months of treatment.

Few studies have systematically examined the relative effects of diets varying in GL (i.e., carbohydrate type and quantity) on weight loss. One 12-week study randomized 129 overweight or obese adults to one of four low-fat energy-restricted diets varying in the percentage of carbohydrate in the diet and GI: (i) diet 1 consisted of 55% energy from carbohydrate and high-GI foods, (ii) diet 2 consisted of 55% energy from carbohydrate and low-GI foods, (iii) diet 3 consisted of 45% energy from carbohydrate and high-GI foods, and (iv) diet 4 consisted of 45% energy from carbohydrate and low-GI foods (166). No significant differences in weight loss were observed among groups. Cardiovascular risk was also examined in this study. Despite similar weight losses, diet 2 (55% carbohydrate, low GI) produced the best overall outcomes, reducing fat mass and LDL cholesterol. Although weight loss was similar among groups, these findings suggest that reducing the GI of the diet may produce some beneficial health effects; however, it is unclear why diet 2 but not diet 4, the diet with the lowest GL, produced the best clinical profile. Similarly, Raatz et al. (163) also reported comparable weight losses among individuals consuming hypocaloric low-GI, high-GI, or high-fat diets for 12 weeks.

Findings from the studies in children and adolescents suggest that ad libitum low-GI diets that provide slightly higher percentages of protein and fat may be more efficacious in reducing weight than standard energy-restricted diets. However, based on these limited findings in adults there appear to be no advantages in terms of weight loss when GI is altered and energy and macronutrient composition are held constant. In addition, the use of table values of GI does not predict GI of composite meals to a degree that justifies its recommendation as a reliable weight loss strategy (167). Findings in adults do suggest however that low-GI diets may play an important role in the prevention and treatment of metabolic and cardiovascular disease.

Implementation of a low-GI diet and safety considerations

Recommendations for this dietary approach are based not only on the GI values of foods but also on the overall nutritional content of the diet (168). Like the low-fat diet, a low-GI diet should consist of a variety of foods that are low in saturated fat and sodium and high in fiber, vitamins, and minerals. The main focus however is increased consumption of low-GI foods such as whole grains, legumes, vegetables, and fruit. Refined and highly processed grains should be replaced with whole grain versions. Unlike the low-carbohydrate diet, this approach allows foods that may be relatively high on the GI scale as long as they are nutrient dense. Individuals following this dietary plan are also encouraged to consume foods low in energy density (e.g., number of calories in a given weight of food) and to recognize that "low fat" does not necessarily mean that a food is healthy. By making wise GI choices, individuals should feel satisfied without having to overly restrict food intake, which should make adherence to this weight loss approach easier (168).

CALCIUM INTAKE AND BODY FATNESS

Observational studies have generally found that an inverse relationship exists between calcium intake and body fatness and that the association is stronger and more consistent for dairy calcium than for supplementary calcium. Most human studies have failed to find any effect of calcium on appetite and energy metabolism (169–171), but there is good evidence to support that dairy calcium increases excretion of fecal fat. Jacobsen et al. compared a low-calcium (500 mg) diet with two different high-calcium diets on the basis of dairy products that differed only in protein content (15 vs. 23% of energy) and found that dairy calcium only increased fecal fat excretion on the diet with the normal protein content (6 vs. 14 g/day). They also found a significant difference between fecal fat excretion on the habitual diet of the subjects and the low-calcium condition, which was consistent with the high habitual dairy calcium intake of this group of subjects (1200 mg/day), and their normal protein intake (14% of energy). However, it is not known whether it is the protein or other factors accompanying protein that is responsible for the inhibition of the calcium binding to fat.

Several short-term controlled dietary intervention trials have been conducted, and they quite consistently demonstrate that an increasing calcium intake increases fecal fat and energy excretion. A few of the studies found nonsignificant increases (171), but none found numerically a decreased or unchanged fecal fat excretion. From the most well-controlled trials, it appears that increasing the intake of dairy calcium from around 500 to ~2000 mg may increase the fecal fat excretion in the order of 5 to 7 g fat/day. A number of factors need to be considered before conclusions on the quantitative effect on fecal fat excretion can be made.

FUTURE DIRECTIONS

Popular dietary approaches for weight loss have generated widespread interest and considerable debate. Despite the publicity surrounding the myriad of dietary approaches, very little is known about their comparative short- and long-term effects. It appears that in our result-oriented society more attention has been devoted to the potential

for "success" of various weight loss approaches, traditionally measured by the general public in terms of pounds lost, rather than their potential health effects and long-term sustainability. For example, a sustained weight loss of 3 to 5 kg in obese individuals is sufficient to reduce the incidence of type 2 diabetes by 40% to 60% (172,173); however, individuals generally do not view a weight loss such as this as successful. The 10% weight loss associated with both behavioral and pharmacological treatments is nearly 6% less than the weight loss (15.6%), which participants described, before treatment, as "could not be viewed as successful in any way" and less than half of the weight loss (24.5%) that was characterized as one "that I would not be particularly happy with . . . but could accept" (174). As such, overweight and obese individuals often find themselves in a vicious cycle of weight loss and regain looking for the next "best" diet.

More effective weight loss options are needed that incorporate healthy and sustainable eating behaviors. Energy balance remains the cornerstone of weight control (i.e., calories still count). Randomized controlled weight loss trials have been designed to assess which diet is best but perhaps researchers have been asking the wrong question. The "winner takes all" mentality does not serve the field or patients well. Rather than asking which is the best diet, investigators should be asking for which type of patients do certain diets work best. Future research might focus more on how macronutrients affect cravings, satiety, hunger, and other behavioral factors that often undermine dieters in the long term. These studies will require large samples that will allow for examination of various behavioral and metabolic subtypes.

REFERENCES

1. Wadden TA, Foster GD. Behavioral treatment of obesity. Med Clin North Am 2000; 84(2):441–461.
2. National Institute of Health/National Heart Lung and Blood Institute. Clinical Guidelines on the Identification, Evaluation, and Treatment of Overweight and Obesity in Adults. The Evidence Report, National Institutes of Health, 1998:1–228.
3. Lauber RP, Sheard NF. American Heart Association. The American Heart Association Dietary Guidelines for 2000: a summary report. Nutr Rev 2001; 59(9):298–306.
4. Tanasescu M, Cho E, Manson JE, et al. Dietary fat and cholesterol and the risk of cardiovascular disease among women with type 2 diabetes. Am J Clin Nutr 2004; 79:999–1005.
5. Wolfram G. Dietary fatty acids and coronary heart disease. Eur J Med Res 2003; 8:321–324.
6. Minehira K, Tappy L. Dietary and lifestyle interventions in the management of the metabolic syndrome: present status and future perspective. Eur J Clin Nutr 2002; 56(7):1262–1267.

7. Wadden TA, Brownell KD, Foster GD. Obesity: responding to the global epidemic. J Consult Clin Psychol 2002; 70(3):510–525.

8. Stender S, Dyerberg J, Astrup A. High levels of industrially produced trans fat in popular fast foods. N Engl J Med. 2006; 354(15):1650–1652.

9. Henkin Y, Shai I. Dietary treatment of hypercholestrolemia: can we predict long-term success? J Am Coll Nutr 2003; 22(6):555–561.

10. Jakobsen MU, Overvad K, Dyerberg J, et al. Dietary fat and risk of coronary heart disease: possible effect modification by gender and age. Am J Epidemiol 2004; 160(2): 141–149.

11. Hu FB, Manson JE, Willett WC. Types of dietary fat and risk of coronary heart disease: a critical review. J Am Coll Nutr 2001; 20(1):5–19.

12. Wardlaw GM. Perspectives in Nutrition. 4th ed. Boston, MA, McGraw-Hill Co., 1999:1–31.

13. Bray GA, Popkin BM. Dietary fat intake does affect obesity! Am J Clin Nutr 1998; 68(6):1157–1173.

14. Nasser J. Taste, food intake and obesity. Obes Rev 2001; 2(4):213–218.

15. Glanz K, Basil M, Maibach E, et al. Why Americans eat what they do: taste, nutrition, cost, convenience, and weight control concerns as influences on food consumption. J Am Diet Assoc 1998; 98(10):1118–1126.

16. Rolls BJ, Kim-Harris S, Fischman MW, et al. Satiety after preloads with different amounts of fat and carbohydrate: implications for obesity. Am J Clin Nutr 1994; 60(4): 476–487.

17. Blundell JE, MacDiarmid JI. Passive overconsumption. Fat intake and short-term energy balance. Ann N Y Acad Sci 1997; 827:392–407.

18. Blundell JE, MacDiarmid JI. Fat as a risk factor for overconsumption: satiation, satiety, and patterns of eating. J Am Diet Assoc 1997; 97(suppl 7):S63–S69.

19. Green SM, Burley VJ, Blundell JE. Effect of fat- and sucrose-containing foods on the size of eating episodes and energy intake in lean males: potential for causing overconsumption. Eur J Clin Nutr 1994; 48(8):547–555.

20. Green SM, Wales JK, Lawton CL, et al. Comparison of high-fat and high-carbohydrate foods in a meal or snack on short-term fat and energy intakes in obese women. Br J Nutr 2000; 84(4):521–530.

21. Green SM, Blundell JE. Effect of fat- and sucrose-containing foods on the size of eating episodes and energy intake in lean dietary restrained and unrestrained females: potential for causing overconsumption. Eur J Clin Nutr 1996; 50(9):625–635.

22. Tremblay A, Lavallee N, Almeras N, et al. Nutritional determinants of the increase in energy intake associated with a high-fat diet. Am J Clin Nutr 1991; 53(5): 1134–1137.

23. Johnson J, Vickers Z. Effects of flavor and macronutrient composition of food servings on liking, hunger and subsequent intake. Appetite 1993; 21(1):25–39.

24. Institutes of Medicine. Dietary Reference Intakes for Energy, Carbohydrate, Fiber, Fat, Fatty Acids, Cholesterol, Protein, and Amino Acids. National Academy Press, 2002:465–608.

25. Smit E, Nieto FJ, Crespo CJ, et al. Estimates of animal and plant protein intake in US adults: results from the Third National Health and Nutrition Examination Survey, 1988–1991. J Am Diet Assoc 1999; 99(7):813–820.

26. St Jeor ST, Howard BV, Prewitt TE, et al. Dietary protein and weight reduction. Circulation 2001; 104:1869–1874.

27. Gums JG. Magnesium in cardiovascular and other disorders. Am J Health Syst Pharm 2004; 61:1569–1576.

28. McCarron DA, Reusser ME. Are low intakes of calcium and potassium important causes of cardiovascular disease? Am J Hypertens 2001; 14:206S–212S.

29. Knight EL, Stampfer MJ, Hankinson SE, et al. The impact of protein intake on renal function decline in women with normal renal function or mild renal insufficiency. Ann Intern Med 2003; 138(6):460–467.

30. Mahan LK, Arlin MT. Krause's Food, Nutrition & Diet Therapy. 8th ed. Philadelphia, PA, WB Saunders Co., 1992:29–43.

31. National Research Council. Recommended Dietary Allowances. 10th ed. Washington, D.C., National Academy Press, 1989:52–77.

32. Reid M, Hetherington M. Relative effects of carbohydrate and protein on satiety-a review of methodology. Neurosci Biobehav Rev 1997; 21(3):295–308.

33. Rolls BJ, Hetherington M, Burley VJ. The specificity of satiety: the influence of foods of different macronutrient content on the development of satiety. Physiol Behav 1988; 43:145–153.

34. Holt SH, Miller JC, Petocz P, et al. A satiety index of common foods. Eur J Clin Nutr 1995; 49(9):675–690.

35. Holt SH, Brand Miller JC, Petocz P. Interrelationships among postprandial satiety, glucose and insulin responses and changes in subsequent food intake. Eur J Clin Nutr 1996; 50(12):788–797.

36. Latner JD, Schwartz M. The effects of a high-carbohydrate, high-protein or balanced lunch upon later food intake and hunger ratings. Appetite 1999; 33:119–128.

37. Cummings DE, Overduin J. Gastrointestinal regulation of food intake. J Clin Invest 2007; 117(1):13–23.

38. Arora S, Anubhuti. Role of neuropeptides in appetite regulation and obesity—a review. Neuropeptides 2006; 40(6):375–401.

39. Schwartz MW, Woods SC, Seeley RJ, et al. Is the energy homeostasis system inherently biased toward weight gain? Diabetes 2003; 52(2):232–238.

40. Schwartz MW, Morton GJ. Obesity: keeping hunger at bay. Nature 2002; 418:595–597.

41. Weigle DS, Cummings DE, Newby PD, et al. Roles of leptin and ghrelin in the loss of body weight caused by a low fat, high carbohydrate diet. J Clin Endocrinol Metab 2003; 88(4):1577–1586.

42. Orr J, Davy B. Dietary influences on peripheral hormones regulating energy intake: potential applications for weight management. J Am Diet Assoc 2005; 105(7):1115–1524.

43. Monteleone P, Bencivenga R, Longobardi N, et al. Differential responses of circulating ghrelin to high-fat or

high-carbohydrate meal in healthy women. J Clin Endocrinol Metab 2003; 88(11):5510–5514.

44. Greenman Y, Golani N, Gilad S, et al. Ghrelin secretion is modulated in a nutrient- and gender-specific manner. Clin Endocrinol (Oxf) 2004; 60(3):382–388.

45. Overduin J, Frayo RS, Grill HJ, et al. Role of the duodenum and macronutrient type in ghrelin regulation. Endocrinology 2005; 146(2):845–850.

46. Bowen J, Noakes M, Trenerry C, et al. Energy intake, ghrelin, and cholecystokinin after different carbohydrate and protein preloads in overweight men. J Clin Endocrinol Metab 2006; 91(4):1477–1483.

47. Erdmann J, Lippl F, Schusdziarra V. Differential effect of protein and fat on plasma ghrelin levels in man. Regul Pept 2003; 116(1–3):101–107.

48. Erdmann J, Töpsch R, Lippl F, et al. Postprandial response of plasma ghrelin levels to various test meals in relation to food intake, plasma insulin, and glucose. J Clin Endocrinol Metab 2004; 89(6):3048–3054.

49. Moran LJ, Luscombe-Marsh ND, Noakes M, et al. The satiating effect of dietary protein is unrelated to postprandial ghrelin secretion. J Clin Endocrinol Metab 2005; 90(9):5205–5211.

50. Weigle DS, Breen PA, Matthys CC, et al. A high-protein diet induces sustained reductions in appetite, ad libitum caloric intake, and body weight despite compensatory changes in diurnal plasma leptin and ghrelin concentrations. Am J Clin Nutr 2005; 82(1):41–48.

51. Teff KL, Elliott SS, Tschöp M, et al. Dietary fructose reduces circulating insulin and leptin, attenuates postprandial suppression of ghrelin, and increases triglycerides in women. J Clin Endocrinol Metab 2004; 89(6):2963–2972.

52. Lin L, Martin R, Schaffhauser AO, et al. Acute changes in the response to peripheral leptin with alteration in the diet composition. Am J Physiol Regul Integr Comp Physiol 2001; 280(2):R504–R509.

53. Havel PJ, Townsend R, Chaump L, et al. High-fat meals reduce 24-h circulating leptin concentrations in women. Diabetes 1999; 48(2):334–341.

54. Romon M, Lebel P, Velly C, et al. Leptin response to carbohydrate or fat meal and association with subsequent satiety and energy intake. Am J Physiol 1999; 277(5 pt 1): E855–E861.

55. Malik VS, Schulze MB, Hu FB. Intake of sugar-sweetened beverages and weight gain: a systematic review. Am J Clin Nutr 2006; 84(2):274–288.

56. Welsh JA, Cogswell ME, Rogers S, et al. Overweight among low-income preschool children associated with the consumption of sweet drinks: Missouri, 1999–2002. Pediatrics 2005; 115(2):e223–e229.

57. Bray GA, Nielsen SJ, Popkin BM. Consumption of high-fructose corn syrup in beverages may play a role in the epidemic of obesity. Am J Clin Nutr 2004; 79(4):537–543.

58. Berkey CS, Rockett HR, Field AE, et al. Sugar-added beverages and adolescent weight change. Obes Res 2004; 12(5):778–788.

59. Schulze MB, Manson JE, Ludwig DS, et al. Sugar-sweetened beverages, weight gain, and incidence of type 2 diabetes in young and middle-aged women. JAMA 2004; 292(8):927–934.

60. Ludwig DS, Peterson KE, Gortmaker SL. Relation between consumption of sugar-sweetened drinks and childhood obesity: a prospective, observational analysis. Lancet 2001; 357(9255):505–508.

61. Mattes RD. Beverages and positive energy balance: the menace is the medium. Int J Obes Relat Metab Disord 2006; 30:560–565.

62. DiMeglio DP, Mattes RD. Liquid versus solid carbohydrate: effects on food intake and body weight. Int J Obes Relat Metab Disord 2000; 24(6):794–800.

63. Dietz WH. Sugar-sweetened beverages, milk intake, and obesity in children and adolescents. J Pediatr 2006; 148(2):152–154.

64. Raben A, Vasilaras TH, Møller AC, et al. Sucrose compared with artificial sweeteners: different effects on ad libitum food intake and body weight after 10 wk of supplementation in overweight subjects. Am J Clin Nutr 2002; 76(4):721–729.

65. Drewnowski A, Bellisle F. Liquid calories, sugar, and body weight. Am J Clin Nutr 2007; 85(3):651–661.

66. Tsuchiya A, Almiron-Roig E, Lluch A, et al. Higher satiety ratings following yogurt consumption relative to fruit drink or dairy fruit drink. J Am Diet Assoc 2006; 106(4):550–557.

67. Rolls BJ, Bell EA. Dietary approaches to the treatment of obesity. Med Clin North Am 2000; 84(2):401–418.

68. Duncan KH, Bacon JA, Weinsier RL. The effects of high and low energy density diets on satiety, energy intake, and eating time of obese and nonobese subjects. Am J Clin Nutr 1983; 37:763–767.

69. Stubbs RJ, Ritz P, Coward WA, et al. Covert manipulation of the ratio of dietary fat to carbohydrate and energy density: effect on food intake and energy balance in free-living men eating *ad libitum*. Am J Clin Nutr 1995; 62:330–337.

70. Rolls BJ, Barnett RA. The Volumetrics Weight Control Plan. New York, NY: HarperCollins Publishers, 2000.

71. Hellstrom PM, Geliebter A, Naslund E, et al. Peripheral and central signals in the control of eating in normal, obese and binge-eating human subjects. Br J Nutr 2004; 92(1 suppl 1):47–57.

72. Gerstein DE, Woodward-Lopez G, Evans AE, et al. Clarifying concepts about macronutrients' effects on satiation and satiety. J Am Diet Assoc 2004; 104: 1151–1153.

73. Geliebter A, Westreich S, Gage D. Gastric distention by balloon and test-meal intake in obese and lean subjects. Am J Clin Nutr 1988; 48:592–594.

74. Rolls BJ, Castellanos VH, Halford JC, et al. Volume of food consumed affects satiety in men. Am J Clin Nutr 1998; 67(6):1170–1177.

75. van Stratum P, Lussenburg RN, van Wezel LA, et al. The effect of dietary carbohydrate: fat ratio on energy intake by adult women. Am J Clin Nutr 1978; 31(2):206–212.

76. Stubbs RJ, Prentice AM. The effect of covertly manipulating the dietary fat: CHO ratio of isoenergetically dense

diets on *ad libitum* intake in "free-living" humans. Proc Nutr Soc 1993; 52:341A.

77. Ornish D. Low-fat diets. N Engl J Med 1998; 338:127.

78. Freedman MR, King J, Kennedy E. Popular diets: a scientific review. Obes Res 2001; 9(1):1S–40S.

79. Ornish D, Scherwitz LW, Billings JH, et al. Intensive lifestyle changes for reversal of coronary heart disease. JAMA 1998; 280:2001–2007.

80. U.S. Department of Health and Human Services and U.S. Department of Agriculture. Dietary Guidelines for Americans, 2005. 6th ed., Washington, DC: U.S. Government Printing Office, January 2005.

81. Johnson RK, Kennedy E. The 2000 dietary guidelines for Americans: what are the changes and why were they made? J Am Diet Assoc 2000; 100:769–774.

82. Irwin T. New dietary guidelines from the American Diabetes Association. Diabetes Care 2002; 25:1262–1263.

83. Kinsella A. American Heart Association issues new dietary guidelines. Home Health Nurse 2002; 20:86–88.

84. Byers T, Nestle M, McTiernan A, et al. American Cancer Society 2001 Nutrition and Physical Activity Guidelines Advisory Committee. American Cancer Society guidelines on nutrition and physical activity for cancer prevention: reducing the risk of cancer with healthy food choices and physical activity. CA Cancer J Clin 2002; 52:92–119.

85. Bray GA, Popkin BM. Dietary fat intake does affect obesity! Am J Clin Nutr 1998; 68(6):1157–1173.

86. Astrup A, Grunwald GK, Melanson EL, et al. The role of low-fat diets in body weight control: a meta-analysis of ad libitum dietary intervention studies. Int J Obes Relat Metab Disord 2000; 24(12):1545–1552.

87. Howard BV, Manson JE Stefanick, ML, et al. Low-fat dietary pattern and weight change over 7 years: the Women's Health Initiative Randomized Controlled Dietary Modification Trial. JAMA 2006; 295(1):39–49.

88. Svetkey LP, Harsha DW, Vollmer WM, et al. Premier: a clinical trial of comprehensive lifestyle modification for blood pressure control: rationale, design and baseline characteristics. Ann Epidemiol 2003; 13(6):462–471.

89. Knowler WC, Barrett-Connor E, Fowler SE, et al. Reduction in the incidence of type 2 diabetes with lifestyle intervention or metformin. N Engl J Med 2002; 346(6):393–403.

90. Lindstrom J, Eriksson JG, Valle TT, et al. Prevention of diabetes mellitus in subjects with impaired glucose tolerance in the Finnish Diabetes Prevention Study: results from a randomized clinical trial. J Am Soc Neph 2003; 14(7):S108–S113.

91. Hamman RF, Wing RR, Edelstein SL, et al. Effect of weight loss with lifestyle intervention on risk of diabetes. Diabetes Care 2006; 29(9):2102–2107.

92. Avenell A, Broom J, Brown TJ, et al. Systematic review of the long-term effects and economic consequences of treatments for obesity and implications for health improvement. Health Technology Assess 2004; 8(21):1–465.

93. Pirozzo S, Summerbell C, Cameron C, et al. Should we recommend low-fat diets for obesity? Obesity Rev 2003; 4:83–90.

94. Swinburn BA, Metcalf PA, Ley SJ. Long-term (5-year) effects of a reduced-fat diet intervention in individuals with glucose intolerance. Diabetes Care 2001; 24(4):619–624.

95. Marques-Vidal P, Ruidavets JB, Cambou JP, et al. Trends in overweight and obesity in middle-aged subjects from southwestern France, 1985–1997. Int J Obes Relat Metab Disord 2002; 26(5):732–734.

96. Willett WC, Sacks F, Trichopoulou A, et al. Mediterranean diet pyramid: a cultural model for healthy eating. Am J Clin Nutr 1995; 61(suppl 6):1402S–1406S.

97. Kok FJ, Kromhout D. AtherosclerosisEpidemiological studies on the health effects of a Mediterranean diet. Eur J Nutr 2004; 43(suppl 1):I2–I5.

98. Trichopoulou A, Costacou T, Bamia C, et al. Adherence to a Mediterranean diet and survival in a Greek population. N Engl J Med 2003; 348(26):2599–2608.

99. Knoops KT, de Groot LC, Kromhout D, et al. Mediterranean diet, lifestyle factors, and 10-year mortality in elderly European men and women: the HALE project. JAMA 2004; 292:1433–1439.

100. Esposito K, Marfella R, Ciotola M, et al. Effect of a Mediterranean-style diet on endothelial dysfunction and markers of vascular inflammation in the metabolic syndrome: a randomized trial. JAMA 2004; 292:1440–1446.

101. McManus K, Antinoro L, Sacks F. A randomized controlled trial of a moderate-fat, low-energy diet compared with a low-fat, low-energy diet for weight loss in overweight adults. Int J Obes Relat Metab Disord 2001; 25(10):1503–1511.

102. Karamanos B, Thanopoulou A, Angelico F, et al. Nutritional habits in the Mediterranean Basin. The macronutrient composition of diet and its relation with the traditional Mediterranean diet. Multi-centre study of the Mediterranean Group for the Study of Diabetes (MGSD). Eur J Clin Nutr 2002; 56(10):983–991.

103. Trichopoulou A, Toupadaki N, Tzonou A, et al. The macronutrient composition of the Greek diet: estimates derived from six case-control studies. Eur J Clin Nutr 1993; 47(8):549–558.

104. Simopoulos AP. The Mediterranean diets: what is so special about the diet of Greece? The scientific evidence. J Nutr 2001; 131(11 suppl):3065S–3073S.

105. Malik VS, Hu FB. Popular weight-loss diets: from evidence to practice. Nat Clin Pract Cardiovasc Med 2007; 4(1):34–41.

106. Estruch R, Martínez-González MA, Corella D, et al. Effects of a Mediterranean-style diet on cardiovascular risk factors: a randomized trial. Ann Intern Med 2006; 145(1):1–11.

107. Due A, Larsen TM, Mu H, et al. Comparison of the "USDA Food Pyramid 2004" versus the new "Healthy Eating Pyramid" versus a Control Diet for Weight Loss Maintenance and Diabetes Risk: A Randomised, Controlled Trial (in press).

108. Kris-Etherton P, Daniels SR, Eckel RH, et al. AHA scientific statement: summary of the Scientific Conference on Dietary Fatty Acids and Cardiovascular Health. Conference summary from the Nutrition Committee of

the American Heart Association. J Nutr 2001; 131(4): 1322–1326.

109. de Lorgeril M, Salen P, Martin JL, et al. Mediterranean diet, traditional risk factors, and the rate of cardiovascular complications after myocardial infarction: final report of the Lyon Diet Heart Study. Circulation 1999; 99(6): 779–785.

110. Eisenstein J, Roberts SB, Dallal G, et al. High-protein weight-loss diets: are they safe and do they work? A review of the experimental and epidemiologic data. Nutr Rev 2002; 1:189–200.

111. Due A, Toubro S, Skov AR, et al. Effect of normal-fat diets, either medium or high in protein, on body weight in overweight subjects: a randomised 1-year trial. Int J Obes Relat Metab Disord 2004; 28:1283–1290.

112. Skov AR, Toubro S, Ronn B, et al. Randomized trial on protein vs carbohydrate in *ad libitum* fat reduced diet for the treatment of obesity. Int J Obes Relat Metab Disord 1999; 23:528–536.

113. Parker B, Noakes M, Luscombe N, et al. Effect of a high-protein, high-monounsaturated fat weight loss diet on glycemic control and lipid levels in type 2 diabetes. Diabetes Care 2002; 25:425–430.

114. Luscombe ND, Clifton PM, Noakes M, et al. Effects of energy-restricted diets containing increased protein on weight loss, resting energy expenditure, and thermic effect of feeding in type 2 diabetes. Diabetes Care 2002; 25: 652–657.

115. Golay A, Eigenheer C, Morel Y, et al. Weight-loss with low or high carbohydrate diet? Int J Obes Relat Metab Disord 1996; 20(12):1067–1072.

116. Farnsworth E, Luscombe ND, Noakes M, et al. Effect of a high-protein, energy-restricted diet on body composition, glycemic control, and lipid concentrations in overweight and obese hyperinsulinemic men and women. Am J Clin Nutr 2003; 78:31–39.

117. Layman DK, Boileau RA, Erickson DJ, et al. A reduced ratio of dietary carbohydrate to protein improves body composition and blood lipid profiles during weight loss in adult women. J Nutr 2003; 133(2):411–417.

118. Piatti PM, Monti F, Fermo I, et al. Hypocaloric high-protein diet improves glucose oxidation and spares lean body mass: comparison to hypocaloric high-carbohydrate diet. Metabolism 1994; 43(12):1481–1487.

119. Krieger JW, Sitren HS, Daniels MJ, et al. Effects of variation in protein and carbohydrate intake on body mass and composition during energy restriction: a meta-regression 1. Am J Clin Nutr 2006; 83(2):260–274.

120. Weigle DS, Breen PA, Matthys CC, et al. A high-protein diet induces sustained reductions in appetite, ad libitum caloric intake, and body weight despite compensatory changes in diurnal plasma leptin and ghrelin concentrations. Am J Clin Nutr 2005; 82(1):41–48.

121. Hoffer LJ, Bistrian BR, Young VR, et al. Metabolic effects of very low calorie weight reduction diets. J Clin Invest 1984; 73(3):750–758.

122. Westerterp-Plantenga MS, Lejeune MP, Nijs I, et al. High protein intake sustains weight maintenance after body

weight loss in humans. Int J Obes Relat Metab Disord 2004; 28(1):57–64.

123. Luscombe-Marsh ND, Noakes M, Wittert GA, et al. Carbohydrate-restricted diets high in either monounsaturated fat or protein are equally effective at promoting fat loss and improving blood lipids. Am J Clin Nutr 2005; 81(4):762–772.

124. Brinkworth GD, Noakes M, Keogh JB, et al. Long-term effects of a high-protein, low-carbohydrate diet on weight control and cardiovascular risk markers in obese hyper-insulinemic subjects. Int J Obes Relat Metab Disord 2004; 28(5):661–670.

125. Westerterp-Plantenga MS, Lejeune MP. Protein intake and body-weight regulation. Appetite 2005; 45(2):187–190.

126. Astrup A. How to maintain a healthy body weight. Int J Vitam Nutr Res 2006; 76(4):208–215.

127. Haulrik N, Toubro S, Dyerberg J, et al. Effect of protein and methionine intakes on plasma homocysteine concentrations: a 6-mo randomized controlled trial in overweight subjects. Am J Clin Nutr 2002; 76(6):1202–1206.

128. Foster GD, Wyatt HR, Hill JO, et al. A randomized trial of a low-carbohydrate diet for obesity. N Engl J Med 2003; 348:2082–2090.

129. Brehm BJ, Seeley RJ, Daniels SR, et al. A randomized trial comparing a very low-carbohydrate diet and a calorie-restricted low-fat diet on body weight and cardio-vascular risk factors in healthy women. J Clin Endocrin Metab 2003; 88:1617–1623.

130. Samaha FF, Iqbal N, Seshadri P et al. A low-carbohydrate as compared with a low-fat diet in severe obesity. N Engl J Med 2003; 348:2074–2081.

131. Stern L, Iqbal N, Seshadri P, et al. The effects of low-carbohydrate versus conventional weight loss diets in severely obese adults: one-year follow-up of a randomized trial. Ann Intern Med 2004; 140:778–785.

132. Yancy WS, Olsen MK, Guyton JR, et al. A low-carbohydrate, ketogenic diet versus a low-fat diet to treat obesity and hyperlipidemia. Ann Intern Med 2004; 140:769–777.

133. Dansinger ML, Gleason JA, Griffith JL, et al. Comparison of the Atkins, Ornish, Weight Watchers, and Zone diets for weight loss and heart disease risk reduction: a randomized trial. JAMA 2005; 293(1):43–53.

134. Gardner CD, Kiazand A, Alhassan S, et al. Comparison of the Atkins, Zone, Ornish, and LEARN diets for change in weight and related risk factors among overweight premenopausal women: the A TO Z Weight Loss Study: a randomized trial. JAMA 2007; 297(9):969–977.

135. Boden G, Sargrad K, Homko C, et al. Effect of a low-carbohydrate diet on appetite, blood glucose levels, and insulin resistance in obese patients with type 2 diabetes. Ann Intern Med 2005; 142(6):403–411.

136. Jeffery RW, Wing RR, Thorson C, et al. Strengthening behavioral interventions for weight loss: a randomized trial of food provision and monetary incentives. J Consult Clin Psychol 1993; 6:1038–1045.

137. Wing RR, Jeffery RW, Burton LR, et al. Food provision vs structured meal plans in the behavioral treatment of obesity. Int J Obes Relat Metab Disord 1996; 20:56–62.

138. Ditschuneit HH, Flechtner-Mors, M. Value of structured meals for weight management: risk factors and long-term weight maintenance. Obes Res 2001; 9(suppl 4): 284S–289S.

139. Ditschuneit HH, Flechtner-Mors M, Johnson TD, et al. Metabolic and weight loss effects of a long-term dietary intervention in obese patients. Am J Clin Nutr 1999; 69:198–204.

140. Rothacker DQ, Staniszewski BA, Ellis PK. Liquid meal replacement vs. traditional food: a potential model for women who cannot maintain eating habit change. J Am Diet Assoc 2001; 101(3):345–347.

141. Ashley JM, St Jeor ST, Perumean-Chaney S, et al. Meal replacements in weight intervention. Obes Res 2001; 9:312S–320S.

142. Nordmann AJ, Nordmann A, Briel M. Effects of low-carbohydrate vs. low-fat diets on weight loss and cardio-vascular risk factors: a meta-analysis of randomized controlled trials. Arch Intern Med 2006; 166(3):285–293.

143. Roberts SB. High-glycemic index foods, hunger, and obesity: is there a connection? Nutr Rev 2000; 58 (6):163–169.

144. Ludwig DS. Dietary glycemic index and obesity. J Nutr 2000; 130:280S–283S.

145. Wolever TM. Carbohydrate and the regulation of blood glucose and metabolism. Nutr Rev 2003; 61(5 pt 2):S40–S48.

146. Ludwig DS. The glycemic index: physiological mechanisms relating to obesity, diabetes, and cardiovascular disease. JAMA 2002; 287(18):2414–2423.

147. Sloth B, Krog-Mikkelsen I, Flint A, et al. No difference in body weight decrease between a low-glycemic-index and a high-glycemic-index diet but reduced LDL cholesterol after 10-wk ad libitum intake of the low-glycemic-index diet. Am J Clin Nutr 2004; 80(2):337–347.

148. Henry CJ, Lightowler HJ, Strik CM, et al. Glycaemic index values for commercially available potatoes in Great Britain. Br J Nutr 2005; 94(6):917–921.

149. Tahvonen R, Hietanen RM, Sihvonen J, et al. Influence of different processing methods on the glycemic index of potato (Nicola). J Food Compos Anal 2006; 19:372–378.

150. Flint A, Moller BK, Raben A, et al. The use of glycaemic index tables to predict glycaemic index of composite breakfast meals. Br J Nutr 2004; 91(6):979–989.

151. Flint A, Møller BK, Raben A, et al. Glycemic and insulinemic responses as determinants of appetite in humans. Am J Clin Nutr 2006; 84(6):1365–1373.

152. Alfenas RC, Mattes RD. Influence of glycemic index/load on glycemic response, appetite, and food intake in healthy humans. Diabetes Care 2005; 28(9):2123–2129.

153. Ludwig DS, Majzoub JA, Al-Zahrani A, et al. High glycemic index foods, overeating, and obesity. Pediatrics 1999; 103:E26.

154. Ball SD, Keller KR, Moyer-Mileur LJ, et al. Prolongation of satiety after low versus moderately high glycemic index meals in obese adolescents. Pediatrics 2003; 111:488–494.

155. Dumesnil JG, Turgeon J, Tremblay A, et al. Effect of a low-glycaemic index-low-fat-high-protein diet on the atherogenic metabolic risk profile of abdominally obese men. Br J Nutr 2001; 86:557–568.

156. Pawlak DB, Ebbeling CB, Ludwig DS. Should obese patients be counseled to follow a low-glycaemic index diet? Yes. Obes Rev 2002; 3:235–243.

157. Raben A. Should obese patients be counseled to follow a low-glycaemic index diet? No. Obes Rev 2002; 3:245–256.

158. Speith LE, Harnish JD, Lenders CM, et al. A low-glycemic index diet in the treatment of pediatric obesity. Arch Pediatr Adolesc Med 2000; 154:947–951.

159. Ebbling CB, Leidig MM, Sinclair KB, et al. A reduced-glycemic load diet in the treatment of adolescent obesity. Arch Pediatr Adolesc Med 2003; 157:773–779.

160. Bouche C, Rizkalla SW, Luo J, et al. Five-week, low-glycemic index diet decreases total fat mass and improves plasma lipid profile in moderately overweight nondiabetic men. Diabetes Care 2002; 25:822–828.

161. Wolever TM, Jenkins DJ, Vuksan V, et al. Beneficial effect of low-glycemic index diet in overweight NIDDM subjects. Diabetes Care 1992; 15:562–564.

162. Pi-Sunyer FX. Glycemic index and disease. Am J Clin Nutr 2002; 76:290S–298S.

163. Raatz SK, Torkelson CJ, Redmon JB. Reduced glycemic index and glycemic load diets do not increase the effects of energy restriction on weight loss and insulin sensitivity in obese men and women. J Nutr 2005; 135(10): 2387–2391.

164. Slabber M, Barnard HC, Kuyl JM, et al. Effects of a low-insulin-response, energy-restricted diet on weight loss and plasma insulin concentrations in hyperinsulinemic obese females. Am J Clin Nutr 1994; 60:48–53.

165. Saris WH, Astrup A, Prentice AM, et al. Randomized controlled trial of changes in dietary carbohydrate/fat ratio and simple vs complex carbohydrates on body weight and blood lipids: the CARMEN study. The Carbohydrate Ratio Management in European National diets. Int J Obes Relat Metab Disord 2000; 24(10):1310–1318.

166. McMillan-Price J, Petocz P, Atkinson F, et al. Comparison of 4 diets of varying glycemic load on weight loss and cardiovascular risk reduction in overweight and obese young adults: a randomized controlled trial. Arch Intern Med 2006; 166(14):1466–1475.

167. Flint A, Møller BK, Raben A, et al. The use of glycaemic index tables to predict glycaemic index of composite breakfast meals. Br J Nutr 2004; 91(6):979–989.

168. Brand-Miller J, Wolever TMS, Foster-Powell K, et al. The New Glucose Revolution. New York, NY: Marlowe & Co., 1996:71–94, 173–195.

169. Jacobsen R, Lorenzen JK, Toubro S, et al. Effect of short-term high dietary calcium intake on 24-h energy expenditure, fat oxidation, and fecal fat excretion. Int J Obes (Lond) 2005; 29(3):292–301.

170. Melanson EL, Donahoo WT, Dong F, et al. Effect of low- and high-calcium dairy-based diets on macronutrient oxidation in humans. Obes Res 2005; 13(12):2102–2112.

171. Boon N, Hul GB, Viguerie N, et al. Effects of 3 diets with various calcium contents on 24-h energy expenditure, fat oxidation, and adipose tissue message RNA expression of lipid metabolism-related proteins. Am J Clin Nutr 2005; 82(6):1244–1252.

172. Knowler WC, Barrett-Connor E, Fowler SE. Reduction in the incidence of type 2 diabetes with lifestyle intervention or metformin. N Engl J Med 2002; 346(6):393–403.

173. Tuomilehto J, Lindström J, Eriksson JG, et al. Prevention of type 2 diabetes mellitus by changes in lifestyle among subjects with impaired glucose tolerance. N Engl J Med 2001; 344(18):1343–1350.

174. Foster GD, Wadden TA, Phelan S, et al. Obese patients' perceptions of treatment outcomes and the factors that influence them. Arch Intern Med 2001; 161(17):2133–2139.

17

Exercise and Weight Management

TIM CHURCH

Laboratory of Preventive Medicine Research, Pennington Biomedical Research Center, Baton Rouge, Louisiana, U.S.A.

INTRODUCTION

The relative importance of exercise in weight management has been a source of confusion and frustration for both the health care professionals and lay people for a constellation of reasons. Individuals are confused by the discrepant and often conflicting recommendations regularly put forth by a variety of private and public health organizations, and the concepts of weight gain prevention, weight loss, and prevention of regain can be confusing even to professionals who are not weight management specialists. This is compounded by the observation that, while updates to exercise recommendations are often specific to weight gain prevention, weight loss, or prevention of regain, this nuance is often lost in translation by the press, and an exercise recommendation for the prevention of weight regain may be incorrectly described as the amount of exercise needed to lose weight. To further complicate the issue, there are exercise recommendations focused specifically on general health, which are not focused on weight management.

This chapter will attempt to bring some clarity to these issues and summarize the relative importance and role of exercise in all phases of weight management. Specifically, the chapter will examine the role of exercise in inducing a negative caloric balance and subsequent weight loss both alone and in combination with caloric restriction. It will explore the role and amount of exercise in the prevention of weight gain, weight loss, and prevention of weight regain as well as the importance of exercise without weight loss in general health. The exercise prescription will be broken down into its individual components, and the minimal screening for safely starting an exercise program will be addressed.

Before examining the role of exercise in weight management, the working definitions of exercise and physical activity need to be examined. In general terms, aerobic exercise is defined as a planned and structured bodily movement resulting in increased oxygen consumption and caloric expenditure. The specific goals of structured aerobic exercise may be improvements in fitness or general well-being, or aerobic exercise may be part of a weight loss (or maintenance) program. Examples include walking, jogging, swimming laps, and participating in an aerobics class. Physical activity is any bodily movement produced by skeletal muscle that results in energy expenditure. Exercise is a type of physical activity, but the most common forms of physical activity are activities of daily living, such as climbing stairs, gardening, and walking the dog. It is important to note that one can be very physically active yet never exercise. This chapter will primarily focus on exercise.

People desire to use weight management for a wide variety of reasons such as vanity, health, social pressures, etc. This chapter is focused on weight loss with the goal of improving health or reducing risk of chronic diseases, which requires a clinically meaningful weight loss. There is substantial evidence demonstrating that 5% to 10% loss of initial weight is sufficient to reduce, at least in the short term, the risk of many health complications associated with obesity including essential hypertension, type 2 diabetes, and dyslipidemia (1,2). For the purposes of this chapter, we will define a clinically meaningful weight loss as at least 5% weight loss.

EXERCISE AND ENERGY BALANCE

Energy balance occurs when energy intake equals energy expenditure. Negative energy balance (energy intake < energy expenditure) results in weight loss and positive energy balance results in weight gain. Energy expenditure is the sum of calories burned by resting metabolic rate (RMR), thermic effect of food (TEF), activities of daily living, and exercise. While the energy balance equation and its role in weight management appear straightforward, the process has proven to be anything but simple. Intervening on any one component of the energy balance equation has been demonstrated to affect other elements of the equation and not always positively. For example, exercise interventions with large doses of supervised exercise have been found to produce less weight loss than expected based on exercise caloric expenditure alone, and very low-calorie meal plans can make increasing levels of activity challenging (3,4). Thus, one must keep in mind that exercise-induced increases in caloric expenditure are but one part of a complex system with multiple feedback loops, and it is this complexity that likely explains the confusing and often conflicting findings related to the role of exercise in weight loss.

EXERCISE AND PREVENTION OF WEIGHT GAIN

The escalation of the prevalence of overweight and obesity is well documented and while the tracking of this modern epidemic is a relatively easy task, identifying the causes is not. It has been suggested that the growing waistlines are due to excess caloric intake because of the plentiful supply of inexpensive, calorically dense food. Others have blamed the problem on the declining energy expenditure brought about by the modernization of the work force, the conveniences of modern life, and shift from outdoor activities to indoor activities across all age groups. While is it is widely accepted that required daily exercise has decreased over the decades and the majority of American citizens lead a sedentary lifestyle, the relative contribution of these reductions in activity to the weight epidemic remain a subject of debate. Understanding the role of exercise in the prevention of weight gain is important because this will provide guidance in the development of exercise guidelines specifically targeting the prevention of weight gain.

Many of the recommendations for physical activity and prevention of weight gain are presented in terms of both minutes per week of activity and individuals' daily physical activity level commonly referred to as PAL. PAL is defined as the ratio of total energy expenditure to 24-hour basal energy expenditure. The higher the PAL the higher the level of daily physical activity performed. While many of the past guidelines for the prevention of weight gain were developed largely from population-based longitudinal studies using self-reported PALs (Table 1), more recent guidelines have been based on studies that directly measured total energy expenditure using doubly labeled water and basal metabolic rate using indirect calorimetry and daily activity levels, resulting in very accurate measures of PAL.

Table 1 Current Recommendations for Prevention of Weight Gain

Expert group (yr)	Recommendation for prevention of weight gain
World Health Organization (1998)	Men and Women should achieve a PAL of 1.75.
U.S. Surgeon General (2001)	Adults should get at least 30 min of moderate physical activity on most days of the week. Children should aim for 60 min.
International Obesity Task Force (2002)	Men and Women should achieve a PAL of 1.8 to prevent unhealthy weight gain. Vigorous activity is more clearly linked to weight stability.
Institute of Medicine (2002)	All adults should accumulate 60 to 90 min of daily physical activity. This corresponds to a PAL greater than 1.6.
Stock conference (2003)	Men and Women should undergo moderate-intensity physical activity for about 45 to 60 min/day to achieve a PAL of 1.7.
USDA Dietary Guidelines (2005)	Engage in approximately 60 min of moderate-to-vigorous intensity activity on most days of the week while not exceeding caloric intake requirements.

Abbreviations: PAL, physical activity level; USDA, United States Department of Agriculture.

Table 2 Physical Activity Level

PAL category	PAL value
Sedentary	1.0–1.39
Low active	1.4–1.59
Active	1.6–1.89
Very active	1.9–2.5

Abbreviation: PAL, physical activity level.

Individuals can be placed into one of four activity categories based on their PAL, which roughly correspond to population quartiles. The sedentary category (lowest 25%) is characterized by a PAL of 1.0 to 1.39 and represents the sum of basal energy expenditure, the TEF, and the energy required for independent living. In other words, the sedentary category represents the minimal basic energy requirements of existence. The low active (PAL 1.4–1.59), active (PAL 1.6–1.89), and very active (PAL 1.9–2.5) categories represent the energy associated with basic existence (sedentary category) combined with increasing amounts of daily activity (Table 2).

The expert recommendations for the prevention of weight gain range from a daily PAL of 1.6 to 1.8 with the recommended minutes of moderate-intensity physical activity ranging from 45 to 90 min/day (Tables 1 and 3). However, it should be noted that there continues to be a debate about the level of activity needed to prevent weight gain with the primary issue being that there is great variability in response to physical activity, and while some individuals may need considerably less than 60 min/day to maintain weight, others may need more. Further, given the many contributing influences to weight, it is somewhat of an oversimplification to address the

Table 3 2005 USDA Dietary Guidelines for American Adults

Chronic disease	Reduce chronic disease risk	Engage in at least 30 min of moderate-intensity physical activity, above usual activity, at work or home on most days of the week.
Prevent weight gain	Manage and prevent weight gain	Engage in approximately 60 min of moderate-to-vigorous intensity activity on most days of the week while not exceeding caloric intake requirements.
Maintenance	Sustain weight loss	Participate in at least 60 to 90 min of daily moderate-intensity physical activity.

prevention of weight gain using increased energy expenditure alone. The relative contribution of energy intake and energy expenditure in the creation of energy balance to prevent weight gain varies from individual to individual, making it impossible for one recommendation to be appropriate for all individuals. For example, one person may opt to eat more but also perform large amounts of exercise resulting in no net weight gain, while another individual may opt to eat less and perform only a moderate amount of exercise to maintain energy balance. The prevention of weight gain is clearly an area in need of further work and understanding.

In summary, though there remains much work to be done in this area, most expert groups recommend individuals achieve on average a daily PAL of 1.6 to 1.8 to prevent weight gain. This level of PAL translates into 45 to 90 min/day of moderate intensity physical activity with the target of 60 min/day being the most commonly cited goal.

EXERCISE AND WEIGHT LOSS

Exercise Alone and Weight Loss

There is sufficient evidence from both individual studies of varying lengths and cumulative reviews to conclude that exercise interventions in absence of dietary intervention produces modest weight loss at best. For example, in a review article Ross et al. reported that in exercise interventions of 16 weeks or less ($n = 20$ studies) the mean weekly weight loss was 0.2 kg with a total weight loss of 2.3 kg ($\approx$ 5 lb) at follow-up assessment (Fig. 1, panel A) (3). It is important to note that the majority of these studies had relatively low weekly energy expenditures ($<$1500 kcal/wk). The magnitude of weight loss change reported by Ross et al. is nearly identical to those reported in the National Institute of Health Clinical Guidelines on the identification, evaluation, and treatment of overweight and obese adults of 2.4 kg (5.3 lb) (2). Tightly controlled studies that utilize large exercise doses ($\geq$3500 kcal/wk) have demonstrated substantial weight loss ($>$1 kg/wk); however, this exercise dose is likely not obtainable for most unfit, overweight, or obese individuals, and even if this dose could be met, the daily time commitment to exercise would be difficult to meet over the long term (3). For example, a common weight loss goal is 1 to 2 lb/wk, which translates into 3500 to 7000 kcal of energy deficit. To meet the goal of 5000 kcal of weekly energy expenditure, a 200-lb individual would have to brisk walk (4 mph, about 7 km/hr) approximately 660 min/wk or 90 minutes every day of the week (Table 4).

The Ross et al. review also reported a dose-response relation between prescribed caloric expenditure and weight loss in studies of 16 weeks or less with 85% of

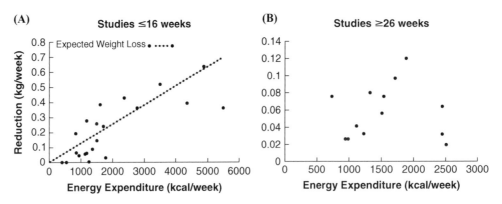

Figure 1 Relationship between energy expenditure and weight loss. (**A**) Studies with a duration of 16 weeks or less and (**B**) studies with a duration of 26 weeks or longer are shown. *Source*: From Ref. 3.

Table 4 Caloric Expenditure Per Minutes for Walking by Weight

									Weight								
		lb:	150	160	170	180	190	200	210	220	230	240	250	260	270	280	290	300
		kg:	68	73	77	82	86	91	95	100	104	109	114	118	123	127	132	136.4
Speed	METS																	
2.0 mph (3.2 kph)	2.5		2.8	3.0	3.2	3.4	3.6	3.8	4.0	4.2	4.4	4.5	4.7	4.9	5.1	5.3	5.5	5.7
2.5 mph (4.0 kph)	3.0		3.4	3.6	3.9	4.1	4.3	4.5	4.8	5.0	5.2	5.5	5.7	5.9	6.1	6.4	6.6	6.8
3.0 mph (4.8 kph)	3.3		3.8	4.0	4.3	4.5	4.8	5.0	5.3	5.5	5.8	6.0	6.3	6.5	6.8	7.0	7.3	7.5
3.5 mph (5.6 kph)	3.8		4.3	4.6	4.9	5.2	5.5	5.8	6.0	6.3	6.6	6.9	7.2	7.5	7.8	8.1	8.3	8.6
4.0 mph (6.4 kph)	5.0		5.7	6.1	6.4	6.8	7.2	7.6	8.0	8.3	8.7	9.1	9.5	9.8	10.2	10.6	11.0	11.4
4.5 mph (7.2 kph)	6.3		7.2	7.6	8.1	8.6	9.1	9.5	10.0	10.5	11.0	11.5	11.9	12.4	12.9	13.4	13.8	14.3

expected weight loss achieved (3). The dose-response relation was not observed in studies of 26 weeks or more (*n* = 12) and achieved weight loss was only 30% of expected. Once again this demonstrates the need to be cautious when extrapolating the result of shorter-term studies to the longer term (Fig. 1, panel B). There are a number of potential causes for longer-term studies failing to produce substantial weight loss including small exercise doses, poor adherence, and even potentially, dietary overcompensation. The concept of exercise-induced dietary overcompensation is important, focusing attention on the complex interactions between exercise-diet and caloric balance, and may in part explain the limited effectiveness of exercise alone in producing weight loss. For example, Donnelly examined the role of exercise only (2000 kcal/wk) on weight loss in men and women over 16 months (Fig. 2) (4). All exercises were supervised, and while both the men and women had good adherence to the exercise intervention, only the men had weight loss

(−6%). The women in the exercise intervention maintained weight during the study period while women in the control group increased weight. Though the men did achieve higher supervised energy expenditure (3300 kcal/wk) than the women (2200 kcal/wk), this does not account for the failure to observe weight loss in the women. The authors have suggested that the source of energy "compensation" is unlikely to be due to decreases in RMR or decreases in spontaneous physical activity, leaving increases in energy intake as the likely cause (5). This study eloquently demonstrates the complexities of the energy balance equation and provides evidence that exercise-induced increases in caloric intake is a topic deserving of additional work.

In summary, exercise without dietary intervention has been found to produce only modest weight loss. There are a number of potential reasons as to why exercise-only studies have resulted in disappointing weight loss, including relatively small exercise-induced caloric expenditure,

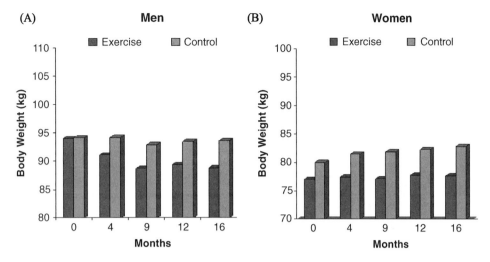

Figure 2 Body weight from baseline to 16 months intervention in men (**A**) and women (**B**) in the exercise and control group. *Source*: From Ref. 4.

poor adherence, and dietary compensation, in response to regular exercise training. Carefully controlled studies that used large exercise doses (>3500 kcal/wk) have demonstrated substantial weight loss. However, these high-dose exercise studies may work for certain individuals or in highly controlled settings, but given the substantial time burden of achieving the exercise dose (≈ 90 minutes or more per day) these interventions have limited clinical utility.

Exercise in Combination with Reduced Caloric Intake in Producing Weight Loss

In studies comparing the effectiveness of exercise alone to diet alone, most found diet alone to be more effective than exercise alone in producing weight loss (1,2,6,7). This finding is not unexpected given that cutting 500 calories out of the daily diet is relatively easier than expending 500 calories through exercise. However, the combination of exercise and diet have been found to be more effective than either alone, and a number of large carefully conducted trials have demonstrated combined exercise and diet interventions to be an effective strategy to produce clinically meaningful weight loss. For example, examining 201 sedentary, obese women, Jakicic et al. explored the interactions of exercise intensity (moderate vs. vigorous) and exercise dose (1000 kcal/wk vs. 2000 kcal/wk) in generating weight loss (8). The four intervention groups were moderate intensity-moderate duration, moderate intensity-high duration, high intensity-moderate duration, and high intensity-high duration. All participants were instructed to reduce calorie intake to between 1200 and 1500 kcal/day and maintain dietary fat between 20% and 30% of total energy intake. All four groups lost at least 6 kg after the one-year intervention with no statistically

significant difference between the groups. Though it appeared that the higher exercise doses achieved greater weight loss (10% vs. 7–8%) compared with the lower doses at one year, this result did not reach statistical significance (Fig. 3). In contrast, the high- and low-intensity groups had nearly identical results within each exercise dose, suggesting that for a given dose of caloric expenditure intensity has no effect on amount of weight lost. This study serves as a good example of how clinically meaningful weight loss can result when diet and exercise are combined. It further demonstrates that even as little as 1000 kcal/wk of exercise when combined with diet can result in clinically meaningful weight loss.

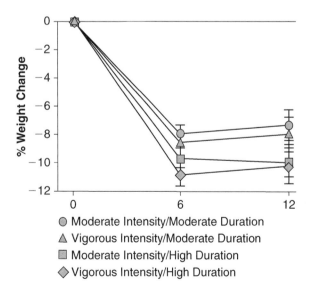

Figure 3 Percentage weight loss after one year of diet and exercise intervention. The exercise intervention was delivery using four different combinations of different intensity and duration. *Source*: From Ref. 8.

Interestingly, while there are a number of expert group recommendations focused on the amount of physical activity needed to prevent weight gain as well as for weigh loss maintenance (discussed below), there are relatively few guidelines which address the optimal exercise dose to induce weight loss in combination with dietary restriction. The American College of Sports Medicine (ACSM) Position Statement titled "Appropriate Intervention Strategies for Weight Loss and Prevention of Weight Regain for Adults" summarizes the literature and provides solid recommendations for combining diet and exercise to promote weight loss. These guidelines recommend reducing daily energy intake by 500 to 1000 kcal with less than 30% of total energy coming from fat. This is combined with a minimum of 150 min/wk of physical activity with the goal increasing to 200 to 300 min/wk ($\geq$2000 kcal) (1). Numerous well-run studies have used diet and exercise plans similar to the ACSM recommendations to successfully produce meaningful weight loss (7). Because of the wide range of suggested daily energy intake reduction (500–100 kcal) combined with a wide range for recommended exercise goals (200–300 minutes), there is a great heterogeneity in the combinations of diet and exercise, which can be used to produce the same weight loss result. For example, Figure 4 demonstrates how the same weight loss goal (1.5 lb lost per week) can be met with either a high-volume exercise or a moderate-volume exercise program due to differences in caloric-intake restriction. This figure demonstrates that there is significant opportunity for individual tailoring of the exercise dose and caloric restriction combination within the weight loss program guidelines.

In summary, the interventions that use both exercise and reduced energy intake have been found to be more effective than either alone in producing clinically significant weight loss. The combination of reducing daily energy intake by 500 to 1000 kcal and a minimum of 150 min/wk of physical activity with the goal increasing to 200 to 300 min/wk ($\geq$2000 kcal) serves as a good foundation for developing effective diet and exercise-based weight loss programs.

Exercise and Maintenance

In some sense, the focus of weight management has changed, and there has been a shift to a greater focus on maintaining weight loss. As detailed above, most weight loss programs grounded in diet and exercise are reasonably successful at producing clinically significant weight loss in the short-to-intermediate term (12 months or less). The challenge has been helping participants maintain the weight loss or prevent weight regain for an extended period of time. For reasons that are not completely understood, regular exercise appears to be critical to the long-term prevention of weight regain. The importance of exercise in prevention of weight regain was first demonstrated in a study using data from the National Weight

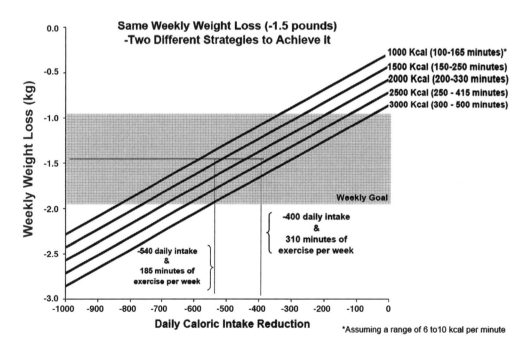

Figure 4 Expected weekly weight loss for different combinations of exercise dose and reduction in caloric intake.

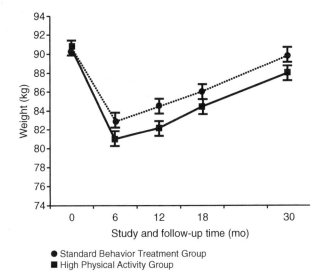

Figure 5 Weight over 30 months in the standard behavior treatment (*circle*) and high physical activity groups (*square*).

● Standard Behavior Treatment Group
■ High Physical Activity Group

Loss Registry (NWLR). It reported that individuals who have lost a substantial amount of weight (≥30 lb) and kept it off for an extended period of time (≥1 year) on average engage in more than 2500 kcal/wk of physical activity for women and almost 3300 kcal/wk for men (9,10). These levels represent more than 300 min/wk of moderate-intensity physical activity.

The data from intervention trials confirm the findings from the NWLR. For example, Tate et al. compared 1000 kcal/wk versus 2500 kcal/wk as part of a behavioral-based weight loss program (Fig. 5) (11). At six months, the 2500-kcal group had greater weight loss and maintained this loss better at 12 and 18 months compared with the 1000-kcal/wk group. Of note is that the participant contact ended at 18 months and by 30 months both groups had regained most of their weight. This intervention trial confirms the findings from the cross-sectional NWLR study that maintaining weight loss likely requires 300 or more minutes per week. Similarly, the 2005 United States Department of Agriculture (USDA) Dietary Guidelines recommended 60 to 90 min/day of moderate-intensity exercise to prevent weight regain.

In summary, exercise plays an important role in the prevention of weight regain after weight loss and data suggest the vast majority of individuals who successfully maintain their weight loss exercise on a regular basis. The available data suggest that to prevent weight regain it requires 300 or more minutes per week of moderate-intensity physical activity. However, as with the prevention of weight gain and promotion of weight loss, the exact amount of exercise required to prevent weight regain is likely to vary greatly from individual to individual.

EXERCISE, FATNESS, AND HEALTH

As noted earlier in the chapter, regular exercise without regard for caloric intake does not produce substantial weight loss. Thus, it is quite possible that an individual may exercise regularly yet remain overweight or obese, resulting in being both fit from cardiorespiratory perspective but overweight or obese. Because people who are physically active also tend to be of lower weight and have fewer comorbidities, there has been great interest in dissecting out the role of weight control in the benefits associated with exercise leading to the question; does exercise have health benefits by itself, or is the weight control (or loss) associated with physical activity responsible for the benefits? In other words, can individuals be both overweight and healthy because they exercise regularly? This has been an area of great debate.

Maximal exercise testing can be used to assess cardiorespiratory fitness, which can serve as a surrogate measure of exercise habits. Examining combinations of fitness and fatness in men from the Aerobics Center Longitudinal Study database (Fig. 6), Wei et al. reported that in normal-weight, overweight, and obese individuals, low fitness was associated with substantially higher risk of cardiovascular disease (CVD) mortality (12). Further, it was also observed that men who were overweight or obese but fit were at lower risk of CVD mortality than men who were of normal weight but unfit. This finding suggested that for CVD mortality risk, it is more important to be fit than to be normal weight. This report received considerable press coverage and led many patients to question their doctors about the importance of losing weight compared with just becoming active.

In a comparison of different combinations of physical activity and fatness in 116,564 women (2370 CVD deaths), Hu et al. reported an inverse relation between self-reported physical activity and risk of CVD death in

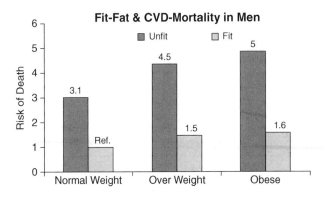

Figure 6 Risk of death in men by fitness and weight categories. *Source*: From Ref. 12.

normal-weight, overweight, and obese women (Fig. 7) (13). However, in direct contrast to the ACLS data in men, in all physical activity categories there was increased risk of CVD mortality with higher BMI. In other words, though higher levels of physical activity had benefit in every weight group, they did not find that higher levels of physical activity negated the effects of excess weight. Given the sharply conflicting data from well-established, large epidemiological studies, the relative importance of fitness and fatness for an individual's health becomes quite confusing.

While the "fitness versus fatness" issue has led to controversy and heated debate that may never be fully resolved, the relative contribution of fitness and fatness to overall health and risk actually may be of little clinical significance because low fitness and excess fatness share the common treatment of increasing regular exercise. Increasing regular exercise results in predictable increases in fitness, and as noted throughout this chapter exercise is a core component of successful weight loss programs and more importantly of long-term weight loss maintenance. In essence, exercise is the common denominator for the clinical treatment of low fitness and excess weight, making the fitness versus fatness debate largely academic (14).

Overweight and obese individuals are at increased risk of diabetes, metabolic syndrome, hypertension, and lipid disorders, and successful weight reduction does not always reverse these conditions. Any strategy to reduce the morbidity and mortality associated with these risk factors has the potential for significant public health impact. For all of these conditions, being a regular exerciser and avoiding low fitness has been associated with lower risk of mortality even when adjusting for weight. For example, Arden et al. examined the benefit of fitness within levels of ATP-III-R risk stratification (15). As

depicted in Figure 8, each level of ATP-III-R risk stratification of CVD mortality was at least twofold higher for unfit individuals compared with fit individuals. Restated even in individuals whose LDL and risk factor profile qualifies them for cholesterol-lowering medication, living an active lifestyle and avoiding being unfit greatly reduce the risk of CVD mortality. Thus, despite the minimal benefit (if any) of regular exercise to LDL cholesterol, those with elevated LDL in a relative sense stand to benefit the most from being physically active. Similar survival benefits associated with exercise without reversal of the risk factor have been shown in individuals with hypertension, diabetes (Fig. 9), and metabolic syndrome (16–19).

The fitness-fatness debate and the demonstrated importance of exercise in individuals with comorbidities provide a good backdrop to discuss the pleiotropic

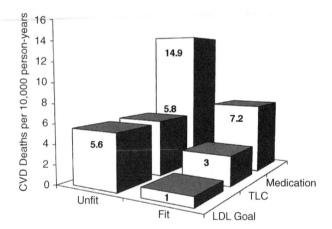

Figure 8 Risk of CVD mortality by combinations of fitness and ATP-III risk stratification. *Abbreviations*: CVD, cardiovascular disease; ATP-III, Adult Treatment Panel III. *Source*: From Ref. 15.

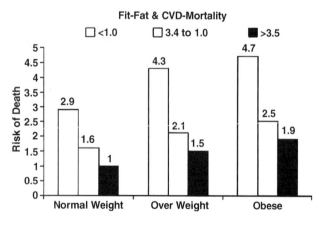

Figure 7 Risk of CVD death in women by physical activity and weight categories. *Abbreviation*: CVD, cardiovascular disease. *Source*: From Ref. 13.

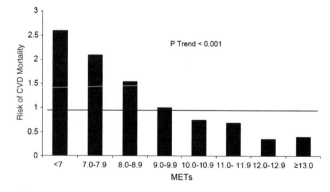

Figure 9 Risk of CVD mortality across levels of fitness with men with diabetes. *Abbreviation*: CVD, cardiovascular disease. *Source*: From Ref. 16.

Table 5 Benefits of Regular Exercise Beyond Weight Loss

Physiological benefits	
Improved heart rate variability	Reduced systemic inflammation
Reduced blood pressure	Improved insulin sensitivity
Improved endothelial function	Decreased myocardial oxygen demand
Increased myocardial function	Maintains lean mass
Decreased platelet aggregation	Increased fibrinolysis
Reduced blood and plasma viscosity	Increased capillary density
Increased mitochondrial density	Reduced visceral adiposity
Better sleep	Improved mood and reduced anxiety

Reduced risk of developing	
Hypertension	Osteoporosis
Metabolic syndrome	Osteoarthritis
Depression	Breast and colon cancer
Type 2 diabetes	Dementia and Alzheimer's disease

benefits of exercise. As summarized in Table 5, exercise improves a variety of physiological measures and risk factors and is associated with reduced risk of a diverse array of important disease conditions. Further, given that this is an active area of research, there are likely to be a number of important medical conditions and physiological measures improved by exercise that have not been identified yet. It should be noted that some of these risk factors such as heart rate variability are improved by exercise even in the absence of weight loss while other variables such as insulin resistance are improved much more by exercise in the presence of weight loss. Given the wide variety of physiological variables and risk factors that exercise improves combined with the great variance in exercise-induced weight loss, it is easy to appreciate the difficulty of dissecting out the relative role of exercise (fitness) and fatness in health. What can be concluded is that regular exercise stands to benefit individuals of every weight but the combination of avoiding excess body weight and participating in regular exercise is the best formula for reducing the risk of developing adverse health conditions.

In summary, the fitness versus fatness debate is largely an academic issue as regular exercise plays a central role in the treatment of low fitness and excess weight. Further, even in individuals with diabetes, hypertension, and/or metabolic syndrome, regular exercise is associated with substantially reduced risk of premature mortality independent of weight. There are health benefits associated with regular exercise that are independent of weight loss but regular exercise combined with maintaining a healthy weight is the best strategy for preventing premature comorbidities and mortality.

Exercise Prescription

As noted earlier, exercise is a type of physical activity, but the most common forms of physical activity are activities of daily living (lifestyle activity), such as climbing stairs, gardening, and walking the dog. While lifestyle activity is an important adjunct to exercise and may be accumulated to meet the daily physical activity requirements, the required caloric expenditure to generate weight loss or prevent weight gain is substantial and likely to require formal exercise to be met.

Exercise prescriptions are generally composed of a combination of type of exercise, intensity of exercise, and amount of exercise, which is the result of frequency and duration. These many variables leave the possibility of a large number of potential options. However, for the purpose of weight loss, the exercise prescription is primarily focused on increased caloric expenditure, making exercise prescription much simpler. The Updated Physical Activity Recommendations for Adults from the ACSM and the American Heart Association is an excellent resource of exercise recommendations and prescriptions (Table 6).

Type

Given the required caloric expenditure, the type of exercise selected for weight management should be aerobic and one that can be safely and comfortably performed for an extended period of time. The most commonly cited type of exercise used by individuals who successfully lose weight and keep it off is walking. This is good news because walking does not require special equipment or

Table 6 Updated Physical Activity Recommendations for Adults from the American College of Sports Medicine and the American Heart Association

1. To promote and maintain good health, adults aged 18–65 yr should maintain a physically active lifestyle.
2. Adults should perform moderate-intensity aerobic (endurance) physical activity for a minimum of 30 min on at least five days each week or vigorous-intensity aerobic activity for a minimum of 20 min on at least three days each week.
3. Combinations of moderate- and vigorous-intensity activity can be performed to meet this recommendation. For example, a person can meet the recommendation by walking briskly for 30 min twice during the week and then jogging for 20 min on two other days.
4. These moderate- or vigorous-intensity activities are in addition to the light-intensity activities frequently performed during daily life (e.g., self-care, washing dishes, using light tools at a desk) or activities of very short duration (e.g., taking out trash, walking to parking lot at store or office).
5. Moderate-intensity aerobic activity, which is generally equivalent to a brisk walk and noticeably accelerates the heart rate, can be accumulated toward the 30-min minimum by performing bouts each lasting 10 or more minutes.
6. Vigorous-intensity activity is exemplified by jogging and causes rapid breathing and a substantial increase in heart rate.
7. In addition, at least twice each week adults will benefit by performing activities using the major muscles of the body that maintain or increase muscular strength and endurance.
8. Because of the dose-response relation between physical activity and health, persons who wish to further improve their personal fitness, reduce their risk for chronic diseases and disabilities or prevent unhealthy weight gain, will likely benefit by exceeding the minimum recommended amount of physical activity.

clothing, does not require membership to a health club, and is associated with minimal risk. (See Table 4 for estimates of calories consumed per minute for different walking paces by body weight.) Note that for a given activity and pace, the more an individual weighs the greater the caloric expenditure for a given pace. This may seem counterintuitive but can be explained by the fact that for a given speed as the weight of the object (in this case a person) goes up so does the required work (caloric expenditure). Other examples of aerobic exercise commonly performed include jogging, cycling, dancing, and swimming.

Though resistance training may provide a number of health benefits in both normal-weight and overweight individuals, there is little evidence that adding resistance training to dietary energy restriction produces additional weight loss (1). Resistance training in overweight individuals may improve strength, which may help mobility and quality of life as well as improve work capacity and thus the ability to perform physical activity. It is often stated that resistance training during active weight loss promotes preservation of lean body mass and subsequently prevents reductions of resting energy expenditure associated with the loss of lean and fat mass. However, there is little evidence to support the idea that performing resistance training during a period of negative energy balance and weight loss promotes maintenance of resting energy expenditure (1). As such, aerobic exercises such as walking are the activity of choice for promoting or maintaining weight loss.

Intensity

While it is possible to exercise at a wide range of intensities from very hard to very light, for the purposes

of weight management the range becomes relatively restricted. Very low intensity activity produces nominal caloric expenditure, resulting in unrealistic exercise time requirements to generate meaningful caloric expenditure, and high intensity or vigorous activity is associated with health risks, leaving moderate intensity as the logical target. Moderate-intensity aerobic activity can be characterized as brisk walking that noticeably accelerates heart rate. Vigorous-intensity activity can be described as jogging that results in rapid breathing and substantial increase in heart rate. Most individuals wishing to lose a substantial amount of weight are not capable of vigorously exercising for an extended period of time. Further, for many overweight/obese individuals, vigorous exercise has substantial health risk including increased risk for acute events of congestive heart failure and orthopedic injury. Thus, vigorous exercise should be avoided in overweight/obese individuals initiating a new exercise program, and those individuals who choose to increase intensity gradually over time should do so with caution and only after discussing this with their health care provider. Thus, moderate intensity should be the target of individuals performing exercise to promote weight loss or prevent weight regain.

Frequency and Duration

Given that both weight loss and the prevention of weight gain require the expenditure of 2000 to 3000 cal/wk through exercise, there are only a limited number of options for different combinations of frequency and duration. It is unlikely that many individuals would try to achieve 200 to 300 minutes of exercise in one or two exercise bouts. It is also unlikely that most individuals want to exercise seven days a week. The most likely combination of frequency and duration is 3 to 5 days/wk for 60 minutes or more per session.

Risks of Exercise

Participation in exercise is not without risk. However, these risks can be minimized with a few basic steps and the risk of serious events (i.e., cardiac event) are rare when appropriate precautions are taken (20). The most common risk of exercise is musculoskeletal injury with the risk increasing with obesity, sedentary lifestyle, amount of exercise, intensity of exercise, and participation in competitive sports. To minimize the risk of injury, the amount (volume) of daily activity should be increased gradually over time. For individuals starting a new exercise program, the importance of starting slow and increasing the amount (time and intensity) gradually over time cannot be over emphasized. This point is often not appreciated by individuals recently motivated to become active, and the importance of gradual progression needs to be strongly reinforced by health care professionals. Risk of serious events such as sudden cardiac death or myocardial infarction acutely increases with participation in higher-intensity activities both in individuals with diagnosed and occult heart disease. As a general rule, the risk of serious events associated with exercise dramatically increases with exercise intensity and number of medical conditions of the exerciser.

Screening/Clearance

For most individuals, it is not necessary to undergo exercise stress testing or receive an extensive clinical examination prior to starting a moderate-intensity exercise program that includes a moderate rate of progression. However, individuals who wish to participate in higher-intensity activities, particularly those with CVD risk factors may need physician clearance prior to participation, and in some cases this should include an exercise test. In brief, in men younger than 45 years and women younger than 55 years with one or less CVD risk factor, exercise testing is not suggested prior to starting an exercise program of any intensity exercise (20,21). Men older than 45 years and women older than 55 years or those with two or more CVD risk factors should have an exercise stress test prior to initiating a high-intensity (vigorous) exercise program (20,21). Individuals with signs or symptoms of CVD or known cardiovascular, pulmonary, or metabolic disease should have a stress test prior to starting a moderate or vigorous exercise program. Thus, the higher the intensity of the proposed exercise program, the older the participant, and the more risk factors/disease present,

the greater the need for an exercise stress test prior to starting. Because many overweight/obese individuals will qualify as moderate or high risk, they should seek clearance from their health care provider prior to starting an exercise program or increasing exercise intensity.

SUMMARY

Regular exercise has meaningful health benefits for individuals of any weight. For the purpose of general health, the goal should be at least 30 min/day, five or more days per week of moderate-intensity activity ($\geq$150 min/wk). However, this amount of activity may be not enough to prevent weight gain in all individuals, leading many expert panels to recommend at least 60 min/day for the purpose of maintaining normal weight. For the purpose of weight loss, the combinations of exercise and reduced energy intake have been found to be more effective than either alone. The combination of reducing daily energy intake by 500 to 1000 kcal and a minimum of 150 min/wk of exercise with the goal increasing to 200 to 300 min/wk ($\geq$2000 kcal) serves as a good foundation for developing effective diet and exercise-based weight loss programs. Regular exercise has been identified as a key behavior in the prevention of weight regain after weight loss and the available data suggest that prevention of weight regain requires 300 or more minutes per week of moderate-intensity exercise. However, it needs to be emphasized that the recommended exercise doses for weight loss and prevention of weight gain or regain are population-based numbers with great individual variation, resulting in some individuals needing more or less than the recommended amounts to achieve the desired weight benefit. As such, these numbers only serve as starting points and should be tailored to meet individuals' specific needs.

REFERENCES

1. Jakicic JM, Clark K, Coleman E, et al. American College of Sports Medicine position stand. Appropriate intervention strategies for weight loss and prevention of weight regain for adults. Med Sci Sports Exerc 2001; 33(12):2145–2156.
2. National Institutes of Health. Clinical guidelines on the identification, evaluation, and treatment of overweight and obesity in adults—the evidence report. Obes Res 1998; 6(suppl 2):51S–209S.
3. Ross R, Janssen I. Physical activity, total and regional obesity: dose-response considerations. Med Sci Sports Exerc 2001; 33(suppl 6):S521–S527.
4. Donnelly JE, Hill JO, Jacobsen DJ, et al. Effects of a 16-month randomized controlled exercise trial on body weight and composition in young, overweight men and women: the Midwest Exercise Trial. Arch Intern Med 2003; 163(11):1343–1350.

5. Donnelly JE, Smith BK. Is exercise effective for weight loss with ad libitum diet? Energy balance, compensation, and gender differences. Exerc Sport Sci Rev 2005; 33(4):169–174.

6. Curioni CC, Lourenco PM. Long-term weight loss after diet and exercise: a systematic review. Int J Obes (Lond) 2005; 29(10):1168–1174.

7. Shaw K, Gennat H, O'Rourke P, et al. Exercise for overweight or obesity. Cochrane Database Syst Rev 2006; (4): CD003817.

8. Jakicic JM, Marcus BH, Gallagher KI, et al. Effect of exercise duration and intensity on weight loss in overweight, sedentary women: a randomized trial. JAMA 2003; 290(10):1323–1330.

9. Klem ML, Wing RR, McGuire MT, et al. A descriptive study of individuals successful at long-term maintenance of substantial weight loss. Am J Clin Nutr 1997; 66(2):239–246.

10. Wing RR, Phelan S. Long-term weight loss maintenance. Am J Clin Nutr 2005; 82(suppl 1):222S–225S.

11. Tate DF, Jeffery RW, Sherwood NE, et al. Long-term weight losses associated with prescription of higher physical activity goals. Are higher levels of physical activity protective against weight regain? Am J Clin Nutr 2007; 85(4):954–959.

12. Wei M, Kampert JB, Barlow CE, et al. Relationship between low cardiorespiratory fitness and mortality in normal-weight, overweight, and obese men. JAMA 1999; 282(16):1547–1553.

13. Hu FB, Willett WC, Li T, et al. Adiposity as compared with physical activity in predicting mortality among women. N Engl J Med 2004; 351(26):2694–2703.

14. Blair SN, Church TS. The fitness, obesity, and health equation: is physical activity the common denominator? JAMA 2004; 292(10):1232–1234.

15. Ardern CI, Katzmarzyk PT, Janssen I, et al. Revised Adult Treatment Panel III guidelines and cardiovascular disease mortality in men attending a preventive medical clinic. Circulation 2005; 112:1481–1488.

16. Church TS, LaMonte MJ, Barlow CE, et al. Cardiorespiratory fitness and body mass index as predictors of cardiovascular disease mortality among men with diabetes. Arch Intern Med 2005; 165(18):2114–2120.

17. Church TS, Cheng YJ, Earnest CP, et al. Exercise capacity and body composition as predictors of mortality among men with diabetes. Diabetes Care 2004; 27(1):83–88.

18. Church TS, Kampert JB, Gibbons LW, et al. Usefulness of cardiorespiratory fitness as a predictor of all-cause and cardiovascular disease mortality in men with systemic hypertension. Am J Cardiol 2001; 88(6):651–656.

19. Katzmarzyk PT, Church TS, Blair SN. Cardiorespiratory fitness attenuates the effects of the metabolic syndrome on all-cause and cardiovascular disease mortality in men. Arch Intern Med 2004; 164(10):1092–1097.

20. Haskell WL, Lee I-M, Pate RR, et al. Physical Activity and Public Health: Updated Recommendation for Adults from the American College of Sports Medicine and the American Heart Association. Med Sci Sports Exerc 2007; 39(8):1423–1434.

21. American College of Sports Medicine, . ACSM's Guidelines for Exercise Testing and Prescription. 7th ed. Philadelphia, Pennsylvania: Lippincott Williams & Wilkins, 2006.

22. Jakicic JM, Winters C, Lang W, et al. Effects of intermittent exercise and use of home exercise equipment on adherence, weight loss, and fitness in overweight women: a randomized trial. JAMA 1999; 282(16):1554–1560.

18

Sibutramine in the Management of Obesity

DONNA H. RYAN

Pennington Biomedical Research Center, Baton Rouge, Louisiana, U.S.A.

INTRODUCTION

Medications can be useful adjuncts to diet and physical activity in helping selected patients achieve and maintain meaningful weight loss. The National Heart, Lung, and Blood Institute report titled "Clinical Guidelines on the Identification, Evaluation, and Treatment of Overweight and Obesity in Adults—the evidence report" (1) emphasizes the need for physicians to address obesity in their patients. The Evidence Report sanctions the clinical use of weight loss drugs approved by the Food and Drug Administration (FDA) for long-term use as part of a concomitant lifestyle modification program. According to these guidelines, appropriate patients for medication include those who have been unsuccessful in previous weight loss attempts, whose body mass index (BMI) exceeds 27 kg/m^2 who have associated conditions such as diabetes, hypertension, or dyslipidemia, or whose BMI exceeds 30 kg/m^2.

There is growing appreciation among medical practitioners for the meaningful health benefits produced by sustained weight loss, even though only 5% to 10% from baseline. Loss of 5% to 10% of body weight by obese individuals can translate into improvement in glycemic control; in blood pressure and hypertension control; in lipid profile; and in symptoms of sleep apnea, arthritis, and other comorbid conditions (1). Furthermore, modest weight loss is arguably the greatest cause of reduction in risk for type 2 diabetes, now rising to epidemic levels around the world. In the Diabetes Prevention Program (DPP), weight loss of 6% to 7% from baseline produced a 58% reduction in risk for developing type 2 diabetes over two to five years in individuals with impaired glucose tolerance (2). Similar diabetes risk reduction with modest weight loss has been demonstrated in the Finnish Diabetes Prevention Study (3).

Sibutramine was approved by the U.S. FDA for use in obesity treatment in 1997. It is one of only two medications (along with orlistat, approved in 1999) approved for long-term use in the United States. The 2007 review of rimonabant by the FDA called for additional neuropsychiatric safety data, and thus sibutramine remains the only centrally acting agent approved for long-term use. This review focuses on the use of sibutramine in medical practices to help obese patients achieve and sustain health benefits through weight loss.

SIBUTRAMINE: PHARMACOLOGY AND MECHANISM OF ACTION

Sibutramine (marketed as Meridia in the United States and Reductil elsewhere) is a selective reuptake inhibitor for norepinephrine, serotonin, and to a lesser extent, dopamine. The drug is rapidly metabolized to two active metabolites, whose half-life is 14 to 16 hours, with the peak concentration at 3 to 4 hours and a plateau from

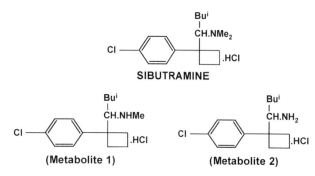

Figure 1 Structural formulas for sibutramine and its two active metabolites. *Source*: From Ref. 5.

3 to 7 hours (4). The chemical structures of sibutramine and those of its two active metabolites are illustrated in Figure 1 (5). The pharmacologic profile allows for once a day dosing, an advantage when appetite regulation is the aim. The drug was first evaluated as a potential antidepressant in three phase II clinical trials with disappointing results in depression (6). However, striking weight loss was observed in the enrolled depressed patients (6), and the drug has since been developed and marketed for weight loss.

The mechanisms by which sibutramine produces its pharmacologic effects are thought to be through the actions of serotonin and norepinephrine in combination, acting within the central nervous system (7). Sibutramine's dopaminergic action is minimal (7).

When administered to experimental animals, sibutramine has dual mechanisms to induce weight reduction: decrease in food intake and increase in energy expenditure (8). The increase in energy expenditure is prominent in rodents, with sustained (> 6 hours) increase in the metabolic rate up to 30%, and is based on sympathetic activation of thermogenesis in brown adipose tissue (8,9). This effect is not prominent in humans, as is discussed later.

In clinical trials with humans, sibutramine decreases food intake in nondieting men (10) and women (11) by increasing meal-induced satiety (10–12). The drug's effect on food intake is more prominent than on energy expenditure, and food intake reduction accounts for the drug's principle mechanism of weight loss.

It takes a carefully designed study to reveal the small acute effects of sibutramine on energy expenditure, such as that by Hansen et al. (12), where energy expenditure was measured for 5.5 hours after dosing with 30-mg sibutramine, and compared with placebo in fed and fasted men. There was a sibutramine-induced increase in energy expenditure of about 3% to 5%. Another study (13) did not show an acute effect of sibutramine, but energy expenditure was only measured for three hours in this study. In a study of the thermogenic effects of sibutramine

when taken over a longer course, Walsh et al. (14) studied obese females receiving 12 weeks of a calorie-reduced diet and either sibutramine 15 mg/day or placebo. The expected decline in resting energy expenditure usually observed with weight loss, and documented in the placebo-treated participants, was blunted in the sibutramine-treated patients. The authors suggest that the sibutramine effect is equivalent to 100 kcal/day, and might be enough to promote weight loss maintenance over the long term.

SIBUTRAMINE: CLINICAL PROFILE

Sibutramine has been extensively evaluated in clinical studies. Overall, clinical data from over 12,000 patients form the basis for the regulatory approval of this drug (15). The first clinical trial with sibutramine lasting eight weeks occurred in 1991 and produced a dose-dependent weight loss with doses of 5 and 20 mg/day (16). Since that time, a number of long-term, randomized, placebo-controlled double-blind clinical trials have been conducted in men and women of all ethnic groups, with ages ranging from 18 to 65 years and with a BMI between 27 and 40 kg/m^2.

Sibutramine has been studied in predominantly overweight and obese healthy adults in comparison to placebo (16–23), different paradigms of weight loss maintenance (24–26), behavioral paradigms (27–29), adolescents (30–32), hypertensive patients (33–37), diabetic patients (38–43), individuals with hyperlipidemia (22), and with binge-eating disorder (44). Sibutramine has been compared with orlistat in randomized clinical trials (45,46) and has been evaluated in populations such as primary care models (47,48). One study (49) reports the results on weight after cessation of sibutramine.

Efficacy of Sibutramine

The experience from these studies reveals issues that are relevant to sibutramine's efficacy characteristics in clinical practice. The first lesson from the clinical trial experience is that the magnitude of weight loss is related to the dose of sibutramine. Second, the intensity of the behavioral component that is used in conjunction with the drug also influences the amount of weight lost with sibutramine. Third, sibutramine is effective in maintaining weight loss for up to two years, or at least as long as it is given. Fourth, initial weight loss predicts long-term success.

Graphic depictions of the dose-response relationship between sibutramine 1, 5, 10, 15, 20, and 30 mg and weight loss is found Figures 2 and 3, which show the results of a double-blind, placebo-controlled study conducted in seven

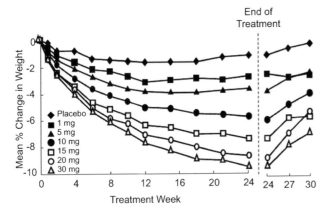

Figure 2 Sequential weight loss in patients completing 24 weeks of treatment, last observation carried forward analysis. (♦) placebo, (■) l-mg sibutramine, (▲) 5-mg sibutramine, (●) 10-mg sibutramine, (□) 15-mg sibutramine, (○) 20-mg sibutramine, (△) 30-mg sibutramine. $p < 0.05$ versus placebo for all time points for sibutramine doses of 5 to 30 mg, nonparametric Williams' test. $N = 87$ to 107 per group. Posttreatment follow-up data are also shown for those patients in whom it was available ($N = 50$–61 per group). *Source*: From Ref. 18.

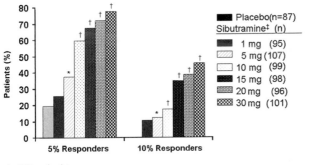

*p<0.01 vs placebo
†p<0.001 vs placebo
‡Recommended dose of sibutramine 10 or 15 mg once daily

Figure 3 Percentage of patients losing at least 5% or 10% of baseline weight after 24 weeks treatment according to dose of sibutramine or placebo. *$p < 0.001$ versus placebo, pairwise Fisher's exact test. *Source*: Adapted from Ref. 18.

centers and enrolling 1047 subjects (18). Figure 2 shows mean weight loss over time displayed graphically for all treatment groups in this trial and demonstrates a clear dose-response relationship. The recommended dose levels for use in clinical practice are 5 to 15 mg/day and these doses produced −3.1%, −4.71%, and −5.8% weight loss from baseline at week 24.

While average weight loss in a clinical trial provides a measure of a drug's activity, the proportion of patients who are exposed to a medication and who achieve meaningful weight loss is another measure of efficacy. In clinical practice, the analysis of data according to proportion of enrollees who achieve >5% or >10% weight loss

is helpful. This gives practicing physicians an idea of what an individual patient's chances are of achieving meaningful weight loss. The percentage of sibutramine-treated patients who achieve >5% weight loss is always greater than placebo.

As can be observed in Figures 2 and 3, the behavioral approach used with pharmacotherapy in this pivotal dose-ranging study was relatively weak, since the mean weight loss associated with placebo was only 0.9% from baseline at 24 weeks, and <20% of patients on placebo achieved ≥5% weight loss from baseline. Weight loss of 5% and 10% from baseline are useful benchmarks because these are associated with significant health benefits. Figure 3 illustrates that 37.4%, 59.6%, and 73% of persons taking sibutramine 5, 10, and 15 mg doses achieved 5% weight loss from baseline, compared to only 19.5% of those taking placebo.

The intensity of the behavioral component of the weight loss program influences the amount of weight lost with sibutramine. Since sibutramine enhances satiety, a dietary program that takes advantage of this mechanism is likely to produce greater weight loss. Wadden et al. (27,29) illustrate the advantage of a good behavioral or lifestyle intervention in combination with sibutramine. The more recent study is a good illustration (29). In this study, 224 obese adults were randomized to one of the following four conditions: (*i*) sibutramine 15-mg daily delivered by the primary care provider in eight visits of 10 to 15 minutes each; (*ii*) lifestyle-modification counseling alone, delivered in 30 group sessions; (*iii*) sibutramine plus 30 group lifestyle-modification sessions (combination therapy); or (*iv*) sibutramine plus brief lifestyle counseling delivered by the primary care provider in eight visits of 10 to 15 minutes each. All subjects received the same recommendations for 1200 to 1500 kcal/day diet and the same exercise regimen recommendations. There was 82% retention over the four arms at 12 months. At one year, as can be observed in Figure 4, the group that received 12 months of sibutramine alone lost 5.0 ± 7.4 kg, while those treated with combined therapy lost 12.1 ± 9.8 kg, and the weight loss for the other two groups was intermediate (6.7 ± 7.9 kg and 7.5 ± 8.0 kg). This study, as illustrated in Figure 4, underscores the importance of using sibutramine as an adjunct to lifestyle measures to achieve weight loss, and demonstrates the benefits of adjunctive pharmacotherapy.

Meta-analysis of Sibutramine's Weight Loss Effects

There are several published meta-analyses (50–53) of the weight loss effects of sibutramine and its effects on blood pressure and other risk factors. In one of these, the meta-analysis of sibutramine reported a mean difference of

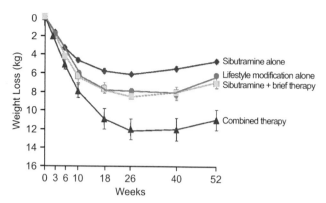

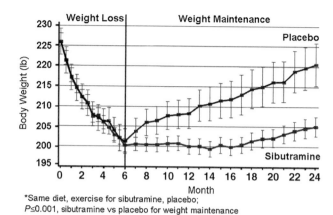

*Same diet, exercise for sibutramine, placebo;
$P \leq 0.001$, sibutramine vs placebo for weight maintenance

Figure 4 Mean (+SE) weight loss in the following four groups is depicted: (*i*) sibutramine alone is sibutramine 15 mg daily prescribed by primary care provider in eight visits of 10 to 15 minutes, (*ii*) lifestyle modification alone—30 group sessions, (*iii*) sibutramine and brief therapy—15-mg sibutramine and brief lifestyle counseling delivered by physician, and (*iv*) combined therapy = 15-mg sibutramine prescribed as in (*i*) and lifestyle therapy as in (*ii*). Subjects receiving combined therapy lost significantly more weight at year one, as well as weeks 18 and 40 than those in the other three groups (*p* < 0.001 by intention-to-treat analysis). *Source*: Adapted from Ref. 29.

Figure 5 Mean (SE) sequential body weight change during weight-loss and weight maintenance phases of the STORM trial for sibutramine and placebo groups. At month 24, mean (SE) kg weight loss was −8.9 (8.1) for sibutramine and −4.0 (5.9) for placebo (*p* < 0.001). *Source*: Adapted from Ref. 25.

4.5 kg weight loss (95% CI, 3.62–5.29 kg) at 12 months (50). However, only five studies (21–24,26,43,47) met the predefined criteria for inclusion in the meta-analysis. A second report produces 12 month weight change with sibutramine of −4.18 kg (95% CI, −5.14 to 3.21 kg) (51). These meta-analyses, despite limitations of small numbers of studies, reinforce the concept that independent of the behavioral intervention, weight loss with sibutramine is modest.

Sibutramine and Weight Loss Maintenance

There are three trials (24–26) that assess sibutramine use as a weight loss *maintenance* agent. After inducing weight loss with very low-calorie liquid diet (24), or with sibutramine (25,26), patients were randomized to placebo or sibutramine for maintenance of weight loss for up to 18 months. All three studies demonstrate sibutramine's efficacy in maintaining weight loss.

The STORM trial (25) illustrates that sibutramine is quite effective for inducing and maintaining weight loss for up to two years (Fig. 5). In this multicenter European study, patients received sibutramine 10 mg and a calorie deficit diet for six months. Of the 605 obese patients who entered the trial, 467 (77%) achieved weight loss of at least 5% from baseline. Those patients were then randomized to receive sibutramine (doses could be titrated from 10 to 20 mg daily) or placebo. Following 24 months of observation, weight loss of the sibutramine-treated group

averaged 10.2 kg below baseline, compared to 4.7 kg for placebo. Practitioners might infer several relevant clinical insights from this study. About three quarters of obese patients who are prescribed sibutramine 10 mg/day with a diet program might be expected to achieve clinically meaningful weight loss (i.e., ≥5% from baseline). If medication is continued, almost half of those will maintain 80% of the weight loss at 18 months follow-up. There is a lesson in the fate of the subjects who were randomized to placebo during the 18-month double-blind portion of the trial. The placebo-treated patients steadily regained weight, maintaining only 20% of their weight loss at the end of the trial. If patients are to be successful to maintain weight loss, the treatment must be continued.

Despite the widespread recognition that weight is regained when treatments are curtailed, recidivism is very common. One approach that should be considered is intermittent therapy or early intervention for relapse. Figure 6 shows the results of an interesting study by Wirth and Krause (26), evaluating an intermittent use of sibutramine. In this study, patients who had lost 2% or 2 kg after four weeks of treatment with sibutramine 15 mg/day were randomized to placebo versus continuous sibutramine versus sibutramine prescribed intermittently (weeks 1–12, 19–30, and 37–48). Both sibutramine treatment regimens gave equivalent results and were significantly better than placebo. The effect of stopping sibutramine is illustrated in Figure 6 by a small increase in weight, which is then reversed when the medication is restarted. This study emphasizes the value of restarting medications before weight regain is advanced, and the necessity of continued therapy for weight loss maintenance. However, another publication by Wirth reports that in 374 patients who had taken sibutramine for at least six months, there was no

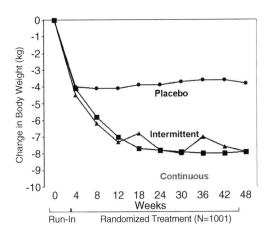

Figure 6 Mean sequential change in body weight during the study period. Patients ($n = 1102$) received sibutramine 15 mg/day for an initial four-week period. Those who lost 2% or 2 kg in four weeks were randomized to placebo ($n = 395$) versus continued sibutramine ($n = 405$) versus intermittent sibutramine (weeks 1–12, 19–30, and 37–48) ($n = 395$). *Source*: Adapted from Ref. 26.

weight regain after an additional six months of observation off sibutramine (49). This is certainly a contradiction to the conventional wisdom and should be interpreted with caution.

Predicting Response to Sibutramine

The chance of an individual achieving meaningful weight loss can be determined by the response to treatment in the first four weeks. In one large trial (18), of the patients who lost 2 kg (4 lb) in the first four weeks of treatment, 60% achieved a weight loss of more than 5%, compared to less than 10% of those who did not lose 2 kg (4 lb) in four weeks (18). It is therefore useful to use "four pounds in four weeks" as a guide to assess efficacy and indication to continue.

Sibutramine Efficacy in Special Populations

Type 2 Diabetes

The obese diabetic and obese hypertensive patients are commonly encountered in primary care practices. There are a number of published studies (38–43) using sibutramine in obese patients with type 2 diabetes. With the exception of the studies by Gokcel et al. (39), Kaukua et al. (42), and the Multicenter Sibutramine Study Group (43), the weight loss observed is somewhat disappointing. In most of the studies, <50% of patients achieved a reduction of 5% body weight on 15 mg/day, which perhaps reflects the frequent comment of clinicians regarding the greater difficulty of achieving weight loss

in patients with diabetes, compared to nondiabetic patients. Still, in all of the studies, the percentage of patients on sibutramine who achieved meaningful weight loss was significantly greater than those on placebo, and the analysis of glycemic control showed benefit corresponding to the degree of weight loss. In the study by Gokcel (39), 60 female patients with diabetes who had poorly controlled glucose levels (HbA1c > 8%) on maximal doses of sulfonylureas and metformin were randomly assigned to sibutramine 10 mg twice daily or placebo. The weight loss at 24 weeks was striking, −9.6 kg in sibutramine-treated patients compared to −0.9 kg with placebo. The improvements in glycemic control were equally striking. In the sibutramine-treated patients, HbA1c fell −2.73%, compared to −0.53% with placebo. Insulin levels fell 5.66 uU/mL compared to 0.68 for placebo, and fasting glucose fell −124.88 mg/dL compared to −15.76 mg/dL for placebo.

In the multicenter study reported by McNulty (43), among 194 metformin-treated diabetic patients, placebo-treated patients lost no weight, but sibutramine 15 mg daily produced 5.3 kg weight loss at six months and 8 kg among 20-mg sibutramine-treated patients, weight at six months. Furthermore, weight loss in both groups was maintained at one year. Glycemic control improved in parallel to weight loss. Weight loss ≥10% was achieved by 14% and 27% of subjects receiving 15 and 20 mg, respectively. For those who lost ≥10%, HbA1c decreased by 1.2 ± 0.4% ($p < 0.0001$).

The Finnish study by Kaukua (42) describes 232 diabetic individuals randomized after a two-week run-in with a low-calorie diet to sibutramine or placebo. The study is remarkable for its high retention: 92% of sibutramine-treated and 89% of the placebo group at 12 months. At 12 months, the sibutramine group lost 7.3% compared to 2.4% for placebo. However, there was no significant change in glycemic control in either group and, furthermore, systolic blood pressure change was 4.1 mmHg and 3.6 mmHg (sibutramine and placebo, respectively), and diastolic blood pressure was 1.7 mmHg and −0.2 mmHg, respectively. These findings may reflect the powerful effect of negative energy balance achieved during the run-in period. The main thrust of this study was assessment of quality of life, which is discussed later.

In one meta-analysis (54) of sibutramine-induced weight loss in patients with type 2 diabetes, there was an overall 0.4% reduction in HbA1c with sibutramine use. In patients who lost 10% of baseline body weight, the HbA1c reduction was 0.7% ($p < 0.003$). In another such (53) meta-analysis, eight clinical trials of sibutramine for weight loss in diabetic patients produced results that reinforce the clinical benefit in terms of weight loss when sibutramine is used, and if weight loss occurs, then glycemic control improves.

Hypertension

Two trials using sibutramine for more than one year in obese hypertensive patients have been reported (33,34), and two additional studies provide data on 12 weeks of treatment (35,36). In all instances, the weight loss pattern favors sibutramine. However, except for one study (36), mean weight loss, though favorable, was associated with small increases in mean blood pressure. McMahon et al. (33) reported a 52-week trial in hypertensive patients whose blood pressure was controlled with calcium channel blockers, with or without β-blockers or thiazides. Sibutramine doses were increased from 5 to 20 mg/day during the first six weeks. Weight loss was significantly greater in the sibutramine-treated patients, averaging −4.4 kg (4.7%) as compared to −0.5 kg (0.7%) in the placebo-treated group. Diastolic blood pressure decreased −1.3 mmHg in the placebo-treated group and increased by 2.0 mmHg in the sibutramine-treated group. The systolic blood pressure increased +1.5 mmHg in the placebo-treated group and by +2.7 mmHg in the sibutramine-treated group. Heart rate was unchanged in the placebo-treated patients, and increased +4.9 beats per minute (bpm) in the sibutramine-treated patients.

A recent study (37) treated 171 obese hypertensive subjects for 16 weeks with sibutramine 15 mg or placebo. There were three antihypertensive therapies being used by the patients (felodipine/ramipril, verapionil/trandolopril, or metaprolol succinate/hydrochlorothiazide). In terms of weight loss, the group taking metaprolol succinate/hydrochlorothiazide had inferior results. This group also had attenuated improvement in glucose tolerance and hypertriglyceridemia. The study suggests that the β-blocker/thiazide diuretic therapy for hypertension may be the least desirable treatment strategy if sibutramine is being used.

Adolescents

There are three reports of sibutramine use in adolescents (30–32). Two of the studies are single center and modest in size, with 82 participants in one (30), and 60 participants (32) in the second, which was conducted in Brazil. Both studies showed superior weight loss and BMI reduction with sibutramine. A large ($n = 498$), 12-month, randomized study (31) conducted in 35 U.S. clinics has recently been published. Participants were 12 to 16 years old and were from multiethnic backgrounds. This study showed a mean BMI reduction of -2.9 kg/m^2 (± 0.15 kg/m^2), compared to -0.3 kg/m^2 for placebo-treated individuals receiving identical behavior therapy. In this study, there were small *decreases* in mean blood pressure and pulse rate observations for both groups, although this was not true with subgroup analysis for those who lost less than 5% BMI where there was 1.8 mmHg increase in blood pressure for sibutramine-treated patients. From all the three studies, one can conclude that sibutramine has cardiovascular activity similar in adolescents as that seen in adults (discussed later, see sec. "Sibutramine and the Cardiovascular System").

Hyperlipidemia

Sibutramine has been used in obese patients with hyperlipidemia. In one study (22), 322 obese men and women with triglycerides ≥250 and ≤1000 mg/dL and serum HDL-cholesterol <40 mg/dL (men) or ≤45 mg/dL (women) were put on a Step 1 American Heart Association diet and randomized to sibutramine 20 mg ($n = 162$) or placebo ($n = 160$). The mean weight loss at 24 weeks favored sibutramine (−4.9 kg vs. 0.6 kg) and 42% of sibutramine-treated patients achieved ≥5% reduction in weight, compared to only 8% of those on placebo. For those patients on sibutramine who achieved ≥5% loss from baseline weight, the serum triglycerides decreased by 33.4 mg/dL and HDL-cholesterol increased by 4.9 mg/dL.

Binge Eating

Sibutramine has been evaluated (55) in 60 obese individuals with binge-eating disorder, diagnosed by *Diagnostic and Statistical Manual for Mental Disorders, Fourth Edition* (DSM-IV) criteria. In this 12-week study at two centers, there was a significant reduction in the number of days with binge episodes, significant weight loss (−7.4 kg vs. −1.4 kg), and improvements in the Beck Depression Inventory and Binge Eating Scale for the sibutramine-treated group.

Sibutramine's Effect on Obesity-Related Risk Factors and Quality of Life

With the exception of resting blood pressure and pulse, the weight loss induced with sibutramine is associated with improvement in all other obesity-related risk factors, including lipids (56), uric acid (25) indices of glycemic control (54), and waist circumference (57). These positive changes are related to weight loss, and the drug does not have an independent effect on these factors.

In addition to improvement in most obesity-related risk factors, weight loss with sibutramine can produce improvements in health-related quality of life (HRQOL). Samsa (58) combined data from four double-blind, randomized controlled trials of sibutramine 20 mg/dL versus placebo. Moderate weight loss (5.01–10%) was associated with a statistically significant improvement in HRQOL. Kaukua et al. (42) evaluated HRQOL in a randomized, controlled trial in 236 diabetic subjects. While sibutramine-treated subjects lost more weight (−7.1 kg) compared to placebo (−2.6 kg, $p < 0.001$), there was no improvement in RAND-36 measures of

HRQOL. This may be explained by the high values of RAND-36 at baseline.

Sibutramine Safety and Tolerability

The cardiovascular side effects of sibutramine are discussed in a separate section later. Sibutramine is available in 5-, 10-, and 15-mg pills, and 10 mg/day as a single daily dose is the recommended starting level, with titration up or down based on response. Doses *above* 15 mg/day are not currently recommended by the FDA.

Sibutramine is not recommended for use in patients with a history of coronary artery disease, congestive heart failure, cardiac arrhythmias, or stroke. It should not be used in patients with poorly controlled hypertension. There should be a two-week interval between termination of monoamine oxidase inhibitors and beginning sibutramine. The latest prescribing recommendations are that sibutramine may be used with caution with selective serotonin reuptake inhibitors. Because sibutramine is metabolized by the cytochrome P_{450} enzyme system (isozyme CYP3A4), when drugs like erythromycin and ketoconazole are taken, there may be competition for this enzymatic pathway, and prolonged metabolism can result. The side effects of sibutramine (insomnia, asthenia, dry mouth, and constipation) are generally mild and transient. Unlike fenfluramine and dexfenfluramine, sibutramine is not associated with valvulopathy (59–61). Although the drug is scheduled as a Class IV substance, there is no evidence for abuse potential, as demonstrated in a study of 31 male recreational stimulant users (62). There is no evidence for a clinically relevant interaction of sibutramine with alcohol in impairment of cognitive function (59).

Sibutramine and the Cardiovascular System (Blood Pressure and Pulse)

If sibutramine acts via central nervous system stimulation of norepinephrine and serotonin, and through the sympathetic nervous system to increase thermogenesis, then cardiostimulatory effects are to be expected. The principle concerns with sibutramine safety have been blood pressure and pulse increases, and a warning required by the FDA that the drug can cause increases in blood pressure and pulse. It is true that the drug is associated with small mean increases in blood pressure and pulse. However, the mean increases do not tell the whole story. This observation is reinforced in a meta-analysis (52), which demonstrates a small effect size on systolic and diastolic blood pressure in sibutramine studies.

Jordan et al. (63) conducted an analysis of two large placebo-controlled clinical trials with a data set of 1336 patients (966 randomized to sibutramine, and 370 to placebo). The data set allowed analysis of normotensive subjects, as well as those with grade I, II, and those with isolated systolic hypertension. There was no difference in blood pressure changes, comparing sibutramine or placebo groups in any five hypertension subgroups. However, despite -8.0 ± 7.2 kg mean weight loss for sibutramine, compared to -3.6 ± 8.0 kg for placebo at 48 weeks, one did not observe the expected mean blood pressure reductions. Systolic blood pressure was -0.1 ± 15.5 mmHg and -0.2 ± 15.2 mmHg for sibutramine and placebo groups, respectively, at 48 weeks. Diastolic measures were 0.3 ± 9.5 and -0.8 ± 9.2 mmHg for the respective groups.

It has been suggested that the blood pressure effects of sibutramine are mitigated by greater weight loss (64). That is, with increasing amounts of weight loss the blood pressure change may actually be a net decrease, albeit less than that observed with similar non-sibutramine weight loss. Thus, for an individual patient who has successfully achieved weight loss with sibutramine, the blood pressure may be reduced from baseline, although the blood pressure reduction may not be as great as that associated with the same degree of weight lost without the medication.

Another strategy (an aerobic exercise program) to deal with the cardiostimulatory effects of sibutramine has been described by Berube-Parent (28) in a small ($n = 8$ men) observational study that should not be extrapolated to a larger, more diverse, population. However, the study did show promise in terms of enhanced weight loss (10.7 kg in 12 weeks), and a benefit in mitigating the blood pressure and pulse side effects of sibutramine with the aerobic exercise component.

When viewed from a population prospective, the small mean increases in blood pressure and pulse are problematic and represent a therapeutic dilemma. Weight loss is usually associated with beneficial effects on risk factors. If sibutramine has mixed effects on risk factors, producing both positive and negative effects, how are we to judge the net result? This may be a moot issue since a recent study has called into question the adversity of sibutramine's blood pressure effects.

Birkenfeld et al. (65) conducted a double-blind, crossover study in 11 healthy men and women comparing placebo to sibutramine effects on cardiovascular response to autonomic reflex tests. In these subjects, there was indeed an increase in supine and upright blood pressure and pulse with sibutramine. The effects were abolished with the β-adrenergic blocker, metaprolol. However, the increase in blood pressure observed with the cold pressor test, and in response to handgrip testing, was attenuated with sibutramine, compared to placebo. These changes are illustrated graphically in Figure 7. Sibutramine was also associated with decreased levels of norepinephrine in the

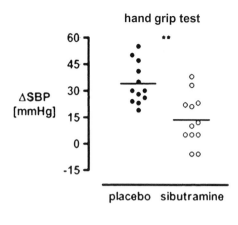

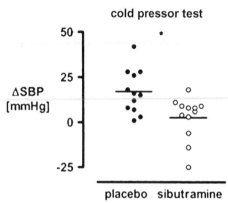

Figure 7 Individual changes in SBP after three minutes' handgrip testing (*top*) and one minute of cold pressor testing on placebo and on sibutramine. Sibutramine blunted response to handgrip and to cold pressor testing. *$p < 0.05$. **$p < 0.01$. *Abbreviation*: SBP, systolic blood pressure. *Source*: From Ref. 65.

plasma while supine. The authors propose that sibutramine may have an inhibitory clonidine-like effect centrally, and a peripheral stimulatory effect. These findings must be investigated further in obese hypertensive and obese nonhypertensive patients before definitive conclusions can be drawn regarding sibutramine's safety profile. Furthermore, ambulatory blood pressure monitoring on these types of individuals may provide additional helpful information regarding this important issue.

Another study (66) reports the multicenter assessment of 195 male and female patients with echocardiographic measurement of left ventricular mass while on sibutramine with a mean reduction at three months of 6.9 ± 0.3 kg on sibutramine and 2.1 ± 0.6 kg on placebo. There were significant decreases in left ventricular mass (-10.9 ± 24.2 g) in sibutramine but not placebo-treated subjects. This study indicates that weight loss may produce cardiovascular benefits even in the presence of the mild blood pressure and pulse effects.

The final story of sibutramine's effect on cardiovascular endpoints may be forthcoming with the SCOUT trial

(Sibutramine Cardiovascular OUTcomes). This large study is conducted globally and assesses cardiovascular events. No results have been presented. Thus, in the mean time, physicians must prescribe thoughtfully in recognition of the drug's potential to raise blood pressure and pulse. Patients on sibutramine should be monitored for blood pressure, and the drug should be discontinued if blood pressure increase occurs to a clinically significant degree.

SIBUTRAMINE'S ROLE IN CLINICAL PRACTICE

The burden of managing obesity (30.5% of Americans in 1999–2000) (67) and metabolic syndrome (24% of Americans in an analysis of the 1996 National Health and Nutrition Examination Survey) (68) mandates that an approach to weight loss be included in routine medical practice. Physicians can help patients lose weight and improve their health risk profile by judicious use of medications for obesity.

Unfortunately, there are few practical, pragmatic studies to guide physicians in the use of medications in clinical practice. One study of sibutramine used in a managed care setting (48) supports that the drug can produce weight lost safely in this setting. The safety and efficacy results are similar to clinical efficacy trials. Another study (47) employed sibutramine or placebo in the practices of 33 general practitioners in Germany. In this study, of the 348 patients, 62% of sibutramine-treated patients lost >5% of their initial weight, which averaged 8.1 ± 8.2 kg (vs. 5.1 ± 6.5 kg for placebo). In both groups, systolic and diastolic blood pressure decreased in those with moderate hypertension and remained unchanged in those with normal blood pressure at baseline.

Questions remain, however. How does sibutramine compare with other medications for weight loss? Several randomized comparisons of sibutramine and orlistat have been published (45–46,69–71). In the study of obese hypertensive individuals (45), 113 individuals completed a four-week run-in, and were randomized to sibutramine or orlistat. Weight loss was equivalent at 12 months for the two groups. Tolerability assessments favored sibutramine, and blood pressure assessments favored orlistat. In another study of 144 obese individuals with diabetes (55), after a four-week reduced energy run-in, they were randomized to either orlistat or sibutramine 10 mg/day At 12 months, 98% of participants were retained. There were equivalent results for improvements in BMI, waist circumference, and measure of glycemic control. Again, blood pressure effects favored orlistat and tolerability profile favored sibutramine.

A study by Gursoy (70) in 182 patients demonstrated superiority for sibutramine over orlistat for weight loss.

Other studies (69,71) have compared orlistat, sibutramine, and the combination. These two studies demonstrated superiority for sibutramine and the combination, but no superiority for the combination over sibutramine alone.

Hopefully, the SCOUT trial will put to rest the unease about sibutramine's cardiovascular effects. Meanwhile, most approaches recommend conservatism. Two authors (64,72) recommend following the Summary of Product Characteristics for clinical management of blood pressure and pulse responses to sibutramine. That recommendation is to withdraw sibutramine treatment if on two consecutive visits there is an increase in systolic or diastolic blood pressure of >10 mmHg from baseline, or >145/90, or heart rate increase >10 bpm, or if there is progressive dyspnea, chest pain, or ankle edema. If any of these criteria are exceeded, sibutramine should be reduced or discontinued.

The duration of therapy is also somewhat uncertain. We are guided by clinical trial data of two years duration. One thing is certain: if initial weight loss does not occur, the drug should be stopped. Sibutramine is an effective agent for maintenance, however, and even intermittent therapy has been demonstrated to sustain weight loss maintenance.

SUMMARY

The modern approach to managing obesity includes medications in the therapeutic armamentarium. Medications are used to produce more weight loss in more patients, and not only to aid in achieving weight loss but also to aid in maintaining weight loss. Sibutramine is an FDA- and CPMP-approved medication with demonstrated efficacy in long-term management of obesity. It is a norepinephrine-serotonin reuptake inhibitor, and produces weight loss by a dual mechanism: primarily by reduction of food intake and possibly by an increase in energy expenditure. Sibutramine is given once daily in doses ranging from 5 to 15 mg. The amount of weight lost with sibutramine is related to both the dose of the drug and the intensity of the behavioral therapy component. Sibutramine produces >5% weight loss from baseline in >75% of patients who are prescribed 15 mg daily and, independent of the behavioral approach, produces additional weight loss that averages about 4% to 5% from baseline. Weight loss with sibutramine is associated with improvement in waist circumference, lipids, glycemic control, uric acid, and HRQOL, and continued weight loss maintenance aided with sibutramine has been demonstrated for two years. The barrier to widespread use of the drug has been that clinical trials with sibutramine demonstrate small increases in mean pulse rate, and sometimes in mean resting blood pressure. The individual blood pressure response is variable, and although weight loss is associated with blood pressure decrease on sibutramine, the

decrease is less than one would expect with that degree of weight loss. Physiologic studies of the blood pressure response to sibutramine have called into question the negative effect of the drug on blood pressure regulation, and a large study with cardiovascular disease endpoints is underway to definitively address the issue. Sibutramine is a useful adjunct to diet and physical activity approaches, and can help selected patients achieve and maintain weight loss with concomitant health benefits.

REFERENCES

1. National Institutes of Health, National Heart, Lung, and Blood Institute. Clinical guidelines on the identification, evaluation, and treatment of overweight and obesity in adults—the evidence report. Obes Res 1998; 6(supp. 2): 51S–210S.
2. Knowler WC, Barrett-Connor E, Fowler SE, et al. Diabetes Prevention Program Research Group. Reduction in the incidence of type 2 diabetes with lifestyle intervention or metformin. N Engl J Med 2002; 346:393–403.
3. Tuomilehto J, Lindstrom J, Eriksson JG, et al. Finnish Diabetes Prevention Study Group. Prevention of type 2 diabetes mellitus by changes in lifestyle among subjects with impaired glucose tolerance. N Engl J Med 2001; 344: 1343–1350.
4. Luque CA, Rey JA. Sibutramine: a serotonin-norepinephrine reuptake-inhibitor for the treatment of obesity. Ann Pharmacother 1999; 33:968–978.
5. Ryan DH, Kaiser P, Bray GA. Sibutramine: a novel new agent for obesity treatment. Obes Res 1995; 3(suppl 4): 553S–559S.
6. Kelly F, Jones SP, Lee JK. Sibutramine weight loss in depressed patients. Int J Obes Relat Metab Disord 1995; 19(suppl 2):P397.
7. Heal DJ, Aspley S, Prow MR, et al. Sibutramine: a novel anti-obesity drug. A review of the pharmacological evidence to differentiate it from d-amphetamine and d-fenfluramine. Int J Obes Relat Metab Disord 1998; 22(suppl 1):S19–S28.
8. Stock MJ. Sibutramine: a review of the pharmacology of a novel antiobesity agent. Int J Obes 1997; 21:S25–S29.
9. Connoley IP, Heal DJ, Stock MJ. A study in rats of the effects of sibutramine on food intake and thermogenesis. Br J Pharmacol 1995; 114:388P.
10. Chapelot D, Marmonier C, Thomas F, et al. Modalities of the food intake-reducing effect of sibutramine in humans. Physiol Behav 2000; 68:299–308.
11. Rolls BJ, Shide DJ, Thorwart ML, et al. Sibutramine reduces food intake in non-dieting women with obesity. Obes Res 1998; 6:1–11.
12. Hansen DL, Toubro S, Stock MJ, et al. Thermogenic effects of sibutramine in humans. Am J Clin Nutr 1998; 68:1180–1186.
13. Seagle HM, Bessessen DA, Hill JO. Effects of sibutramine on resting metabolic rate and weight loss in overweight women. Obes Res 1998; 6(2):115–121.

14. Walsh KM, Leen E, Lean MEJ. The effect of sibutramine on resting energy expenditure and adrenaline-induced thermogenesis in obese females. Int J Obes Relat Metab Disord 1999; 23(10):1009–1015.

15. Gura T. Obesity drug pipeline not so fat. Science 2003; 299:S49–S52.

16. Weintraub M, Rubio A, Golik A, et al. Sibutramine in weight control: a dose-ranging, efficacy study. Clin Pharmacol Ther 1991; 50:330–337.

17. Bray GA, Ryan DH, Gordon D, et al. A double-blind randomized placebo-controlled trial of sibutramine. Obes Res 1996; 4:263–270.

18. Bray GA, Blackburn GL, Ferguson JM, et al. Sibutramine produces dose-related weight loss. Obes Res 1999; 7:189–198.

19. Fanghanel G, Cortinas L, Sanchez-Reyes L, et al. A clinical trial of the use of sibutramine for the treatment of patients suffering essential obesity. Int J Obes 2000; 24: 144–150.

20. Cuellar GEM, Ruiz AM, Monsalve MCR, et al. Six-month treatment of obesity with sibutramine 15 mg; a double-blind, placebo-controlled monocenter clinical trial in a Hispanic population. Obes Res 2000; 8(1):71–82.

21. Smith IG, Goulder MA. Randomized placebo-controlled trial of long-term treatment with sibutramine in mild to moderate obesity. J Fam Pract 2001; 50(6):505–512.

22. Dujovne CA, Zavoral JH, Rowe E, et al. Effects of sibutramine on body weight and serum lipids: a double-blind, randomized, placebo-controlled study in 322 overweight and obese patients with dyslipidemia. Am Heart J 2001; 142(3):489–497.

23. Sanchez-Reyes L, Fanghanel G, Yamamoto J, et al. Use of sibutramine in overweight adult Hispanic patients with type 2 diabetes mellitus: a 12-month, randomized, double-blind, placebo-controlled clinical trial. Clin Ther 2004; 26:1427–1435.

24. Apfelbaum M, Vague P, Ziegler O, et al. Long-term maintenance of weight loss after a very-low-calorie diet: a randomized blinded trial of the efficacy and tolerability of sibutramine. Am J Med 1999; 106:179–184.

25. James WPT, Astrup A, Finer N, et al., STORM Study Group. Effect of sibutramine on weight maintenance after weight loss: a randomized trial. Lancet 2000; 356: 2119–2125.

26. Wirth A, Krause J. Long-term weight loss with sibutramine. JAMA 2001; 286(11):1331–1339.

27. Wadden TA, Berkowitz RI, Sarwer DB, et al. Benefits of lifestyle modification in the pharmacologic treatment of obesity: a randomized trial. Arch Intern Med 2001; 161:218–227.

28. Berube-Parent S, Prud-homme D, St-Pierre S, et al. Obesity treatment with a progressive clinical tri-therapy combining sibutramine and a supervised diet-exercise intervention. Int J Obes Relat Metab Disord 2001; 25(8):1144–1153.

29. Wadden TA, Berkowitz RI, Womble LG, et al. Randomized trial of lifestyle modification and pharmacotherapy for obesity. N Engl J Med 2005; 353:2111–2120.

30. Berkowitz RI, Wadden TA, Tershakovec AM, et al. Behavior therapy and sibutramine for the treatment of adolescent obesity. JAMA 2003; 289:1805–1812.

31. Daniels SR, Long B, Crow S, et al. Cardiovascular effects of sibutramine in the treatment of obese adolescents: results of a randomized, double-blind, placebo-controlled study. Pediatrics 2007; 120(1):e174–e157 (Epub).

32. Godoy-Matos A, Carraro L, Vieira A, et al. Treatment of obese adolescents with sibutramine: a randomized, double-blind controlled study. J Clin Endocrinol Metab 2005; 90:1460–1465.

33. McMahon FG, Fujioka K, Singh BN, et al. Efficacy and safety of sibutramine in obese white and African-American patients with hypertension. Arch Int Med 2000; 160: 2185–2191.

34. McMahon FG, Weinstein SP, Rowe E, et al. Sibutramine is safe and effective for weight loss in obese patients whose hypertension is well controlled with angiotensin-converting enzyme inhibitors. J Hum Hypertens 2002; 16:5–11.

35. Hazenberg BP. Randomized, double-blind, placebo-controlled, multicenter study of sibutramine in obese hypertensive patients. Cardiology 2000; 94:152–158.

36. Sramek JJ, Seiowitz MT, Weinstein SP, et al. Efficacy and safety of sibutramine for weight loss in obese patients with hypertension well controlled by β-adrenergic blocking agents: a placebo-controlled, double-blind, randomized trial. Am J Hypertens 2002; 16:13–199.

37. Scholze J, Grimm E, Herrmann D, et al. Optimal treatment of obesity-related hypertension: the Hypertension-Obesity-Sibutramine (HOS) study. Circulation 2007; 115(15): 1991–1998.

38. Fujioka K, Seaton TB, Rowe E, et al., Sibutramine/Diabetes Clinical Study Group. Weight loss with sibutramine improves glycemic control and other metabolic parameters in obese type 2 diabetes mellitus. Diabetes Obes Metab 2000; 2:1–13.

39. Gokcel A, Karakose H, Ertorer EM, et al. Effects of sibutramine in obese female subjects with type 2 diabetes and poor blood glucose control. Diabetes Care 2001; 24: 1957–1960.

40. Serrano-Rios M, Melchionda N, Moreno-Carretero E, Spanish Investigators. Role of sibutramine in the treatment of obese Type 2 diabetic patients receiving sulphonylurea therapy. Diabet Med 2002; 19(2):119–124.

41. Finer N, Bloom SR, Frost GS, et al. Sibutramine is effective for weight loss and diabetic control in obesity with type 2 diabetes: a randomised, double-blind placebo-controlled study. Diabetes Obes Metab 2000; 2:105–112.

42. Kaukua JK, Pekkarinen TA, Rissanen AM. Health-related quality of life in a randomised placebo-controlled trial of sibutramine in obese patients with type II diabetes. Int J Obes Relat Metab Disord 2004; 28(4):600–605.

43. McNulty SJ, Ur E, Williams G, et al. A randomized trial of sibutramine in the management of obese type 2 diabetic patients treated with metformin. Diabetes Care 2003; 26(1):125–131.

44. Appolinario JC, Bacaltchuk J, Sichieri R, et al. A randomized, double-blind, placebo-controlled study of sibutramine in the treatment of binge-eating disorder. Arch Gen Psychiatry 2003; 60:1109–1116.

45. Derosa G, Cicero AFG, Murdolo G, et al. Efficacy and safety comparative evaluation of orlistat and sibutramine

treatment in hypertensive obese patients. Diabetes Obes Metab 2005; 7(1):47–55.

46. Elfhag K, Rossner S, Barkeling B, et al. Sibutramine treatment in obesity: initial eating behaviour in relation to weight loss results and changes in mood. Pharmacol Res 2005; 51(2):159–163.

47. Hauner H, Meier M, Wendland G, et al. Weight reduction by sibutramine in obese subjects in primary care medicine: the SAT Study. Exp Clin Endocrinol Diabetes 2004; 112:201–207.

48. Porter J, Raebel M, Conner D, et al. The Long-Term Outcomes of Sibutramine Effectiveness on Weight (LOSE Weight) study: evaluating the role of drug therapy within a weight management program in a group-model health maintenance organization. Am J Manag Care 2004; 10:369–376.

49. Wirth A. Sustained weight reduction after cessation of obesity treatment with sibutramine. Dtsch Med Wochenschr 2004; 129:1002–1005.

50. Li Z, Maglione M, Tu W, et al. Meta-analysis: pharmacologic treatment of obesity. Ann Int Med 2005; 142(7): 532–546.

51. Avenell A, Brown TJ, McGee MA, et al. What interventions should we add to weight reducing diets in adults with obesity? A systematic review of randomized controlled trials of adding drug therapy, exercise, behaviour therapy or combinations of these interventions. J Hum Nutr Diet 2004; 17(4):293–316.

52. Kim SH, Lee YM, Jee SH, et al. Effect of sibutramine on weight loss and blood pressure: a meta-analysis of controlled trials. Obes Res 2003; 11(9):1116–1123.

53. Bettor R, Serra R, Fabris R, et al. Effect of sibutramine on weight management and metabolic control in type 2 diabetes: a meta-analysis of clinical studies. Diabetes Care 2005; 28(4):942–949.

54. Krejs GJ. Metabolic benefits associated with sibutramine therapy. Int J Obes Relat Metab Disord 2002; 26(suppl 4): S34–S37.

55. Derosa G, Cicero AFG, Murdolo G, et al. Comparison of metabolic effects or orlistat and sibutramine treatment in Type 2 diabetic obese patients. Diabetes Nutr Metab 2004; 17(4):222–229.

56. Aronne LJ. Treating obesity: a new target of prevention of coronary heart disease. Prog Cardiovasc Nurs 2001; 16(3): 98–106, 115.

57. Van Gaal LF, Wauters M, De Leeuw IH. The beneficial effects of modest weight loss on cardiovascular risk factors. Int J Obes 1997; 21(suppl. 1):S5–S9.

58. Samsa GP, Kolotkin RL, Williams GR, et al. Effect of moderate weight loss on health-related quality of life: an analysis of combined data from 4 randomized trials of

sibutramine vs. placebo. Am J Manag Care 2001; 7(9): 875–883.

59. Bach DS, Rissanen AM, Mendel CM, et al. Absence of cardiac valve dysfunction in obese patients treated with sibutramine. Obes Res 1999; 7(4):363–369.

60. Halpern A, Leite CC, Herszkowicz N, et al. Evaluation of efficacy, reliability, and tolerability of sibutramine in obese patients, with and echocardiographic study. Rev Hosp Clin 2002; 57(3):98–102.

61. Zannad F, Gille B, Grentzinger G, et al. Effects of sibutramine on ventricular dimensions and heart valves in obese patients during weight reduction. Am Heart J 2002; 144:508–515.

62. Cole JO, Levin A, Beake B, et al. Sibutramine: a new weight loss agent without evidence of the abuse potential associated with amphetamines. J Clin Psychopharmacol 1998; 18(3):231–236.

63. Jordan J, Scholze J, Matiba B, et al. Influence of sibutramine on blood pressure: evidence from placebo-controlled trials. Int J Obes Relat Metab Disord 2005; 26(5):509–516; advance online copy.

64. Sharma AM. Sibutramine in overweight/obese hypertensive patients. Int J Obes Relat Metab Disord 2001; 25(suppl 4): S20–S23.

65. Birkenfeld AL, Schroeder C, Boschmann M, et al. Paradoxical effect of sibutramine on autonomic cardiovascular regulation. Circulation 2002; 106:2459–2465.

66. Wirth A, Scholze J, Sharma AM, et al. Reduced left ventricular mass after treatment of obese patients with sibutramine: an echocardiographic multicentre study. Diabetes Obes Metab 2006; 8(6):674–681.

67. Flegal KM, Carroll MD, Ogden CL, et al. Prevalence and trends in obesity among US adults, 1999-2000. JAMA 2002; 288:1723–1727.

68. Ford ES, Giles WH, Dietz WH. Prevalence of the metabolic syndrome among US adults: findings from the third National Health and Nutrition Examination Survey. JAMA 2002; 287:356–359.

69. Sari R, Balci MK, Cakir M, et al. Comparison of efficacy of sibutramine or orlistat versus their combination in obese women. Endocr Res 2004; 30:159–167.

70. Gursoy A, Erdogan MF, Cin MO, et al. Comparison of orlistat and sibutramine in an obesity management program: efficacy, compliance, and weight regain after noncompliance. Eat Weight Disord 2006; 11:e127–e132.

71. Kaya A, Aydin N, Topsever P, et al. Efficacy of sibutramine, orlistat and combination therapy on short-term weight management in obese patients. Biomed Pharmacother 2004; 58:582–587.

72. Narkiewicz K. Sibutramine and its cardiovascular profile. Int J Obes Relat Metab Disord 2002; 26(4):S38–S41.

19

Drugs That Modify Fat Absorption and Alter Metabolism

GEORGE A. BRAY

Pennington Biomedical Research Center, Baton Rouge, Louisiana, U.S.A.

LUC F. VAN GAAL

Department of Diabetology, Metabolism and Clinical Nutrition, Antwerp University Hospital and Faculty of Medicine, Antwerp, Belgium

INTRODUCTION

There is growing evidence that obesity, and particularly central obesity, has an important impact on predisposing risk factors for coronary heart disease, including dyslipidemia, glucose intolerance, insulin resistance, and elevated blood pressure (1,2). Reversal of these metabolic abnormalities associated with obesity is one of the most important targets in the clinical management of obesity.

Although diet and lifestyle remain the cornerstones of therapy for obesity (3,4), weight losses are often small and long-term success is extremely disappointing. Despite the availability of a variety of dietary manipulations ranging from calorie restriction to fat restriction and very low-calorie diets (VLCD), the long-term maintenance of clinically significant weight loss, defined as a loss of 10% of initial body weight, remains uncommon (3). Over the last two decades, obesity research has been focused on the exploration of new biochemical pathways and on new pharmacological intervention possibilities.

The use of pharmacological agents for long-term treatment of obesity may play a useful role as part of an overall weight-reduction program that includes diet, physical exercise, and behavioral support (5,6). The use of drugs to treat obesity may be considered for people with body mass index (BMI) > 30 kg/m^2, or BMI > 27 kg/m^2, when additional complicating factors are present. Although not endorsed by American or European drug agencies, subjects with a recent onset of obesity and a rather sudden weight gain of 10 to 15 kg may also qualify for pharmacological treatment.

Large-scale, long-term clinical trials lasting up to four years have demonstrated that pharmacological agents, including orlistat and sibutramine, are able to induce significant weight loss over and above that produced in the control group. Important reductions in comorbidities are usually observed as well. These drugs allow the maintenance of reduced body weight for at least one to two years. The weight loss that can be attributed to these drugs is in general modest, i.e., <10%. However, the reduction of up to 25% in most of the well-known comorbid risk factors can be more than the magnitude of the weight loss. This chapter will deal with drugs to treat obesity that affect metabolism or nutrient partitioning.

PREABSORPTIVE DRUGS

Orlistat

Due to their high energy content and low potential for inducing satiety, high-fat diets are conducive to over-consumption and to weight gain, particularly in individuals who are relatively inactive. Indeed, humans are much more likely to become obese through excessive consumption of dietary fat than through excess consumption of carbohydrate (7). It is reasonable, therefore, to decrease the proportion of fat as well as the total number of calories. By reducing fat absorption after ingestion, a continued calorie deficit may be maintained more easily over the long term than by dieting alone. Lipase inhibition may help in this strategy to reduce fat absorption.

Pharmacology

Orlistat is the hydrogenated derivative of lipstatin that is produced by the bacterium *Streptococcus toxytricini* (8,9). It has an α-lactone ring structure that is essential for activity, since opening this ring destroys it. This compound is highly lipophilic and is a potent inhibitor of most, if not all, mammalian lipases (8–10). Pancreatic lipase is a 449 amino acid enzyme that shares with other lipases a folded structure that is inactive. In the folded state, the N-terminal domain contains the catalytic site that includes serine, histidine, and aspartate. Binding of the enzyme to triglyceride is facilitated by colipase in the presence of bile salts. This interaction serves to expose the active site by opening the lid. One view of this is as though a lid were moved away from the active site by the interaction of colipase and triglyceride in the bile salt milieu. Orlistat attaches to the active site of the lipase once the lid is opened and in doing so creates an irreversible inhibition at this site. In contrast to its inhibition of lipases, orlistat does not inhibit other intestinal enzymes, including hydrolases, trypsin, pancreatic phospholipase A_2, phosphoinositol-specific phospholipase C, acetylcholinesterase, or nonspecific liver carboxyesterase. Because of its very low absorption (11,12), it has no effect on systemic lipases.

During short-term treatment with orlistat, fecal fat loss rises during the days of treatment and then returns to control levels after discontinuing medication, as would be expected from an inhibitor of intestinal lipase (11,13,14). With volunteers eating a 30% fat diet, there is a dose-related increase in fecal fat loss that increases rapidly with doses up to 200 mg/day and then reaches a plateau with doses above 400 to 600 mg/day. The plateau is at approximately 32% of dietary fat lost into the stools. Because the drug partially inhibits triglyceride digestion, it is possible that nutrients or drugs might be less well absorbed (11). Because of its lipid solubility, less than

1% of an oral dose is absorbed and degraded into two major metabolites (15).

Pharmacodynamic studies suggest that orlistat does not affect the pharmacokinetic properties of digoxin (16), phenytoin (16), warfarin (17), glyburide (17), oral contraceptives (18), or alcohol (8). Orlistat also does not affect a single dose of four different antihypertensive drugs: furosemide, captopril, nifedipine (16), or atenolol (19). Absorption of vitamin A, E, and β-carotene may be slightly reduced (15,16), and this may require vitamin therapy in a small number of patients. After oral administration of a single dose of 360 mg ^{14}C-labeled orlistat to healthy or obese volunteers, peak plasma radioactivity levels were reached approximately six to eight hours after the dose (15,20). Plasma concentrations of intact orlistat were small, indicating negligible systemic absorption of the drug (15). Pooled data from five long-term clinical trials with orlistat lasting six months to two years at doses of 180 to 720 mg/day in obese patients indicated that there was a dose-related increase in plasma concentrations of orlistat. However, these plasma concentrations were low and generally below the level of assay detection (21).

Clinical Trials

Short-term clinical trials

A number of initial short-term trials have revealed that orlistat promotes weight loss and improves hypercholesterolemia in obese patients. The weight-reducing effect of orlistat was further confirmed in a short-term dose-ranging study involving almost 200 healthy obese subjects. Weight reduction was statistically significant in those subjects receiving orlistat 120 mg three times a day (t.i.d.) compared with those receiving diet and placebo (22,23).

A dose-ranging study of orlistat 30 to 240 mg t.i.d., in 676 obese male and female subjects, resulted in a dose-dependent reduction in body weight. Orlistat 120 mg t.i.d. represents the optimal dosing regimen (24). In absolute terms, mean weight loss reached 9.8% in the 120 mg t.i.d. orlistat group. More orlistat-treated patients lost more than 10% of initial body weight than those who received placebo (37% of the 120 mg t.i.d. group vs. 19% of the placebo group) (25). Daily fecal fat excretion also increased from the baseline value in a dose-dependent manner up to 18.5 g/day in those treated with orlistat 120 mg t.i.d.

Long-term clinical trials

Several double-blind randomized placebo-controlled trials lasting one to four years have been published. Table 1 summarizes these data. A one-year multicenter placebo-controlled study, designed to assess the efficacy and tolerability of orlistat administered for 52 weeks, indicated that at six months the orlistat-treated patients lost 8.6 kg,

Table 1 Effect of Orlistat in Clinical Trials of One and Two Years Duration

Author (reference)	Yr	Number of subjects Placebo	Number of subjects Drug	Dose (mg t.i.d.)	Duration of study (wk)	Run in (wk)	Diet	Initial wt (kg) Placebo	Initial wt (kg) Drug	Wt loss (kg or %) Placebo	Wt loss (kg or %) Drug	Met criteria FDA	Met criteria CPMP	Comments
Drent and van der Veen (22)	1993	19	20	50	12	4	500 kcal/day deficit	81.9	85.5	−2.1 kg	−4.3 kg	No	No	Single site
Drent et al. (23)	1995	46			12	4	500 kcal/day deficit							Multicenter dose-ranging
			48	30				90.0	92.1	−2.98kg	−3.61 kg	No	No	
			45	60					92.6		−3.69 kg	No	No	
			47	120					94.1		−4.74 kg	No	No	
Drent and van der Veen (146)	1995	7	7	120	12	4	500 kcal/day deficit	86.8	89.8	−2.8kg	−4.2 kg	No	No	Substudy of 821
James et al. (25)	1997	23	23	120	52	4	600 kcal/day deficit	99	100	−2.6kg −2.6kg	−8.4 kg −8.4 kg	Yes	No	Wt loss at 12 mo
Finer et al. (38)	2000	108	110		52	4	600 kcal/day deficit	98.4	97.9	−5.4%	−8.5%	No	No	British1 yr
Van Gaal et al. (24)	1998	125			24	4	500 kcal/day deficit	35 BMI		−6.5%				Multicenter dose-ranging
			122	30					35		−8.5%	No	No	
			124	60					34		−8.8%	No	No	
			122	120					35		−9.8%	No	±	
			120	240					34		−9.3%	No	±	
Sjostrom et al. (27)	1998	340	343	120	104	4	600 kcal/day deficit (yr 1) maintenance (yr 2)	99.8	99.1	−6.1kg	−10.3 kg	No	Yes	European multicenter cross-over 52-wk data
Hollander et al. (43)	1998	159	162	120	52	5	500 kcal/day deficit 30% fat	99.7	99.6	−6.1% −4.3 kg	−10.2% −6.2 kg	No No	Yes No	U.S. diabetic study
Davidson et al. (28)	1999	223	657	120	104	4	600 kcal/day deficit (yr 1) maintenance (yr 2) 30% fat	100.6	100.7	−5.8 kg −4.3%	−8.8 kg −6.2%	No	No	U.S. multicenter cross-over 52-wk data
Torgerson et al. (30)	2004	1637	1640	120	208	—	800 kcal/day deficit 30% fat adjusted 6-monthly	110.6	110.4	−3.0 kg	−5.8 kg	No	Yes	XENDOS 4-yr trial. Max weight loss: −10.2 in orlistat, −6.2 in placebo at 1 yr
Richelsen et al. (32)	2007	156	153	120	156	600–800 kcal/day VLED for 8 wk	600 kcal/day deficit	112	110	−7.2 kg −6.4%	−9.4 kg −8.3%	No	No	European 3-yr weight-maintenance trial following very low energy diet

versus 5.5 kg on placebo, a net additional loss in body weight of 0.13 kg/wk (25).

The design of the trials lasting two years followed two formats. They all included a four- to five-week single-blind run-in period, after which subjects were stratified into those losing ≥2 kg or <2 kg. Orlistat was given at a dose of 60 or 120 mg before each of the three meals. The diet contained 30% fat and was designed to produce a mild hypocaloric deficit of 500 to 600 kcal/day during the first year. During the second year, patients were placed on a "eucaloric" diet to evaluate the effect of orlistat on weight maintenance. Weight loss at one year varied from 5.5% to 6.6% of the initial body weight in the placebo group and 8.5% to 10.2% in the orlistat-treated group. During the second year, patients were kept on the same drug regimen as in the first year in two trials (26), and in the other two trials (27,28), patients were re-randomized to placebo or active drug in a crossover design. The percentage of patients losing >5% weight ranged from 23% to 49.2% in the placebo-treated group and 49% to 68.5% in those treated with orlistat. Using a criterion of >10% weight loss, 17.7% to 25% of placebo-treated patients reached this goal compared with the more successful 38.8% to 43% of those treated with orlistat. Nearly two-thirds of the enrolled patients completed year 1.

Data on the second year of treatment are available from four studies. In one study (26), subjects remained on the same treatment for two years. At the end of the second year, weight loss from baseline was –7.6% ± 7.0% for those receiving orlistat compared with –4.5% ± 7.6% for the placebo-treated group. At one year, the corresponding losses were –9.7% ± 6.3% and –6.6% ± 6.8%. In the two other studies, the orlistat subjects were re-randomized at the end of one year to placebo or orlistat 60 or 120 mg t.i.d. (25,28).

Those remaining on orlistat for two years regained 32.5% from the end of year 1 to the end of year 2 but were still –8.8% ± 7.6% below baseline. The patients who continued on orlistat with the maintenance diet regained half as much weight (2.5 kg or 2.6% regain) than those who switched from orlistat to placebo (5.7 kg or 52% regain). In this trial, subjects who received orlistat in the second year and placebo in the first year lost an average of 0.9 kg more. These data show that initial weight loss is greater and that weight regain is slowed by orlistat. The two-year U.S. Prevention of Weight Regain Study treated patients who had lost more than 8% of their initial weight by dieting with orlistat 30, 60, or 120 mg t.i.d. (28). At the end of one year the placebo-treated group had regained 56% of the weight they had lost, in contrast to a regain of 32.4% in the group treated with orlistat 120 mg t.i.d.

Initial successful weight loss, both during the initial 4 weeks run-in phase and during the active treatment period of 8 to 12 weeks, predicted the final outcome. Subjects who were not able to lose significant amounts of weight during these periods were considered as non-responders, whereas those who lost more than 5% of initial body weight after three months of therapy lost >16% of body weight after one year (29).

The results of a three-year and a four-year double-blind, randomized, placebo-controlled trial with orlistat have also been reported (30). A total of 3304 overweight patients were included in the four-year Swedish trial, of which 21% had impaired glucose tolerance (IGT).

The lowest body weight—more than –11% below baseline—was achieved during the first year in the orlistat-treated group and 6% below baseline in the placebo-treated group. Over the remaining three years of the trial, there was a small regain in weight, such that by the end of four years, the orlistat-treated patients were –6.9% below baseline, compared with –4.1% for those receiving placebo. The trial also showed a 37% reduction in the conversion of patients from IGT to diabetes; essentially all of this benefit occurred in patients with IGT at enrollment in the trial.

Weight maintenance with orlistat has been evaluated in two studies (31,32). In the one-year study (31), patients were enrolled if they had lost more than 8% of their body weight over six months while eating a 1000 kcal/day (4180 kJ/day) diet. These 729 patients were randomized to receive placebo or orlistat at 30, 60, or 120 mg t.i.d. for 12 months. At the end of this period, the placebo-treated patients had regained 56% of their body weight, compared with 32.4% in the group treated with orlistat 120 mg t.i.d. The other two doses of orlistat were no different from placebo in preventing the regain of weight. A three-year randomized clinical trial of weight regain and effects of cardiovascular risk factors enrolled 383 overweight patients (BMI 30–45 kg/m^2). Out of these, 309 patients who successfully lost >5% of their body weight when eating a diet of 600 to 800 kcal/day for eight weeks were randomized to placebo or orlistat 120 mg t.i.d. while eating a 600-kcal/day deficit diet. After eight weeks, patients randomized to placebo had lost an average of 14.3 ± 2.0 kg compared with 14.5 ± 2.1 kg in the orlistat group. After 36 months, the orlistat-treated patients had regained less weight (4.6 ± 8.6 kg) than the placebo-treated patients (7.0 ± 7.1 kg). Over the three years, fewer orlistat-treated patients (5.2%) developed diabetes than those in the placebo group (10.9%) (32).

An assessment of clinical use of orlistat in French medical practices was done by a study of 714 general practitioners who provided information on 6801 patients (33). Only 40% were treated with orlistat and monitored for an average of 11 months with a maximum of 23 months. Between 64% and 77% stopped taking orlistat, primarily because of its higher cost. The average weight loss was 5% after 3 months and 9% after 12 months of treatment.

Studies in Special Populations

Effects of orlistat on lipids and lipoproteins

The modest weight reduction observed with orlistat treatment may have a beneficial effect on lipids and lipoproteins (34). A 10% weight loss usually results in modest improvement of total and LDL cholesterol (LDL-C) (–5 to –10%), a reduction of up to 30% in triglycerides, and a favorable increase of 8% to 10% in HDL cholesterol (HDL-C). In addition, a beneficial effect has been observed in concentrations of small, dense lipoprotein particles (35).

These improvements in lipid profile are in agreement with a meta-analysis conducted by Dattilo and Kris-Etherton (36) on the effects of weight loss on plasma lipids and lipoproteins. It was estimated that for every 1 kg reduction in body weight, there is 0.05, 0.02, and 0.015 mmol/L decrease in TC, LDL-C, and TG, respectively. In addition, for every 1 kg decrease in body weight, a 0.007 mmol/L increase in HDL-C occurred in subjects at stabilized, reduced body weight. Baseline risk factors, the magnitude of weight loss, and exercise can influence the degree of change in lipid profile.

Orlistat seems to have an independent effect on LDL-C. From a meta-analysis of the data relating orlistat to lipids, orlistat-treated subjects had almost twice as much reduction in LDL-C as their placebo-treated counterparts for the same weight loss category reached after one year.

One study was designed to evaluate the effects of orlistat on weight loss and cardiovascular risk factors, particularly serum lipids, in obese patients with hypercholesterolemia (37). The main findings were that orlistat promoted clinically significant weight loss and reduced LDL-C in obese patients with elevated cholesterol levels more than could be attributed to weight loss alone. These data support previous controlled trials that concluded that partial inhibition of dietary fat absorption with the gastrointestinal (GI) lipase inhibitor, in conjunction with a hypocaloric diet, promotes weight loss of 6% to 10% in at-risk patients (26,28,38,39).

Weight loss and modification of dietary fat appear to have independent and additive effects on the reduction in serum lipids: The net favorable effect of weight loss seems to be greater than that of dietary fat modification, as weight loss per se is responsible for about 60% and 70% of decrease in LDL-C and TG, respectively.

The ObelHyx study examined the effects of orlistat on cardiovascular risk factors and demonstrated an additional 10% lowering of LDL-C in obese subjects with baseline-elevated LDL-C levels compared to placebo (37).

Table 2 provides mean percentage changes in LDL-C after 24 weeks of double-blind treatment in three two-year controlled trials, where the majority of patients were normocholesterolemic at baseline. These data indicate

Table 2 Effect on LDL-Cholesterol: Comparison of Three Studies

Study (reference)	Mean percent change	
	Placebo	Orlistat 120 mg t.i.d.
Sjostrom et al., 1998 (27)	−1.2	11.9
Rössner et al., 2000 (26)	−2.2	−10.3
Muls et al., 2001 (37)	−7.6	−17.6

that the difference in mean percentage change in LDL-C between orlistat and placebo is roughly 10% to 12% in all studies, whether this difference is computed as change from the start of the single-blind placebo dietary run-in or from the start of double-blind treatment. It is noteworthy that LDL-C levels continued to decline after the start of double-blind treatment in orlistat-treated subjects in all trials, but that LDL-C either remained largely unchanged or increased during double-blind therapy in placebo-treated recipients, despite further weight loss (Table 2). These data are in agreement with the 10% LDL-C decrease previously seen with orlistat 120 mg t.i.d. in nonobese patients with primary hyperlipidemia, who were kept on a weight-maintenance diet. This independent cholesterol-lowering effect probably reflects a reduction in intestinal absorption of cholesterol (40). Since lipase inhibition by orlistat prevents the absorption of approximately 30% of dietary fat, the prescribed diet of 30% of energy from fat would thus become, in effect, a 20% to 24% of the available fat in the diet when associated with orlistat treatment. It has been hypothesized that inhibition of GI lipase activity may lead to retention of cholesterol in the gut through a reduction in the amount of fatty acids and monoglycerides absorbed from the gut, and/or lead to sequestration of cholesterol within a more persistent oil phase in the intestine. Partial inhibition of intestinal fat and cholesterol absorption probably leads to decreased hepatic cholesterol and saturated fatty acid concentration, upregulation of hepatic LDL receptors, and decreased LDL-C levels. The decrease in LDL-C observed in the study with hypercholesterolemic subjects (37) is comparable to the 14% LDL-C reduction that was previously achieved with a plant stanol ester-containing margarine but is of a lesser magnitude than the LDL-C-lowering effects that are commonly observed with fibrate or statin drugs (41,42).

Studies in diabetics

The efficacy of orlistat in patients with type 2 diabetes has been demonstrated in three six-month and four one-year studies (43–46). One study randomized 550 insulin-treated patients to receive either placebo or orlistat 120 mg t.i.d.

for one year. Weight loss in the orlistat-treated group was $-3.9\% \pm 0.3\%$ compared to $-1.3\% \pm 0.3\%$ in the placebo-treated group. Hemoglobin A_{1c} (HbA_{1c}) was reduced by -0.62% in the orlistat-treated group, but only by -0.27% in the placebo group. The required dose of insulin decreased more in the orlistat group, as did plasma cholesterol (44). According to the data from a retrospective analysis of seven multicenter, double-blind trials enrolling overweight or obese patients (BMI 28–43 kg/m^2) with type 2 diabetes and treated with metformin, sulfonylurea (SU), and/or insulin, orlistat-treated patients had significantly greater improvements in HbA_{1c} and fasting plasma glucose (FPG) than placebo-treated patients (43). The improvements in HbA_{1c} and FPG achieved with orlistat were similar across the diabetic medication subgroups. Orlistat-treated patients had least square mean differences from placebo in HbA_{1c} of -0.34% ($p = 0.0007$), -0.42% ($p < 0.0001$), and -0.35% ($p = 0.002$) in the metformin, SU, and insulin groups, respectively. Orlistat, in combination with diet, represents a clinically beneficial adjunct to antidiabetic therapy for overweight or obese patients with type 2 diabetes (43).

Effects of orlistat on glucose tolerance and diabetes

The orlistat-treated subjects in trials lasting for at least one year were analyzed by Heymsfield and coworkers (47), who found that orlistat reduced the conversion of IGT to diabetes and also the transition from normal to IGT in subjects treated with orlistat for one year. In orlistat-treated subjects, the conversion from normal glucose tolerance to diabetes occurred in 6.6% of patients, whereas approximately 11% of placebo-treated patients had a similar worsening of glucose tolerance. Conversion from IGT to diabetes was less frequent in orlistat-treated patients than in placebo-treated obese subjects, by 3.0% and 7.6%, respectively (47). Although these data are based on a retrospective analysis of one-year trials in which data on glucose tolerance were available, it shows that modest weight reduction—with pharmacotherapy—may lead to an important risk reduction for the development of type 2 diabetes.

The effect of orlistat in preventing diabetes has been assessed in a four-year study (30). In this trial, weight was reduced by 2.8 kg (95% CI, 1.1–4.5 kg) compared to placebo, and the conversion rate of diabetes was reduced from 9% to 6% for a relative risk reduction of 0.63 (95% CI, 0.46–0.86) (48). The incidence of new cases of diabetes was also reduced from 10.9% to 5.2% ($p = 0.041$) during a three-year period in which overweight patients were treated with orlistat and lifestyle or with lifestyle alone (32).

There are studies on more than 2500 diabetic subjects treated for six months to one year with orlistat who received different antidiabetic medications. Orlistat has been proven, in spite of the limited weight loss in diabetics (43), to improve metabolic control with a reduction of up to 0.53% in HbA_{1c} and a decrease in the concomitant ongoing antidiabetic therapy. More patients treated with orlistat achieve clinically beneficial changes in HbA_{1c}, particularly those with baseline levels of HbA_{1c} >8%. Concomitant reduction in the requirement for antidiabetic medication has been also observed. Independent effects of orlistat on lipids were also shown in this study (43). Orlistat also has an acute effect on postprandial lipemia in overweight patients with type 2 diabetes (45). By lowering both remnant-like particle cholesterol and free fatty acids (FFA) in the postprandial period, orlistat may contribute to a reduction in atherogenic risk (46).

Metabolic syndrome and lipids

In a further analysis, patients who had participated in previously reported studies of orlistat were divided into the highest and lowest quintiles for triglyceride and HDL-C levels (49). Those with high triglyceride and low HDL-C levels were labeled as having "syndrome X," and those with the lowest triglyceride levels and highest HDL-C levels were labeled as "non-syndrome X" controls. In this classification, there were almost no men in the non-syndrome X group, compared with an equal sex breakdown in the syndrome X group. In addition, the syndrome X group had slightly higher systolic and diastolic blood pressure levels and a nearly twofold higher level of fasting insulin. Other than weight loss, the only difference between the placebo- and the orlistat-treated patients was the decrease in LDL-C levels in patients treated with orlistat. However, the syndrome X subgroup showed a significantly greater decrease in triglyceride and insulin levels than those without syndrome X. Levels of HDL-C increased more in the syndrome X group, but LDL-C levels showed a smaller decrease than in the non-syndrome X group. All of the clinical studies with orlistat have shown significant decreases in serum cholesterol and LDL-C levels that usually are greater than can be accounted for by weight loss alone (6). One study showed that orlistat reduces the absorption of cholesterol from the GI tract, thus providing a mechanism for clinical observations (40).

Studies in children

Adolescents have participated in two trials with orlistat. A multicenter trial tested the effect of orlistat in 539 obese adolescents (50). Subjects were randomized to placebo or orlistat 120 mg t.i.d. and a mildly hypocaloric diet containing 30% fat. By the end of the study, BMI had decreased by 0.55 kg/m^2 in the drug-treated group, but had increased by 0.31 kg/m^2 in the placebo group ($p < 0.05$). By the end of the study, weight had increased by only 0.51 kg in the orlistat-treated group, compared with

3.14 kg in the placebo-treated group. This difference was due to differences in body fat. In a follow-up, these authors showed that weight loss in the first 12 weeks was predictive of weight loss at the end of one year (51). The side effects were GI in origin as expected from the mode of action of orlistat. A second, small, six-month randomized clinical trial from a single site failed to find a difference resulting from treatment with orlistat in a population of 40 adolescents (52). In a smaller six-month trial, 40 adolescents were randomized to treatment with orlistat or placebo. Both groups lost weight, but there was no statistically significant difference between treatments.

Meta-analyses of Orlistat Studies

Several meta-analyses of orlistat have been published (53–56). By pooling six studies, Haddock and colleagues (53) estimated the weight loss in patients treated with orlistat as –7.1 kg (range –4.0 to –10.3 kg) compared to –5.02 kg (range –3.0 to –6.1 kg) for the placebo-treated groups, or a difference of 2.1 kg. In the meta-analysis of Li and colleagues (54), the overall mean weighted difference after 12 months of therapy in 22 studies was –2.70 kg (95% CI, –3.79 to –1.61 kg). Since this analysis included both diabetic and nondiabetic subjects, we have summarized the data from the five two-year studies in Table 3. In another meta-analysis of orlistat (Table 4) including eight one-year-long studies, only one of which was on diabetics,

the overall effect of orlistat on weight loss at 12 months using the weighted mean difference (WMD) was –3.01 kg (95% CI, –3.48 to –2.54 kg). This meta-analysis also examined the effects of weight loss at one and two years on various laboratory and clinical responses. After 24 months, the overall effect of orlistat on weight loss was –3.26 kg (95% CI, –4.15 to –2.37 kg). In terms of weight maintenance, the overall effect of orlistat after 12 months was –0.85 kg (95% CI, –1.50 to –0.19 kg) (26,28,31,57). The pooled data show significant overall effects after one year of treatment on the change in cholesterol [–0.34 mmol/L (95% CI, –0.41 to –0.27) (N = 7 studies)], the change in LDL-C [–0.29 mmol/L (95% CI, –0.34 to –0.24) (N = 7 studies)], the change in HDL-C [–0.03 mmol/L (95% CI, –0.05 to –0.01) (N = 6 studies)], the change in triglycerides [0.03 mmol/L (95% CI, –0.04 to 0.10) (N = 6 studies)], the change in HbA$_{1c}$ [–0.17% (95% CI, –0.24 to –0.10) (N = 3 studies)] (43,58,59), the change in SBP [–2.02 mmHg (95% CI, –2.87 to –1.17) (N = 7 studies)], and the change in DBP [–1.64 mmHg (95% CI, –2.20 to –1.09) (N = 7 studies)]. In a meta-analysis focused on the use of orlistat in diabetics, Norris and colleagues (56) reported a WMD in favor of orlistat of –2.6 kg (95% CI, –3.2 to –2.1) after 52 to 57 weeks of treatment. Another systematic review identified 28 studies comparing orlistat and placebo (60). The WMD in body weight was 3.86 kg favoring orlistat in low-risk patients, 2.50 kg favoring orlistat in diabetic patients, and 2.04 kg favoring orlistat in high-risk patients. In a meta-analysis of weight loss in adults with type 2 diabetes mellitus (56), orlistat produced a WMD in weight loss of 2.0 kg (95% CI, 1.3–2.8) for trials lasting 12 to 57 weeks.

Nonalcoholic fatty liver disease

In a six-month randomized clinical trial, Zelber-Sagi and colleagues (61) randomized 52 patients to placebo or orlistat. Both groups lost weight and improved their liver function tests, with no significant differences between groups. However, there was a significantly greater improvement in liver fat by ultrasound in the orlistat-treated group.

Table 3 Meta-analysis of Studies with Long-term Use of Orlistat

Author, yr (reference)	Mean (95% CI)
Davidson et al., 1999 (28)	–2.95 (95% CI, –4.45 to –1.45)
Hauptman, 2000 (57)	–3.80 (95% CI, –5.37 to –2.23)
Rössner et al., 2000 (26)	–3.00 (95% CI, –4.17 to –1.83)
Sjostrom et al., 1998 (27)	–4.20 (95% CI, –5.26 to –3.14)
Torgerson et al., 2004 (30)	–4.17 (95% CI, –4.60 to –3.74)

Source: Adapted from Ref. 54.

Table 4 Meta-analysis of Studies Using Orlistat

Author (reference)	Yr	Treatment		Placebo		Wt %	WMD (95% CI)
		N	Mean SD	N	Mean SD		
Sjostrom et al. (27)	1998	343	–8.10 ± 8.21	340	–3.90 ± 7.02	11.1	–4.20 (–5.35 to –3.05)
Hollander et al. (43)	1998	156	–3.84 ± 5.00	151	–1.43 ± 5.10	11.4	–2.41 (–3.54 to –1.29)
Davidson et al. (28)	1999	657	–8.76 ± 9.48	223	–5.81 ± 10.01	6.5	–2.95 (–4.45 to –1.45)
Rössner et al. (26)	2000	241	–8.13 ± 8.22	236	–5.23 ± 7.40	7.4	–2.90 (–4.30 to –1.50)
Hauptman (57)	2000	210	–5.40 ± 7.44	212	–1.41 ± 6.31	8.4	–3.99 (–5.31 to –2.67)
Lindegarde (59)	2000	190	–4.20 ± 7.03	186	–2.90 ± 6.74	7.5	–1.30 (–2.69 to 0.09)
Finer et al. (38)	2000	110	–3.29 ± 6.85	108	–1.31 ± 6.29	4.8	–1.98 (–3.73 to –0.23)
Broom et al. (58)	2002	259	–5.80 ± 8.50	163	–2.30 ± 6.40	8.7	–3.50 (–4.79 to –2.21)

Source: Adapted from Ref. 55.

Orlistat as an Over-the-Counter Preparation

Orlistat has been approved by the U.S. Food and Drug Administration for use in a 60-mg capsule to be taken three times a day for up to six months as an aid in weight control for individuals with BMI > 25 kg/m^2. In a clinical trial comparing placebo with this dose of orlistat and a packaged weight loss program, the orlistat-treated individuals lost 50% more weight during the four-month trial (62).

Side Effects and Safety Considerations

Orlistat is not absorbed to any significant degree, and its side effects are thus related to the blockade of triglyceride digestion in the intestine (63). Fecal fat loss and related GI symptoms are common initially, but they subside as patients learn to use the drug (6). The quality of life in patients treated with orlistat may improve despite concerns about GI symptoms.

Orlistat can cause small but significant decreases in fat-soluble vitamins. Levels usually remain within the normal range, but a few patients may need vitamin supplementation. In a six-month European dose-ranging study, mean levels of vitamin A, D, E, and β-carotene were evaluated; the results showed that vitamin levels remained within the clinical reference range in all treatment groups and rarely required supplementation (24). Some patients need supplementation with fat-soluble vitamins that can be lost in stools. Because it is impossible to predict which patients need such supplements, a multivitamin can be provided with instructions to take it before bedtime. Absorption of other drugs does not seem to be significantly affected by orlistat (6). In some studies, there was some trend toward a decrease in lipid-soluble vitamin levels, but only the decrease in vitamin E levels was statistically significant, while remaining within normal windows.

One case of renal oxalate stones in a patient treated with orlistat has been reported. The renal oxalate resolved when treatment was discontinued (64).

No pharmacodynamic or pharmacokinetic interactions were observed with orlistat 360 mg/day and warfarin (15) or glyburide (20) in healthy volunteers or with pravastatin in patients with mild hypercholesterolemia (65). No pharmacokinetic interactions were reported with orlistat and digoxin (16), nifedipine (66), or phenytoin (67). Orlistat did not interfere with oral contraceptive medication in healthy women (68). It had no clinically significant effects on the pharmacokinetics of captopril, nifedipine, atenolol, or furosemide in healthy volunteers (69). It does reduce the absorption of cyclosporin. Short-term treatment with orlistat had no effect on ethanol pharmacokinetics, nor did ethanol interfere with the ability of orlistat to inhibit dietary fat absorption in healthy male volunteers (21,69).

Other pivotal functions such as blood pressure and heart rate are influenced positively by orlistat.

Cetilistat, A Lipase Inhibitor

Although one lipase inhibitor, orlistat, is already approved for the treatment of overweight people, cetilistat (ATL-962), another GI lipase inhibitor, is in development. A five-day trial of ATL-962 in 90 normal volunteers was conducted on an inpatient unit. There was a three- to sevenfold increase in fecal fat that was dose dependent, but only 11% of the subjects had more than one oily stool. This suggested that this lipase inhibitor may have fewer GI adverse events than orlistat (70).

In a 12-week double-blind randomized trial in 372 patients comparing placebo with doses of 60, 120, or 240 mg of cetilistat t.i.d., the drug-treated patients lost between 3.5 and 4 kg compared with a 2-kg loss in the placebo-treated group (71). In a second phase II study, doses of 40, 80, and 120 mg t.i.d. were given to type 2 diabetics who showed a dose-related reduction in body weight and in HbA$_{1c}$ (71).

Intestinal Amylase Inhibitors

Obese individuals have impaired starch tolerance due to their insulin resistance. Berchtold and Kiesselbach reported that an amylase inhibitor, BAY e 4609, improved insulin and glucose during a starch-tolerance test, but did not cause weight loss in a controlled trial of 59 obese humans (72). Nevertheless, commercial preparations of amylase inhibitors were sold in the early 1980s with the claim that when taken in tablet form 10 minutes before meals, they would block the digestion of 100 g of starch in the diet. Garrow et al. tested this claim with starch enriched with ^{13}C and found that these "starch blockers" do not affect starch digestion or absorption in vivo (73).

In 1979, Hillebrand and colleagues reported that acarbose, an α-glucosidase inhibitor, reduced the insulin and glucose response to a mixed meal (74,75). Puls et al. reported a dose-related inhibition of weight gain in both Wistar and Zucker rats (76). Similar findings and a reduction in visceral adipose tissue was demonstrated with another α-glucosidase inhibitor, voglibose (AO-128), suggesting that these effects are related to this class of compounds (77–79). William-Olsson treated 24 weight-reduced women with acarbose, showing that such treatment was able to inhibit weight regain (80). Wolever and colleagues have recently reported a one-year, double-blind, randomized, placebo-controlled study in 354 subjects with type 2 diabetes. Subjects on acarbose lost 0.46 kg while the placebo group gained 0.33 kg, which was a small, but statistically significant, difference ($p = 0.027$) (81).

We conclude that α-amylase inhibitors usually have no place in the treatment of obesity without concomitant diabetes. Acarbose gives only a small weight loss and is not indicated as an obesity treatment, but it certainly deserves consideration in treating obese type 2 diabetic subjects who have failed treatment with diet and exercise. Also the more recent molecule miglitol, a second-generation α-glucosidase inhibitor, has been shown to improve metabolic control in type 2 diabetics. In a combination trial with metformin, in patients insufficiently treated with the biguanide alone, addition of miglitol led to an improvement of metabolic control (placebo subtracted; −0.43% in HbA$_{1c}$) but also to a weight reduction of 2.5 kg over 28 weeks of treatment (82). Although this was not significant when compared to placebo, weight reduction during active therapy for glucose control always has to be considered as a success, in view of the known weight effects in U.K. Prospective Diabetes Study (UKPDS) (83).

POSTABSORPTIVE MODIFIERS OF NUTRIENT METABOLISM

Growth Hormone

Human growth hormone is a 191 amino acid peptide composed of a single chain with two disulfide bonds (84). It is of interest in relation to obesity because obese individuals secrete less growth hormone (85), and because growth hormone enhances lipolysis (86), increases metabolic rate, and leads to changes in fat patterning in hypopituitary children treated with growth hormone (87). On the basis of these observations, early studies with growth hormone showed that it would enhance mobilization of fat, stimulate oxygen consumption (88), and lead to reduced protein loss in obese people (89). When given to fasting obese subjects on a metabolic ward, it accelerated ketosis by increasing fatty acid mobilization (90). More recently, treatment of adult growth hormone deficiency has been shown to reduce body fat (91), whereas lowering growth hormone after treatment of acromegaly, a condition with high growth hormone secretion, increases fat (92).

The nitrogen-sparing effects of growth hormone in human subjects on a reduced-calorie diet were investigated in a series of studies using different levels of caloric restriction (93–100). In all of these studies, growth hormone increased the concentration of FFA in the circulation, increased IGF-1, and increased insulin and C-peptide. In most studies, growth hormone preserved nitrogen and increased fat loss or the loss of fat relative to body weight loss. Table 5 summarizes these data and other clinical trials

in obese subjects. Most of the studies have been relatively short term, with treatment lasting from 21 days to 5 weeks (90,95,99), but a few have lasted from 11 to 39 weeks (93,94,101–103). Most of the subjects were women. Metabolic rate is increased where measured, and respiratory exchange rate (RER) is reduced, indicating that more fat is being oxidized. IGF-I and FFA both increased, and the rate of fat loss relative to protein loss increased. The only long-term study has lasted nine months and used continuous daily injections of growth hormone. There were 15 men in each arm of the randomized double-blind placebo-controlled clinical trial (102). In these men, growth hormone enhanced fat loss, with a larger percentage of this fat coming from the visceral than from the subcutaneous compartment (Table 5). A number of side effects, including cardiac changes, were noted (99), which reduce the enthusiasm for its use.

Metformin

Metformin is a biguanide that is approved for the treatment of diabetes mellitus, a disease that is exacerbated by obesity and weight gain. Although the cellular mechanisms for the effects of metformin are poorly understood, it has three effects at the clinical level (104–110). First, it reduces hepatic glucose production, which is a major source of circulating glucose. Mainly among overweight and obese subjects, metformin also reduces intestinal absorption of glucose, which is an additional source of circulating glucose. Finally, metformin increases the sensitivity to insulin, mainly in obese individuals, thus increasing peripheral glucose uptake and utilization.

Metformin has been associated with significant weight loss when compared to SUs or placebo. Campbell and colleagues (106) compared metformin and glipizide in a randomized double-blind study of type 2 diabetic individuals who had failed on diets. The 24 subjects on metformin lost weight and had better diabetic control of fasting glucose and glycohemoglobin than did the glipizide group. The glipizide group gained weight, and the difference in weight between the two groups at the end of the study was highly significant. In a double-blind, placebo-controlled trial in subjects with the insulin-resistance syndrome, metformin also increased weight loss. Fontbonne and colleagues (107) reported the results from the BIGPRO study, a one-year French multicenter study that compared metformin with placebo in 324 middle-aged subjects with upper-body obesity and the insulin-resistance syndrome. The subjects on metformin lost significantly more weight (1–2 kg) than did the placebo group, and the study concluded that metformin may have a role in the primary prevention of type 2 diabetes (107). In a meta-analysis of three of these studies, Avenell et al. (55)

Table 5 Clinical Studies with Growth Hormone in Obesity

Author (reference)	Yr	Number of subjects Placebo	Number of subjects Drug	Dose of medication	Duration	Diet	Weight loss (kg) Placebo	Weight loss (kg) Drug	Fat loss (kg or %) Placebo	Fat loss (kg or %) Drug	Comments
Bray et al. (89)	1971	4F, (hGH – N = 2), (hGH + T$_3$ N = 4)		5 mg/day	hGH alone: 30 days, hGH + T: 15 days	900 kcal/day, formula diet	211 g/day 523 g/day 550 g/day T$_3$	337 g/day 240 g/day 380 g/day T$_3$+hGH			Metabolic ward
Clemmons et al. (93)	1987	5F, 3M		0.1 mg/kg, IBW every other day, wk 3–5, wk 8–10	11 wk	24 kcal/kg IBW, 1.0 prot/kg IBW	−4.16	−3.42	−2.64 ± 1.08	−3.06 ± 1.39	Metabolic ward, cross-over study or IGF-1 ↑, nitrogen balance improved
Snyder et al. (94)	1988	8F 2M	8F 2M	0.1 mg/kgIBW every other day wk 2–12	13 wk	18 kcal/kg IBW 1.2 g prot/kg IBW	−15.2 ± 3.8	−13.9 ± 3.0	−7.5 ± 1.5%	−8.1 ± 2.4%	Metabolic ward, parallel arm study; nitrogen balance positive but less with time IGF-1 ↑, FFA ↑
Snyder et al. (95)	1989	11F		0.1 mg/kg IBW every other day wk 2–4	two 5-wk periods, 5-wk washout	12 kcal/kg IBW 1.0 g prot/kg IBW diet I: 72% Carb diet II: 20% Carb	−8.5 ± 1.7 −8.2 ± 0.7	−7.4 ± 1.9 −7.5 ± 1.8	−2.8 ± 0.7%	−3.7 ± 1.0% −3.8 ± 0.9% −3.6 ± 1.2%	Metabolic unit study; GH ↑ fat loss as % wt loss from 64% to 81%
Snyder et al. (96)	1990	8F		0.1 mg/kg daily	Two 5-wk periods, 5-wk washout	12 kcal/kg IBW	−7.2 ± 2.3	−6.3 ± 5.0	−3.6 ± 1.1%	−3.5 ± 1.1%	Cross-over; improved N$_2$ balance ↑ IGF-I

Reference	Year	Subjects	Dose	Duration	Diet					Comments
Richelson et al. (97)	1994	9F premenopausal	0.03 mg/kg IBW/day	Two 5-wk periods, 5-wk washout	Not specified			+3.0 ± 0.13	−2.1 ± 0.06kg	Cross-over; visceral fat LPL ↓; FFA ↑; C-peptide ↑
Jorgensen et al. (98)	1994	10F Premenopausal	0.03 mg/kg IBW/day	Two 5-wk periods, 5-wk washout	Not specified		Data not given, subjects may overlap with paper above	Data not given, subjects may overlap with paper above		Cross-over T$_3$ ↑; EE ↑; FFA ↓; RER ↓; IGF-I ↑
Snyder et al. (99)	1995	11	0.05 mg/kg	4 wk	15 kcal/kg	−8.4 ± 1.4	−7.3 ± 1.4	−2.6 ± 1.0%	−3.4 ± 0.9%	Cross-over IGF-1↑
Drent et al. (100)	1995	7F; 6F 2M	6 µg/day	8 wk	VLCD + exercise	−12.8 ± 5.0	−13.8 ± 4.0			IGF-1↑; IGFBP-3↑
Johannsson et al. (101)	1997	15M	9.5 µg/kg daily	39 wk	Not specified	+0.7	FFM +2.0		−9.2 ± 2.4%	Parallel arm
Karlsson et al. (102)	1998	15M	9.5 µg/kg daily	39 wk	Not specified	+0.5	−1.0	−0.1 kg	−3.0 kg	Parallel arm, same patients as in report, BMR ↑; leptin ↓; visceral fat ↓ 68.1%
Thompson et al. (103)	1998	7		12 wk	500 kcal/day deficit					Parallel arm
		9	GH 0.025 mg/kg BW/day			−3.7	−4.2	−3.5 kg	−6.3 kg	
		9	IGI1 0.015 mg/kg/day				−3.5		−4.0 kg	
		10	GH+IGFI				−5.6		−8.4 kg	

Abbreviation: hGH, human growth hormone.

reported a weight loss of –1.09 kg at 12 months (95% CI, –2.29 to 0.11 kg).

The package insert for metformin (108) describes a 29-week double-blind study comparing glyburide 20 mg/day with metformin 2.5 g/day and their combination in 632 type 2 diabetic subjects who had inadequate glucose control. The metformin group lost 3.8 kg compared to a loss of 0.3 kg in the glyburide group and a gain of 0.4 kg in the combined group. The package insert also describes a double-blind controlled study in poorly controlled type 2 diabetic subjects comparing metformin 2.5 m/day to placebo. Weight loss in the placebo group was 1.1 kg, compared with 0.64 kg in the metformin group. Lee and Morley (109) compared 48 type 2 diabetic women in a double-blind controlled trial, randomizing subjects to metformin 850 mg twice a day (b.i.d.) or a placebo. Subjects on metformin lost 8.8 kg over 24 weeks, compared to only 1.0 kg in the placebo group, a highly significant difference ($p < 0.001$).

The Diabetes Prevention Program trial to prevent or delay the conversion of individuals with IGT to diabetes mellitus is the most recent and largest trial with metformin. Of the slightly more than 1000 individuals treated with medication, half received metformin and the other half took placebo. Nearly 75% of each group took their pills for the average 2.8 years of follow-up. Weight loss in the metformin group was significantly greater than placebo with a nadir at six months, but with weight remaining below baseline for the remainder of the trial. Metformin was effective in men and women and all ethnic groups. It was more effective in younger individuals and in those who were more overweight (110). Although metformin may not give enough weight loss to receive an indication from the U.S. Food and Drug Administration for treating obesity, it certainly deserves consideration in obese type 2 diabetic individuals who have failed diet and exercise treatment for their diabetes, and it has been used in children (111).

Hydroxycitrate

Another compound, (–)–hydroxycitrate, inhibits citrate lyase, the first extra-mitochondrial step in fatty acid synthesis from glucose. This compound causes weight loss by decreasing calorie intake (112). Although the mechanism of this inhibition of food intake is not clear, studies by Hellerstein and Xie (113) suggest that it may be through trioses such as pyruvate. In a double-blind trial of 60 subjects who were randomized to hydroxycitric acid 1320 mg/day or placebo and a 1200-calorie diet for eight weeks, the hydroxycitrate group lost 6.4 kg, whereas the placebo group lost only 3.8 kg ($p < 0.001$) (114). Garcinia cambogia, an herbal product containing hydroxycitrate, has been com-

pared to placebo in a double-blind randomized clinical trial (115). The herbal product was given t.i.d. in a dose to provide 500 mg each time. The subjects treated with hydroxycitrate lost no more weight than those receiving placebo.

Human Chorionic Gonadotropin

Injection of small doses of human chorionic gonadotropin (HCG) daily for six weeks or more has been used in the treatment of obesity following the introduction of this treatment for undescended testes and its use with alleged success in patients with what was termed "Frohlich's" syndrome. A number of controlled clinical trials have been done to evaluate the use of HCG, and these have recently been reviewed (116,117) (Table 6).

Lijesen and colleagues (116) evaluated 16 uncontrolled and eight controlled studies found through a literature search. All studies were graded on a 100-point scale, and those making a score of 50 or greater were evaluated. Of these studies, only one concluded that HCG was a useful adjunct to a weight loss program compared to a placebo. Table 6 is a summary of the double-blind, placebo-controlled, randomized trials that have been published in the past 30 years (118–127). We conclude that HCG is no more effective than placebo, but we also note that all of these studies used a VLCD that gave a significant weight loss in both groups.

Androgens

For this discussion, androgens will be divided into two groups, the "weak" androgenic compounds including androsterone, dehydroepiandrosterone, Δ^4-androstenedione, and anabolic steroids; and the potent androgens, testosterone and dihydrotestosterone (DHT).

Dehydroepiandrosterone

Dehydroepiandrosterone (DHEA = Δ^5-androsten-3-β-ol-17-one) is a product of the adrenal gland. In human beings, this steroid and its sulfated derivative are the most abundant steroids produced by the adrenal. In experimental animals, the quantities are much lower, and in rodents they are just above the threshold for detection. In spite of their high concentration in the circulation and abundance as adrenal products, no clear function has been identified. DHEA levels decline with age in men and women (128). In contrast with the limited relationship between DHEA and body weight or total fat, there is a clearer relation with fat distribution (129) and hyperinsulinemia (128). Animal studies have shown that DHEA may be immuno-suppressive and have antiatherogenic and antitumor effects

Table 6 Clinical Trials with Injections of Human Chorionic Gonadotropin for the Treatment of Obesity

Author	Yr	Number of subjects		Diet (kcal/day)	Design	Wt loss (kg)		Wt loss (%)		Comments
		Placebo	Drug			Placebo	Drug	Placebo	Drug	
Carne (118)	1961	13/12		500	Diet + HCG		−9.5		−12.5	Injections were better than no injections, but HCG was not better than saline.
		12/10			Diet + Vehicle	−8.6		−10.3		
		11/8			Diet + Vehicle	−10.1		−12.2		
		10/7			Diet Only	−8.0		−11.3		
Craig et al. (119)	1963	11/9		550	Randomized double-blind	−3.0	−4.0			HCG had no demonstrable effect. Weight loss due to diet.
Frank (120)	1964	63/30		500	Double-blind 3 injections/wk	−5.6	−5.2			Changes in body measurements and rating of hunger were the same in both groups. HCG had no effect.
Asher and Harper (122)	1973	20/13	20/17	500	Modified double-blind (3 patients from each vial)	−9.0	−5.0	−6.8	−11.5	HCG possibly effective. Five of placebo group and none of HCG group received fewer than 21 injections.
Stein et al. (123)	1976	26/21	25/20	500	Double-blind, randomized, placebo-controlled	−7.0	−7.2	−9.3	−9.5	No difference in weight loss, waist or hip circumference, or hunger rating between HCG and placebo.
Greenway and Bray (117)	1977	20/20		500	Double-blind, randomized, placebo-controlled	−8.1	−8.8	−10.2	−10.9	No difference in weight loss, hunger rating, mood or body circumference between HCG and placebo.
Shetty and Kalkhoff (124)	1977	5/5	6/6	500	Double-blind inpatient study lasting 30 days	−9.4	−9.3	−9.5	−9.1	No difference in weight loss, fat redistribution, hunger or well-being.
Bosch et al. (125)	1990	20/16	20/17	1190 (5000 kJ)	Double-blind, randomized	−4.6	−3.2	−4.9	−3.4	No difference in weight loss, fat redistribution, hunger or well-being.

Abbreviations: HCG, human chorionic gonadotropin.

(130). It is a fact that mice, rats, cats, and dogs fed with DHEA lose weight, which has led to its evaluation as a potential treatment for obesity. A recent structure-function analysis by Lardy and colleagues (131) has shown that the biological effect of DHEA-related steroids on body fat was greatest with 7-oxo-DHEA derivatives.

Several clinical studies with DHEA have been done and are reviewed by Clore (130). In a study lasting 28 days with 10 normal-weight volunteers, DHEA at 1600 mg/day (near the limit where hepatic toxicity is a risk) had no effect on body weight or on insulin sensitivity as assessed by the euglycemic-hyperinsulinemic clamp (132). A similar study showed no effect of DHEA on energy expenditure, body composition, or protein turnover (133). After 28 days of treatment with DHEA, obese male volunteers showed no improvement in body fat or insulin sensitivity (134). In obese female volunteers, there was likewise no change in body fat, but there was a decrease in insulin sensitivity (135). On the basis of these negative studies in both lean and obese human subjects, it would appear that DHEA is ineffective in human obesity. The study with DHEA was also conducted in older men and women. Fifty-six elderly men and women aged 65 to 78 years were randomly assigned to either placebo or 50 mg/day of DHEA for six months. Compliance with the intervention was 97%. After six months of treatment, body weight declined by −0.9 kg in the DHEA-treated group compared with a small gain of 0.6 kg in the placebo-treated group. Visceral fat decreased by −13 cm^2 in the DHEA-treated group, corresponding to a 10.2% reduction for women and 7.4% for men, compared with a small gain of +0.3 cm^2 ($p < 0.001$) in the placebo-treated group. There were similar changes in subcutaneous fat (−13 cm^2 in the DHEA group and +2 cm^2 in the placebo group $p < 0.003$). The insulin response after an oral glucose-tolerance test was improved in the DHEA group and glucose response was unchanged, indicating improved insulin sensitivity after treatment with DHEA (136). Thus, DHEA can have significant effects on visceral fat.

Testosterone and Dihydrotestosterone

Testosterone is the principal product of the testis and is responsible for masculinization. Testosterone is converted to DHT in peripheral androgenic tissues and converts the "soft" hair to the terminal hair in male androgenic areas. Testosterone can also be produced by the adrenal, by the ovary, and by conversion in peripheral tissues (137). In females, 25% of testosterone comes from the ovary, 25% from the adrenals, and 50% from peripheral conversion. In human subjects, the concentration of testosterone is positively related to the level of visceral fat in women and negatively correlated with visceral fat in men (138,139). A

recent report suggests that androstane-3-β,17-α-diol may be a correlate of visceral obesity (140).

The inverse relationship between testosterone and visceral fat in men suggested the possibility that visceral fat might be reduced by treatment with testosterone. Marin and colleagues (141–143) have evaluated this in two trials using men with low-normal circulating testosterone levels (<20 nmol/L) and a BMI > 25 kg/m^2. In the first trial, testosterone 80 mg b.i.d. was given orally as the undecenoate. The 11 men who received testosterone had a significant decrease in visceral fat mass as measured by computed tomography compared with the 12 men who received placebo for eight months. No changes were observed in body mass, subcutaneous fat mass, or lean body mass, but insulin sensitivity was improved (141).

In a second trial (142), 31 men were randomly allocated to three groups receiving placebo, testosterone, or DHT. The testosterone was given as a gel (5 g) containing 125 mg of testosterone applied to the arms daily. The DHT was applied in a similar gel at the same dose. The placebo group received only the gel. After nine months, the testosterone-treated group showed a significant decrease in waist circumference and visceral fat. In contrast, the DHT-treated group showed an increase in visceral fat. Testosterone was increased in the group treated with the testosterone. Treatment with DHT reduced testosterone and increased DHT levels. Insulin sensitivity was also improved by treatment with testosterone (143,144).

Two additional studies have examined the effects of anabolic steroids in men and women (144,145). The first was a nine-month trial on 30 healthy overweight men with mean BMI values of 33.8 to 34.5 kg/m^2 and testosterone values between 2 and 5 ng/mL (145). During the first three months, when an oral anabolic steroid (oxandrolone) was given daily, there was a significantly greater decrease in subcutaneous fat and a greater reduction in visceral fat than in the groups treated with placebo or testosterone enanthate injected every two weeks. Because of the drop in HDL-C, which is a known side effect of oral anabolic steroids (144), the anabolic steroid group was changed to an injectable drug, nandrolone decanoate. The effects were similar to those of testosterone enanthate. The data with testosterone given as a biweekly injection did not replicate the data of Marin and colleagues (141,142), and the biweekly injections of nandrolone failed to maintain the difference seen with daily treatment with oxandrolone. This suggests that to obtain the visceral effects with steroids, frequent if not daily administration may be needed.

In a second nine-month trial with 30 postmenopausal overweight women, Lovejoy and colleagues (145) randomized subjects to nandrolone decanoate, spironolactone, or placebo. The weight loss was comparable in all three groups, but the women treated with nandrolone decanoate gained lean mass and visceral fat and lost more total body fat. Women treated with the antiandrogen spironolactone lost significantly more visceral fat. The conclusion from the four studies described above is that visceral and total body fat can be manipulated separately, and that testosterone plays an important role in this differential fat distribution in both men and women.

CONCLUSION

In this chapter, we have examined the use of drugs that affect fat absorption and post-absorptive metabolism. The effects of lipase inhibitors are modest, but consistent across studies. Weight reduction improves risk factors for diabetes and cardiovascular disease, when present. The metabolic drugs, including steroids, have not been approved for treatment of obesity. Growth hormone and anabolic steroids are particularly interesting because they preferentially modulate visceral fat. A separate chapter (chap. 21) discusses the drugs based on hormones from the gut (glucagon-like peptide-1) or pancreas (amylin), which reduce weight. From the vantage point of the year 2007, the future looks good for agents to modulate total and visceral fat through peripheral mechanisms.

REFERENCES

1. Adams KF, Schatzkin A, Harris TB, et al. Overweight, obesity, and mortality in a large prospective cohort of persons 50 to 71 years old. N Engl J Med 2006; 355(8): 763–778.
2. Bray GA. The Metabolic Syndrome and Obesity. Totowa, NJ: Humana Press, 2007.
3. Dansinger, ML, Tatsioni A, Wong JB, et al. Meta-analysis: The effect of dietary counseling for weight loss. Ann Int Med 2007; 147:41–50.
4. Douketis JD, Macie C, Thabane L, et al. Systematic review of long-term weight loss studies in obese adults: clinical significance and applicability to clinical practice. Int J Obes (Lond) 2005; 29(10):1153–1167.
5. Bray GA, Greenway FL. Pharmacological treatment of the overweight patient. Pharmacol Rev 2007; 59(2):151–184.
6. Bray GA, Ryan DH. Drug treatment of the overweight patient. Gastroenterology 2007; 132(6):2239–2252.
7. Bray GA, Popkin BM. Dietary fat intake does affect obesity! Am J Clin Nutr 1998; 68(6):1157–1173.
8. Guerciolini R. Mode of action of orlistat. Int J Obes Relat Metab Disord 1997; 21(suppl 3):S12–S23.
9. Hadvary P, Lengsfield H, Wolfer H. Inhibition of pancreatic lipase in vitro by the covalent inhibitor tetrahydrolipstatin. Biochem J 1988; 256:357–361.
10. Lookene A, Skottova N, Olivecrona G. Interactions of lipoprotein lipase with the active-site inhibitor tetrahydrolipstatin (orlistat). Eur J Biochem 1994; 222:395–403.

11. Zhi J, Melia AT, Guerciolini R, et al. Retrospective population-based analysis of the dose-response (fecal fat excretion) relationship of orlistat in normal and obese volunteers. Clin Pharmacol Ther 1994; 56:82–85.
12. Reitsma JB, Castro Cabezas M, de Bruin TW, et al. Relationship between improved postprandial lipemia and low-density lipoprotein metabolism during treatment with tetrahydrolipstatin, a pancreatic lipase inhibitor. Metabolism 1994; 43:293–298.
13. Hauptman JB, Jeunet FS, Hartmann D. Initial studies in humans with the novel gastrointestinal lipase inhibitor Ro 18-0647 (tetrahydrolipstatin). Am J Clin Nutr 1992; 55(suppl 1), 309S–313S.
14. Hussain Y, Guzelhan C, Odink J, et al. Comparison of the inhibition of dietary fat absorption by full versus divided doses of orlistat. J Clin Pharmacol 1994; 34:1121–1125.
15. Zhi J, Melia AT, Funk C, et al. Metabolic profiles of minimally absorbed orlistat in obese/overweight volunteers. J Clin Pharmacol 1996; 36:1006–1011.
16. Melia AT, Zhi J, Koss-Twardy SG, et al. The influence of reduced dietary fat absorption induced by orlistat on the pharmacokinetics of digoxin in healthy volunteers. J Clin Pharmacol 1995; 35:840–843.
17. Zhi J, Melia AT, Koss-Twardy SG, et al. The influence of orlistat on the pharmacokinetics and pharmacodynamics of glyburide in healthy volunteers. J Clin Pharmacol 1995; 35:521–525.
18. Guzelhan C, Odink J, Niestijl Jansen-Zuidema JJ, et al. Influence of dietary composition on the inhibition of fat absorption by orlistat. J Int Med Res 1994; 22:255–265.
19. Weber C, Tam YK, Schmidtke-Schrezenmeier G, et al. Effect of the lipase inhibitor orlistat on the pharmacokinetics of four different antihypertensive drugs in healthy volunteers. Eur J Clin Pharmacol 1996; 51:87–90.
20. Zhi J, Melia AT, Eggers H, et al. Review of limited systemic absorption of orlistat, a lipase inhibitor, in healthy human volunteers. J Clin Pharmacol 1995; 35: 1103–1108.
21. Hvizdos KM, Markham A. Orlistat: a review of its use in the management of obesity. Drugs 1999; 58:743–760.
22. Drent ML, van der Veen EA. Lipase inhibition: a novel concept in the treatment of obesity. Int J Obes Relat Metab Disord 1993; 17:241–244.
23. Drent ML, Larsson I, William-Olsson T, et al. Orlistat (Ro 18-0647), a lipase inhibitor, in the treatment of human obesity: a multiple dose study. Int J Obes Relat Metab Disord 1995; 19:221–226.
24. Van Gaal LF, Broom JI, Enzi G, et al. Efficacy and tolerability of orlistat in the treatment of obesity: a 6-month dose-ranging study. Eur J Clin Pharmacol 1998; 54:125–132.
25. James WP, Avenell A, Broom J, et al. A one-year trial to assess the value of orlistat in the management of obesity. Int J Obes Relat Metab Disord 1997; 21(suppl 3):S24–S30.
26. Rössner S, Sjöstrom L, Noack R, et al. Weight loss, weight maintenance and improved cardiovascular risk factors after 2 years treatment with orlistat for obesity. European Orlistat Obesity Study Group. Obes Res 2000; 8:49–61.

27. Sjostrom L, Rissanen A, Andersen T, et al. Randomized placebo-controlled trial of orlistat for weight loss and prevention of weight regain in obese patients. European Multicentre Orlistat Study Group. Lancet 1998; 352:167–172.

28. Davidson MH, Hauptman J, DiGirolamo M, et al. Weight control and risk factor reduction in obese subjects treated for 2 years with orlistat: a randomized controlled trial. JAMA 1999; 281(3):235–242.

29. Rissanen A, Lean M, Rossner S, et al. Predictive value of early weight loss in obesity management with orlistat: an evidence-based assessment of prescribing guidelines. Int J Obes Relat Metab Disord 2003; 27:103–109.

30. Torgerson JS, Hauptman J, Boldrin MN, et al. XENical in the prevention of diabetes in obese subjects (XENDOS) study: a randomized study of orlistat as an adjunct to lifestyle changes for the prevention of type 2 diabetes in obese patients. Diabetes Care 2004; 27(1):155–161.

31. Hill JO, Hauptman J, Anderson JW, et al. Orlistat, a lipase inhibitor, for weight maintenance after conventional dieting: a 1-y study. Am J Clin Nutr 1999; 69(6):1108–1116.

32. Richelsen B, Tonstad S, Rossner S, et al. Effect of orlistat on weight regain and cardiovascular risk factors following a very-low-energy diet in abdominally obese patients: a 3-year randomized, placebo-controlled study. Diabetes Care 2007; 30(1):27–32.

33. Vray M, Joubert JM, Eschwege E, et al. [Results from the observational study EPIGRAM: management of excess weight in general practice and follow-up of patients treated with orlistat]. Therapie 2005; 60(1):17–24.

34. Tonstad S, Pometta D, Erkelens DW, et al. The effects of gastrointestinal lipase inhibitor, orlistat, on serum lipids and lipoproteins in patients with primary hyperlipidaemia. Eur J Clin Pharmacol 1994; 46:405–410.

35. Van Gaal LF, Wauters M, De Leeuw IH. The beneficial effects of modest weight loss on cardiovascular risk factors. Int J Obes 1997; 21(suppl 1):S5–S9.

36. Dattilo AM, Kris-Etherton PM. Effects of weight reduction on blood lipids and lipoproteins: a meta-analysis. Am J Clin Nutr 1992; 56:320–328.

37. Muls E, Kolanowski J, Scheen A, et al. The effects of orlistat on weight and on serum lipids in obese patients with hypercholesterolemia: a randomized, double-blind, placebo-controlled, multicenter study. Int J Obes Relat Metab Disord 2001; 25:1713–1721.

38. Finer N, James WP, Kopelman PG, et al. One-year treatment of obesity: a randomized, double-blind, placebo-controlled, multicentre study of orlistat, a gastrointestinal lipase inhibitor. Int J Obes Relat Metab Disord 2000; 24:306–313.

39. Zavoral JH. Treatment with orlistat reduces cardiovascular risk in obese patients. J Hypertens 1998; 16:2013–2017.

40. Mittendorfer B, Ostlund RE Jr., Patterson BW, et al. Orlistat inhibits dietary cholesterol absorption. Obes Res 2001; 9(10):599–604.

41. Linton MF, Fazio S. Re-emergence of fibrates in the management of dyslipidemia and cardiovascular risk. Curr Atheroscler Rep 2000; 2:29–35.

42. Maron DJ, Fazio S, Linton MF. Current perspectives on statins. Circulation 2000; 101:207–213.

43. Hollander PA, Elbein SC, Hirsch IB, et al. Role of orlistat in the treatment of obese patients with type 2 diabetes. A 1-year randomized double-blind study. Diabetes Care 1998; 21(8):1288–1294.

44. Kelley DE, Bray GA, Pi-Sunyer FX, et al. Clinical efficacy of orlistat therapy in overweight and obese patients with insulin-treated type 2 diabetes: a 1-year randomized controlled trial. Diabetes Care 2002; 25(6):1033–1041.

45. Tan MH. Current treatment of insulin resistance in type 2 diabetes mellitus. Int J Clin Pract Suppl 2000; 113:54–62.

46. Ceriello A. The postprandial state and cardiovascular disease: relevance to diabetes mellitus. Diabetes Metab Res Rev 2000; 16:125–132.

47. Heymsfield SB, Segal KR, Hauptman J, et al. Effects of weight loss with orlistat on glucose tolerance and progression to type 2 diabetes in obese adults. Arch Intern Med 2000; 160:1321–1326.

48. Padwal R, Majumdar SR, Johnson JA, et al. A systematic review of drug therapy to delay or prevent type 2 diabetes. Diabetes Care 2005; 28(3):736–744.

49. Reaven G, Segal K, Hauptman J, et al. Effect of orlistat-assisted weight loss in decreasing coronary heart disease risk in patients with syndrome X. Am J Cardiol 2001; 87(7):827–831.

50. Chanoine JP, Hampl S, Jensen C, et al. Effect of orlistat on weight and body composition in obese adolescents: a randomized controlled trial. JAMA 2005; 293(23):2873–2883.

51. Chanoine J-P, Hauptman J, Boldin M. Weight reduction in overweight adolescents achieving early response to orlistat. Obes Rev 2006; 7(suppl 2):318.

52. Maahs D, de Serna DG, Kolotkin RL, et al. Randomized, double-blind, placebo-controlled trial of orlistat for weight loss in adolescents. Endocr Pract 2006; 12(1):18–28.

53. Haddock CK, Poston WS, Dill PL, et al. Pharmacotherapy for obesity: a quantitative analysis of four decades of published randomized clinical trials. Int J Obes Relat Metab Disord 2002; 26(2):262–273.

54. Li Z, Maglione M, Tu W, et al. Meta-analysis: pharmacologic treatment of obesity. Ann Intern Med 2005; 142(7):532–546.

55. Avenell A, Brown TJ, McGee MA, et al. What interventions should we add to weight reducing diets in adults with obesity? A systematic review of randomized controlled trials of adding drug therapy, exercise, behaviour therapy or combinations of these interventions. J Hum Nutr Diet 2004; 17(4):293–316.

56. Norris SL, Zhang X, Avenell A, et al. Efficacy of pharmacotherapy for weight loss in adults with type 2 diabetes mellitus: a meta-analysis. Arch Intern Med 2004; 164(13):1395–1404.

57. Hauptman J. Orlistat: selective inhibition of caloric absorption can affect long-term body weight. Endocrine 2000; 13(2):201–206.

58. Broom I, Wilding J, Stott P, et al., UK Multimorbidity Study Group. Randomised trial of the effect of orlistat on body weight and cardiovascular disease risk profile in obese patients. UK Multimorbidity Study. Int J Clin Pract 2002; 56(7):494–499.

59. Lindgarde F. The effect of orlistat on body weight and coronary heart disease risk profile in obese patients: the Swedish Multimorbidity Study. J Intern Med 2000; 248(3): 245–254.

60. Hutton B, Fergusson D. Changes in body weight and serum lipid profile in obese patients treated with orlistat in addition to a hypocaloric diet: a systematic review of randomized clinical trials. Am J Clin Nutr 2004; 80(6): 1461–1468.

61. Zelber-Sagi S, Kessler A, Brazowsky E, et al. A double-blind randomized placebo-controlled trial of orlistat for the treatment of nonalcoholic fatty liver disease. Clin Gastroenterol Hepatol 2006; 4(5):639–644.

62. Anderson JW, Schwartz SM, Hauptman J, et al. Low-dose orlistat effects on body weight of mildly to moderately overweight individuals: a 16 week, double-blind, placebo-controlled trial. Ann Pharmacother 2006; 40:1717–1723.

63. Zhi J, Mulligan TE, Hauptman JB. Long-term systemic exposure of orlistat, a lipase inhibitor, and its metabolites in obese patients. J Clin Pharmacol 1999; 39(1):41–46.

64. Singh A, Sarkar SR, Gaber LW, et al. Acute oxalate nephropathy associated with orlistat, a gastrointestinal lipase inhibitor. Am J Kidney Dis 2007; 49(1):153–157.

65. Oo CY, Akbari B, Lee S, et al. Effect of orlistat, a novel anti-obesity agent, on the pharmacokinetics and pharmacodynamics of pravastatin in patients with mild hypercholesterolaemia. Clin Drug Invest 1999; 17:217–223.

66. Melia AT, Mulligan TE, Zhi J. Lack of effect of orlistat on the bioavailability of a single dose of nifedipine extended-release tablets (Procardia XL) in healthy volunteers. J Clin Pharmacol 1996; 36:352–355.

67. Melia AT, Mulligan TE, Zhi J. The effect of orlistat on the pharmacokinetics of phenytoin in healthy volunteers. J Clin Pharmacol 1996; 36:654–658.

68. Hartmann D, Guzelhan C, Zuiderwijk PB, et al. Lack of interaction between orlistat and oral contraceptives. Eur J Clin Pharmacol 1996; 50:421–424.

69. Melia AT, Zhi J, Zelasko R, et al. The interaction of the lipase inhibitor orlistat with ethanol in healthy volunteers. Eur J Clin Pharmacol 1998; 54:773–777.

70. Dunk C, Enunwa M, De La Monte S, et al. Increased fecal fat excretion in normal volunteers treated with lipase inhibitor ATL-962. Int J Obes Relat Metab Disord 2002; 26(suppl):S135.

71. Kopelman P, Bryson A, Hickling R, et al. Cetilistat (ATL-962), a novel lipase inhibitor: a 12-week randomized, placebo-controlled study of weight reduction in obese patients. Int J Obes (Lond) 2007; 31(3):494–499.

72. Berchtold P, Kiesselbach NHK. The clinical significance of the alpha-amylase inhibitors Bay d 7791 and Bay e 4609. In: Berchtold P, Cairella M, Jacobelli A, et al., eds. Regulators of Intestinal Absorption in Obesity, Diabetes and Nutrition. Proceedings of Satellite Symposium 7, Third International Congress on Obesity. Siena, Italy: October 13–15, 1980. Vol. 1. Roma: Societa Editrice Universo, 1981:181–200.

73. Garrow JS, Scott PF, Heels S, et al. A study of "starch blockers" in man using 13C-enriched starch as a tracer. Hum Nutr Clin Nutr 1983; 37:301–305.

74. Hillebrand I, Boehme K, Frank G, et al. The effects of the alpha-glucosidase inhibitor BAY g 5421 (acarbose) on meal-stimulated elevations of circulating glucose, insulin, and triglyceride levels in man. Res Exp Med (Berl) 1979; 175:81–86.

75. Hillebrand I, Boehme K, Frank G, et al. The effects of the alpha-glucosidase inhibitor BAY g 5421 (acarbose) on postprandial blood glucose, serum insulin, and triglyceride levels: dose–time–response relationships in man. Res Exp Med (Berl) 1979; 175:87–94.

76. Puls W, Keup U, Krause HP, et al. Pharmacological significance of glucosidase inhibitors (acarbose). In: Berchtold P, Cairella M, Jacobelli A, et al., eds. Regulators of Intestinal Absorption in Obesity, Diabetes and Nutrition. Proceedings of Satellite Symposium 7, Third International Congress on Obesity. Siena, Italy: October 13–15, 1980. Vol. 1. Roma: Societa Editrice Universo, 1981:231–260.

77. Goto Y, Yamada K, Ohyama T, et al. An alpha-glucosidase inhibitor, AO-128, retards carbohydrate absorption in rats and humans. Diabetes Res Clin Pract 1995; 28:81–87.

78. Ikeda H, Odaka H. AO-128, alpha-glucosidase inhibitor: antiobesity and antidiabetic actions in genetically obese diabetic rats, Wistar family. Obes Res 1995; 3(suppl 4): 617S–621S.

79. Kobatake T, Matsuzawa Y, Tokunaga K, et al. Metabolic improvements associated with a reduction of abdominal visceral fat caused by a new alpha-glucosidase inhibitor, AO-128, in Zucker fatty rats. Int J Obes 1989; 13:147–154.

80. William-Olsson T. Alpha-glucosidase inhibition in obesity. Acta Med Scand Suppl 1985; 706:1–39.

81. Wolever TM, Chiasson JL, Josse RG, et al. Small weight loss on long-term acarbose therapy with no change in dietary pattern or nutrient intake of individuals with non-insulin-dependent diabetes. Int J Obes Relat Metab Disord 1997; 21:756–763.

82. Van Gaal L, Maislos M, Schernthaner G, et al. Miglitol combined with metformin improves glycaemic control in type 2 diabetes. Diabetes Obes Metab 2001; 3:326–331.

83. UK Prospective Diabetes Study (UKPDS) Group. Effect of intensive blood-glucose control with metformin on complications in overweight patients with type 2 diabetes (UKPDS 34). Lancet 1998, 352(9131):854–865.

84. Daughaday WH. Growth hormone, insulin-like growth factors, and acromegaly. In: DeGroot LJ, Besser M, Burger HG, et al., eds. Endocrinology. 3rd ed. Philadelphia: W.B. Saunders Company, 1995:303–329.

85. Veldhuis JD, Liem AY, South S, et al. Differential impact of age, sex steroid hormones, and obesity on basal versus pulsatile growth hormone secretion in men as assessed in an ultrasensitive chemiluminescence assay. J Clin Endocrinol 1995; 80:3209–3222.

86. Gertner JM. Effects of growth hormone on body fat in adults. Horm Res 1993; 40:10–15.

87. Gertner JM. Growth hormone actions on fat distribution and metabolism. Horm Res 1992; 38(suppl 2):41–43.

88. Bray GA. Calorigenic effect of human growth hormone in obesity. J Clin Endocrinol Metab 1969; 29:119–122.

89. Bray GA, Raben MS, Londono J, et al. Effects of triiodothyronine, growth hormone and anabolic steroids

on nitrogen excretion and oxygen consumption of obese patients. J Clin Endocrinol Metab 1971; 33:293–300.

90. Felig P, Marliss EB, Cahill GF Jr. Metabolic response to human growth hormone during prolonged starvation. J Clin Invest 1971; 50:411–421.

91. Bengtsson BA, Eden S, Lonn L, et al. Treatment of adults with growth hormone (GH) deficiency with recombinant human GH. J Clin Endocrinol Metab 1993; 76:309–317.

92. Brummer RJ, Lonn L, Kvist H, et al. Adipose tissue and muscle volume determination by computed tomography in acromegaly, before and 1 year after adenomectomy. Eur J Clin Invest 1993; 23:199–205.

93. Clemmons DR, Snyder DK, Williams R, et al. Growth hormone administration conserves lean body mass during dietary restriction in obese subjects. J Clin Endocrinol Metab 1987; 64:878–883.

94. Snyder DK, Clemmons DR, Underwood LE. Treatment of obese, diet-restricted subjects with growth hormone for 11 weeks: effects on anabolism, lipolysis, and body composition. J Clin Endocrinol Metab 1988; 67:54–61.

95. Snyder DK, Clemmons DR, Underwood LE. Dietary carbohydrate content determines responsiveness to growth hormone in energy-restricted humans. J Clin Endocrinol Metab 1989; 69:745–752.

96. Snyder DK, Underwood LE, Clemmons DR. Anabolic effects of growth hormone in obese diet-restricted subjects are dose dependent. Am J Clin Nutr 1990; 52:431–437.

97. Richelsen B, Pederson SB, Borglum JD, et al. Growth hormone treatment of obese women for 5 wk: effect on body composition and adipose tissue LPL activity. Am J Physiol 1994; 266:E211–E216.

98. Jorgensen JO, Pedersen SB, Borglum J, et al. Fuel metabolism, energy expenditure, and thyroid function in growth hormone-treated obese women: a double-blind placebo-controlled study. Metabolism 1994; 43:872–877.

99. Snyder DK, Underwood LE, Clemmons DR. Persistent lipolytic effect of exogenous growth hormone during caloric restriction. Am J Med 1995; 98:129–134.

100. Drent ML, Wever LD, Ader HJ, et al. Growth hormone administration in addition to a very low calorie diet and an exercise program in obese subjects. Eur J Endocrinol 1995; 132:565–572.

101. Johannsson G, Marin P, Lonn L, et al. Growth hormone treatment of abdominally obese men reduces abdominal fat mass, improves glucose and lipoprotein metabolism, and reduces diastolic blood pressure. J Clin Endocrinol Metab 1997; 82:727–734.

102. Karlsson C, Stenlof K, Johannsson G, et al. Effects of growth hormone treatment on the leptin system and on energy expenditure in abdominally obese men. Eur J Endocrinol 1998; 138:408–414.

103. Thompson JL, Butterfield GE, Gylfadottir UK, et al. Effects of human growth hormone, insulin-like growth factor I, and diet and exercise on body composition of obese postmenopausal women. J Clin Endocrinol Metab 1998; 83:1477–1484.

104. McAlpine LG, McAlpine CH, Waclawski ER, et al. A comparison of treatment with metformin and gliclazide in

patients with non-insulin-dependent diabetes. Eur J Clin Pharmacol 1988; 34:129–132.

105. Josephkutty S, Potter JM. Comparison of tolbutamide and metformin in elderly diabetic patients. Diabetes Med 1990; 7:510–514.

106. Campbell IW, Menzies DG, Chalmers J, et al. One year comparative trial of metformin and glipizide in type 2 diabetes mellitus. Diabet Metab 1994; 20:394–400.

107. Fontbonne A, Charles MA, Juhan-Vague I, et al. The effect of metformin on the metabolic abnormalities associated with upper-body fat distribution. BIGPRO Study Group. Diabetes Care 1996; 19:920–926.

108. Scheen AJ, Letiexhe MR, Lefebvre PJ. Short administration of metformin improves insulin sensitivity in android obese subjects with impaired glucose tolerance. Diabetes Med 1995; 12:985–989.

109. Lee A, Morley JE. Metformin decreases food consumption and induces weight loss in subjects with obesity with type II non-insulin-dependent diabetes. Obes Res 1998; 6:47–53.

110. Knowler WC, Barrett-Connor E, Fowler SE, et al. Reduction in the incidence of type 2 diabetes with lifestyle intervention or metformin. N Engl J Med 2002; 346: 393–403.

111. Lutjens A, Smit JL. Effect of biguanide treatment in obese children. Helv Paediatr Acta 1977; 31:473–480.

112. Sullivan AC, Triscari J, Hamilton JG, et al. Effect of (-)-hydroxycitrate upon the accumulation of lipid in the rat: II. Appetite. Lipids 1974; 9:129–134.

113. Hellerstein MK, Xie Y. The indirect pathway of hepatic glycogen synthesis and reduction of food intake by metabolic inhibitors. Life Sci 1993; 53:1833–1845.

114. Thom E. Hydroxycitrate in the treatment of obesity. Int J Obes Relat Metab Disord 1996; 20(suppl 4):75.

115. Heymsfield SB, Allison DB, Vasselli JR, et al. Garcinia cambogia (hydroxycitric acid) as a potential antiobesity agent: a randomized controlled trial. JAMA 1998; 280:1596–1600.

116. Lijesen GK, Theeuwen I, Assendelft WJ, et al. The effect of human chorionic gonadotropin (HCG) in the treatment of obesity by means of the Simeons therapy: a criteria-based meta-analysis. Br J Clin Pharmacol 1995; 40:237–243.

117. Greenway FL, Bray GA. Human chorionic gonadotropin (HCG) in the treatment of obesity: a critical assessment of the Simeons method. West J Med 1977; 127:461–463.

118. Carne S. The action of chorionic gonadotrophin in the obese. Lancet 1961; 2:1282–1284.

119. Craig LS, Ray RE, Waxler SH, et al. Chorionic gonadotropin in the treatment of obese women. Am J Clin Nutr 1963; 12:230–234.

120. Frank BW. The use of chorionic gonadotropin hormone in the treatment of obesity. A double-blind study. Am J Clin Nutr 1964; 14:133–136.

121. Lebon P. Treatment of overweight patients with chorionic gonadotropin: follow-up study. J Am Geriatr Soc 1966; 14: 116–125.

122. Asher WL, Harper HW. Effect of human chorionic gonadotrophin on weight loss, hunger and feeling of well-being. Am J Clin Nutr 1973; 26:211–218.

123. Stein MR, Julis RE, Peck CC, et al. Ineffectiveness of human chorionic gonadotropin in weight reduction: a double-blind study. Am J Clin Nutr 1976; 29:940–948.

124. Shetty KR, Kalkhoff RK. Human chorionic gonadotropin (HCG) treatment of obesity. Arch Intern Med 1977; 137:151–155.

125. Bosch B, Venter I, Stewart RI, et al. Human chorionic gonadotrophin and weight loss. A double-blind, placebo-controlled trial. S Afr Med J 1990; 77:185–189.

126. Young RL, Fuchs, RJ, Woltjen MJ. Chorionic gonadotropin in weight control. A double-blind crossover study. JAMA 1976; 236:2495–2497.

127. Miller R, Schneiderman LJ. A clinical study of the use of human chorionic gonadotropin in weight reduction. J Fam Pract 1977; 4:445–448.

128. Svec F, Porter JR. The actions of exogenous dehydroepiandrosterone in experimental animals and humans. Proc Soc Exp Biol Med 1998; 218:174–191.

129. Williams DP, Boyden TW, Pamenter RW, et al. Relationship of body fat percentage and fat distribution with dehydroepiandrosterone sulfate in premenopausal females. J Clin Endocrinol Metab 1993; 77:80–85.

130. Clore JN. Dehydroepiandrosterone and body fat. Obes Res 1995; 3(suppl 4):613S–616S.

131. Lardy H, Kneer N, Wei Y, et al. Ergosteroids II: biologically active metabolites and synthetic derivatives of dehydroepiandrosterone. Steroids 1998; 63:158–165.

132. Nestler JE, Barlascini CO, Clore JN, et al. Dehydroepiandrosterone reduces serum low density lipoprotein levels and body fat but does not alter insulin sensitivity in normal men. J Clin Endocrinol Metab 1998; 66:57–61.

133. Welle S, Jozefowicz R, Statt M. Failure of dehydroepiandrosterone to influence energy and protein metabolism in humans. J Clin Endocrinol Metab 1990; 71:1259–1264.

134. Usiskin KS, Butterworth S, Clore JN, et al. Lack of effect of dehydroepiandrosterone in obese men. Int J Obes 1990; 14:457–463.

135. Mortola JF, Yen SS. The effects of oral dehydroepiandrosterone on endocrine-metabolic parameters in postmenopausal women. J Clin Endocrinol Metab 1990; 71:696–704.

136. Villareal DT, Holloszy JO. Effect of DHEA on abdominal fat and insulin action in elderly women and men: a randomized controlled trial. JAMA 2004; 292(18):2243–2248.

137. Handelsman DJ. Testosterone and other androgens: physiology, pharmacology and therapeutic use. Endocrinology 1995; 3:2351–2361.

138. Evans DJ, Hoffmann RG, Kalkoff RK, et al. Relationship of androgenic activity to body fat topography, fat cell morphology, and metabolic aberrations in premenopausal women. J Clin Endocrinol Metab 1983; 57:304–310.

139. Seidell JC, Bjorntorp P, Sjostrom L, et al. Regional distribution of muscle and fat mass in men—new insight into the risk of abdominal obesity using computed tomography. Int J Obes 1989; 13:289–303.

140. Tchernof A, Labrie F, Belanger A, et al. Androstane-3-α, 17-β-diol glucuronide as a steroid correlate of visceral obesity in men. J Clin Endocrinol Metab 1997; 82:1528–1534.

141. Marin P, Holmang S, Jonsson L, et al. The effects of testosterone treatment on body composition and metabolism in middle-aged obese men. Int J Obes Relat Metab Disord 1992; 16:991–997.

142. Marin P, Holmang S, Gustafsson C, et al. Androgen treatment of abdominally obese men. Obes Res 1993; 1:245–251.

143. Marin P. Testosterone and regional fat distribution. Obes Res 1995; 3(suppl 4):609S–612S.

144. Lovejoy JC, Bray GA, Breeson CS, et al. Oral anabolic steroid treatment, but not parenteral androgen treatment, decreases abdominal fat in obese, older men. Int J Obes Relat Metab Disord 1995; 19:614–624.

145. Lovejoy JC, Bray GA, Bourgeois MO, et al. Exogenous androgens influence body composition and regional body fat distribution in obese postmenopausal women—a clinical research center study. J Clin Endocrinol Metab 1996; 81:2198–2203.

146. Drent ML, van der Veen EA. First clinical studies with orlistat: a short review. Obes Res 1995; 3:S623–S625.

20

Cannabinoid Receptor Antagonists as Potential Antiobesity Agents

GEORGE A. BRAY

Pennington Biomedical Research Center, Baton Rouge, Louisiana, U.S.A.

INTRODUCTION

At present, only two drugs, orlistat and sibutramine, are approved by the U.S. Food and Drug Administration for long-term use in the treatment of obesity, and four others are approved for short-term use. In contrast, there are a large number of very good drugs to treat hypertension and diabetes. Thus, the development of a new class of drugs, as exemplified by the cannabinoid receptor 1 antagonist, is very welcome. At the time of writing, one of these drugs, rimonabant, has been approved by the European Committee on Proprietary Medicinal Products (CPMP) for use in Europe and by several other countries. Although a good deal of basic and clinical data has been published on rimonabant, other cannabinoid receptor antagonists are known to be in clinical trial. Thus, this area is deserving of careful review.

MECHANISM OF ACTION

There are two cannabinoid receptors, CB-1 (470 amino acids in length) and CB-2 (360 amino acids in length). The CB-1 receptor includes almost all the amino acids that comprise the CB-2 receptor and additional amino acids at both the N-terminal and C-terminal ends. CB-1 receptors are distributed throughout the brain in the areas related to feeding as well as on fat cells, liver, pancreas, muscle, and gastrointestinal tract. The CB-2 receptors are primarily found on immune cells.

Marijuana and tetrahydrocannabinol, which is purified from this plant, stimulate the CB-1 receptor, resulting in an increase in the consumption of high-fat and high-sweetness foods. Fasting increases the levels of endocannabinoids.

Once the exogenous cannabinoids were identified, the search was on for endogenous cannabinoids or endocannabinoids. There are two primary endocannabinoids, anandamide and 2-arachidonoyl-glycerol. These products are both formed in the cell membrane from arachidonic acid. They are not stored in cellular vesicles, like many neurotransmitters, and thus their synthesis is stimulated "on demand." When released into the interneural cleft, they act retrogradely on the presynaptic cannabinoid receptor (CB-1), a seven-membrane-spanning G-coupled receptor. Activation of this receptor by endogenous or exogenous cannabinoid inhibits the release of γ-aminobutyric acid and thus removes an inhibitory influence of "satiety" signals, allowing the positive feedback for palatable food to drive eating. Blockade of the CB-1 receptors turns this system off and induces satiety. The brain content of the endogenous 2-arachidonoyl-glycerol is reduced in fed animals where satiation has occurred and is high in "hungry" animals who want to eat. As anticipated, these endogenous cannabinoids will stimulate food intake.

Table 1 RIO Pivotal Phase III Clinical Trials

Study name (reference)	Population	Number of subjects	Design
RIO-Europe (7)	Obese or overweight with/without comorbidities (except diabetes)	1507	2 yr with 4-wk run-in
RIO-North America (8)	Obese or overweight with/without comorbidities (except diabetes)	3405	1 + 1 yr Re-randomized; 4-wk run-in
RIO-Lipids (9)	Obese or overweight with untreated dyslipidemia (diabetes excluded)	1036	1 yr with 4-wk run-in
RIO-Diabetes (10)	Obese or overweight with type 2 diabetes	1045	1 yr with 4-wk run-in

Abbreviation: RIO, Rimonabant in Obesity.

The rewarding properties of cannabinoid agonists are mediated through the mesolimbic dopaminergic system. Rimonabant is a specific antagonist of the CB-1 receptor and inhibits sweet food intake in marmosets as well as palatable, high-fat food intake in rats but not in rats fed standard rat chow, which is not very palatable. In addition to being specific in inhibiting highly palatable food intake, pair-feeding experiments in diet-induced obese rats show that the rimonabant-treated animals lost 21% of their body weight compared with 14% in the pair-fed controls. This suggests, at least in rodents, that rimonabant increases energy expenditure in addition to reducing food intake. CB-1 receptor knockout mice are lean and resistant to diet-induced weight gain. CB-1 receptors are upregulated on adipocytes in diet-induced obese mice, and rimonabant increases adiponectin, a fat cell hormone associated with insulin sensitivity (1–4).

In human studies, rimonabant reduces the craving for food and the motivation to eat with either high-fat or low-fat meals (5). Rimonabant is orally absorbed and has a half-life of several days.

CLINICAL TRIALS

Short-Term Clinical Studies

A 16-week dose-ranging randomized clinical trial of rimonabant at doses of 5, 10, and 20 mg/day has been reported (6). During treatment, the placebo group lost 1.1 kg compared with 3.5 kg with the 5-mg dose, 3.9 kg with the 10-mg dose, and 4.4 kg with the 20-mg dose. On the basis of these data, the phase III program compared 5- and 20-mg/day doses of rimonabant with placebo.

Long-Term Clinical Studies

The results of four long-term phase III clinical trials with rimonabant for the treatment of overweight have been published. The set of trials are called Rimonabant in

Obesity, or RIO, with a specific title relating to the specific study site or topic. Some features of these trials are shown in Table 1.

The first trial published, called RIO-Europe, was reported in 2005 (7) and was intended to be conducted in Europe, but slow recruitment led to inclusion of 276 subjects from the United States. This was a two-year trial with one-year results reported in this paper. A total of 1057 patients with a body mass index (BMI) >30 kg/m^2 without comorbidities, or >27 kg/m^2 with hypertension or dyslipidemia, were stratified on whether they lost more or less than 2 kg during run-in and then were randomized in a ratio of 1:2:2 to receive placebo, rimonabant 5 mg/day, or rimonabant 20 mg/day. The energy content of the diet was calculated by subtracting 600 kcal/day from the energy requirements as estimated from the Harris-Benedict equation. The trial consisted of a four-week run-in period followed by 52 weeks of treatment. Of those who started, 61% (920) completed the first year. Weight loss was 2% in the placebo group and 8.5% in the 20-mg/day-rimonabant group. Baseline weight was between 98.5 kg (placebo group) and 102 kg (for the rimonabant 20-mg dose). During run-in there was a mean -1.9-kg weight loss. During the next 52 weeks, the participants in the placebo group who completed the trial lost an additional -2.3 kg, the low-dose rimonabant group lost -3.6 kg, and the high-dose group lost -8.6 kg. On an intent-to-treat (ITT) basis, these numbers were a weight loss of -1.8 kg for the placebo group, -3.4 kg for the 5-mg/day group, and -6.6 kg for the 20-mg/day group. Expressing the data as a responder analysis, the authors reported that 30.5% of the placebo group lost 5% or more, compared with 44.2% for the 5-mg/day and 67.4% for the 20-mg/day dose of rimonabant. When a weight loss of 10% or more was considered, the numbers were 12.4% for the placebo group, 15.3% for the 5-mg/day group, and 39% for the 20-mg/day dose of rimonabant. Waist circumference was also reduced by treatment. With the ITT analysis, waist declined 2.4 cm in the placebo group, 3.9 cm in the 5-mg/day group, and 6.5 cm with the 20-mg/day dose, i.e., almost

1 cm for each kilogram of weight loss. Triglycerides were reduced by 6.8% in the 20-mg/day group compared with a rise of 8.3% in the placebo group. High-density lipoprotein (HDL) cholesterol was improved. It increased by 22.3% compared with 13.4% in the placebo group. These changes in metabolic parameters were reflected in a change in the prevalence of the metabolic syndrome. Among the completers there was a 33.9% reduction in the prevalence of the metabolic syndrome, compared with 34.8% in the 5-mg/day-dose group and 64.8% in the rimonabant 20-mg/day-dose group. In the 20-mg/day group the low-density lipoprotein (LDL) particle size increased, adiponectin increased, glucose decreased, insulin decreased, C-reactive protein decreased, and the metabolic syndrome prevalence was cut in half. There was no significant change in blood pressure or pulse between groups.

The two-year randomized, double-blind, placebo-controlled study called RIO-North America (8) started with 3045 overweight subjects with a BMI >30 kg/m^2 or with a BMI >27 kg/m^2 with treated or untreated hypertension or dyslipidemia but without diabetes (Table 1). They were randomized to placebo, 5-mg rimonabant, or 20-mg rimonabant. Participants were instructed in a 600-kcal/day-deficit diet. Randomization and baseline occurred after a four-week run-in period when subjects had lost an average of -1.9 kg. They were thus stratified by whether they lost more or less than 2 kg during run-in. At one year, half of the patients in each drug group were switched to placebo, on the basis of their initial randomization. The trial was conducted at 64 American and eight Canadian centers. At one year, completion rates were 51% to 55% for the three arms. Weight loss was evident in all groups. During the first year, weight loss was -2.8 kg in the placebo group and -8.6 kg in the 20-mg rimonabant group. Weight loss declined steadily until week 36, after which it reached a plateau. For the second year, those individuals who were switched from rimonabant to placebo regained weight at almost the mirror image of the rate at which they lost it during the first year. At the end of the study, they were still slightly lighter, but no different from the group treated with placebo for the full two years. In the group receiving 20 mg/day, waist circumference decreased and the percentage with the metabolic syndrome decreased from 34.8% at baseline to 21.2% at trial end of the study compared with the small reduction from 31.7% to 29.2% in the placebo-treated group. HDL-cholesterol rose more in the rimonabant group treated with 20 mg/day than in the placebo group, and triglycerides fell more in the participants receiving the higher dose of rimonabant. Patients with depression were not included in this study. Adverse events leading to discontinuation of the study were higher in the rimonabant-treated than in the placebo-treated participants. This said, the profile and effectiveness of this agent appear very promising for treatment of obesity and the physical and laboratory findings that make up the metabolic syndrome.

Studies in Special Populations

Dyslipidemia

The study in dyslipidemic patients is called the RIO-Lipids study (Table 1) (9). This was a 12-month, randomized, double-blind, placebo-controlled trial of rimonabant at two doses versus placebo in overweight subjects eating a 600-kcal/day-deficit diet. It was conducted at 67 sites in eight countries. As a lipids trial, the inclusion criteria were a BMI of 27 to 40 kg/m^2, elevated fasting triglycerides (150–700 mg/dL), ratio of cholesterol to HDL-cholesterol >5 in men and >4.5 in women, and no more than 5 kg variation in body weight in the previous three months. Subjects were stratified at run-in by triglycerides below or above 400 mg/dL and at the end of run-in by a weight loss of more or less than 2 kg. Randomization was on a 1:1:1 basis of placebo:5-mg/day rimonabant:20-mg/day rimonabant. Following the end of the four-week run-in, participants were randomized and treated for 12 months—the dropout rate was about 40% by the end of 12 months. Weight losses in this trial were almost identical to those in the RIO-Europe trial. After an approximate 2-kg weight loss during run-in, the placebo-treated patients in the completers group lost an additional -2.3 kg, compared with -4.2 kg in the 5-mg/day-dose group and -8.8 kg in the 20-mg/day-dose group of rimonabant. Waist circumference also showed a dose-dependent reduction by 3.4 cm in the placebo group, 4.9 cm in the 5-mg/day-dose group, and 9.1 cm in the 20-mg/day-dose group.

A number of other metabolic parameters also responded to the drug or weight loss. They included a decrease in triglycerides, an increase in HDL-cholesterol, a decrease in peak size of LDL-cholesterol particles, an increase in adiponectin, a decline in fasting insulin, a fall in leptin, and a decrease in C-reactive protein. Several liver enzymes fell with treatment, suggesting improvement in nonalcoholic steatosis. Blood pressure decreased significantly in RIO-Lipids in contrast with RIO-Europe. As might be expected from these metabolic changes, the prevalence of the metabolic syndrome in those who met the ATP-III criteria at randomization fell to 25.8% in the 20-mg/day group, to 40% in the 5-mg/day group, and to 41% in the placebo group.

Diabetic Patients

The final large-scale study, called RIO-Diabetes (10), randomized 1045 diabetic subjects in 151 centers from 11 countries to treatment for one year with placebo or rimonabant 5 or 20 mg/day (Table 1). These diabetic patients could be treated with diet, metformin, or

Table 2 Comparison of Effects Between Placebo and Rimonabant 20 mg/day

Outcome	Number of studies	Number of participants	Effect size
Weight change (kg)	4	4105	−4.64 (−4.99, −4.28)
Waist circumference change (cm)	4	4105	−3.84 (−4.26, −3.42)
Systolic blood pressure change (mmHg)	3	2279	−1.57 (−2.59, −0.55)
Diastolic blood pressure change (mmHg)	3	2279	−1.16 (−1.86, −0.47)
Triglycerides change (mg/dL)	4	4105	−19.8 (−24.1, −15.6)
HDL-cholesterol change (mg/dL)	4	4105	3.51 (2.99, 4.04)
Adverse effects (general)	3	3417	1.05 (1.01, 1.08)
Adverse effects (serious)	4	4105	1.37 (1.04, −1.80)

Source: Adapted from Ref. 12.

sulfonylurea drugs. Weight loss in the placebo group was −1.4 kg, compared with −2.3 kg in the 5-mg/day group and −5.3 kg in the 20-mg/day group. Triglycerides and blood pressure declined more in the subjects treated with 20 mg/day of rimonabant. During treatment with 20 mg/day of rimonabant, 55.9% of completers lost >5% of body weight, compared with 19.5% in the placebo-treated group.

A second trial in drug-naive diabetics has been reported in abstract form (11). Called the SERENADE trial (Study Evaluating Rimonabant Efficacy in Drug-NAive DiabEtic Patients), it randomized 131 diabetics to placebo and 130 diabetics to 20 mg/day of rimonabant. Body weight decreased −2.7 kg in the placebo group versus −6.7 kg in the rimonabant group and the waist circumference showed a nearly 1-cm change for each 1 kg of weight loss, giving the rimonabant group a significant greater decrease in waist circumference. Hemoglobin A1C also decreased significantly (−0.3% in placebo vs. −0.8% in rimonabant group). HDL-cholesterol increased slightly in the placebo group (3.2 mg/dL) but more in the rimonabant group (10.1 mg/dL). Triglycerides fell by −4.4 in the placebo group and −16.3 in the rimonabant group. Systolic blood pressure did not show a significant difference in response between groups, but there was a small decrease in both groups.

Meta-analysis and Systematic Reviews

There have been two reviews of rimonabant as a clinical agent. The first is a Cochrane Data Base analysis by

Curioni and Andre (Table 2) (12). Table 2 shows the data from the meta-analysis by Curioni and Andre comparing the placebo and 20-mg/day dose. It is clear that there is a significant effect of rimonabant on body weight and waist circumference, favoring the drug. In the analysis in Table 2, the weighted mean weight loss was −4.64 kg. However, there was significant heterogeneity between studies. Eliminating the RIO-Diabetes studies reduced this heterogeneity, and in the other three studies, the mean weighted effect size was −4.9 kg, a better reflection of drug action on the general obese population. There are also significant positive effects on triglycerides and HDL-cholesterol, but not on blood pressure. When the general and serious adverse events were examined, there was a significant effect favoring the placebo.

The results of the second analysis by Gadde and Allison (6) are summarized in Table 3. Treatment with rimonabant showed improvements in many of the comorbidities associated with the improvement in weight in the treated patients. After one year of treatment, there was improvement in weight, waist circumference, triglycerides, and HDL-cholesterol.

SAFETY CONSIDERATIONS

Because this drug "dampens" the feedback systems for pleasurable responses, there is concern about its behavioral effects. Table 4 summarizes the side effects. Discontinuation for adverse events was similar, but the

Table 3 Effect of Rimonabant on Various Outcomes After One Year of Treatment

Variable	RIO-Europe	RIO-NA	RIO-Lipids	RIO-Diabetes
Weight loss (kg)	−4.7	−4.7	−5.4	−3.9
Change in waist circumference (cm)	−4.2	−3.6	−4.7	−3.3
Systolic blood pressure (mmHg)	−1.2	−0.2	−1.7	−2.3
Triglycerides (percent change)	−15.1	−13.2	−12.4	−16.4
HDL-cholesterol (percent change)	+8.9	+7.2	+8.1	+8.4

Abbreviations: RIO, Rimonabant in Obesity; RIO-NA, Rimonabant in Obesity–North America; HDL, high-density lipoprotein.
Source: Adapted from Ref. 6.

Table 4 Side Effects Observed in the Placebo and Rimonabant Groups

	Placebo N = 2474 (%)	Rimonabant 20 mg N = 2742 (%)
Any event	81.4	86.3
Gastrointestinal disorders		
Nausea	4.7	13.6
Diarrhea	5.8	7.7
Vomiting	2.3	4.7
Nervous system disorders		
Dizziness	4.1	7.3
Psychiatric disorders		
Anxiety	2.1	5.9
Insomnia	3.4	5.8
Mood alterations with depressive symptoms	2.8	4.7
Depressive disorders	1.7	3.9
Others		
Influenza	9.1	10.3
Asthenia/fatigue	4.4	6.1
Gastroenteritis	3.5	4.5
Contusion	1.1	3.1
Hot flush	0.8	2

reasons were different. Among placebo-treated patients, it was for lack of weight loss. With the higher dose of rimonabant (20 mg/day), depressed mood disorders, nausea, vomiting, diarrhea, headache, dizziness, and anxiety were all more common in the rimonabant 20-mg/day-dose group than in the placebo group. The scores on the Hospital Anxiety and Depression Scale were not significantly different between treatment groups.

Slightly more patients withdrew for drug-related adverse events in the 5-mg/day-dose group and even more with the 20-mg/day dose relative to placebo. The major reasons for withdrawal were psychiatric, nervous system, and gastrointestinal track symptoms. The complaints that occurred with more than 5% frequency in the drug-treated patients included upper respiratory tract infection, nasopharyngitis, nausea, influenza, diarrhea, arthralgia, anxiety, insomnia, viral gastroenteritis, dizziness, depressed mood, and fatigue in the 20-mg/day-dose group (8).

STATUS OF RIMONABANT

Rimonabant was submitted in June 2005 for review by the CPMP, the medication approval agency for the European Union. It was approved by the CPMP and eventually in 37 countries. It is already marketed in up to 18 of these countries.

In the United States, the application for approval received an approvable letter and on June 13, 2007, the U.S. Food and Drug Administration Endocrinologic and Metabolic Drugs Advisory Committee met to review the corporate and agency presentations. Sanofi-Aventis presented a plan to minimize use of the drug by potentially high-risk individuals, since rimonabant may not be appropriate for people with a history of depression and/or suicidal thoughts, or who have been diagnosed with depression or are taking antidepressant medication, and proposed a novel "risk-management action plan" for physicians. The Advisory Committee, however, did not recommend approval of rimonabant to the U.S. Food and Drug Administration for use in obese and overweight patients with associated risk factors because of continuing concerns about increased risk of suicidality related events, psychiatric events, neurologic events, and seizures. The Advisory Committee felt that there were not enough safety data and that the Company had failed to demonstrate that the drug's benefits outweighed its risks. Following this decision, Sanofi-Aventis announced on June 29, 2007, that it is withdrawing its U.S. marketing application for rimonabant and that it plans to resubmit at a future date.

A recent paper has performed a meta-analysis of the safety of rimonabant using the published clinical trials (13). The patients treated with rimonabant lost significantly greater (4.7 kg) weight after one year. But rimonabant caused significantly more side effects than placebo. There were 1.4 times as many serious adverse events, and patients taking rimonabant were 2.5 times as likely to discontinue treatment because of depressive mood disorders and three times more likely to discontinue because of anxiety than the placebo groups. It is thus clear that rimonabant at 20 mg/day increases the risk of psychiatric adverse events.

OTHER CANNABINOID ANTAGONISTS

Several other cannabinoid antagonists or inverse agonists are also under investigation, indicating the potential interest in this pharmacologic mechanism. These include Taranabant, which is being developed by Merck and Company in phase III trials. Abstracts about this drug indicate that it reduces food intake and increases energy expenditure. Pfizer & Company has CP 945,598 in phase III trials, and two other modulators of this receptor are in phase II trials.

CONCLUSION

The cannabinoid antagonists present an interesting approach to modulation of food intake. This physiological promise has been clouded by the concern about side effects of rimonabant presented to the Food and Drug Administration. The principal question for this new class of drugs is whether these effects are the response to the receptors that are being inhibited or whether these effects can be significantly attenuated by molecular modifications in the receptor antagonists. Time will tell.

REFERENCES

1. Bensaid M, Gary-Bobo M, Esclangon A, et al. The cannabinoid CB1 receptor antagonist SR141716 increases Acrp30 mRNA expression in adipose tissue of obese fa/fa rats and in cultured adipocyte cells. Mol Pharmacol 2003; 63(4):908–914.
2. Pagotto U, Marsicano G, Cota D, et al. The emerging role of the endocannabinoid system in endocrine regulation and energy balance. Endocr Rev 2006; 27(1):73–100.
3. Kirkham TC. Endocannabinoids in the regulation of appetite and body weight. Behav Pharmacol 2005; 16(5–6):297–313.
4. Juan-Picó P, Fuentes E, Bermúdez-Silva FJ, et al. Cannabinoid receptors regulate Ca(2+) signals and insulin secretion in pancreatic beta-cell. Cell Calcium 2006; 39(2):155–162.
5. Blundell JE, Jebb SA, Stubbs RJ, et al. Effect of rimonabant on energy intake motivation to eat and body weight with or without hypocaloric diet: the REBA study. Obes Rev 2006; 7(suppl 2):104.
6. Gadde KM, Allison D. Cannabinoid Receptor-1 antagonist, rimonabant, for management of obesity and related risks. Circulation 2006; 114(9):974–984.
7. Van Gaal, LF, Rissanen AM, Scheen AJ, et al. Effects of the cannabinoid-1 receptor blocker rimonabant on weight reduction and cardiovascular risk factors in overweight patients: 1-year experience from the RIO-Europe study. Lancet 2005; 365(9468):1389–1397.
8. Pi-Sunyer FX, Aronne LJ, Heshmati HM, et al. Effect of rimonabant, a cannabinoid-1 receptor blocker, on weight and cardiometabolic risk factors in overweight or obese patients: RIO-North America: a randomized controlled trial. JAMA 2006; 295(7):761–775.
9. Despres JP, Golay A, Sjostrom L, et al. Effects of rimonabant on metabolic risk factors in overweight patients with dyslipidemia. N Engl J Med 2005; 353(20):2121–2134.
10. Scheen AJ, Finer N, Hollander P, et al., and RIO-Diabetes Study Group. Efficacy and tolerability of rimonabant in overweight or obese patients with type 2 diabetes: a randomized controlled study. Lancet 2006; 368:1660–1672.
11. Iranmanesh A, Rosenstock J, Hollander P. Presented at the 19th World Diabetes Congress, December 3–7, 2006, Cape Town, South Africa (abstr 637b).
12. Curioni C, Andre C. Rimonabant for overweight or obesity. Cochrane Database Syst Rev 2006; 18(4):CD006162.
13. Christensen R, Kristensen PK, Bartels EM, et al. Efficacy and safety of the weight-loss drug rimonabant: a meta-analysis of randomized trials. Lancet 2007; 370:1706–1713.

21

Integrated Neurohormonal Approach to the Treatment of Obesity: The Amylin Agonist Pramlintide and Its Interactions with Leptin and PYY Signaling Pathways

JONATHAN D. ROTH, CHRISTINE MACK, and DAVID G. PARKES
In Vivo Pharmacology, Amylin Pharmaceuticals, Inc., San Diego, California, U.S.A.

NICOLE C. KESTY
Medical Affairs, Amylin Pharmaceuticals, Inc., San Diego, California, U.S.A.

CHRISTIAN WEYER
Clinical Research, Amylin Pharmaceuticals, Inc., San Diego, California, U.S.A.

INTRODUCTION

Over the past decade, advances in endocrine and neurosciences research have revolutionized our understanding of the biological basis underlying the complex regulation of glucose and energy homeostasis. These advances include not only the discovery and characterization of numerous novel hormones but also a much deeper understanding of how various peripheral endocrine signals are integrated within the central nervous system (CNS) to regulate energy homeostasis. It is widely recognized that hormonal signals secreted from pancreatic islets [e.g., glucagon, insulin, amylin, and pancreatic polypeptide (PP)], the gut [e.g., glucagon-like peptide-1 (GLP-1), glucose-dependent insulinotropic polypeptide, cholecystokinin (CCK), and peptide YY (PYY)], and white adipose tissue (e.g., leptin and adiponectin) collectively play a pivotal role in the physiological regulation of glucose metabolism, food intake, and body weight (1).

Scientific advances in our understanding of the complex, multihormonal regulation of energy homeostasis and body weight have yet to translate into successful peptide hormone therapeutics approved for the treatment of obesity. Most antiobesity compounds previously approved or advanced to late-stage clinical development are small-molecule agents, the majority of which were discovered by serendipity (most were originally developed for various neuropsychiatric indications) (2). Over the past five decades, centrally acting small-molecule monotherapies for obesity have repeatedly been hampered not only by modest efficacy but also by recurring safety issues that have left lingering concerns among physicians and patients regarding the use of weight loss medications (2,3). Increased efficacy beyond monotherapy was achieved by coadministration of fenfluramine and phentermine, a widely used combination in the 1990s that clearly demonstrated the potential of combinatorial treatment (4,5). However, the detection of treatment-related cardiac valvulopathy, leading to the withdrawal of fenfluramine (and dexfenfluramine), has increased scrutiny over the safety of small-molecule anorectics, whether used alone or in combination (3,6). Due to the potentially increased efficacy of combinatorial therapies, other small-molecule combinations are now being tested (7–9).

There is a pressing need for alternative weight loss products with improved efficacy and safety profiles. Peptide hormone therapeutics can be regarded as one promising approach. This is not only because of their ability to enhance, activate, and integrate intact, naturally occurring, and feeding-related signaling pathways but also because of their reduced potential for inducing idiosyncratic toxicities.

Peripheral circulating neurohormones involved in body weight regulation include orexigenic peptides (ghrelin) and a vast array of anorexigenic peptides, which are commonly classified into long-term adiposity and short-term satiety signals (10,11).

Adiposity signals, such as leptin and insulin, are thought to be long-term (tonic) signals that act primarily on the hypothalamus (arcuate nucleus) and inform the central neurocircuitry of changes in the body's energy reserves (i.e., the amount of body fat stored) (12,13). Consistent with this hypothesis, fasting plasma concentrations of these hormones are proportionate to the degree of adiposity and change gradually in response to weight gain or weight loss (12,13). The predominant centrally mediated response to a diet-induced fall in circulating leptin levels is a multifaceted counterregulatory response (comprised of changes in appetite, metabolic rate, fuel efficiency, and fat oxidation), aimed at defending the initial body weight (14,15).

Satiety signals, such as amylin, PYY_{3-36}, CCK, and GLP-1, are thought to be short-term (episodic) signals that act primarily on the hindbrain (area postrema and nucleus tractus solitarii) to convey information on the amount of food ingested (1,16). To fulfill this physiological role, plasma concentrations of these hormones increase acutely with each meal, in proportion to meal size (1,16). The predominant centrally mediated response to an acute, meal-related rise in short-term satiety signals is thought to be meal termination (satiation) and/or subsequent suppression of hunger and food intake during the intermeal period (satiety) (17,18).

While the aforementioned model of long-term adiposity and short-term satiety signals provides a basic framework for the neurohormonal regulation of food intake and body weight, it has become increasingly clear that the homeostatic regulation is in fact more complex. For instance, there is growing evidence that leptin exerts important extrahypothalamic effects, acting directly or indirectly on the hindbrain to amplify the effect of short-term satiety signals (19). Hormones, such as amylin, whose effect on appetite was previously attributed solely to direct satiety signaling, are in addition emerging as regulators of hypothalamic and hindbrain circuits to enhance, respectively, the action of leptin and other satiety signals, such as PYY_{3-36} or CCK

(20–23). Hence, the antiobesity effects of a given neurohormone may be multifaceted, resulting partly from a direct effect to reduce food intake and partly from an augmentation of other neurohormonal signals.

On the basis of this integrated neurohormonal regulation of food intake and body weight, several promising approaches to the development of peptide hormone therapeutics for obesity exist.

First, a single peptide hormone therapeutic (monotherapy) could be developed, such as a pharmaceutically optimized analog of the naturally occurring hormone. Although this approach has not been successful with some hormone classes (e.g., CCK, leptin), it may be quite promising for others. For example, a peptide hormone therapeutic might have therapeutic utility as a monotherapy for obesity if it were to enhance the signaling of other endogenous neurohormones in the obese state, which in turn could strengthen the overall appetite control system. In this chapter, we illustrate this monotherapy approach by reviewing preclinical and clinical studies with the amylin analog pramlintide, which is currently approved as an adjunctive treatment to insulin for patients with type 2 or type 1 diabetes and is in late-stage development as a potential treatment for obesity.

Secondly, one might contemplate the development of a combination of peptide hormone therapeutics, such as a combination of a long-term adiposity and a short-term satiety signal. Such an integrated neurohormonal therapeutic regimen might lead to increased weight loss by harnessing naturally occurring synergies and by preventing or minimizing weight loss counterregulation. This combinatorial approach is consistent with the concept that simultaneous changes in the secretion of multiple hormones may be an important mechanism contributing to the marked weight loss seen after Roux-en-Y gastric bypass surgery (24,25). In the second part of this chapter, we review nonclinical studies demonstrating how amylin agonism interacts with both PYY_{3-36} and leptin to produce marked, additive/synergistic weight loss in diet-induced obese (DIO) rodents.

AMYLIN, PYY_{3-36}, AND LEPTIN: BASIC PHYSIOLOGY

Peripheral Secretory Profiles

The secretion of peripheral signals derived from pancreatic β-cells, gastrointestinal L cells, and white adipocytes (amylin, PYY, and leptin, respectively) differs with respect to 24-hour diurnal profiles (Fig. 1) as well as with respect to the key determinants of secretion.

Amylin

Secretion

Amylin is a 37 amino acid peptide hormone cosecreted with insulin by pancreatic β cells (26,27). Amylin was

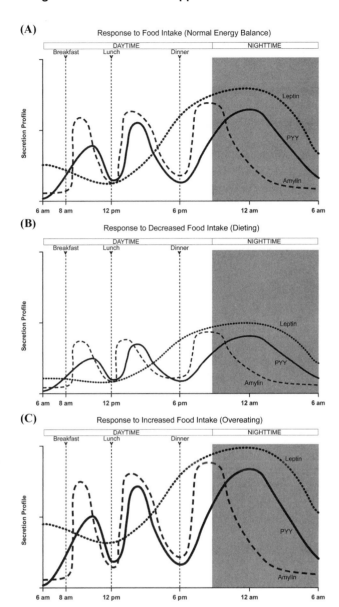

Figure 1 Secretion of amylin, PYY, and leptin. Schematic representing approximate 24-hour secretion profiles (6 AM to 6 AM) of amylin, PYY, and leptin under normal conditions (**A**), periods of reduced food intake (**B**), and periods of increased food intake (**C**). In lean healthy individuals the peak plasma response is approximately 20 pM for amylin (35), 24 pM for PYY (40), and 12 ng/mL for leptin (49,51,57). Arrows represent timing of meals (breakfast, lunch, and dinner). *Abbreviation*: PYY, peptide YY.

first isolated, purified, and chemically characterized in 1987 from amyloid deposits in the islets of Langerhans from patients with type 2 diabetes (28). The structure of amylin, which is highly preserved across mammalian species, has some similarities to calcitonin gene-related peptide, calcitonins, and adrenomedullin (29,30). Amylin is most widely expressed in pancreatic β cells (28,31), where the peptide is colocalized with insulin in the same

secretory granules (32). Consequently, the secretion of amylin is anatomically linked to insulin secretion, and the diurnal profiles of amylin and insulin plasma concentrations are almost superimposable (33,34).

Secretory profile

As pancreatic β cells are uniquely equipped to sense even small rises in circulating nutrients, most notably glucose, plasma amylin concentrations rise rapidly and severalfold in response to meals (Fig. 1A) (33,35). As is the case with insulin, plasma amylin concentrations peak approximately 30 minutes after a meal and typically return to baseline levels between meals after approximately two hours (33,35). This secretory profile is consistent with a potential role of amylin in mediating meal-related satiation.

Determinants of secretion

Fasting plasma amylin concentrations increase in response to weight gain, and like insulin, are elevated in most individuals with obesity and insulin resistance (33,35,36). Postprandial amylin secretion is proportionate to meal size. Hence, amylin secretion is augmented in response to large meals (e.g., overeating), while diminished in response to small meals (e.g., dieting) (Fig. 1B, C).

Peptide YY$_{3\text{-}36}$

Secretion

PYY, in addition to neuropeptide Y (NPY) and PP, is a member of the PP family of peptides. PYY is primarily expressed in and secreted by gastrointestinal L cells in the distal ileum, colon, and cecum (37). The same L cells also express proglucagon, the precursor of GLP-1, GLP-2, and oxyntomodulin, which are other gastrointestinal hormones secreted in response to meals. Following secretion, full length PYY (PYY$_{1\text{-}36}$) is proteolytically cleaved by dipeptidyl peptidase-IV to PYY$_{3\text{-}36}$, a predominant circulating form of PYY shown to possess anorexigenic activity (38–41).

Secretory profile

Secretion of PYY in response to meals is biphasic and dependent on meal size and macronutrient content (Fig. 1A) (37). Early secretion appears to be primarily mediated by the vagus nerve, while late secretion is thought to result from direct contact of ingested nutrients with the luminal side of L cells in the intestine (42). Plasma total PYY levels increase within 15 minutes postprandially, peak at approximately 90 to 120 minutes, and remain elevated for up to five hours depending on meal size and composition (Fig. 1) (37). This secretory profile is consistent with a potential role of PYY in mediating satiety (i.e., the suppression of hunger during intermeal intervals).

Determinants of secretion

Although some authors have reported that fasting plasma total PYY concentrations are reduced in obese individuals (40,43), this finding remains controversial. It seems clear, however, that fasting PYY concentrations do not increase with increasing body mass index (BMI), in contrast to amylin and leptin. Similar to amylin, postprandial PYY responses are proportionate to meal size (Fig. 1B, C). Dietary fat is the strongest nutritive stimulus for PYY secretion (37,44).

Leptin

Secretion

Leptin is a cytokine encoded by the *obese* (*ob*) gene that was identified through genetic analysis of profoundly obese (*ob/ob*) mice (45). Leptin is predominantly expressed and secreted by adipocytes, particularly white adipose tissue (46), with small amounts secreted also by the stomach (47). The soluble leptin receptor isoform, which lacks the intracellular and transmembrane domains, serves as the key binding protein for plasma leptin and acts to prolong the hormone's circulating half-life (48). Enlarged hypertrophic adipocytes, as observed after periods of excess food intake and weight gain, secrete significantly more leptin than do small hypotrophic adipocytes, the latter being characteristic of marked weight loss, such as that following bariatric surgery (49,50).

Secretory profile

Leptin secretion follows a diurnal rhythm, with relatively low levels during daytime, followed by a nocturnal rise (Fig. 1A) (51). Although the mechanistic basis and physiological significance of this pattern is still not fully understood, some authors have suggested that the nocturnal rise in leptinemia is a delayed response to the amount of food consumed during the preceding day (52–55). Some studies have also indicated that leptin concentrations may increase postprandially, albeit to a much lesser extent than with amylin or PYY (56,57). Overall, the diurnal secretory profile is consistent with a potential role of leptin in integrating cumulative food intake over the course of the day, thereby signaling short-term episodes of overeating or undereating to the CNS.

Determinants of secretion

In addition to the day-to-day changes in leptinemia resulting from short-term energy excess or deficits that are dissociated from fat mass, leptin levels also change in proportion to long-term changes in energy stores, with a gradual lasting increase in response to weight gain and a fall in response to weight loss (Fig. 1B, C) (58). Across the population, fasting leptin levels increase in proportion to body size (BMI, fat mass, adiposity). For any given BMI, females have higher plasma leptin concentrations compared with males, even after accounting for differences in body fat (59–61). Other factors such as cytokines and other hormones, including insulin, cortisol, and sex steroids, have also been implicated as possible determinants of leptin secretion (52,56,59,60,62).

Overall, the aforementioned secretory pattern is consistent with a role for leptin as a long-term adiposity signal, where rising levels signal excess fat storage and falling levels signal diminishing fat stores, the latter teleologically serving as an early warning signal of starvation.

The relevance of leptinemia as a predictor of leptin responsiveness is complex and still not fully understood. On one hand, it is well established that complete leptin deficiency due to leptin gene defect (*ob/ob* genotype) results in a rare phenotype of severe hyperphagia and obesity that is profoundly improved by administration of exogenous leptin (63). On the other hand, the vast majority of obese individuals are not leptin deficient and show little if any weight loss following treatment with exogenous leptin or leptin agonists (64,65). Although this suggests that diet-induced obesity is generally associated with reduced leptin responsiveness, the degree of leptinemia does not appear to be a reliable marker of the degree of leptin resistance (66).

Integrated Neurohormonal Signaling of Amylin, PYY$_{3-36}$, and Leptin

The aforementioned peripheral neurohormones interact within the CNS via signaling between the main hindbrain, midbrain, and forebrain regions involved in the regulation of food intake and body weight (Fig. 2).

The CNS regulates and maintains long-term energy balance by receiving, integrating, and responding to feedback from numerous peripheral signals. This includes balancing recent nutritional state signals [e.g., relating the form of absorbed nutrients (fat, carbohydrates, protein)], neuronal signals (e.g., from vagal afferents), and signals from several neurohormones secreted from the endocrine pancreas, the gut, and adipose tissue.

The organization of these homeostatic neuroregulatory systems is hierarchical (67). Hindbrain structures (nucleus of the solitary tract, area postrema) and hypothalamic nuclei (arcuate, paraventricular, ventromedial, and lateral hypothalamus) receive and monitor satiety and adiposity signals (vagal, neurohormonal, and nutritive), representing the neuroanatomical process for the homeostatic control of food intake (Fig. 2). Neuronal projections between the hindbrain and hypothalamus are bidirectional, providing a neuroanatomical basis for interaction between the

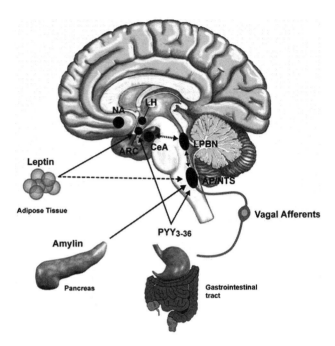

Figure 2 Neurobiology of amylin, PYY, and leptin. Schematic representing hormone-mediated neuronal activation in the CNS. Model based on animal studies. Amylin's effects on food intake, body weight, and gastric emptying are mediated through binding of amylin to the AP. Peripherally administered amylin stimulates c-Fos in the AP, NTS, and CeA. Acute and sustained amylin administration alters mRNA expression for hypothalamic peptides. The physiological role of the dense amylin-binding sites in the NA remains to be elucidated. The anorexigenic effects of PYY_{3-36} appear mediated through NPY receptors in the ARC. Although the physiological role is unclear, PYY_{3-36} also binds to receptors in the AP. Leptin receptors are expressed in the ARC, NA, and AP, representing possible points of convergence between amylin, PYY-36, and leptin signaling. *Abbreviations*: PYY, peptide YY; CNS, central nervous system; NA, nucleus accumbens; ARC, arcuate nucleus of hypothalamus; LH, lateral hypothalamus; CeA, central nucleus of the amygdala; LPBN, lateral parabrachial nucleus; NTS, nucleus tractus solitarii; AP, area postrema.

CNS and peripheral hormones acting as long-term adiposity and short-term satiety signals. In addition, cortico-limbic structures (sensory and orbitofrontal cortex, hippocampus, amygdala, and nucleus accumbens) mediate powerful emotive aspects of feeding, contributing to the hedonic control of food intake. Collectively, this distributed neural network controls a coordinated set of autonomic and neuroendocrine outputs affecting ingestive behavior, metabolic rate, and nutrient partitioning.

In the following section, we briefly review the neurobiology of amylin, PYY_{3-36}, and leptin, including possible points of convergence in the signaling pathways of these neurohormonal signals.

Amylin

A major binding site for amylin is the area postrema, a circumventricular organ that lacks a blood-brain barrier, which is thus exposed to acute and tonic changes of a multitude of circulating nutrients and hormones (Fig. 2). Within the area postrema, amylin binds to specific amylin receptors that emerge from the dimerization of the calcitonin receptor with certain receptor activity modifying proteins (RAMP1, RAMP2, and RAMP3) (68–71). Peripherally administered amylin stimulates neuronal activation in area postrema neurons that coexpress calcitonin receptor and RAMP3 (72).

The area postrema serves an important role in the reception and integration of peripheral (humoral and vagal afferent) satiety signals (1,18,73). Several lines of evidence suggest that the area postrema plays a primary role in mediating the anorexigenic effect of amylin. First, area postrema lesions completely abolish the anorexigenic effect of peripherally administered amylin (74). Secondly, administration of low doses of amylin directly into the third ventricle potently reduces food intake (75,76). Finally, the anorexigenic effect of peripheral amylin is fully preserved after bilateral vagotomy, which abrogates the effects of amylin on gastrointestinal motility (77). Hence, amylin's effect on gastric emptying is not required to achieve a reduction in food intake.

c-Fos, a marker of neural activation, has been used to map amylin-activated brain regions rostral/upstream to the hindbrain (area postrema). Peripheral administration of amylin was found to activate the area postrema/nucleus tractus solitarii, the lateral parabrachial nucleus, and the central nucleus of the amygdala (Fig. 2) (78,79). Structures within this circuit play a key role in the integration of gustatory and visceral information and share rich bidirectional projections with hypothalamic nuclei (80). Although it remains unclear whether amylin has direct effects on hypothalamic neurons, amylin administration has clearly been shown to modulate hypothalamic activity in a manner similar to that seen after ingestion of food. Specifically, neuronal activation in the lateral hypothalamus induced by food deprivation was reversible either by refeeding the animal or by peripheral administration of amylin to fasted animals (81). Consistent with these findings, a single injection of amylin downregulated lateral hypothalamic mRNA levels of the food intake-stimulating peptidergic neurotransmitter orexin (82).

Rich amylin binding has also been demonstrated in the nucleus accumbens, a key brain region mediating food reward (83) (Fig. 2). Because the nucleus accumbens lies within the blood-brain barrier, it is unlikely that circulating amylin accesses these receptors. The physiological significance of these amylin-binding sites, as well as the source of their cognate ligand, remains to be established. It is conceivable however that amylin signaling may influence the hedonic response to food. Of interest in this regard are findings from food choice experiments, which showed that decreased food choice experiments, which showed decreased preference for highly palatable (high-fat and/or sucrose) foods in amylin-treated rats (84) (detailed in the sect. "Amylin Agonism: Monotherapy").

Collectively, these functional neuroanatomical findings suggest that peripheral amylin (secreted from pancreas or pharmacologically administered) binds neurons in the area postrema thereby activating a transsynaptic circuit that includes the nucleus tractus solitarii, the lateral parabrachial nucleus, and the central nucleus of the amygdala, ultimately influencing activation of and peptide levels of neurons in the lateral hypothalamus (Fig. 2).

PYY$_{3-36}$

While the exact mechanisms underlying the effect of peripherally administered PYY$_{3-36}$ on food intake remain to be elucidated, most evidence suggests that the anorexigenic effects are mediated through hypothalamic NPY receptors (Fig. 2). Specifically, PYY$_{3-36}$ is a selective agonist at Y2 receptors, an NPY receptor subtype expressed on NPY [but not pro-opiomelanocortin (POMC)], containing neurons within the arcuate nucleus (85). Batterham et al. (41) proposed that PYY$_{3-36}$ acts on presynaptic Y2 receptors on arcuate NPY neurons to reduce food intake. Subsequent electrophysiological mapping confirmed this hypothesis, implicating a neural circuit wherein activation of NPY Y2 neurons stimulates apposing POMC neurons by decreasing release of NPY and γ-aminobutyric acid onto POMC neurons (86). This would ultimately favor an increase in the release of α-melanocyte-stimulating hormone, a potent anorexigen at other hypothalamic sites. However, because POMC gene knockout mice are still responsive to the anorexigenic effects of PYY$_{3-36}$, other contributory pathways are likely involved as well (87).

The roles of hindbrain nuclei and the vagus nerve in the anorexigenic effect of PYY$_{3-36}$ have also been investigated, but studies have not been conclusive. Y2 receptors have been identified within the dorsal vagal complex (88,89). It is known that effects of PYY$_{3-36}$ on gastrointestinal motility are mediated through brain stem Y2 receptors (90,91). PYY$_{3-36}$ has also been shown to bind within the area postrema (92). However, unlike amylin, animals with lesions of the area postrema are still responsive, or even hyperresponsive, to the anorexigenic effects of peripherally administered PYY$_{3-36}$ (93). In rats, abdominal vagotomy abolished the anorexigenic effect of PYY$_{3-36}$ as well as its ability to stimulate arcuate c-Fos expression (94). In mice, however, an intact vagus does not appear to be

essential for the inhibition of feeding imposed by PYY$_{3-36}$ (95), suggesting that there may be species differences.

Despite some of the inconsistencies that have emerged regarding the mechanism of action of PYY$_{3-36}$, the key observations that (*i*) peripherally administered PYY$_{3-36}$ in rodents reduces food intake (41) and body weight (39), (*ii*) PYY$_{3-36}$ is transported (by nonsaturable mechanisms) across the blood-brain barrier (96), and (*iii*) PYY$_{3-36}$ is a selective agonist for Y2 receptors and does not inhibit feeding in Y2 deficient mice (41) support the hypothesis that PYY$_{3-36}$ is a centrally acting anorexigenic neurohormone.

Leptin

Leptin is a peripherally secreted circulating neurohormonal signal that has been reported to be transported across the blood-brain barrier (73,97). Additionally, leptin may reach the CNS via the median eminence, a circumventricular organ with close proximity to the hypothalamus (66). Within the CNS, leptin binds to long-form leptin receptors on hypothalamic neurons, chiefly in the arcuate nucleus (Fig. 2). Within the arcuate nucleus, leptin exerts both immediate electrophysiological effects of rapid depolarization of POMC neurons and hyperpolarization of NPY neurons, as well as long-term effects on gene expression, such as reducing mRNA expression of the potent orexigens, NPY, and agouti-related protein, while increasing the expression of the anorexigens POMC and cocaine- and amphetamine-regulated transcript (66,98,99).

In rodents with diet-induced obesity (DIO), several abnormalities in leptin neurobiology have been described that could underlie the marked leptin resistance observed in that model. These abnormalities include defects in leptin transport across the blood-brain barrier (100), as well as impaired intracellular signaling, most notably in the arcuate nucleus (101). The latter includes a marked diminution of pSTAT-3 signaling, as well as increased expression of suppressor of cytokine signaling 3, an intracellular protein that suppresses leptin signaling (102). Leptin receptors are abundantly expressed in other hypothalamic regions, such as the ventromedial hypothalamus (103), where diminished signaling has also been observed with diet-induced obesity (100).

The importance of extrahypothalamic leptin receptors has also received increased recognition in recent years (104,105). Intriguingly, these extrahypothalamic sites of leptin action include the nucleus accumbens and hindbrain, presenting possible points of convergence between amylin, PYY$_{3-36}$, and leptin signaling (Fig. 2). Within the accumbens, leptin receptor signaling has been linked to the regulation of food intake, food hedonics, and locomotor behaviors (104,105). Long-form leptin receptors are also widely distributed within the caudal brain stem (e.g., within the nucleus tractus solitarii) (106–108). Several findings indicate that hindbrain leptin signaling is involved in the short-term regulation of satiety and meal size. First, administration of leptin into the fourth cerebroventricle of lean rats slows gastric emptying and reduces food intake and body weight (108). Secondly, leptin may act directly on neurons within the caudal nucleus tractus solitarii to potentiate the effects of gastric distension on food intake (109). Finally, leptin appears to modulate signaling within the brain stem to increase the ability of satiety peptides, such as CCK, GLP-1, and bombesin, to activate dorsal vagal complex neurons (19,110–112). Collectively these findings suggest that leptin can interact with multiple levels of the neuraxis to regulate energy homeostasis.

Convergence of Signaling: Amylin, PYY$_{3-36}$, and Leptin

Direct caudal brain stem activation is an attribute shared by all three neurohormones. As mentioned above, an intact area postrema is required for the expression of amylin's effect on food intake and body weight, and both the area postrema and the nucleus tractus solitarii express robust neuronal activation following amylin administration (78). Long-form leptin receptors are expressed on neurons within the nucleus tractus solitarii (106,108). The nucleus tractus solitarii in particular may be an important site for the interaction of leptin signals of gastric distension (109). Though it remains to be formally determined whether amylin and leptin receptors are colocalized on area postrema neurons and/or whether leptin receptors are coexpressed on amylin-activated nucleus tractus solitarii neurons, the caudal brain stem is clearly a direct site of convergence for these signals. Likewise, while the contribution of PYY$_{3-36}$ to signaling within this region remains to be fully interrogated, it is reasonable to imagine a maximal amplification of hindbrain satiety center signaling with the coadministration of all three neurohormones.

While amylin is not known to have direct effects on hypothalamic neurons, the actions of leptin and PYY$_{3-36}$ are believed to be attributable to direct effects on the arcuate nucleus of the hypothalamus. The observation that 40% to 80% of NPY neurons, which are thought to contain Y2 receptors, within the arcuate nucleus express leptin receptors, coupled with the report that direct application of PYY$_{3-36}$ inhibits electrophysiological responsiveness of NPY neurons (113) points to a potentially rich neural population for direct convergence of signaling between leptin and PYY$_{3-36}$.

Although direct convergence is a possibility, it is also likely that interactions between these neurohormones arise via indirect projection pathways. While this concept raises the potential for many possible permutations for conver-gence, there is emerging literature on amylin-specific effects at the area postrema influencing upstream hypothalamic signaling. For example, acute peripheral amylin injections inhibit fasting-induced neuronal activation within the lateral hypothalamic area and downregulate mRNA expression levels for the food intake-stimulating peptide orexin (72,81). Likewise, sustained administration of amylin (but not pair-feeding) increased arcuate POMC levels, consistent with amylin restoring hypothalamic responsiveness to leptin (114).

AMYLIN AGONISM: MONOTHERAPY

Nonclinical Studies with Amylin in Rodents

Food Intake

In a review of the nonclinical literature, Lutz noted that amylin fulfills the main criteria for a peripheral satiety signal (115). Amylin is secreted in response to food intake, with plasma concentrations being proportional to the size of the meal. Furthermore, its anorexigenic effect is short-acting, evident at near-physiological doses, and is not associated with signs of malaise.

Specifically, peripherally administered amylin in rodents reduces meal size and increases the postmeal interval/meal size ratio (17,84). Conversely, blockade of endogenous amylin signaling in non-food-deprived rats led to a dose-dependent, severalfold increase in food intake, which was mediated by increased meal size (81). Collectively, these results suggest that amylin agonism may have a physiological role in the regulation of both satiation (meal termination) and intermeal satiety.

Three different behavioral assays provide strong evidence that amylin-induced reductions in food intake are not due to malaise or to the induction of competing behaviors. Amylin did not induce taste aversion learning in rats or mice (75,116). Agents with emetic properties also produce pica behavior, the ingestion of nonnutritive substances such as the synthetic white clay kaolin. Doses of peripherally administered amylin that robustly decrease food intake failed to elicit pica behavior (84). Lastly, at doses that decrease food intake, peripheral amylin also had no effect on locomotor activity (84). Together, the failure of amylin to produce taste aversion learning, elicit pica behavior, or change locomotor activity points to a satiety-specific effect that is independent of malaise or competing behaviors incompatible with food intake.

Several findings suggest that amylin agonism also elicits an effect on food preference. During 11 weeks of amylin infusion via subcutaneously implanted osmotic pumps, self-selecting rats displayed a durable difference in food preference, compared with controls, from a palatable diet (58% kcal from fat) to a standard chow diet (6% kcal from fat) (84). Similarly, subcutaneous infusion of amylin in rats subjected to restraint stress decreased the percentage of sucrose calories ingested, and increased the percentage of standard chow calories, compared with controls (117). Consistent with these results, chocolate intake was reduced and standard chow intake was increased in mice injected peripherally with the amylin receptor agonist salmon calcitonin (118).

Body Weight

Rushing et al. (76) initially found that amylin delivered centrally as a continuous 10-day infusion significantly decreased body weight by the fourth day of infusion, with this effect being maintained for the duration of the infusion period. Retroperitoneal fat pad weight, an indicator of total body adiposity, was reduced by approximately 20% in amylin-treated rats relative to vehicle controls (76). Amylin knockout mice displayed a greater rate of weight gain compared with wild-type mice (119,120), pointing to a role of endogenous amylin in body weight regulation.

Perhaps more informative of the therapeutic antiobesity potential of amylin are studies in which amylin was administered peripherally to DIO rats, a model displaying many characteristics of human obesity [increases in fat mass and obesity-related disturbances (e.g., dyslipidemia, hyperinsulinemia), while lacking genetic disruption of key feeding-related central signaling pathways] (121). Importantly, amylin's antiobesity effects are preserved in DIO prone rats (114). In a recent study, the effects of amylin on body weight and metabolic parameters relative to pair-fed controls were characterized in male DIO prone rats (114). Peripherally administered rat amylin (300 µg/kg/day for 22 days) reduced food intake (by ~28%) and slowed weight gain (by ~10%), similar to pair-fed controls (Fig. 3A, B) (114). While food intake reduction (Fig. 3B) was the predominant mode of action for overall weight loss, the composition of weight loss was notably different across treatment groups. In amylin-treated rats, weight loss was attributable to a reduction in fat mass, with relative preservation of lean mass (Fig. 3C, D). In

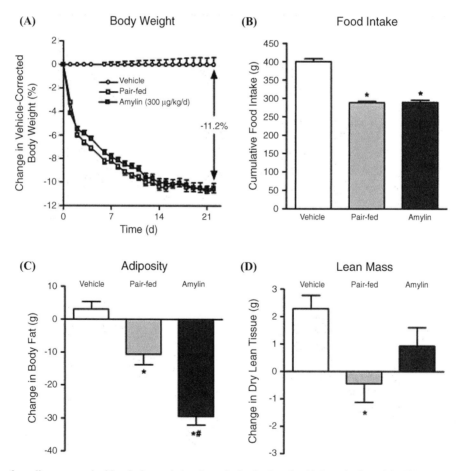

Figure 3 Effects of amylin compared with caloric restriction (by pair-feeding) and vehicle on body weight (**A**), cumulative food intake (**B**), and changes in body composition (**C** and **D**) in DIO prone rats. Amylin (300 µg/kg/day) or vehicle was administered for three weeks via subcutaneously implanted osmotic minipump. Body composition (**C** and **D**) was determined by NMR following treatment. Mean ± SE, $^*p < 0.05$ amylin versus Vehicle; $^\#p < 0.05$ amylin versus pair-fed controls. *Abbreviation*: DIO, diet-induced obese. *Source*: From Ref. 114.

contrast, pair-fed control animals experienced reductions in both fat and lean body masses. Amylin-induced changes in body weight and composition are durable, persisting even across 11 weeks of administration (84).

Importantly, amylin-induced weight loss was not associated with counterregulatory decreases in energy expenditure, and energy expenditure was maintained during periods of active weight loss (84,114). In fact, energy expenditure increased with amylin treatment, an effect that is most likely attributable to relative increases in lean mass and not to the induction of specific amylin-induced thermogenesis (84,114).

Clinical Studies: Antiobesity Effects of the Amylin Analog Pramlintide in Humans

The clinical relevance of the aforementioned findings in rodents has been confirmed in clinical studies, providing solid proof of concept that amylin agonism reduces food intake and body weight in obese individuals.

Clinical use of human amylin as a pharmacological agent is impractical because the native peptide is unstable in solution and has a propensity to aggregate and adhere to surfaces. Pramlintide is a stable, soluble, nonaggregating, nonadhesive, fully active, and equipotent synthetic analog of human amylin (122,123). The undesired physicochemical properties of native human amylin have been overcome in pramlintide by replacing three amino acid residues (25Ala, 28Ser, and 29Ser) with prolines (123).

Pramlintide has been extensively studied in a clinical development program for a diabetes indication, and it was approved in March 2005 in the United States as pramlintide acetate injection, to be given at mealtimes as an adjunct to mealtime insulin therapy in certain patients with type 1 and type 2 diabetes in doses specific for each type of diabetes (124). In addition, pramlintide is in development as a potential treatment for obesity.

Effect of Pramlintide on Satiety, Food Intake, and Control of Eating in Obese Humans

The acute effect of pramlintide on satiety and food intake in obese subjects without diabetes was assessed in a randomized, double-blind, placebo-controlled crossover study, utilizing a well-established buffet meal design (125). Compared with placebo injection, a single subcutaneous injection of pramlintide (120 μg) elicited a significant 16% reduction in ad libitum food intake (Fig. 4A). Concomitant assessment of subjective hunger, fullness, and nausea ratings provided evidence that the reduction in food intake was accompanied by enhanced meal-related satiation and was clearly dissociated from the occurrence of nausea. Specifically, pramlintide decreased the amount

of food required to suppress hunger ratings and elicited a significant 58% increase in the satiety quotient (an integrated measure of food intake and hunger suppression) (Fig. 4B) (125). The effects of pramlintide on satiety do not appear to be mediated by changes in plasma concentrations of other orexigenic or anorexigenic gut peptides assessed to date (Fig. 4C, D). Pramlintide did not exert a significant effect on changes in plasma concentrations of ghrelin, nor did it enhance the postprandial CCK, GLP-1, or PYY response in these subjects. If anything, postprandial PYY plasma concentrations were diminished following pramlintide administration, possibly as a result of the significant reduction in food intake.

Similar reductions in food intake with pramlintide have also been documented in patients with type 2 diabetes and in healthy normal-weight volunteers (125,126). In normal-weight volunteers, a low dose of pramlintide (30 μg), estimated to approximately replicate the physiological increases in amylin during the postprandial period, elicited a significant 14% reduction in ad libitum food intake and a reduction in meal duration. This finding further supports the concept that amylin agonism may have a physiological role in meal-related satiation (125,126).

To obtain a more comprehensive assessment of pramlintide on human eating behavior, we next assessed the effect of pramlintide on 24-hour food intake and control of eating in obese subjects in a six-week randomized, placebo-controlled parallel group study (127). Compared with placebo injection, six weeks of treatment with pramlintide (180 μg three times a day, t.i.d.) elicited progressive weight loss that was accompanied by sustained reductions in 24-hour food intake. The reduction in 24-hour food intake (assessed during carefully controlled inpatient conditions) averaged approximately 500 to 750 kcal/day (15–20%) and was evident early and at the end of the study ($p < 0.01$) (Fig. 5A). The reduction in food intake with pramlintide was evident at each major meal, but not at the ad libitum evening snack prior to which no study medication was administered (Fig. 5B). Moreover, consistent with nonclinical findings that amylin preferentially reduced the intake of highly palatable high-fat food (84), pramlintide treatment elicited acute and sustained reductions in food intake in a "fast-food challenge," which comprised of pizza, ice cream, and sugar-containing soft drinks (Fig. 5C). Finally, compared with placebo, pramlintide-mediated weight loss in this study was also accompanied by a significant 45% reduction in binge eating score ($p < 0.01$) (Fig. 5D). Collectively, these results suggest that pramlintide-mediated weight loss in obese subjects is mediated by multiple effects to prevent overeating and help reduce food consumption, including sustained reductions in 24-hour food intake, portion sizes, "fast-food" intake, and binge eating tendencies (127).

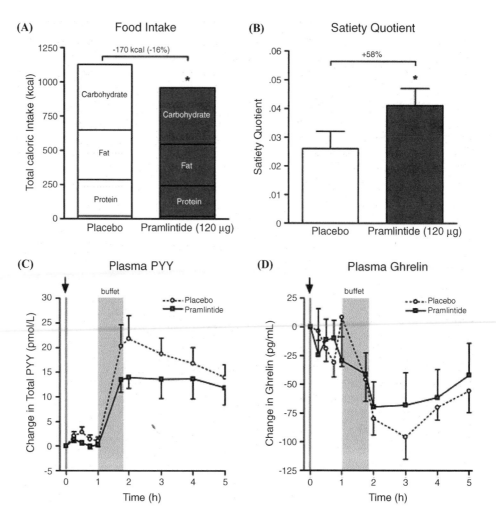

Figure 4 Acute effect of pramlintide on food intake and postprandial hormonal analyte excursions in a crossover study in obese subjects (evaluable $N = 15$). Total caloric intake (**A**) and satiety (**B**) measured at an ad libitum buffet meal following a single injection of pramlintide (120 μg) or placebo. Overall column height represents total caloric intake, while subcolumn height represents macronutrient intake. Incremental changes in plasma concentrations of total PYY (**C**) and ghrelin (**D**) measured following administration of treatment medication. Arrow/gray line indicates injection of study medication; shaded area indicates the time during which the buffet meal was offered. Mean ± SE; $^*p < 0.05$ pramlintide versus placebo. *Abbreviation*: PYY, peptide YY. *Source*: From Ref. 125.

Effect of Pramlintide on Body Weight in Obese Humans

The effect of pramlintide on body weight in obese subjects was assessed in two randomized, double-blind, placebo-controlled phase 2 studies, each of 16-week duration.

In a phase 2A dose-escalation study, pramlintide was given t.i.d. at doses up to 240 μg in the absence of any new lifestyle intervention (LSI) (128). Pramlintide was initiated at a low dose and gradually escalated, in a nonforced manner, on the basis of individual tolerability. Pramlintide was well tolerated, with approximately 90% of subjects able to escalate to 240 μg t.i.d. The most common adverse event with pramlintide was mild, transient nausea (38% vs. 22% with placebo). Pramlintide-

treated subjects experienced progressive weight loss (3.6% ± 0.6% vs. placebo, $p < 0.0001$) (Fig. 6A), which was accompanied by a reduction in waist circumference (3.4 ± 1.1 cm, placebo-corrected $p < 0.003$). Weight loss was not due to nausea, as evidenced by the fact that pramlintide-treated subjects not reporting nausea experienced weight loss similar to those who did (3.6% ± 0.5% and 3.9% ± 0.5%, respectively). Instead, in a blinded, nonvalidated, end-of-study questionnaire, a greater proportion of pramlintide- than placebo-treated subjects reported that use of study medication improved their ability to control their appetite (Fig. 6C). Thirty-one percent of pramlintide-treated subjects (vs. 2% placebo) achieved >5% weight loss ($p < 0.0001$) (Fig. 6B). In the subgroup of >5% responders, weight loss had a rapid

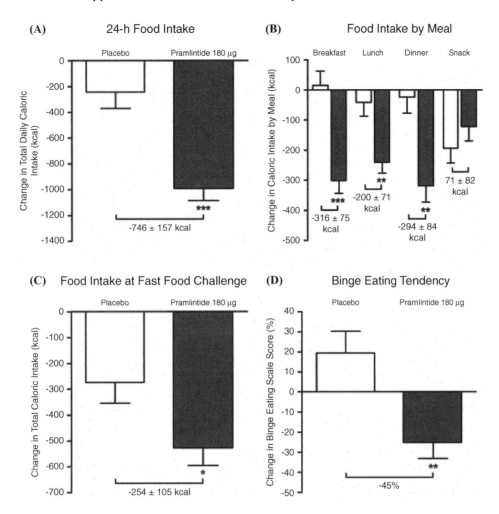

Figure 5 Effect of pramlintide on food intake and binge eating in obese subjects (evaluable $N = 84$). Subjects were treated with pramlintide (180 μg t.i.d.) or placebo for six weeks. Changes in 24-hour total caloric intake (**A**) and caloric intake by meal (**B**) from placebo lead-in (day 1) to day 3 at three ad libitum buffets. No treatment medication was administered prior to the snack. (**C**) Changes in total caloric intake during the ad libitum "fast food" lunch meal from placebo lead-in (day 2) to day 4. (**D**) Change in Binge Eating Scale score from baseline to day 42. Mean ± SE; $^*p < 0.05$, $^{**}p < 0.01$, $^{***}p < 0.001$ pramlintide versus placebo. *Source*: From Ref. 127.

onset (∼3% after 4 weeks), averaged approximately 7.8% at week 16, and was accompanied by a 21% reduction in plasma leptin (Fig. 6D).

In a subsequent phase 2B dose-ranging study utilizing a structured LSI program, 408 obese subjects were randomly assigned to four months of LSI plus treatment with either pramlintide (120, 240, 360 μg, b.i.d./t.i.d.) or placebo administered 15 minutes before meals (129). By four months, weight loss from baseline in the pramlintide arms ranged from 3.8 ± 0.7 to 6.1 ± 0.8 kg, and several of the pramlintide dosage arms (120 μg t.i.d., 240 μg b.i.d., 360 μg b.i.d./t.i.d.) achieved statistical significance compared with placebo (2.8 ± 0.8 kg, $p < 0.05$). Overall, this study showed that pramlintide treatment induced weight loss above and beyond that achieved with LSI alone and that twice daily dosing (at higher doses) was sufficient to induce significant sustained weight loss. The most

common adverse event was nausea, which occurred more often in pramlintide-treated (9–29%) than placebo-treated subjects (2%).

To assess the effect of pramlintide on body weight beyond four months of treatment, a placebo-controlled extension protocol to the aforementioned study was instituted (130). Of evaluable subjects completing the initial study, 75% of subjects opted to continue treatment in the extension. Throughout the extension, LSI was geared toward weight maintenance (not loss). Initial weight loss was largely regained during the extension in the placebo group, but was fully maintained in all but one pramlintide group (120 μg b.i.d.). By 12 months, subjects treated with 120 μg t.i.d. and 360 μg b.i.d. pramlintide experienced significant weight loss compared with placebo (6.9 ± 1.7 kg and 8.0 ± 2.0 kg vs. 0.8 ± 1.3 kg, $p < 0.01$), with 40% and 43% of subjects, respectively, achieving ≥10% weight loss

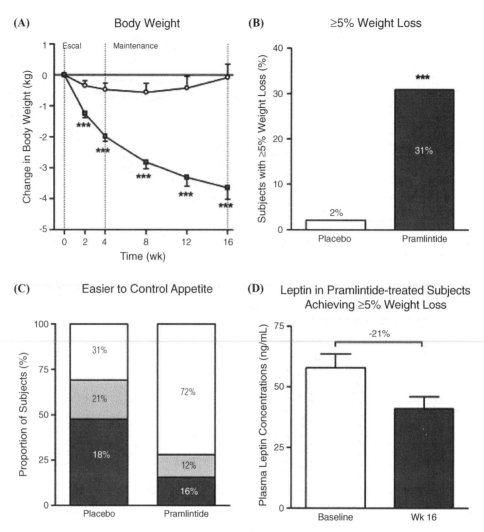

Figure 6 Effect of pramlintide (up to 240 µg t.i.d.) or placebo on body weight and appetite control in obese subjects (evaluable $N =$ 145). (**A**) Change from baseline in body weight (kg) for pramlintide- and placebo-treated subjects during the escalation and maintenance periods. (**B**) Proportion of evaluable subjects achieving ≥5% reduction in weight by week 16. (**C**) Subject responses in a nonvalidated, end-of-study questionnaire to the statement: "I feel that using the study medication made it easier for me to control my appetite." Data presented as proportions of placebo- and pramlintide-treated subjects (%) who responded Strongly Disagree/Disagree (*pooled in black*), Neutral (*gray*), and Strongly Agree/Agree (*pooled in white*). (**D**) Changes in leptin concentrations in subset of pramlintide-treated subjects achieving ≥5% weight loss by week 16. Mean ± SE; ***$p < 0.001$ pramlintide versus placebo. *Source*: From Ref. 128.

(vs. 12% for placebo). The pramlintide-mediated reduction in body weight was accompanied by a significant reduction in waist circumference. During the extension study, the incidence of nausea was generally low and not different between pramlintide and placebo (0–9% vs. 0%). There were no clinically significant adverse changes in vital signs or laboratory parameters with pramlintide treatment.

Collectively, these studies with pramlintide in obese humans are consistent with nonclinical evidence to support a role of amylin agonism in the regulation of food intake and body weight. Furthermore, available clinical study data indicate that amylin agonists, such as pramlintide, have the potential to become peptide hormone therapeutics for obesity.

PYY$_{3\text{-}36}$ AND LEPTIN AGONISM: POTENTIAL AS MONOTHERAPIES VS. AS ADJUNCTS TO AMYLIN AGONISM

Even though amylin agonists hold promise as monotherapies for obesity, the full potential of peptide hormone therapeutics for obesity treatment may not be realized if each neurohormone is evaluated in isolation only. Greater weight loss could conceivably be achieved with neuropeptide combinatorial regimens, especially by identifying and harnessing naturally occurring neurohormonal synergies. In this section, we review results from a comprehensive nonclinical research program designed to assess the interaction between amylin, leptin, and PYY$_{3\text{-}36}$ in the

DIO rat, a model that has been reasonably predictive of clinical efficacy of antiobesity monotherapies.

PYY$_{3-36}$ Agonism

PYY$_{3-36}$ Monotherapy: Nonclinical Studies

In the first experiments testing the anorexigenic effects of PYY$_{3-36}$, continuous infusion of PYY$_{3-36}$ (100 or 300 μg/day) for four weeks significantly reduced cumulative food intake, but not body weight gain, in Zucker diabetic fatty rats (131). However, infusion of PYY$_{3-36}$ (100 μg/kg/day) for eight weeks in obese nonfatty Zucker rats reduced body weight gain compared with vehicle (132). Subsequent reports confirmed that peripheral administration of PYY$_{3-36}$ via subcutaneous injections or infusion reduced food intake, body weight, and adiposity in rodent models (39,41,133). Administration of PYY$_{3-36}$ to DIO mice also increased utilization of fat stores, resulting in decreased adiposity (134). However, the antiobesity effects of PYY$_{3-36}$ remain controversial in that several other groups have failed to demonstrate significant reductions in food intake and/or body weight in various rodent models (135). In rhesus monkeys, twice daily or continuous intravenous infusion of PYY$_{3-36}$ reduced food intake at the morning meal but not at the evening meal, and it did not reduce cumulative 24-hour intake. With twice daily infusions of PYY$_{3-36}$ for two weeks, modest but significant reductions in body weight were observed ($\sim 1.9\%$) (136). Overall, it appears that PYY$_{3-36}$ agonism exerts antiobesity effects in certain nonclinical models, but the effect seems to be less consistent and reproducible than with amylin agonism.

PYY$_{3-36}$ Monotherapy: Clinical Studies

While data with PYY$_{3-36}$ in humans are limited and the route of PYY$_{3-36}$ administration has varied between clinical trials, small studies have revealed statistically significant reductions in food intake in lean and obese humans (40,41). In two crossover studies, infusion of PYY$_{3-36}$ in lean and obese subjects reduced caloric intake at an ad libitum buffet by approximately 30% (40,41). Prior to the buffet meal, visual analog scores demonstrated reductions in hunger following infusion of PYY$_{3-36}$ (41,137). Other investigators have reported similar findings (138). Consistent with these infusion studies, results from a phase 1 study in lean and obese subjects demonstrated that a single subcutaneous injection of synthetic PYY$_{3-36}$ resulted in a trend toward greater hunger suppression and satiety quotients one hour after ingestion of a standardized breakfast (137). However, in a phase 2 randomized, placebo-controlled study of nasally administered PYY$_{3-36}$, 12 weeks of treatment with 200 μg led to only a marginal nonsignificant reduction in body weight compared with placebo (139). With the higher-tested dose (600 μg), no conclusions could be drawn regarding weight loss efficacy due to the low completion rate (26% compared with 88% with placebo). In the 600 μg dose group, 59% withdrew because of nausea and vomiting. With the exception of the nasally administered 600 μg treatment arm, PYY$_{3-36}$ was generally well-tolerated over a wide range of doses. Nausea was the most frequently reported adverse event.

PYY$_{3-36}$ Agonism as an Adjunctive Treatment to Amylin

To explore the potential of PYY$_{3-36}$ as an adjunct to amylin agonism, several nonclinical studies have examined the combined effects of both neurohormones in DIO rats. After two weeks, PYY$_{3-36}$ (1000 μg/kg/day) and amylin monotherapy (100 μg/kg/day) significantly reduced food intake (27% and 27%, $p < 0.05$ vs. vehicle) and body weight (9% and 7%, $p < 0.05$ vs. vehicle). Coadministration of amylin and PYY$_{3-36}$ induced marked additive antiobesity effects, including a 55% inhibition of food intake and a 15% reduction in body weight (140). Treatment with amylin plus PYY$_{3-36}$ was lean sparing and significantly decreased adiposity from 15% to 8% ($p < 0.05$ vs. vehicle). When a range of doses of PYY$_{3-36}$ and amylin were tested alone and in combination (using a 4 × 3 factorial design), the statistical analyses and predicted response surface formally confirmed that amylin and PYY$_{3-36}$ have additive effects on weight loss, mediated in part via a synergistic suppression of food intake (140).

Leptin Agonism

Leptin Monotherapy: Nonclinical Studies

In leptin-deficient rodents, leptin treatment elicits remarkable metabolic effects. Peripheral administration of leptin to (ob/ob) mice resulted in profound reductions in food intake, body weight, and adiposity, and normalized hyperglycemia and hyperlipidemia (63,98,141). Likewise, leptin administration reversed many of the abnormalities, such as insulin resistance and fatty liver, which are characteristics of the severely hypoleptinemic rat models of lipodystrophy (A-ZIP and SCREBP1−/−) (142,143). However, when a hyperleptinemic state was induced by high-fat feeding (DIO mice or rats), administration of murine leptin elicited only marginal weight loss (144).

Leptin Monotherapy: Clinical Studies

The profound effects of leptin in murine models of genetic leptin deficiency (ob/ob) and lipodystrophy (A-ZIP and SCREBP1−/−) were replicated in the corresponding human conditions (145,148). In children and adults with congenital leptin deficiency, leptin replacement therapy resulted in profound and sustained reductions in body weight (145,146,149). Likewise, in clinical trials, leptin has been shown to alleviate the profound hyperglycemia, dyslipidemia, insulin resistance, and hepatosteatosis of patients with severe lipodystrophy (147,150). Hence, with respect to leptin deficiency (*ob/ob*, lipodystrophy), rodent models have been highly predictive of the leptin response seen in the corresponding human conditions. Moreover, the fact that patients with *ob/ob* and severe lipodystrophy have been successfully treated with leptin for several years suggests that leptin has the potential of becoming a chronic treatment for severe lipodystrophy.

With respect to DIO, results in rodents are also highly consistent with findings obtained with leptin monotherapy in obese humans. Hence, in keeping with the lack of leptin responsiveness in DIO rats, leptin monotherapy does not appear efficacious in eliciting weight loss in obese subjects, even at pharmacological doses (64, 65, data on file Amylin Pharmaceuticals, Inc.).

Studies by Rosenbaum and Leibel suggest that leptin's primary role on weight control may not lie in the induction of weight loss using high pharmacological doses, but, rather, in the prevention of weight loss counterregulation and maintenance of weight loss (14,15). Indeed, in relatively short-term studies (weeks to months), administration of replacement doses of leptin prevented many of the metabolic counterregulatory adaptations (decline in metabolic rate, reduced thyroid hormone levels, increased muscle work efficiency) induced by 10% weight loss following a very low-calorie diet (14,15). These mechanistic studies notwithstanding, available clinical trial data suggest that leptin monotherapy may not induce meaningful weight loss in the broad obese target population.

Leptin as an Adjunctive Treatment to Amylin

As part of our nonclinical program to explore neurohormonal interactions in obesity, leptin-resistant DIO rats were concurrently treated with amylin and leptin. Consistent with previous nonclinical studies, amylin monotherapy (100 µg/kg/day) significantly decreased food intake and body weight, while leptin (500 µg/kg/day) monotherapy at a dose efficacious in lean rats had minimal effects on weight or food intake (21). Amylin plus leptin combination treatment resulted in significant synergistic reductions in food intake and body weight (12%, $p < 0.05$ vs. all groups), which exceeded that predicted by the sum of amylin and leptin monotherapy. The observed weight loss synergy was dissociable from amylin's anorexigenic properties, as leptin administration to rats pair-fed to the amylin-treated group did not elicit weight loss greater than that achieved by pair-feeding alone. Treatment with amylin plus leptin, while sparing lean mass, specifically decreased adiposity. Additionally, amylin plus leptin increased light cycle fat oxidation and dark cycle energy expenditure (corrected for lean mass), effects not observed with either treatment alone (21). A response surface analysis (similar to that conducted

for amylin plus PYY_{3-36}) formally confirmed that the weight-reducing effects of the amylin plus leptin combination are statistically synergistic (20). The synergism between these agents may be due in part to amylin's effects on neural leptin responses. Specifically, amylin pretreatment partially restored leptin signaling within the ventromedial hypothalamus and augmented leptin's effects in the hindbrain, as detected by pSTAT-3 immunoreactivity, an accepted marker of leptin receptor activation (20). Collectively, these findings are consistent with amylin restoring responsiveness to peripheral leptin in leptin-resistant DIO rats.

In another study, where DIO leptin-resistant rats were pretreated with amylin for two weeks and then treated with amylin or leptin monotherapy or the combination of amylin and leptin for four weeks, amylin- plus leptin-treated rats achieved a significantly greater vehicle-corrected weight loss (15%) than with amylin (9%) or leptin alone (8%) (Fig. 7) (21). Importantly, the response to leptin alone in this study (8%) was significantly greater than that achievable with leptin treatment (2–3%) in the face of no pretreatment with amylin.

The relevance of these nonclinical findings to human obesity was recently demonstrated in a 24-week, randomized, double-blind, clinical proof-of-concept study in overweight/obese subjects. In this study, subjects initially followed a 40% caloric-deficit diet in conjunction with pramlintide (180 µg b.i.d. for 2 weeks, then 360 µg b.i.d. for 2 weeks). Following the lead-in period, subjects either remained on pramlintide or received metreleptin monotherapy or the combination of pramlintide and metreleptin for 20 weeks. At week 20, coadministration of pramlintide and metreleptin elicited 12.7% mean weight loss, significantly more than was observed with pramlintide (8.4%) or leptin alone (8.2%) (Fig. 7) (21). The most common side effects seen with pramlintide plus metreleptin combination treatment were injection site adverse events and nausea, which were mostly mild to moderate and transient in nature.

While metreleptin monotherapy failed to elicit significant weight loss (2% or less) in clinical studies in general obesity (65, data on file Amylin Pharmaceuticals, Inc., San Diego, California, U.S.), in this clinical study the combination of pramlintide and metreleptin recapitulated preclinical observations and provided evidence that responsiveness to exogenous leptin can be, at least partially, restored by amylin agonism. These data provide the first clinical evidence that it may be feasible to safely achieve greater than 10% weight loss using an integrated neurohormonal approach to obesity pharmacotherapy.

Triple Combination Regimen with Amylin, Leptin, and PYY—Nonclinical Studies in Rodents

Given the weight loss additivity/synergism observed with dual combination regimens, we next examined a regimen

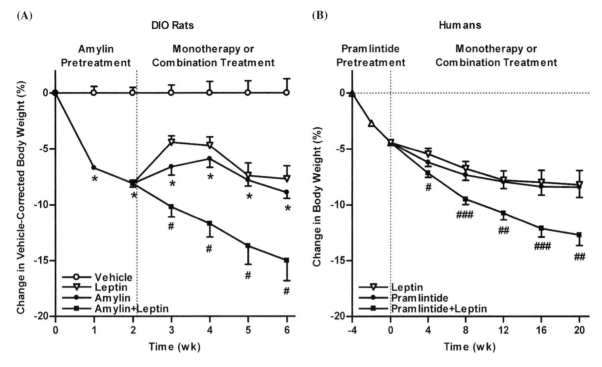

Figure 7 Effects of amylin and leptin agonism on body weight in (**A**) DIO leptin-resistant rats and (**B**) overweight/obese humans. (**A**) DIO rats were pretreated with amylin (100 μg/kg/day) administered by continuous subcutaneous infusion for two weeks and were then treated for four weeks with amylin, leptin (500 μg/kg/day), vehicle, or amylin plus leptin combination treatment. (**B**) Change in weight from enrolment (week 4) for subjects pretreated with pramlintide (titrated from 180 μg to 360 μg b.i.d.) for two weeks and then treated with pramlintide (360 μg b.i.d.), metreleptin (5 mg b.i.d.), or pramlintide plus metreleptin combination treatment. Mean ± SE; *$p < 0.05$ versus vehicle; #$p < 0.05$ versus monotherapies. *Abbreviation*: DIO, diet-induced obesity. *Source*: From Ref. 21.

consisting of all three neurohormones in combination. In a four-week study in DIO rats, the effects of monotherapy with amylin, PYY$_{3-36}$, or leptin were compared with a group of rats that received all three neurohormones in combination, at 50% of the respective monotherapy doses (22). Consistent with previous studies, leptin monotherapy did not decrease food intake or body weight, while monotherapy with either amylin or PYY$_{3-36}$ significantly reduced food intake ($\sim$25%, respectively) and body weight (8% and 5%, respectively) ($p < 0.05$ vs. vehicle). Compared with the monotherapies, the triple combination resulted in significantly greater vehicle-corrected reductions in body weight (17% $p < 0.05$) and food intake ($\sim$50%, $p < 0.05$). Consistent with our findings with dual-combination regimens, the half-dose triple-combination regimen significantly reduced adiposity ($p < 0.05$ vs. monotherapies) but not lean mass, and was not accompanied by compensatory decreases in the metabolic rate. These findings demonstrate that the combination of amylin, PYY$_{3-36}$, and leptin results in enhanced signaling, which elicits marked, fat-specific weight loss in DIO rats, and suggest that the combinatorial approach may prevent counterregulatory adaptations that can limit pharmacological efficacy in maintaining a clinically significant reduction in body weight.

SUMMARY AND CONCLUSIONS

As reviewed in this chapter, peripherally secreted islet-, gut-, and adipocyte-derived neurohormones are known to play an important role in the complex physiological regulation of food intake and body weight. Peptide hormone therapeutics based on these advances in obesity research and neuroscience may thus offer a promising alternative approach to obesity pharmacotherapy. The effects of amylin, PYY$_{3-36}$, and leptin monotherapies and combination therapies on food intake and body weight in DIO rats and obese humans are summarized in Table 1.

The antiobesity properties of amylin in DIO rodents include sustained reductions in food intake and restoration of leptin sensitivity. Amylin-mediated weight loss is fat-specific and does not appear to be accompanied by compensatory reductions in energy expenditure or fat oxidation. In obese humans, treatment with the amylin agonist pramlintide led to sustained reductions in 24-hour food intake, meal size, and body weight. There was no evidence of neuropsychiatric or idiosyncratic side effects; the most common adverse event was mild transient nausea that decreased over several weeks of treatment.

In addition to the antiobesity effects seen with monotherapy, amylin agonism in DIO rats consistently elicits

Table 1 Effects of Amylin, PYY$_{3-36}$, and Leptin Monotherapies and Combination Therapies on Food Intake and Body Weight in DIO Rats and Obese Humans: Consistency Between Nonclinical and Clinical Data

	Regimen	Nonclinical	Clinical
Monotherapy	Amylin/pramlintide		
	Food intake	↓	↓
	Body weight	↓	↓
	PYY$_{3-36}$		
	Food intake	↓	↓
	Body weight	↓	TBD
	Leptin		
	Food intake	↔	↔
	Body weight	↔	↔
Combination therapy	Amylin + PYY$_{3-36}$		
	Food intake	↓↓ (Synergy)	TBD
	Body weight	↓↓ (Additive)	TBD
	Amylin + leptin		
	Food intake	↓↓ (Synergy)	TBD
	Body weight	↓↓ (Synergy)	TBD
	Amylin + PYY$_{3-36}$ + leptin		
	Food intake	↓↓↓ (Reversal of DIO)	TBD
	Body weight	↓↓↓ (Reversal of DIO)	TBD

Abbreviation: DIO, diet-induced obesity; TBD, to be determined.

marked additive/synergistic reductions in food intake (by up to 55%) and body weight (by up to 17%) when used in combination with the gut-derived hormone PYY$_{3-36}$ and the adipocyte-derived hormone leptin. These nonclinical findings, coupled with the recent clinical study results of pramlintide+metreleptin combination treatment, provide growing evidence that combinatorial regimens of peptide hormone therapeutics may have the potential to become innovative medicine that offer marked weight loss in a safe, physiological rational manner.

This integrated neurohormonal treatment for obesity may offer an innovative approach to obesity pharmacotherapy that harnesses naturally occurring synergies among adipocyte-, islet-, and gut-derived signals.

As reviewed in this chapter, peptide hormone therapeutics hold promise as more physiological alternatives to existing small-molecule agents for obesity. Recent progress in peptide/protein chemistry (aimed at designing analogs that optimize the efficacy, potency, and pharmaceutical properties of naturally occurring hormones) and drug delivery research (aimed at developing more convenient delivery systems, such as long-acting release formulations) may further unleash the therapeutic potential of peptide hormone therapeutics.

Ultimately, through the pharmaceutical development of peptide hormone therapeutics, it may be possible to translate some of the important advances in basic obesity research into innovative therapies. If that were achieved, obesity could follow a similar path to that of diabetes drug development where peptide hormone therapeutics,

such as insulin, glucagon, GLP-1, and amylin agonists, have already become an integral part of the therapeutic armamentarium.

REFERENCES

1. Badman MK, Flier JS. The gut and energy balance: visceral allies in the obesity wars. Science 2005; 307 (5717):1909–1914.
2. Bray GA. Drug insight: appetite suppressants. Nat Clin Pract Gastroenterol Hepatol 2005; 2(2):89–95.
3. Colman E. Anorectics on trial: a half century of federal regulation of prescription appetite suppressants. Ann Intern Med 2005; 143(5):380–385.
4. Weintraub M, Sundaresan PR, Schuster B, et al. Long-term weight control study. III (weeks 104 to 156). An open-label study of dose adjustment of fenfluramine and phentermine. Clin Pharmacol Ther 1992; 51(5):602–607.
5. Steel JM, Munro JF, Duncan LJ. A comparative trial of different regimens of fenfluramine and phentermine in obesity. Practitioner 1973; 211(262):232–236.
6. Connolly HM, Crary JL, McGoon MD, et al. Valvular heart disease associated with fenfluramine-phentermine. N Engl J Med 1997; 337(9):581–588.
7. Greenway F, Anderson J, Atkinson R, et al. Bupropion and zonisamide for the treatment of obesity. Obesity 2006; 14(suppl 9):A17 (abstr 52-OR).
8. Gadde KM, Yonish GM, Foust MS, et al. A 24-week randomized controlled trial of VI-0521, a combination weight loss therapy, in obese adults. Obesity 2006; 14 (suppl 9):A17–A18 (abstr 55-OR).

9. Devlin MJ, Goldfein JA, Carino JS, et al. Open treatment of overweight binge eaters with phentermine and fluoxetine as an adjunct to cognitive-behavioral therapy. Int J Eat Disord 2000; 28(3):325–332.

10. Morton GJ, Cummings DE, Baskin DG, et al. Central nervous system control of food intake and body weight. Nature 2006; 443(7109):289–295.

11. Cummings DE, Overduin J. Gastrointestinal regulation of food intake. J Clin Invest 2007; 117(1):13–23.

12. Niswender KD, Schwartz MW. Insulin and leptin revisited: adiposity signals with overlapping physiological and intracellular signaling capabilities. Front Neuroendocrinol 2003; 24(1):1–10.

13. Benoit SC, Clegg DJ, Seeley RJ, et al. Insulin and leptin as adiposity signals. Recent Prog Horm Res 2004; 59: 267–285.

14. Rosenbaum M, Murphy EM, Heymsfield SB, et al. Low dose leptin administration reverses effects of sustained weight-reduction on energy expenditure and circulating concentrations of thyroid hormones. J Clin Endocrinol Metab 2002; 87(5):2391–2394.

15. Rosenbaum M, Goldsmith R, Bloomfield D, et al. Low-dose leptin reverses skeletal muscle, autonomic, and neuroendocrine adaptations to maintenance of reduced weight. J Clin Invest 2005; 115(12):3579–3586.

16. Wynne K, Stanley S, McGowan B, et al. Appetite control. J Endocrinol 2005; 184(2):291–318.

17. Halford JC, Blundell JE. Pharmacology of appetite suppression. Prog Drug Res 2000; 54:25–58.

18. Halford JC, Cooper GD, Dovey TM. The pharmacology of human appetite expression. Curr Drug Targets 2004; 5(3): 221–240.

19. Emond M, Schwartz GJ, Ladenheim EE, et al. Central leptin modulates behavioral and neural responsivity to CCK. Am J Physiol 1999; 276(5 pt 2):R1545–R1549.

20. Roth JD, Roland B, Cole R, et al. Responsiveness to leptin restored by amylin in diet induced obese (DIO) rats: magnitude and mechanisms of synergy. Diabetes 2007; 56(suppl 1):A72 (abstr 0277-OR).

21. Roth JD, Roland BL, Cole RL, et al. Leptin responsiveness restored by amylin agonism in diet-induced obesity: evidence from nonclinical and clinical studies. Proc Natl Acad Sci USA 2008 (in press).

22. Roth J, Barnhill S, Lei C, et al. Multihormonal treatment with amylin, PYY (3-36), and leptin elicited marked, fat-specific weight loss in diet-induced obese (DIO) rats. Obesity 2006; 14(suppl 9):A57–A58 (abstr 177-P).

23. Bhavsar S, Watkins J, Young A. Synergy between amylin and cholecystokinin for inhibition of food intake in mice. Physiol Behav 1998; 64(4):557–561.

24. le Roux CW, Bloom SR. Why do patients lose weight after Roux-en-Y gastric bypass? J Clin Endocrinol Metab 2005; 90(1):591–592.

25. Korner J, Bessler M, Cirilo L, et al. Effects of Roux-en-Y gastric bypass surgery on fasting and postprandial concentrations of plasma ghrelin, peptide YY, and insulin. J Clin Endocrinol Metab 2005; 90(1):359–365.

26. Ogawa A, Harris V, McCorkle SK, et al. Amylin secretion from the rat pancreas and its selective loss after streptozotocin treatment. J Clin Invest 1990; 85(3):973–976.

27. Moore CX, Cooper GJS. Co-secretion of amylin and insulin from cultured islet beta-cells: modulation by nutrient secretagogues, islet hormones and hypoglycemic agents. Biochem Biophys Res Commun 1991; 179(1):1–9.

28. Cooper GJS, Willis AC, Clark A, et al. Purification and characterization of a peptide from amyloid-rich pancreases of type 2 diabetic patients. Proc Natl Acad Sci USA 1987; 84(23):8628–8632.

29. Young AA, Wang MW, Gedulin B, et al. Diabetogenic effects of salmon calcitonin are attributable to amylin-like activity. Metabolism 1995; 44(12):1581–1589.

30. Kitamura K, Kangawa K, Kawamoto M, et al. Adrenomedullin: a novel hypotensive peptide isolated from human pheochromocytoma. Biochem Biophys Res Commun 1993; 192(2):553–560.

31. Leffert JD, Newgard CB, Okamoto H, et al. Rat amylin: cloning and tissue-specific expression in pancreatic islets. Proc Natl Acad Sci USA 1989; 86(9):3127–3310.

32. Badman MK, Shennan KIJ, Jermany JL, et al. Processing of pro-islet amyloid polypeptide (proIAPP) by the prohormone convertase PC2. FEBS Lett 1996; 378(3): 227–231.

33. Koda JE, Fineman M, Rink TJ, et al. Amylin concentrations and glucose control. Lancet 1992; 339(8802): 1179–1180.

34. Weyer C, Maggs DG, Young AA, et al. Amylin replacement with pramlintide as an adjunct to insulin therapy in type 1 and type 2 diabetes mellitus: a physiological approach toward improved metabolic control. Curr Pharm Des 2001; 7(14):1353–1373.

35. Koda JE, Fineman MS, Kolterman OG, et al. 24 hour plasma amylin profiles are elevated in IGT subjects vs. normal controls. Diabetes 1995; 44(suppl 1):238A (abstr 876).

36. Makimattila S, Fineman MS, Yki-Jarvinen H. Deficiency of total and nonglycosylated amylin in plasma characterizes subjects with impaired glucose tolerance and type 2 diabetes. J Clin Endocrinol Metab 2000; 85(8):2822–2827.

37. Adrian TE, Ferri GL, Bacarese-Hamilton AJ, et al. Human distribution and release of a putative new gut hormone, peptide YY. Gastroenterology 1985; 89(5):1070–1077.

38. Grandt D, Schimiczek M, Beglinger C, et al. Two molecular forms of peptide YY (PYY) are abundant in human blood: characterization of a radioimmunoassay recognizing PYY 1-36 and PYY 3- 36. Regul Pept 1994; 51(2): 151–159.

39. Pittner RA, Moore CX, Bhavsar SP, et al. Effects of PYY [3-36] in rodent models of diabetes and obesity. Int J Obes Relat Metab Disord 2004; 28(8):963–971.

40. Batterham RL, Cohen MA, Ellis SM, et al. Inhibition of food intake in obese subjects by peptide YY3-36. N Engl J Med 2003; 349(10):941–948.

41. Batterham RL, Cowley MA, Small CJ, et al. Gut hormone PYY(3-36) physiologically inhibits food intake. Nature 2002; 418(6898):650–654.

42. Anini Y, Fu-Cheng X, Cuber JC, et al. Comparison of the postprandial release of peptide YY and proglucagon-derived peptides in the rat. Pflugers Arch 1999; 438(3): 299–306.

43. le Roux CW, Batterham RL, Aylwin SJ, et al. Attenuated peptide YY release in obese subjects is associated with reduced satiety. Endocrinology 2006; 147(1):3–8.

44. Lin HC, Chey WY. Cholecystokinin and peptide YY are released by fat in either proximal or distal small intestine in dogs. Regul Pept 2003; 114(2–3):131–135.

45. Zhang Y, Proenca R, Maffei M, et al. Positional cloning of the mouse obese gene and its human homologue. Nature 1994; 372(6505):425–432.

46. Klein S, Coppack SW, MohamedAli V, et al. Adipose tissue leptin production and plasma leptin kinetics in humans. Diabetes 1996; 45(7):984–987.

47. Bado A, Levasseur S, Attoub S, et al. The stomach is a source of leptin. Nature 1998; 394(6695):790–793.

48. Huang L, Wang Z, Li C. Modulation of circulating leptin levels by its soluble receptor. J Biol Chem 2001; 276(9): 6343–6349.

49. Lonnqvist F, Nordfors L, Jansson M, et al. Leptin secretion from adipose tissue in women. Relationship to plasma levels and gene expression. J Clin Invest 1997; 99(10): 2398–2404.

50. Lofgren P, Andersson I, Adolfsson B, et al. Long-term prospective and controlled studies demonstrate adipose tissue hypercellularity and relative leptin deficiency in the postobese state. J Clin Endocrinol Metab 2005; 90(11): 6207–6213.

51. Sinha MK, Ohannesian JP, Heiman ML, et al. Nocturnal rise of leptin in lean, obese, and non-insulin-dependent diabetes mellitus subjects. J Clin Invest 1996; 97(5):1344–1347.

52. Chan JL, Heist K, DePaoli AM, et al. The role of falling leptin levels in the neuroendocrine and metabolic adaptation to short-term starvation in healthy men. J Clin Invest 2003; 111(9):1409–1421.

53. Mars M, de Graaf C, de Groot CP, et al. Fasting leptin and appetite responses induced by a 4-day 65%-energy-restricted diet. Int J Obes 2006; 30(1):122–128.

54. Dubuc GR, Phinney SD, Stern JS, et al. Changes of serum leptin and endocrine and metabolic parameters after 7 days of energy restriction in men and women. Metabolism 1998; 47(4):429–434.

55. Keim NL, Stern JS, Havel PJ. Relation between circulating leptin concentrations and appetite during a prolonged, moderate energy deficit in women. Am J Clin Nutr 1998; 68(4):794–801.

56. Kolaczynski JW, Nyce MR, Considine RV, et al. Acute and chronic effect of insulin on leptin production in humans: studies in vivo and in vitro. Diabetes 1996; 45(5):699–701.

57. Kolaczynski JW, Ohannesian JP, Considine RV, et al. Response of leptin to short-term and prolonged overfeeding in humans. J Clin Endocrinol Metab 1996; 81(11): 4162–4165.

58. Weigle DS, Cummings DE, Newby PD, et al. Roles of leptin and ghrelin in the loss of body weight caused by a low fat, high carbohydrate diet. J Clin Endocrinol Metab 2003; 88(4):1577–1586.

59. Saad MF, Damani S, Gingerich RL, et al. Sexual dimorphism in plasma leptin concentration. J Clin Endocrinol Metab 1997; 82(2):579–584.

60. Rosenbaum M, Nicolson M, Hirsch J, et al. Effects of gender, body composition, and menopause on plasma concentrations of leptin. J Clin Endocrinol Metab 1996; 81(9):3424–3427.

61. Kennedy A, Gettys TW, Watson P, et al. The metabolic significance of leptin in humans: gender-based differences in relationship to adiposity, insulin sensitivity, and energy expenditure. J Clin Endocrinol Metab 1997; 82(4):1293–1300.

62. Licinio J, Mantzoros C, Negrao AB, et al. Human leptin levels are pulsatile and inversely related to pituitary-adrenal function. Nat Med 1997; 3(5):575–579.

63. Halaas JL, Gajiwala KS, Maffei M, et al. Weight-reducing effects of the plasma protein encoded by the obese gene. Science 1995; 269(5223):543–546.

64. Hukshorn CJ, Saris WH, Westerterp-Plantenga MS, et al. Weekly subcutaneous pegylated recombinant native human leptin (PEG-OB) administration in obese men. J Clin Endocrinol Metab 2000; 85(11):4003–4009.

65. Heymsfield SB, Greenberg AS, Fujioka K, et al. Recombinant leptin for weight loss in obese and lean adults: a randomized, controlled, dose-escalation trial. JAMA 1999; 282(16):1568–1575.

66. Hamann A, Matthaei S. Regulation of energy balance by leptin. Exp Clin Endocrinol Diabetes 1996; 104(4): 293–300.

67. Berthoud HR. Interactions between the "cognitive" and "metabolic" brain in the control of food intake. Physiol Behav 2007; 91(5):486–498.

68. Christopoulos G, Perry KJ, Morfis M, et al. Multiple amylin receptors arise from receptor activity-modifying protein interaction with the calcitonin receptor gene product. Mol Pharmacol 1999; 56(1):235–242.

69. Hay DL, Christopoulos G, Christopoulos A, et al. Amylin receptors: molecular composition and pharmacology. Biochem Soc Trans 2004; 32(pt 5):865–867.

70. Muff R, Bühlmann N, Fischer JA, et al. An amylin receptor is revealed following co-transfection of a calcitonin receptor with receptor activity modifying proteins-1 or -3. Endocrinology 1999; 140(6):2924–2927.

71. Sexton PM, Morfis M, Tilakaratne N, et al. Complexing receptor pharmacology: modulation of family B G protein-coupled receptor function by RAMPs. Ann N Y Acad Sci 2006; 1070:90–104.

72. Barth SW, Riediger T, Lutz TA, et al. Peripheral amylin activates circumventricular organs expressing calcitonin receptor a/b subtypes and receptor-activity modifying proteins in the rat. Brain Res 2004; 997(1):97–102.

73. Fry M, Hoyda TD, Ferguson AV. Making sense of it: roles of the sensory circumventricular organs in feeding and regulation of energy homeostasis. Exp Biol Med 2007; 232(1):14–26.

74. Lutz TA, Senn M, Althaus J, et al. Lesion of the area postrema nucleus of the solitary tract (AP/NTS) attenuates the anorectic effects of amylin and calcitonin gene-related peptide (CGRP) in rats. Peptides 1998; 19(2):309–317.

75. Rushing PA, Seeley RJ, Air EL, et al. Acute 3rd-ventricular amylin infusion potently reduces food intake but does not produce aversive consequences. Peptides 2002; 23(5): 985–988.

76. Rushing PA, Hagan MM, Seeley RJ, et al. Amylin: a novel action in the brain to reduce body weight. Endocrinology 2000; 141(2):850–853.

77. Jodka C, Green D, Young A, et al. Amylin modulation of gastric emptying in rats depends upon an intact vagus nerve. Diabetes 1996; 45(suppl 2):235A (abstr 867).

78. Rowland NE, Crews EC, Gentry RM. Comparison of Fos induced in rat brain by GLP-1 and amylin. Regul Pept 1997; 71(3):171–174.

79. Riediger T, Schmid HA, Lutz T, et al. Amylin potently activates AP neurons possibly via formation of the excitatory second messenger cGMP. Am J Physiol Regul Integr Comp Physiol 2001; 281(6):R1833–R1843.

80. Rinaman L, Baker EA, Hoffman GE, et al. Medullary c-Fos activation in rats after ingestion of a satiating meal. Am J Physiol 1998; 275(1 pt 2):R262–R268.

81. Riediger T, Zuend D, Becskei C, et al. The anorectic hormone amylin contributes to feeding-related changes of neuronal activity in key structures of the gut-brain axis. Am J Physiol Regul Integr Comp Physiol 2004; 286(1): R114–R122.

82. Barth SW, Riediger T, Lutz TA, et al. Differential effects of amylin and salmon calcitonin on neuropeptide gene expression in the lateral hypothalamic area and the arcuate nucleus of the rat. Neurosci Lett 2003; 341(2):131–134.

83. Kelley AE, Baldo BA, Pratt WE, et al. Corticostriatal-hypothalamic circuitry and food motivation: integration of energy, action and reward. Physiol Behav 2005; 86(5): 773–795.

84. Mack C, Wilson J, Athanacio J, et al. Pharmacological actions of the peptide hormone amylin in the long-term regulation of food intake, food preference, and body weight. Am J Physiol Regulatory Integrative Comp Physiol 2007; 293:1855–1863.

85. Broberger C, Landry M, Wong H, et al. Subtypes Y1 and Y2 of the neuropeptide Y receptor are respectively expressed in pro-opiomelanocortin- and neuropeptide-Y-containing neurons of the rat hypothalamic arcuate nucleus. Neuroendocrinology 1997; 66(6):393–408.

86. Jobst EE, Enriori PJ, Cowley MA. The electrophysiology of feeding circuits. Trends Endocrinol Metab 2004; 15(10):488–499.

87. Challis BG, Coll AP, Yeo GS, et al. Mice lacking pro-opiomelanocortin are sensitive to high-fat feeding but respond normally to the acute anorectic effects of peptide-YY3-36. Proc Natl Acad Sci USA 2004; 101(13):4695–4700.

88. McLean KJ, Jarrott B, Lawrence AJ. Neuropeptide Y gene expression and receptor autoradiography in hypertensive and normotensive rat brain. Brain Res Mol Brain Res 1996; 35(1–2):249–259.

89. Lynch DR, Walker MW, Miller RJ, et al. Neuropeptide Y receptor binding sites in rat brain: differential autoradiographic localizations with 125I-peptide YY and 125I-neuropeptide Y imply receptor heterogeneity. J Neurosci 1989; 9(8):2607–2619.

90. Chen CH, Stephens RL Jr., Rogers RC. PYY and NPY: control of gastric motility via action on Y1 and Y2 receptors in the DVC. Neurogastroenterol Motil 1997; 9(2):109–116.

91. Browning KN, Travagli RA. Neuropeptide Y and peptide YY inhibit excitatory synaptic transmission in the rat

dorsal motor nucleus of the vagus. J Physiol 2003; 549(3):775–785.

92. Dumont Y, St-Pierre JA, Quirion R. Comparative autoradiographic distribution of neuropeptide Y Y1 receptors visualized with the Y1 receptor agonist. Neuroreport 1996; 7(4):901–904.

93. Cox JE, Randich A. Enhancement of feeding suppression by PYY(3-36) in rats with area postrema ablations. Peptides 2004; 25(6):985–989.

94. Koda S, Date Y, Murakami N, et al. The role of the vagal nerve in peripheral PYY3-36-induced feeding reduction in rats. Endocrinology 2005; 146(5):2369–2375.

95. Halatchev IG, Cone RD. Peripheral administration of PYY (3-36) produces conditioned taste aversion in mice. Cell Metab 2005; 1(3):159–168.

96. Nonaka N, Shioda S, Niehoff ML, et al. Characterization of blood-brain barrier permeability to PYY3-36 in the mouse. J Pharmacol Exp Ther 2003; 306(3):948–953.

97. Banks WA, Kastin AJ, Huang WT, et al. Leptin enters the brain by a saturable system independent of insulin. Peptides 1996; 17(2):305–311.

98. Schwartz MW, Baskin DG, Bukowski TR, et al. Specificity of leptin action on elevated blood glucose levels and hypothalamic neuropeptide Y gene expression in ob/ob mice. Diabetes 1996; 45(4):531–535.

99. Mizuno TM, Mobbs CV. Hypothalamic agouti-related protein messenger ribonucleic acid is inhibited by leptin and stimulated by fasting. Endocrinology 1999; 140(2): 814–817.

100. Levin BE, Dunn-Meynell AA, Banks WA. Obesity-prone rats have normal blood-brain barrier transport but defective central leptin signaling prior to obesity onset. Am J Physiol Regul Integr Comp Physiol 2004; 286(1):R143–R150.

101. Munzberg H, Flier JS, Bjorbaek C. Region-specific leptin resistance within the hypothalamus of diet-induced obese mice. Endocrinology 2004; 145(11):4880–4889.

102. Bjorbaek C, Elmquist JK, Frantz JD, et al. Identification of SOCS-3 as a potential mediator of central leptin resistance. Mol Cell 1998; 1(4):619–625.

103. Elmquist JK, Maratos-Flier E, Saper CB, et al. Unraveling the central nervous system pathways underlying responses to leptin. Nat Neurosci 1998; 1(6):445–450.

104. Hommel JD, Trinko R, Sears RM, et al. Leptin receptor signaling in midbrain dopamine neurons regulates feeding. Neuron 2006; 51(6):801–810.

105. Fulton S, Pissios P, Manchon RP, et al. Leptin regulation of the mesoaccumbens dopamine pathway. Neuron 2006; 51(6):811–822.

106. Mercer JG, Moar KM, Hoggard N. Localization of leptin receptor (Ob-R) messenger ribonucleic acid in the rodent hindbrain. Endocrinology 1998; 139(1):29–34.

107. Hosoi T, Kawagishi T, Okuma Y, et al. Brain stem is a direct target for leptin's action in the central nervous system. Endocrinology 2002; 143(9):3498–3504.

108. Grill HJ, Schwartz MW, Kaplan JM, et al. Evidence that the caudal brainstem is a target for the inhibitory effect of leptin on food intake. Endocrinology 2002; 143(1): 239–246.

109. Huo L, Maeng L, Bjorbaek C, et al. Leptin and the control of food intake: neurons in the nucleus of the solitary tract

are activated by both gastric distension and leptin. Endocrinology 2007; 148(5):2189–2197.

110. Matson CA, Wiater MF, Kuijper JL, et al. Synergy between leptin and cholecystokinin (CCK) to control daily caloric intake. Peptides 1997; 18(8):1275–1278.

111. Ladenheim EE, Emond M, Moran TH. Leptin enhances feeding suppression and neural activation produced by systemically administered bombesin. Am J Physiol Regul Integr Comp Physiol 2005; 289(2):R473–R477.

112. Williams KW, Smith BN. Rapid inhibition of neural excitability in the nucleus tractus solitarii by leptin: implications for ingestive behavior. J Physiol 2006; 573 (pt 2):395–412.

113. Baskin DG, Figlewicz Lattemann D, Seeley RJ, et al. Insulin and leptin: dual adiposity signals to the brain for the regulation of food intake and body weight. Brain Res 1999; 848(1–2):114–123.

114. Roth JD, Hughes H, Kendall E, et al. Anti-obesity effects of the β-cell hormone amylin in diet induced obese rats: effects on food intake, body weight, composition, energy expenditure and gene expression. Endocrinology 2006; 147(12):5855–5864.

115. Lutz TA. Pancreatic amylin as a centrally acting satiating hormone. Curr Drug Targets 2005; 6(2):181–189.

116. Chance WT, Balasubramaniam A, Chen X, et al. Tests of adipsia and conditioned taste aversion following the intrahypothalamic injection of amylin. Peptides 1992; 13(5):961–964.

117. Laugero KD, Mack C, Hankey M, et al. Rat amylin prevents stress-related feeding behavior. Society for Neuroscience: Abstract Viewer/Itinerary Planner 2005, Program No. 530.17 (abstr).

118. Eiden S, Daniel C, Steinbrueck A, et al. Salmon calcitonin—a potent inhibitor of food intake in states of impaired leptin signalling in laboratory rodents. J Physiol 2002; 541(pt 3):1041–1048.

119. Gebre-Medhin S, Mulder H, Pekny M, et al. Increased insulin secretion and glucose tolerance in mice lacking islet amyloid polypeptide (amylin). Biochem Biophys Res Commun 1998; 250(2):271–277.

120. Devine E, Young AA. Weight gain in male and female mice with amylin gene knockout. Diabetes 1998; 47 (suppl 1):A317 (abstr 1224).

121. Levin BE, Dunn-Meynell AA, Balkan B, et al. Selective breeding for diet-induced obesity and resistance in Sprague-Dawley rats. Am J Physiol 1997; 273(2 pt 2):R725–R730.

122. Janes S, Gaeta L, Beaumont K, et al. The selection of pramlintide for clinical evaluation. Diabetes 1996; 45 (suppl 2):235A (abstr 865).

123. Young AA, Vine W, Gedulin BR, et al. Preclinical pharmacology of pramlintide in the rat: comparisons with human and rat amylin. Drug Dev Res 1996; 37(4):231–248.

124. SYMLIN®. Available at: www.symlin.com. Accessed May 2007.

125. Chapman I, Parker B, Doran S, et al. Effect of pramlintide on satiety and food intake in obese subjects and subjects with type 2 diabetes. Diabetologia 2005; 48(5):838–848.

126. Chapman I, Parker B, Doran S, et al. Low-dose pramlintide reduced food intake and meal duration in healthy, normal weight subjects. Obesity 2007; 15(5):1179–1186.

127. Smith SR, Blundell JE, Burns C, et al. Pramlintide-treatment reduces 24-hour caloric intake and meal sizes, and improves control of eating in obese subjects: a 6-week translational research study. Am J Physiol Endocrinol Metab 2007; 293:620–627.

128. Aronne L, Fujioka K, Aroda V, et al. Progressive reduction in body weight following treatment with the amylin analog pramlintide in obese subjects: a phase 2, randomized, placebo-controlled, dose-escalation study. J Clin Endocrinol Metab 2007; 92(8):2977–2983.

129. Wadden T, Klein S, Aronne L, et al. Pramlintide treatment in obesity elicited progressive weight loss when used with a structured lifestyle intervention program: a randomized controlled trial. Obes Rev 2006; 7(suppl 2):112–113 (abstr PP0056).

130. Smith S, Klein E, Burns C, et al. Sustained weight loss following 1-y pramlintide treatment as an adjunct to lifestyle intervention in obesity. Diabetes 2007; 56(suppl 1):A88 (abstr 0335-OR).

131. Bhavsar S, Parkes D, Hoyt J, et al. PYY[3-36] decreases food consumption and improves glycemic control in Zucker Diabetes Fatty (ZDF) rats. Diabetes 2002; 51 (suppl 2):A418–A419 (abstr 1717-P).

132. Bhavsar S, Hoyt J, Paterniti JR, et al. Continuous infusion of PYY[3-36] reduces food consumption and body weight in Fatty Zucker (fa/fa) rats. Diabetes 2002; 51(suppl 2):A602. (abstr 2499-PO).

133. Challis BG, Pinnock SB, Coll AP, et al. Acute effects of PYY(3-36) on food intake and hypothalamic neuropeptide expression in the mouse. Biochem Biophys Res Commun 2003; 311(4):915–919.

134. Adams SH, Lei C, Jodka CM, et al. PYY[3-36] administration decreases the respiratory quotient and reduces adiposity in diet-induced obese mice. J Nutr 2006; 136(1):195–201.

135. Tschop M, Castaneda TR, Joost HG, et al. Physiology: does gut hormone PYY3-36 decrease food intake in rodents? Nature 2004; 430 (6996). Available at: http://www.nature.com/nature/journal/v430/n6996/full/nature02665.html. Accessed June 2007.

136. Koegler FH, Enriori PJ, Billes SK, et al. Peptide YY$_{(3-36)}$ inhibits morning, but not evening, food intake and decreases body weight in rhesus macaques. Diabetes 2005; 54(11):3198–3204.

137. Lush C, Chen K, Hompesch M, et al. A phase 1 study to evaluate the safety, tolerability, and pharmacokinetics of rising doses of AC162352 (synthetic human PYY$_{3-36}$) in lean and obese subjects. Obes Rev 2005; 6(suppl 1):21 (abstr O051).

138. Degen L, Oesch S, Casanova M, et al. Effect of peptide YY$_{3-36}$ on food intake in humans. Gastroenterology 2005; 129(5):1430–1436.

139. Gantz I, Erondu N, Mallick M, et al. Efficacy and safety of intranasal peptide YY3-36 for weight reduction in obese adults. J Clin Endocrinol Metab 2007; 92(5):1754–1757.

140. Roth JD, Coffey T, Jodka CM, et al. Combination therapy with amylin and peptide YY[3 36] in obese rodents: anorexigenic synergy and weight loss additivity. Endocrinology 2007; 148:6054–6061.

141. Farooqi IS. Leptin and the onset of puberty: insights from rodent and human genetics. Semin Reprod Med 2002; 20(2):139–144.

142. Shimomura I, Hammer RE, Ikemoto S, et al. Leptin reverses insulin resistance and diabetes mellitus in mice with congenital lipodystrophy. Nature 1999; 401 (6748):73–76.

143. Asilmaz E, Cohen P, Miyazaki M, et al. Site and mechanism of leptin action in a rodent form of congenital lipodystrophy. J Clin Invest 2004; 113(3):414–424.

144. Halaas JL, Boozer C, Blair-West J, et al. Physiological response to long-term peripheral and central leptin infusion in lean and obese mice. Proc Natl Acad Sci USA 1997; 94(16):8878–8883.

145. Farooqi IS, Matarese G, Lord GM, et al. Beneficial effects of leptin on obesity, T cell hyporesponsiveness, and neuroendocrine/metabolic dysfunction of human congenital leptin deficiency. J Clin Invest 2002; 110(8): 1093–1103.

146. Farooqi IS, Jebb SA, Langmack G, et al. Effects of recombinant leptin therapy in a child with congenital leptin deficiency. N Engl J Med 1999; 341(12):879–884.

147. Oral EA, Simha V, Ruiz E, et al. Leptin-replacement therapy for lipodystrophy. N Engl J Med 2002; 346(8): 570–578.

148. Ebihara K, Kusakabe T, Hirata M, et al. Efficacy and safety of leptin-replacement therapy and possible mechanisms of leptin actions in patients with generalized lipodystrophy. J Clin Endocrinol Metab 2007; 92(2): 532–541.

149. Licinio J, Caglayan S, Ozata M, et al. Phenotypic effects of leptin replacement on morbid obesity, diabetes mellitus, hypogonadism, and behavior in leptin-deficient adults. Proc Natl Acad Sci USA 2004; 101(13):4531–4536.

150. Javor ED, Cochran EK, Musso C, et al. Long-term efficacy of leptin replacement in patients with generalized lipodystrophy. Diabetes 2005; 54(7):1994–2002.

22

Neuropeptide Y in the Management of Obesity

IRA GANTZ and NGOZI E. ERONDU

Clinical Research, Metabolism, Merck Research Laboratories, Rahway, New Jersey, U.S.A.

INTRODUCTION

Neuropeptide Y (NPY) was initially identified as an orexigenic neuropeptide more than two decades ago. Since then, numerous pharmacological, neuroanatomical, and genetic studies indicate that an NPY energy regulatory system consisting of NPY neurons in the hypothalamus and brain stem, mediating their actions through the NPY Y1 and Y5 receptors (NPY1R and NPY5R), constitutes a pivotal anabolic pathway in mammals, promoting positive energy balance by increasing food intake and decreasing energy expenditure. Consistent with its role in energy balance, NPY synthesis and release is controlled by nutrients and hormones, which transmit the acute and chronic status of peripheral energy stores. On the basis of these data, the NPY1R and NPY5R have been considered potential targets for antiobesity drug development. In this chapter, we will first provide an overview of the NPY family of peptides and cognate receptors, followed by a review of pharmacological, neuroanatomical, and genetic studies that support the role of this system in the regulation of energy homeostasis. We will conclude by describing clinical trials that have been conducted to examine the efficacy of NPY5 receptor blockade for the treatment of obesity.

NPY FAMILY OF PEPTIDES

NPY is one of three evolutionarily and structurally related peptides, which include peptide YY (PYY) and pancreatic polypeptide (PP). These peptides were discovered utilizing a strategy designed to isolate C-terminally amidated peptides; a strategy that was based on the knowledge that several brain-gut peptide hormones known at the time were amidated (1–4). The nomenclature (NPY and PYY) derives from the presence of a tyrosine residue (abbreviated by the letter Y in the single-letter amino acid code) at both ends of these molecules.

NPY RECEPTORS

NPY, PYY, and PP act upon the same family of G-protein-coupled seven transmembrane receptors, which are classified together as NPY receptors (5). NPY Y1, Y2, Y4, Y5, and y6 receptors have been cloned and characterized pharmacologically. Of note, the y6 receptor is only functionally expressed in mice (6–8). The y6 gene is absent in the rat and is a nonfunctional pseudogene in rabbits and primates. The restricted presence of the y6 receptor in mice has the potential to confound studies of the NPY system in that species. The existence of a y3 receptor is based on circumstantial pharmacological evidence since it has not been cloned and no specific agonists or antagonists have been identified to date (9,10). The NPY5R is largely restricted to the central nervous system (CNS) (11), whereas the NPY1R has been detected in multiple rodent and human tissues including brain, heart, kidney, and gastrointestinal tract (12).

With regard to endogenous agonists, the NPY Y1, Y2, and Y5 receptors preferentially bind NPY and PYY, whereas the NPY4R preferentially binds PP. Relative to NPY1R and NPY4R, the NPY2R and NPY5R are also potently activated by NPY_{3-36} and PYY_{3-36} (13–16). Both NPY_{3-36} and PYY_{3-36} are believed to be derived from dipeptidyl peptidase IV processing of the native peptides (17). The primary consequence of this cleavage is to significantly diminish the affinity of PYY_{3-36} at the NPY1R compared with PYY_{1-36}. However, PYY_{3-36} retains approximately the same affinity for the NPY2R and has only slightly diminished affinity at the NPY5R compared with PYY_{1-36}. This affinity profile has potential relevance to the development of PYY_{3-36} as an antiobesity drug since a narrow therapeutic window might be encountered between activation of the anorexigenic NPY2R and the orexigenic NPY5R (18).

THE NPY SYSTEM IN ENERGY HOMEOSTASIS

NPY was first identified as an orexigenic factor more than two decades ago (19–21), and since that time data from numerous pharmacological, neuroanatomical, and genetic studies have supported the hypothesis that an NPY system consisting of NPY, NPY1R, and NPY5R is an important energy homeostatic pathway in mammals. This chapter will focus on preclinical and clinical advances related to the development of NPY1R and NPY5R antagonists. Attempts to develop anorexigenic PYY_{3-36}, PP, or NPY2/4R agonists for the management of obesity are beyond the scope of this chapter since these are not components of the anabolic NPY system.

Pharmacological Studies

Substantial experimental evidence indicates that NPY mediates its effects on energy homeostasis through both the NPY1R and NPY5R (13,22–24). The selective NPY1R agonists, [D-Arg^{25}]NPY and [D-His^{26}]NPY potently stimulate feeding behavior (25). Conversely, the selective NPY1R antagonist, J-115814, suppresses NPY-induced feeding in satiated rats and attenuates spontaneous feeding in C57BL6 and genetically obese db/db mice (26). Oral administration of the NPY1R antagonist J-104870 (6-(5-ethyl-1,3-thiazol-2-ylthio-

methyl)-2-[3-methoxy-5-(2-propenyloxycarbonylamino) benzyl-amino]-4 morpholinopyridine) significantly suppresses daily food intake and body weight gain of *fatty* Zucker rats. Although food intake in this experiment gradually returned to near the control levels, the body weight of the treated animals remained significantly less than that of controls (27).

Similarly, studies have demonstrated that the selective NPY5R agonists, [Ala^{31}, Aib^{32}]NPY (28) and [D-Trp^{34}] NPY (29) potently stimulate food intake in rats. The effect of [D-Trp^{34}]NPY was blocked by the selective NPY5R antagonist, CGP 71683A. CGP 71683A also potently antagonizes NPY-induced food intake in lean satiated, fasted, and streptozotocin diabetic rats and decreases body weight over 28 days in free-feeding lean rats (30). However, off-target effects of CGP 71683A have also been reported (31). The selective NPY5R antagonist GW438014 was reported to reduce NPY-induced and normal overnight food intake in rats and to decrease weight gain in *fatty* Zucker rats (32). Another highly selective NPY5R antagonist L-152804 (3,3-dimethyl-9-(4,4-dimethyl-2,6-dioxocyclohexyl-1-oxo-1,2,3,4-tetrahydroxanthene) was demonstrated to block [D-Trp^{34}]NPY-induced hyperphagia and weight gain in mice (33), to ameliorate diet-induced obesity in mice, and was efficacious in inducing weight loss in a nonhuman primate (rhesus macaque) diet-induced obese model (34). However, it had no effect on lean mice fed a regular diet or on genetically obese db/db mice (27). In contrast to pair-fed DIO rats who showed reduced body temperature, those receiving the NPY5R antagonist had unaltered body temperature and upregulation of uncoupling protein mRNA in brown and white adipose tissue, which is consistent with modulation of energy expenditure in addition to suppression of food intake (35). On the other hand, it was reported that the selective antagonist NPY5RA-972 had no significant effect on food intake in free-feeding Wistar rats or obese Zucker rats and that its chronic administration had no effect on body weight in free-feeding Wistar or diet-induced obese rats (36).

The NPY5R antagonist MK-0557, *trans-N*-[1-(2-fluorophenyl)-3-pyrazolyl]-3-oxospiro-[6 azaisobenzofuran-1 (3*H*), 1′-cyclohexane]-4′-carboxamide, is particularly important since it is the first compound to be used in clinical studies to examine the NPY system. MK-0557, is a high affinity ($K_i = 1.3$ nM), orally bioavailable NPY5R antagonist, which has greater than 7500-fold selectivity for the NPY5R versus the other cloned NPYR subtypes (37). MK-0557 was demonstrated to induce weight loss and suppress body weight gain in rodents and to potently antagonize the effects of the NPY5R-selective agonist, D-Trp^{34}NPY, on body weight gain and hyperphagia in C57BL/6J mice (38). When lean mice were switched from regular chow to a medium high-fat diet (4.2 kcal/g) (Oriental BioService, Tsukuba, Japan: 53.4% energy as carbohydrate, 15.3% as protein and 31.3% as fat), treatment with MK-0557 at 30 mg/kg PO q.d. induced a 40% reduction in body weight gain at day 35 ($p < 0.05$ vs. control). In addition to this effect on body weight, there was a reduction of $\sim 30\%$ in retroperitoneal fat pad weight ($p < 0.05$), $\sim 22\%$ in epididymal and mesenteric fat pad weights (n.s.), and $\sim 36\%$ in leptin levels ($p < 0.05$). There was also a $\sim 5\%$ reduction in cumulative food intake compared with controls (n.s.).

While the above referenced pharmacological studies strongly implicate both the NPY1R and NPY5R in energy regulation, they do not define the relative contribution of these receptors to NPY-mediated energy regulation. Whether the NPY1R or NPY5R represents a better target for antiobesity drug development has been (and remains) controversial. In an attempt to answer this question, NPY1R $-/-$ and NPY5R $-/-$ mice were generated on a similar genetic background and compared (39). In this study, NPY-induced food intake was markedly reduced in NPY1R $-/-$ mice but not in NPY5R $-/-$ mice, suggesting that the NPY1R has a dominant role in NPY-induced feeding. However, the potential limitations of genetic approaches (see below) and the fact that rodent results do not necessarily predict human outcomes, limit the conclusions that can be drawn from this study.

Neuroanatomical Studies

NPY is widely expressed in the central and peripheral nervous system (40–43). In the CNS, NPY neuronal cell bodies are primarily found in the brain stem (locus coeruleus and nucleus of the solitary tract) and hypothalamus (arcuate nucleus, ARC) (41,44). NPY neurons in both the ARC and brain stem appear to play a role in energy homeostasis (45–50).

Evidence supporting a role for brain stem NPY neurons in energy regulation is both anatomical and physiological. Brain stem NPY neurons send projections that innervate a number of hypothalamic nuclei involved in energy regulation, including the ARC, ventromedial nucleus (VMN), dorsomedial nucleus (DMN), and paraventricular nucleus (PVN), and contribute substantially to the NPY present in those nuclei. For example, studies in rats involving neural transections at the level of the dorsal tegmentum in the mesencephalon demonstrated marked (50–60%) reduction in NPY levels in four hypothalamic sites, including the PVN and the DMN (45). Furthermore, these neural transections made rats hypersensitive to the effects of NPY presumably due to denervation-induced hyperresponsiveness (51). Finally, it is worth noting that brain stem NPY neurons coproduce several other orexigenic transmitters, including norepinephrine, epinephrine, and galanin (52).

The cytoarchitecture of the ARC is notable in that it contains two physiologically opposing neuronal populations, the anorexigenic/catabolic pro-opiomelanocortin (POMC) neurons in the ventrolateral and dorsomedial ARC and the orexigenic/anabolic NPY neurons in the ventromedial ARC (46,48,49,53). Notably, NPY neurons in the ARC coproduce the orexigenic protein agouti-related protein (AgRP) (54,55) and the inhibitory neurotransmitter γ-aminobutyric acid (GABA) (56). AgRP is an inverse agonist at the anorexigenic melanocortin-3 and -4 receptors (57) and is believed to be an important modulator of melanocortin system tone. Since NPY neurons in the ARC are the only NPY neurons in the CNS that produce AgRP, this peptide has conveniently served experimentally as a means of identifying NPY fibers originating exclusively from the ARC.

In contrast, POMC neurons produce the anorexigenic melanocortin peptides α-, β-melanocyte-stimulating hormone (MSH) and the anorexigenic protein, cocaine- and amphetamine-regulated transcript (CART) (58–61). POMC/CART neurons also produce GABA (62). NPY neurons have been shown to contact nearby POMC neurons and inhibit them through the release of GABA (63). Interestingly, the inhibition of POMC neurons by NPY appears to be unidirectional, suggesting an asymmetry in the ARC circuitry that favors orexigenic drive (49).

Consistent with its prominent regulatory role in energy balance, NPY synthesis and release by the NPY neuron is controlled by hormones that transmit the status of peripheral energy stores, including insulin (64–66), ghrelin (67–70), and PYY$_{3-36}$ (71). NPY neurons are also likely modulated by circulating nutrients such as glucose (72,73) and long-chain fatty acids (74).

As would be anticipated for a neuronal population that plays a crucial role in energy regulation, ARC NPY neurons are interconnected with other hypothalamic nuclei/areas and regulatory systems involved in energy homeostasis. Several examples illustrating this point are described in the ensuing paragraphs.

ARC NPY neurons project to the PVN (75,76), where they come in close contact with corticotropin-releasing hormone (CRH) (77) and thyrotropin-releasing hormone (TRH) (78,79) neurons. It should be noted that the majority of NPY innervation of PVN CRH neurons apparently originates outside the ARC (80). Both CRH and TRH are anorexigenic (48) and also have profound influences on metabolism through the pituitary-adrenal axis and autonomic nervous system (CRH) (81) and hypothalamic-pituitary-thyroid axis (TRH).

ARC NPY neurons innervate two neuronal populations in the lateral hypothalamic area (LHA), which have a prominent role in feeding behavior—melanin-concentrating hormone (MCH) and orexin (also referred to as hypocretin) neurons (82,83). Moreover, there is a heavy reciprocal innervation of ARC NPY neurons by orexin terminals from the LHA (84). Orexins have been reported to have a stimulatory action on NPY neurons (85), constituting one mechanism through which orexins may increase food intake. This is supported by studies showing that orexin-stimulated feeding in satiated rats is inhibited by Y1R and Y5R antagonists (86,87).

Neurons in both the LHA and PVN are known to send projections to autonomic nervous system–related structures in the brain stem and spinal cord (46,88). Therefore, by modulating target neurons in the PVN and LHA, NPY neurons have the potential to decrease energy expenditure by affecting autonomic outflow to peripheral organs.

ARC NPY neurons also innervate the DMN, which is recognized to be a nucleus involved in energy regulation (89). Actually, the DMN contains neurons that normally produce a small amount of NPY and under certain physiological conditions such as lactation, DMN NPY mRNA may be upregulated (90–92).

Finally, the NPY system interacts with the anorexigenic serotonin system (93–95) and the potential relevance of this interaction is discussed later in this chapter in the context of a clinical study (the coadministration study).

The distribution of the NPY1R and NPY5R is consistent with their role and the role of NPY in energy homeostasis. As described below, the distribution of these receptors is consistent with an inhibition of the melanocortin system by the NPY system in the ARC and a dueling counterregulatory circuitry of the NPY and melanocortin systems in the PVN.

NPY1R are expressed in multiple hypothalamic nuclei and in several extrahypothalamic forebrain and hindbrain sites involved in feeding and/or autonomic regulation. (96). In this regard, it is particularly notable that NPY1R are expressed by the anorexigenic POMC neuron in the ARC (53,97). In the PVN, NPY1R colocalize with melanocortin-4 receptors (96) and are expressed by TRH neurons (96,98).

The NPY5R is highly expressed in the human hypothalamus, including those nuclei/areas associated with energy homeostasis such as the ARC, PVN, DMN, VMN, and LHA (99,100). In the mouse, β-gal-positive staining, which served as a proxy for NPY5R expression in NPY5R −/− mice, was found in ARC neurons that expressed β-endorphin (presumably indicating POMC neurons as POMC is the precursor prohormone for β-endorphin) (101). In the PVN, the NPY5R is expressed by a subpopulation of CRH neurons (102). This is in contrast to the NPY1R, which apparently is not expressed by the CRH neuron (77,98).

Genetic Studies

Initial genetic studies using a germ line knockout approach to investigate the role of NPY in energy homeostasis raised doubt about the essential role of NPY in the

regulation of body weight. NPY knockout (NPY −/−) mice were observed to have normal food intake and body weight, although NPY −/− mice bred to *ob/ob* leptin-deficient mice demonstrated partial reduction of the *ob/ob* obese phenotype (103,104). NPY1R −/− mice had only slightly diminished spontaneous and NPY-stimulated feeding and paradoxically developed late onset mild obesity (105,106). Similarly, NPY5R −/− mice had normal feeding response and developed late onset mild obesity (107). However, more recent genetic investigations, which have approached the question of the role of NPY in the regulation of body weight by examining hypothalamic NPY expression in adult mice, have generated results that are consistent with a critical role for NPY in energy homeostasis. Expression of antisense cRNA in the ARC of adult male rats led to a 40% less weight gain than controls at the end of the 50-day study, and cumulative food intake was significantly lower from day 23 (108). Similarly, a transgenic neurotoxin approach, which led to a 20% to 47% ablation of AgRP neurons by 16 weeks of age, resulted in a significantly reduced body weight and food intake (109). Even more convincingly, acute ablation of NPY/AgRP neurons in adult mice, using a toxin receptor-mediated cell ablation strategy, led to significant reduction in food intake and body weight (110,111). These studies also suggest that developmental compensation might account for the relatively small impact observed in earlier genetic studies.

CLINICAL TRIALS

Significant efforts to develop antagonists to the NPY1R and NPY5R for the treatment of obesity have been underway in the pharmaceutical industry for a number of years. A detailed description of the structurally diverse NPY1R and NPY5R antagonists reported in the scientific and patent literature is beyond the scope of this chapter (112). To date, no weight loss trials have been reported with NPY1R antagonists, and it is unclear if any NPY1R antagonists have been administered to subjects in phase I studies. The development of NPY5R antagonists is more advanced. Recently, the results of clinical studies that examined the efficacy of the NPY5R antagonist, MK-0557, to induce weight loss and prevent weight regain in overweight and obese patients were published (38,113). In addition, there was a press release of the results of clinical trials with another NPY5R antagonist, S-2367 (114). The results of these studies are discussed below.

Long-Term Weight Loss Study with MK-0557

This 52-week study was preceded by two studies (described below), which established the brain receptor occupancy (RO) as well as the proof of principle for MK-0557, a selective antagonist of the NPY5R. In all these studies, MK-0557 was generally safe and well tolerated.

MK-0557 Receptor Occupancy Studies

To assist dose selection for clinical trials, positron-emission tomography (PET) studies were conducted in healthy volunteers using the selective PET ligand, [^{11}C]MK-0233, which has a similar structure and NPY5R affinity as MK-0557. Compared with predose baseline, NPY5R occupancies (RO) 24 hours after a single oral 125-, 5-, or 1.25-mg dose of MK-0557 were (mean ± SD) 107 ± 5%, 105 ± 3%, and 98 ± 5%, respectively. The RO, five days after a single oral dose 5 mg, remained fairly high, with a mean (±SD) value of 69 ± 24%, while placebo subjects had a RO of 3 ± 9%. These data were consistent with essentially complete receptor occupancy at the relatively small (1.25 mg), single dose of MK-0557.

MK-0557 Proof-of-Concept/Dose Range Finding Study

This multicenter, double-blind, randomized, placebo-controlled study included a six-week diet and exercise run-in, the last two weeks of which subjects were dosed a single-blind placebo, followed by 12 weeks of double-blind drug treatment and 12 weeks of off-drug follow-up period. Five hundred and forty-seven subjects were randomized in a 1:1:1:1:1 ratio to placebo or 0.2-, 1-, 5- or 25-mg MK-0557; 402 subjects completed the 12-week double-blind treatment period while 354 subjects completed the entire study. There were no significant differences in patient discontinuations between the treatment groups. The primary analysis population was a modified intention to treat (MITT) population, defined as those subjects who received at least one dose of double-blind study medication and had at least one postrandomization weight measurement.

As shown in Table 1, the mean change from baseline body weight after 12 weeks in the MITT population was −0.6, −1.3, −1.9, −1.7, and −2.0 kg for subjects treated with placebo or 0.2-, 1-, 5-, and 25-mg MK-0557, respectively. The 1-, 5-, and 25-mg dose groups were significantly different from placebo ($p \leq 0.001$), while the 0.2-mg dose group was not significantly different from placebo ($p = 0.054$). There were no statistically significant differences between the 1-, 5-, and 25-mg dose groups, consistent with a plateau in the dose-response curve. For subjects who completed 12 weeks of double-blind treatment with no major protocol violations, all dose groups were significantly different from placebo ($p \leq 0.001$ for 1-, 5-, and 25 mg, and $p = 0.036$ for 0.2 mg). Subjects, who entered the off-drug period, generally maintained the weight loss induced during the 12-week treatment phase.

Table 1 Analysis of Weight (kg) Change with MK-0557 or Placebo

LS mean (95% CI)	MITT	Per protocol completers
Proof-of-concept/dose ranging study[a]		
Placebo	−0.6 (−1.1, −0.1)	−0.7 (−1.3, −0.0)
0.2 mg	−1.3 (−1.8, −0.8)	−1.6 (−2.3, −1.0)
1 mg	−1.9 (−2.4, −1.4)	−2.2 (−2.9, −1.5)
5 mg	−1.7 (−2.3, −1.2)	−2.1 (−2.7, −1.4)
25 mg	−2.0 (−2.5, −1.4)	−2.3 (−3.0, −1.7)
Long-term study[b]		
Placebo	−1.1 (−1.5, −0.6)	−1.8 (−2.6, −1.0)
1 mg	−2.2 (−2.5, 1.8)	−3.4 (−4.0, −2.8)

[a]12 weeks of treatment.
[b]52 weeks of treatment.
Source: From Ref. 38.

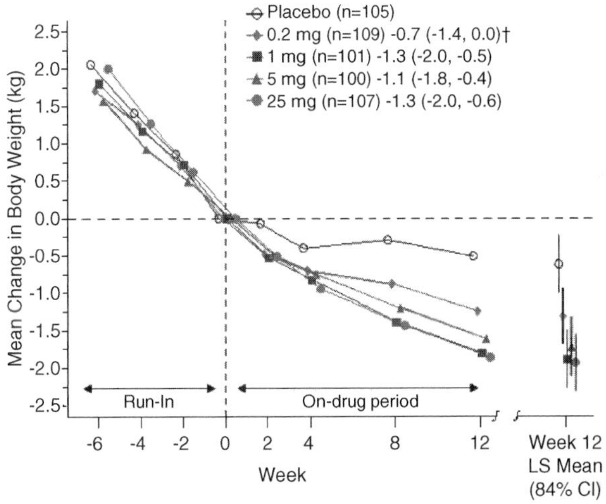

Figure 1 Change in body weight (kg) during the run-in and on-drug period in the MK-0557 proof-of-concept study/dose ranging study (MITT population). *Abbreviation*: MITT, modified intention to treat. *Source*: From Ref. 38.

On the basis of the absence of a plateau (over time) in the weight loss over the 12-week treatment period (Figure 1), the possibility that continued weight loss might be observed over a longer treatment period could not be ruled out.

MK-0557 Long-Term Weight Loss Study

This 52-week, multicenter, double-blind, randomized, placebo-controlled study included a 2-week diet and exercise single-blind placebo run-in followed by the randomization in a 1:2 ratio of 1661 patients to placebo or 1-mg MK-0557. Similar to the 12-week study, the primary analysis was conducted in a MITT population, consisting of 1555 patients (106 patients were excluded because of a lack of postbaseline data). A total of 832 patients (∼49%

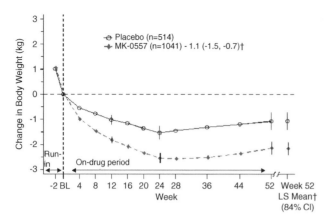

Figure 2 Change in body weight (kg) during run-in and on-drug phase in the MK-0557 long-term study (MITT population). The symbol † indicates LS mean estimates and 84% CI based on Analysis of Covariance (ANCOVA) model with terms for treatment, baseline body weight, center, and run-in weight change. Eighty-four percent CI on the observed means shown at weeks 12, 24, and 52. Last observation carried forward. *Abbreviations*: MITT, modified intention to treat; BL, baseline; LS, least squares; CI, confidence interval. *Source*: From Ref. 38.

of patients randomized to placebo and 51% of patients randomized to MK-0557) completed the study without major protocol violations.

The results of this study are summarized in Table 1 and Figure 2. After 52 weeks, the mean change from baseline (95% CI) for the MITT population was −1.1 (−1.5, −0.6) kg and −2.2 (−2.5, 1.8) kg for patients on placebo and 1-mg MK-0557, respectively. In the per protocol completers, defined as patients who completed the 52-week treatment period without major protocol violations, the mean weight loss from baseline was −1.8 (−2.6, −1.0) kg and −3.4 (−4.0, −2.8) kg for patients on placebo and 1-mg MK-0557, respectively. In the two analysis populations, the difference in mean weight loss between the treatment groups was significant ($p < 0.001$). There was also a significant difference in the percent of patients who lost ≥5% (5% responders) or ≥10% (10% responders) of their baseline body weight. The proportion of 5% responders was 17.5% and 23.3% for patients treated with placebo and MK-0557, respectively; with an adjusted odds ratio (95% CI) of 1.5 (1.1, 2.0), $p = 0.006$, while the proportion of 10% responders was 5.6% and 8.7% for patients treated with placebo and MK-0557, respectively; with an adjusted odds ratio (95% CI) of 1.7(1.1, 2.6), $p = 0.022$. No significant differences were observed in obesity related comorbidity endpoints such as blood pressure, glycemic parameters, or lipid parameters.

The results of the long-term weight loss study described above indicate that the degree of weight loss observed with MK-0557, while statistically significant, was not clinically meaningful and was significantly less than that observed

for several other weight loss drugs (orlistat, sibutramine, rimonabant). On the basis of the results of the PET ligand and proof-of-concept/dose range finding studies, the 1-mg dose of MK-0557 used in the long-term study should have been adequate to test the hypothesis that the NPY5R was a useful target for antiobesity drug monotherapy in humans. The modest degree of statistically significant weight loss achieved does appear to validate the NPY5R as one component in the regulation of energy homeostasis in humans. One possible explanation for the modest weight loss efficacy observed with NPY5R blockade is that compensation by another orexigenic system (or the NPY1R component of the NPY system) may have overridden the effect of NPY5R antagonism.

Concurrent with the long-term weight loss study, two additional studies were conducted with MK-0557 to examine the effects on weight regain when administered after a very low calorie diet (VLCD) and to evaluate the weight loss efficacy when coadministered with sibutramine or orlistat (113,115).

Prevention of Weight Regain (Post-VLCD) Study with MK-0557

In this multicenter, double-blind, randomized, placebo-controlled study, 502 eligible patients aged 18 to 65 years with a body mass index (BMI) 30 to 43 kg/m² were placed on a liquid VLCD (800 kcal/day) for six weeks. Those patients who lost at least 6% of their initial body weight ($n = 359$) were randomized to 1 mg/day MK-0557 or placebo and were maintained on a hypocaloric diet (300 kcal below weight maintenance requirements) for 52 weeks. Seventy-three percent of patients in the placebo group and 70% of patients in the MK-0557-treated group completed 52 weeks of the post-VLCD phase.

During the VLCD phase, patients had an average weight loss of 9.1 kg. However, after 12 weeks of double-blind treatment, weight began to gradually increase for both placebo and MK-0557-treated patients (Figure 3). The mean body weight change (95% CI) from baseline at the end of the VLCD to week 52 was +3.1 (2.1, 4.0) kg and +1.5 (0.5, 2.4) kg for patients treated with placebo and MK-0557, respectively. Although treatment with MK-0557 prevented 50% of the post-VLCD weight regain observed in the placebo group and the difference of 1.6 kg between the two groups was statistically significant ($p = 0.014$), the magnitude of the effect was deemed small and not clinically meaningful (113). It should be noted that the efficacy of MK-0557 in preventing weight regain observed in this study is similar to the degree of efficacy observed in the long-term weight loss study described above. Consistent with the long-term weight loss study, these results indicate that the NPY5R plays a role in human energy homeostasis.

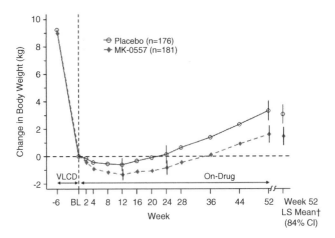

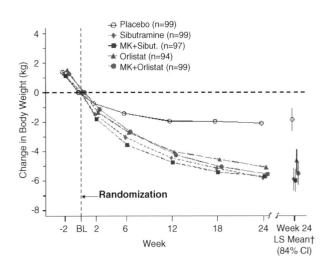

Figure 3 Change in body weight (kg) in the MK-0557 prevention of weight regain (post-VLCD) study (all patients treated population). The symbol † indicates LS mean estimates and 84% CI based on ANCOVA model with terms for treatment, baseline measurement, center, and run-in weight change. Eighty-four percent CI on the observed means shown at weeks 12, 24, and 52. *Abbreviations*: VLCD, very low calorie diet; BL, baseline; LS, least squares; CI, confidence interval. *Source*: From Ref. 113.

Figure 4 Mean change in body weight (kg) in the MK-0557 coadministration study with orlistat and sibutramine (MITT population). The symbol † indicates LS mean estimates (84% CI) based on ANCOVA model with terms for treatment, baseline body weight, center, and run-in weight change. *Abbreviations*: MITT, modified intention to treat; LS, least squares; CI, confidence interval. *Source*: From Ref. 115.

Coadministration (with Orlistat and Sibutramine) Study with MK-0557

The objective of this double-blind, placebo-controlled study was to evaluate whether MK-0557 might potentiate the weight loss effects of sibutramine and orlistat, two drugs that are currently approved for the treatment of obesity (115).

Four hundred and ninety-seven obese patients (BMI 30–43 kg/m^2) were randomized to one of five treatment arms: placebo, sibutramine 10 mg q.d., MK-0557 1-mg q.d. plus sibutramine 10 mg q.d., orlistat 120 mg t.i.d., and MK-0557 1 mg q.d. plus orlistat 120 mg t.i.d. Seventy-one percent in the placebo, 76% of patients in the sibutramine alone, 79% in the MK-0557 plus sibutramine, 69% in the orlistat alone, and 76% in the MK-0557 plus orlistat groups completed the study. As shown in Figure 4, MK-0557 did not induce significant weight loss when coadministered with sibutramine ($p = 0.892$) or with orlistat ($p = 0.250$), although there appeared to be a trend for greater weight loss in the MK-0557 plus orlistat group versus the orlistat alone group. The least squares (LS) mean difference (95% CI) in body weight change from baseline between MK-0557 plus orlistat and orlistat alone was -0.9 (-2.4, 0.6) kg and between MK-0557 plus sibutramine and sibutramine alone was -0.1 (-1.6, 1.4) kg.

Given the limited efficacy observed in the long-term and VLCD studies described above, the results of the coadministration study are not entirely surprising. Although the lack of statistical significance especially

for the orlistat component probably reflects the limited power of the study due to small sample size, the observed additional weight loss was quite small and not clinically meaningful. On the basis of the results of a pharmacokinetic interaction study, malabsorption of MK-0557 when coadministered with orlistat is an unlikely explanation for the lack of additional weight loss observed.

The interaction between the serotonin (5-HT) and NPY pathways could be one possible explanation for the lack of additional weight loss with MK-0557 plus sibutramine versus sibutramine alone. For example, fenfluramine (a serotonergic drug) reduces food intake and increases NPY levels in the VMN, DMN, and LH (95). Studies in rats have also shown that methysergide (a 5-HT antagonist) stimulates feeding and increases NPY mRNA levels and secretion in the PVN (93), while mCPP (m-chlorophenylpiperazine, a 5-HT$_{1B/2C}$ receptor agonist) reduces food intake and NPY levels in the PVN (94). Finally, sibutramine has been shown to dose-dependently reduce feeding caused by NPY microinjection into the PVN (116). Therefore, it is possible that sibutramine treatment, by increasing brain serotonin levels, could have reduced the orexigenic effects mediated by the NPY pathway to a sufficient extent such that NPY5R antagonism by MK-0557 had no additional effect.

Short-Term Weight Loss Study with S-2367

Recently, Shionogi announced results from a phase IIa study with S-2367, a selective NPY5R antagonist (114). In this study, 342 obese patients were randomized into two arms referred to as the delayed weight reduction (DWR) arm in which patients were given a four-week low-calorie diet (900–950 kcal/day) and the second referred to as the immediate weight reduction (IWR) arm. In the DWR arm, S-2367 was reported to induce a statistically significant decrease in body weight versus placebo over a 12-week treatment period following LCD. Patients on 1600 mg of S-2367 lost an additional 2.2 kg of baseline body weight versus no weight change for those on placebo ($p < 0.0001$). Results from the IWR treatment arm were not statistically significant at the end of the 12-week treatment period, but were reported to have shown a trend of enhanced weight loss versus placebo. Subjects in the high-dose group lost an average of 3.6 kg over 12 weeks, or 3.7% of baseline weight, versus a loss of 2.4 kg or 2.4% of baseline weight for placebo ($p = 0.0638$). A repeated measures analysis of the IWR arm was reported to have a statistically significant difference at the high dose ($p = 0.0479$).

Although Shionogi has not disclosed full data from this study, the results appear to be consistent with those conducted with MK-0557 in that treatment with an NPY5R antagonist only produced very modest weight loss. Although limited data prevents a careful comparison, it is interesting to note that in the MK-0557 VLCD study and the Shionogi DWR group, slightly more weight loss occurred in the active drug group than placebo during the 12 weeks following completion of the diet phase of the study (Figure 3). In the case of MK-0557, weight regain began after 12 weeks and this might represent when counter regulatory mechanisms are activated.

CONCLUSION

The past two decades have been a time of enormous advances in our understanding of the molecular pharmacology, neuroanatomy, and genetics of the NPY system with respect to its role in mammalian energy regulation. Although most of our current knowledge is derived from studies in rodents and nonhuman primates, recent clinical studies (described herein) have begun to explore blockade of the NPY system for the treatment of obesity. Although the results indicate that the NPY5R indeed plays a role in human energy balance, it appears that blockade of the NPY5R is unlikely to be successful as monotherapy for obesity. However, these clinical experiments represent the early stages of what will ultimately be necessary to thoroughly evaluate the utility of the NPY system as a target for antiobesity therapy in humans.

Since these clinical studies only examined one component of the NPY system, it would be premature to discount the importance of the NPY system in human feeding behavior. Similarly, one cannot conclude that the observed clinical results indicate the dominance of the NPY1R component of the NPY system until the efficacy of a suitable NPY1R antagonist is examined in a randomized clinical trial. If other orexigenic regulatory pathways are able to compensate for blockade of a single orexigenic receptor or pathway, it is possible that a similar modest weight loss will be observed with an NPY1R antagonist. It will be important in the future to examine the efficacy of simultaneous blockade of the NPY1R and NPY5R. Although purely speculative, it is likely that any therapy narrowly directed at a single orexigenic or anorexigenic pathway will not result in robust weight loss efficacy.

The results of the NPY5R antagonist studies described above appear to indicate that an appropriate safety and tolerability profile can be achieved with this class of drugs. The human safety profile of an NPY1R antagonist remains to be elucidated. NPY1R have been reported to be involved in diverse physiological functions besides energy regulation, including regulation of blood pressure (117), mood (118), reproductive function (119), and pain, and may be involved in other activities such as seizures, any or all of which could conceivably prove to be clinical liabilities.

Discoveries during the past decade indicate that energy homeostasis involves multiple redundant anabolic and catabolic pathways. On the basis of the enormous volume of preclinical data and the more limited clinical data, the obesity research community has begun to embrace the notion that effective pharmacotherapy of obesity will likely require a multidrug regimen, as is commonly employed for diseases such as hypertension or diabetes. An exciting challenge of the future will be to design rational combinations of drugs that provide adequate weight loss efficacy with an acceptable safety and tolerability profile. The possibility remains that blockade of the NPY system will play a part in those combination strategies.

ACKNOWLEDGMENT

The authors would like to thank Drs. Akio Kanatani and Douglas J. MacNeil for their helpful comments.

REFERENCES

1. Tatemoto K, Mutt V. Isolation of two novel candidate hormones using a chemical method for finding naturally occurring polypeptides. Nature 1980; 285(5764):417–418.
2. Tatemoto K, Carlquist M, Mutt V. Neuropeptide Y—a novel brain peptide with structural similarities to peptide YY and pancreatic polypeptide. Nature 1982; 296(5858): 659–660.

3. Eberlein GA, Eysselein VE, Schaeffer M, et al. A new molecular form of PYY: structural characterization of human PYY (3-36) and PYY (1-36). Peptides 1989; 10(4): 797–803.

4. Larhammar D. Evolution of neuropeptide Y, peptide YY and pancreatic polypeptide. Regul Pept 1996; 62(1):1–11.

5. Michel MC, Beck-Sickinger A, Cox H, et al. XVI. International Union of Pharmacology recommendations for the nomenclature of neuropeptide Y, peptide YY, and pancreatic polypeptide receptors. Pharmacol Rev 1998; 50(1): 143–150.

6. Matsumoto M, Nomura T, Momose K, et al. Inactivation of a novel neuropeptide Y/peptide YY receptor gene in primate species. J Biol Chem 1996; 271(44): 27217–27220.

7. Gregor P, Feng Y, DeCarr LB, et al. Molecular characterization of a second mouse pancreatic polypeptide receptor and its inactivated human homologue. J Biol Chem 1996; 271(44):27776–27781.

8. Burkhoff A, Linemeyer DL, Salon JA. Distribution of a novel hypothalamic neuropeptide Y receptor gene and its absence in rat. Brain Res Mol Brain Res 1998; 53(1–2): 311–316.

9. Herzog H, Hort YJ, Shine J, et al. Molecular cloning, characterization, and localization of the human homolog to the reported bovine NPY Y3 receptor: lack of NPY binding and activation. DNA Cell Biol 1993; 12(6): 465–471.

10. Jazin EE, Yoo H, Blomqvist AG, et al. A proposed bovine neuropeptide Y (NPY) receptor cDNA clone, or its human homologue, confers neither NPY binding sites nor NPY responsiveness on transfected cells. Regul Pept 1993; 47(3):247–258.

11. Bischoff A, Michel MC. Emerging functions for neuropeptide Y5 receptors. Trends Pharmacol Sci 1999; 20(3): 104–106.

12. International Union of Pharmacology Database. Available at: http://www.iuphar-db.org/GPCR/. Accessed July 2007.

13. Gerald C, Walker MW, Criscione L, et al. A receptor subtype involved in neuropeptide-Y-induced food intake. Nature 1996; 382(6587):168–171.

14. Wyss P, Stricker-Krongrad A, Brunner L, et al. The pharmacology of neuropeptide Y (NPY) receptor-mediated feeding in rats characterizes better Y5 than Y1, but not Y2 or Y4 subtypes. Regul Pept 1998; 75–76: 363–371.

15. Dumont Y, Cadieux A, Doods H, et al. BIIE0246, a potent and highly selective non-peptide neuropeptide Y Y (2) receptor antagonist. Br J Pharmacol 2000; 129(6): 1075–1088.

16. Bonaventure P, Nepomuceno D, Mazur C, et al. Characterization of N-(1-acetyl-2,3-dihydro-1H-indol-6-yl)-3-(3-cyano-phenyl)-N-[1- (2-cyclopentyl-ethyl)-piperidin-4yl]acrylamide (JNJ-5207787), a small molecule antagonist of the neuropeptide Y Y2 receptor. J Pharmacol Exp Ther 2004; 308(3):1130–1137.

17. Mentlein R, Dahms P, Grandt D, et al. Proteolytic processing of neuropeptide Y and peptide YY by dipeptidyl peptidase IV. Regul Pept 1993; 49(2):133–144.

18. Gantz I, Erondu N, Mallick M, et al. Efficacy and Safety of Intranasal Peptide YY$_{3-36}$ for Weight Reduction in Obese Adults. J Clin Endocrinol Metab 2007; 92:1754–1757.

19. Clark JT, Kalra PS, Crowley WR, et al. Neuropeptide Y and human pancreatic polypeptide stimulate feeding behavior in rats. Endocrinology 1984; 115(1):427–429.

20. Stanley BG, Leibowitz SF. Neuropeptide Y: stimulation of feeding and drinking by injection into the paraventricular nucleus. Life Sci 1984; 35(26):2635–2642.

21. Levine AS, Morley JE. Neuropeptide Y: a potent inducer of consummatory behavior in rats. Peptides 1984; 5(6): 1025–1029.

22. Larhammar D, Blomqvist AG, Yee F, et al. Cloning and functional expression of a human neuropeptide Y/peptide YY receptor of the Y1 type. J Biol Chem 1992; 267(16): 10935–10938.

23. Hu Y, Bloomquist BT, Cornfield LJ, et al. Identification of a novel hypothalamic neuropeptide Y receptor associated with feeding behavior. J Biol Chem 1996; 271(42): 26315–26319.

24. Inui A. Neuropeptide Y feeding receptors: are multiple subtypes involved? Trends Pharmacol Sci 1999; 20(2): 43–46.

25. Mullins D, Kirby D, Hwa J, et al. Identification of potent and selective neuropeptide Y Y (1) receptor agonists with orexigenic activity in vivo. Mol Pharmacol 2001; 60(3): 534–540.

26. Kanatani A, Hata M, Mashiko S, et al. A typical Y1 receptor regulates feeding behaviors: effects of a potent and selective Y1 antagonist, J-115814. Mol Pharmacol 2001; 59(3):501–505.

27. Ishihara A, Kanatani A, Okada M, et al. Blockade of body weight gain and plasma corticosterone levels in Zucker fatty rats using an orally active neuropeptide Y Y1 antagonist. Br J Pharmacol 2002; 136(3):341–346.

28. Cabrele C, Langer M, Bader R, et al. The first selective agonist for the neuropeptide YY5 receptor increases food intake in rats. J Biol Chem 2000; 275(46):36043–36048.

29. Parker EM, Balasubramaniam A, Guzzi M, et al. [D-Trp (34)] neuropeptide Y is a potent and selective neuropeptide Y Y (5) receptor agonist with dramatic effects on food intake. Peptides 2000; 21(3):393–399.

30. Criscione L, Rigollier P, Batzl-Hartmann C, et al. Food intake in free-feeding and energy-deprived lean rats is mediated by the neuropeptide Y5 receptor. J Clin Invest 1998; 102(12):2136–2145.

31. Della Zuana O, Sadlo M, Germain M, et al. Reduced food intake in response to CGP 71683A may be due to mechanisms other than NPY Y5 receptor blockade. Int J Obes Relat Metab Disord 2001; 25(1):84–94.

32. Daniels AJ, Grizzle MK, Wiard RP, et al. Food intake inhibition and reduction in body weight gain in lean and obese rodents treated with GW438014A, a potent and selective NPY-Y5 receptor antagonist. Regul Pept 2002; 106(1–3):47–54.

33. Mashiko S, Ishihara A, Iwaasa H, et al. A pair-feeding study reveals that a Y5 antagonist causes weight loss in diet-induced obese mice by modulating food intake and energy expenditure. Mol Pharmacol 2007; 71:602–608.

34. MacNeil DJ, Rogers I, Weekley B, et al. A Y5 antagonist causes weight loss in diet-induced obese rhesus monkeys. Keystone Symposium: Gut Hormones and Other Regulators of Appetite, Satiety and Energy Expenditure, Santa Fe, New Mexico, March 24, 2006.

35. Mashiko S, Ishihara A, Iwaasa H, et al. Characterization of neuropeptide Y (NPY) Y5 receptor-mediated obesity in mice: chronic intracerebroventricular infusion of D-Trp (34)NPY. Endocrinology 2003; 144(5):1793–1801.

36. Turnbull AV, Ellershaw L, Masters DJ, et al. Selective antagonism of the NPY Y5 receptor does not have a major effect on feeding in rats. Diabetes 2002; 51:2441–2449.

37. Fukami T, Kanatani A, Ishihara A, et al. (2004) Spiro Compounds. US Patent 6,723,847.

38. Erondu N, Gantz I, Musser B, et al. Neuropeptide Y5 receptor antagonism does not induce clinically meaningful weight loss in overweight and obese adults. Cell Metab 2006; 4(4):275–282.

39. Kanatani A, Mashiko S, Murai N, et al. Role of the Y1 receptor in the regulation of neuropeptide Y-mediated feeding: comparison of wild-type, Y1 receptor-deficient, and Y5 receptor-deficient mice. Endocrinology 2000; 141: 1011–1016.

40. Lundberg JM, Terenius L, Hokfelt T, et al. Neuropeptide Y (NPY)-like immunoreactivity in peripheral noradrenergic neurons and effects of NPY on sympathetic function. Acta Physiol Scand 1982; 116(4):477–480.

41. Chronwall BM, DiMaggio DA, Massari VJ, et al. The anatomy of neuropeptide-Y-containing neurons in rat brain. Neuroscience 1985; 15(4):1159–1181.

42. Grundemar L, Hakanson R. Multiple neuropeptide Y receptors are involved in cardiovascular regulation. Peripheral and central mechanisms. Gen Pharmacol 1993; 24(4):785–796.

43. McDermott BJ, Millar BC, Piper HM. Cardiovascular effects of neuropeptide Y: receptor interactions and cellular mechanisms. Cardiovasc Res 1993; 27(6):893–905.

44. Kalra SP, Dube MG, Pu S, et al. Interacting appetite-regulating pathways in the hypothalamic regulation of body weight. Endocr Rev 1999; 20(1):68–100.

45. Sahu A, Kalra SP, Crowley WR, et al. Evidence that NPY-containing neurons in the brainstem project into selected hypothalamic nuclei: implication in feeding behavior. Brain Res 1988; 457(2):376–378.

46. Sawchenko PE. Toward a new neurobiology of energy balance, appetite, and obesity: the anatomists weigh in. J Comp Neurol 1998; 402(4):435–441.

47. Kalra SP, Kalra PS. Is neuropeptide Y a naturally occurring appetite transducer? Curr Opin Endocrinol Diabetes 1996; 3:157–163.

48. Schwartz MW, Woods SC, Porte D Jr., et al. Central nervous system control of food intake. Nature 2000; 404(6778):661–671.

49. Abizaid A, Gao Q, Horvath TL. Thoughts for food: brain mechanisms and peripheral energy balance. Neuron 2006; 51(6):691–702.

50. Schwartz GJ. Integrative capacity of the caudal brainstem in the control of food intake. Philos Trans R Soc Lond B Biol Sci 2006; 361(1471):1275–12780.

51. Sahu A, Dube MG, Kalra SP, et al. Bilateral neural transections at the level of mesencephalon increase food intake and reduce latency to onset of feeding in response to neuropeptide Y. Peptides 1988; 9(6):1269–1273.

52. Holets VR, Hokfelt T, Rokaeus A, et al. Locus coeruleus neurons in the rat containing neuropeptide Y, tyrosine hydroxylase or galanin and their efferent projections to the spinal cord, cerebral cortex and hypothalamus. Neuroscience 1988; 24(3):893–906.

53. Broberger C, Landry M, Wong H, et al. Subtypes Y1 and Y2 of the neuropeptide Y receptor are respectively expressed in pro-opiomelanocortin- and neuropeptide-Y-containing neurons of the rat hypothalamic arcuate nucleus. Neuroendocrinology 1997; 66(6):393–408.

54. Hahn TM, Breininger JF, Baskin DG, et al. Coexpression of Agrp and NPY in fasting-activated hypothalamic neurons. Nat Neurosci 1998; 1(4):271–272.

55. Broberger C, Johansen J, Johansson C, et al. The neuropeptide Y/agouti gene-related protein (AgRP) brain circuitry in normal, anorectic, and monosodium glutamate-treated mice. Proc Natl Acad Sci U S A 1998; 95 (25):15043–15048.

56. Horvath TL, Bechmann I, Naftolin F, et al. Heterogeneity in the neuropeptide Y-containing neurons of the rat arcuate nucleus: GABAergic and non-GABAergic subpopulations. Brain Res 1997; 756(1–2):283–286.

57. Ollmann MM, Wilson BD, Yang YK, et al. Antagonism of central melanocortin receptors in vitro and in vivo by agouti-related protein. Science 1997; 278(5335):135–138.

58. Elias CF, Lee C, Kelly J, et al. Leptin activates hypothalamic CART neurons projecting to the spinal cord. Neuron 1998; 21(6):1375–1385.

59. Lee YS, Challis BG, Thompson DA, et al. A POMC variant implicates beta-melanocyte-stimulating hormone in the control of human energy balance. Cell Metab 2006; 3(2):135–140.

60. Biebermann H, Castaneda TR, van Landeghem F, et al. A role for beta-melanocyte-stimulating hormone in human body-weight regulation. Cell Metab 2006; 3(2):141–146.

61. Cone RD. Anatomy and regulation of the central melanocortin system. Nat Neurosci 2005; 8(5):571–578.

62. Hentges ST, Nishiyama M, Overstreet LS, et al. GABA release from proopiomelanocortin neurons. J Neurosci 2004; 24(7):1578–1583.

63. Cowley MA, Smart JL, Rubinstein M, et al. Leptin activates anorexigenic POMC neurons through a neural network in the arcuate nucleus. Nature 2001; 411(6836):480–484.

64. Schwartz MW, Sipols AJ, Marks JL, et al. Inhibition of hypothalamic neuropeptide Y gene expression by insulin. Endocrinology 1992; 130(6):3608–3616.

65. Stephens TW, Basinski M, Bristow PK, et al. The role of neuropeptide Y in the antiobesity action of the obese gene product. Nature 1995; 377(6549):530–532.

66. Baskin DG, Breininger JF, Schwartz MW. Leptin receptor mRNA identifies a subpopulation of neuropeptide Y neurons activated by fasting in rat hypothalamus. Diabetes 1999; 48(4):828–833.

67. Dickson SL, Luckman SM. Induction of c-fos messenger ribonucleic acid in neuropeptide Y and growth hormone

(GH)-releasing factor neurons in the rat arcuate nucleus following systemic injection of the GH secretagogue, GH-releasing peptide-6. Endocrinology 1997; 138(2):771–777.

68. Willesen MG, Kristensen P, Romer J. Co-localization of growth hormone secretagogue receptor and NPY mRNA in the arcuate nucleus of the rat. Neuroendocrinology 1999; 70(5):306–316.

69. Kumarnsit E, Johnstone LE, Leng G. Actions of neuropeptide Y and growth hormone secretagogues in the arcuate nucleus and ventromedial hypothalamic nucleus. Eur J Neurosci 2003; 17(5):937–944.

70. Riediger T, Traebert M, Schmid HA, et al. Site-specific effects of ghrelin on the neuronal activity in the hypothalamic arcuate nucleus. Neurosci Lett 2003; 341(2):151–155.

71. Batterham RL, Cowley MA, Small CJ, et al. Gut hormone PYY (3-36) physiologically inhibits food intake. Nature 2002; 418(6898):650–654.

72. Muroya S, Yada T, Shioda S, et al. Glucose-sensitive neurons in the rat arcuate nucleus contain neuropeptide Y. Neurosci Lett 1999; 264(1–3):113–116.

73. Levin BE. Glucosensing neurons do more than just sense glucose. Int J Obes Relat Metab Disord 2001; 25(suppl 5): S68–S72.

74. Morgan K, Obici S, Rossetti L. Hypothalamic responses to long-chain fatty acids are nutritionally regulated. J Biol Chem 2004; 279(30):31139–31148.

75. Wilson BD, Bagnol D, Kaelin CB, et al. Physiological and anatomical circuitry between Agouti-related protein and leptin signaling. Endocrinology 1999; 140(5):2387–2397.

76. Haskell-Luevano C, Chen P, Li C, et al. Characterization of the neuroanatomical distribution of agouti-related protein immunoreactivity in the rhesus monkey and the rat. Endocrinology 1999; 140(3):1408–1415.

77. Li C, Chen P, Smith MS. Corticotropin releasing hormone neurons in the paraventricular nucleus are direct targets for neuropeptide Y neurons in the arcuate nucleus: an anterograde tracing study. Brain Res 2000; 854(1–2):122–129.

78. Legradi G, Lechan RM. Agouti-related protein containing nerve terminals innervate thyrotropin-releasing hormone neurons in the hypothalamic paraventricular nucleus. Endocrinology 1999; 140(8):3643–3652.

79. Mihaly E, Fekete C, Tatro JB, et al. Hypophysiotropic thyrotropin-releasing hormone-synthesizing neurons in the human hypothalamus are innervated by neuropeptide Y, agouti-related protein, and alpha-melanocyte-stimulating hormone. J Clin Endocrinol Metab 2000; 85(7):2596–2603.

80. Mihaly E, Fekete C, Lechan RM, et al. Corticotropin-releasing hormone-synthesizing neurons of the human hypothalamus receive neuropeptide Y-immunoreactive innervation from neurons residing primarily outside the infundibular nucleus. J Comp Neurol 2002; 446(3): 235–243.

81. Carrasco GA, Van de Kar LD. Neuroendocrine pharmacology of stress. Eur J Pharmacol 2003; 463(1–3): 235–272.

82. Elias CF, Saper CB, Maratos-Flier E, et al. Chemically defined projections linking the mediobasal hypothalamus and the lateral hypothalamic area. J Comp Neurol 1998; 402(4):442–459.

83. Broberger C, De Lecea L, Sutcliffe JG, et al. Hypocretin/ orexin- and melanin-concentrating hormone-expressing cells form distinct populations in the rodent lateral hypothalamus: relationship to the neuropeptide Y and agouti gene-related protein systems. J Comp Neurol 1998; 402(4):460–474.

84. Horvath TL, Diano S, van den Pol AN. Synaptic interaction between hypocretin (orexin) and neuropeptide Y cells in the rodent and primate hypothalamus: a novel circuit implicated in metabolic and endocrine regulations. J Neurosci 1999; 19(3):1072–1087.

85. de Lecea L, Kilduff TS, Peyron C, et al. The hypocretins: hypothalamus-specific peptides with neuroexcitatory activity. Proc Natl Acad Sci U S A 1998; 95(1):322–327.

86. Dube MG, Horvath TL, Kalra PS, et al. Evidence of NPY Y5 receptor involvement in food intake elicited by orexin A in sated rats. Peptides 2000; 21:1557–1560.

87. Jain MR, Horvath TL, Kalra PS, et al. Evidence that NPY Y1 receptors are involved in stimulation of feeding by orexins (hypocretins) in sated rats. Reg Peptides 2000; 87:19–24.

88. Uyama N, Geerts A, Reynaert H. Neural connections between the hypothalamus and the liver. Anat Rec A Discov Mol Cell Evol Biol 2004; 280(1):808–820.

89. Bai FL, Yamano M, Shiotani Y, et al. An arcuato-paraventricular and -dorsomedial hypothalamic neuropeptide Y-containing system which lacks noradrenaline in the rat. Brain Res 1985; 331(1):172–175.

90. Guan XM, Yu H, Trumbauer M, et al. Induction of neuropeptide Y expression in dorsomedial hypothalamus of diet-induced obese mice. Neuroreport 1998; 9(15): 3415–3419.

91. Pu S, Dube MG, Xu B, et al. Induction of neuropeptide Y (NPY) gene expression in novel hypothalamic sites in association with transient hyperphagia and body weight gain. Program of the 80th Annual Meeting of The Endocrine Society, New Orleans, LA, 1998:435 (abstr P3–236).

92. Li C, Chen P, Smith MS. Neuropeptide Y (NPY) neurons in the arcuate nucleus (ARH) and dorsomedial nucleus (DMH), areas activated during lactation, project to the paraventricular nucleus of the hypothalamus (PVH). Regul Pept 1998; 75–76:93–100.

93. Dryden S, Wang Q, Frankish HM, et al. The serotonin (5-HT) antagonist methysergide increases neuropeptide Y (NPY) synthesis and secretion in the hypothalamus of the rat. Brain Res 1995; 699(1):12–18.

94. Dryden S, Wang Q, Frankish HM, et al. Differential effects of the 5-HT 1B/2C receptor agonist mCPP and the 5-HT1A agonist flesinoxan on hypothalamic neuropeptide Y in the rat: evidence that NPY may mediate serotonin's effects on food intake. Peptides 1996; 17(6): 943–949.

95. Rogers P, McKibbin PE, Williams G. Acute fenfluramine administration reduces neuropeptide Y concentrations in specific hypothalamic regions of the rat: possible implications for the anorectic effect of fenfluramine. Peptides 1991; 12(2):251–255.

96. Kishi T, Aschkenasi CJ, Choi BJ, et al. Neuropeptide Y Y1 receptor mRNA in rodent brain: distribution and

colocalization with melanocortin-4 receptor. J Comp Neurol 2005; 482(3):217–243.

97. Fuxe K, Tinner B, Caberlotto L, et al. NPY Y1 receptor like immunoreactivity exists in a subpopulation of beta-endorphin immunoreactive nerve cells in the arcuate nucleus: a double immunolabelling analysis in the rat. Neurosci Lett 1997; 225(1):49–52.

98. Broberger C, Visser TJ, Kuhar MJ, et al. Neuropeptide Y innervation and neuropeptide-Y-Y1-receptor-expressing neurons in the paraventricular hypothalamic nucleus of the mouse. Neuroendocrinology 1999; 70(5):295–305.

99. Nichol KA, Morey A, Couzens MH, et al. Conservation of expression of neuropeptide Y5 receptor between human and rat hypothalamus and limbic regions suggests an integral role in central neuroendocrine control. J Neurosci 1999; 19(23):10295–10304.

100. Jacques D, Tong Y, Shen SH, et al. Discrete distribution of the neuropeptide Y Y5 receptor gene in the human brain: an in situ hybridization study. Brain Res Mol Brain Res 1998; 61(1–2):100–107.

101. Fetissov SO, Byrne LC, Hassani H, et al. Characterization of neuropeptide Y Y2 and Y5 receptor expression in the mouse hypothalamus. J Comp Neurol 2004; 470(3):256–265.

102. Campbell RE, ffrench-Mullen JM, Cowley MA, et al. Hypothalamic circuitry of neuropeptide Y regulation of neuroendocrine function and food intake via the Y5 receptor subtype. Neuroendocrinology 2001; 74(2):106–119.

103. Erickson JC, Clegg KE, Palmiter RD. Sensitivity to leptin and susceptibility to seizures of mice lacking neuropeptide Y. Nature 1996; 381(6581):415–421.

104. Erickson JC, Hollopeter G, Palmiter RD. Attenuation of the obesity syndrome of ob/ob mice by the loss of neuropeptide Y. Science 1996; 274(5293):1704–1707.

105. Pedrazzini T, Seydoux J, Kunstner P, et al. Cardiovascular response, feeding behavior and locomotor activity in mice lacking the NPY Y1 receptor. Nat Med 1998; 4(6):722–726.

106. Kushi A, Sasai H, Koizumi H, et al. Obesity and mild hyperinsulinemia found in neuropeptide Y-Y1 receptor-deficient mice. Proc Natl Acad Sci U S A 1998; 95(26):15659–15664.

107. Marsh DJ, Hollopeter G, Kafer KE, et al. Role of the Y5 neuropeptide Y receptor in feeding and obesity. Nat Med 1998; 4(6):718–721.

108. Gardiner JV, Kong WM, Ward H, et al. AAV mediated expression of anti-sense neuropeptide Y cRNA in the arcuate nucleus of rats results in decreased weight gain and food intake. Biochem Biophys Res Commun 2005; 327(4):108810–108893.

109. Bewick GA, Gardiner JV, Dhillo WS, et al. Post-embryonic ablation of AgRP neurons in mice leads to a lean, hypophagic phenotype. FASEB J 2005; 19(12):1680–1682.

110. Luquet S, Perez FA, Hnasko TS, et al. NPY/AgRP neurons are essential for feeding in adult mice but can be ablated in neonates. Science 2005; 310(5748):683–685.

111. Gropp E, Shanabrough M, Borok E, et al. Agouti-related peptide-expressing neurons are mandatory for feeding. Nat Neurosci 2005; 8(10):1289–1291.

112. Ishihara A, Moriya M, MacNeil DJ, et al. Neuropeptide Y receptors as targets of obesity treatment. Expert Opin Ther Patents 2006; 16(12):1701–1712.

113. Erondu, N, Wadden T, Gantz I, et al. Effect of NPY5R antagonist MK-0557 on weight regain after VLCD-induced weight loss. Obesity 2007; 15:895–905.

114. Shionogi Co Ltd. Available at: http://www.shionogi.co.jp/ir_en/news/index.html. Accessed July 2007.

115. Erondu N, Addy C, Lu K, et al. NPY5R antagonism does not augment the weight loss efficacy of orlistat or sibutramine. Obesity 2007; 15:2027–2042.

116. Grignaschi G, Fanelli E, Scagnol I, et al. Studies on the role of serotonin receptor subtypes in the effect of sibutramine in various feeding paradigms in rats. Br J Pharmacol 1999; 127(5):1190–1194.

117. Pons J, Lee EW, Li L, et al. Neuropeptide Y: multiple receptors and multiple roles in cardiovascular diseases. Curr Opin Investig Drugs 2004; 5(9):957–962.

118. Wettstein JG, Earley B, Junien JL. Central nervous system pharmacology of neuropeptide Y. Pharmacol Ther 1995; 65(3):397–414.

119. Markiewicz W, Jaroszewski JJ, Bossowska A, et al. NPY: its occurrence and relevance in the female reproductive system. Folia Histochem Cytobiol 2003; 41(4):183–192.

23

Serotonin Receptor Modulation in the Treatment of Obesity

JASON C.G. HALFORD

Laboratory for the Study of Human Ingestive Behaviour, School of Psychology, University of Liverpool, Liverpool, U.K.

JOHN E. BLUNDELL

Institute of Psychological Sciences, University of Leeds, Leeds, U.K.

INTRODUCTION: EPISODIC AND TONIC SIGNALS TO THE CENTRAL NERVOUS SYSTEM AND THEIR IMPORTANCE IN THE CONTROL OF APPETITE EXPRESSION

Although experienced as a subjective state, appetite can be considered as an expression of numerous regulatory processes. These processes not only determine the initiation and termination of meals, but also the amount and types of foods consumed, meal length and frequency, and the duration of between-meal intervals. The very act of consuming food determines the expression of appetite. Before the act of ingestion anticipatory physiological and psychological events occur, preparing the body for the eating event and reinforcing eating behavior. Once consumption commences, powerful signals are generated that inhibit further intake. These pre-, during-, and postmeal processes are critical to the experience of appetite and underpin our experiences of hunger and satiety. It is in this flux between hunger and satiety that serotonin (5-HT, 5-hydroxytryptamine) plays a critical role in appetite regulation (1).

Here it is useful to draw a distinction between the short-term satiety signals produced by the physiological consequences of meal intake (episodic) and the longer-term signals created by the body's constant metabolic need for energy (tonic). The former are a crucial factor in the meal-by-meal regulation of energy intake. Episodic signals are critical to oscillations in appetite and fluctuations in the pattern of eating behavior observed throughout the day.

Tonic inhibitory signals, by contrast, are not a result of this flux of meal-generated signals but are instead primarily generated by the storage and metabolism of energy. These constitute separate aspects of appetite regulation. Episodic and tonic signals are generated by markedly distinct processes (1–3). However, both ultimately act to adjust food intake via common hypothalamic circuitry. The roles of the central nervous system (CNS) in appetite regulation and of tonic signals in energy regulation are dealt with elsewhere in this book. But it is worth examining the process that underpins the episodic control of feeding behavior in greater detail.

Serotonergic drugs have been shown to decrease hunger and strengthen indices of satiety. Hunger can be defined as the motivation to seek and consume food, and it initiates a period of feeding behavior. The process that brings this period of eating (or meal) to an end is termed satiation. Satiation processes ultimately lead to the state of satiety in which the hunger drive and, consequently, eating behavior are inhibited. The process of satiation determines the meal size, and the state of satiety determines the length of the postmeal interval. The net effect of these systems can be considered as before (preprandial or cephalic phase), during (prandial), and after (postprandial) a meal. Preconsumption physiological signals are generated by the sight and smell of the food, preparing the body for the ingestion of food. Such afferent sensory information, carried to the brain stem via cranial nerves, stimulates hunger before eating and into the initial stages of consumption (the prandial phase) (2).

For CNS 5-HT to be involved in episodic appetite regulation, it must receive input from the periphery during and after consumption. These signals can be classified by their origin (i.e., stimulus and location). During the prandial phase, the CNS receives postingestive sensory afferent input from the gut, reflecting both the amount of food eaten and the earliest representations of its nutrient content. Firstly, mechanoreceptors in the gut detect the distension of gut lining caused by the presence of food, contributing to the estimation of the volume of food consumed. Secondly, gut chemoreceptors detect the chemical presence of various nutrients in the gastrointestinal tract providing information on the composition (and possible energy content) of the food consumed. Finally, prandial and postprandial signals are generated by the detection of nutrients that were absorbed from the gastrointestinal tract and then entered the circulation in the periphery (postabsorptive satiety signals). Circulating nutrients are either metabolized in the periphery (e.g., liver) and activate CNS receptors (e.g., in brain stem) or they enter and affect the brain directly and act as postabsorptive metabolic satiety signals (2,3). Such afferent information must ultimately affect CNS 5-HT functioning.

The CNS therefore has a rich source of episodic signals through which the nutritional status of the organism can be assessed. Here the signals are integrated and influence the expression of eating behavior. At these sites of integration, potential antiobesity drugs can be used to influence subjective feelings of appetite experiences before, during, and after food intake. In the last 14 years, a tremendous amount of research has uncovered orexigenic and anorexigenic systems in the CNS, particularly in the brain stem and the hypothalamic region, critical to energy regulation and the control of feeding behavior. However, prior to that, the role of CNS 5-HT in the control of appetite was already very well established (4,5).

The Serotonin (5-HT) System, Its Receptors, and Their Role in Satiation and Satiety

Serotonin is a classic monoamine neurotransmitter found extensively in the periphery where it is not limited to neurons. In the periphery, the majority of 5-HT is located in enterochromaffin cells within the gut wall where it is involved in gastric motility. 5-HT is also found in high concentrations in blood platelets involved in the process of platelet aggregation (blood clotting). Within the CNS, 5-HT is found in particularly high concentration in the midbrain. CNS 5-HT has been linked to mood, hallucinations, wakefulness and sleep, control of sensory transmission, as well as the regulation of feeding behavior. As 5-HT cannot cross the blood-brain barrier, neuronal 5-HT must be synthesized within the CNS (6,7).

The cell bodies of many 5-HT containing neurons are grouped in the upper medulla and the pons in an area termed the Raphe nuclei (i.e., between the mid and hindbrain). Projections from these neurons ascend into the forebrain to a number of sites where they release the transmitter. Some of these forebrain sites, such as the hypothalamus, are critical to appetite control. 5-HT-releasing neurons projecting into appetite regulatory sites probably possess numerous receptors along their length for anorexigenic (reducing food intake) and orexigenic (promoting food intake) factors. This would allow the integration of various peripheral episodic appetite signals. For instance, ascending afferent vagal signals from gut or liver and peptides crossing over from the periphery or those secreted within the CNS could all stimulate or inhibit axonal receptors. This in turn would stimulate or inhibit 5-HT release in areas such as the hypothalamus.

Neuronal 5-HT is synthesized from the essential amino acid tryptophan. Tryptophan of dietary origin, in the plasma, crosses the blood-brain barrier through an active uptake process. Here, it competes along with other large neutral amino acids (LNAAs) for entry into the CNS. Once in the CNS, it circulates and reaches the cytoplasm of the neuronal cell body. Within a neuron, the enzyme tryptophan hydroxylase hydroxylates the tryptophan to 5-hydroxytryptophan (5-HTP). This hydroxylation is regarded as the rate-limiting step in 5-HT synthesis. 5-HTP is then rapidly decarboxylated at the terminal by the enzyme I-amino acid decarboxylase to produce 5-HT (Fig. 1). The majority of 5-HT produced is taken up via a vesicle membrane transport mechanism and stored in presynaptic vesicles. After release, synaptic 5-HT continues to stimulate pre- and postsynaptic receptors until it is either converted to 5-hydoxyindole acetic acid (5-HIAA) by monoamine oxidase or reabsorbed into the presynaptic neuron for reuse (a sodium-dependent process) (6–8).

It is interesting to note that many early studies in rodents demonstrated that depletion of dietary tryptophan causes marked reduction in CNS 5-HT levels (5,9–11). Moreover, these early studies also demonstrated that dietary carbohydrate and protein differentially affected LNAA ratios, which in turn influenced the rate of tryptophan entry into the CNS (5,9–11). This gave rise to the notion that the central 5-HT system was not only sensitive

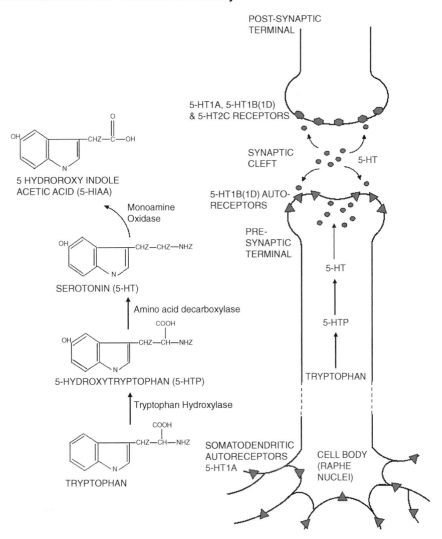

Figure 1 5-HT synthesis.

to macronutrient ingestion but also controlled appetite for specific macronutrients. While this notion has receded in recent years, this body of data still demonstrates that endogenous 5-HT is sensitive to the nutritional status of the organism. In humans, dieting reduces circulating tryptophan (12,13). Moreover, in animals that are malnourished, significant reductions in CNS 5-HT levels are apparent (14–16). Thus, endogenous 5-HT levels may be profoundly reduced by energy deficit. It would be logical that levels of a powerful hypophagic neurotransmitter would be dramatically reduced in situations of severe energy deficit.

Serotonin was linked to the control of food intake and feeding behavior 30 years ago (4). Prior to this, initial studies demonstrated that 5-HT precursors (tryptophan and 5-HTP) potently affected CNS 5-HT levels and also produced significant reduction in the food intake in rodents. Similarly, the direct administration of 5-HT into the CNS produced the same hypophagic response (17–20).

Conversely, preventing 5-HT synthesis or destroying 5-HT neurons resulted in not only a prevention of 5-HT-induced hypophagia but also an increase in food intake (21). Therefore, even with the crude pharmacological tools available at the time, it was evident that CNS 5-HT was implicated in the control of food intake.

Through analysis of feeding behavior, Blundell (4) proposed that 5-HT was a key satiety factor, adjusting the expression of appetite in a manner similar to that of food ingestion itself. Since those early studies and Blundell's subsequent review, a wealth of data on the effects of serotonergic drugs on appetite and body weight have been collected. It is probably fair to state that for no other target (peripheral or central) do such a wealth of data on the effects of pharmacological targeting one system exist. Even at the time of writing this chapter, there are more published data available on the effects of 5-HT drugs on human appetite than for any other system involved in appetite regulation (22,23).

Over a decade ago, there were significant advances in the discovery and identification of novel 5-HT receptors (6,7). Cloning and radioligand techniques allowed the subdivision of 5-HT receptors into up to 14 distinct subtypes. Currently, the core receptor subtypes appear to be 5-HT$_{1A}$, 5-HT$_{1B}$, 5-HT$_{1D}$, 5-HT$_{2A}$, 5-HT$_{2B}$, 5-HT$_{2C}$, 5-HT$_3$, 5-HT$_4$, 5-HT$_5$, 5-HT$_6$, and 5-HT$_7$. Generally, all 5-HT receptors are G-protein-coupled seven transmembrane receptors, with the exception of the 5-HT$_3$ receptor, which is a ligand-gated ion channel. The ongoing identification of new 5-HT receptor subtypes consequently led to research to determine which of these 5-HT receptors were involved in the processes of satiety (6,7). The 5-HT receptors currently thought to be most directly implicated in the feeding control mechanisms are 5-HT$_{1A}$, 5-HT$_{1B}$, and 5-HT$_{2C}$. Agonism or antagonism of other receptors subtypes can also produce potent effects on food intake; however, the changes in feeding behavior they produce are not always consistent with a primary effect on satiety (24).

Serotonin and Other Orexigenic and Anorexigenic Pathways

To regulate appetite, a variety of structures within the CNS integrate multiple signals to assess the biological need for energy, to generate or inhibit conscious experiences of hunger, and to subsequently initiate the appropriate behavioral action. Given that CNS 5-HT is a key satiety system, its functioning must somehow be regulated by peripheral episodic signals. It is assumed that afferent signals from the periphery stimulate brain stem 5-HT neurons, projecting into the hypothalamic area. Preabsorptive signals, such as ingested nutrients, generate powerful satiety signals in response to the physical and chemical presence of food in the gastrointestinal tract. Potent effects on human appetite are produced by the release of gastrointestinal factors such as cholecystokinin (CCK) and enterostatin from stomach and proximal gut (duodenum), glucagon-like peptide, oxyntomodulin and apoplipoprotein-iv from the distal gut (ileum), and peptide YY from the distal gut and large intestine.

Of these factors, the interaction between 5-HT and gut peptide CCK, which is released in response to the presence of fat and protein in the stomach, has been researched most extensively. 5-HT and CCK functioning have been experimentally linked (25). Earlier in this chapter, we detailed evidence that CNS 5-HT levels vary in accordance with the nutritional state of the organism (9–11). Not only is the availability of the 5-HT precursor dietary tryptophan dependent on ingestion, but its transport across the blood-brain barrier is affected by dietary composition. Increasing carbohydrate does alter the plasma tryptophan: LNAA ratio potentially increasing CNS 5-HT levels (26).

Similarly, if the CNS 5-HT system is affected by peripheral signals, these in turn must influence CNS systems critical to energy regulation and the control of feeding behavior. The discovery of the adiposity signal leptin (27) led to the subsequent identification of various anabolic (stimulate the intake and suppress expenditure of energy) and catabolic (stimulate expenditure and inhibit intake of energy) circuits within the CNS. Within this neural circuitry, numerous neuropeptides, both orexigenic (stimulate food intake) and anorexigenic (inhibit food intake), were discovered. Of particular interest have been the inhibitory and stimulatory neurons that project from the arcuate nucleus (ARC) to the paraventricular nucleus (PVN) and to other hypothalamic nuclei (28). These "first order" neurons, such as the anorexigenic pro-opiomelanocortin/cocaine- and amphetamine-regulating transcript (POMC/CART) containing neurons and the stimulatory orexigenic neuropeptide Y/agouti-related peptide (NPY/AgRP) containing neurons, are a key convergence point for peripherally generated episodic and tonic signals (such as leptin, ghrelin, insulin, and corticosteroids) (28).

Until quite recently, it was not clear how 5-HT is integrated into these various orexigenic and anorexigenic pathways. The extent to which 5-HT-induced hypophagia involves other neuropeptide signaling systems linked to the hypothalamic regulation of appetite is not yet really understood. An antagonistic relationship between 5-HT and the food intake stimulating NPY was established a number of years ago. NPY-induced hyperphagia was shown to be blocked by the 5-HT drug fenfluramine, and hypothalamic NPY peptide levels have been reported to decrease after treatment with 5-HT agonists as well as to increase after administration of 5-HT antagonists (29–31).

Recent data also suggest that the hypothalamic melanocortin (MC) system may be required for 5-HT drugs to alter feeding behavior and presumably for feeding-induced changes in endogenous 5-HT to influence appetite (32–34). Presynaptic MC3R and MC4R receptors in the PVN have been shown to be critical in mediating the effects of the tonic signal leptin downstream of these first order neurons. The MC system is of particular interest as these receptors not only have an endogenous agonist, alpha-melanocyte-stimulating hormone (αMSH), which when released by the POMC neurons decreases food intake, but the MC system also possesses an endogenous antagonist AgRP which, when released by AgRP neurons, increases food intake.

Heisler and colleagues have recently demonstrated the inhibition of AgRP neuron and the inhibition of the AgRP axonal projection by 5-HT through 5-HT$_{1B}$ receptor action. Thus, 5-HT inhibits orexigenic neurons. This is in addition to the activation of the POMC neuron through the 5-HT$_{2C}$ receptor. Thus, 5-HT stimulates anorexigenic neurons. The net result of the 5-HT receptor agonism of

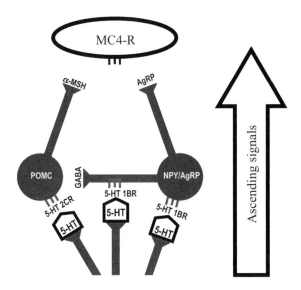

Figure 2 Interaction of 5-HT with other neurotransmitters. *Source*: Courtesy of Nina Laidlaw

first order neurons in the ARC is the stimulation of αMSH and the inhibition of AgRP release in the PVN. This increases activation of the downstream anorexigenic MC system (Fig. 2).

Beyond mechanistic considerations, there is an implication of clinical relevance. These data suggest that the MC system within the PVN is a critical juncture for the integration of episodic signals mediated by the 5-HT system and tonic signals such as leptin within the CNS. Some studies have shown that both leptin deficiency and fasting decrease CNS αMSH levels while increasing those of AgRP (28). These changes would normally bring about a robust increase in food intake. It is plausible that during weight loss, dieting-induced reductions in circulating leptin could reduce PVN αMSH releases and increase AgRP releases. Individuals would experience this as an increase in hunger.

Given this point of convergence between the leptin and 5-HT systems, these potentially unhelpful effects on appetite could be counteracted by serotonergic drugs. The drug would act on these key ARC 5-HT$_{2C}$ and 5HT$_{1B}$ receptors, and in doing so, it would amplify the episodic inhibitory input, in essence strengthening the satiety impact of reduced caloric intake, thereby compensating for any weight loss–induced fall in the tonic signal. Obviously, this has yet to be demonstrated in the rodent model.

THE EFFECT OF SEROTONERGIC DRUGS ON FEEDING BEHAVIOR AND APPETITE EXPRESSION

Given the raphe 5-HT projections into the hypothalamus and the location of key 5-HT receptors on key energy regulatory neurones in the ARC that project into the PVN,

it is not surprising that the serotonergic drugs produce robust effects on food intake and the structure of feeding behavior. The first studies in rodents with drugs such as fenfluramine (a 5-HT releaser) and, later, D-fenfluramine helped establish the role of 5-HT in the behavioral expression of appetite. Subsequent research employed various selective 5-HT receptor antagonists to find the 5-HT receptor subtypes mediating this response. Over the past 20 years, a considerable body of research has demonstrated that the hypophagic effects of D-fenfluramine in either rats or mice are mediated by 5-HT$_{2C}$ and 5-HT$_{1B}$ receptors within the hypothalamic area (35–39). Similarly, the hypophagic effects of the selective serotonin reuptake inhibitors such as fluoxetine and sertraline appear to be mediated by the same receptors (40–42).

The direct agonism of these 5-HT receptors in rodents also produces reductions in food intake in rodents (24,43–51). Similarly, the recent ability to breed animals lacking functional receptor 5-HT subtypes has allowed researchers to examine the role of the endogenous 5-HT system in appetite and body weight regulation. Mice lacking functional 5-HT$_{2C}$ receptors demonstrate a phenotype characterized by marked hyperphagia and the eventual development of excess adiposity when compared with their wild-type littermates (52,53). Similarly, 5-HT$_{1B}$ receptor knockout mice are significantly heavier than wild types, an effect again associated with significantly greater food consumption (54). These data again support the notion that a functional CNS 5-HT system is critical for appetite control and body weight regulation and also confirm the important role of these two receptor subtypes.

What has been critical to establishing the role of 5-HT in the natural expression of appetite is that agonism of these receptor subtypes have produced changes in feeding behavior consistent with the natural development of satiety. From the earliest research, it was important to establish that serotonergic drugs reduced food intake by exerting an effect on natural satiety mechanisms (4), not on those that cause a reduction in food intake by inducing nausea, sedation, hyperactivity, or malaise (24). To achieve this, the effects of various 5-HT drugs on the macro and microstructure of rodent feeding behavior were examined. These data are reviewed elsewhere, but to summarize the findings, numerous studies have shown that drugs that either stimulate 5-HT release or inhibit 5-HT reuptake produce appropriate changes in the organization of feeding behavior, as measured by the Behavioral Satiety Sequence or other behavioral assays (24).

Serotonergic releasers and reuptake inhibitors such as fenfluramine, D-fenfluramine; selective serotonin reuptake inhibitors (SSRIs) such as sertraline and fluoxetine; and sibutramine (a noradrenergic and 5-HT reuptake inhibitor) have all been shown to adjust rodent feeding behavior in a manner consistent with the operation of satiety (24). Similarly, selective agonists of 5-HT$_{2C}$ and 5-HT$_{1B}$ particularly also produce changes in feeding behavior consistent with the operation of satiety (24,51,47). However, agonism of other 5-HT receptors can disrupt the expression of feeding behavior (24,43).

As with rodents, the first human studies into the effects of 5-HT drugs on human feeding behavior employed racemic fenfluramine and then later D-fenfluramine. These studies demonstrated that these drugs enhanced the within-meal development of satiation, while strengthening between-meal satiety. Thus, individuals ate less at meals but did not compensate by increasing the number or size of subsequent eating episodes. Rogers and Blundell (55) demonstrated that an acute single dose of fenfluramine (60 mg) reduced food intake of a lunchtime meal by 789 kJ (26%) in lean healthy men. The drug also reduced eating rate and desire to eat (an effect noted prior to the test meal). Foltin et al. (56) demonstrated that fenfluramine (40 mg) could reduce total daily caloric intake in lean healthy participants. The drug reduced meal size rather than the number of meals, indicating an enhancement of within-meal satiation.

With regard to D-fenfluramine, Goodall and Silverstone (57) gave a 30-mg dose to normal-weight males. This reduced both total meal intake and eating rate, an effect associated with a reduction in premeal hunger. Blundell and Hill (58) also noted that D-fenfluramine produced significant reductions in hunger prior to a meal in normal and obese participants. In a free-living environment, Drent et al. (59) demonstrated that chronic D-fenfluramine (30 mg daily) treatment reduced energy intake and meal and snack size but not the number of eating occasions in the clinically obese. This again suggests D-fenfluramine strengthened between-meal satiety as well as reduced the intake at each eating occasion.

Earlier researchers were also able to use the SSRI fluoxetine in clinical feeding studies to understand the role of 5-HT in the expression of human appetite. A number of groups carried out 14-day dosing crossover design studies, examining the effects of fluoxetine 60 mg/ day on eating behavior (60–62). Participants would be given the drug or placebo to take over 14 days and they would come into the laboratory during and at the end of this treatment to have the effects of the drug on intake and appetite directly measured. Typically, in these studies the participants lost a significant amount of weight during the drug treatment phase, either compared with baseline or against placebo. The weight loss varied between 1 and 3 kg over the two-week dosing period. In all the three studies, the drug produced significant reductions in food intake, and these changes in intake were accompanied by reductions in hunger.

In the only fluoxetine study in obese participants, Lawton et al. (62) found that over the two-week treatment period, significantly more weight was lost in the drug condition than the control (1.93 kg). During test days, at ad libitum evening meals, fluoxetine produced a 27% (198 kcal) reduction in energy consumption, an effect associated with reduction in hunger. During the rest of the treatment period, participants also reported 22.4% reduction in energy intake outside the laboratory. While fluoxetine is not used as an obesity treatment, these clinical data do suggest that 5-HT reuptake inhibition can produce potent effects on caloric intake, and this occurs through an action on satiety.

The net effect of increased 5-HT release or reuptake inhibition is an increase in 5-HT receptor activation. As detailed earlier, the receptors linked with 5-HT and satiety are the 5-HT$_{1B}$ and 5-HT$_{2C}$ subtypes. To date, most of the clinical studies using direct agonists of 5-HT receptors have used m-chlorophenylpiperazine (mCPP). mCPP is a powerful 5-HT$_{1B/2C}$ receptor preferential agonist rather than a highly selective agonist of either receptor subtype, producing changes in rodent food intake and feeding behavior consistent with the development of satiety (24). A number of studies have shown mCPP reduces food intake in humans (63,64), an effect associated with a significant reduction in hunger. In obese subjects treated for 14 days with mCPP, significant reductions in weight and hunger have been observed (65). However, mCPP also produces transient increases in blood pressure and heart rate (66). Consequently, this drug would be problematic in a clinical population with a high risk of cardiovascular events. Another receptor subtype implicated in satiety, the 5-HT$_{1B}$ receptor, sumatriptan, a novel 5-HT$_{1B/1D}$ receptor agonist, has also been shown to produce a significant reduction in food intake in healthy women (67). This effect was not associated with any significant changes in appetite. These data suggest that selective agonists of 5-HT$_{1B}$ and/or 5-HT$_{2C}$ receptors do produce changes in appetite and the expression of feeding behavior consistent with satiety.

Finally, it is also worth considering the effect of some drugs with actions not restricted to the 5-HT system, but with effects on appetite that are consistent with a serotonergic mechanism of action (24). Sibutramine is a 5-HT, and serotonin-noradrenaline reuptake inhibitor currently globally licensed for the treatment of obesity. It is reviewed extensively elsewhere in this book (chap. 18). Considering sibutramine's effects on appetite in clinical studies, it has been shown to reduce food intake (68) and appetite (69). These effects were first characterized in the obese by Rolls et al. (70) in a design similar to the early fluoxetine studies (60–62). Sibutramine (30 mg/day) significantly reduced food intake and body weight, and when only prelunch ratings were included in the analysis, a significant reduction in appetite was also observed. It is interesting to note that the magnitude of the drug's initial effects on food intake appears to be associated with subsequent weight loss (71). Moreover, even after 10 months of treatment and significant weight loss, the hypophagic effects of the drug are still very much apparent (71). These data show that sibutramine does have a potent effect on feeding behavior and possibly appetite expression. However, the doses employed in these studies (15 or 30 mg) were in general far higher than doses most commonly used in the clinical population.

Considering the clinical prescribed dose, in a recent clinical trial, the effects of sibutramine 10 mg/day on feeding behavior and appetite expression were assessed in a group of obese participants (72). In this randomized, placebo-controlled, crossover trial, the participants received placebo or 10 mg or 15 mg of sibutramine in each study phase. After seven days of dosing, at the end of each phase, the participants' eating behavior within a test meal was monitored through the use of a hidden set of scales under the food plate. Results showed that 10 mg of sibutramine produced a 16% reduction in test meal intake. The drug reduced eating rate during the meal, rather than meal length, suggesting that satiation started to develop early in the meal (Fig. 3). To confirm that these were appetite-specific effects, ratings taken during the meal showed that the drug enhanced feelings of fullness and reduced the feeling of hunger earlier in the meal (Fig. 4). These data confirm that sibutramine-induced hypophagia is accompanied by appropriate changes in appetite in the obese. Whether this effect is entirely dependent on the

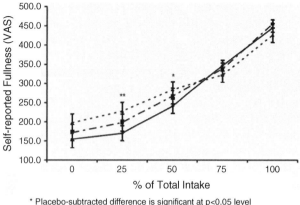

* Placebo-subtracted difference is significant at p<0.05 level
** Placebo-subtracted difference is significant at p<0.01 level

———◆——— Placebo
———■——— 10 mg Sibutramine
———▲——— 15 mg Sibutramine

Figure 4 The effects of sibutramine 10 and 15 mg on mean within-meal VAS ratings of fullness during an ad libitum meal on a universal eating monitor.

mechanism of 5-HT reuptake inhibition is yet to be determined.

THE EFFECT OF 5-HT DRUGS ON BODY WEIGHT, BODY COMPOSITION, AND RISK FACTORS FOR CARDIOMETABOLIC DISEASE

The efficacy of various 5-HT drugs for treating obesity has been assessed at various times over the past 40 years. As with the food intake and appetite, the earliest clinical data on 5-HT drugs and weight loss originate from studies employing fenfluramine and later D-fenfluramine and fluoxetine. Clinical data on the effects of fenfluramine on body weight have been published since the late 1960s (20). Reviewing these early studies shows that despite variations in the dose of fenfluramine given, the duration of the trial, and the additional dietary advice/regime given to the participants, fenfluramine-induced weight loss was a robust clinical effect. This has been confirmed by a recent meta-analysis of published clinical trials, which suggests that fenfluramine produced an average placebo-subtracted weight loss of 2.41 kg in these studies (73).

The efficacy of D-fenfluramine, the more selective and potent isomer of the parent compound, was assessed during the 1980s and 1990s. This drug was ultimately withdrawn from the market soon after its launch in 1997, due to a critical side effect issue. Despite this withdrawal, clinical studies have been published on the efficacy of this drug. The key D-fenfluramine study, the European INDEX (International DEXfenfluramine study) trial, demonstrated that the drug could produce a placebo-subtracted weight loss of 7.15 kg (74,75). However, recent meta-analysis of

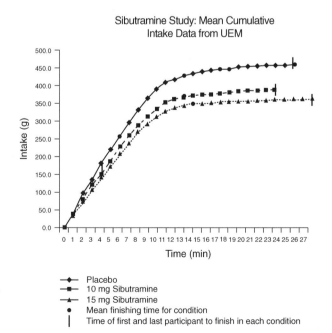

Figure 3 The effect of sibutramine 10 and 15 mg on mean cumulative intake in female obese participants offered an ad libitum meal on a universal eating monitor.

D-fenfluramine trials suggests that placebo-subtracted weight loss is in fact a little more modest at 3.82 kg (73). D-Fenfluramine was not the only drug assessed in clinical trials during this time. Given the effects of fluoxetine on food intake and appetite, its effect on body weight was also assessed in trials of varying lengths. While the data from the short-term studies suggested fluoxetine could produce effects on body weight equivalent to those produced by D-fenfluramine, in the trials of longer duration, it was evident that weight regain occurred within 6 to 12 months of treatment (76).

Currently, there is no clearly selective serotonergic antiobesity compound licensed to treat obesity. However, the 5-HT and noradrenergic reuptake inhibitor sibutramine was licensed for the treatment of obesity in the late 1990s. The data required by regulatory authorities for approval have ensured that there is a comparative wealth of published data on its efficacy. This is dealt with in far more detail in chapter 18. However, it is worth noting again the classic weight control study of sibutramine, Sibutramine Trial of Obesity Reduction and Maintenance (STORM). Obese patients were prescribed a 10-mg dose of sibutramine in addition to a low-calorie diet over six months, and they lost 11.3 kg (77). Following the open label run-in period, patients were entered into an 18-month placebo controlled study. During this second phase, little weight regain was seen in the group that continued on sibutramine. However, weight regain appeared in those switched to placebo. Subsequently, a number of other one and two year studies have demonstrated the weight loss-inducing efficacy of sibutramine (78–80), and meta-analyses have shown that sibutramine produces a placebo-subtracted weight loss of 4.45 kg (81,82). This appears to be similar to and possibly even superior to D-fenfluramine (74) and nearly equivalent to the novel endocannabinoid antiobesity drug rimonabant (83) (see chap. 20).

With regard to the effect of 5-HT drugs on cardiometabolic risk factors, the data from studies prior to the late 1990s are somewhat limited. Certainly, the large-scale multisite clinical trials in obese populations with D-fenfluramine were focused far more on weight loss rather than on specific key risk factors (75). At the time, it was argued that the drug-induced weight loss observed in these studies was of sufficient magnitude to be considered medically significant for reducing risk factors for "some diseases associated with obesity" (75,84). However, D-fenfluramine studies in specific patient populations (i.e., those with obesity related comorbidities) did demonstrate the beneficial effects of the drug. For instance, a number of studies were conducted in obese type 2 diabetics. These showed that D-fenfluramine produced beneficial changes in glycemic control as well as weight loss (85–87). At least some of these beneficial changes were independent of weight loss (85). With regard to cardiovascular disease, the effects of D-fenfluramine were examined in morbidly obese and obese hypertensive patients (88,89). Together with weight loss, beneficial changes in the risk factors for cardiovascular events were found in these studies. No D-fenfluramine long-term outcome study on cardiovascular events (the actual likelihood of suffering or dying from stroke or heart attack during treatment) has been published. Given the drug's early withdrawal, any such trial would have had to be abandoned.

A large body of published clinical literature demonstrates that sibutramine-induced weight loss produces beneficial effects on key risk factors for noncommunicable diseases (see chap. 18). However, it is worth noting here that sibutramine increases sympathetic nervous system activity, raising issues of safety in patients with severe cardiovascular problems, such as congestive heart failure, coronary artery disease, hypertension, stroke, and arrhythmia. From a meta-analysis of 21 placebo-controlled studies, it has been concluded that sibutramine does raise blood pressure slightly (90). These effects are likely due to the noradrenergic rather than serotonergic actions of the drug, although agonism of some 5-HT receptor subtypes can also produce similar effects. Nonetheless, McMohan et al. (78), demonstrated that sibutramine is both safe and effective in patients with controlled hypertension (i.e., taking other medication), producing only a small and transient increase in pulse rate and blood pressure. Moreover, sibutramine-induced weight loss can reduce blood pressure in hypertensive patients in the long term (91).

Despite the issues around blood pressure and heart rate, sibutramine treatment does produce beneficial reductions in serum triglyceride levels and increases high-density lipoprotein cholesterol concentrations (77,78,82,92–94), both key risk factors for the development of cardiovascular problems. With regard to diabetes, numerous studies have demonstrated that sibutramine-induced weight loss is associated with improved glycemic control and a reduction in other diabetes risk factors (blood pressure, insulin sensitivity, fasting blood glucose levels, triglyceride levels, and low-density lipoprotein cholesterol) (95–99).

A long-term cardiovascular events outcome study with sibutramine is ongoing (100). This five-year study [Sibutramine Cardiovascular Morbidity and Mortality OUTcome Study (SCOUT)] is being conducted in a high-risk patient population, which has either an established cardiovascular risk factor or has suffered a cardiovascular event. During the six-week lead-in phase, sibutramine appeared to be safe in this at-risk hypertensive population and even produced a reduction in blood pressure from baseline (101,102).

These clinical data suggest that 5-HT drugs are effective at producing clinically significant weight loss in patient populations. They appear to be able to reduce cardiometabolic risk factors in general and to produce beneficial changes to cardiovascular function and diabetes control in specific patent populations. The weight loss–inducing effects of sibutramine appear to be equivalent to the novel nonserotonergic antiobesity drug rimonabant. Whether sibutramine can produce changes in cardiometabolic risk factors independent of weight loss is unclear. However, this may have been a property of D-fenfluramine and is certainly a therapeutic benefit unlikely to be limited to endocannabinoid antiobesity drugs (chap. 20). It is not clear whether the new generation of selective 5-HT drugs will be equally effective but probably they will lack the side effect profiles that led to the removal of D-fenfluramine from the market and limited the use of sibutramine as a treatment in at-risk populations.

THE EFFECT OF 5-HT DRUGS ON ABERRANT EATING BEHAVIOR

Disordered eating, as seen in clinical disorders such as bulimia nervosa, has been observed in the obese. This observation has led to the development of the diagnostic criteria for binge eating disorder (BED), which is dealt with in chapter 36. What is worth mentioning here is that a sizeable proportion of obese individuals may display subclinical binge eating, i.e., the frequent consumption of abnormally large amounts of food in single meals, even if the full symptomatology is not shown. While not all the obese binge and not all bingers are chronically overweight, binge eating is a distinctive characteristic in the eating patterns of many obese individuals. This is not really surprising since binge eating was first characterized in the obese nearly 50 years ago (103). Consequently, the beneficial effects of 5-HT drug treatment on binge eating are worthy of mention here.

The functioning of endogenous 5-HT system has been linked to psychopathology of a variety of disorders, such as depression and obsessive-compulsive disorders, and as such has been studied for a number of years. Many of these disorders are currently treated with serotonergic drugs such as the SSRI fluoxetine, including disorders characterized by binge eating. Polymorphisms of 5-HT$_{2A}$ receptor genes are associated with conditions such as bulimia nervosa (104–106), behavioral traits such as impulsiveness (105,107), susceptibility to weight gain (108,109), and even differences in children's caloric intake (110), suggesting some common underlying origin.

For a number of years, bulimic symptomatology has been explained in terms of a dysregulation of 5-HT function (111–113). Like dieting (9,12,13), repeated bingeing may also alter CNS 5-HT receptor sensitivity and functioning. Therefore, it seems possible that an inherited

vulnerability in the 5-HT system (e.g., polymorphisms in 5-HT$_{2A}$ receptor genes) and neurochemical responses to caloric restriction (fall in CNS 5-HT levels) may perpetuate aberrant eating behavior. Recently, it has been argued that disturbances in eating and impulsiveness reflect 5-HT dysregulation specifically in the cortical and limbic 5-HT system. These disturbances could also affect the hedonic (rather than just regulatory) aspects of feeding (107). This in turn could disrupt normal appetite regulation, disinhibiting eating behavior. This topic is covered in extensive detail in chapter 7.

The use of 5-HT drugs in the treatment of bulimia preceded the evaluation of their effects on binge eating in obese. Ten years ago, there were few studies demonstrating that 5-HT drugs had any effect on BED (8). However, as SSRIs had been shown to be effective in reducing binge eating in bulimia, it seemed logical they would be of some benefit in BED (8). Since then the beneficial effects of 5-HT drugs on aberrant eating behavior in the obese have been demonstrated in a number of studies. For instance, fluoxetine reduces the frequency of binge episodes in the obese binge eaters (114). Other SSRIs such as fluvoxamine and sertraline have also been shown to be effective in treating binge eating disorder (115,116). Similarly, the serotonin-noradrenaline reuptake inhibitor sibutramine has also been shown to reduce the size of binge eating episodes, the number of days on which bingeing occurred, and also self-reported binge eating psychopathology (117–119).

These data demonstrate that we should consider wider aspects of appetite control than just satiety when evaluating the behavioral effect of appetite-suppressing antiobesity drugs. Their ability to strengthen the impact of food on appetite and to reduce incidents of impulsive and uncontrolled eating may be clinically important attributes. Such actions would help patients in adhering to dietary advice by reducing the likelihood of disinhibition and binge eating. These data also demonstrate the central role of CNS 5-HT in controlling the expression of feeding behavior, not only in strengthening satiety but also by inhibiting the impulse to consume.

THE NEW GENERATION OF SEROTONERGIC ANTIOBESITY DRUGS: 5-HT$_{2C}$ RECEPTOR AGONISTS AND 5-HT$_6$ RECEPTOR ANTAGONISTS

Recently, pharmaceutical companies have focused on developing 5-HT$_{2C}$ receptor agonists. As described above, research has shown the critical role of this receptor in the regulation of appetite, and specifically in the processes of satiation and satiety. Importantly, 5-HT$_{2C}$ receptors are not thought to be widely distributed outside the CNS. This is fairly critical as D-fenfluramine (Redux) was voluntarily withdrawn in 1997 because of primary pulmonary hypertension, an effect linked with peripheral 5-HT receptors (120). A drug that is a selective agonist for the 5-HT_{2C} receptor obviously avoids the issue of primary pulmonary hypertension, as well as targeting one of the key 5-HT satiety receptors (120). Numerous selective 5-HT_{2C} agonists have passed into clinical trials. However, their effects on food intake and potential clinical efficacy remain unknown, as do the reasons for failing to progress into the clinic (8). However, lorcaserin hydrochloride, also known as APD356 (Arena Pharmaceuticals, San Diego, California, U.S.), is a highly selective 5-HT_{2C} receptor agonist known to be currently undergoing phase 3 clinical trials for obesity (121). The structure of lorcaserin is undisclosed, but it is likely to have come from a series of novel 3-benzazepine derivatives (122). The results of a 12-week phase 2 dose-ranging study of lorcaserin have been presented (123). A total of 459 male and female subjects with a body mass index between 29 and 46 kg/m^2 with an average weight of 100 kg were enrolled in a randomized, double-blind, controlled trial comparing placebo, against 10 and 15 mg given once daily and 10 mg given twice daily (20 mg/day). Over the 12 weeks of the trial, the placebo group gained +0.32 kg ($N = 88$ completers) compared with -1.8 kg in the 10-mg/day dose given once daily ($N = 86$), -2.6 kg in the 15-mg/day dose ($N = 82$ completers), and -3.6 kg in the 10-mg dose given twice daily (20 mg total) ($N = 77$ completers). Side effects that were higher in the active treatment groups than the placebo group were headache, nausea, dizziness, vomiting, and dry mouth. No cardiac valvular changes were noted (124).

SUMMARY

It has been over 30 years since it became apparent that serotonergic systems were involved in mediating episodic signaling for the control of food intake. Since then, evidence has accumulated to confirm the role of specific 5-HT receptors in the modulation of the pattern of feeding. Animal studies identified an action of 5-HT in the modulation of satiation and the control of meal size leading to a decrease in food consumed. Importantly, in the presence of 5-HT activation, the reduced food intake did not lead to any weakening of satiety. Consequently, 5-HT systems were acknowledged to exert a notable inhibition of the willingness to eat, mediated through actions on satiation and satiety. Drugs acting on autoreceptors, which initially appeared to have produced paradoxical findings, actually confirmed the mechanism of action underlying the inhibition of intake. Importantly, a number of pharmacological tools allowed serotonergic interventions to be carried out in humans. Here, the inhibition of appetite was a significant feature of increasing the availability of serotonin or activation of postsynaptic receptors.

Antiobesity drugs based on these actions generated a clear suppression of energy intake and a body weight reduction of 6 to 10 kg over one year. Receptors critically involved in the mediation of appetite suppression are 5HT_{2C} and 5HT_{1B} receptors. Recently, the 5-HT_6 receptor has also shown some therapeutic potential in preclinical models (124,125); however, its effect on appetite and behavior are completely unknown. A more pervasive influence of 5-HT may be occurring since polymorphisms of 5-HT receptors have been associated with obesity (108,109,125–129) and eating disorders (104–108,130,131). Important research has indicated an interaction between leptin and 5-HT, thus providing a mechanism for the influence of tonic modulation over episodic signaling. This integration also involves an interrelationship between 5-HT appetite inhibition and the MC system in the PVN. These data have provided a bridge between the serotoninergic appetite signaling system and the peptide regulation of energy homeostasis.

REFERENCES

1. Halford JCG, Blundell JE. Separate systems for serotonin and leptin in appetite control. Ann Med 2000; 32:222–232.
2. Blundell JE, Goodson S, Halford JCG. Regulation of appetite; role of leptin in signaling systems for drive and satiety. Int J Obes Relat Metab Disord 2001; 25(s1): s29–s34.
3. Blundell JE. Pharmacological approaches to appetite suppression. Trends Pharmacol Sci 1991; 12:147–157.
4. Blundell JE. Is there a role for serotonin (5-hydroxytryptamine) in feeding? Int J Obes 1977; 1:15–42.
5. Blundell JE. Serotonin and the biology of feeding. Am J Clin Nutr 1992; 55:1555–1595.
6. Barnes NM, Sharp T. A review of central 5-HT receptors and their function. Neuropharmacology 1999; 38(8): 1083–1152.
7. Hoyer D, Hannon JP, Martin GR. Molecular, pharmacological and functional diversity of 5-HT receptors. Pharmacol Biochem Behav 2002; 71:533–554.
8. Blundell JE, Halford JCG. Serotonin and appetite regulation: implications for the pharmacological treatment of obesity. CNS Drugs 1998; 9:473–495.
9. Wurtman RJ, Fernstorm JD. Effects of diet on brain neurotransmitters. Nutr Rev 1974; 32(7):193–200.
10. Wurtman JJ, Wurtman RJ. Drugs that enhance central serotoninergic transmission diminish elective carbohydrate consumption by rats. Life Sci 1977; 24:895–904.
11. Wurtman JJ, Wurtman RJ. Fenfluramine and fluoxetine spare protein consumption while suppressing caloric intake by rats. Science 1977; 198:1178–1180.
12. Walsh AE, Oldman AD, Franklin M, et al. Dieting decreases plasma tryptophan and increases the prolactin response to D-fenfluramine in women but not men. J Affect Disord 1995; 33:89–97.

13. Wolfe BW, Metzger ED, Stollar C. The effects of dieting on plasma tryptophan concentration and food intake in healthy women. Physiol Behav 1997; 61:537–541.

14. Barrafan-Majia MG, Castilla-Serna L, Calderon-Guzman D, et al. Effect of nutritional status and ozone exposure on rat brain serotonin. Arch Med Res 2002; 33:15–19.

15. Xie QW. Experimental studies on changes of neuroendocrine functions during starvation and refeeding. Neuroendocrinology 1991; 53:52–59.

16. Nishimura F, Nishihara M, Torii K, et al. Changes in responsiveness to serotonin on rat ventromedial hypothalamic neurons after food deprivation. Physiol Behav 1996; 60:7–12.

17. Bray GA, York DA. Studies on food intake of genetically obese rats. Am J Physiol 1972; 233:176–179.

18. Jesperson S, Scheel-Kruger J. Evidence for a difference in mechanism of action between fenfluramine- and amphetamine-induced anorexia. J Pharm Pharmacol 1973; 25: 49–54.

19. Barrett AM, McSherry L. Inhibition of drug-induced anorexia in rats by methysergide. J Pharm Pharmacol 1975; 27:889–895.

20. Pinder BM, Brogden RN, Sawyer PR, et al. Fenfluramine: a review of its pharmacological properties and therapeutic efficacy in obesity. Drugs 1975; 10:241–323.

21. MacKenzie RG, Hoebel BG, Ducret RP. Hyperphagia following intraventricular p-chlorophenylalanine-, leucine- or tryptophan-methyl esters: lack of correlation with whole brain serotonin levels. Pharmacol Biochem Behav 1979; 10:951–955.

22. Halford JCG, Dovey TM, Cooper GD. Pharmacology of human appetite expression. Curr Drug Targets 2004; 5: 221–240.

23. Halford JCG, Harrold JA, Boyland EJ et al. Serotonergic drugs: effects on appetite expression and use for the treatment of obesity. Drugs 2007; 67(1):27–55.

24. Halford JCG, Wanninayake SCD, Blundell JE. Behavioural satiety sequence (BSS) for the diagnosis of drug action on food intake. Pharmacol Biochem Behav 1998; 61:159–168.

25. Cooper SJ. Cholecystokinin modulation of serotonergic control of feeding behavior. Ann N Y Acad Sci 1996; 780:213–222.

26. Teff KL, Young SN, Blundell JE. The effect of protein or carbohydrate breakfasts on subsequent plasma amino acid levels, satiety and nutrient selection in normal males. Pharmacol Biochem Behav 1989; 34:410–417.

27. Zhang Y, Proenca R, Maffei M. et al. Positional cloning of the mouse obese gene and its human homologue. Nature 1994; 372:425–432.

28. Harrold JA. Hypothalamic control of energy balance. Curr Drug Targets 2004; 5:207–219.

29. Rogers P, McKibbin PE, Williams G. Acute fenfluramine administration reduces neuropeptide Y concentrations in specific hypothalamic regions of the rat: possible implications for the anorectic effect of fenfluramine. Peptides 1991; 12:251–255.

30. Compan V, Dusticier N, Nieoullon A, et al. Opposite changes in striatal neuropeptide Y immunoreactivity after partial and complete serotonergic depletion in the rat. Synapse 1996; 24:87–96.

31. Currie PJ. Integration of hypothalamic feeding and metabolic signals: focus on neuropeptide Y. Appetite 2003; 41:335–337.

32. Heisler LK, Cowley MA, Tecott LH, et al. Activation of central melanocortin pathways by fenfluramine. Science 2002; 297:609–611.

33. Heisler LK, Cowley MA, Kishi T, et al. Central serotonin and melanocortin pathways regulating energy homeostasis. Ann N Y Acad Sci 2003; 994:169–174.

34. Heilser LK, Jobst EE, Sutton GM, et al. Serotonin reciprocally regulated melanocortin neurons to modulate food intake. Neuron 2006; 51:239–249.

35. Neill JC, Cooper SJ. Evidence that d-fenfluramine anorexia is mediated by 5-HT$_1$ receptors. Psychopharmacology 1989; 97:213–218.

36. Samanin R, Mennini T, Bendotti C, et al. Evidence that central 5-HT$_{2C}$ receptors do not play an important role in anorectic activity of d-fenfluramine in the rat. Neuropharmacology 1989; 28:465–469.

37. Neill JC, Bendotti C, Samanin R. Studies on the role of 5-HT receptors in satiation and the effect of d-fenfluramine in the runway test. Eur J Pharmacol 1990; 190:105–112.

38. Simansky KJ, Nicklous DM. Parabrachial infusion of D-fenfluramine reduces food intake: blockade by the 5-HT$_{1B}$ antagonist SB-216641. Pharmacol Biochem Behav 2002; 71:681–690.

39. Vickers SP, Dourish CT, Kennett GA. Evidence that hypophagia induced by d-fenfluramine and d-norfenfluramine in the rat is mediated by 5-HT$_{2C}$ receptors. Neuropharmacology 2001; 41:200–209.

40. Lee MD, Clifton PG. Partial reversal of fluoxetine anorexia by the 5-HT antagonist metergoline. Psychopharmacology 1992; 107:359–364.

41. Halford JCG, Blundell JE. Metergoline antagonizes fluoxetine induced suppression of food intake but not changes in the behavioural satiety sequence. Pharmacol Biochem Behav 1996; 54:745–751.

42. Lucki I, Kreider MS, Simansky KJ. Reduction of feeding behaviour by the serotonin uptake inhibitor sertraline. Psychopharmacology 1988; 96:289–295.

43. Hewitt KN, Lee MD, Dourish CT, et al. Serotonin 2C receptor agonists and the behavioural satiety sequence in mice. Pharmacol Biochem Behav 2002; 71:691–700.

44. Kennett GA, Curzon G. Evidence that the hypophagia induced by mCPP and TFMPP requires 5-HT$_{1C}$ and 5-HT$_{1B}$ receptors; hypophagia induced by RU-24969 only requires 5-HT$_{1B}$ receptors. Psychopharmacology 1988; 96:93–100.

45. Kennett GA, Curzon G. Evidence that mCPP may have behavioural effects mediated by central 5-HT$_{1C}$ receptors. Br J Pharmacol 1988; 94:137–147.

46. Kennett GA, Curzon G. Potencies of antagonists indicate that 5-HT$_{1C}$ receptors mediate 1-3(chlorophenyl)piperazine-induced hypophagia. Br J Pharmacol 1991; 10:2016–2020.

47. Halford JCG, Blundell JE. The 5-HT$_{1B}$ receptor agonist CP-94,253 reduces food intake and preserves the behavioural satiety sequence. Physiol Behav 1996; 60:933–939.

48. Lee MD, Simansky KJ. CP-94,253: a selective serotonin$_{1B}$ (5-HT$_{1B}$) agonist that promotes satiety. Psychopharmacology 1997; 131:264–270.

49. Schreiber R, Selbach K, Asmussen M, et al. Effects of serotonin$_{1/2}$ receptor agonists on dark-phase food and water intake in rats. Pharmacol Biochem Behav 2000; 67:291–305.

50. Clifton PG, Lee MD, Dourish CT. Similarities in the action of Ro 60-0175, a 5-HT$_{2C}$ receptor agonist, and d-fenfluramine on feeding patterns in the rat. Psychopharmacology 2000; 152:256–267.

51. Lee MD, Kennett GA, Dourish CT, et al. 5-HT$_{1B}$ receptors modulate components of satiety in the rat: behavioural and pharmacological analyses of the selective serotonin$_{1B}$ agonist CP-94,253. Psychopharmacology 2002; 164:49–60.

52. Tecott LH, Sun LM, Akanna SF, et al. Eating disorder and epilepsy in mice lacking 5-HT$_{2C}$ serotonin receptors. Nature 1995; 374:542–546.

53. Nonogaki K, Abdullah L, Goulding EH, et al. Hyperactivity and reduced energy cost of physical activity in serotonin 5-HT$_{2C}$ receptor mutant mice. Diabetes 2003; 52:315–320.

54. Bouwknecht JA, van der Guten J, Hijsenm TH, et al. Male and female 5-HT$_{1B}$ receptor knockout mice have higher body weights than wildtypes. Physiol Behav 2001; 74:507–516.

55. Rogers PJ, Blundell JE. Effect of anorexic drugs on food intake and the micro-structure of eating in human subjects. Psychopharmacology 1979; 66:159–165.

56. Foltin RW, Haney M, Comer S, et al. Effect of fenfluramine on food intake, mood, and performance of humans living in a residential laboratory. Physiol Behav 1996; 59:295–305.

57. Goodall E, Silverstone T. Differential effect of d-fenfluramine and metergoline on food intake in human subjects. Appetite 1988; 11:215–288.

58. Blundell JE, Hill AJ. Sensitivity of the appetite control system in obese subjects to nutritional and serotoninergic challenges. Int J Obes 1990; 14:219–233.

59. Drent ML, Zelissen PMJ, Kopperchaar HPF, et al. The effect of dexfenfluramine on eating habits in a Dutch ambulatory android overweight population with an over consumption of snacks. Int J Obes Relat Metab Disord 1995; 19:299–304.

60. McGuirk J, Silverstone T. The effect of 5-HT re-uptake inhibitor fluoxetine on food intake and body weight in healthy male subjects. Int J Obes 1990; 14:361–372.

61. Pijl H, Koppeschaar HPF, Willekens FLA, et al. Effect of serotonin re-uptake inhibition by fluoxetine on body weight and spontaneous food choice in obesity. Int J Obes 1991; 15:237–242.

62. Lawton CL, Wales JK, Hill AJ, et al. Serotoninergic manipulation, meal-induced satiety and eating patterns. Obesity Res 1995; 3:345–356.

63. Walsh AE, Smith KA, Oldman AD. M-Chlorophenylpiperazine decreases food intake in a test meal. Psychopharmacology 1994; 116:120–122.

64. Cowen PJ, Sargent PA, Williams C, et al. Hypophagic, endocrine and subjective responses to m-chlorophenylpiperazine in healthy men and women. Hum Psychopharmacol 1995; 10:385–391.

65. Sargent PA, Sharpley AL, Williams C, et al. 5-HT$_{2C}$ receptor activation decreases appetite and body weight in obese subjects. Psychopharmacology 1997; 133:309–312.

66. Ghaziuddin N, Welch K, Greden J. Central serotonergic effects of m-chlorophenylpiperazine (mCPP) among normal control adolescents. Neuropsychopharmacology 2003:28:133–139.

67. Boeles S, Williams C, Campling GM, et al. Sumatriptan decreases food intake and increases plasma growth hormone in healthy women. Psychopharmacology 1997; 129(pt 2):179–182.

68. Chapelot D, Mamonier C, Thomas F, et al. Modalities of the food intake-reducing effect of sibutramine in humans. Physiol Behav 2000; 68:299–308.

69. Hansen DL, Toubro S, Stock MJ, et al. Thermogenic effects of sibutramine in humans. Am J Clin Nutr 1998; 68:1180–1186.

70. Rolls BJ, Shide DJ, Thorward ML, et al. Sibutramine reduces food intake in non-dieting women with obesity. Obesity Res 1998; 6:1–11.

71. Barkeling B, Elfhag K, Rooth P, et al. Short-term effects of sibutramine (Reductil^{TM}) on appetite and eating behaviour and the long-term therapeutic outcome. Int J Obes Relat Metab Disord 2003; 27:693–700.

72. Halford JCG, Boyland E, Dovey TM, et al. A double-blind, placebo-controlled crossover study to quantify the effects of sibutramine on energy intake and energy expenditure in obese subjects during a test meal using a Universal Eating Monitor (UEM) method. Int J Obes Relat Metab Disord 2007; 31(suppl 1):T3PO.188, s151.

73. Haddock CK, Poston WSC, Dill PL, et al. Pharmacotherapy for obesity: a quantitative analysis of four decades of published randomized clinical trials. Int J Obes Relat Metab Disord 2002; 26:262–273.

74. Guy-Grand B, Apfelbaum M, Creoaldi C, et al. International trial of long-term dexfenfluramine in obesity. Lancet 1989; 2:1142–1145.

75. Guy-Grand B. Clinical studies with d-fenfluramine. Am J Clin Nutr 1992; 55:173s–176s.

76. Goldstein DJ, Rampey AH, Enas GG, et al. Fluoxetine: a randomized clinical trial in the treatment of obesity. Int J Obes Relat Metab Disord 1994; 18:129–135.

77. James WPT, Astrup A, Finer N, et al. Effect of sibutramine on weight maintenance after weight loss: a randomised trial. Lancet 2000; 356:2119–2125.

78. McMohan FG, Fujioja K, Singh BN, et al. Efficacy and safety of sibutramine in obese White and African American patients with hypertension: a 1-year, double-blind, placebo-controlled multicenter trial. Arch Intern Med 2000; 160:2185–2191.

79. Smith IG, Goulder MA. Randomized placebo-controlled trial of long-term treatment with sibutramine in mild to moderate obesity. J Fam Pract 2001; 50:505–512.

80. McNulty SJ, Ur E, Williams G. A randomized trial of sibutramine in the management of obese type 2 diabetic patients treated with metformin. Diabetes Care 2003; 26:125–133.

81. Poston WSC, Reeves RS, Haddock CK, et al. Weight loss in obese Mexican Americans treated for 1-year with orlistat and lifestyle modification. Int J Obes Relat Metab Disord 2003; 27:1486–1493.

82. Arterburn DE, Crane PK, Veenstra DL. The efficacy and safety of sibutramine for weight loss: a systematic review. Arch Intern Med 2004; 164:994–1003.

83. Curioni C, Andre C. Rimonabant for overweight or obesity. Cochrane Database Syst Rev 2006; 4:CD006162.

84. Goldstein DJ. Beneficial health effects of modest weight loss. Int J Obes Relat Metab Disord 1992; 16:1–19.

85. Scheen AJ, Paolisso G, Salvatore T, Lefebvre P. Dexfenfluramine reduces insulin resistance independently of weight reduction in obese type II diabetic patients. Diabetes Care 1991; 14:325–332.

86. Stewart GO, Stein GR, Davis TM, et al. Dexfenfluramine in type 2 diabetes: effect on weight and diabetes control. Med J Aust 1993; 158:167–169.

87. Willey KA, Molyneaux LM, Overland JE, et al. The effects of dexfenfluramine on blood glucose in patients with type II diabetes. Diabet Med 1992; 9:341–343.

88. Kolanowski J, Younis R, Vanbustele R, et al. Effect of dexfenfluramine on body weight, blood pressure, and noradrenergic activity in obese hypertensive patients. Eur J Clin Pharmacol 1992; 42:599–606.

89. Mathus-Vliegen EM, Van de Woord K, Kak AM, et al. Dexfenfluramine in the treatment of severe obesity: a placebo controlled study of the effect on weight loss, cardiovascular risk factors food intake and eating behaviour. J Intern Med 1992; 232:119–127.

90. Kim, SH, Lee YM, Jee HJ, et al. Effect of sibutramine on weight loss and blood pressure: a meta-analysis of controlled trials. Obes Res 2003; 11:1116–1123.

91. Sharma AM. Sibutramine in overweight/obese hypertensive patients. Int J Obes Relat Metab Disord 2001; 25(s4): s20–s23.

92. Apfelbaum M, Vague P, Zieler O, et al. Long-term maintenance of weight loss after a very-low calorie diet: a randomised blinded trial of the efficacy and tolerability of sibutramine. Am J Med 1999; 106:179–184.

93. Dujovne CA, Zavoral JH, Rowe A, et al. Effect of sibutramine on body weight and serum lipids: a double-blind, randomised, placebo-controlled study in 322 overweight and obese patients with dyslipidemia. Am Heart J 2001; 142:489–497.

94. Wirth A, Krause J. Long-term weight loss with sibutramine: a randomized controlled trial. JAMA 2001; 286:1331–1339.

95. Finer N, Bloom SR, Frost GS, et al. Sibutramine is effective for weight loss and diabetic control in obesity with type 2 diabetes: a randomised, double-blind, placebo-controlled study. Diabetes Obes Metab 2000; 2:105–112.

96. Fujioka K, Seaton TB, Rowe E, et al. Weight loss with sibutramine improves glycaemic control and other metabolic parameters in obese patients with type 2 diabetes mellitus. Diabetes Obes Metab 2000; 2:175–187.

97. Van Gaal LF, Peiffer FW. The importance of obesity in diabetes and its treatment with sibutramine. Int J Obes Relat Metab Disord 2001; 25(s4):s24–s28.

98. Gokcel A, Gumurdulu Y, Karakose H, et al. Evaluation of the safety and efficacy of sibutramine, orlistat and metformin in the treatment of obesity. Diabetes Obes Metab 2002; 4:49–55.

99. Redmon JB, Kwong CA, Raatz SK, et al. One year outcome of a combination of weight loss therapies for subjects with type 2 diabetes. Diabetes Care 2003; 26: 2505–2511.

100. James WPT. The SCOUT study: risk-benefit profile of sibutramine in overweight high-risk cardiovascular patients. Eur Heart J Suppl 2007; 7:L44–L48.

101. Maggioni A, Caterson I, Coutinho W, et al. Safety profile of sibutramine during a 6-week treatment period in high-risk patients with cardiovascular disease and/or diabetes—an analysis of the Sibutramine Cardiovascular Outcomes (SCOUT) Trial. Int J Obes Relat Metab Disord 2007; 31: S167–S167.

102. Sharma A, Caterson I, Coutinho W, et al. Six-week treatment period with sibutramine reduces blood pressure in high-risk hypertensive patients—an analysis of the sibutramine cardiovascular outcomes (SCOUT) trial. Int J Obes Relat Metab Disord 2007; 31:S168–S168.

103. Stunkard AJ. Eating patterns in obesity. Psychiatr Q 1959; 33:284–292.

104. Hinney A, Resmschmidt H, Hebebrand J. Candidate gene polymorphisms in eating disorders. Eur J Pharmacol 2000; 410:147–159.

105. Bruce KR, Steiger H, Joober R, et al. Association of the promoter—polymorphism1438G/A of the 5-HT2A receptor gene with behavioral impulsiveness and serotonin function in women with bulimia nervosa. Am J Med Genet B 2005; 137B:40–44.

106. Kaye WH, Frank GK, Bailer UF, et al. Serotonin alterations, in anorexia and bulimia nervosa: new insights from imaging studies. Physiol Behav 2005; 85:73–81.

107. Nomura M, Nomura Y. Psychological, neuroimaging, and biochemical studies on functional association between impulsive behavior and the 5-HT2A receptor gene polymorphism in humans. Ann N Y Acad Sci 2003; 1066:134–143.

108. Hinney A, Ziegler A, Nothen MM, et al. 5-HT2A receptor gene polymorphisms, anorexia nervosa, and obesity. Lancet 1997; 350(9087):1324–1325.

109. Aubert R, Betoulle D, Herbeth B, et al. 5-HT2A receptor gene polymorphism is associated with food and alcohol intake in obese people. Int J Obes Relat Metab Disord 2000; 24(7):920–924.

110. Herbeth B, Aubry E, Fumeron F, et al. Polymorphism of the 5-HT2A receptor gene and food intakes in children and adolescents: the Stanislas Family Study. Am J Clin Nutr 2005; 82:467–470.

111. Brewerton TD, George MS. Is migraine related to the eating disorders? Int J Eat Disord 1993; 14:75–79.

112. Brewerton TD, Mueller EA, Lesam MD, et al., Neuroendocrine responses to m-chlorophenylypiperazine and l-tryptophan in bulimia. Arch Gen Psychiatr 1992; 49: 852–861.

113. Brewerton TD. Toward a unified theory of serotonin dysregulation in eating and related disorders. Psychoneuroendocrinology 1995; 20:561–590.

114. Arnold LM, McElroy SL, Hudson JI, et al. A placebo-controlled, randomized trial of fluoxetine in the treatment of binge-eating disorder. J Clin Psychiatr 2002; 63: 1028–1033.

115. Carter WP, Hudson JI, Lalonde JK, et al. Pharmacologic treatment of binge eating disorder. Int J Eat Disord 2003; 34:s74–s88.

116. Appolinario JC, McElroy SL. Pharmacological approaches in the treatment of binge eating disorder. Curr Drug Targets 2004; 5:301–307.

117. Appolinario JC, Godoy-Matos A, Fontenelle LF, et al. An open-label trial of sibutramine in obese patients with binge-eating disorder. J Clin Psychiatr 2002; 63:28–30.

118. Appolinario JC, Bacaltchuk J, Sichieri R et al. A randomized, double-blind, placebo-controlled study of sibutramine in the treatment of binge-eating disorder. Arch Gen Psychiatr 2003; 60:1109–1116.

119. Mitchell JE, Gosnell BA, Roerig JL et al. Effects of sibutramine on binge eating, hunger, and fullness in a laboratory human feeding paradigm. Obes Res 2003; 11:599–602.

120. Bays HE. Current and investigational antiobesity agents and obesity therapeutic treatment targets. Obes Res 2004; 12:1197–1211.

121. Halford JC. Obesity drugs in clinical development. Curr Opin Investig Drugs 2006; 7:312–318.

122. Smith BM, Smith JM, Tsai JH, et al., Discovery and SAR of new benzazapines and potent and selective 5-HT2C receptor agonist for the treatment of obesity. Bioorg Med Chem Lett 2005; 12:1467–1470.

123. Smith SR, Prosser W, Donahue D, et al. APD356, an orally-active selective 5HT2c agonist reduces body weight in obese men and women. Diabetes Metab 2006; 55(suppl 1):A80.

124. Smith S, Anderson J, Frank A, et al. The effects of APD356, a selective 5-HT2C agonist, on weight loss in a 4 week study in healthy obese patients. Obes Res 2005; 13(suppl) (abstr 101-OR).

125. Harrold JA, Orbach P, Shacham S, et al. Reductions in food intake and body weight induced by PRX-07020, a novel 5-HT$_6$ receptor antagonist. Obes Rev 2006; 7(suppl 2): PO0808, 339.

126. Fisas A, Codony X, Romero G, et al. Chronic 5-HT6 receptor modulation by E-6837 induces hypophagia and sustained weight loss in diet-induced obese rats. Br J Pharmacol 2006; 48:973–983.

127. Rosmond R, Bouchard C, Bjorntorp P. Increased abdominal obesity in subjects with a mutation in the 5-HT2A receptor gene promoter. Ann N Y Acad Sci 2002; 967: 571–575.

128. Rosmond R, Bouchard C, Bjorntorp P. 5-HT2A receptor gene promoter polymorphism in relation to abdominal obesity and cortisol. Obes Res 2002; 10(7):585–589.

129. Pooley EC, Fairburn CG, Cooper Z, et al. A 5-HT2C receptor promoter polymorphism (HTR2C-759C/T) is associated with obesity in women, and with resistance to weight loss in heterozygotes. Am J Med Genet Part B 2004; 126B(1):124–127.

130. Hu X, Giotakis O, Li T, et al. Association of the 5-HT2c gene with susceptibility and minimum body mass index in anorexia nervosa. Neuroreport 2003; 14(6):781–783.

131. Ricca V, Nacmias B, Cellini E, et al. 5-HT2A receptor gene polymorphism and eating disorders. Neurosci Lett 2003; 323(2):105–108.

24

Melanocortin-4 Receptor as a New Target for Drug Development

TUNG M. FONG

Department of Metabolic Disorders, Merck Research Laboratories, Rahway, New Jersey, U.S.A.

ALISON STRACK

Department of Pharmacology, Merck Research Laboratories, Rahway, New Jersey, U.S.A.

INTRODUCTION

The discovery of the link between melanocortin-4 receptor (MC4R) and obesity followed a long history of investigations in an entirely different area, the coat color of mice. The agouti gene in mouse chromosome 2 normally functions to influence coat color of mice. Several naturally occurring mutations in the agouti gene caused a number of dominant effects, including yellow coat color and obesity (1,2). The most notable mutation is the lethal yellow A^y allele. Subsequent studies documented that that mutation in the A^y allele leads to ectopic expression of the agouti protein in many tissues, including the brain. A pivotal study demonstrated that the agouti protein is an antagonist at the MC4R (3), which led to the subsequent pharmacological study demonstrating reduction of food intake by nonselective melanocortin agonist melanotan-II (MT-II) (4) and genetic study demonstrating the obese phenotype of MC4R knockout mice (5). The combined pharmacological and genetic studies firmly established the MC4R as a potential target for antiobesity drug development.

BIOLOGY

MC4R and Its Ligands

MC4R is one of five receptors whose endogenous ligands include α-melanocyte-stimulating hormone (α-MSH), β-MSH, γ-MSH, and adrenocorticotropic hormone (ACTH). These peptides ligands are encoded by the proopiomelanocortin (POMC) gene and are generated through posttranslational processing (Fig. 1). The five melanocortin receptors are encoded by five distinct genes and are involved in a wide spectrum of biological functions (6–8). MC1R is primarily involved in pigmentation. Variation in MC1R activity or melanocortin level or agouti protein level leads to various skin color, hair color, and eye color (9–11). MC2R is expressed in the adrenal gland and regulates the biosynthesis of steroids. MC2R is uniquely different from the other four receptors in that ACTH is the only potent endogenous ligand for MC2R (12). MC5R is predominantly expressed in exocrine glands (13). Both MC3R and MC4R are involved in energy balance, although the MC4R appears to have a

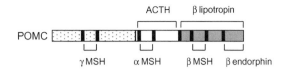

Receptor	Primary Ligands	Function
MC1R	α MSH, ACTH	Pigmentation
MC2R	ACTH	Steroidogenesis
MC3R	α MSH, γ MSH, ACTH	Energy balance
MC4R	α MSH, ACTH	Energy balance, Erectile function
MC5R	α MSH, ACTH	Exocrine function

Figure 1 Peptides encoded by the POMC gene and the five melanocortin receptors. *Abbreviation*: POMC, pro-opiomelanocortin.

more prominent role. The MC4R knockout mice are extremely obese while the MC3R knockout mice are only subtly obese (5,14,15), suggesting that activating the MC4R may be required to maintain the lean phenotype.

Besides the endogenous peptide agonists, melanocortin receptors are also inhibited by endogenous antagonists. The agouti protein is normally expressed in the skin and functions as an endogenous antagonist of MC1R. When ectopically expressed as in agouti yellow mice, agouti protein has the potential to antagonize MC2R, MC3R, MC4R, and MC5R to various extents (3,16). In addition, the agouti-related protein (AGRP) is expressed in the arcuate neurons of the hypothalamus (17), and AGRP has been shown to antagonize MC3R and MC4R (18,19). Further mutational analysis and modeling suggested that a small loop within AGRP appears to bind to the same binding pocket of MC4R for α-MSH, hence providing a molecular basis for the antagonist activity of AGRP at MC4R (20).

Neuroanatomy and Neurophysiology of MC4R

MC4R distribution is widespread. Its localization was first described in 1990 using in situ hybridization. All analyses since then have made use either of mRNA distribution or receptor binding because of the difficulties that have existed in generating MC4R antibodies. Table 1 illustrates regions of the central nervous system (CNS) and peripheral nervous system (PNS) in which substantial levels of MC4R mRNA are found. Of particular note for this discussion are those that may potentially be involved in regulation of energy balance. The hypothalamus, a region that significantly modulates both feeding and energy expenditure, has high levels of MC4R in the ventromedial hypothalamus (VMH), dorsomedial hypothalamus (DMH), and lateral hypothalamic area (LHA). Lower levels, but which are also likely key, are those MC4R-containing neurons in the paraventricular nucleus (PVN). The limbic system, which has been implicated in the reward circuit, also contains MC4R mRNA expressing neurons, among them the nucleus accumbens, the central nucleus of the amygdala, and the basolateral nucleus of the amygdala. More caudally, MC4R mRNA-containing neurons in the dorsal motor nucleus of the vagus nerve (DMX) and the lateral parabrachial nucleus have been implicated in melanocortin-mediated feeding. The DMX may also be involved, directly or indirectly, in energy expenditure similar to the MC4R-containing neurons of the sympathetic preganglionic neurons of the spinal cord.

The activation of melanocortin receptors in the hypothalamus was shown to reduce the neuronal firing rate in the slice preparation (21). In addition, inhibitory synaptic

Table 1 Neural Regions with Moderate to High MC4R mRNA Level in Rats

Area	Representative subregion	Age	References
Forebrain	Auditory cortex, anterior olfactory n., taenia tecta, olfactory tubercle, piriform area; dorsal peduncular cortex, visual cortex, entorhinal cortex, caudoputamen	adult	59,60
Limbic system	n. accumbens, central n. amygdala, medial amygdala, cortical n., lateral septal n., septohippocampal n., subfornical organ	adult	59,60
Hypothalamus	Medial preoptic n., anterior hypothalamic n., VMH, DMH, tuberomammillary n., LHA, median preoptic n., suprachiasmatic nucleus, periventricular n., anteroventral periventricular n., SON, n. circularis, PVNp, PVNm, ventromedial preoptic n.	adult	59,60
Midbrain, pons, and medulla	Superior colliculus, n. optic tract, DMNX, lateral. parabrachial n., NTS, red n., paragigantocellular reticular n.	adult	59,60
Spinal cord	Dorsal horn, IML n.	adult	59,60
Peripheral nervous system	Superior cervical ganglion, paravertebral ganglion, celiac ganglion, vagus nerve	fetus	61

Abbreviations: n., nucleus; VMH, ventromedial hypothalamus; DMH, dorsomedial hypothalamus; LHA, lateral hypothalamic area; SON, supra optic nucleus; PVNp, paraventricular nucleus (parvocellular part); PVNm, paraventricular nucleus (magnocellular part); IML, intermediolateral.

transmission can be increased by melanocortin agonist (22). Both of these electrophysiological effects provide a cellular basis for the way that MC4R agonists may modulate brain neural functions related to the control of energy balance.

Genetics of MC4R and the Obesity Association

Following the discovery that the agouti protein is an antagonist of MC4R and the ectopic expression of agouti protein in the brain may be responsible for the obesity phenotype of the A^y mice (3), MC4R knockout mice were generated which proved that MC4R deficiency does indeed lead to obesity, as a result of increased food intake and reduced energy expenditure (5,23). These studies also demonstrated that heterozygous mice carrying only one copy of the intact MC4R gene developed an intermediate obesity phenotype, suggesting that varying degrees of MC4R activation should lead to a gradation of lean phenotype. Further supporting the important role of the melanocortin pathway in energy balance are the POMC knockout mice, which also exhibit an obesity phenotype (24).

Human genetic studies led to the identification of many MC4R variants in some obese subjects, and these variants are associated with varying degree of obesity (25). All loss-of-function MC4R variants are associated with obesity. On the other hand, some MC4R variants do not significantly affect the function of MC4R, and yet they are associated with obesity. It is likely that the sequence variation may influence the delivery of MC4R to the plasma membrane, indirectly controlling MC4R signaling. In vitro studies do support that this is the case at least for some of the variants that have been evaluated (26,27). While most MC4R variants lead to monogenic obesity, two variants (V103I and I251L) are associated with a lean phenotype (28–30). These genetic data strongly imply that modulating the function of MC4R can affect body weight in both lean and obese directions.

Consistent with rodent genetic studies, POMC variants have also been identified in humans, and carriers of these variants exhibit a significant obesity phenotype (31–34). Because the POMC gene encodes additional peptides, including ACTH, certain POMC variants are also associated with impaired hormone functions (33).

Since MC4R is broadly distributed in the CNS, MC4R may affect various components of energy balance regulation. By blocking the transcription of MC4R in all regions and then reactivating the transcription only in selective regions, Balthasar et al. showed that restoration of MC4R in paraventricular hypothalamus and a subpopulation of amygdala neurons can prevent the hyperphagia, but not reduced energy expenditure due to MC4R inactivation

(35). These data suggest that while MC4R activation affects both food intake and energy expenditure, these two components appear to be regulated by MC4R in distinct neuronal populations. This intriguing finding may stimulate future research to distinguish the contribution from different brain regions, although at the present time, all drugs designed to be brain penetrating will not achieve region-specific targeting.

DEVELOPMENT OF MC4R SELECTIVE AGONISTS

Extensive efforts have been devoted to the development of MC4R selective agonists by many groups. Early efforts focused on peptide ligands, including nonselective agonists and selective agonists (7,36,37). These encouraging results in peptide research suggested the feasibility of developing nonpeptide, orally bioavailable agonists. One of the first nonpeptide MC4R selective agonists is THIQ (38). Subsequently, many more MC4R agonists have been discovered by various groups (39,40). In general, these compounds are excellent agonists in vitro and exhibit in vivo efficacy in rodent studies. The challenges in the future are to optimize these molecules and demonstrate their effectiveness and appropriate therapeutic margin in humans.

REGULATION OF ENERGY BALANCE

Following the initial demonstration that nonselective melanocortin agonists can reduce body weight and adiposity in rodents (41) and the genetic association between MC4R variants and obesity, selective MC4R agonists were developed and tested in diet-induced obese (DIO) rodents. In DIO rats, one MC4R selective agonist was shown to cause weight loss over 14 days of oral administration (42), thus validating the MC4R as a potential antiobesity target. To further understand the mechanism of MC4R agonist-induced weight loss, various studies were performed to determine which component of the energy balance equation is affected by MC4R agonists.

MC4R and Food Intake

Fan et al. first demonstrated that the nonselective melanocortin agonist MT-II reduces food intake in rodents (4). The resultant decrease of food intake as a consequence of activation of MC4R could stem from multiple sites of action. In the hypothalamus, region-specific injections of [Nle4, D-Phe7]-alpha-MSH decreased food intake to the greatest degree in the PVN, and significant decreased food intake in other areas including the DMH, medial preoptic (MPO), arcuate nucleus and LHA. Interestingly, AGRP caused increases in feeding in most of those regions, but not in the arcuate nucleus or the LHA (43).

Studies with an MC4R selective agonist Ro-3225 have been used to address the question as to whether MC4R activation results in food intake suppression via direct effects on food intake (e.g., satiety, satiation, and motivation) or due to other effects such as malaise or sickness. Ro-3225, when administered to rats, does not cause signs of illness behavior in sodium chloride intake, or pica assays, or in a conditioned taste aversion assay. However, it does decrease food intake in both rats and *db/db* mice (44). In contrast, studies with the nonselective melanocortin agonist, MT-II, do show formation of conditioned taste aversion when given to rats, implicating MC3R as a player in the aversive effects of nonselective agonists (45). A caveat in interpreting the conditioned taste aversion assay is that all known drugs of abuse produce taste aversion in rodents, yet these drugs are highly reinforcing and do not usually cause sickness behavior in humans (46).

Further investigations demonstrated that selective MC4R agonists can produce significant food intake reduction in a mechanism based manner in rodents. Ye et al. discovered a selective MC4R agonist RY764, which is effective in reducing food intake in wild type mice but not in MC3R-MC4R double knockout mice (47). The combination of a pharmacological agent with MC4R knockout mice provided convincing evidence that the anorexic effect is MC4R-mediated rather than from some structure-based nonspecific mechanism. Another MC4R agonist MK-0493 was reported in a single dose human food intake study, in which MK-0493 at 500 mg caused a small nonsignificant reduction of 24-hour total caloric intake (48). Further studies are necessary to fully evaluate the potential of MC4R agonists in reducing food intake in humans.

MC4R and Metabolic Rate

In addition to the anorexic effect, melanocortin agonists also increase energy expenditure in rodents. Chen et al. showed that the nonselective agonist MT-II increases metabolic rate only in wild type mice but not in the MC4R knockout mice (49). These data are consistent with the results obtained from the MC4R knockout mice, which exhibit a hypometabolic phenotype (23,35), and suggest that MC4R selective agonists should increase energy expenditure.

MC4R and Other Biological Functions

Melanocortin agonists have been shown to affect glucose metabolism. Centrally administered MT-II lowers plasma insulin level acutely, which can be blocked by α-adrenergic receptor antagonism (50). Centrally administered MT-II also enhances insulin sensitivity of glucose disposal in 24 hours (51). These effects on glucose metabolism along with the metabolic rate–enhancing effect appear to result from melanocortins acting in the hypothalamus and influencing peripheral tissue metabolism via the autonomic nervous system. Since MC4R selective agonists have not yet been evaluated in the assays of insulin sensitivity, future studies will need to address which MC receptor specifically influences glucose metabolism.

Cardiovascular (CV) functions may also be affected by MC receptors. Central administration of MT-II for 10 days leads to increased mean arterial pressure in rats (52). It is not yet clear whether MC4R selective agonists may produce similar effect. On the other hand, MC4R knockout mice are normotensive despite obesity and hyperleptinemia (53), while MC3R knockout mice develop high salt-dependent hypertension (54). MC3R has been proposed to play a role in CV functions (55,56). Elucidating the complex interplay between melanocortins and CV functions will require further studies utilizing both genetic and pharmacological tools.

Expression pattern studies demonstrated that MC4R is associated with a number of tissues linked to regulation of sexual function, including sites in the brain and spinal cord, pelvic ganglia, and the penis itself. MC4R is localized in the nerve fibers within the corpus and glans penis (38). In situ hybridization studies demonstrate that the MC4R is in two sensory endings, the end bulb of Krause and the Raffini nerve ending. These endings are thought to be associated with stretch sensations. MC4R agonists have been shown to exhibit pro-erectile activity in wild type mice but not in MC4R knockout mice (38), substantiating the role of MC4R in rodent sexual function. While selective MC4R agonists have not been reported in human testing, nonselective agonist MT-II and its analog have been shown to produce erectile activity in patients with erectile dysfunction (57,58).

SUMMARY

MC4R represents a novel target that may lead to a new generation of antiobesity therapeutics. Human and mouse genetic data and rodent pharmacological data provide strong support for this approach. As illustrated in the studies of Y5R antagonist and CB1R inverse agonist (Chapter 22 and Chapter 20) rodent efficacy may or may not quantitatively predict the magnitude of human efficacy. A clear understanding of any potential species difference in neuroanatomy and neurochemistry will be critical in interpreting future studies of MC4R agonists. In the case of the melanocortin system, the presence of AGRP as an endogenous MC4R antagonist in the brain clearly represents a factor in determining the relative efficacy of MC4R agonists. Do humans have similar basal and stimulated release level of AGRP as rodents? Does MC4R in humans receive similar input from AGRP and POMC neurons? How does one determine the level of MC4R occupancy with MC4R agonist treatment in humans? These questions may not be easy to answer with current technology. Thus, clinical studies with innovative design will be critical in determining whether MC4R can be successfully used in the treatment of obesity.

REFERENCES

1. Siracusa LD. The agouti gene: turned on to yellow. Trends Genet 1994; 10:423–428.
2. Klebig ML, Wilkinson JE, Woychik RP. Molecular analysis of the mouse agouti gene and the role of sominant agouti-locus mutations in obesity and insulin resistance. In: Bray GA, Ryan DH, eds. Molecular and Genetic Aspects of Obesity. Baton Rouge: Louisiana State University Press, 1996:120–158.
3. Lu D, Willard D, Patel IR, et al. Agouti protein is an antagonist of the melanocortin-stimulating hormone receptor. Nature 1994; 371:799–802.
4. Fan W, Boston BA, Kesterson RA, et al. Role of melanocortinergic neurons in feeding and the agouti obesity syndrome. Nature 1997; 385:165–168.
5. Huszar D, Lynch CA, Fair-Huntress V, et al. Targeted disruption of the melanocortin-4 receptor results in obesity in mice. Cell 1997; 88:131–141.
6. Cone RD. Anatomy and regulation of the central melanocortin system. Nat Neurosci 2005; 8:571–578.
7. Hadley ME, Hruby VJ, Jiang J, et al. Melanocortin receptors: identification and characterization by melanotropic peptide agonists and antagonists. Pigment Cell Res 1996; 9:213–234.
8. Gantz I, Fong TM. The melanocortin system. Am J Physiol Endocrinol Metab 2003; 284:E468–E474.
9. Sturm RA, Teasdale RD, Box NF. Human pigmentation genes: identification, structure and consequences of polymorphic variation. Gene 2001; 277:49–62.
10. Wong TH, Rees JL. The relation between melanocortin 1 receptor (MC1R) variation and the generation of phenotypic diversity in the cutaneous response to ultraviolet radiation. Peptides 2005; 26:1965–1971.
11. Schaffer JV, Bolognia JL. The melanocortin-1 receptor: red hair and beyond. Arch Dermatol 2001; 137:1477–1485.
12. Clark AJ, Metherell LA. Mechanisms of disease: the adrenocorticotropin receptor and disease. Nat Clin Pract Endocrinol Metab 2006; 2:282–290.
13. Chen W, Kelly MA, Opitz-Araya X, et al. Exocrine gland dysfunction in MC5-R-deficient mice: evidence for coordinated regulation of exocrine gland function by melanocortin peptides. Cell 1997; 91:789–798.
14. Chen AS, Marsh DJ, Trumbauer ME, et al. Inactivation of the mouse melanocortin-3 receptor results in increased fat mass and reduced lean body mass. Nat Genet 2000; 26: 97–102.
15. Butler AA, Kesterson RA, Khong K, et al. A unique metabolic syndrome causes obesity in the melanocortin-3 receptor-deficient mouse. Endocrinology 2000; 141:3518–3521.
16. Yang YK, Ollmann MM, Wilson BD, et al. Effects of recombinant agouti-signaling protein on melanocortin action. Mol Endocrinol 1997; 11(3):274–280.
17. Shutter JR, Gramham M, Kinsey AC, et al. Hypothalamic expression of ART, a novel gene related to agouti, is upregulated in obese and diabetic mutant mice. Genes Dev 1997; 11:593–602.
18. Fong TM, Mao C, MacNeil T, et al. ART (protein product of agouti-related transcript) as an antagonist of MC3 and MC4 receptors. Biochem Biophys Res Commun 1997; 237:629–631.
19. Ollmann MM, Wilson BD, Yang Y-K, et al. Antagonism of central melanocortin receptors in vitro and in vivo by agouti-related protein. Science 1997; 278:135–138.
20. Tota MR, Smith TS, Mao C, et al. Molecular interaction of agouti protein and agouti-related protein with human melanocortin receptors. Biochemistry 1999; 38:897–904.
21. Fong TM, Van der Ploeg LH. A melanocortin agonist reduces neuronal firing rate in rat hypothalamic slices. Neurosci Lett 2000; 283:5–8.
22. Cowley MA, Pronchuk N, Fan W, et al. Integration of NPY, AGRP and melanocortin signals in the hypothalamic paraventricular nucleus. Neuron 1999; 24:155–168.
23. Ste Marie L, Miura GI, Marsh DJ, et al. A metabolic defect promotes obesity in mice lacking melanocortin-4 receptors. Proc Natl Acad Sci U S A 2000; 97(22):12339–12344.
24. Yaswen L, Diehl N, Brennan MB, et al. Obesity in the mouse model of pro-opiomelanocortin deficiency responds to peripheral melanocortin. Nat Med 1999; 5(9):1066–1070.
25. Farooqi IS, O'Rahilly S. Monogenic obesity in humans. Annu Rev Med 2005; 56:443–458.
26. Lubrano-Berthelier C, Durand E, Dubern B, et al. Intracellular retention is a common characteristic of childhood obesity-associated MC4R mutations. Hum Mol Genet 2003; 12:145–153.
27. Nijenhuis WA, Garner KM, van Rozen RJ, et al. Poor cell surface expression of human melanocortin-4 receptor mutations associated with obesity. J Biol Chem 2003; 278:22939–22945.
28. Stutzmann F, Vatin V, Cauchi S, et al. Non-synonymous polymorphisms in melanocortin-4 receptor protect against obesity: the two facets of a Janus obesity gene. Hum Mol Genet 2007; 16(15):1837–1844.
29. Bronner G, Sattler AM, Hinney A, et al. The 103I variant of the melanocortin 4 receptor is associated with low serum triglyceride levels. J Clin Endocrinol Metab 2006; 91(2): 535–538.
30. Young EH, Wareham NJ, Farooqi S, et al. The V103I polymorphism of the MC4R gene and obesity: population based studies and meta-analysis of 29 563 individuals. Int J Obes (Lond) 2007; 31(9):1437–1441.
31. Coll AP, Farooqi IS, Challis BG, et al. Proopiomelanocortin and Energy Balance: Insights from Human and Murine Genetics. J Clin Endocrinol Metab 2004; 89:2557–2562.

32. Hinney A, Becker I, Heibult O, et al. Systematic mutation screening of the pro-opiomelanocortin gene: identification of several genetic variants including three different insertions, one nonsense and two missense point mutations in probands of different weight extremes. J Clin Endocrinol Metab 1998; 83:3737–3741.

33. Krude H, Biebermann H, Luck W, et al. Severe early-onset obesity, adrenal insufficiency and red hair pigmentation caused by POMC mutations in humans. Nat Genet 1998; 19:155–157.

34. Krude H, Biebermann H, Schnabel D, et al. Obesity due to proopiomelanocortin deficiency: three new cases and treatment trials with thyroid hormone and ACTH4-10. J Clin Endocrinol Metab 2003; 88:4633–4640.

35. Balthasar N, Dalgaard LT, Lee CE, et al. Divergence of melanocortin pathways in the control of food intake and energy expenditure. Cell 2005; 123(3):493–505.

36. Hruby VJ, Lu D, Sharma SD, et al. Cyclic lactam alpha-melanocortin analogs Ac-Nle4-cyclo[Asp5, D-Phe7, Lys10] alpha-melanocyte stimulating hormone-(4-10)-NH2 with bulky aromatic amino acids at position 7 show high antagonist potency and selectivity at specific melanocortin receptors. J Med Chem 1995; 38:3454–3461.

37. Schioth HB, Mutulis F, Muceniece R, et al. Discovery of novel melanocortin4 receptor selective MSH analogues. Br J Pharmacol 1998; 124:75–82.

38. Van der Ploeg LHT, Martin WJ, Howard AD, et al. A role for the melanocortin 4 receptor in sexual function. Proc Natl Acad Sci U S A 2002; 99:11381–11386.

39. Nargund RP, Strack AM, Fong TM. Melanocortin-4 receptor (MC4R) agonists for the treatment of obesity. J Med Chem 2006; 49(14):4035–4043.

40. Sebhat I, Ye Z, Bednarek M, et al. Melanocortin-4 receptor agonists and antagonists: chemistry and potential therapeutic utilities. Annu Rep Med Chem 2003; 38:31–40.

41. Pierroz DD, Ziotopoulou M, Ungsunan L, et al. Effects of acute and chronic administration of the melanocortin agonist MTII in mice with diet-induced obesity. Diabetes 2002; 51(5):1337–1345.

42. Van der Ploeg LHT, Kanatani A, MacNeil D, et al. Design and synthesis of (ant)-agonists that alter appetite and adiposity. Prog Brain Res 2006; 153:107–118.

43. Kim MS, Rossi M, Abusnana S, et al. Hypothalamic localization of the feeding effect of agouti-related peptide and alpha-melanocyte-stimulating hormone. Diabetes 2000; 49(2):177–182.

44. Benoit S, Schwartz M, Lachey J, et al. A novel selective melanocortin-4 receptor agonist reduces food intake in rats and mice without producing aversive consequences. J Neurosci 2000; 20(9):3442–3448.

45. Thiele TE, Van Dijk G, Yagaloff KA, et al. Central infusion of melanocortin agonist MTII in rats: assessment of c-Fos expression and taste aversion. Am J Physiol Regul Integr Comp Physiol 1998; 274(1 pt 2):R248–R254.

46. Grigson PS, Twining RC, Carelli RM. Heroin-induced suppression of saccharin intake in water-deprived and water-replete rats. Pharmacol Biochem Behav 2000; 66(3):603–608.

47. Ye Z, Guo L, Barakat KJ, et al. Discovery and activity of (1R, 4S, 6R)-N-[(1R)-2-[4-cyclohexyl-4-[[(1, 1-dimethylethyl) amino]carbonyl]- 1-piperidinyl]-1-[(4-fluorophenyl)methyl]-2-oxoethyl]-2-methyl-2-azabicycl o[2.2.2]octane-6-carboxamide (3, RY764), a potent and selective melanocortin subtype-4 receptor agonist. Bioorg Med Chem Lett 2005; 15:3501–3505.

48. Stevens C, Maganti L, Zhu H, et al. Effects of an MC4R agonist on food intake in overweight/obese men. In: 7th Annual Scientific Sessions of ADA. Chicago, IL: American Diabetes Association, 2007 (abstr 1829-P).

49. Chen AS, Metzger JM, Trumbauer ME, et al. Role of the melanocortin-4 receptor in metabolic rate and food intake in mice. Transgenic Res 2000; 9:145–154.

50. Fan W, Dinulescu DM, Butler AA, et al. The central melanocortin system can directly regulate serum insulin levels. Endocrinology 2000; 141:3072–3079.

51. Heijboer AC, van den Hoek AM, Pijl H, et al. Intracerebroventricular administration of melanotan II increases insulin sensitivity of glucose disposal in mice. Diabetologia 2005; 48:1621–1626.

52. Silva AA, Kuo JJ, Tallam LS, et al. Does obesity induce resistance to the long-term cardiovascular and metabolic actions of melanocortin 3/4 receptor activation? Hypertension 2006; 47(2):259–264.

53. Tallam LS, Stec DE, Willis MA, et al. Melanocortin-4 receptor-deficient mice are not hypertensive or salt-sensitive despite obesity, hyperinsulinemia, and hyperleptinemia. Hypertension 2005; 46:326–332.

54. Ni X-P, Pearce D, Butler AA, et al. Genetic disruption of {gamma}-melanocyte-stimulating hormone signaling leads to salt-sensitive hypertension in the mouse. J Clin Invest 2003; 111(8):1251–1258.

55. Mioni C, Giuliani D, Cainazzo MM, et al. Further evidence that melanocortins prevent myocardial reperfusion injury by activating melanocortin MC3 receptors. Eur J Pharmacol 2003; 477:227–234.

56. Li SJ, Varga K, Archer P, et al. Melanocortin antagonists define two distinct pathways of cardiovascular control by alpha- and gamma-melanocyte-stimulating hormones. J Neurosci 1996; 16:5182–5188.

57. Rosen RC, Diamond LE, Earle DC, et al. Evaluation of the safety, pharmacokinetics and pharmacodynamic effects of subcutaneously administered PT-141, a melanocortin receptor agonist, in healthy male subjects and in patients with an inadequate response to Viagra. Int J Impot Res 2004; 16:135–142.

58. Wessells H, Gralnek D, Dorr R, et al. Effect of an alpha-melanocyte stimulating hormone analog on penile erection and sexual desire in men with organic erectile dysfunction. Urology 2000; 56:641–646.

59. Mountjoy K, Mortrud M, Low M, et al. Localization of the melanocortin-4 receptor (MC4-R) in neuroendocrine and autonomic control circuits in the brain. Mol Endocrinol 1994; 8(10):1298–1308.

60. Kishi T, Aschkenasi CJ, Lee CE, et al. Expression of melanocortin 4 receptor mRNA in the central nervous system of the rat. J Comp Neurol 2003; 457:213–235.

61. Mountjoy K, Wild J. Melanocortin-4 receptor mRNA expression in the developing autonomic and central nervous systems. Dev Brain Res 1998; 107(2):309–314.

25

Histamine H₃ Receptor Antagonists in the Treatment of Obesity

KARIN RIMVALL

Section of Diabetes and Obesity, AstraZeneca R&D, Mölndal, Sweden

ROLF HOHLWEG

Department of Patent Information, Novo Nordisk Library, Novo Nordisk A/S, Bagsværd, Denmark

KJELL MALMLÖF

Department of Anatomy, Physiology and Biochemistry, Faculty of Veterinary Medicine, SLU, Uppsala, Sweden

INTRODUCTION

During the past 10 to 15 years, new knowledge relating to mammalian appetite and body weight regulation has accumulated and various central nervous system (CNS) receptors, e.g., the NPY_2, NPY_5, and MC_4, have been targeted in attempts to identify chemical entities that could potentially be used for the pharmacological treatment of obesity in the clinic. In this process, relatively little attention has been paid to the involvement of neuronal histamine in the regulation of food intake and body weight. However, much preclinical data is now available in the literature that clearly establish that the neuronal central H_1 and H_3 receptors are central players in the regulation of energy homeostasis and metabolism. This chapter reviews the role played by the central histaminergic neurotransmitter system in the regulation of food intake and body weight in rodents and in higher mammalian species. Following a brief overview of the morphology and function of the central histaminergic system, we will discuss how this system can be modulated to obtain beneficial metabolic effects. Previously unpublished data obtained in animal models of obesity will be presented. These data add further support to the concept that increased central histamine levels may have a great potential in the clinical treatment of human obesity and associated metabolic disorders.

HISTAMINE AND ITS RECEPTORS

Overview

The monoamine histamine plays a role in a variety of biological processes in the mammalian body. Its effects range from transmitting neural signals in the central and peripheral nervous systems (CNS and PNS), to inducing, e.g., inflammatory responses, gastric acid secretion, and smooth muscle contraction (Table 1).

The work presented here was conducted at Novo Nordisk A/S in Denmark.

Table 1 Overview of the Four Histamine Receptor's Expression and Examples of Physiological Effects

Receptor subtype	Histamine 1	Histamine 2	Histamine 3	Histamine 4
Expression	Peripheral tissues CNS	Peripheral tissues CNS	PNS CNS	Peripheral tissues
Function	**Peripheral** H_1 receptors mediate allergic manifestations induced by histamine released from peripheral mast cells	**Peripheral** H_2 receptors mediate gastric acid secretion	**Central** histamine H_3 receptors as well as those expressed on **peripheral nerve endings** modulate synthesis and release of histamine and other neurotransmitters	**Peripheral** H_4 receptors in the hemopoetic system mediate histamine's immunomodulatory effects
	Central H_1 receptors mediate histamine-induced arousal, cognitive enhancement, and inhibition of appetite	**Central** H_2 receptors mediate fetal brain development?		

Abbreviations: CNS, central nervous system; PNS, peripheral nervous system.

In the rat CNS, immunocytochemical studies show that histaminergic neurons are exclusively located in the tuberomammillary nucleus (TMN) in the lateral part of the posterior hypothalamus (1,2). These neurons project widely to many different areas of the rat brain (3), and histamine-immunoreactive fibers are numerous within and between those hypothalamic nuclei that are involved in the regulation of food intake and energy expenditure (4).

It is established that histamine mediates its actions through four distinct histamine receptors, the histamine H_1, H_2, H_3, and H_4 receptors. They are all G-protein-coupled receptors but have a fairly low level of homology between them (5). In the following section, the four histamine receptors will be described in somewhat more detail with emphasis on the H_1 and the H_3 receptors as these are the two histamine receptors that are of interest in relation to control of food intake.

H_1 Receptor

The H_1 receptor was cloned in 1991 (6) and is found both in the CNS and in most peripheral tissues. In the periphery, the H_1 receptor mediates the histamine-induced contraction of smooth musculature and mediates the effects of the histamine released from mast cells in allergic reactions. In the brain, the H_1 receptor has a widespread distribution (7). In the hypothalamus it is highly expressed in the ventromedial hypothalamus (VMH), moderately expressed in the paraventricular nucleus (PVN), and is also expressed at low levels in the arcuate nucleus and in the lateral and posterior hypothalamic nuclei. In the CNS, the H_1 receptor mediates histamine's arousing and cognitive effects (8), and in the hypothalamus it is responsible

for the inhibitory effects on food intake that have frequently been observed following increases in central histamine levels. This is elaborated in more detail later in this chapter.

H_2 Receptor

The H_2 receptor was also cloned in 1991 (9) and, like the H_1 receptor, it is expressed both in the CNS and in peripheral tissues. In the periphery, the H_2 receptor mediates, for example, the histamine-induced gastric acid secretion in the stomach. An example of an H_2 receptor antagonist used clinically is the "antacid" cimetidine. The role of the H_2 receptor in the CNS is not quite clear, but it may be involved in mediating neuroendocrine processes (10) and in fetal brain development and excitability of brain cells (11). There is no evidence that the H_2 receptor is of importance in the histaminergic regulation of food intake or body weight and no expression of the H_2 receptor mRNA can be found in monkey hypothalamus (12).

H_3 Receptor

The H_3 receptor in the CNS was identified pharmacologically in 1983 as a presynaptic receptor that influences neurotransmission (13). These authors demonstrated that histamine-induced activation of the presynaptic H_3 autoreceptor lead to a decreased synthesis of histamine as well as to a decreased release of this transmitter from synaptosomes (13,14). The histaminergic activation of H_3 heteroreceptors, situated on presynaptic terminals of, e.g., noradrenergic, cholinergic, dopaminergic, and serotonergic neurons, also inhibit the release of these neurotransmitters (15). The molecular cloning of the H$_3$ receptor was not achieved until 1999 (16). H$_3$ mRNA expression is most abundant in the CNS, and only little H$_3$ mRNA expression can be seen in peripheral organs (17,18). It has been pharmacologically characterized as being present on sympathetic nerve endings in, e.g., the nasal mucosa (19) and the heart (20). In the hypothalamus, the density of binding sites for the iodinated, selective H$_3$ receptor agonist ^{125}I-iodoproxyfan is highest in the TMN (21). Dense binding also appears in the PVN and in the VMH. Since the H$_3$ receptor mediates histamine's negative feedback inhibition of its own synthesis and release, this histamine receptor is a major player in the histaminergic system's regulation of food intake and body weight.

H$_4$ Receptor

The H4 receptor was cloned by several laboratories in 2000 (22), and it is mainly expressed peripherally, in blood-cells, and in cells in the spleen and bone marrow (5). In addition, there are some indications that it is also expressed at low levels in the mouse hippocampus (23). It is not considered to be of importance in mediating any of histamine's effects on food intake and metabolism.

REGULATION OF FOOD INTAKE

Rodents

Experimental data supporting the importance of the histaminergic system in food intake regulation in rodents have recently been the subject of several reviews (24–26). However, the very first study demonstrating the effects of histamine levels on food intake was already published in 1973 when Clineschmidt and Lotti observed that injections of histamine into the lateral ventricles of the cat suppressed food intake (27).

Histamine levels in the CNS can be experimentally modulated by administration of histidine (the precursor of histamine), metoprine (an inhibitor of histamine breakdown), and H$_3$ receptor antagonists. The latter type of compounds increases histamine synthesis and release into synapses. Many researchers have come to the conclusion that increased histamine levels in the CNS inhibit food intake in rodents regardless of how histamine levels are raised (28–31). Using the three selective H$_3$ receptor antagonists, ciproxifan (32), NNC 0038-0000-1049 (33), and NNC 0038-0000-1202 (34), we have demonstrated very good correlations between histamine levels in the PVN and acute effects on food intake in rodents.

As indicated previously, several lines of evidence clearly suggest that it is the hypothalamic H$_1$ receptor that mediates the inhibitory effects on food intake elicited by increased histamine levels.

- Administration of the H$_1$ receptor *agonist* 2-(3-trifluoromethylphenyl)histamine (FMPH) *decreased* food intake in rodents (35).
- Administration of a specific H$_1$ receptor antagonist *increases* feeding (29,36).
- H$_1$ receptor knockout mice are obese, in particular if they are crossed with the ob/ob mouse (37).
- The degree of increase in food intake in rodents treated with tricyclic antidepressants is related to these compounds' affinities for the H$_1$ receptor (38).

Thus, we conclude that there is a large body of evidence available suggesting that increased histamine levels in the CNS exert an inhibitory effect on food intake that is mediated by the histamine H$_1$ receptors.

In summary, the degree of activation of the H$_1$ receptor together with the H$_3$ receptor–mediated control of intrasynaptic concentrations of histamine both seem to be of importance for the anorectic signal. Consequently, there is a strong interest in finding pharmacological approaches to increase signal transmission through the histamine H$_1$ receptor (26). This could be achieved either with an H$_1$ or with an H$_3$ receptor antagonist. As already mentioned above, the peripheral H$_1$ receptor mediates the effects of histamine that is released in allergic manifestations and as it would be virtually impossible to synthesize an H$_1$ receptor agonist that does not target the peripheral H$_1$ receptor but only the central H$_1$ receptor, the most safe and promising way of achieving an increased signaling through the central H$_1$ receptor is with an H$_3$ receptor antagonist that raises intrasynaptic histamine levels. Our, and others', efforts have consequently focused on identifying selective H$_3$ receptor antagonists for the treatment of obesity.

Pigs and Rhesus Monkeys

Since rodents are night-active animals and histamine has been shown to be involved in the control of circadian rhythms (39), it has been important for us to demonstrate that also higher mammalian species decrease their food intake after administration of a H$_3$ antagonist. We have done so both in pigs and obese rhesus monkeys using the selective H$_3$ antagonist NNC 0038-0000-1202 (40). In pigs, an oral dose of 15 mg/kg reduced daily caloric intake by 55%, and in obese rhesus monkeys, a reduction of 40% was recorded following a subcutaneous dose of 0.1 mg/kg. In the monkey study, the reduction of food intake was seen in both females and males. In this connection, it is worth mentioning that the human and monkey variants of the histamine H3 receptor show a 98.4%

identity (40). In addition, the supposed binding regions are identical (18). Obviously, these observations increase the probability that H3 antagonists that are able to reduce food intake in monkeys would do so also in humans.

HISTAMINE H₃ RECEPTOR ANTAGONISTS AND THEIR POTENTIAL ROLE IN TREATMENT OF OBESITY

H₃ Receptor Antagonists and Effects on Body Weight and Metabolism in Rodents

The first study demonstrating that increased histamine levels in the CNS not only affects food intake acutely but also induces body weight loss after longer treatment in rodents appeared in 2004 when the Abbott research team published work using their H₃ antagonist A-331440 in a mouse model of diet-induced obesity (DIO) (41). After administration of 5-mg/kg A-331440 perorally (PO) to DIO mice for four weeks, a significant weight loss and loss of fat depots was achieved. The weight loss was attributed not only to decreased food intake but also to maintained energy expenditure. Normally a decrease in caloric intake results in decreased energy expenditure. The fact that the H₃ receptor antagonist prevented this decrease further promoted the establishment of the negative energy balance that is a prerequisite for a decrease in body weight. In addition, A-331440 improved insulin tolerance in these mice. This compound was subsequently put into preclinical development, but unfortunately failed due to in vitro genotoxicity (42).

Recently published data from our own laboratory confirm and extend the Abbott group's data to rats and, partly, to pigs and monkeys. Novo Nordisk's two compounds NNC 0038-0000-1049 and NNC 0038-0000-1202 were the first potent, selective H₃ receptor antagonists identified by us that had sufficiently good pharmacokinetic properties to make them useful for in vivo studies. Both these compounds are unsuitable for clinical development, but we have used them as tools to demonstrate beneficial effects on food intake in rats, pigs, and rhesus monkeys and on body weight in DIO rats. Using these two compounds, we were able to confirm that sustained administration of H₃ antagonists over several weeks indeed causes a significant body weight loss of approximately 5% to 7% (33,34). In addition, more recent data with a third, potent (K_i at hH₃ receptor ~2.3 nM) and selective H₃ antagonist from our laboratory, NNC 0038-0000-1718, show that the H₃ antagonist-induced weight loss in DIO rats (for experimental details see Ref. 34) is also dose dependent and that up to 20% of body weight is lost in three weeks with the highest oral dose used (6.4 mg/kg) (Fig. 1A). This weight loss is represented mainly by fat (Fig. 1B). In fact, after administration of 5 mg/kg PO of

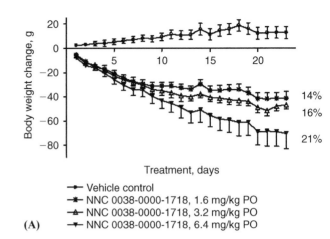

(A)

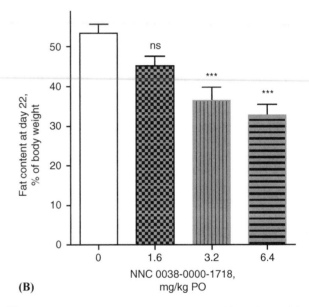

(B)

Figure 1 The H₃ antagonist NNC 0038-0000-1718, administered orally at 1.6, 3.2, and 6.4 mg/kg PO for three weeks, dose dependently decreased body weight (**A**) and fat depots (**B**) in DIO rats. *Abbreviation*: DIO, diet-induced obesity.

NNC 0038-0000-1718 for three weeks, body weight was normalized down to the level of age-matched rats that were never obese as they were never fed a high-fat diet (previously unpublished; Fig. 2). The lowest effective dose of NNC 0038-0000-1718 to cause a significant, ~5% weight loss was 0.32 mg/kg PO (not shown). The NNC 0038-0000-1718–induced weight loss was also reversible (Fig. 3) and not associated with any adverse effects whatsoever at any doses.

In addition to the weight-reducing effects, beneficial effects on metabolic parameters were obtained by treating DIO rats with histamine H₃ receptor antagonists for ~20 days. At the end of the 20-day treatment with our

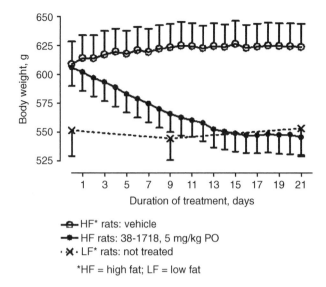

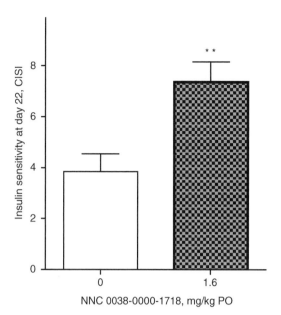

Figure 2 The H₃ antagonists NNC 0038-0000-1718, administered at 5 mg/kg PO for three weeks, reduced body weight of DIO rats to the level of age-matched rats that had never been fed high-fat feed. The weight loss in this experiment corresponded to ~17%. *Abbreviation*: DIO, diet-induced obesity.

Figure 4 Insulin sensitivity is improved in DIO rats after three weeks' treatment with NNC 0038-0000-1718 (1.6 mg/kg PO). *Abbreviations*: DIO, diet-induced obesity; CISI, composite insulin sensitivity index. *Source*: From Ref. 43.

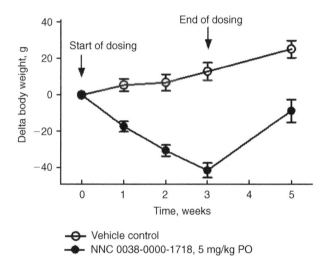

Figure 3 The weight loss achieved with a three week treatment with NNC 0038-0000-1718 of DIO rats is reversed upon termination of treatment. *Abbreviation*: DIO, diet-induced obesity.

data agree very well with those obtained with our more efficacious H₃ antagonists NNC 0038-0000-1718. With this compound, we also observed that insulin sensitivity was improved after three weeks' treatment (Fig. 4).

At the present stage, it is difficult to draw any conclusions as to whether the effects on metabolic parameters, like plasma lipid, insulin, and glucose levels, are mainly due to the weight decrease or whether other factors, like increased sympathetic output from the CNS, also play a role and induce weight-independent effects on the metabolism. It has been suggested that histidine or histamine injected into the PVN and preoptic area (POA) of the hypothalamus increase the firing of the sympathetic nervous system innervating brown adipose tissue in rats (44,45). Furthermore, there are data suggesting that administration of histamine H₃ receptor antagonists not only increases the sympathetic output from the CNS but also promotes peripheral lipolysis in rodents (46). An investigation of the dynamics of such a process will be needed to clarify this issue.

Human Relevance

The data reviewed above clearly demonstrate that oral administration of a histamine H₃ receptor antagonist inhibits food intake in rodents, pigs, and rhesus monkeys and that this inhibition of food intake in DIO rats is associated with a normalization of body weight, body composition, plasma triglycerides levels, and insulin

compounds NNC 0038-0000-1049 and NNC 0038-0000-1202, which induced 5% to 7% weight loss, we observed reduced plasma triglycerides and increased plasma free fatty acids and β-hydroxybutyrate levels, indicating a sustained negative energy balance over the three-week treatment period. In line with this, we also observed an increase in whole-body lipid oxidation, and despite the weight loss, energy expenditure was maintained also with these two H₃ receptor antagonist (33,34). These sensitivity, as well as an increased lipid oxidation. In the coming years it will be shown whether this is a concept that also can be used clinically for the treatment of human obesity and associated metabolic disturbances.

There are three lines of evidence that suggest that an increased histaminergic tone in the CNS will be of relevance and use also in the human situation. First, it is well known that clinical treatment with tricyclic antidepressants (47) and atypical antipsychotics (48,49) induce weight gain, and it has been shown that a high affinity for the H_1 receptor is correlated to these compounds' capability to induce excessive body weight gain (48). Second, clinical treatment with H_1 receptor antagonists, i.e. "antihistamines," for allergic conditions like hayfever and urticaria, often induce unwanted body weight gain in humans (50,51). Third, promising data from clinical weight loss trials with the amylin analog Symlin® (52) have also provided indirect evidence for the potential importance of the histaminergic CNS system in regulation of body weight in humans. Amylin is a pancreatic peptide with well-documented effects on food intake and body weight in rodents (53–55), but interestingly, amylin's anorectic effects appear to a large extent to be mediated by the histaminergic system. For instance, amylin does not affect food intake in mice lacking the H_1 receptor (56), and its effect in rats is strongly attenuated by administration of H_1 receptor antagonists into the VMH (57). Furthermore, administration of H_3 *agonists*, which decrease histamine levels in the CNS, also attenuates the effects of peripherally administered amylin (58). There are also data available in the literature that add neuroanatomical support for the observations that amylin requires an intact histaminergic system in the CNS in order to exert its anorectic effects (59).

The conclusion that can be drawn from these clinical and preclinical observations is that the H_1 receptor probably is involved in body weight regulation also in humans and this makes it likely that a safe H_3 antagonist can be of use also in the treatment of human obesity and related metabolic disorders.

When the first human trials with an H_3 receptor antagonist for obesity treatment are initiated, there will of course be an increased focus on potential mechanism-related side effects and safety issues. In the coming section, we will briefly review what peripheral side effects that might potentially occur and also address the question of what we know about other effects, apart from those on food intake and body weight that increased CNS levels of histamine may have.

Potential Side Effects with H_3 Antagonists

Potential Peripheral Side Effects

H_3 receptor mRNA expression is most abundant in the CNS, and only little expression have been observed in peripheral organs (17,18). For example, a recently published study showed the complete absence of both H_3 receptor mRNA and protein in the human gastrointestinal tract and in the human enteric nervous system (60). However, the H_3 receptor has been pharmacologically characterized as being present on sympathetic nerve endings, for example, in the human nasal mucosa (19) as well as in the human heart (20,61). In in vitro heart preparations, a stimulation of the H_3 receptors on the sympathetic nerve endings with H_3 agonists attenuate the release of noradrenalin. It has in fact been suggested that H_3 agonists could be of clinical use in treatment of heart failure, myocardial ischemia, and other conditions associated with an increased, local noradrenalin release from sympathetic nerve endings (62). However, the functional significance of these H_3 receptors in *human* heart is not quite clear, and even less clear is the potential pharmacological in vivo effects of an H_3 antagonist.

From this it seems unlikely that an H_3 receptor antagonist administered to humans would have any serious, mechanism related, peripheral side effects. Nevertheless, it would be valuable to test H_3 antagonist compounds in in vivo heart disease models prior to clinical trials in order to minimize the risk of potential negative effects of H_3 antagonism in such disease states.

Potential CNS Side Effects

As mentioned above, neither the H_3 nor the H_1 receptor are expressed exclusively in the hypothalamus, i.e., in the area of the brain relevant for regulation of ingestive behavior, but they have a broad distribution in the CNS (7). Furthermore, the presynaptic H_3 receptor controls not only the synthesis and release of histamine but also of other neurotransmitters (15). Thus, it is not surprising that compounds acting at these two receptors also have effects that are not related to regulation of food intake and body weight. For example, the central H_1 receptor is known to mediate histamine's arousing effects as well as its effects on cognitive functions and sleep patterns (8). Consequently, many pharmaceutical companies are currently developing H_3 antagonists as "cognition enhancers" for diseases like attention deficit and hyperactivity disorder (ADHD), Alzheimer's disease and Schizophrenia (8,63,64), as well as for narcolepsy (65). The first human data from these trials are eagerly awaited! However, from this also follows that insomnia may be a possible side effect for a H_3 receptor antagonist, for the very same reason that it may have positive effects on arousal and narcolepsy.

The potential involvement of histamine H_1 and H_3 receptors in anxiety is not quite clear as studies investigating the role of histamine in this condition give contradictory results. Beneficial effects of H_3 antagonism on emotional memory/contextual fear conditioning have been demonstrated (66). Using the H$_3$ antagonist thioperamide, Yuzurihara and coworkers showed that it had anxiogenic properties in a light-dark test, but only when it is coadministered with an H$_2$ antagonist (67). These authors claim that H$_1$ receptors mediate histamine's anxiogenic effects, while H$_2$ receptors mediate histamine's anxiolytic effects. The net effect of an H$_3$ antagonist that increases levels of histamine that can act on both H$_1$ and H$_2$ receptors is of course quite difficult to predict. Bongers and coworkers (68) also reported increased anxiety with thioperamide in mice, while Perez-Garcia and coworkers (69) reported that neither the H$_3$ antagonist thioperamide nor the H$_3$ agonist R-α-methylhistamine (RAMHA) had any anxiogenic or anxiolytic effects in a rat elevated plus-maze test. Thus, no clear consensus yet appears to have been reached regarding the anxiogenic/anxiolytic potential of H$_3$ antagonism. However, clinical human trials with H$_3$ antagonist compounds will have to be designed to carefully assess their anxiogenic potential.

The overall conclusion from this is that H$_3$ antagonist administration, as part of obesity treatment, may also induce mechanism-related effects on sleeping behavior, cognition, and anxiety that may or may not be regarded as negative side effects.

CONCLUSIONS

The histaminergic system in the hypothalamus is highly integrated in the control of food intake and metabolism. Currently, the use of safe, selective H$_3$ receptor antagonists appears to be a promising approach to produce sustained reduction in food intake and body weight and an improvement in the metabolic status in rodents and even in higher mammalian species. We firmly believe that the positive results obtained with H$_3$ receptor antagonist in animals are promising and warrant future clinical studies to evaluate whether this principle is effective in the treatment of human obesity.

REFERENCES

1. Reiner PB, Heimrich B, Keller F, et al. Organotypic culture of central histamine neurons. Brain Res 1988; 442:166–170.
2. Panula P, Yang HYT, Costa E. Histamine-containing neurons in the rat hypothalamus. Proc Natl Acad Sci U S A 1984; 81:2572–2576.
3. Haas H, Panula P. The role of histamine and the tuberomamillary nucleus in the nervous system. Nat Rev Neurosci 2003; 4:121–130.
4. Panula P, Pirvola U, Auvinen S, et al. Histamine-immunoreactive nerve fibers in the rat brain. Neuroscience 1989; 28:585–610.
5. Hough LB. Genomics meets histamine receptors: new subtypes, new receptors. Mol Pharmacol 2001; 59:415–419.
6. Yamashita M, Fukui H, Sugama K, et al. Expression cloning of a cDNA encoding the bovine histamine H1 receptor. Proc Natl Acad Sci U S A 1991; 88:11515–11519.
7. Palacios JM, Wamsley JK, Kuhar MJ. The distribution of histamine H1-receptors in the rat brain: an autoradiographic study. Neuroscience 1981; 6:15–37.
8. Hancock AA, Fox GB. Perspectives on cognitive domains, H3 receptor ligands and neurological disease. Expert Opin Investig Drugs 2004; 13(10):1237–1248.
9. Gantz I, Munzert G, Tashiro T, et al. Molecular cloning of the human histamine H2 receptor. Biochem Biophys Res Commun 1991; 178:1386–1392.
10. Hatton GI, Yang QZ. Ionotropic histamine receptors and H-2 receptors modulate supraoptic oxytocin neuronal excitability and dye coupling. J Neurosci 2001; 21: 2974–2982.
11. Karlstedt K, Senkas A, Ahman M, et al. Regional expression of the histamine H(2) receptor in adult and developing rat brain. Neuroscience 2001; 102:201–208.
12. Honrubia MA, Vilaro MT, Palacios JM, et al. Distribution of the histamine H2 receptor in monkey brain and its mRNA localization in monkey and human brain. Synapse (New York) 2000; 38:343–354.
13. Arrang J, Garbarg M, Schwartz J. Auto inhibition of brain histamine release mediated by a novel class of H-3 of histamine receptor. Nature (London) 1983; 302:832–837.
14. Arrang JM, Garbarg M, Schwartz JC. Autoinhibition of histamine synthesis mediated by presynaptic H3-receptors. Neuroscience 1987; 23:149–157.
15. Schlicker E, Malinowska B, Kathmann M, et al. Modulation of neurotransmitter release via histamine h-3 heteroreceptors. Fund Clin Pharm 1994; 8:128–137.
16. Lovenberg TW, Roland BL, Wilson SJ et al. Cloning and functional expression of the human histamine H-3 receptor. Mol Pharmacol 1999; 55:1101–1107.
17. Lovenberg TW, Pyati J, Chang H, et al. Cloning of rat histamine H-3 receptor reveals distinct species pharmacological profiles. J Pharmacol Exp Ther 2000; 293: 771–778.
18. Hancock AA, Esbenshade TA, Krueger KM, et al. Genetic and pharmacological aspects of histamine H-3 receptor heterogeneity. Life Sci 2003; 73:3043–3072.
19. Varty LM, Gustafson E, Laverty M, et al. Activation of histamine H-3 receptors in human nasal mucosa inhibits sympathetic vasoconstriction. Eur J Pharmacol 2004; 484:83–89.
20. Silver RB, Mackins CJ, Smith NCE, et al. Coupling of histamine H-3 receptors to neuronal Na$^+$/H$^+$ exchange: a novel protective mechanism in myocardial ischemia. Proc Natl Acad Sci U S A 2001; 98:2855–2859.
21. Pillot C, Heron A, Cochois V, et al. A detailed mapping of the histamine H-3 receptor and its gene transcripts in rat brain. Neuroscience 2002; 114:173–193.
22. Oda T, Morikawa N, Saito Y, et al. Molecular cloning and characterization of a novel type of histamine receptor preferentially expressed in leukocytes. J Biol Chem 2000; 275(47):36781–36786.

23. Zhu Y, Michalovich D, Wu HL, et al. Cloning, expression, and pharmacological characterization of a novel human histamine receptor. Mol Pharmacol 2001; 59:434–441.

24. Malmlöf K, Hohlweg R, Rimvall K. Targeting of the central histaminergic system for treatment of obesity and associated metabolic disorders. Drug Dev Res 2006; 67(8):651–665.

25. Hancock AA, Brune ME. Assessment of pharmacology and potential anti-obesity properties of H-3 receptor antagonists/inverse agonists. Expert Opin Investig Drugs 2005; 14(3):223–241.

26. Masaki T, Yoshimatsu H. The hypothalamic H-1 receptor: a novel therapeutic target for disrupting diurnal feeding rhythm and obesity. Trends Pharm Sci 2006; 27(5): 279–284.

27. Clineschmidt BV, Lotti VJ. Histamine: intraventricular injection suppresses ingestive behavior of the cat. Arch Int Pharmacodyn Ther 1973; 206:288–298.

28. Lecklin A, Tuomisto L. The blockade of H_1 receptors attenuates the suppression of feeding and diuresis induced by inhibition of histamine catabolism. Pharmacol Biochem Behav 1998; 59:753–758.

29. Orthen-Gambill N. Antihistaminic drugs increase feeding, while histidine suppresses feeding in rats. Pharmacol Biochem Behav 1988; 31:81–86.

30. Vaziri P, Dang K, Anderson GH. Evidence for histamine involvement in the effect of histidine loads on food and water intake in rats. J Nutr 1997; 127:1519–1526.

31. Lecklin A, Tuomisto L, Macdonald E. Metoprine, an inhibitor of histamine N-methyltransferase but no catechol-O-methyltransferase, suppresses feeding in sated and in food deprived rats. Methods Find Exp Clin Pharmacol 1995; 17:47–52.

32. Bjenning C, Juul A-G, Lange KZ, et al. Peripherally administered ciproxifan elevates hypothalamic histamine levels and potently reduces food intake in the Sprague Dawley rat. In: Watanabe T, Timmerman H, Yanai K, eds. Histamine Research in the New Millennium. Amsterdam: Elsevier, 2001:449–450.

33. Malmlöf K, Zaragoza F, Golozoubova V, et al. Influence of a selective histamine H-3 receptor antagonist on hypothalamic neural activity, food intake and body weight. Int J Obes 2005; 29(12):1402–1412.

34. Malmlöf K, Golozoubova V, Peschke B, et al. Increase of neuronal histamine in obese rats is associated with decreases in body weight and plasma triglycerides. Obesity 2006; 14:2154–2162.

35. Lecklin A, Etuseppala P, Stark H, et al. Effects of intra-cerebroventricularly infused histamine and selective h-1, h-2 and h-3 agonists on food and water-intake and urine flow in wistar rats. Brain Res 1998; 793:279–288.

36. Sakata T, Ookuma K, Fukagawa K, et al. Blockade of the histamine H1-receptor in the rat ventromedial hypothalamus and feeding elicitation. Brain Res 1988; 441:403–407.

37. Morimoto T, Yamamoto Y, Mobarakeh JI et al. Involvement of the histaminergic system in leptin-induced suppression of food intake. Physiol Behav 1999; 67:679–683.

38. Ookuma K, Sakata T, Fujimoto K. Evidence for feeding elicited through antihistaminergic effects of tricyclic

39. antidepressants in the rat hypothalamus. Psychopharmacology 1990; 101:481–485.

39. Tuomisto L, Lozeva V, Valjakka A, et al. Modifying effects of histamine on circadian rhythms and neuronal excitability. Behav Brain Res 2001; 124(2):129–135.

40. Malmlöf K, Hastrup S, Wulff BS, et al. Antagonistic targeting of the histamine H3 receptor decreases caloric intake in higher mammalian species. Biochem Pharmacol 2007; 73:1237–1242.

41. Hancock AA, Bennani YL, Bush EN, et al. Antiobesity effects of A-331440, a novel non-imidazole histamine H3 receptor antagonist. Eur J Pharmacol 2004; 487:183–197.

42. Hancock AA. The challenge of drug discovery of a GPCR target: analysis of preclinical pharmacology of histamine H_3 antagonists/inverse agonists. Biochem Pharmacol 2006; 71(8):1103–1113.

43. Matsuda M, DeFronzo RA. Insulin sensitivity indices obtained from oral glucose tolerance testing: comparison with the euglycemic insulin clamp. Diabetes Care 1999; 22(9):1462–1470.

44. Yasuda T, Masaki T, Chiba S, et al. L-Histidine stimulates sympathetic nerve activity to brown adipose tissue in rats. Neurosci Lett 2004; 362:71–74.

45. Yasuda T, Masaki T, Sakata T, et al. Hypothalamic neuronal histamine regulates sympathetic nerve activity and expression of uncoupling protein 1 mRNA in brown adipose tissue in rats. Neuroscience 2004; 125(3):535–540.

46. Tsuda K, Yoshimatsu H, Niijima A, et al. Hypothalamic histamine neurons activate lipolysis in rat adipose tissue. Exp Biol Med 2002; 227(3):208–213.

47. Berken GH, Weinstein DO, Stern WC. Weight gain. A side-effect of tricyclic antidepressants. J Affect Disord 1984; 7:133–138.

48. Baptista T, Zarate J, Joober R, et al. Drug induced weight gain, an impediment to successful pharmacotherapy: focus on antipsychotics. Curr Drug Targets 2004; 5:279–299.

49. Kraus T, Zimmermann U, Schuld A, et al. On the pathophysiology of weight regulation during treatment with psychotropic drugs. Forschritte Neurol Psychiatr 2001; 69:116–137.

50. Van Ganse E, Kaufman L, Derde MP, et al. Effects of antihistamines in adult asthma: a meta-analysis of clinical trials. Eur Respir J 1997; 10:2216–2224.

51. Horak F, Stubner UP. Comparative tolerability of second generation antihistamines. Drug Safety 1999; 20:385–401.

52. http://www.media.corporate-ir.net/media_files/IROL/10/101911/Lehman_2007_v3_FINAL. pdf.

53. Reda TK, Geliebter A, Pi-Sunyer FX. Amylin, food intake, and obesity. Obes Res 2002; 10:1087–1091.

54. Rushing PA, Hagan MM, Seeley RJ, et al. Inhibition of central amylin signaling increases food intake and body adiposity in rats. Endocrinology 2001; 142:5035–5038.

55. Roth JD, Hughes H, Kendall E, et al. Antiobesity effects of the beta-cell hormone amylin in diet- induced obese rats: effects on food intake, body weight, composition, energy expenditure, and gene expression. Endocrinology 2006; 147(12):5855–5864.

56. Mollet A, Lutz TA, Meier S, et al. Histamine H-1 receptors mediate the anorectic action of the pancreatic hormone

amylin. Am J Physiol Regul Integr Comp Physiol 2001; 281:R1442–R1448.

57. Mollet A, Meier S, Riediger T, et al. Histamine H1 receptors in the ventromedial hypothalamus mediate the anorectic action of the pancreatic hormone amylin. Peptides 2003; 24:155–158.

58. Lutz TA, Del Prete E, Walzer B, et al. The histaminergic, but not the serotoninergic, system mediates amylin's anorectic effect. Peptides 1996; 17:1317–1322.

59. D'Este L, Wimalawansa SJ, Renda TG. Distribution of amylin-immunoreactive neurons in the monkey hypothalamus and their relationships with the histaminergic system. Arch Histol Cytol 2001; 64:295–303.

60. Sander LE, Lorentz A, Sellge G, et al. Selective expression of histamine receptors H1R, H2R, and H4R, but not H3R, in the human intestinal tract. Gut 2006; 55(4):498–504.

61. Imamura M, Seyedi N, Lander HM, et al. Functional identification of histamine H3-receptors in the human heart. Circ Res 1995; 77(1):206–210.

62. Mackins CJ, Levi R. Therapeutic potential of H(3)-receptor agonists in myocardial infarction. Expert Opin Investig Drugs 2000; 9(11):2537–2542.

63. Witkin JM, Nelson DL. Selective histamine H-3 receptor antagonists for treatment of cognitive deficiencies and other disorders of the central nervous system. Pharmacol Ther 2004; 103:1–20.

64. Passani MB, Lin JS, Hancock A, et al. The histamine H-3 receptor as a novel therapeutic target for cognitive and sleep disorders. Trends Pharm Sci 2004; 25(12):618–625.

65. Barbier AJ, Berridge C, Dugovic C, et al. Acute wake-promoting actions of JNJ-5207852, a novel, diamine-based H-3 antagonist. Br J Pharmacol 2004; 143(5):649–661.

66. Passani MB, Cangioli L, Baldi E, et al. Histamine H-3 receptor-mediated impairment of contextual fear conditioning and in-vivo inhibition of cholinergic transmission in the rat basolateral amygdala. Eur J Neurosci 2001; 14:1522–1532.

67. Yuzurihara M, Ikarashi Y, Ishige A, et al. Effects of drugs acting as histamine releasers or histamine receptor blockers on an experimental anxiety model in mice. Pharmacol Biochem Behav 2000; 67(1):145–150.

68. Bongers G, Leurs R, Robertson J, et al. Role of H-3-receptor-mediated signaling in anxiety and cognition in wild-type and Apoe(−/−) mice. Neuropsychopharmacology 2004; 29:441–449.

69. Perez-Garcia C, Morales L, Cano MV, et al. Effects of histamine H-3 receptor ligands in experimental models of anxiety and depression. Psychopharmacology 1999; 142:215–220.

26

Drugs with Thermogenic Properties

ARNE ASTRUP

Department of Human Nutrition, Faculty of Life Sciences, University of Copenhagen, Frederiksberg C, Denmark

SØREN TOUBRO

Reduce aps - Research Clinic of Nutrition, Hvidovre Hospital, Hvidovre, University of Copenhagen, Copenhagen, Denmark

INTRODUCTION

Currently available drugs used to treat obesity exert their main action on energy balance by reducing energy intake or by inhibiting intestinal fat absorption. However, some of the drugs that reduce food intake also possess thermogenic properties that contribute to their clinical efficacy in terms of loss of body fat and of weight maintenance. A number of other pharmaceutical compounds possess thermogenic effects but are used for indications other than obesity. Specific thermogenic agents developed for the treatment of obesity and diabetes are still in the first phases of clinical development. Compounds are reviewed in this chapter irrespective of whether they are approved for use in obesity treatment by the U.S. Food and Drug Administration (FDA), the European Committee for Proprietary Medicinal Products (CPMP), or by other regulatory bodies.

RATIONALE FOR STIMULATING ENERGY EXPENDITURE

Daily energy expenditure (EE) represents one side of the energy balance equation. Over a longer period, total energy expenditure should be in equilibrium with total energy intake to ensure weight stability. The inability to ensure this balance is the overall background for the prevalent weight gain in the population and the current obesity epidemic. The average weight gain in the population has been estimated to be due to a 50 to 100 kcal daily surplus. Many efforts are exerted to produce weight loss and subsequently, to maintain energy balance at the reduced body size by adjustments of both dietary energy intake and physical exercise, but this strategy is unfortunately successful only in a small proportion of obese subjects. The rapidly increasing prevalence of obesity in most countries must be due to changes in environmental factors, but there is increasing evidence that some of those who gain weight when exposed to these environmental factors have a genetic susceptibility. It is interesting that receptors and proteins important for regulation of substrate and energy metabolism, such as the β-adrenergic receptors (β_2 and β_3), and the uncoupling proteins 1, 2, and 3 may be such susceptible genes. This knowledge, and the lack of efficacy of lifestyle changes in reducing body weight and maintaining weight loss, supports the development of a pharmacological strategy to "normalize" energy and substrate metabolism as a tool to improve the results of obesity management. There is evidence to support the hypothesis that a low-energy output phenotype predisposes individuals to weight gain and obesity, the low-energy output being caused by a low resting metabolic rate (RMR), a low nonexercise activity thermogenesis, physical inactivity, or combinations thereof (1). Among the potential mechanisms are low T3, low sympathetic nervous system (SNS) activity, and perhaps gene variants in the above mentioned genes or in some other relevant genes. Increased energy metabolism and fat oxidation are logical and attractive targets because they may counteract a depressed RMR, and perhaps even diminish the hunger that accompanies weight loss, thereby allowing people to maintain food intake at more tolerable and socially acceptable levels. In addition, any increase in energy expenditure not fully counteracted by a similar increase in energy intake (2), irrespective of whether the increased energy output is achieved through increased exercise or pharmacologically would be desirable (3). Even a slightly sustained increase of 2% to 3% in daily energy expenditure may have clinical relevance, particularly in preventing the compensatory decline in RMR following weight loss but also in decreasing the risk of weight regain following weight loss.

Energy expenditure can be stimulated pharmacologically by interference with several steps in the regulatory system. These can be activation of the central leptin receptor, the CNS regulatory systems, peripheral efferent neurons of the SNS, the adrenergic receptors, the thyroid and growth hormones, or cellular mechanisms responsible for thermogenic futile mechanisms such as those associated with uncoupling proteins.

Physiological Rationale for the Sympathoadrenal System as a Drug Target

RMR comprises 50% to 80% of daily energy expenditure (4). The remaining expended energy is mainly derived from the cost of physical activity and, to a lesser degree, meal-induced thermogenesis, mental stress, cold, and thermogenic stimulants in food and beverages (nicotine, caffeine and its derivatives, catechins in green tea, and capsaicin in hot chilies). About 70% to 80% of the variance of RMR can be accounted for by differences in fat-free mass, fat mass, age, and sex (4,5). However, an additional 5% to 8% of the variance in RMR is accounted for by family membership, which strongly supports the existence of influence by genetic factors. Some of this variance can be explained by individual differences within the normal physiological range in sympathetic tone, thyroid hormone levels, and polymorphisms in β-receptor and uncoupling protein (UCP) genes (5–8). Other components of 24-hour EE are influenced by the sympathetic tone. Meal ingestion is accompanied by an increased SNS

activity, and studies using β-blockade have demonstrated a facultative, β-adrenergically mediated component (9).

Physical activity also seems to be stimulated by sympathetic activity. The positive relationship between spontaneous physical activity and norepinephrine appearance rate is consistent with the idea that SNS activity is a determinant of individual differences in the level of spontaneous physical activity, i.e., how much people move around, change position, and fidget, all of which contribute to total energy expenditure. So "fidgeters" seem either to have a constitutionally higher SNS activity (5) or to possess certain functional polymorphisms in genes controlling the activity of β-adrenoceptors and uncoupling proteins (7,8).

The contribution of the sympathoadrenal system to 24-hour EE has been addressed using measurements in whole-body calorimeters. Administration of 5 to 10 mg of the nonspecific β-antagonist propranolol causes a 2% to 4% decrease in 24-hour EE, suggesting that a total blockade of the β-mediated pathways of the sympathoadrenal system may suppress 24-hour EE by as much as 4% to 6%, equivalent to 50 to 150 kcal/day (5). This is consistent with observations from meta-analyses of clinical trials showing that treatment with β-adrenoceptor antagonists produces weight gain (10). SNS activity also influences the mixture of substrates oxidized, and norepinephrine increases intracellular lipolysis and nonesterified fatty acid (NEFA) uptake in muscle (11), which seem to be impaired in some obese subjects (12). The stimulatory effect of β-adrenergic agonists on fat oxidation is well established. β-Antagonists have the opposite effect; that is, they decrease energy expenditure and the relative rate of fat oxidation.

Role of Low Energy Expenditure in the Development of Obesity

Several studies support the idea that a low RMR is associated with weight gain. A low metabolic rate has been shown to precede body weight gain in infants, children, and in adult Pima Indians and Caucasians (5). On the basis of the assumption that formerly obese, weight-reduced subjects exhibit the metabolic characteristics that predisposed them to obesity, it has been found in a meta-analysis that formerly obese subjects have a 3% to 5% lower mean RMR than never-obese control subjects (13). Studies of the contribution of the sympathoadrenal activity to a low RMR have yielded conflicting results, probably because comparisons of lean and obese subjects provide only very limited information about the role of the SNS in the etiology of obesity (5). Furthermore, they do not discern between the causes and the consequences of weight gain. However, longitudinal studies both in

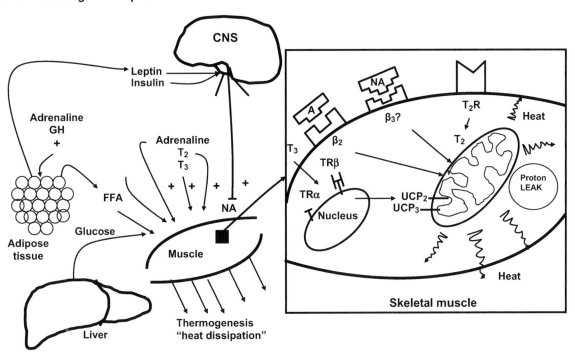

Figure 1 Where can thermogenesis be stimulated pharmacologically in humans? Model of the effector side of decreased metabolic efficiency in humans. Thyroid hormones, growth hormones, circulating catecholamines, and sympathetic nerves stimulate thermogenesis, fat oxidation, and uncoupling in skeletal muscle and liver.

Pima Indians and Caucasians have shown a relationship between both low urinary norepinephrine excretion, low T3 levels and weight gain, and a relationship between low urinary epinephrine excretion and the development of central obesity (5). These results strongly suggest that a low SNS activity is also a risk factor for weight gain in humans. SNS activity increases in response to weight gain, thereby attenuating the original impairment.

THYROID HORMONES AND DERIVATIVES

Thyroid hormones are the physiological controllers of basal metabolism. Hypothyroid and hyperthyroid states are associated with predictable changes in energy expenditure and in body weight and composition. Mean body weight and fat mass are normally decreased by 15% in hyperthyroidism, and hypothyroid patients weigh 15% to 30% more than in their euthyroid states. These perturbations in thyroid hormone metabolism are good examples of primary changes in energy expenditure that are not fully compensated for by corrective adjustments in energy intake. Normal physiological variations in T_3 concentrations have also been shown to be responsible for differences between individuals in daily energy expenditure as much as 150 kcal/day (6), and a low T3 level is a risk factor for subsequent weight gain (14). Moreover, among morbidly obese subjects, 20% have overt or subclinical hypothyroidism (15). The short-term thermogenic effect of thyroid hormone involves a direct interaction between T_2 and mitochondrial enzymes with an onset after six hours and lasting for two days, whereas the long-term effects are mediated by T_3 through nuclear receptors (TR$_\alpha$ and TR$_\beta$) (16). The long-term effects require binding to the regulatory regions of the genes. Effects are seen after 30 hours and last up to 60 days (16). Thyroid hormones produce actions as a result of interactions with several genes controlling energy metabolism, and many of these effects result in increased energy production and utilization of fat as substrate. One of the important effects of T_3 is upregulation of the uncoupling proteins (Fig. 1), which subsequently leads to heat dissipation without synthesis of adenosine triphosphate (ATP). In hypothyroidism, UCP$_3$ levels are decreased threefold and they are increased sixfold in hyperthyroidism, but the expression of the UCP$_3$ gene is also influenced by energy balance, leptin, and β_3-adrenoceptors. Although obesity is not normally characterized by subnormal T_3 levels, the receptors responsible for T_3 actions remain attractive targets for enhancing energy expenditure.

Clinical Trials with Thyroid Hormone Therapy in Euthyroid Obese Subjects

Thyroid hormones have been used to treat obesity for more than a century (17). Initially thyroid extracts were used, but after the identification of T_4, and later T_3, several studies of the specific actions of these components were conducted in the 1960s and 1970s. Desiccated thyroid extract, T_4, and T_3 have all been used in clinical trials, but the design of many of these studies was not optimal, and the outcome was therefore variable. More recent trials using T_3 in controlled designs generally support that T_3 is effective in producing substantial weight loss in obese euthyroid subjects (for complete review see Ref. 17), with most of the studies using high doses varying from 0.15 to 2.00 mg/day (18). High doses of T_3 caused several side effects, serious cardiac problems, and muscle weakness, all of which can probably be attributed to excessive loss of lean body tissue (18–22). Recent studies using T_3 treatment following a very low-calorie diet where endogenous T_3 levels are suppressed have failed to find excessive urinary nitrogen loss or changes in leucine or lysine kinetics (23–25). Although there is a widespread use of T_3 supplementation among overweight and obese subjects, this is not endorsed by the existing data on efficacy and safety. Clinical trials with current state-of-the-art design and methodology are required (16,17), but recent experimental evidence shows that even mild hyperthyroidism has adverse effects (26).

Selective Thyroid Receptor Analogs

Selective agonists at the TR_β have been developed and have been shown in animal models to have fewer side effects than T_3 (27). In comparison with T_3, one of these agonists, GC-1 [3,5-dimethyl-4-(4'-hydroy-3'-isopropylbenzyl)-phenoxy acid], has more marked lipid-lowering effect, does not increase heart rate, and has less positive inotropic effect (28). Ribeiro et al. (29) have shown that TR_α is essential for thyroid hormone to restore the levels of a factor in the norepinephrine signaling pathway, downstream of the adrenergic receptors, that is limiting for the norepinephrine action in hypothyroidism. Grover et al. have reported promising findings using a TR_β agonist (KB-141) in lowering body weight and blood cholesterol levels in various animal models (30).

This effect is seen in several tissues and could be a way to increase thermogenesis. Compounds taking advantage of the fact that thyroid-induced thermogenesis is thyroid hormone receptor isoform-specific may be promising for the treatment of obesity and the metabolic syndrome, but no human data are yet in the public domain.

CONTROLLED UNCOUPLERS

2,4-Dinitrophenol

Mitochondria are the cellular organelles that convert food energy to carbon dioxide, water, and ATP, and they are fundamental in mediating effects on energy dissipation. Mitochondria are responsible for 90% of cellular oxygen consumption and the majority of ATP production. However, not all of the available energy is coupled to ATP synthesis. Much is lost by uncoupled reactions when protons move from the cytosol back into the mitochondrial matrix via pathways that circumvent the ATP synthase and other uses of the electrochemical gradient (28). Proton cycling has been estimated to account for 20% to 25% of resting metabolic rate, and there is very good evidence to support the concept that drugs can further stimulate it. 2,4-Dinitrophenol (DNP) is an artificial uncoupler that acts as a protonophore because it can cross membranes protonated, lose its proton, and return as the anion, then reprotonate and repeat the cycle. By this mechanism DNP increases the basal proton conductance of mitochondria and uncouples. DNP was introduced as a drug in the 1930s and was used with enormous success for weight loss purposes. The ability of DNP to produce effective weight loss without dieting led to widespread use, but several problems occurred due to its low therapeutic index (31). Owing to a steep dose dependence of metabolic rate, a number of people were literally "cooked to death" in the 1930s because of accidental or deliberate overdose (32). Reports of cataracts and deaths from overdose led to its withdrawal from the market by the FDA in 1938 (31). Currently, pharmaceutical companies are developing derivatives of DNP with a less steep dose-response relationship and with a built-in inhibition that limits the uncoupling process.

Uncoupling Proteins

Uncoupling protein UCP_2 and UCP_3 are proteins that can uncouple ATP production from mitochondrial respiration, thereby dissipating energy as heat and reducing energy metabolism efficiency (31,33). In rodents, brown adipose tissue (BAT) functions to dissipate energy in the form of heat through the action of UCP_1. Heat production by brown adipocytes results from a controlled uncoupling of oxidative phosphorylation by an UCP_1-mediated proton conductance pathway in the inner mitochondrial membrane. In animal models, the β_3-receptor stimulates lipolysis in white adipose tissue (WAT) and BAT, and in BAT both activates UCP and upregulates the UCP gene, both of which result in a further increase in energy expenditure. BAT is abundant in rodents but has no functional role in adult humans (34), and the β_3-receptor is a questionable drug target (see sect. "β_3-Adrenoceptor Agonists"). In humans, however, the major site of catecholamine-induced thermogenesis is skeletal muscle, which can account for 50% to 60% of the whole-body response (35).

In contrast to UCP$_1$, which is only present in BAT, UCP$_2$ has a wide tissue distribution, whereas UCP$_3$ is expressed predominantly in skeletal muscle. Linkage and association studies have provided some evidence of a role for UCPs in modulating metabolic rate in human studies. Until recently, the cellular thermogenic mechanisms were unknown, but the discovery of both UCP$_2$ and UCP$_3$ expressed in skeletal muscle offers a plausible mechanism for heat dissipation (36). Treatment with thyroid hormone increases expression of the UCP$_2$ and UCP$_3$ genes. Other regulators of UCP$_2$ and UCP$_3$ gene expression are β$_3$-adrenergic agonists and glucocorticoids. The UCP$_3$ and UCP$_2$ genes are located adjacent to each other in a region implicated in linkage studies as contributing to obesity (37,38), and a polymorphism in the gene I encoding for both UCP$_2$ and UCP$_3$ has been associated with reduced RMR and fat oxidation (7,8,37). However, it is still controversial whether UCP$_2$ and UCP$_3$ are real uncoupling proteins similar to that of UCP$_1$, which is induced by unidentified agonists. Indeed, recent studies suggest that both UCP$_2$ and UCP$_3$ are functional (36,39). Other promising drug targets for uncoupling are the adenine nucleotide transporters responsible for uncoupling by free fatty acids and adenosine monophosphate (AMP) (31).

THERMOGENIC PROPERTIES OF ENHANCERS OF SYMPATHETIC ACTIVITY

Leptin

Animals and humans, with a genetic deficiency in the adipocyte-derived hormone leptin or its receptor, exhibit extreme obesity (40). Leptin acts on the hypothalamus to suppress appetite and increase energy expenditure, and the negative energy balance produced by exogenous administration of leptin in deficient animals is partly mediated by increased SNS outflow to several organs, including BAT. Accordingly, rodents with defective leptin biosynthesis or receptor function (*ob/ob* mouse, *db/db* mouse, *or fa/fa* rat) exhibit severely reduced SNS activity, gain weight rapidly, and become obese. Leptin deficiency is extremely rare in humans and has only rarely been identified as a cause of obesity in patients. By contrast, serum concentrations of leptin increase with body fat in all the obese persons who do not have this mutation in the gene encoding for leptin. The high leptin levels in obese individuals suggest leptin insensitivity and pose questions about the potential for leptin in the treatment of simple obesity. However, observational studies in humans suggest that leptin, in humans as in animals, stimulates SNS and energy expenditure (41,42). Recombinant leptin has indeed proved to be very effective in two children with leptin deficiency, although the investigators did not detect any stimulatory impact of leptin on energy expenditure,

which could easily have been blurred by the pronounced concomitant decrease in body weight (43). However, physical activity level index increased from 1.6 to 1.9 after 12 months of treatment, which is most probably due to movement being less restrained with less adiposity and is thus not a direct effect of leptin. In normal-weight subjects and in leptin-intact obese subjects, injections of recombinant leptin produced only a modest reduction in weight and fat loss over 24 weeks (44). Moreover, a recent study of Hukshorn et al. did not find any effect of subcutaneous pegylated recombinant native human leptin treatment on body fat, energy expenditure, or substrate utilization in obese men (45). Leptin and analogs are therefore not potential thermogenic agents for the induction of weight loss, but may be used to counteract the suppression of SNS and thyroid activity that accompanies weight loss, and that are responsible for the suppression of metabolic rate accompanying weight loss. Leibel's group has shown that this adaptation to a low energy intake can be abolished by leptin administration in obese humans (46). Studies of longer duration are required to determine whether chronic reactivation of the leptin axis following weight reduction enhances weight maintenance.

Ephedrine/Caffeine

Numerous studies have shown that ephedrine (E) as monotheraphy decreases body fat in obese subjects by a combined action of suppression of appetite and stimulation of energy expenditure (47). Adenosine antagonists such as caffeine (C) potentiate the thermogenic and clinical effects. Dose-response studies found that the combination of ephedrine 20 mg and caffeine 200 mg produced the best synergistic effect on thermogenesis (48). Ephedrine is both an indirect sympathomimetic, causing release of norepinephrine from the sympathetic nerve endings (35), and a direct agonist on β-receptors. Experimental human studies suggest that not only β$_1$ and β$_2$ but also β$_3$ is involved in its peripheral thermogenic effect (49).

Combinations of E + C have been shown to be effective for treatment of obesity for up to 50 weeks (Fig. 2). In a study including 180 obese patients, it was found that E + C (20 mg/200 mg t.i.d.) produced a larger weight loss than placebo, caffeine, or ephedrine, in combination with a hypoenergetic diet over 24 weeks (50). After 24 weeks, the placebo group had lost 13.2 kg, and E + C further increased the weight loss by 3.4 kg to a total loss of 16.6 kg. Also, more patients in the E + C group than in the placebo group lost >5% and 10% of the initial body weight. Breum et al. tested E + C against dexfenfluramine in a double-blind placebo-controlled trial, and found E + C produced a greater weight loss than dexfenfluramine in subjects with a body mass index (BMI) of >30 kg/m^2 (51).

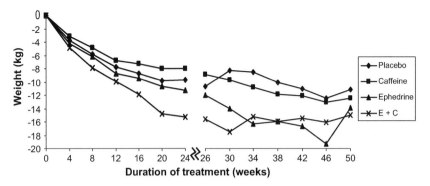

Figure 2 Effect of a combination of 20-mg ephedrine and 200-mg caffeine t.i.d. as adjuvant to a hypocaloric diet on weight loss and weight maintenance for 1 year. The first 24 months involved a randomized, double-blind, placebo-controlled study, whereas all groups received E + C from week 26 to 50. *Abbreviations*: E, ephedrine; C, caffeine. *Source*: Adapted from Refs. 50,56.

The reductions in pulse rate and blood pressure were similar to the two treatments. E + C has also been evaluated for prevention of weight gain after smoking cessation. The double-blind placebo-controlled trial included 225 subjects, and after 12 weeks weight gain was less in the E + C group than in placebo group (52).

Notably, E + C increases blood pressure and heart rate slightly with the first exposure (50). However, during chronic treatment tachyphylaxis develops to the cardiovascular effects of the compound, but not to the anorectic and thermogenic (50). In the largest trial of E + C, only a slight increase in blood pressure and heart rate could be detected when the treatment was initiated, but after 12 weeks, the reductions in blood pressure were similar in the E + C group to those in the placebo group (50). A hypothetical cardiovascular safety concern could be raised by the combination of E + C and exercise. However, Stich et al. studied the metabolic and hemodynamic responses to submaximal exercise before and after three days of E + C treatment in obese patients and found no indications of an enhanced exercise-induced increase in blood pressure and heart rate as compared with placebo (53). With more extensive measurement of cardiovascular function by thoracic impedance, automatic sphygmomanometry, and continuous electrocardiographic recording, Waluga et al. concluded that E + C had no undesirable effects on cardiovascular function in obese subjects (54). E + C has also been tested in overweight subjects with controlled hypertension (55). Treatment with E + C produced a larger weight loss than placebo, and reduced systolic blood pressure 5.5 mmHg more than placebo, and the antihypertensive effect of β-blockers was not reduced by E + C (55).

The clinical studies of E + C clearly show that the compound is effective in the treatment of obesity for up to one year (56). However, owing to the limited number of patients enrolled in these trials the total evidence does not meet the efficacy and safety requirements of the American FDA or the European Medicines Agency (EMEA) for licensing E + C as a prescription compound. Dietary supplements that contain the herbal alkaloid ephedra have been banned in the United States since April 2004. The FDA banned the products after it concluded that ephedra poses an unreasonable risk to those who use it.

A recent systematic review concluded that the risks of E + C are outweighed by the benefits of achieving and maintaining a healthy weight (47). Unfortunately, the pharmaceutical industry does not invest in a compound that is difficult to protect.

Thermogenic Properties of Sibutramine

Sibutramine is a serotonin and norepinephrine reuptake inhibitor, and it causes weight loss in laboratory animals through effects on both food intake and metabolic rate (57). Controlled trials conducted in obese patients have consistently shown dose-related weight loss and optimal weight loss at 10 to 15 mg sibutramine (58). Typically, weight loss was 3 to 5 kg greater than placebo at 24 weeks, and the loss was sustained for two years. The Sibutramine Trial of Obesity Reduction and Maintenance (STORM) trial demonstrates that sibutramine is also more effective in maintaining two-year weight loss than placebo (59). Sibutramine causes dose-dependent inhibition of daily food intake in rats owing to the enhancement of satiety, whereas eating patterns and other behaviors remain similar to those exhibited by control animals. Sibutramine also stimulates thermogenesis in rats, producing sustained (>6 hours) elevation of energy expenditure of up to 30% (57). The thermogenic effect of sibutramine results from central stimulation of efferent sympathetic activity because it is inhibited by ganglionic blockade and by high doses of nonselective β-adrenergic antagonists. Sibutramine also decreases food intake in humans by increasing meal-induced satiety (60,61).

The thermogenic properties of sibutramine have been tested in a number of acute tests and in one long-term trial using indirect calorimetry. Seagle et al. evaluated the thermogenic response to sibutramine in 44 obese women on a hypocaloric diet and receiving either placebo, 10 or 30 mg sibutramine for eight weeks (62). There was no difference in the thermogenic response to sibutramine and placebo measured three hours after acute dosing. However, the active metabolite of sibutramine does not peak in plasma before 3 to 3.5 hours after oral intake, and it is possible that Seagle et al. missed the thermogenic effect by their early termination of the measurements. Having taken the pharmacokinetic profile of sibutramine and its active metabolites into consideration, Hansen et al. found that sibutramine increased basal metabolic rate, the thermic effect of meals and core temperature more than placebo in normal-weight males (63). The increased energy expenditure was covered by higher levels of both glucose and fat utilization and was linked to enhanced sympathoadrenal activity. The contribution of the thermogenic effect of sibutramine to weight loss was examined in two trials. Hansen et al. studied the chronic effect of sibutramine in 32 obese subjects randomized to eight weeks of treatment with either 15 mg of sibutramine daily or placebo in a double-blind design (61). Twenty-four-hour EE was measured before the start and on the last day of treatment. Weight loss was 2.4 kg in the sibutramine group versus 0.3 kg in the placebo group ($p < 0.001$). Despite larger losses of both fat-free mass and fat mass in the sibutramine-treated group, 24-hour EE did not decrease more than in the placebo group (-2.6% vs. -2.5%, NS). As expected, the reduction in body weight during the eight weeks was associated with a decrease in 24-hour EE ($r = 0.42$, $p < 0.01$). When the body weight changes were taken into account, 24-hour EE decreased less in the sibutramine than in the placebo group (0.8% vs. 3.8%, $p < 0.02$). In a trial by Walsh et al., 19 obese females were instructed to consume a hypocaloric diet for 12 weeks and, in a double-blind design, received 15 mg sibutramine or placebo daily. RMR was measured before and after 12 weeks of treatment (64). After RMR was adjusted for weight loss, there was a tendency toward sibutramine blunting the decline in RMR, although this was not statistically significant. Trials in obese adolescents have found similar results, suggesting a weak thermogenic effect of sibutramine (65), and these studies demonstrate that sibutramine possesses mild thermogenic properties in humans, sufficient to prevent the decline in 24-hour EE that normally occurs in obese subjects during energy restriction and weight loss. It can be estimated that the thermogenic effect of sibutramine could account for ~23% of the fat loss induced during eight weeks of treatment (64). Future studies should carefully consider the pharmacokinetics of sibutramine and its active metabolites, and study designs should possess sufficient statistical power to detect differences in 24-hour EE of the order of 2% to 4% (66).

β_2-Adrenoceptor Agonists

The β_2-adrenoceptor is involved in several regulatory systems, such as vasodilatation and bronchodilatation, but also in lipolysis in adipose tissue and skeletal muscle metabolism (glucose uptake, thermogenesis, and muscle anabolism). Genetic studies have addressed the importance of this receptor subtype for body weight regulation and obesity by looking at a common polymorphism (Gln27Glu) in the gene encoding for the receptor. The amino acid substitution has been shown to have a functional impact on the biological response to receptor stimulation, and the genetic studies suggest that those bearing the Glu allele are more likely to be obese if they have a sedentary lifestyle (67,68). The sedentary behavior may actually be linked to the effect of the polymorphism. Larsen et al. found that individuals with the Gln/Gln genotype had a 7% higher daily spontaneous physical activity than those bearing the Glu allele (69). β_2-Agonists, such as terbutaline and salbutamol, are used in the treatment of asthma, but they have been shown to be thermogenic, to increase insulin-mediated glucose disposal, and to increase the ratio of T_3 to T_4 (70). In a six-week crossover trial, Acheson et al. studied the impact of treatment with terbutaline versus placebo in healthy volunteers (71). They found that terbutaline increased fat oxidation and T_3/T_4 ratio and decreased nitrogen excretion. These results support that β_2-adrenoceptor stimulate repartitioning in man with reduction of fat mass and increase in the lean tissue mass. The clinical value for obesity treatment is limited due to the effect on heart rate, tremor, and the uterus.

β_3-Adrenoceptor Agonists

Sympathomimetic agents are widely used in the treatment of obesity due to their appetite suppressant activity and thermogenic effect (e.g., ephedrine, sibutramine). However, the use of unselective β-adrenoceptor stimulants is associated with adverse effects such as palpitations, tremor, and insomnia attributable to β_1 and β_2 stimulation. A unique β-adrenergic receptor subtype, termed β_3, has been identified. This receptor is pharmacologically distinct from the classical β_1- and β_2-receptor. In animal models, the β_3-receptor stimulates lipolysis in WAT and BAT, and in BAT it activates UCP_1 and upregulates the UCP_1 gene, both of which result in a further increase in energy expenditure (72). BAT is abundant in rodents and in neonatal humans, where it is important for thermoregulation, but it also appears that chronic β_3-adrenergic stimulation in WAT increases the expression of UCP_2 and UCP_3 and a "reawakening" of dormant brown adipocytes. In humans, the presence of β_3-adrenergic receptor mRNA has been demonstrated in brown and white adipose tissue, gallbladder, colon, stomach, small intestine, prostate gland (73,74), and more recently also in human brain, gastrocnemius muscle, and right atrium (75,76). A functional role for the β_3-receptor in adipocyte lipolysis has been suggested by studies in isolated human omental and subcutaneous fat cells (77–79), and in in vivo microdialysis studies with such agonists (79–81). However, these drugs are not available for use in humans, usually because of additional β_{1+2} antagonism (e.g., CGP 12177), so their thermogenic efficacy is unknown. Indirect studies, using combinations of different sympathomimetics and blockers to dissect out the contribution of the β-receptor to human thermogenesis have yielded inconsistent results (82–84).

Shortly after their discovery in the early 1980s, β_3-agonists were found to possess potent antiobesity and antidiabetic properties in rodents. Despite these promising qualities, several pharmaceutical problems and theoretical concerns have slowed the development of these products as therapeutic agents in humans during the last 20 years. Initial problems were due to disregarded differences between rodent and human β_3-receptors and to the difficulty in finding a compound with sufficient bioavailability while being highly selective and a full agonist at the human receptor (85). Most of these problems were solved with the cloning of the human β_3-receptor, which has made it possible to develop novel compounds directly and specifically aimed at the human receptor. A few companies have been successful in developing compounds fulfilling these criteria. These compounds appear to have the bioavailability necessary to increase systemic levels sufficiently and to produce an optimal biological stimulation of the human β_3-receptor.

From Rodent to Human Agonist

Examples of the first generation of β_3-agonists are ZD7114, ZD2079, and CL316243, compounds that are all found to be without thermogenic effect in human clinical trials (86–89). Despite the failure of the first generation compounds in man, their proven acute effects on metabolic rate and insulin action suggest that the β_3-adrenoceptor is a valid target. It might be argued that the acute effects of BRL-26830, BRL-35135, and ZD-2079 after first exposure in man were due to stimulation of β_2- or even β_1-adrenoceptor. Indeed, 60% of the thermogenic effect of BRL-35135 was resistant to blockade with the β_1/β_2-adrenoceptor antagonist nadolol, but the remaining activity appears nevertheless to be mediated by the β_3-adrenoceptor (90). In humans, treatment with CL 316,243 for eight weeks, in spite of limited bioavailability, induced marked plasma concentration-dependent increases in insulin sensitivity, lipolysis, and fat oxidation in lean volunteers, without causing β_1- or β_2-mediated side effects (87).

However, the compound had no effect on 24-hour EE. This finding may be explained by a low intrinsic activity at the human β_3-receptor (85).

L-796568 (Merck) is a more recently developed β_3-adrenergic receptor agonist with high affinity ($EC_{50} = 3.6$ nM) and efficacy (94% of maximal cAMP accumulation by isoprenaline) for the human β_3-adrenoceptor (91). L-796568 is a weak partial agonist at the human β_1- and β_2-receptor, with EC_{50}s of 4.8 and 2.4 μM, respectively, and efficacy of 25% of isoprenaline activity (92). The first study conducted was a randomized placebo-controlled trial in which obese patients were exposed acutely to either 250- or 1000-mg L-796568, or placebo (92). During the four-hour postdose period, energy expenditure increased after the 1000-mg dose (~8%), and this was accompanied by an increase in plasma glycerol and free fatty acid concentrations. Systolic blood pressure also increased by 12 mmHg with 1000 mg, but no changes occurred in heart rate, diastolic blood pressure, core temperature, plasma catecholamine, or potassium. This is the first study to demonstrate such an effect of β_3-adrenergic receptor agonists in humans, without significant evidence for β_2-adrenergic receptor involvement. In the second study, the effect of 28 days daily oral dosing with 375-mg L-796568 on 24-hour EE, substrate oxidations, and body composition was studied in 20 obese subjects (93). Twenty-four-hour EE change from baseline did not differ between L-796568 and placebo ($+92 \pm 586$ vs. $+86 \pm 512$ kJ/24 hr). Likewise, no effect could be found on body weight and composition, 24-hour nonprotein respiratory quotient, or glucose tolerance, but triacylglycerides were decreased by L-796568. However, fat loss was correlated with plasma L-796568 concentration in the L-796568 group ($r = -0.69$, $p < 0.03$).

Other human β_3-agonists are in preclinical development. A single dose of LY-377604 (Lilly), which has been reported as having >20% oral bioavailability, increased metabolic rate by 17.5% at the highest dose used (120 mg) in normal-weight and obese subjects (94). This compound did not move on to clinical tests because of toxicological problems. A compound from Takeda (AJ-9677) has shown body fat-reducing properties in dogs and could go into clinical human trials. AJ-9677 is structurally similar to the first generation compounds BRL-37344 (active metabolite of BRL-35135) and, although its selectivity is 100-fold, it retains some β_1- and β_2-adrenoceptor agonist activity (85). It remains to be to be seen whether it overcomes the efficacy and selectivity problems of the first generation of compounds.

The Future of β_3-Receptor as a Drug Target

BAT is abundant in rodents and in neonatal humans, where it is important for thermoregulation, but no apparent functional BAT remains in adult humans (34).

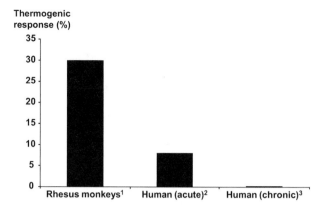

Figure 3 Thermogenic effects of the highly selective human β_3-adrenergic receptor agonist L-796,568 (L-755,507) in rhesus monkeys, and in humans following acute and chronic exposure. Thermogenic response is expressed as increased above resting metabolic rate (%). Superscripted number 1 indicates the thermogenic response in rhesus monkeys after acute intravenous bolus administration of 0.1 mg/kg (95), 2 indicates after oral intake of 100 mg (92), and 3 the change in placebo-subtracted 24-hour energy expenditure after 28 days of daily treatment with 375-mg 1-796,568 in 20 obese subjects (93).

However, recent morphological and functional studies in humans have found small pockets of BAT dispersed in WAT (46). The observation that patients with the catecholamine-secreting adrenal tumor pheochromocytoma display an increase in metabolic rate and weight loss in conjunction with the appearance of BAT demonstrates the potential for recruitment and activation of BAT in adult humans and other primates (95) under certain circumstances. But why does the highly selective β_3-agonist L-796568 possess pronounced lipolytic and thermogenic efficacy following the first exposure in humans, but no efficacy after 28 days of chronic treatment? (Fig. 3). Clearly, the plasma concentrations achieved during the chronic study were 20- to 30-fold higher than the EC_{50} for stimulation of the human β_3-adrenoceptor (93). It cannot entirely be ruled out that the thermogenic effect observed in the acute dosing study was mediated by β^{1+2} receptors, and tachyphylaxia to this effect developed during chronic treatment. In this scenario, there would be insufficient β_3-adrenoceptors in the adult human to achieve a measurable thermogenic effect. It is also likely that recruitment of BAT requires an initial, sustained β_1 stimulation, as described in rodents. This prerequisite may explain why an enhanced thermogenic response to β-adrenergic stimulation can be achieved in humans following chronic nonselective β stimulation (96).

There are several reports to the effect that the Trp64Arg polymorphism in the β_3-adrenoceptor gene is associated with increased body weight, clinical features of insulin resistance, and early development of type 2 diabetes in several populations, and these findings have provided support for the theory that the receptor is of physiological importance also in humans. However, two different meta-analyses based on almost the same studies have provided conflicting conclusions about whether this polymorphism is associated with BMI (97,98).

In conclusion, on the basis of studies of the latest highly selective and potent agonists, the human β_3-adrenoceptor does not yet seem to be a promising drug target for antiobesity compounds.

OTHER THERMOGENIC COMPOUNDS

Hormones such as testosterone and growth hormone have been used to treat obesity, and it is likely that both have thermogenic effects (17). Growth hormone increases lean body mass and reduces body fat through stimulation of thermogenesis and fat oxidation (99,100).

However, due to serious side effects its use is restricted to growth hormone-deficient patients. A number of thermogenic compounds with other modes of action are currently being tested in animal studies, and some in human phase I studies. These include derivatives of thyroid hormone, $PPAR_r$ coactivator, PCC-1 (33), new uncouplers related to dinitrophenol, capsaicin from hot chilies (101), and polyphenols from green tea (102,103). None of them had gone into clinical trials as of mid-2007 and therefore we do not expect thermogenic compound to be marketed within the next five years.

ACKNOWLEDGMENT

Supported by grants from Desiree and Niels Yde's Foundation, Denmark.

REFERENCES

1. Astrup A. Macronutrient balances and obesity: the role of diet and physical activity. Public Health Nutr 1980; 2: 314–347.
2. Bray GA. The MONA LISA hypothesis: most obesities known are low in sympathetic activity. In: Oomura Y, Inoue S, Shimazu T, eds. Progress in Obesity Research. London: John Libbey, 1990:61–74.
3. Grujic D, Susulic VS, Harper M-E, et al. β_3-Adrenergic receptors on white and brown adipocytes mediate β_3-selective agonist-induced effects on energy expenditure, insulin secretion, and food intake. J Biol Chem 1997; 28: 17686–17693.
4. Ravussin E, Lillioja S, Anderson TE, et al. Determinants of 24-hour energy expenditure in man. J Clin Invest 1986; 78:1568–1578.

5. Snitker S, Macdonald I, Ravussin E, et al. The sympathetic nervous system and obesity: role in etiology and treatment. Obes Rev 2000; 1:5–15.

6. Toubro S, Sørensen TIA, Rønn B, et al. Twenty-four-hour energy expenditure: the role of body composition, thyroid status, sympathetic activity and family membership. J Clin Endocrinol Metab 1996; 81:2670–2674.

7. Astrup A, Toubro S, Dalgaard LT, et al. Impact of the v/v 55 polymorphism of the uncoupling protein 2 gene on 24-hour energy expenditure. Int J Obes 1999; 23:1030–1034.

8. Bnemann B, Schierning B, Toubro S, et al. The association between the VAL/ALA-55 polymorphism of the uncoupling protein 2 gene and exercise efficiency. Int J Obes 2001; 25:467–471.

9. Astrup A, Simonsen L, Billow J, et al. Epinephrine mediates facultative carbohydrate induced thermogenesis in human skeletal muscle. Am J Physiol 1989; 257: E340–E345.

10. Sharma AM, Pischon T, Hardt S, et al. β-Adrenergic receptor blockers and weight gain. A systematic analysis. Hypertension 2001; 37:250–254.

11. Snitker S, Tataranni PA, Ravussin E. Respiratory quotient is inversely associated with muscle sympathetic nerve activity. J Clin Endocrinol Metab 1998; 83:3977–3979.

12. Ranneries C, Bülow J, Buemann B, et al. Fat metabolism in formerly obese women: effect of exercise on substrate oxidation and adipose tissue lipolysis. Am J Physiol (Endocrinol Metab) 1998; 274:155–161.

13. Astrup A, Gøtzsche PC, van de Werken K, et al. Meta-analysis of resting metabolic rate in formerly obese subjects. Am J Clin Nutr 1999; 69:1117–1122.

14. Ortega E, Pannacciulli N, Bogardus C, et al. Plasma concentrations of free triiodothyronine predict weight change in euthyroid persons. Am J Clin Nutr 2007; 85: 440–445.

15. Michalaki MA, Vagenakis AG, Leonardou AS, et al. Thyroid function in humans with morbid obesity. Thyroid 2006; 16(1):73–78.

16. Krotkiewski M. Thyroid hormones and treatment of obesity. Int J Obes 2000; 24(suppl 2):S116–S119.

17. Bray GA, Greenway FL. Current and potential drugs for treatment of obesity. Endocr Rev 1999; 20:805–875.

18. Hollingsworth DR, Amatruda TT, Schei R. Quantitative and qualitative effects of L-triiodothyronine in massive obesity. Metabolism 1970; 19:934–945.

19. Moore R, Grant AN, Howard AN, et al. Treatment of obesity with triiodothyronine and a very-low calorie liquid formula diet. Lancet 1980; 1:233–226.

20. Koppeschaar HPF, Meinders AE, Schwarz F. Metabolic responses in grossly obese subjects treated with a very-low-calorie diet with and without triiodothyronine treatment. Int J Obes 1983; 7:133–141.

21. Burman KD, Wartofsky L, Dinterman RE, et al. The effect of T3 and reverse T3 administration on muscle protein catbolism during fasting as measured by 3-methylhistindine excretion. Metabolism 1979; 28:805–813.

22. Abraham RR, Densen JW, Davies P, et al. The effects of triiodothyronine on energy expenditure, nitrogen balance and rates of weight and fat loss in obese patients during prolongued caloric restriction. Int J Obes 1985; 9:433–442.

23. Byerley LO, Heber D. Metabolic effects of triiodothyronine replacement during fasting in obese subjects. J Clin Endocrinol Metab 1996; 81:968–976.

24. Nair KS, Halliday D, Ford GC, et al. Effect of triiodothyronine on leucine kinetics, metabolic rate, glucose concentration and insulin secretion rate during two weeks fasting in obese women. Int J Obes 1989; 13:487–496.

25. Wilson JH, Lamberts SW. The effect of triiodothyronine on weight loss and nitrogen balance of obese patients on a very-low calorie liquid-formula diet. Int J Obes 1981; 5: 279–282.

26. Lovejoy JC, Smith SR, Bray GA, et al. A paradigm of experimentally induced mild hyperthyroidism: effects on nitrogen balance, body composition, and energy expenditure in healthy young men. J Clin Endocrinol Metab 1997; 82:765–770.

27. Trost SU, Swanson E, Gloss B, et al. The thyroid hormone receptor-beta-selective agonist GC-1 differentially affects plasma lipids and cardiac activity. Endocrinology 2000; 141:3055–3056.

28. Wagner RL, Huber BR, Shiau AK, et al. Hormone selectivity in thyroid hormone receptors. Mol Endocrinol 2001; 15:398–410.

29. Ribeiro MO, Carvalho SD, Schultz JJ, et al. Thyroid hormones-sympathetic interaction and adaptive thermogenesis are thyroid hormone receptor isoform-specific. J Clin Invest 2001; 108:97–105.

30. Grover GJ, Mellstrom K, Malm J. Development of the thyroid hormone receptor beta-subtype agonist KB-141: a strategy for body weight reduction and lipid lowering with minimal cardiac side effects. Cardiovasc Drug Rev 2005; 23(2):133–148.

31. Harper JA, Dickinson K, Brand MD. Mitochondrial uncoupling as a target for drug development for the treatment of obesity. Obes Rev 2001; 2:255–265.

32. Tainter ML, Cutting WC, Stickton AB. Use of dinitrophenol in nutritional disorders: a critical survey of clinical results. Am J Public Health 1934; 24:1045–1053.

33. Lowell BB, Spiegelman BM. Towards a molecular understanding of adaptive thermogenesis. Nature 2000; 404:652–677.

34. Astrup A. Thermogenesis in human brown adipose tissue and skeletal muscle induced by sympathomimetic stimulation. Acta Endocrinol Scand 1986; 112:1–32.

35. Astrup A, Bülow J, Madsen J, et al. Contribution of brown adipose tissue and skeletal muscle to thermogenesis induced by ephedrine in man. Am J Physiol 1985; 248: E507–E515.

36. Simoneau JA, Kelley DE, Neverova M, et al. Overexpression of muscle uncoupling protein protein 2 content in human obesity associates with reduced skeletal muscle lipid utilization. FASEB J 1998; 12:1739–1745.

37. Argyropoulos G, Brown AM, Willi SM, et al. Effects of mutations in the human uncoupling protein 3 gene on respiratory quotient and fat oxidation in severe obesity and type 2 diabetes. J Clin Invest 1998; 102:1345–1351.

38. Esterbauer H, Schneitler C, Oberkofler H, et al. A common polymorphism in promoter of UCP2 is associated with decreased risk of obesity in middle-aged humans. Nat Genet 2001; 28:178–183.

39. Schrauwen P, Troost FJ, Xia J, et al. Skeletal muscle UCP2 and UCP3 expression in trained and untrained male subjects. Int J Obes 1999; 23:966–972.

40. Montague CT, Farooqi IS, Whitehead J-P. Congential leptin deficiency is associated with severe early-onset obesity in humans. Nature 1997; 387:903–908.

41. Salbe AD, Nicolson M, Ravussin E. Total energy expenditure and the level of physical activity co-relates with plasma leptin concentrations in five-year-old children. J Clin Invest 1997; 99:592–595.

42. Verdich C, Toubro S, Buemann B, et al. Leptin levels are associated with fat oxidation and dietary-induced weight loss in obesity. Obes Res 2001; 9:452–61.

43. Farooqi IS, Jebb SA, Langmack G, et al. Effects of recombinant leptin therapy in a child with congenital leptin deficiency. N Engl J Med 1999; 341:879–884.

44. Heymsfield SB, Greenberg AS, Fujioka K, et al. Recombinant leptin for weight loss in obese and lean adults. JAMA 1999; 282:1568–1575.

45. Hukshorn CJ, Saris WH, Westerterp-Plantenga MS, et al. Weekly subcutaneous pegylated recombinant native human leptin (PEG-OB) administration in obese men. J Clin Endocrinol Metab 2000; 85:4003–4009.

46. Nedergaard J, Bengtsson T, Cannon B. Unexpected evidence for active brown adipose tissue in adult humans. Am J Physiol Endocrinol Metab 2007; 293(2):E444–E452.

47. Greenway FL. The safety and efficacy of pharmaceutical and herbal caffeine and ephedrine use as a weight loss agent. Obes Rev 2001; 2:199–211.

48. Astrup A, Toubro S. Thermogenic, metabolic and cardiovascular responses to ephedrine and caffeine in man. Int J Obes 1993; 17:S41–S43.

49. Liu Y-L, Toubro S, Astrup A, et al. Contribution of β_3-adrenoceptor activation to ephedrine-induced thermogenesis in humans. Int J Obes 1995; 19:678–685.

50. Astrup A, Breum L, Toubro S, et al. The effect and safety of an ephedrine/caffeine compound compared to ephedrine, caffeine and placebo in obese subjects on an energy restricted diet. A double blind trial. Int J Obes 1992; 16:269–277.

51. Breum L, Pedersen JK, Ahlstrom F, et al. Comparison of an ephedrine/caffeine combination and dexfenfluramine in the treatment of obesity. A double-blind multi-centre trial in general practice. Int J Obes 1994; 18:99–103.

52. Norregaard J, Jorgensen S, Mikkelsen KL, et al. The effect of ephedrine plus caffeine on smoking cessation and post-cessation weight gain. Clin Pharmacol Ther 1996; 60(6):679–686.

53. Stich V, Hainer V, Kunesova M. Effect of ephedrine/caffeine mixture on metabolic response to exercise in obese subjects. Int J Obes 1993; 17:31.

54. Waluga M, Janusz M, Karpel E, et al. Cardiovascular effects of ephedrine, caffeine and yo-himbine measured by thoracic electrical bioimpedance in obese women. Clin Physiol 1998; 18:69–76.

55. Svendsen TL, Ingerslev J, Mork A. Is Letigen contraindicated in hypertension? A double-blind, placebo controlled multipractice study of Letigen administered to normotensive and adequately treated patients with hypersensitivity. Ugeskr Laeger 1998; 160:4073–4075.

56. Toubro S, Astrup A, Breum L, et al. Safety and efficacy of long-term treatment with ephedrine, caffeine and an ephedrine/caffeine mixture. Int J Obes 1993; 17:S69–S72.

57. Stock MJ. Sibutramine: a review of the pharmacology of a novel anti-obesity agent. Int J Obes 1997; 21:25–29.

58. Bray GA, Ryan DH, Gordon D, et al. A double-blind randomized placebo-controlled trial of sibutramine. Obes Res 1996; 4:263–270.

59. James WPT, Astrup A, Finer N, et al. Effect of sibutramine on weight maintenance after weight loss: a randomised trial. Lancet 2000; 356:2119–2125.

60. Rolls BJ, Thorwart ML, Shide DJ, et al. Sibutramine reduces food intake in non-dieting women with obesity. Obes Res 1998; 6:1–11.

61. Hansen DL, Toubro S, Stock MJ, et al. The effect of sibutramine on energy expenditure and appetite during chronic treatment without dietary restriction. Int J Obes 1999; 23:1016–1024.

62. Seagle HM, Bessesen DH, Hill JO. Effects of sibutramine on resting metabolic rate and weight loss in overweight women. Obes Res 1998; 6:115–121.

63. Hansen DL, Toubro S, Stock MJ, et al. Thermogenic effects of sibutramine in humans. Am J Clin Nutr 1998; 68:1180–1186.

64. Walsh KM, Leen E, Lean MEJ. The effect of sibutramine on resting energy expenditure and adrenaline-induced thermogenesis in obese females. Int J Obes 1999; 23:1009–1015.

65. Van Mil EG, Westerterp KR, Kester AD, et al. The effect of sibutramine on energy expenditure and body composition in obese adolescents. J Clin Endocrinol Metab 2007; 92(4):1409–1414.

66. Danforth E. Sibutramine and thermogenesis in humans. Int J Obes 1999; 23:1007–1008.

67. Meirhaeghe A, Helbecque N, Cottel D, et al. Beta2-adrenoceptor gene polymorphism, body weight, and physical activity. Lancet 1999; 353:896.

68. Large V, Hellstrom L, Reynisdottir S, et al. Human beta-2 adrenoceptor gene polymorphisms are highly frequent in obesity and associate with altered adipocyte beta-2 adrenoceptor function. J Clin Invest 1997; 100:3005–3013.

69. Larsen TM, Buemann B, Toubro S, et al. β_2-Receptor polymorphism Gln27Glu associated with 24hr spontaneous physical activity. Int J Obes 2001; 25(suppl 2):S13.

70. Scheidegger K, O'Connell M, Robbins DC, et al. Effects of chronic beta-receptor stimulation on sympathetic nervous system activity, energy expenditure, and thyroid hormones. J Clin Endocrinol Metab 1984; 58:895–903.

71. Acheson KJ, Tavussin E, Schoeller DA, et al. Two-week stimulation or blockade of the sympathetic nervous system in man: influence on body weight, body composition, and twenty-four hour energy expenditure. Metabolism 1988; 37:91–98.

72. Van Baak MA. The peripheral sympathetic nervous system in human obesity. Obes Rev 2001; 2:3–14.

73. Krief S, Lönnqvist F, Raimbault S, et al. Tissue distribution of β_3-adrenergic receptor mRNA in man. J Clin Invest 1993; 91:344–349.

74. Berkowitz DE, Nardone NA, Smiley RM, et al. Distribution of β_3-adrenoceptor mRNA in human tissues. Eur J Pharmacol 1995; 289:223–228.

75. Rodriguez M, Carillon C, Coquerel A, et al. Evidence for the presence of beta$_3$-adrenergic receptor mRNA in the human brain. Brain Res Mol Brain Res 1995; 29: 369–375.

76. Chamberlain PD, Jennings KH, Paul F, et al. The tissue distribution of the human β-adrenoceptors studied using a monoclonal antibody: direct evidence of the β-adrenoceptor in human adipose tissue, atrium and skeletal muscle. Int J Obes 1999; 23:1057–1065.

77. Lönnqvist F, Krief S, Strosberg AD, et al. Evidence for a functional β3-adrenoceptor in man. Br J Pharmacol 1993; 110:929–936.

78. Hoffstedt J, Shimizu M, Sjöstedt S, et al. Determination of β3-adrenoceptor mediated lipolysis in human fat cells. Obes Res 1995; 3:447–457.

79. Enocksson S, Shimizu M, Lönnqvist F, et al. Demonstration of an in vivo functional β3-adrenoceptor in man. J Clin Invest 1995; 95:2239–2245.

80. Barbe P, Millet L, Galitzky J, et al. In situ assessment of the role of the β−, β2 and βs adrenoceptors in the control of lipolysis and nutritive blood flow in human subcutaneous adipose tissue. Br J Pharmacol 1996; 117:907–913.

81. Tavernier G, Barbe P, Galitzky J, et al. Expression of β3-adrenoceptor with low lipolytic action in human subcutaneous white adipocytes. J Lipid Res 1996; 37:87–97.

82. Wheeldpn NM, McDevitt DG, Lipworth BJ. Do β 3-adrenoceptors mediate metabolic responses to isoprenaline. Q J Med 1993; 86:595–600.

83. Blaak EE, Saris WHM, Van Baak MA. Adrenoceptor subtypes mediating catecholamine-induced thermogenesis in man. Int J Obes 1993; 17(suppl 3):S78–S81.

84. Schiffelers SLH, Blaak EE, Saris WHM, et al. In vivo β 3-adrenergic stimulation of human ther-mogenesis and lipid use. Clin Pharmacol Ther 2000; 67:558–566.

85. Arch JRS, Wilson S. Prospects for β-adrenoceptor agonists in the treatment of obesity and diabetes. Int J Obes 1996; 20:191–199.

86. Weyer C, Gautier JF, Danforth E Jr. Development of beta 3-adrenoceptor agonists for the treatment of obesity and diabetes—an update. Diabetes Metab 1999; 25:11–21.

87. Weyer C, Tataranni PA, Snitker S, et al. Increase in insulin action and fat oxidation after treatment with CL-316,243, a highly selectiv beta 3-adrenoceptor agonist in humans. Diabetes 1998; 47:1555–1561.

88. Buemann B, Toubro S, Astrup A. Effects of the two β 3-agonists, XD7114 and ZD2079, on 24-hour energy expenditure and respiratory quotient in obese subjects. Int J Obes 2000; 24:1553–1560.

89. Melnyk A, Zingaretti MC, Ceresi E, et al. Transformation of some unilocular (UL) into multilocular (ML) adipocytes in white adipose tissue (WAT) of CL 316,243(CL)-treated rats. Obes Res 1999; 7:74.

90. Wheeldon NM, McDevitt DG, McFarlane LC, et al. β-Adrenoceptor subtypes mediating the metabolic effects of BRL 35135 in man. Clin Sci 1994; 86:331–337.

91. Mathvink RJ, Tolman JS, Chitty D, et al. Discovery of a potent, orally bioavailable β3adrenergic receptor agonist, (R)-N-[4-[2-[[2-hydroxy-2-(3-piridinyl)ethyl]amino]ethyl]-phenyl]-4-[4-[4-(trifluoromethyl)phenyl]thiazol-2-yl]benzenesulfonamide. J Med Chem 2000; 43:3832–3836.

92. Van Baak MA, Hul GBJ, Toubro S, et al. Acute effect of L-796568, aβ 3-adrenergic receptor agonist, on energy expenditure in obese men. Clin Pharmacol Ther 2002; 71: 272–279.

93. Larsen TM, Toubro S, Van Baak MA, et al. The effect of 28 days treatment with L-796568, a novel β_3-adrenoceptor agonist, on energy expenditure and body composition in obese men. Am J Clin Nut 2002; 76:780–788.

94. Harada H, Kato S, Kawashima H, et al. A new β_3-adrenergic agonist: synthesis and biological activity of indole derivatives. 214th Meeting of the American Chemical Society, Las Vegas, Medi 208, 1997.

95. Fisher MH, Amend AM, Bach TJ, et al. A selective human β_3 adrenergic receptor agonist increases metabolic rate in rhesus monkeys. J Clin Invest 1998; 101:2387–2393.

96. Astrup A, Lundsgaard C, Madsen J, et al. Enhanced thermogenic responsiveness during chronic ephedrine treatment in man. Am J Clin Nutr 1985; 42:83–94.

97. Fujisawa T, Ikegami H, Kawaguchi Y, et al. Meta-analysis of the association of Trp^{64}Arg polymorphism of β_3-adrenergic receptor gene with body mass index. J Clin Endocrinol Metab 1998; 83:2441–2444.

98. Allison DB, Heo M, Faith MS, et al. Meta-analysis of the association of the Trp^{64}Arg polymorphism in the beta3 adrenergic receptor with body mass index. Int J Obes 1998; 22:559–566.

99. Karlsson C, Stenlof K, Johannsson G, et al. Effects of growth hormone treatment on the leptin system and on energy expenditure in abdominally obese men. Eur J Endocrinol 1998; 138:408–414.

100. Møller N, Jørgensen JO, Møller N, et al. Growth hormone enhances effects of endurance training on oxidative muscle metabolism in elderly women. Am J Physiol 2000; 279:E989–E996.

101. Yoshioka M, St-Pierre S, Suzuki M, et al. Effects of red pepper added to high-fat and high-carbohydrate meals on energy metabolism and substrate utilization in Japanese women. Br J Nutr 1998; 80:503–510.

102. Dulloo AG, Duret C, Rohrer D, et al. Efficacy of a green tea extract rich in catechin polyphenols and caffeine in increasing 24-h energy expenditure and fat oxidation in humans. Am J Clin Nutr 1999; 70:1040–1045.

103. Astrup A. Thermogenic drugs as a strategy for treatment of obesity. Endocrine 2000; 13:207–212.

27

Strategies to Reduce Calories in Food

ALEXANDRA G. KAZAKS and JUDITH S. STERN
Department of Nutrition, University of California, Davis, California, U.S.A.

INTRODUCTION

Weight reduction is accomplished by reducing energy intake below energy expenditure (1). Reducing food consumption, or dieting, is often associated with hunger, restricting preferred foods, eventual diet failure, guilt, and weight regain. In most people, the pleasure of eating satisfying amounts of favorite foods wins over the deprivation and denial needed to stay on a diet. While there are many factors that contribute to control of food intake, the weight and volume of food ingested are important short-term signals (2). This chapter explores existing methods and emerging technologies that the food industry uses to reduce calories in food and how these reduced-calorie products contribute to weight management. Throughout the chapter, the term "calories" represents 1 kcal or 4.18 kJ.

Question: How can people reduce energy intake, and reduce weight, without giving up the quantity of foods they prefer?

Answer: Eat foods that have low energy density. These foods provide high-volume, low-calorie value and increased satiety.

Energy density is defined as the amount of energy in a given weight of food or the ratio of calories per gram of food (3). Rich desserts or fried meats are high in energy density. Fat contributes the greatest amount of energy per gram; therefore high-fat foods have high energy density. They provide a large number of calories in a small volume of food. In contrast, fresh vegetables and fruits and lean meats have low energy density. They provide fewer calories in a larger portion size. These items are low in fat and concentrated starches and sugars and high in fiber and water content. Water and fiber provide weight, but are energy-dilute. Low-energy-density foods provide volume and weight that contribute to satiation and satiety (Table 1) (4). In a clinical trial, individuals who ate low-energy-dense foods were more successful at weight loss than those who restricted fat and portion sizes. Eating satisfying portions of low-energy-dense food helped to enhance satiety and allowed the participants to reduce energy intake without counting calories (5).

Barriers to weight management exist when individuals do not know about, do not like, or do not have the time to prepare low-energy-dense foods. Consumers want low-cost, convenient food that also supports good health and tastes good. In a 2005 survey by the Grocery Manufacturers

Table 1 Definition of Psychological and Physiological Cues that Affect Eating Behavior

---

Satiation—Occurs during eating. Satiation refers to the processes that control size, duration, and termination of a meal.

Satiety—Occurs after eating. Satiety refers to the effects of food (often described as a preload) on subsequent intake, meal frequency, and feeling of fullness.

Appetite—Associated with sensory experiences or aspects such as the sight and aroma of food, emotional cues, social situations, and cultural conventions; desire to eat.

Hunger—The physiological need for food as fuel.

Source: From Refs. 30, 31.

of America, 73% of shoppers said they were purchasing more nutritious and healthy foods and beverages than in the past (6). Specifically, consumers wanted more products that contain the following:

- Whole, unrefined grains
- Low fat
- Low calorie
- Sugar free and low carbohydrate

The food industry plays a major role in the "energy in, energy out" equation. As it responds to market forces and consumer demands, the industry, in turn, shapes consumer eating habits. The current result is that lower-energy-density convenience foods are increasingly available in the marketplace.

METHODS TO REDUCE CALORIES IN PROCESSED FOODS

Calories in processed foods can be reduced by the following methods:

- Reducing sugars and fat
- Increasing fiber and water

Manufacturers of prepared food products have already been successful in manipulating energy density. Reduced-calorie foods such as low-fat milk, diet sodas, sugar substitutes, and lower-fat dressings and spreads are a popular and an accepted part of our national diet. Calorie reduction in beverages is relatively easy. Concentrated sugars are replaced with no-calorie or low-calorie sweeteners. Calorie reduction in structurally complex food products with a higher level of solids, such as baked goods and dairy-based desserts, is more difficult. Besides taste, fat and sugars have multiple functions in food products. Along with sweetness, sugars also provide bulk, increased shelf-life and browning in baked foods. Fats provide a rich mouth feel and are responsible for a whole host of flavors. They impart creaminess, transmit

heat rapidly, and provide crisping. In a low-fat product, several ingredients are usually needed to replace the functional and sensory characteristics of a full-fat food. Low-fat foods were very popular a few years ago when hundreds of new products appeared in the market. However, many brands of reduced-fat cookies, cakes, crackers, snack foods, and cheese are no longer sold, because they did not meet consumer expectations for taste and value. In addition, some of the fat-reduced foods had large amounts of sugars added to maintain flavor, so there was no calorie savings. Food technology for fat and calorie reduction has been steadily evolving. Today, manufacturers aim to produce better tasting reduced-calorie foods that allow consumers to reduce energy intake and continue to consume the quality—and quantity—of foods they prefer.

Reducing Energy from Sugars: High-Intensity Sweeteners and Sugar Substitutes

High-Intensity Sweeteners

Replacing sugar (4 kcal/g) is a common practice for weight management. High-intensity sweeteners are 160 to 13,000 times sweeter than sucrose. Only a small amount of the product adds enormously to sweetness. Five high-intensity sweeteners are currently approved for use in the United States:

- Aspartame
- Acesulfame K
- Saccharin
- Sucralose
- Neotame

These sweeteners are regulated as food additives. They must be approved as safe for consumption before they are marketed. The typical use of each of these artificial sweeteners is within the "acceptable daily intake," or level that can be consumed safely every day over a lifetime. While there has been controversy over potential health risks related to their consumption, each of these products has undergone rigorous scientific testing (7) (Table 2).

Sugar Substitutes and Bulking Agents: Inulin, Polyols, Polydextrose

These ingredients replace the "bulk" or physical weight and volume lost when sugar is removed. They also provide properties like texture, viscosity, and mouth feel. Since they provide little or no sweetness, they are often blended with high-intensity sweeteners.

Inulin

Extracted from chicory root, inulin is a mixture of oligomers and polymers of fructose that have a variety

Table 2 Characteristics and Safety of High-Intensity Sweeteners

Sweetener	Brand names	Sweetness	Use in food	Safety and Structure
Acesulfame K	Sunett, Sweet One	200 times sweeter than sucrose	A general purpose sweetener; can be used in baked goods	According to the FDA, its safety is backed by more than 90 studies. Acesulfame K is a potassium salt of 5,6-dimethyl-1,2,3-oxathiazine-4(3H)-1-2,2-dioxide. Its structure is similar to saccharin.
Saccharin	Sweet 'N Low, Sugar Twin, others	200–700 times sweeter than sucrose	Used in tabletop sweeteners, baked goods, soft drinks, and chewing gum	In 1977 the FDA proposed a ban on saccharin because a study linked saccharin to bladder cancer in rats. The case against the sweetener was dropped when it was disclosed that the rats had consumed saccharin equivalent to 800 cans of diet soda a day for a lifetime. Since then, the National Cancer Institute and the FDA have concluded that saccharin use is not a major risk for bladder cancer in humans. The chemical name for saccharin is 2,3-dihydro-3-oxobenzisosulfonazole and is used in the ammonium saccharin, calcium saccharin, and sodium saccharin forms.
Aspartame	Nutra-Sweet, Equal	200 times sweeter than sucrose	A general purpose sweetener in all foods and drinks. Aspartame loses its sweetness when heated	The American Medical Association and the FDA have concluded that aspartame is safe at recommended levels. However, people with PKU should avoid it because they cannot metabolize the amino acid phenylalanine. Aspartame-containing foods must display a PKU warning. Aspartame is the methyl ester of the dipeptide aspartyl phenylalanine.
Sucralose	Splenda	600 times sweeter than sucrose	A general purpose sweetener. Splenda can be directly substituted for sugar in baking and cooking	According to the FDA, its safety is backed by more than 110 animal and human studies. Sucralose is manufactured by the selective chlorination of sucrose, in which three of the hydroxyl groups are replaced with chlorine atoms to produce 1,6-dichloro-1,6-dideoxy-β-D-fructo-furanosyl 4-chloro-4-deoxy-α-D-galactopyranoside or $C_{12}H_{19}Cl_3O_8$.
Neotame	Neotame is made by the same company that produces NutraSweet (aspartame)	7,000–13,000 times sweeter than sucrose	At this time, neotame is not available directly to consumers. Neotame is used in the same types of foods and beverages as aspartame and acesulfame K	According to the FDA, neotame's safety is backed by more than 100 animal and human studies. Similarly to aspartame, neotame's structure is based on the phenylalanine and aspartic acid dipeptide (N-[N-(3,3-dimethylbutyl)-L-α-aspartyl]-L-phenylalanine-1-methyl ester). Because it is metabolized differently from aspartame, products containing neotame are not required to carry the PKU warning.

Abbreviation: PKU, phenylketonuria.

of caloric contents, ranging from 1.0 kcal/g to 1.5 kcal/g. Inulin resists digestion in the upper gastrointestinal tract. It is fermented by bacteria in the colon, which produce short-chain fatty acids that are absorbed and metabolized in other parts of the body. Colonic fermentation is a way that a small part of energy content is captured from inulin and other digestion-resistant products (8).

Polyols

This group of reduced-calorie sweeteners, also known as sugar alcohols (5 or 6 carbon structures), not only replaces bulk but provides some sweetness. All polyols are absorbed slowly and incompletely, which is why they have fewer calories (1.6–3.0 kcal/g) than sugar. However, this property can also cause gas and diarrhea. Products containing large amounts of polyols must be labeled with the warning, "Excess consumption may have a laxative effect." Despite this warning, it is possible for consumers to experience these symptoms if they consume a variety of products containing polyols. Some of these products are listed in the ingredients as sorbitol, mannitol, xylitol, erythritol, and D-tagatose.

Combination products

Polydextrose is an example of a multifunctional ingredient that can replace both fat and sugar while also adding fiber. It is a combination of high-molecular-weight polysaccharides that supply the smooth mouth feel of fat and lower-molecular-weight oligosaccharides that simulate the functionality of sugars. Polydextrose is only partially metabolized, provides 1 kcal/g, and may have a laxative effect at high levels. Because polydextrose is about 90% fiber, it can help a product earn "source of fiber" labeling. It is found in a broad range of applications including cereals, beverages, candies, salad dressings, frozen desserts, and baked goods.

Reducing Energy from Fats: Decrease and Replace

As a nutrient, fat is a multitasker. It provides nutrition, physical structure, and unique sensory characteristics. Fat provides essential fatty acids and fat-soluble vitamins. Functionally, fat content controls the melting point, viscosity, and spreadability of many foods. Fat provides moistness in baked goods, creamy texture in ice cream, and crispiness in chips and crackers.

While people enjoy the flavors, aromas, and creamy rich textures that fat gives to food, reducing fat is the most efficient way to reduce calories. At 9 kcal/g, fat has higher energy content than protein or carbohydrates at 4 kcal/g. The food industry offers consumers a wide variety of fat-free and low-fat products. New and existing methods and ingredients are used to reduce and replace fat, while maintaining at least some of the flavors and textures of full-fat foods. Fat reduction is accomplished in a number of ways.

Use Less Fat

Skim milk and low-fat dressings and cheeses can have constituent fat removed with no replacement. Prepared foods can be processed without fat. For example, potato chips may be baked instead of fried. These products do not taste the same as the full-fat types, but consumers have generally accepted the altered versions.

Use Fat Replacers

Fat replacers are hydrophobic substances that provide some of the characteristics of fat. They fall into three

Table 3 Fat Reduction Ingredients Used in Common Food Products

Fat reduction ingredients	Energy contribution (kcal/g)	Food application examples
Carbohydrate based		
Carrageenan, cellulose, gelatin, gels, guar gum, maltodextrins, polydextrose, xanthin gum, modified dietary starches	0–4	Baked goods, frozen desserts, puddings, salad dressings, sauces, sour cream, yogurt, cheese, ground beef
Protein based		
Whey protein concentrate, microparticulated egg white, soy and milk protein	1–4	Baked goods, butter, cheese, frozen desserts, mayonnaise, salad dressings, sour cream
Fat based		
Caprenin, salatrim, mono- and diglycerides,	5	Baked goods, cheese, chocolate, frozen desserts, candy coatings, margarine, spreads, chips, and crackers
Olestra	0	

Source: From Ref. 19.

main categories: carbohydrates, proteins, and reduced-calorie fats. Most carbohydrate and protein fat replacers are ingredients already approved by the Food and Drug Administration (FDA) for other uses in food. They are familiar ingredients used in new ways. For instance, some conventional starches such as rice, corn, potato, and tapioca have traditionally been used as thickeners and stabilizers (9) (Table 3).

Carbohydrate-based fat replacers

Digestible carbohydrate, such as modified starches and dextrins, supply 4 kcal/g. Although these carbohydrates contribute some energy, it is significantly less than the energy from fat. These ingredients replace the bulk of fat, add viscosity, and add a pleasing mouth feel to fat-reduced foods. They cannot be used for frying and they do not melt, but they work well in emulsions, such as salad dressings. Carbohydrate-based fat replacers are listed on food labels as maltodextrin, cellulose, guar and locust bean gum, carrageenan, alginate, pectin, and xanthan gum.

Use Protein-Based Fat Replacers

Proteins commonly found in foods, including egg white, soy, or milk proteins, can function as fat replacers. These proteins are digested and absorbed and contribute 1 to 4 cal/g.

However, only small amounts are needed, which reduces the calorie content overall. Because they can form colloidal gels that simulate the body and mouth feel of fat, they provide a perception of fat without the extra calories. Proteins can be processed to give them fat-like properties. An example is Simplesse®, which is made from whey or egg protein. The proteins are "microparticulated," or formed into tiny beads that roll over each other, imitating the creaminess of fat. Simplesse gives richness to frozen desserts, cheese spreads, sour cream, and yogurt.

Use Reduced-Calorie Fats

The majority of reduced-calorie fats are either triglycerides with modified configurations, or substances with chemical structures that prevent their absorption in the intestine. Salatrim, sold under the trade name Benefat®, is a triglyceride composed of both long- and short-chain fatty acids. Because of its unusual structure, it contributes only 5 kcal/g. It has the properties of a shortening-type fat and is used in baked goods and frozen desserts. Some fat-based replacers, such as olestra, pass through the body unabsorbed. Olestra is heat-stable and can replace both the functionality and flavor of traditional fats. There has been concern about its safety because of reports from individuals who experienced gastrointestinal problems, such as cramps and loose stools after consuming large amounts of olestra. However, a review of more than 100 studies has shown that consumption of olestra-containing food does not affect gastric emptying or bowel transit times. Occurrence of gastrointestinal symptoms under ordinary snacking conditions is comparable following consumption of snacks fried in regular fats and oils with those made with olestra. Olestra does cause a decrease in the availability of lipid-soluble vitamins A, D, E, and K, and carotenoids such as β-carotene, lycopene, and lutein (10,11). To attempt to offset this effect, the FDA requires manufacturers to add vitamins A, D, E, and K to products containing olestra. In an olestra diet study in 2005, vitamin supplementation prevented decreases in vitamin A and E, but carotenoid levels of subjects were significantly lower than the control or low-fat diet groups (12). Since a growing body of evidence indicates that carotenoids are associated with health benefits, further research should evaluate whether olestra's effect on reduction of serum carotenoid levels is clinically meaningful.

Enhancing Fiber

Weight-conscious consumers are often encouraged to add fiber to their diets. Dietary fiber products are typically derived from plant sources that are completely or partially resistant to human digestive enzymes. They provide 0 to 3 kcal/g. Common sources of fiber include the cereals, fruits, and vegetables recommended by the U.S. Department of Agriculture's (USDA) dietary guidelines (13). However, most people do not eat enough of these foods to meet daily fiber requirements (14). Consumers now have additional options with the wide variety of fiber-enhanced foods and beverages new to the market. These foods have an added benefit—as they replace fat and reduce calories, they also are a source of dietary fiber.

Commercial fiber-based fat replacers can be produced from low-cost agricultural by-products such as hulls of oats, rice, corn, soybean, and peas. During processing, their cellular structure disintegrates so they become fine powders that form gels when mixed with water. These fibers can replace fat because of their ability to hold water and provide a smooth mouth feel (15).

Products Using Multiple Replacements

Since fats and sweeteners have several functions in complex food products, it usually requires a systems approach to maintain food quality and consumer satisfaction when these ingredients are reduced or removed. The strategy is to match the properties of the higher-calorie ingredients with those of the substitute ingredients to provide reduced energy density, good taste, a satisfying volume, and increased satiety.

IMPACT OF REDUCED-CALORIE PRODUCTS ON BODY WEIGHT

Will people lose weight snacking on fat-free chips and sugar-free pudding? Or, will they just feel free to eat more of everything? Are the numerous new and existing products that reduce food energy effective in weight loss and long-lasting maintenance?

Sugar Replacement Studies

Although it seems to make sense that replacing high-calorie sweeteners with sugar substitutes could help control weight, there is no scientific consensus regarding their usefulness. In a review of evidence from laboratory, clinical and epidemiological studies, artificial sweeteners were associated with only modest weight loss. Overall, the intense sweeteners did not suppress appetite and consequent consumption. It was suggested that their major benefit occurs when they are integrated into a reduced energy diet (16). A study by Raben et al. suggested that overweight individuals should consider choosing beverages containing artificial sweeteners, rather than sucrose, to prevent weight gain. Overweight subjects who consumed 28% of energy from sucrose, mostly as beverages, had increased energy intake, body weight, and fat mass after 10 weeks when compared with subjects who used artificial sweeteners (17).

While some investigators have concluded that artificial sweeteners do enhance weight loss, others have proposed that these sweeteners actually increase body weight. This idea is based on studies such as one in France that showed that people who regularly consume artificial sweeteners in place of sucrose have a higher body mass index (18). Instead of suggesting a causal relationship between artificial sweeteners and increased body weight, these data may reflect populations in which subjects were using artificial sweeteners to reduce calories for weight reduction because they were already overweight. Little is known about the long-term impact of sweetener replacements on energy intake and body weight.

Fat Replacement Studies

The American Heart Association and the American Dietetic Association report that fat substitutes provide flexibility in food choices and can have a substantial impact on weight reduction as long as they lower total calorie intake (9,19). A study described as "long term" concluded that reduced fat products contribute to lower energy consumption when compared with full-fat products (20). However, one cannot reach conclusions about the "longer-term" health effects of fat replacements when a study lasts only six months. Studies of the long-term health benefits of dietary constituents must last for a number of years such as the Women's Health Initiative study that lasted more than seven years (21).

Olestra has been studied more than many other fat substitutes. The fact that olestra-based foods have the potential to deliver the sensory qualities of real fat suggests that these foods may be helpful for consumers with a sensory preference for dietary fat. A review of works on the effects of olestra on appetite and energy intake in humans included both lean and obese men and women under a variety of conditions ranging from the laboratory to real life. A three-month study showed that including olestra-based foods did not induce dietary energy deficits, but significant weight gain was limited compared to that seen with full-fat diet controls (22). In a nine-month randomized, feeding trial, 45 healthy overweight men consumed a diet in which one-third of the dietary fat was replaced with olestra to provide 25% available fat. They were compared with men on a control diet (33% fat) or a fat-reduced diet (25%). The results showed that replacement of dietary fat with olestra reduced body weight and total body fat more than the 25% fat diet or a control diet containing 33% fat (23). Another study examined the effects of replacing dietary fat with olestra on body composition and weight change in men and women. Replacement of 1/3 of dietary fat with olestra for up to 10 weeks resulted in weight loss that was

significantly different from a control diet (24). In these studies weight loss occurred because total energy intake was reduced. It is significant that compensation for the reduced energy intake did not occur when olestra replaced dietary fat. Fat replacers can be valuable in reducing energy density of many foods. However, if total energy density in a person's diet is not decreased, the benefit of fat-reduced foods for weight management is limited.

Fiber Additions

Dietary fiber, regardless of the source, has also been linked to weight regulation. A review summarizing the effects of high- versus low-fiber diet interventions found that the high-fiber diets increased satiety and decreased subsequent appetite. Mean values for published studies indicate that consumption of an additional 14 g/day fiber is associated with a 10% decrease in energy intake and body weight loss of 1.9 kg over about four months. Changes in energy intake and body weight occur both when the fiber is naturally occurring in foods and when it is from a fiber supplement. Since the average dietary fiber intake in the United States is approximately half the USDA recommendation of 25 to 30 g/day, increasing dietary fiber in individuals consuming <25 g/day may help to decrease the prevalence of obesity (14). Again, it is the short-term studies that suggest fiber additions can lower energy density and have the potential to lower body weight. Longer studies are necessary to determine lasting weight and health effects.

Example of Research Study in Detail: Chitosan

Here is a detailed examination of research findings related to chitosan, a nonnutritive, high-fiber carbohydrate. Chitosan is produced commercially by deacetylation of chitin, which is the structural element in the exoskeleton of crustaceans such as crabs, shrimp, and lobsters. It is a linear polysaccharide with interspersed D-glucosamine, and acetyl-D-glucosamine units. Chitosan's strong positive charge allows it to bind to fats and cholesterol. As a food ingredient, chitosan can impart viscosity and form gels and is used in applications such as thickening of chocolate milk drinks. Chitosan also has been approved by the FDA for use as an edible film to protect foods from dehydration. Like other forms of fiber, such as oat bran, chitosan is not well digested by the human body. As it passes through the digestive tract, it has been purported to bind with ingested fat and carry it out of the digestive tract. For this reason, it has been suggested as an agent for reducing weight. In Japan, several foods including soybean paste, potato chips, and noodles have added chitosan as cholesterol-lowering functional foods. It is also used in

Choco Lady, a sweet chocolate pellet that contains a crispy chitosan-enriched center. The pellets are claimed to prevent fat absorption and help with weight loss. The product description states,

> For maximum effect, the consumer is advised to eat 5 pellets before each meal.
>
> … targeted towards men and women who tend to eat greasy meals (25).

Apart from its role as a food additive, chitosan is sold as a dietary supplement that will block the absorption of significant amounts of dietary fat and lead to rapid weight loss. In support of the fat-blocking claim was a demonstration aired on the QVC television channel. A beaker was filled with oil and a water-based liquid to simulate what happens in a person's gastrointestinal tract, even though a beaker clearly does not simulate human digestion. When the oil and water do not mix, chitosan is added to the concoction. The TV camera shows clumps of chitosan. This demonstration is offered as proof that chitosan combines with fat, prevents it from being absorbed by the body, and will lead to rapid weight loss.

If chitosan worked as claimed, there should be increased fat in the feces when a person consumes chitosan along with meals containing fat. We published a series of three studies that measured the amount of fat in feces of a total of 104 men and women taking chitosan (26–28). These data were compared to a control period. Three different brands of chitosan were tested. Research for our first study was funded, in part, by the Consumer Affairs Division of the District Attorney's Office in Napa County. The greatest amount of fat that was malabsorbed in men was 1.8 g/day or 16 kcal. We calculated that it would take more than 15 months to lose 1 kg of body fat using chitosan. This is not "rapid weight loss." Furthermore, it did not block the absorption of any fat in women (Table 4) (28). In addition to our studies, a systematic review of randomized controlled trials of chitosan indicated that the effect of chitosan on body weight was minimal and unlikely to be of clinical significance (29).

The overall results from studies of sugar and fat replacers and increased dietary fiber indicate that some products used to reduce energy density are helpful in obesity management, while others do not make a significant contribution. The essential factor that determines effectiveness of modified food products is that total energy density in a person's diet must be decreased.

CLINICAL PRACTICE: REDUCED CALORIE PRODUCTS AND WEIGHT MANAGEMENT

Realities

1. Calories do count. Calories consumed must equal calories expended even with low-energy-density foods.
2. Use low-calorie products as *substitutes* for higher-calorie foods, not *in addition* to a regular diet. A reduced-calorie food label is not a license to eat unlimited amounts guilt-free.
3. Consumers want lower-calorie foods, but they also want food that tastes good. Not all reduced-calorie products provide desirable flavors, aromas, and textures.
4. Although the calorie-reducing products have undergone rigorous testing, individuals may be concerned or confused about the safety of these food additives.

Promises

1. Reducing energy intake is easier and less painful when the taste and qualities of sugars and fats are provided in reduced-calorie versions of foods.
2. The volume of food in low-energy-density products can increase satiety and help control appetite.
3. With high-volume, reduced-energy-density foods, consumers may be satisfied with smaller portions at each meal, and consequently, fewer calories overall.

Final Considerations

Low-energy-density foods provide volume, weight, and satisfying portions that contribute to satiety. Whether low energy density is a characteristic of a naturally occurring

Table 4   Results from Studies of the Effect of Chitosan on Excretion of Dietary Fat

Subjects (reference)	Chitosan (g/day)	Fecal fat (g/day) no supplement	Fecal fat (g/day) with supplement	Difference (g) of fecal fat	Extra fat calories excreted (kcal/day)
7 men (26)	5.25	6.9	6.8	−0.1	−0.9
15 men (27)	4.50	6.1	7.2	+1.1	+10
12 men (28)	2.50	5.0	6.9	+1.8	+16
12 men (28)	2.50	3.7	3.7	0	0

Manufacturers claim that a chitosan supplement, when taken as directed, will prevent the absorption of up to 120 g of dietary fat per day.

food like an apple, or is a product of food technology such as fat-free frozen yogurt, it will contribute to weight management only if total energy consumed is balanced by energy expenditure.

REFERENCES

1. Jakicic JM, Clark K, Coleman E, et al. American College of Sports Medicine position stand. Appropriate intervention strategies for weight loss and prevention of weight regain for adults. Med Sci Sports Exerc 2001; 33(12):2145–556.

2. de Castro JM. Macronutrient and dietary energy density influences on the intake of free-living humans. Appetite 2006; 46(1):1–5.

3. Rolls BJ, Drewnowski A, Ledikwe JH. Changing the energy density of the diet as a strategy for weight management. J Am Diet Assoc 2005; 105(5 suppl 1):S98–S103.

4. Ledikwe JH, Blanck HM, Kettel Khan L, et al. Dietary energy density is associated with energy intake and weight status in US adults. Am J Clin Nutr 2006; 83(6):1362–1368.

5. Ello-Martin JA, Ledikwe JH, Rolls BJ. The influence of food portion size and energy density on energy intake: implications for weight management. Am J Clin Nutr 2005; 82(suppl 1):236S–241S.

6. Whole grains and low-fat food top consumers' grocery lists. Grocery Manufacturers of America, 2005. Available at: http://www.gmabrands.com/news/docs/NewsRelease.cfm?DocID=1462. Accessed May 10, 2007.

7. Artificial sweeteners: no calories … sweet!, 2006. Available at: http://www.ncbi.nlm.nih.gov/entrez/query.fcgi?cmd=Retrieve&db=PubMed&dopt=Citation&list_uids=17243285. Accessed May 10, 2007.

8. Roberfroid MB. Caloric value of inulin and oligofructose. J Nutr 1999; 129(suppl 7):1436S–1437S.

9. Wylie-Rosett J. Fat substitutes and health: an advisory from the Nutrition Committee of the American Heart Association. Circulation 2002; 105(23):2800–2804.

10. Hunt R, Zorich NL, Thomson AB. Overview of olestra: a new fat substitute. Can J Gastroenterol 1998; 12(3):193–197.

11. Thomson AB, Hunt RH, Zorich NL. Olestra and its gastrointestinal safety. Aliment Pharmacol Ther 1998; 12(12):1185–1200.

12. Tulley RT, Vaidyanathan J, Wilson JB, et al. Daily intake of multivitamins during long-term intake of olestra in men prevents declines in serum vitamins A and E but not carotenoids. J Nutr 2005; 135(6):1456–1461.

13. Dietary Guidelines for Americans, 2005. 6th ed. U.S. Government Printing Office, 2005. Available at: http://www.health.gov/dietaryguidelines/dga2005/document/. Accessed May 10, 2007.

14. Howarth NC, Saltzman E, Roberts SB. Dietary fiber and weight regulation. Nutr Rev 2001; 59(5):129–139.

15. Filling in for fat—redesigned fat replacers create more options, June 2004. Available at: http://www.ffnmag.com/ASP/articleDisplay.asp?strArticleId=498&strSite=FFNSITE&Screen=CURRENTISSUE.

16. Bellisle F, Drewnowski A. Intense sweeteners, energy intake and the control of body weight. Eur J Clin Nutr 2007; 61(6):691–700.

17. Raben A, Vasilaras TH, Moller AC, et al. Sucrose compared with artificial sweeteners: different effects on ad libitum food intake and body weight after 10 wk of supplementation in overweight subjects. Am J Clin Nutr 2002; 76(4):721–729.

18. West JA, de Looy AE. Weight loss in overweight subjects following low-sucrose or sucrose-containing diets. Int J Obes Relat Metab Disord 2001; 25(8):1122–1128.

19. JADA. Position of the American Dietetic association: fat replacers. J Am Diet Assoc 2005; 105(2):266–275.

20. Lovejoy JC, Bray GA, Lefevre M, et al. Consumption of a controlled low-fat diet containing olestra for 9 months improves health risk factors in conjunction with weight loss in obese men: the Ole' study. Int J Obes Relat Metab Disord 2003; 27(10):1242–1249.

21. Caan B, Neuhouser M, Aragaki A, et al. Calcium plus vitamin d supplementation and the risk of postmenopausal weight gain. Arch Intern Med 2007; 167(9):893–902.

22. Stubbs RJ. The effect of ingesting olestra-based foods on feeding behavior and energy balance in humans. Crit Rev Food Sci Nutr 2001; 41(5):363–386.

23. Bray GA, Lovejoy JC, Most-Windhauser M, et al. A 9-mo randomized clinical trial comparing fat-substituted and fat-reduced diets in healthy obese men: the Ole Study. Am J Clin Nutr 2002; 76(5):928–934.

24. Roy HJ, Most MM, Sparti A, et al. Effect on body weight of replacing dietary fat with olestra for two or ten weeks in healthy men and women. J Am Coll Nutr 2002; 21(3):259–267.

25. Choco Lady (Japan) 2006. Available at: http://www.asiafoodjournal.com/print.asp?id=3580. Accessed May 10, 2007.

26. Gades MD, Stern JS. Chitosan supplementation does not affect fat absorption in healthy males fed a high-fat diet, a pilot study. Int J Obes Relat Metab Disord 2002; 26(1):119–122.

27. Gades MD, Stern JS. Chitosan supplementation and fecal fat excretion in men. Obes Res 2003; 11(5):683–638.

28. Gades MD, Stern JS. Chitosan supplementation and fat absorption in men and women. J Am Diet Assoc 2005; 105(1):72–77.

29. Mhurchu CN, Dunshea-Mooij C, Bennett D, et al. Effect of chitosan on weight loss in overweight and obese individuals: a systematic review of randomized controlled trials. Obes Rev 2005; 6(1):35–42.

30. Blundell JE, Halford JC. Regulation of nutrient supply: the brain and appetite control. Proc Nutr Soc 1994; 53(2):407–418.

31. Strubbe JH, Woods SC. The timing of meals. Psychol Rev 2004; 111(1):128–141.

28

Herbal and Alternative Approaches to Obesity

FRANK GREENWAY

Pennington Biomedical Research Center, Baton Rouge, Louisiana, U.S.A.

DAVID HEBER

Center for Human Nutrition, UCLA School of Medicine, Los Angeles, California, U.S.A.

INTRODUCTION

The use of herbal and alternative medicines has increased in the last two decades in the United States, and is now the subject of clinical and basic science investigations supported by the NIH Office of Dietary Supplements Research and the National Center for Complementary and Alternative Medicine. The Dietary Supplements Health Education Act (DSHEA) of 1994 enables manufacturers to market these approaches without proving efficacy or safety. The Food and Drug Administration (FDA) has limited resources for policing claims and relies on adverse effects reporting to monitor safety. This method has significant drawbacks in terms of scientifically examining the causative relationship of a particular herbal or alternative approach to a reported side effect.

The most widely used herbal approach to weight loss was dietary supplements that contained ephedra alkaloids (sometimes called ma huang). Ephedra was declared an adulterant by the FDA and was taken off the market for safety concerns (1). Since this combination of ephedra with caffeine containing herbs was widely used, its use will be reviewed. The evidence for efficacy of the herbal approaches remaining after the removal of ephedra from the market are much less, but will also be reviewed.

There are biological rationales for the actions of the different alternative medical and herbal approaches to weight loss discussed in detail below. First, thermogenic aids such as ephedra and caffeine, synephrine, tea catechins, and chili pepper capsaicin are directed at increasing fat burning or metabolism during dieting. Many individuals attempting to lose weight believe that their metabolism is abnormally slow. The adaptive decrease in metabolism which occurs in response to caloric restriction is 10% to 15% of resting metabolic rate. The popularity of stimulants suggests that they have some effects on weight loss reviewed below, and there is some evidence that these agents can affect metabolism. In addition, the same principles have been applied to the development of topical fat reduction creams. Second, a number of supplements and herbs claim to result in nutrient partitioning so that ingested calories will be directed to muscle rather than fat. This diverse group includes a herb (*Garcinia cambogia*), a lipid which is the product of bacterial metabolism (conjugated linoleic acid), a mineral (chromium), a hormone precursor (dehydroepiandrosterone), and an amino acid metabolite (β-hydroxymethylbutyrate). Third, a number of approaches attempt to influence food intake and satiety through effects on noradrenergic, serotoninergic, or dopaminergic mechanisms including tyrosine, phenylalanine, and 5-hydroxytryptophan (5-HTP). Fourth, a series of approaches attempt to physically affect gastric satiety by filling the stomach. Fiber swells after ingestion and has been found to result in increased satiety. A binding resin (chitosan) has the ability to precipitate fat in the laboratory, and is touted for its ability to bind fat in the intestines so that it is not absorbed. However, there has been some success noted with the use of a gastric pacemaker or detection of stomach fullness through a waist cord. Finally, psychophysiological approaches including hypnosis and aromatherapy have been evaluated. For the most part, the discussion has been restricted to methods of weight reduction for which some clinical or basic research could be found. However, there may be other methods, including traditional herbal medicines from other cultures, which remain to be discovered and studied in the future.

Clearly, one attraction of alternative obesity treatments to consumers is the lack of any required professional assistance with these approaches. For those obese individuals who cannot afford to see a physician, these approaches often represent a more accessible solution. For many others, these approaches represent alternatives to failed attempts at weight loss using more conventional approaches. These consumers are often discouraged by previous failures, and are likely to combine approaches or use these supplements at doses higher than recommended doses.

HERBAL THERMOGENIC AIDS

Herbal Caffeine and Ephedrine

Herbal ephedra was declared an adulterant by the FDA in 2004 due to safety concerns (2). In 2005, a U.S. district court ruled that 10 mg/day of ephedra alkaloids was not restricted by the FDA ban on ephedra, but in 2006 the Tenth Circuit Court of Appeals reinstated the full FDA ban on all ephedra-containing supplements regardless of dose (3). Herbal ephedra, however, remains the one efficacious dietary herbal supplement for the treatment of obesity. Thus, it deserves mention for two reasons. One is for its historical value, and the other is that prescription ephedrine remains available to medical practitioners.

In 1972, Dr. Erikson, a Danish general practitioner in Elsinore, Denmark, noted unintentional weight loss when he prescribed a compound containing ephedrine, caffeine, and phenobarbital to patients he was treating for asthma. As he pursued his observation, rumor spread from his patients to the rest of the country. By 1977, over 70,000 patients were taking the "Elsinore Pill," and one Danish pharmaceutical house was producing one million tablets a week.

During the time that the Elsinore Pill was used for the treatment of obesity, there were more skin rashes, some serious, reported. These were most likely due to the phenobarbital in the Elsinore Pill. In 1977, the Danish Institute of Health issued a warning to doctors not to prescribe the compound due to the increased incidence of skin rashes, and Dr. Erikson was harshly criticized in the public and scientific press.

The Elsinore Pill without phenobarbital was compared to the appetite suppressant diethylpropion and to a placebo in 132 subjects in a 12-week double-blind trial. Diethylpropion 25 mg three times a day (t.i.d.) and the Elsinore Pill without phenobarbital (caffeine 100 mg and ephedrine 40 mg t.i.d.) gave 8.4 and 8.1 kg weight loss, respectively, which were not different from each other, but greater than the placebo weight loss of 4.1 kg ($p < 0.01$). Tremor and agitation were more frequent on the Elsinore Pill, but were transient and the withdrawal for side effects was equal in the diethylpropion and Elsinore Pill groups. There was no increase in blood pressure, pulse rate, or laboratory parameters. The authors concluded that ephedrine and caffeine had the advantage over diethylpropion because of its lower cost with equivalent safety and efficacy (4).

Other early studies of ephedrine and caffeine also used commercial asthma preparations. Theophylline and caffeine are both methylxanthines and have the same pharmacological actions. One milligram of theophylline is equivalent to 2 mg of caffeine (5). Ephedrine with theophylline was the primary treatment for asthma in the 1960s and 1970s (6). Ephedrine with caffeine was the most widely sold prescription weight loss medication in Denmark for more than a decade and held 80% of the market share even when dexfenfluramine was available.

To support the approval of caffeine and ephedrine as a prescription drug in Denmark, a combination of 20-mg ephedrine with 200-mg caffeine given t.i.d. was studied in 180 obese subjects randomized to ephedrine 20 mg t.i.d., caffeine 200 mg t.i.d., ephedrine 20 mg with caffeine 200 mg t.i.d., or placebo for a 24-week double-blind trial. Weight loss with caffeine and ephedrine was greater than placebo from eight weeks to the end of the trial. Ephedrine alone and caffeine alone were not different than placebo. The caffeine with ephedrine group lost 17.5% of their body weight in the 24-week trial. Side effects of tremor, insomnia, and dizziness reached the levels of placebo by eight weeks, and blood pressure fell similarly in all four groups. Heart rate rose in a statistically significant manner in the ephedrine group compared to placebo, but fell below the baseline value in the caffeine and ephedrine group (7). Two weeks after cessation of the 24-week trial, headache and tiredness were more frequent in the group that had taken caffeine with ephedrine. At the end of the two-week washout period, all subjects were given the opportunity to participate in an additional 24-week open-label trial using caffeine with ephedrine. Those subjects remaining on caffeine with ephedrine maintained their weight loss to the end of trial at week 50 (8). Seventy-five percent of the weight loss was explained by anorexia and 25% was explained by increased thermogenesis (9). Since acute treatment with caffeine 200 mg and ephedrine 20 mg t.i.d. had cardiovascular and metabolic effects, the chronic effects were evaluated in the 24-week trial. By week 12, the blood pressure had dropped 4 to 11 mmHg below baseline and remained similar to the placebo group. The pulse rate dropped 1 to 2 bpm from baseline during the trial, and reductions in plasma glucose, cholesterol, and triglycerides were not different between the groups at the end of the 24-week double-blind trial (10).

The effect of caffeine 200 mg with ephedrine 20 mg t.i.d. on body composition has been studied using bioimpedance analysis. At the end of eight weeks, weight loss was not different, but the group on caffeine and ephedrine lost 4.5 kg more fat and 2.5 kg less lean tissue than the placebo group, a significant difference. As one might expect, the fall in energy expenditure was 13% in the placebo group and only 8% in the group treated with caffeine and ephedrine (11). Treatment with caffeine and ephedrine over eight weeks also prevented the expected drop in HDL cholesterol. Since HDL cholesterol protects from atherogenesis, this finding suggests that caffeine and ephedrine may have the potential to reduce atherosclerotic cardiovascular disease. The placebo group experienced the drop in HDL cholesterol routinely reported with diet-induced weight loss (12).

Ephedrine with or without a methylxanthine was evaluated in adolescents. The effect of ephedrine in stimulating thermogenesis was lost after one week of treatment, but was restored by combining it with aminophylline for one week (13). This would explain why the trials with ephedrine alone give more weight loss than placebo early in trial that decreases with time unless combined with a methylxanthine. The same group reported a 20-week, double-blind, placebo-controlled, and randomized clinical trial of caffeine and ephedrine in 32 adolescents age of 16 ± 1 years and Tanner stage III–V (14). Subjects less than 80 kg were given one tablet containing 100-mg caffeine and 10-mg ephedrine t.i.d. and subjects more than 80 kg were given two pills t.i.d. The loss of initial body weight was 14.4% and 2.2% in the caffeine with ephedrine and placebo groups, respectively ($p < 0.01$). All three dropouts were in the placebo group and adverse events were described as negligible. After the first four weeks the adverse events in the caffeine group were not different than placebo.

Selling caffeine and ephedrine, in herbal form, for weight loss, became a large industry after the DSHEA law was passed in 1994. Caffeine in the herbal products was the same chemical contained in pharmaceutical caffeine. Herbal ephedra has four isomers, but the

pharmaceutical grade product contains the most potent of these (15). Therefore, the herbal form of ephedrine contained less of the most potent isomer. Ephedrine products were sold without a prescription for the treatment of asthma with a recommended dosage up to 150 mg/day. Caffeine is sold without a prescription as a stimulant with a recommended dose of up to 1600 mg/day. The herbal products containing caffeine and ephedrine for weight loss had dosage recommendations up to 100 mg of ephedrine equivalent per day as ephedra. The caffeine content of these herbal products containing caffeine and ephedrine varied, but was less than 600 mg/day. The most popular and widely sold herbal product containing caffeine and ephedra had 240 mg of caffeine per day.

One of the concerns regarding herbal caffeine and ephedrine, as with other dietary herbal supplements, is the lack of uniform quality. Standardization of the extracts used in herbal dietary supplements for their levels of active ingredients or marker compounds is not universal. In addition, most of the products sold as herbal dietary supplements contain many other herbal ingredients. These other ingredients had no proven efficacy or safety for treating obesity, and raised issues of potential drug interactions.

Herbal dietary supplements containing caffeine 20 or 60 mg with ephedrine 10 or 24 mg were shown to increase oxygen consumption acutely in man compared to placebo using a ventilated hood system (16,17). Using a whole room indirect calorimeter, another study compared ephedra 24 mg, caffeine 80 mg, and chromium 225 µg given t.i.d. to a placebo (18). There was a 3.5% increase in oxygen consumption, a 5 bpm increase in pulse rate, and a decrease in calorie intake in the ephedra, caffeine, and chromium group compared to placebo ($p < 0.01$). There were clinical trials comparing herbal caffeine and ephedrine with placebo. The caffeine and ephedrine gave greater weight loss than placebo (Table 1). Side effects greater in the caffeine and ephedrine group were dry mouth, heartburn, insomnia, and diarrhea (19). The higher dose of caffeine in the pharmaceutical grade product may have been responsible for the decrease in pulse and blood pressure not seen with the herbal product (7). Shekelle et al. reviewed the trials with herbal and pharmaceutical ephedrine with or without caffeine. Trials with ephedrine ($n = 5$), ephedrine and caffeine ($n = 12$), ephedra ($n = 1$), and ephedra and caffeine ($n = 4$) gave weight losses greater than placebo of 0.6, 1, 0.8, and 1 kg/mo, respectively (20).

Concerns relative to the safety of herbal supplements containing caffeine and ephedrine were fueled by a report in which the adverse events reported to the FDA MedWatch program were analyzed (1). The adverse events associated with herbal caffeine and ephedrine were hypertension, palpitations, tachycardia, stroke, and seizures. Although such a surveillance registry is unable to

Table 1 Efficacy of Herbal Caffeine and Ephedrine

Reference	Start D/P	End D/P	Dose (E/C)	Study length	Kg lost D/P	% wt lost D/P	Comments
16	6/6	6/6	10/20 mg/dose	2 days	N/A	N/A	Crossover trial—E/C increased 2 hr RMR
18	17/17	17/17	72/240 mg/day and Cr 225 μg/day	2 days	N/A	N/A	Metabolic chamber increased EE and pulse/decreased EI
269	35/32	24/24	72/240 mg/day	8 wk	4.0/0.8	4.4/0.9	E/C gave more fat loss/ higher pulse rate
19	83/84	46/41	90/192 mg/day	6 mo	7.0/3.1	8.0/3.5	E/C gave more fat loss/ higher pulse rate
270	52/52	44/42	30/180 mg/day	12 wk	2.1/0.46	2.2/0.5	E/C dose 50% of that claimed
17	20/20	12/19	72/180 mg/day	12 wk	3.5/0.8	4.2/1.0	8% and gave more fat loss
271	29/32	19/23	40/100 mg/day	9 mo	7.2/2.3	8.1/2.7	E/C gave more fat loss

The table lists the human herbal caffeine (C) and ephedrine (E) studies by number in the reference list. The number of subjects who started and finished the studies in the drug (D) and placebo (P) groups are listed. The study length is given, and the weight lost in kilograms and/or percent initial body weight lost is also given. The comment section lists special aspects of the various studies.
Abbreviations: Cr, chromium, N/A, not applicable, EE, energy expenditure, EI, energy intake.

determine the frequency of adverse events, an estimate of the relative frequency compared to other nonprescription medications is possible. Three billion doses of ephedra-containing dietary herbal supplements were sold in 1999, equivalent to one adverse event per 70 million doses (21). By comparison, ibuprofen produced one adverse event, mostly gastrointestinal, per 25 million 200-mg doses sold. Adverse events with low-dose aspirin use are one to three times higher than with ibuprofen (19,22). Although it would appear that ephedra supplements were at least as safe as other nonprescription medication, there continued to be safety concerns, and the Rand Corporation was commissioned to review the safety data. That meta-analysis of the published and some unpublished studies ($n = 50$) of ephedrine and ephedra with and without caffeine revealed a 2.2- to 3.6-fold increase in the odds of psychiatric, autonomic, gastrointestinal, and heart palpitations (20). This analysis leads to the decision by the FDA to declare ephedra an adulterant removing it from the dietary herbal supplement market.

Green Tea Catechins

Green tea prepared by heating or steaming the leaves of *Camellia sinensis* is widely consumed on a regular basis throughout Asia. However, the most widely consumed tea is black tea consumed by over 80% of the world's population (23). Black tea is made by allowing the green tea leaves to auto-oxidize enzymatically leading to the conversion of a large percentage of green tea catechins to theaflavins. The catechins are a family of compounds, which include epigallocatechin gallate, most potent

antioxidant in the family. Drinking one cup of tea per day has been reported to decrease the odds ratio of suffering a myocardial infarction to 0.56 compared to non-tea drinkers (24). In vitro, a green tea extract containing both catechins and caffeine was more potent in stimulating brown adipose tissue thermogenesis than equimolar concentrations of caffeine alone (25). The use of ephedrine to release norepinephrine increased the thermogenic effect noted with green tea catechins. Catechins from green tea inhibit catechol-*O*-methyl transferase at the level of the fat cell, the hormone that degrades norepinephrine while the caffeine it contains slows the breakdown of cyclic AMP by inhibiting phosphodiesterase. Ten healthy men spent three nights in a respiratory chamber. On one occasion they took two capsules of AR25 (50 mg of caffeine and 90 mg of epigallocatechin gallate) t.i.d., on another occasion they took the caffeine contained in the AR25 and on the third occasion they took a placebo. The 24-hour energy expenditure increased 4% ($p < 0.01$), and the respiratory quotient fell ($p < 0.001$), but only in the AR25 group (26). The net effect attributable to AR25 was ~80 kcal/day. An open label three-month study of AR25 in obese subjects gave a weight loss of 4.6% of initial body weight and a 4.5% reduction of waist circumference (27). A weight maintenance study randomized subjects to a green tea-caffeine mixture (270 mg epigallocatechin gallate with 150 mg of caffeine per day) or placebo after a one-month weight loss period using a very low energy diet. During the weight loss phase those who drank more than 360 mg of caffeine per day lost significantly more weight, but during the three-month maintenance phase they regained as much as the placebo group. The group drinking less than 360 mg of caffeine per day continued to lose weight in the maintenance phase. Subjects lost an average of 7% of body weight during the weight loss phase (6.7 kg in the high caffeine intake group and 5.1 kg in both groups combined). In the maintenance phase the high-caffeine consumers regained 41% of their lost weight compared to an additional 11% loss in the low-caffeine consumers ($p < 0.01$) (28). Thus, the evidence for catechins giving weight loss is weak and dependent, in part, upon the level of chronic caffeine intake. More studies are clearly indicated.

Synephrine from *Citrus aurantium*

Since ephedra was declared an adulterant by the FDA, the dietary herbal supplement makers have been substituting *C. aurantium*, which is an extract of the essential oils from the Seville orange. *C. aurantium* contains indirect acting β-sympathomimetics including synephrine, hordenine, octopamine, tyramine, and *N*-methyltyramine (29). Women have a lower thermic effect of food than men, and a study demonstrated that *C. aurantium* increased this 29% in women, but not in men in a single-dose experiment (29). Colker et al. reported that a combination of *C. aurantium* and St. John's Wort gave more weight loss than placebo, but the difference was not statistically significant (30). A crossover study showed a 0.94 kg weight loss over two weeks and a significantly different 2.4 kg weight loss in the second two weeks when the nine subjects were switched to *C. aurantium* (30). Two eight-week pilot studies, one with *C. aurantium* and one with phenylephrine, showed an acute rise in metabolic rate that was not sustained over the eight weeks and there was no weight loss compared to the placebo (31). Phenylephrine has been found to be a notable component of the marketed *C. aurantium* and there is a case report of an association with syncope and a prolonged QT interval in a healthy 22-year-old woman (32). However, a larger study with 18 healthy men with *C. aurantium* standardized to 27 mg of synephrine gave no change in the QT interval (33). There is also a case report of a 55-year-old woman who presented with a lateral myocardial infarction associated with a lesion in the left main coronary artery after taking 300 mg of *C. aurantium* extract daily for a year (34). Thus, there is some suggestion of possible toxicity from *C. aurantium* and very little evidence of efficacy. Further studies are needed to draw any firm conclusions.

Capsaicin and Analogs

Capsaicin, which activates the vanilloid type-1 receptor, has been studied in 3T3-L1 murine preadipocytes. Capsaicin stimulates calcium influx to visceral adipose tissue through the vanilloid type-1 receptor and prevents adipogenesis (35). Capsaicin also stimulates the release of reactive oxygen species, which activates AMP kinase leading to the inhibition of differentiation in preadipocytes and stimulation of apoptosis in mature adipocytes (36). Capsaicin also causes the loss of mitochondrial membrane potential, which induces apoptosis, stimulates caspace-3, and inhibits intracellular triglycerides by inhibiting PPARγ (37).

Capsaicin has been shown to increase satiety and energy expenditure in humans (38). The effect seems more robust in the lean than in the obese (39). The effect also seems to be greater when the capsaicin is contained in food such as tomato juice rather than in capsules, suggesting that an effect on the gastrointestinal tract is involved (40). Combination products containing capsaicin seem to have efficacy. A product containing 0.4 mg of capsaicin, 625 mg of green tea, and 800 mg of chicken essence gave a decrease in body fat and an increase in energy expenditure over a two-week treatment period (41). Another combination product contained capsaicin 1.2 mg, L-tyrosine 1218 mg, caffeine 302 mg, and calcium carbonate 3890 mg daily. Eighty subjects were randomized to the combination product or placebo. The significant increase in energy expenditure was maintained for eight weeks of treatment and there was significant fat loss in the combination group compared to the placebo. The combination product was well tolerated (42).

It was initially thought that the pungent (spicy hot) nature of capsaicin was integral to its action. There are related compounds, however, that seem to stimulate the same receptor and are not pungent. Capsiate is a nonpungent capsaicin analog that is found in the CH-19 sweet red pepper cultivar. Two weeks of treatment with this analog increased metabolic rate, increased fat oxidation, and increased the levels of UCP-1 protein and mRNA in brown adipose tissue of mice (43). Evodiamine is a nonpungent vanilloid receptor agonist that comes from the fruit of the Evodia rutaecarpa. Evodiamine has no taste and increases fat loss in rodents (44). Raspberry ketone is similar in structure to capsaicin, prevents fatty liver, improves obesity, and increases norepinephrine-induced lipolysis in white adipocytes of rodents (45). A four-week study of capsiate was conducted in 44 human subjects randomized to 10 mg/day, 3 mg/day, or a placebo. The 10 mg/day dose significantly increased oxygen consumption, resting energy expenditure, and fat oxidation in those with a body mass index (BMI) >25 kg/m^2 (46).

Fucoxanthin from Seaweed

Fucoxanthin is a major carotenoid found in edible seaweed such as *Undaria pinnatifida* and *Hijikia fusiformis*. Fucoxanthin fed to rats reduced white adipose tissue weight and increased UCP-1 protein and mRNA in the white adipose tissue (47). Fucoxanthin is converted to fucoxanthinol within 3T3-L1 murine preadipocytes.

Fucoxanthinol is more potent in inhibiting lipid accumulation and differentiation of the 3T3-L1 preadipocytes. This inhibition seems to take place through downregulation of PPARγ (48).

1,3-Diacylglycerol Oil

1,3-Diacylglycerol oil, a cooking oil used to reduce body fat in Japan (classified in Japan as a food for a designated health use), has been introduced into the United States by Archer–Daniel–Midland in partnership with Kao under the trade name of Econa^{TM} and is generally regarded as safe (GRAS) by the U.S. FDA (49). 1,3-Diacylglycerol is present in various vegetable oils in small amounts, but is made enzymatically so that the vegetable oil will contain 70% of this component. 1,3-Diglyceride is handled differently metabolically due to the lack of a 2-fatty acid. It is the 2-fatty acid that is used by the enzyme as a pivot when breaking down or resynthesizing triglycerides (50). Thus, the 1,3-diglyceride which has the same caloric value as triglyceride, goes to the liver where it is oxidized without being stored as fat (51).

1,3-Diacylglycerol has been shown to increase fat oxidation and to decrease hunger (52). 1,3-Diacylglycerol also decreases total body fat, subcutaneous fat, and visceral fat compared to a triglyceride control (53). The largest double-blind clinical trial randomized 131 overweight and obese subjects to 24 weeks of treatment with food containing 1,3-diacylglyceride or identical food made with triacylglyceride. Body weight and body fat decreased 3.6% and 8.3%, respectively, in the 1,3-diacylglycerol group compared to 2.5% and 5.6% in the triacylglycerol group ($p <$ 0.04) (54). 1,3-Diacylglycerol also decreased body fat and leptin in children seven to 17 years of age over five months compared to a triglyceride control (55). 1,3-Diacylglycerol was safe in dose up to 0.5 mg/kg/day over 12 weeks (56). The rise in triglycerides after a meal was blunted by 1,3-diacylglyceride compared to a triglyceride control and this effect was greater in those with insulin resistance or lipoprotein lipase deficiency (57–59). In addition to decreasing the postprandial rise in triglycerides, 1,3-diacylglycerol has other positive effects in type 2 diabetes. Glycohemoglobin decreased 9.7% compared to a triglyceride control over 12 weeks (6.41 $\pm$ 1.15 to 5.79 $\pm$ 0.85 vs. 6.88 $\pm$ 0.53 to 6.65 $\pm$ 0.73), and 1,3-diacylglycerol delayed the progression of renal failure in type 2 diabetic subjects with nephropathy (60,61).

Pinellia ternata

P. ternata is a herb used in Korean traditional medicine. An extract of this herb was fed to Zucker fatty rats in a dose of 400 mg/kg/day for six weeks. The extract lowered blood triglyceride and free fatty acids. The body weight was reduced slightly, UCP1 mRNA in brown fat was increased as was PPARα, and PGC1α mRNA in white adipose tissue (62). No human reports of this herb for the treatment of obesity exist in the medical literature.

FAT METABOLISM AND NUTRIENT PARTITIONING

Conjugated Linoleic Acid

The *cis*-9, *trans*-11 isomer of conjugated linoleic acid (63) is formed naturally in the rumen of cattle (64), and supplementation of cattle feed with linoleic or linolenic acids increases the amount of conjugated linoleic acid in milk (65). Synthetic conjugated linoleic acid is a mixture of the *cis*-9, *trans*-11 isomer and *trans*-10, *cis*-12 isomer (66). The 9-11 isomer is thought to be responsible for the anticancer activity of conjugated linoleic acid (67) while the 10-12 isomer is thought to be responsible for the body compositional changes observed in animals (68,69).

Mice fed a diet supplemented with 0.5% conjugated linoleic acid at constant calories develop 60% less body fat than animals fed a control diet (70). This decrease in body fat is most likely due to a combination of reduced fat deposition, increased lipolysis, and increased fat oxidation. These findings were confirmed by West et al. who demonstrated that conjugated linoleic acid reduced energy intake, growth rate, carcass lipid, and carcass protein in mice (71). Metabolic rate was increased and nocturnal respiratory quotient was decreased in these mice. On a high-fat diet, however, DeLany et al. showed that conjugated linoleic acid decreased body fat without suppressing energy intake in mice (72). In this study, there was a marked decrease in body fat, and increase in body protein and without changes in food intake. Rats also respond to conjugated linoleic acid with a decrease in body fat (73).

Conjugated linoleic acid induces apoptosis of adipocytes and results in a form of lipodystrophy in which there is a decrease in white adipose tissue with the development of insulin resistance and enlargement of the liver (74). The mechanism is far from certain, however. Satory and Smith postulate a reduction in fat accumulation in growing animals by inhibition of stromal vascular preadiposite hyperplasia (75). Azain et al. found a reduction in fat cell size rather than a change in fat cell number (76).

Despite some encouraging findings in animals, the human trials have been inconsistent. A recent review concluded that the consensus from 17 published studies in human subjects suggests that conjugated linoleic acid does not affect body weight or body composition (77). Although a 12-month human trial with 6 g of conjugated linoleic acid per day found no change in body composition, the racemic mixture was judged to be safe (78).

Another 12-month study to prevent weight regain in 122 obese subjects showed no difference between conjugated linoleic acid and placebo (79). Even those studies that reported a weight loss, the difference from placebo was only ~2 kg over 12 months (80,81). A study with the *cis*-9, *trans*-11 isomer at 3 g/day for three months decreased insulin sensitivity by 15% and increased lipid peroxidation compared to placebo (82). Studies with the *trans*-10, *cis*-12 isomer for 12 weeks increased insulin sensitivity 19%, increased blood sugar, increased proinsulin, and decreased HDL cholesterol (83,84). Other studies reported a decrease in appetite, a decrease in sagittal diameter, a decrease in total cholesterol and a 2% increase in lean body tissue, but none reported an effect on body composition (85–87). Thus, in humans, conjugated linoleic acid does not appear to give clinically meaningful changes in body composition and may have detrimental effects on insulin resistance, which is associated with many of the medical liabilities linked with obesity.

G. cambogia (Hydroxycitric Acid)

G. cambogia contains hydroxycitric acid (HCA) which is extracted from the rind of the brindall berry. HCA is one of 16 isomers of citric acid and the only one that inhibits citrate lyase, the enzyme that catalyzes the first step in fatty acid synthesis outside the mitochondrion. HCA was studied by Roche Pharmaceuticals in rodents in the 1970s. Those studies, using the sodium salt of HCA, demonstrated weight reduction in three rodent models of obesity, the mature rat, the goldthioglucose-induced obese mouse and the ventromedial hypothalamic lesioned obese rat. Food intake, body weight gain, and body lipid content were all reduced with no change in body protein (88). Three clinical trials have evaluated the efficacy and safety of HCA. The first trial evaluated a product containing both HCA from *G. cambogia* and chromium picolinate. This single-arm open-label trial of eight weeks in 77 adults, 500 mg of *G. cambogia* extract was combined with 100 μg of chromium picolinate taken t.i.d. A 5.5% weight loss was seen in women and 4.9% weight loss in men (89). HCA is also sold as an herbal supplement containing the calcium salt for which the dose is 3 g/day as a treatment for obesity. Two human clinical trials have evaluated the safety and efficacy of this marketed product. The first trial used 10 males acting as their own controls in a crossover trial evaluating energy expenditure and substrate oxidation. There was no difference in respiratory quotient, energy expenditure, glucose, insulin, glucagon, lactate, or β-hydroxybutyrate at rest or during exercise (90). The second trial randomized 135 obese adults using a double-blind placebo-controlled design. HCA 1500 mg/day was administered daily for 12 weeks, and both groups were given a low fat, high fiber diet. In this trial, there was no

significant difference in the weight loss observed between the two groups (3.2 ± 3.3 for HCA group vs. 4.1 ± 3.9 kg for placebo, $p = 0.14$) (91).

Two trials evaluated the effect of HCA on appetite and on 24-hour energy intake. In the first trial there was no difference in appetite compared to placebo, but the HCA group did lose a significant 1.3 kg more than placebo over three months (92). In the second study, there was no difference in 24-hour energy intake in the HCA group compared to placebo (93). It has been suggested that the calcium salt of HCA may not be bioavailable due to its poor solubility (94). Preuss summarized two trials using a mixture of calcium and potassium HCA at 2.8 g/day compared to a placebo. The HCA group lost 5.4% of body weight over eight weeks compared to 1.7% in the placebo group, and serotonin genes were upregulated (95,96). High doses of HCA cause testicular toxicity in rats, but the no observed adverse effect level (NOAEL) was judged to be 389 mg/kg/day, which suggests that the doses presently used are safe (97). Thus, the calcium salt of HCA appears to be ineffective, but studies with a more bioavailable HCA salt appear more promising.

Guggul

Guggul is a resin produced by the mukul mirth tree. Guggulipid is extracted from guggul and contains plant sterols (guggulsterones) that are believed to be its bioactive compounds. There have been four trials comparing guggul or guggul derivatives to placebo for obesity. None gave a statistically superior weight loss compared to placebo. Bhatt et al., in a trial of 58 subjects given guggulipid 1.5 g t.i.d. for one month showed only a trend toward weight loss in those over 90 kg (98). Sidhu et al. gave 4 g/day of guggul gum to 60 subjects for four weeks and saw a trend toward weight loss in the guggul group (99). Kotiyal et al. and Antonio et al. conducted trials of 85 and 20 subjects, respectively, and neither demonstrated more weight loss in the guggul groups (100,101). In another clinical randomized clinical trial a preparation containing Triphala guggul was assessed for obesity. Patients in the treated group lost between 7.9 and 8.2 kg, which was significantly greater than placebo (102). Thus, the evidence to support the use of guggul for weight loss is weak (102).

Cissus quadrangularis

C. quadrangularis is commonly used in the folk medicine of India to aid the healing of bone fractures, and has been used in Africa and Asia for a variety of ailments. Oben et al. evaluated *C. quadrangularis* standardized to 2.5% phytosterols and 15% soluble plant fibers combined with green tea extract (22% epigallocatechin gallate and 40% caffeine), niacin bound chromium, selenium (0.5% L-selenomethionine), pyridoxine, folic acid, and cyanocobalamin compared to placebo in a double-blind clinical trial with 123 subjects. In this eight-week study obese subjects lost 7.2% of initial body weight compared to 2.5% for placebo, and overweight subjects lost 6.3% of initial body weight ($p < 0.05$). In addition there was a significant reduction in waist circumference and body fat compared to placebo ($p < 0.01$). There was an 18% to 26% reduction in LDL cholesterol, a 15% to 37% reduction in triglycerides, a 16% to 21% reduction in CRP, an 11% to 13% reduction in glucose, and a 20% to 50% increase in HDL cholesterol ($p < 0.5$ compared to placebo) (103). In a second study Oben et al. compared *C. quadrangularis* standardized to 5% ketosteroids to placebo in 64 obese subjects. In this six-week trial the placebo group gained 1% of initial body weight and the *C. quadrangularis* group lost 4% of body weight. There were improvements of antioxidant status and parameters of the metabolic syndrome compared to placebo that were similar to the first study with the combination product. Side effects were greater in the placebo group compared to the *C. quadrangularis* group. (104). The weight loss in these studies projected to a presumed plateau at six months would give more than a 5% weight loss compared to placebo which is felt to be medically significant.

Evening Primrose Oil

Evening primrose oil contains γ-linolenic acid and has been proposed as a treatment for obesity. Haslett et al. compared evening primrose oil and placebo in 100 obese women by giving two capsules four t.i.d. plus a weight reduction diet. There was no difference in weight loss over the 12 weeks of the study between the groups (105). Thus, there is no reason to believe that evening primrose oil is effective in the treatment of obesity.

Hoodia gordonii

H. gordonii is a cactus that grows in Africa. It has been eaten by bushmen to decrease appetite and thirst on long treks across the desert. The active ingredient is steroidal glycoside called P57AS3 or just P57. P57 injected into the third ventricle of animals increases the ATP content of hypothalamic tissue by 50% to 150% ($p < 0.05$) and decreases food intake by 40% to 60% over 24 hours ($p < 0.05$) (106,107). Phytopharm is developing P57 in partnership with Unilever. Information on the Phytopharm website describes a double-blind 15-day trial in which 19 overweight males were randomized to P57 or placebo. Nine subjects in each group completed that study. There

was a statistically significant decrease of 1000 kcal/day by day 15 in calorie intake and body fat decreased with good safety (107). Since *Hoodia* is a rare cactus in the wild and cultivation is difficult, it is not clear what the dietary herbal supplements claiming to contain *Hoodia* actually contain or if they are effective in causing weight loss.

Caralluma fimbriata

C. fimbriata is an edible cactus, like *Hoodia*, and was used by Indians to suppress appetite. *C. fimbriata* extract was tested in a placebo-controlled trial in which 50 overweight or obese subjects were randomized to receive 1 g/day of extract or a placebo for 60 days. *C. fimbriata* extract reduced appetite and waist circumference compared to placebo, but there was no difference in body weight (108).

Pyruvate

Pyruvate or mixtures of pyruvate and dihydroxyacetone at 15% to 20% of dietary calories accelerate weight loss on a calorie-restricted diet and slow weight regain after weight loss (109,110). Pyruvate sold as a dietary herbal supplement is sold as a calcium salt and is taken at 3 to 6 g/day for weight loss. A six-week study that randomized 26 subjects to pyruvate 6 g/day or placebo for six weeks showed no difference between pyruvate and placebo (111). A second study that randomized 23 females to pyruvate 5 g/day or a placebo with an exercise program showed no changes in body composition (112). Thus, at the doses and/or in the form pyruvate is sold as a dietary herbal supplement, it appears not to be efficacious for the treatment of obesity.

Yohimbine

There are two conflicting studies on the efficacy of yohimbine in the treatment of obesity. One study randomized 20 subjects to yohimbine 20 mg/day or a placebo and a 1000 kcal/day diet. Over the three-week study the yohimbine group lost 3.55 kg compared to 2.21 kg in the placebo group ($p < 0.005$) (113). The second study randomized 47 men to yohimbine 43 mg/day or placebo for six months. There was no change in body weight, body fat, visceral fat, or any other parameter (114). The preponderance of evidence suggests that yohimbine is not efficacious for the treatment of obesity.

Dehydroepiandrosterone

Dehydroepiandrosterone (DHEA) and its sulfate are the most abundant circulating steroids in humans. They originate in the adrenal gland and gonads and are weak androgens. However, they can be converted into estrogens by enzymes found in many tissues. In lower animals, DHEA acts as an antiobesity agent (115) in amounts manyfold greater than those naturally produced in these animals. The mechanism of this effect has not been established. DHEA has been tested for the treatment of obesity in humans, and has been sold as a dietary supplement for weight loss. The reduction of endogenous DHEA production with aging and with malnutrition or illness has suggested that DHEA may be more effective in elderly obese subjects. However, the evidence of any efficacy is minimal.

Abrahamsson and Hackl treated obese women with 200-mg DHEA enanthate per day. Half of the women lost more than 1 kg/mo, and these women were older with lower levels of urinary ketosteroids (116). Nestler et al. treated normal men with DHEA 1600 mg/day orally for one month. The percent body fat decreased 31% by skinfold measures without weight change (117). Mortola and Yen performed a similar study in older women without a change in body weight or body fat by underwater weighing (118). Usiskin et al. tried to repeat the study in men performed by Nestler et al. using the more sensitive method of underwater weighing. They could not confirm a loss of fat and weight did not change (119). Welle et al. also treated men with DHEA 1600 mg for one month without a change in body weight or indices of lean body mass (120).

Since DHEA is known to decrease through life, Morales et al. treated aging humans with 50 mg of DHEA once a day for six months. There was no change in body fat (121). The same group treated aging humans for one year with DHEA 100 mg/day and placebo for six months each in a crossover design. DHEA supplementation restored youthful levels of the hormone. Body fat by dual energy X-ray absorptiometry (DEXA) decreased by 1 kg in men during the DHEA treatment but not in women. Women gained 1.4 kg of body mass but men did not (122). Another study randomized 56 elderly individuals (mean age 71 years) to 50 mg/day of DHEA or a placebo for six months. There was a significant 1.5 kg difference in weight compared to the placebo and there was also a significant decrease in visceral fat and subcutaneous fat with a significant increase in insulin sensitivity that was similar in both genders (123). DHEA sulfate has also been shown to upregulate adiponectin gene expression in omental adipocytes (124). Taken in total, these studies suggest that DHEA may have a positive impact on insulin sensitivity, but its effect on body fat or body weight in humans is minimal and clinically insignificant.

Chromium Picolinate

Chromium picolinate is a dietary supplement that has gained popularity for both weightlifters and people desiring weight loss (125). The concept is that it enhances the effectiveness of insulin and has been called "glucose tolerance factor." Page et al. reported an increased percentage of muscle and a decreased percentage of fat in swine supplemented with chromium picolinate during growth from 55 to 119 kg, a phase of growth called finishing (126). These findings were confirmed by Mooney and Cromwell as well as by Lindemann et al. who also demonstrated an increased litter size in chromium treated reproducing sows (127–129). Boleman et al. demonstrated that the chromium picolinate effect on body composition was limited to supplementation during the finishing phase of growth and was not seen when the chromium picolinate supplementation was given throughout growth from 19 to 106 kg (130). Myers et al. could not confirm the effects of chromium picolinate on body composition, but gave the supplementation throughout growth from 20 to 90 kg (131). Evock-Clover et al., who supplemented with chromium picolinate during growth from 30 to 60 kg, demonstrated a lowering of glucose and insulin concentrations, but failed to find an effect on body composition (132). Bunting et al., while studying cattle, demonstrated an increased rate of glucose clearance with chromium picolinate supplementation (133).

Although the animal literature is encouraging, studies in humans have not confirmed the experience in swine. Hasten et al. studied the effect of 200 µg/day of chromium as chromium picolinate compared to placebo and administered to students of both sexes beginning a 12-week weight training class using a randomized double-blind design. Although there was an increase in circumferences and a decrease in skinfolds in all groups, the only significant difference seen was a greater increase in body weight in the females supplemented with chromium picolinate compared to the other three groups (134). These findings were confirmed by Grant et al. who studied 43 obese women using 400 µg/day of chromium. Women taking chromium picolinate gained weight unless engaged in exercise, which lowered weight and the insulin response to glucose (135).

Clancy et al. performed a double-blind placebo-controlled study in football players attending a nine-week spring training. There was no effect of 200 µg/day of chromium as picolinate on strength or body composition, but the group taking chromium picolinate had urinary chromium that was five times higher than the placebo group (136). Trent and Thieding-Cancel studied obese U.S. Navy personnel (>than 22% fat for men and >30% fat for women by skinfolds) in a double-blind placebo-controlled protocol utilizing 400 µg/day of chromium picolinate. The 95 out of 212 military personnel who completed the 16-week study lost a small amount of weight and body fat but no effect of chromium picolinate was demonstrated (137).

Lukaski et al. compared chromium chloride and chromium picolinate to placebo in an eight-week double-blind study in 36 men on a weight program. Serum and urine chromium increased equally in both chromium supplemented groups, but the transferrin saturation decreased more in the chromium picolinate group than in the chromium chloride or the placebo groups. There was no effect of chromium supplementation on strength or body composition by DEXA (138). Bahadori et al. compared 200 µg/day of chromium picolinate with 200 µg/day of chromium as yeast in 36 obese subjects during an eight-week very low calorie diet (VLCD) and an 18-week follow-up. Chromium picolinate, but not chromium as yeast, increased lean body mass without altering weight loss (139).

Pasman et al. compared 200 µg/day chromium picolinate to fiber, caffeine, and 50 g of carbohydrate in 33 obese subjects during a 16-month weight loss study the first two months of which included a VLCD. Chromium had no effect on body composition (140). Walker et al. compared 200 µg of chromium picolinate with placebo in 20 wrestlers over 14 weeks. There was no effect of chromium on body composition or performance (141). Campbell et al. evaluated the effect of chromium picolinate 200 µg/day in 18 men between 56 and 69 years of age during a resistance-training program (142). Chromium had no effect on body composition or strength. Volpe et al. evaluated 44 women randomized to 400 µg/day of chromium picolinate for 12 weeks of exercise. Chromium had no effect on body composition (143) (Table 2).

Although chromium picolinate 200 and 400 µg/day has no effect upon body composition in humans, it has a significant effect on lipids, blood pressure, and glucose tolerance. Press et al. found that chromium picolinate 200 µg/day reduced LDL cholesterol, apolipoprotein B, and increased apolipoprotein A-1 in 28 subjects in a double-blind, placebo-controlled, crossover trial (144). Lee and Reasner demonstrated a significant 17% drop of triglycerides in 30 non-insulin-dependent diabetic subjects using a similar design (145). Chromium ameliorates sucrose-induced blood pressure elevations in hypertensive rats and improves insulin sensitivity in man (146,147). The extent to which this is due to urinary losses of chromium and depletion of chromium stores in diabetic patients has not been evaluated. Chromium also reduces glycohemoglobin in diabetic subjects (148).

The toxicity of chromium, and chromium picolinate in particular, has been questioned. Evans and Bowman compared the effect of chromium chloride, chromium nicotinate, and chromium picolinate on insulin, glucose, and leucine internalization in cultured cells. Increased internalization was specific to chromium picolinate since the other chromium salts and zinc picolinate did not have an effect. This was attributed to the demonstrated effect of chromium picolinate on the membrane fluidity in synthetic microsomal membranes (149). Chromium picolinate has been shown to produce chromosomal damage in Chinese hamster ovary cells, an effect attributed to the picolinate (150). Although not demonstrated, it has been postulated that with the use of dietary supplements of chromium picolinate over extended periods, levels could become high enough to damage DNA in humans (151).

Toxicology testing in animals, however, suggests that chromium supplements have a wide margin of safety

Table 2 Double-Blind, Placebo-Controlled Chromium Picolinate Studies on Body Composition in Humans

Reference	Yr	Duration	Dose (µg/day)	Number of drug/placebo	Comments
134	1994	12 wk	200	30 and 29	Weight training females on Cr gained weight
135	1997	9 wk	400	22 and 21	Obese women gained weight on Cr
136	1994	9 wk	200	19 and 19	Football players on Cr no change in body comp
132	1995	16 wk	400	106 and 106	Obese Navy personnel on Cr no change on body comp
138	1996	8 wk	200	18 and 18	Cr no effect on strength or body comp in men
139	1997	26 wk	200	18 and 18	Cr picolinate not as yeast increased lean mass after VLCD
140	1997	16 mo	200	11 and 22	Obese Cr no effect on body comp
141	1998	14 wk	200	10 and 10	Cr no effect on body comp or performance
142	1999	13 wk	200	9 and 9	Men 56–69 yr Cr no effect on body comp or strength
143	2001	12 wk	400	22 and 22	Women 27–51 yr no effect on body comp

(152). The effect of chromium upon insulin resistance is mediated through the oligopeptide, chromodulin that binds chromium. The chromium-chromodulin complex binds the insulin receptor and activates tyrosine kinase (153). Regardless of other beneficial uses, chromium picolinate does not alter body composition in humans, and as such is not helpful for the treatment of obesity.

Calcium

Nearly 20 years ago, McCarron et al. reported that there was a negative relationship between BMI and dietary calcium intake in the data collected by the National Center for Health Statistics (154). More recently, Zemel et al. found that there was a strong inverse relationship between calcium intake and the risk of being in the highest quartile of BMI (155). These studies have prompted a re-evaluation of studies measuring calcium intake or giving calcium orally.

The relationship of calcium and body weight is the most confusing, and there is a patent issued for the effects of dairy products for producing weight loss issued to one of the proponents of this approach. Moreover, there is inconsistency in both the animal and human studies.

In one small clinical trial, increasing dietary intake of calcium by adding 800 mg/day of supplemental calcium to a diet containing 400 to 500 mg/day was claimed to augment weight loss and fat loss on reducing diets (156). In two small studies in African-American adults, Zemel et al. claimed that substitution of calcium-rich foods in isocaloric diets reduced adiposity and improved metabolic profiles during a 24-week trial (157). In another small study, Zemel et al. randomized 34 subjects to receive a control calcium diet with 400 to 500 mg/day ($N = 16$) or a yogurt supplemented diet ($N = 18$) for 12 weeks. In this small, short duration study, fat loss was greater on the yogurt diet (-4.43 kg) than the control diet (-2.75 kg). On the basis of this data they claim that yogurt enhances central fat loss (158). In a large multi-center trial that enrolled nearly 100 subjects, the same authors claim that a hypocaloric diet with calcium supplemented to the level of 1400 mg/day did not significantly improve weight loss or body composition when compared to a diet with lower calcium intake (600 mg/day), whereas a diet with three servings per day of dairy products augmented weight and fat loss (157). The same group demonstrated in a study that of 90 obese subjects that 800 mg/day of dairy calcium gave equivalent weight loss to 1400 mg of dairy calcium (159,160). A study in 54 women by a different research group estimated that a 1 g/day increase in dairy calcium would cause losses of 3.3 and 4.3 kg of weight and fat, respectively, over a two-year period (161).

Increasing supplemental calcium from zero to nearly 2000 g/day was associated with a reduction in BMI of about 5 BMI units (162). These data might suggest that low calcium intake was playing a role in the current epidemic of overweight. However, five controlled clinical trials have failed to show an effect of calcium on weight loss, leaving the issue unresolved (160,163–166). The first of these studies, Shapses et al., however, gave trends toward weight loss with 1 g/day calcium supplement for six months of 0.8 kg of weight and 1 kg of fat (163). Thus, there appears to be an effect of calcium and particularly dairy calcium to reduce body weight, but the magnitude of this effect appears controversial. There are no major concerns regarding adverse events due to supplementation with dairy calcium.

β-Hydroxy-β-Methylbutyrate

β-Hydroxy-β-methylbutyrate (HMB) is a metabolite of leucine that is sold as a supplement to burn fat and builds both strength and muscle tissue. Nissen et al. reported that HMB supplementation at 1.5 to 3 g/day reduced muscle catabolism and increased fat free mass during a weight lifting program of two to six weeks duration (167). These effects were not seen, however, in trained athletes (168). A study of 3 g/day in college students for five weeks or in football players for four weeks gave no change in body composition (169,170). An eight-week study in 70-year-old adults exercising five days per week, HMB caused more fat loss by skinfolds (171). Although supplementation with HMB has been shown to be safe in studies lasting three to eight weeks, it has not yet been tested for efficacy in the treatment of obesity (172).

Topical Fat Reduction

The goal of local fat reduction is the cosmetic benefit to individuals who are dissatisfied with the distribution of their fat tissue. The primary cosmetic concerns with fat topography have come from women who have a concentration of fat in the thigh area with a dimply appearance that has been termed cellulite (173). The actual cause of the dimpling is an increased growth of fibrous boundaries in the subcutaneous fat tissue occurring in the third and fourth decades of life. This is usually associated with childbearing and postpregnancy weight gain, but can also occur in women with a primarily gynoid fat distribution in the second decade of life. The cosmetic goal of reducing and smoothing thigh fat can be approached with topical treatment which will be discussed here, and liposuction, which, being a cosmetic surgical procedure is beyond the scope of this chapter.

The lipolytic threshold in various fat tissues is determined by the balance of stimulatory and inhibitory GTP binding proteins (G-proteins) on the cell surface influencing the activity of adenylate cyclase. Women have more α-2 receptors in the thigh area with inhibitory effects on the lipolytic β-2 receptors due to their higher levels of circulating estrogen. Adenosine receptors are also inhibitory G-protein receptors, and phosphodiesterase, by degrading adenylate cyclase, also plays an inhibitory role in the lipolytic process (174–178).

Local application of substances to the fat cells that stimulate the lipolytic process have the potential to reduce the size of the treated fat cells. Using one thigh as a control, isoproterenol injections (a β-receptor stimulator), forskolin ointment (a direct stimulator of adenylate cyclase), yohimbine ointment (an α-2 receptor inhibitor), and aminophylline (an inhibitor of phosphodiesterase and the adenosine receptor) gave more girth loss from the treated than the control thigh. Treatments were given once daily, five days a week, for one month (179).

A six-week study with 10% aminophylline ointment in 23 subjects, a five-week study with 2% aminophylline cream in 11 subjects, and a five-week study with 0.5% aminophylline cream in 12 subjects confirmed these findings. None of the creams were more effective than the 0.5% aminophylline, which had more than a 3 cm difference between the treated and untreated thighs (180). Another study by Collis et al., however, was unable to reproduce these results in a 12-week study of aminophylline cream using a similar design (181).

There seem to be alternative mechanisms to effect local fat reduction that do not involve the adrenergic innervation of the fat cell. Armanini et al. used a 2.5% glycyrrhetinic acid cream on one thigh of nine women and treated the other thigh and nine control women with the cream base. The thigh circumference and the thigh fat thickness by ultrasound decreased significantly in the treated thigh compared to the control thigh and the control women. This study demonstrates that inhibiting 11β-hydroxysteroid dehydrogenase is another mechanism by which a cream can effect local fat reduction. Polylactide-co-glycolide microspheres injected into fat pads also caused local fat reduction in rodents by increasing fat cell apoptosis (182). Recently, a low energy laser has been shown to lyse fat cells releasing fat into the lymphatic drainage system, but a controlled trial has yet to be reported (183).

An oral product containing *Ginkgo biloba*, sweet clover, seaweed, grape seed oil, lecithins, and evening primrose oil has been marketed orally for the treatment of cellulite. In a two-month placebo-controlled trial, there was no reduction in body weight, fat content, thigh circumference, hip circumference, or dimply appearance of the fat (184).

The other area of cosmetic concern is the waist for those with a central fat distribution. A study was performed in 50 men and women who were randomized in a 1:1 ratio to aminophylline 0.5% cream twice a day for 12 weeks or no treatment along with a calorie-restricted diet. The groups were well-matched at baseline and had equal weight losses, but the group using the aminophylline cream lost 11 cm from the waist compared to only 5 cm in the group not receiving the cream which was a highly significant difference (185). This demonstrates that altering the lipolytic threshold in a specific area causes local fat reduction and the effect is not limited to the thigh.

AMINO ACIDS AND NEUROTRANSMITTER MODULATION

5-Hydroxytryptophan

Changes in plasma amino acid levels can modify food intake by affecting the brain availability of neurotransmitter precursors (186,187). Both theoretical and experimental data support a role for serotonin in the central nervous system regulation of satiety. Wurtman has suggested that serotonin may also play a role in the selection of carbohydrate-rich foods contributing to so-called "carbohydrate craving" (188). Blundell and Leshem reported in 1975 that food intake could be reduced in hyperphagic rats through the parenteral administration of 5-HTP, the metabolic precursor of serotonin (189). 5-HTP is used based on the rationale that high brain tryptophan concentrations can facilitate the conversion of tryptophan to serotonin by stimulating the reduced activity of 5-tryptophan hydroxylase, the enzyme that forms 5-HTP from L-tryptophan (190). Osborne-Mendel rats have reduced activity of 5-tryptophan hydroxylase (191) and a genetic predisposition to obesity.

There have been two studies in humans from the same group evaluating the effects of 5-HTP on weight loss (192,193). In 19 obese women in a randomized, controlled double-blind crossover study comparing 5-HTP and placebo without diet instruction, a small but significant difference in weight loss was noted over five weeks between subjects treated with 5-HTP at a dose of 8 mg/kg/day and placebo. In a second study, 20 of 28 subjects completed a 12-week study in which there was no dietary instruction in the first six weeks and a 1200-calorie diet in the second six weeks. Subjects on 5-HTP lost ~5% of starting weight in the trial, more than was observed in subjects treated with placebo with 2 kg additional lost in the first six weeks and 3 kg additional lost in the next six weeks. The high dropout rate and small size of this trial supports preliminary data that 5-HTP is effective, but further studies must be done to establish this as a reasonable adjunct to weight loss therapies.

L-Tyrosine

L-tyrosine administration to rats increases the rate at which brain neurons synthesize and release catecholamine neurotransmitters (194). If a similar mechanism was operative in humans then L-tyrosine could be used to increase catecholamine synthesis and affect satiety. Administration of 100 mg/kg/day of tyrosine led to increased CSF tyrosine concentrations in nine patients with Parkinson's disease changing from 3.5 ± 1.9 to 5.9 ± 3.4 μg/mL (194). In mice undergoing caloric restriction to 40% of usual intake, there was impairment of cognitive functions evaluated in a maze not seen at 60% of usual intakes. However, when 100 mg/kg/day of tyrosine was injected into the mice, no decrease in cognitive function was seen at 40% of usual intake (195). While there are no studies of weight loss in humans taking tyrosine, these observations suggest that this might be useful in restoring normal well-being during dietary restriction.

Notwithstanding these observations suggesting a benefit of L-tyrosine supplementation, the enzyme tyrosine hydroxylase has been thought to be the rate-limiting step in the synthesis of norepinephrine, not the availability of the substrate L-tyrosine. Hull and Maher have suggested that this relationship might change in the presence of drugs that release catecholamines. The anorectic activity of phenylpropanolamine, ephedrine, and amphetamine are increased in food deprived rats from 37% to 50% by L-tyrosine supplementation in a dose dependent manner (25–400 mg/kg). This enhanced anorectic activity is mediated by catecholamines, and was not seen with direct acting beta agonists (196). Hull and Maher also demonstrated that the effect of tyrosine to enhance the anorectic effect of drugs that release catecholamines was limited to the central nervous system. The peripheral actions of these drugs such as blood pressure elevation were not enhanced by tyrosine supplementation (197,198). Although these studies suggest a role for tyrosine supplementation in enhancing the anorectic effect of centrally acting anorectic medications that release catecholamines without increasing side effects, evaluation of this possibility in humans has not been reported.

Methionine Restriction

Restriction of L-methionine for the life of a rat from the normal 0.86% to 0.17% of the diet extends life 30%. Methionine restriction, unlike calorie restriction which also extends life to the same extent, increases food intake while reducing body weight (199). A 17-week trial in which eight cancer patients without cachexia followed a diet restricted to 2 mg/kg/day, methionine restriction gave a weight loss of 0.5 kg/wk with an increase in food intake and no toxicity (200). Trials in obesity have yet to be reported.

FIBERS AND ALGAE

Spirulina

Spirulina is a cyanobacteria or blue-green algae that grows in warm waters and is usually grown in controlled conditions which reduces the chances of contamination. A single trial by Becker et al. evaluated 200-mg spirulina tablets compared to 200-mg spinach tablets. Fifteen subjects took 14 tablets t.i.d. for four weeks. There was no difference in weight between the two groups. There was a statistically significant decrease in body weight from baseline in the spirulina group that did not occur in the placebo group (201). Although there was no evidence for weight loss efficacy comparing spirulina with placebo, the small number of study subjects and the difference in weight from baseline only in the spirulina group suggest the study may have been underpowered to detect a difference, if it exists.

Soluble and Insoluble Dietary Fibers

It has been suggested that the increase in obesity in Western countries since 1900 may be related to changes in dietary fiber. The fiber associated with starchy foods has decreased while the fiber associated with fruits and vegetables has increased (202). Efforts to evaluate the association of dietary fiber with body weight regulation began in the 1980s. Guar gum, a water-soluble fiber, was shown to reduce hunger and weight more effectively than water-insoluble bran-fiber in the absence of a prescribed diet (203). When given with a calorie-restricted diet, guar gum reduced hunger and increased satiety compared to a control (204).

Glucomannan, another water-soluble fiber supplemented at 20 g/day over eight weeks gave a 5.5 lb. weight loss with no prescribed diet (205). These results were confirmed in a two-month study using the same fiber with a calorie-restricted diet (206). In a two-week trial, 45 subjects on psyllium, a third water-soluble fiber, were compared to 40 subjects on bran, a water-insoluble fiber, and a control without a specific diet. There was no difference in weight but hunger was reduced in both fiber groups (207).

In an effort to further define the physiology of fiber, 31 normal males and 19 overweight males were given a 5.2 or 0.2 g fiber preload. The high fiber preload increased fullness in both normal and overweight subjects, but only overweight decreased food intake at the subsequent meal (208). Another study confirmed the ability of fiber to decrease appetite (209). The relationship between appetite and fiber was further defined by a study using two doses of water-soluble fiber. During one week of supplementation (40 g/day) without calorie restriction, food intake was reduced without change in appetite. During one week of supplementation (20 g/day) with calorie restriction, hunger was suppressed without a change in food intake (210).

Baron et al. compared two 1000 kcal/day diets in 135 subjects, one low in carbohydrate and fiber, and the other higher in both these components. In contrast to subsequent studies, there was significantly more weight loss (5.0 vs. 3.7 kg) over three months on the lower fiber diet (211). In a trial of 52 overweight subjects randomized to 7 g of fiber per day or a placebo with a calorie-restricted diet for six months, the fiber-supplemented group lost more weight (5.5 vs. 3.0 kg) and had less hunger (212).

Solum et al. randomized 60 overweight women to dietary fiber tablets or placebo and a weight reducing diet for 12 weeks. The group on fiber lost more (8.5 vs. 6.7 kg) than those on placebo (213). An eight-week study compared fiber tablets (5 g/day) with placebo on a calorie-restricted diet in 60 obese females. The fiber group lost significantly more weight (7.0 vs. 6.0 kg). This finding was confirmed in a second study of 45 obese females. The group on 7 g of fiber per day lost more weight than the placebo (6.2 vs. 4.1 kg) (214). Birketvedt et al. randomized 53 women to 6 g of fiber supplement vs. control for 24 weeks. The fiber group lost 8 kg vs. 5.8 kg for the control (215).

Specific foods higher in fiber have been evaluated for satiety or weight loss. Lupin flour enriched bread has been shown to decrease hunger at a meal and a subsequent meal (216). A higher fiber Goami No. 2 rice gave a significant 1 kg more weight loss than a normal rice control over four weeks (217). Oligofructose is a fermentable dietary fiber that increases gut peptides associated with the reduction of energy intake in rats. Oligofructose increased satiety more than dextrine maltose when given for two weeks in a crossover trial (218). Increasing fiber to a goal of 30 g/day by increasing the intake of fruits and vegetables in survivors of breast cancer over a four-year period did not change body weight despite success in increasing fiber intake (219).

There has been an attempt to look at different fibers. Agar supplementation in 36 type 2 diabetic subjects for 12 weeks gave 2.8 kg of weight loss compared to 1.3 kg in the 36 subjects randomized to be controls (220). Another study compared three dietary supplements in 176 subjects with a 1200 kcal/day diet over five weeks. Glucomannan gave equivalent weight loss of ~4 kg to glucomannan with guar gum or to glucomannan with guar gum and alginate (221).

Because of its safety, dietary fiber supplementation has been evaluated in obese children. There was no difference between a 15 g/day supplement and control during a four-week trial (222). Longer term trials in adults were conducted as well. Ninety obese females were randomly assigned to a 6 to 7 g/day dietary supplement or placebo and a 1200 to 1600 kcal/day diet in a one-year double-blind

trial. The fiber group lost 3.8 kg (4.9% of initial body weight) compared to 2.8 kg (3.6%), a statistically significant difference (223).

Fiber 30 g/day has been supplemented in a very low-calorie diet in a four-week crossover trial. Weight loss was not different but hunger was less during the supplementation with fiber (224). In a two-month trial of a very low-calorie diet followed by a 12-month maintenance phase, 20 obese subjects and 11 obese controls, there was no difference in weight loss between the groups supplemented with 20 g guar gum/day compared to placebo (225).

The relationship between obesity and fiber has also been evaluated epidemiologically. Using food frequency questionnaires, obese men and women had significantly more fat and less fiber in their diets than lean men and women (226). These findings were confirmed using three-day food diaries. Total fiber intake was higher in the lean than the obese group and grams of fiber per 1000 kcal was inversely related to BMI (227).

In summary, the bulk of evidence suggests that dietary fiber decreases food intake and decreases hunger. Water-soluble fiber may be more efficient than water-insoluble fiber for weight loss. Dietary fiber supplements (5–40 g/day) lead to small (1–3 kg) weight losses greater than placebo (Table 3). Although the weight loss obtained with dietary fiber is less than the 5% of initial body weight felt to confer clinically significant health benefits, the safety of dietary fiber and its other potential benefits on cardiovascular risk factors recommend it for inclusion in weight reduction diets.

Chitosan

Chitosan is acetylated chitin from the exoskeletons of crustaceans such as shrimp. The product has a molecular weight of more than a million Daltons, and is designed to bind to intestinal lipids including cholesterol and triglycerides. Originally developed as a lipid binding resin in the 1970s based on its properties as a charged nonabsorbable carbohydrate, chitosan has received a great deal of attention as a potential weight loss aid working through a "fat blocker" mechanism. In public demonstrations, chitosan is mixed with corn oil in a glass and the precipitation of the oil and clarification of the solution is emphasized as a mechanism which would result in fat malabsorption and weight loss in humans. This promises individuals that they can eat the fatty foods they desire without gaining weight.

Mice fed a high-fat diet with 3% to 15% chitosan for nine weeks had less weight gain, hyperlipidemia, fatty liver, and higher fecal fat excretion than high-fat diet fed controls. These changes were shown to be the result of chitosan binding of dietary fat rather than through the inhibition of fat digestion (228).

Table 3 Controlled Studies of Dietary Fiber for the Treatment of Obesity

Reference	Number fiber (Control)	Time	Weight loss (Fiber vs. Control)	Water soluble	Water insoluble	Diet	Hunger	Comment
207	95 (23)	2 wk	4.6 vs. 4.2 kg (NS)	Psyllium (45)	Bran (40)	No	Less	20 g fiber/day
205	10 (10)	8 wk	5.5 vs. −1.5	Glucomannan 3 g/day		No		3 g fiber/day
203	5 (5)	1 meal	NS	Guar 20 g/day		No	Less	Blood sugar 10% less
211	169 (66)	3 mo	3.7 vs. 5.0 kg			Yes		20 vs. 27 g fiber/day
213	30 (30)	3 mo	8.5 vs. 6.7 kg	10%	90%	Yes		6 g fiber/day
214	30 (30)	3 mo	7.0 vs. 6.0 kg	10%	90%	Yes		5 g fiber/day
	45	3 mo	6.2 vs. 4.1 kg	10%	90%	Yes		7 g fiber/day
222	9 (9)	8 wk	NS	10%	90%	Yes		Children 15 g fiber/ day
223	45 (45)	52 wk	3.8 vs. 2.8 kg	10%	90%	Yes		6–7 g fiber/day
224	22 (22)	4 wk	NS			VLCD	Less	
212	26 (26)	6 mo	5.5 vs. 3.0	10%	90%	Yes	Less	7 g fiber/day
206	15 (15)	2 mo		Glucomannan		Yes	Less	
225	20 (11)	14 mo	NS	Guar gum 20 g/day		VLCD		20 g fiber/day
216	28 (28)	2 wk	NS	100%	0%	VLCD	Less	2.8 g modified guar
217	21	4 wk	0.9 vs. −0.1			No		Goami #2 rice
215	53	24 wk	8 kg vs. 5.8 kg			Yes		6 g fiber/day
216	16	1 day				No	Less	Bread w/lupin flour
218	10	2 wk				No	Less	Oligofructose
219	52	4 yr	0	Fruit/vegetables 30 g/day		No		Breast cancer survivors
220	76	12 wk	2.8 vs. 1.3			Yes		Agar fiber
221	176	5 wk	4 kg all groups	3 water-soluble fibers		Yes		Glucomannan/others

Two double-blind clinical trials evaluated the effect of chitosan 1200 to 1600 mg orally twice a day. One trial included 51 obese women who were treated for eight weeks without any reduction in weight (229). The second trial included 34 overweight men and women who were treated for 28 days without any weight reduction relative to control (230). There were no serious adverse events or changes in safety laboratory in either trial, and no changes in fat-soluble vitamins or iron metabolism were seen. Another trial compared the fecal fat excretion of orlistat 120 mg and chitosan 890 mg taken t.i.d. The effect of chitosan on fecal fat was not different than placebo, but the orlistat had a significant increase in fecal fat (231). Two larger trials compared chitosan 3 g/day with placebo. The first trial had 150 participants and the chitosan group lost 1.3 kg compared to 0.04 kg in the placebo group over eight weeks which was statistically significant (232). The second trial had 250 subjects randomized equally to chitosan or placebo for 24 weeks. The chitosan group lost 0.4 kg compared to a gain of 0.2 kg in the placebo group which was statistically significant (233). It would appear that chitosan, in the doses used clinically, does not bind dietary fat and gives a weight loss of less than a kilogram over 8 to 24 weeks.

PHYSICAL AGENTS

Jaw Wiring

Jaw wiring has been used for the treatment of obesity since the 1970s. Rodgers et al. wired the jaws of 17 subjects with resistant obesity. The mean weight loss was 25.3 kg in six months which is comparable to obesity surgery over the same period of time. The majority of subjects regained weight after the wires were removed (234). Kark and Burke, who wired the jaws of nine subjects for six to eight months, confirmed this observation. Their subjects lost 28.8 kg making gastric bypass surgery less difficult (235).

Castelnuovo-Tedesco et al. attempted jaw wiring in 14 self-referred obese women who were immature and had passive-dependent or passive-aggressive personalities. Only one-third completed the six-month study and most of those regained weight (235). Ross et al. confirmed that psychologically frail subjects do not tolerate this procedure well, and demonstrated that one could predict success of the jaw wiring with a psychological questionnaire (236). They also demonstrated that subjects with panic or fear did not tolerate jaw wiring well (237).

Garrow demonstrated that weight is almost inevitably regained when the jaw wires are removed by following a group of nine subjects who lost 30.3 kg in nine months of jaw wiring (238). Discouraged by these results, 10 subjects with jaw wiring were compared to 10 subjects treated with milk-based liquid diets. The group with jaw wiring lost twice the amount of weight as the group on the milk-based diets, demonstrating that compliance was enhanced by jaw wiring (239). Pacy et al. confirmed these results by comparing diet advice to jaw wiring in 17 obese individuals followed for more than a year. The dietary advice group lost 17 kg compared to 33 kg in the jaw-wiring group (240).

Ramsey-Stewart and Martin treated 10 subjects with jaw wiring who lost an average 85% of their excess body weight in 16 to 40 weeks. Five of these subjects then underwent gastric reduction surgery and continued to lose further weight. Four of the five subjects who did not have surgery regained their weight, and only one subject maintained a significant weight loss after removal of the jaw wires. These authors concluded that jaw wiring has no place as a stand-alone treatment for obesity. It can, however, be useful for inducing a rapid weight loss safely, if it is sustained by an effective weight maintenance strategy (241).

Waist Cord

Seven subjects with an average weight of 107 kg had jaw wiring for an average of 9.3 months (time limited by dental considerations) and lost an average of 38.1 kg. When these seven subjects had the jaw wires removed, a 2-mm nylon cord was placed around their waists and left permanently in place. The group with the waist cord regained only 5.6 kg in an average of 7.8 months compared to 15 kg in the control group. The difference between the two groups was statistically significant ($p < 0.05$) (238).

Simpson et al. compared two groups of obese subjects for weight loss and weight maintenance, one with a waist cord that was progressively tightened as weight was lost and the other group without a waist cord. Both groups were treated with four-week periods of very low calorie dieting alternating with four-week periods of 1200 kcal/day high-fiber dieting. At 18 to 20 weeks the two groups lost 7.7 and 7.8 kg, which was not significantly different. At the end of the 48-week study 14 of 27 subjects remained in the waist cord group and 7 of 19 remained in the group without a waist cord. The group with a waist cord lost 16 kg and regained 1.2 kg compared with a regain of 6.6 kg in the group not treated with a waist cord ($p < 0.01$). This suggests that a waist cord can be a useful tool for weight maintenance, but does not improve weight loss (242).

Garrow subjected a series of 38 subjects to jaw wiring for weight loss. Twenty-six of these 38 subjects tolerated the jaw wiring and completed the weight loss phase losing

43 kg and had a waist cord applied. The waist cord was removed in 12 subjects for pregnancy, abdominal operations or personal reasons. The 14 subjects continuing to wear the waist cord maintained a 33 kg weight loss at three years of follow-up, 77% of the weight loss achieved with jaw wiring (243).

Garrow also described three subjects who achieved a weight loss of 41.7 kg by conventional dieting followed by the application of a waist cord (244). These three subjects maintained a 33 kg weight loss at 21 months of follow-up, 79% of the weight lost with dieting. This suggests that the maintenance of large weight losses using the waist cord is achievable with diet-induced weight loss. The waist cord is believed to provide a feedback signal whenever weight gain occurs, triggering behaviors designed to result in prevention of weight gain (245).

A new design for the fastener of the waist cord was proposed in which the patient could adjust the tightness within limits. This new design also allowed for the cord to be tightened during weight loss (246). Although this new design was claimed to be better tolerated and successful clinically, trials with this new design have not been published.

PSYCHOPHYSIOLOGICAL APPROACHES

Hypnosis

Hypnosis consists of relaxing subjects so that they are prone to carrying out posthypnotic suggestions. The majority of the psychiatric literature suggests that this methodology is only useful in a subset of patients suggestible enough to be hypnotized. Hypnosis was evaluated by Kirsch et al. in a meta-analysis of 18 studies in which cognitive behavior therapy was compared with and without hypnosis (247). Kirsch concluded that, averaged across posttreatment and follow-up periods, the hypnosis groups lost 5.14 kg compared to 2.73 kg in the non-hypnosis groups. At the last assessment period, the weight loss in the hypnosis group was 6.73 kg compared to 2.73 kg in the nonhypnosis group suggesting that the benefits of hypnosis increased with time (248). Allison and Faith, on the other hand, performed a meta-analysis on the same studies and found that by eliminating one questionable study, the statistical significance between the hypnosis and nonhypnosis groups was no longer present (249). These studies suggest that hypnosis is only useful in some subjects and on balance is not better than cognitive-behavioral therapy.

Since these meta-analyses were done, Johnson and Karkut reported a lack of difference in weight loss between hypnosis with and without aversive therapy (250). Johnson reported an uncontrolled study describing weight loss with hypnotherapy (251). Stradling et al.

treated obese subjects with sleep apnea using hypnotherapy compared to dietary advice. Weight loss was equal at three months but the hypnotherapy group maintained a significant 3.8 kg weight loss at 18 months that was not present in the dietary group (252).

With the exception of a report citing adverse reactions to hypnotherapy in developing adolescents, hypnotherapy for obesity appears to be a safe treatment (253). Schoenberger, in a review of the literature on hypnosis as an adjunct to cognitive-behavioral psychotherapy, states that although the studies cite benefits, the numbers are relatively small and many have methodological limitations suggesting the need for well-designed randomized clinical trials (254). Therefore, although promising, the place of hypnotherapy in the treatment of obesity remains unresolved.

Aromatherapy

The lay literature has suggested aromatherapy may be effective in the treatment of obesity. We could find only one controlled trial to assess this approach. This was an eight-week treatment program in which one group had 25 selected foods paired with noxious odors each week while the control group had air paired with these foods. The 14 subjects in the group given noxious odors lost significantly more weight (2.14 kg) compared to the air group (1.64 kg). Weight returned to baseline in both groups eight weeks after treatment, suggesting that aromatherapy has limited potential to treat obesity, which is a chronic disease (255).

Acupuncture

Acupuncture has been suggested as a treatment for obesity. Using acupuncture points that stimulate the auricular branch of the vagus nerve in the ear, appetite suppression has been postulated. There is intriguing information from animal studies that acupuncture alters level of serotonin related neurotransmitter levels in the brain and data in humans that suggests acupuncture points increase in temperature in proportion to the weight lost with acupuncture (256,257). There have been nine controlled trials to evaluate this claim. Mok et al. randomized 24 overweight subjects in a single-blind trial to acupuncture needles placed for nine weeks in active or inactive auricular sites. These needles were stimulated before eating. The treatment was safe but there was no difference in weight loss between the groups. A simultaneous trial was run in six guinea pigs with no change in weight (258). Mazzoni et al. randomized 40 subjects to weekly acupuncture or superficial acupuncture on points lateral to the treatment points and found no difference in weight loss over 12 weeks, but the dropout rate in both groups was very high (259).

Bahadori et al. reported an eight-week study in which 14 women treated with acupuncture and diet lost 7.7 kg vs. 3.6 kg in the diet only group ($p < 0.005$) (260). Steiner et al. randomized 78 subjects to sham acupuncture, acupuncture, behavior modification, or wait list. The subjects receiving acupuncture for eight weeks lost 2.7 kg, which was greater than 1.2 kg loss in the sham acupuncture group, but the behavior modification lost 4.3 kg in the same period (261). Cabioglu and Ergene reported two trials in which they randomized 55 women to electroacupuncture to the ear 30 min/day, diet and a not treatment control for 20 days or 40 women to the same electroacupuncture regimen vs. a diet control. The electroacupuncture group lost 4.8% body weight compared to 2.5% in the diet treated group in the first trial and 4.5% compared to 3.1% in the diet group in the second trial (262,263). Hsu et al. compared electroacupuncture to sit-up exercise over 13 weeks in 54 obese women. The electroacupuncture group lost 1.8 kg compared to 0.4 kg in the sit-up group ($p < 0.001$) (264).

Richards and Marley randomized 60 overweight subjects in a four-week trial to a transcutaneous nerve stimulator device placed on the auricular branch of the vagus nerve in the ear or on the thumb as a control. Appetite was suppressed in a higher percentage of the active (ear) group ($p < 0.05$), and there was greater weight loss in the active group (2.98 kg vs. 0.62 kg, $p < 0.05$) (265).

Allison et al. randomized 96 obese subjects to an acupressure device that was massaged before each meal for 12 weeks. The active device fit into the ear like a hearing aide putting pressure on the auricular branch of the vagus nerve. The inactive device was placed on the wrist. The treatment was safe but there was no significant difference in weight loss, fat loss, or blood pressure between the groups (266).

Three of nine human studies using acupuncture with good clinical trial designs and one animal study gave no significant weight loss. One of the positive studies used a transcutaneous nerve stimulation approach. In this study, there was less than a 2.5 kg difference between the active and inactive groups. The positive acupuncture studies gave 1.4 to 4.1 kg or 2.3% to 2.4% greater weight losses than the control, but behavior modification which is less invasive gave greater weight loss than acupuncture. Although there were no adverse events in these studies, the efficacy of using stimulation of the auricular branch of the vagus nerve for weight loss appears to be modest and less efficacious than behavior modification therapy.

Homeopathy

Helianthus tuberoses D1 was investigated in a randomized controlled trial for three months where those receiving the active ingredient lost −7.1 kg which was significantly more than in the placebo group (267). The second trial gave a single oral dose of Thyroidinum 30cH to fasting patients who had stagnated on a weight loss program, but Thyroidinum 30cH was no more effective than placebo (268).

EFFICACY AND SAFETY ASSESSMENT

While many of the studies presented above are not conclusive, and others are incomplete or poorly controlled, there are some general conclusions which can be drawn as to the safety and efficacy of the herbal and alternative approaches reviewed above (Table 4).

One of the key problems in this assessment is that only those agents found to be effective have had adequate clinical studies performed to begin to look at safety. Even in these cases, it may be that adverse effect reports

will be obtained in the field. It is sometimes difficult to assess whether the effects are caused by the agent being used. This problem will require careful documentation, but this work is only likely to be done with the most effective agents that become widely used.

CONCLUSION

The opportunities for additional research in this area are plentiful. Unfortunately, there has been relatively limited funding by comparison to funding for research on pharmaceuticals. However, botanical dietary supplements often contain complex mixtures of phytochemicals that have additive or synergistic interactions. For example, the tea catechins include a group of related compounds with effects demonstrable beyond those seen with epigallocatechin gallate (EGCG), the most potent catechin. The metabolism of families of related compounds may be

Table 4   Efficacy and Safety of Herbal/Alternative Approaches to Obesity Treatment

Herbal/alternative approach	Evidence of efficacy	Evidence of safety
Caffeine and ephedra	Good—clinical trial	Good
Green tea catechins	Weak	Excellent
Synephrine	Weak	Excellent
Capsaicin	Modest	Excellent
Fucoxanthin from seaweed	Weak—preclinical	Good
1,3-Diacylglycerol	Good—clinical trial	Excellent
Pinellia ternata	Weak—preclinical	Good
Conjugated linoleic acid	Weak—clinical trial	Questionable
Garcinia cambogia	Modest—clinical trial	Good
Guggul	Weak—clinical trial	Good
Cissus quadrangularis	Good—clinical trial	Excellent
Evening primrose	Ineffective—clinical trial	Good
Hoodia gordonii	Modest—clinical trial	Good
Caralluma fimbriata	Weak—clinical trial	Good
Pyruvate	Ineffective—clinical trial	Good
Yohimbine	Weak—clinical trial	Good
Dehydroepiandrosterone	Minimal, if any—clinical trial	Questionable
Chromium picolinate	Ineffective—clinical trial	Good
Calcium	Modest—clinical trial	Excellent
β-Hydroxymethylbutyrate	Ineffective for weight loss	Good
Topical fat reduction	Cosmetic only	Excellent
5-Hydroxytryptophan	Modest—clinical trial	Excellent
L-Tyrosine	Weak—preclinical	Excellent
Methionine restriction	Good—clinical trial	Good
Spirulina		
Dietary fiber	Good—clinical trial	Excellent
Chitosan	Weak—clinical trial	Excellent
Jaw wiring	Effective	Dental problems
Waist cord	Effective maintenance	Safe
Hypnosis	Ineffective	Safe
Aromatherapy	Ineffective	Safe
Acupuncture	Good—clinical trial	Safe
Homeopathy	Weak—clinical trial	Safe

different than the metabolism of purified crystallized compounds. Herbal medicines in some cases may be simply less purified forms of single active ingredients, but in other cases represent unique formulations of multiple related compounds that may have superior safety and efficacy compared to single ingredients.

Obesity is a global epidemic, and traditional herbal medicines may have more acceptance than prescription drugs in many cultures with emerging epidemics of obesity. A large number of ethnobotanical studies have found herbal treatments for diabetes, and similar surveys, termed bioprospecting, for obesity treatments may be productive.

Unfortunately, there have been a number of instances where unscrupulous profiteers have plundered the resources of the obese public with nothing to show for it. While Americans spend some $30 billion per year on weight loss aids, our regulatory and monitoring capability as a society are woefully inadequate. Without adequate resources, the FDA has resorted to "guilt by association" adverse events reporting which often results in the loss of potentially helpful therapies without adequate investigation of the real causes of the adverse events being reported. Scientific investigations of herbal and alternative therapies represent a potentially important source for new discoveries in obesity treatment and prevention. Cooperative interactions in research between the Office of Dietary Supplements, the National Center for Complementary and Alternative Medicine, and the FDA could lead to major advances in research on the efficacy and safety of the most promising of these alternative approaches.

REFERENCES

1. Haller CA, Benowitz NL. Adverse cardiovascular and central nervous system events associated with dietary supplements containing ephedra alkaloids. New Engl J Med 2000; 343:1833–1838.
2. Final rule declaring dietary supplements containing ephedrine alkaloids adulterated because they present an unreasonable risk. Final rule. Fed Regist 2004; 69: 6787–6854.
3. Inchiosa M. Letter to the Editor. Concerning ephedra alkaloids for weight loss. Int J Obes 2007; 31(9):1481.
4. Malchow-Moller A, Larsen S, Hey H, et al. Ephedrine as an anorectic: the story of the 'Elsinore pill'. Int J Obes 1981; 5:183–187.
5. Goodman L. The Pharmacological Basis of Therapeutics. 7th ed. New York: Macmillan Publishing Company, 1985.
6. Drug Topics Red Book. Montvale, NJ: Medical Economics Company, Inc., 2000.
7. Astrup A, Breum L, Toubro S, et al. The effect and safety of an ephedrine/caffeine compound compared to ephedrine, caffeine and placebo in obese subjects on an energy-restricted diet. A double blind trial. Int J Obes Relat Metab Disord 1992; 16:269–277.
8. Toubro S, Astrup A, Breum L, et al. The acute and chronic effects of ephedrine/caffeine mixtures on energy expenditure and glucose metabolism in humans. Int J Obes Relat Metab Disord 1993; 17(suppl 3):S73–S77.
9. Astrup A, Toubro S, Christensen NJ, Quaade F. Pharmacology of thermogenic drugs. Am J Clin Nutr 1992; 55:246S–248S.
10. Astrup A, Toubro S. Thermogenic, metabolic, and cardiovascular responses to ephedrine and caffeine in man. Int J Obes Relat Metab Disord 1993; 17(suppl 1):S41–S43.
11. Astrup A, Buemann B, Christensen NJ, et al. The effect of ephedrine/caffeine mixture on energy expenditure and body composition in obese women. Metabolism 1992; 41:686–688.
12. Buemann B, Marckmann P, Christensen NJ, et al. The effect of ephedrine plus caffeine on plasma lipids and lipoproteins during a 4.2 MJ/day diet. Int J Obes Relat Metab Disord 1994; 18:329–332.
13. Molnar D. Effects of ephedrine and aminophylline on resting energy expenditure in obese adolescents. Int J Obes Relat Metab Disord 1993; 17(suppl 1):S49–S52.
14. Molnar D, Torok K, Erhardt E, et al. Safety and efficacy of treatment with an ephedrine/caffeine mixture. The first double-blind placebo-controlled pilot study in adolescents. Int J Obes Relat Metab Disord 2000; 24:1573–1578.
15. Vansal SS, Feller DR. Direct effects of ephedrine isomers on human beta-adrenergic receptor subtypes. Biochem Pharmacol 1999; 58:807–810.
16. Greenway FL, Raum WJ, DeLany JP. The effect of an herbal dietary supplement containing ephedrine and caffeine on oxygen consumption in humans. J Altern Complement Med 2000; 6:553–555.
17. Greenway FL, de Jonge L, Blanchard D, et al. Effect of a dietary herbal supplement containing caffeine and ephedra on weight, metabolic rate, and body composition. Obes Res 2004; 12:1152–1157.
18. Gwirtsman H, Virts K, Chen K, et al. An ephedrine, caffeine, and chromium compound acutely increases energy expenditure in healthy obese adults: a placebo-controlled, crossover study. Obes Res 1999; 7:117S.
19. Boozer CN, Daly PA, Homel P, et al. Herbal ephedra/caffeine for weight loss: a 6-month randomized safety and efficacy trial. Int J Obes Relat Metab Disord 2002; 26:593–604.
20. Shekelle PG, Hardy ML, Morton SC, et al. Efficacy and safety of ephedra and ephedrine for weight loss and athletic performance: a meta-analysis. JAMA 2003; 289:1537–1545.
21. Dietary Supplement Market View. Washington D.C., 2000.
22. Moore N, Noblet C, Breemeersch C. Focus on the safety of ibuprofen at the analgesic–antipyretic dose. Therapie 1996; 51:458–463.
23. Steele VE, Kelloff GJ, Balentine D, et al. Comparative chemopreventive mechanisms of green tea, black tea and selected polyphenol extracts measured by in vitro bioassays. Carcinogenesis 2000; 21:63–67.
24. Sesso HD, Gaziano JM, Buring JE, et al. Coffee and tea intake and the risk of myocardial infarction. Am J Epidemiol 1999; 149:162–167.

25. Dulloo A, Seydoux J, Giradier L. Tealine and thermo-genesis: interactions between polyphenols, caffeine and sympathetic activity. Int J Obes 1996; 20:71.

26. Dulloo AG, Duret C, Rohrer D, et al. Efficacy of a green tea extract rich in catechin polyphenols and caffeine in increasing 24-h energy expenditure and fat oxidation in humans. Am J Clin Nutr 1999; 70:1040–1045.

27. Chantre P, Lairon D. Recent findings of green tea extract AR25 (Exolise) and its activity for the treatment of obesity. Phytomedicine 2002; 9:3–8.

28. Westerterp-Plantenga MS, Lejeune MP, Kovacs EM. Body weight loss and weight maintenance in relation to habitual caffeine intake and green tea supplementation. Obes Res 2005; 13:1195–1204.

29. Gougeon R, Harrigan K, Tremblay JF, et al. Increase in the thermic effect of food in women by adrenergic amines extracted from citrus aurantium. Obes Res 2005; 13:1187–1194.

30. Colker C, Kalman D, Torina G, et al. Effects of citrus aurantium extract, caffeine and St. John's wort on body fat loss, lipid levels and mood state in overweight healthy adults. Curr Ther Res 1999; 60:145–153.

31. Greenway F, de Jonge-Levitan L, Martin C, et al. Dietary herbal supplements with phenylephrine for weight loss. J Med Food 2006; 9:572–578.

32. Nasir JM, Durning SJ, Ferguson M, et al. Exercise-induced syncope associated with QT prolongation and ephedra-free Xenadrine. Mayo Clin Proc 2004; 79:1059–1062.

33. Min B, Cios D, Kluger J, et al. Absence of QTc-interval-prolonging or hemodynamic effects of a single dose of bitter-orange extract in healthy subjects. Pharmacotherapy 2005; 25:1719–1724.

34. Nykamp DL, Fackih MN, Compton AL. Possible association of acute lateral-wall myocardial infarction and bitter orange supplement. Ann Pharmacother 2004; 38:812–816.

35. Zhang LL, Yan Liu D, Ma LQ, et al. Activation of transient receptor potential vanilloid type-1 channel prevents adipogenesis and obesity. Circ Res 2007; 100:1063–1070.

36. Hwang JT, Park IJ, Shin JI, et al. Genistein, EGCG, and capsaicin inhibit adipocyte differentiation process via activating AMP-activated protein kinase. Biochem Biophys Res Commun 2005; 338:694–699.

37. Hsu CL, Yen GC. Effects of capsaicin on induction of apoptosis and inhibition of adipogenesis in 3T3-L1 cells. J Agric Food Chem 2007; 55:1730–1736.

38. Doucet E, Tremblay A. Food intake, energy balance and body weight control. Eur J Clin Nutr 1997; 51:846–855.

39. Matsumoto T, Miyawaki C, Ue H, et al. Effects of capsaicin-containing yellow curry sauce on sympathetic nervous system activity and diet-induced thermogenesis in lean and obese young women. J Nutr Sci Vitaminol (Tokyo) 2000; 46:309–315.

40. Westerterp-Plantenga MS, Smeets A, Lejeune MP. Sensory and gastrointestinal satiety effects of capsaicin on food intake. Int J Obes (Lond) 2005; 29:682–688.

41. Tsi D, Nah AK, Kiso Y, et al. Clinical study on the combined effect of capsaicin, green tea extract and essence of chicken on body fat content in human subjects. J Nutr Sci Vitaminol (Tokyo) 2003; 49:437–441.

42. Belza A, Frandsen E, Kondrup J. Body fat loss achieved by stimulation of thermogenesis by a combination of bioactive food ingredients: a placebo-controlled, double-blind 8-week intervention in obese subjects. Int J Obes (Lond) 2007; 31:121–130.

43. Masuda Y, Haramizu S, Oki K, et al. Upregulation of uncoupling proteins by oral administration of capsiate, a nonpungent capsaicin analog. J Appl Physiol 2003; 95:2408–2415.

44. Kobayashi Y, Nakano Y, Kizaki M, et al. Capsaicin-like anti-obese activities of evodiamine from fruits of Evodia rutaecarpa, a vanilloid receptor agonist. Planta Med 2001; 67:628–633.

45. Morimoto C, Satoh Y, Hara M, et al. Anti-obese action of raspberry ketone. Life Sci 2005; 77:194–204.

46. Inuoe N, Matsunaga Y, Satoh H, et al. Enhancement of energy expenditure and fat oxidation in human subjects by ingestion of novel and nonpungent capsaicin analogues (capsinoids). Obesity 2006; 14:A67.

47. Maeda H, Hosokawa M, Sashima T, et al. Fucoxanthin from edible seaweed, *Undaria pinnatifida,* shows antiobesity effect through UCP1 expression in white adipose tissues. Biochem Biophys Res Commun 2005; 332:392–397.

48. Maeda H, Hosokawa M, Sashima T, Takahashi N, Kawada T, Miyashita K. Fucoxanthin and its metabolite, fucoxanthinol, suppress adipocyte differentiation in 3T3-L1 cells. Int J Mol Med 2006; 18:147–152.

49. Liao HF, Tsai WC, Chang SW, et al. Application of solvent engineering to optimize lipase-catalyzed 1,3-diglyacylcerols by mixture response surface methodology. Biotechnol Lett 2003; 25:1857–1861.

50. Rudkowska I, Roynette CE, Demonty I, et al. Diacylglycerol: efficacy and mechanism of action of an anti-obesity agent. Obes Res 2005; 13:1864–1876.

51. Taguchi H, Nagao T, Watanabe H, et al. Energy value and digestibility of dietary oil containing mainly 1,3-diacylglycerol are similar to those of triacylglycerol. Lipids 2001; 36:379–382.

52. Kamphuis MM, Mela DJ, Westerterp-Plantenga MS. Diacylglycerols affect substrate oxidation and appetite in humans. Am J Clin Nutr 2003; 77:1133–1139.

53. Nagao T, Watanabe H, Goto N, et al. Dietary diacylglycerol suppresses accumulation of body fat compared to triacylglycerol in men in a double-blind controlled trial. J Nutr 2000; 130:792–797.

54. Maki KC, Davidson MH, Tsushima R, et al. Consumption of diacylglycerol oil as part of a reduced-energy diet enhances loss of body weight and fat in comparison with consumption of a triacylglycerol control oil. Am J Clin Nutr 2002; 76:1230–1236.

55. Matsuyama T, Shoji K, Watanabe H, et al. Effects of diacylglycerol oil on adiposity in obese children: initial communication. J Pediatr Endocrinol Metab 2006; 19:795–804.

56. Yasunaga K, Glinsmann WH, Seo Y, et al. Safety aspects regarding the consumption of high-dose dietary

diacylglycerol oil in men and women in a double-blind controlled trial in comparison with consumption of a triacylglycerol control oil. Food Chem Toxicol 2004; 42:1419–1429.

57. Taguchi H, Watanabe H, Onizawa K, et al. Double-blind controlled study on the effects of dietary diacylglycerol on postprandial serum and chylomicron triacylglycerol responses in healthy humans. J Am Coll Nutr 2000; 19:789–796.

58. Ai M, Tanaka A, Shoji K, et al. Suppressive effects of diacylglycerol oil on postprandial hyperlipidemia in insulin resistance and glucose intolerance. Atherosclerosis 2006; 195(2):398–403.

59. Yamamoto K, Asakawa H, Tokunaga K, et al. Effects of diacylglycerol administration on serum triacylglycerol in a patient homozygous for complete lipoprotein lipase deletion. Metabolism 2005; 54:67–71.

60. Yamamoto K, Asakawa H, Tokunaga K, et al. Long-term ingestion of dietary diacylglycerol lowers serum triacylglycerol in type II diabetic patients with hypertriglyceridemia. J Nutr 2001; 131:3204–3207.

61. Yamamoto K, Tomonobu K, Asakawa H, et al. Diet therapy with diacylglycerol oil delays the progression of renal failure in type 2 diabetic patients with nephropathy. Diabetes Care 2006; 29:417–419.

62. Kim YJ, Shin YO, Ha YW, et al. Anti-obesity effect of *Pinellia ternata* extract in Zucker rats. Biol Pharm Bull 2006; 29:1278–1281.

63. Choi Y, Kim YC, Han YB, et al. The *trans*-10, *cis*-12 isomer of conjugated linoleic acid downregulates stearoyl-CoA desaturase 1 gene expression in 3T3-L1 adipocytes. J Nutr 2000; 130:1920–1924.

64. Griinari JM, Corl BA, Lacy SH, et al. Conjugated linoleic acid is synthesized endogenously in lactating dairy cows by Delta(9)-desaturase. J Nutr 2000; 130:2285–2291.

65. Dhiman TR, Satter LD, Pariza MW, et al. Conjugated linoleic acid (CLA) content of milk from cows offered diets rich in linoleic and linolenic acid. J Dairy Sci 2000; 83:1016–1027.

66. Kritchevsky D. Antimutagenic and some other effects of conjugated linoleic acid. Br J Nutr 2000; 83:459–465.

67. MacDonald HB. Conjugated linoleic acid and disease prevention: a review of current knowledge. J Am Coll Nutr 2000; 19:111S–118S.

68. Pariza MW, Park Y, Cook ME. Conjugated linoleic acid and the control of cancer and obesity. Toxicol Sci 1999; 52:107–110.

69. Park Y, Storkson JM, Albright KJ, et al. Evidence that the *trans*-10, *cis*-12 isomer of conjugated linoleic acid induces body composition changes in mice. Lipids 1999; 34:235–241.

70. Park Y, Albright KJ, Liu W, et al. Effect of conjugated linoleic acid on body composition in mice. Lipids 1997; 32:853–858.

71. West DB, Delany JP, Camet PM, et al. Effects of conjugated linoleic acid on body fat and energy metabolism in the mouse. Am J Physiol 1998; 275:R667–R672.

72. DeLany JP, Blohm F, Truett AA, et al. Conjugated linoleic acid rapidly reduces body fat content in mice without affecting energy intake. Am J Physiol 1999; 276: R1172–R1179.

73. Yamasaki M, Mansho K, Mishima H, et al. Dietary effect of conjugated linoleic acid on lipid levels in white adipose tissue of Sprague-Dawley rats. Biosci Biotechnol Biochem 1999; 63:1104–1106.

74. Tsuboyama-Kasaoka N, Takahashi M, Tanemura K, et al. Conjugated linoleic acid supplementation reduces adipose tissue by apoptosis and develops lipodystrophy in mice. Diabetes 2000; 49:1534–1542.

75. Satory DL, Smith SB. Conjugated linoleic acid inhibits proliferation but stimulates lipid filling of murine 3T3-L1 preadipocytes. J Nutr 1999; 129:92–97.

76. Azain MJ, Hausman DB, Sisk MB, et al. Dietary conjugated linoleic acid reduces rat adipose tissue cell size rather than cell number. J Nutr 2000; 130:1548–1554.

77. Tricon S, Burdge GC, Williams CM, et al. The effects of conjugated linoleic acid on human health-related outcomes. Proc Nutr Soc 2005; 64:171–182.

78. Whigham LD, O'Shea M, Mohede IC, et al. Safety profile of conjugated linoleic acid in a 12-month trial in obese humans. Food Chem Toxicol 2004; 42:1701–1709.

79. Larsen TM, Toubro S, Gudmundsen O, et al. Conjugated linoleic acid supplementation for 1 y does not prevent weight or body fat regain. Am J Clin Nutr 2006; 83: 606–612.

80. Gaullier JM, Halse J, Hoye K, et al. Conjugated linoleic acid supplementation for 1 y reduces body fat mass in healthy overweight humans. Am J Clin Nutr 2004; 79:1118–1125.

81. Gaullier JM, Halse J, Hoye K, et al. Supplementation with conjugated linoleic acid for 24 months is well tolerated by and reduces body fat mass in healthy, overweight humans. J Nutr 2005; 135:778–784.

82. Riserus U, Vessby B, Arnlov J, et al. Effects of *cis*-9, *trans*-11 conjugated linoleic acid supplementation on insulin sensitivity, lipid peroxidation, and proinflammatory markers in obese men. Am J Clin Nutr 2004; 80: 279–283.

83. Riserus U, Arner P, Brismar K, et al. Treatment with dietary *trans*-10 *cis*-12 conjugated linoleic acid causes isomer-specific insulin resistance in obese men with the metabolic syndrome. Diabetes Care 2002; 25:1516–1521.

84. Riserus U, Vessby B, Arner P, et al. Supplementation with *trans*-10 *cis*-12-conjugated linoleic acid induces hyper-proinsulinaemia in obese men: close association with impaired insulin sensitivity. Diabetologia 2004; 47: 1016–1019.

85. Riserus U, Berglund L, Vessby B. Conjugated linoleic acid (CLA) reduced abdominal adipose tissue in obese middle-aged men with signs of the metabolic syndrome: a randomised controlled trial. Int J Obes Relat Metab Disord 2001; 25:1129–1135.

86. Kamphuis MM, Lejeune MP, Saris WH, et al. Effect of conjugated linoleic acid supplementation after weight loss on appetite and food intake in overweight subjects. Eur J Clin Nutr 2003; 57:1268–1274.

87. Desroches S, Chouinard PY, Galibois I, et al. Lack of effect of dietary conjugated linoleic acids naturally

incorporated into butter on the lipid profile and body composition of overweight and obese men. Am J Clin Nutr 2005; 82:309–319.

88. Sullivan C, Triscari J. Metabolic regulation as a control for lipid disorders. I. Influence of (–)-hydroxycitrate on experimentally induced obesity in the rodent. Am J Clin Nutr 1977; 30:767–776.

89. Badmaev V, Majeed M. Open field, physician-controlled evaluation of botanical weight loss formula citrin. Presented at Nutracon: Nutraceuticals, Dietary Supplements and Functional Foods. Las Vegas, NV, 1995.

90. Kriketos AD, Thompson HR, Greene H, et al. (–)-Hydroxycitric acid does not affect energy expenditure and substrate oxidation in adult males in a post-absorptive state. Int J Obes Relat Metab Disord 1999; 23:867–873.

91. Heymsfield SB, Allison DB, Vasselli JR., et al. *Garcinia cambogia* (hydroxycitric acid) as a potential antiobesity agent: a randomized controlled trial. JAMA 1998; 280:1596–1600.

92. Mattes RD, Bormann L. Effects of (–)-hydroxycitric acid on appetitive variables. Physiol Behav 2000; 71:87–94.

93. Kovacs EM, Westerterp-Plantenga MS, de Vries M, Brouns F, et al. Effects of 2-week ingestion of (–)-hydroxycitrate and (–)-hydroxycitrate combined with medium-chain triglycerides on satiety and food intake. Physiol Behav 2001; 74:543–549.

94. Downs BW, Bagchi M, Subbaraju GV, et al. Bioefficacy of a novel calcium–potassium salt of (–)-hydroxycitric acid. Mutat Res 2005; 579:149–162.

95. Preuss HG, Garis RI, Bramble JD, et al. Efficacy of a novel calcium/potassium salt of (–)-hydroxycitric acid in weight control. Int J Clin Pharmacol Res 2005; 25:133–144.

96. Roy S, Rink C, Khanna S, et al. Body weight and abdominal fat gene expression profile in response to a novel hydroxycitric acid-based dietary supplement. Gene Expr 2004; 11:251–262.

97. Saito M, Ueno M, Ogino S, et al. High dose of *Garcinia cambogia* is effective in suppressing fat accumulation in developing male Zucker obese rats, but highly toxic to the testis. Food Chem Toxicol 2005; 43:411–419.

98. Bhatt AD, Dalal DG, Shah SJ, et al. Conceptual and methodologic challenges of assessing the short-term efficacy of Guggulu in obesity: data emergent from a naturalistic clinical trial. J Postgrad Med 1995; 41:5–7.

99. Sidhu L, Sharma K, Puri A, et al. Effect of gum guggul on body weight and subcutaneous tissue folds. J Res Indian Med Yoga Hom 1976; 11:16–22.

100. Kotiyal P, Singh D, Bisht D. Gum guggulu (Commiphora mukul) fraction "A" in obesity: a double-blind clinical trial. J Res Ayur Siddha 1985; 6:20–35.

101. Antonio J, Colker C, Torina G, et al. Effects of a standardized guggulsterone phosphate supplement on body composition in overweight adults: a pilot study. Curr Ther Res 1999; 60:220–227.

102. Paranjpe P, Patki P, Patwardhan B. Ayurvedic treatment of obesity: a randomised double-blind, placebo-controlled clinical trial. J Ethnopharmacol 1990; 29:1–11.

103. Oben J, Kuate D, Agbor G, et al. The use of a *Cissus quadrangularis* formulation in the management of weight loss and metabolic syndrome. Lipids Health Dis 2006; 5:24.

104. Oben JE, Enyegue DM, Fomekong GI, et al. The effect of *Cissus quadrangularis* (CQR-300) and a Cissus formulation (CORE) on obesity and obesity-induced oxidative stress. Lipids Health Dis 2007; 6:4.

105. Haslett C, Douglas JG, Chalmers SR, et al. A double-blind evaluation of evening primrose oil as an antiobesity agent. Int J Obes 1983; 7:549–553.

106. MacLean DB, Luo LG. Increased ATP content/production in the hypothalamus may be a signal for energy-sensing of satiety: studies of the anorectic mechanism of a plant steroidal glycoside. Brain Res 2004; 1020:1–11.

107. Phytopharm. Hoodia Factfile. Available at: http://www.phytopharm.co.uk/hoodiafactfile/. Accessed October 1, 2007.

108. Kuriyan R, Raj T, Srinivas SK, et al. Effect of *Caralluma fimbriata* extract on appetite, food intake and anthropometry in adult Indian men and women. Appetite 2007; 48:338–344.

109. Stanko RT, Tietze DL, Arch JE. Body composition, energy utilization, and nitrogen metabolism with a 4.25-MJ/day low-energy diet supplemented with pyruvate. Am J Clin Nutr 1992; 56:630–635.

110. Stanko RT, Arch JE. Inhibition of regain in body weight and fat with addition of 3-carbon compounds to the diet with hyperenergetic refeeding after weight reduction. Int J Obes Relat Metab Disord 1996; 20:925–930.

111. Kalman D, Colker CM, Wilets I, et al. The effects of pyruvate supplementation on body composition in overweight individuals. Nutrition 1999; 15:337–340.

112. Koh-Banerjee PK, Ferreira MP, Greenwood M, et al. Effects of calcium pyruvate supplementation during training on body composition, exercise capacity, and metabolic responses to exercise. Nutrition 2005; 21:312–319.

113. Kucio C. Does yohimbine act as a slimming drug?. Isr J Med Sci 1991; 27, 550–556.

114. Sax L. Yohimbine does not affect fat distribution in men. Int J Obes 1991; 15:561–565.

115. Clore JN. Dehydroepiandrosterone and body fat. Obes Res 1995; 3(suppl 4):613S–616S.

116. Abrahamsson L, Hackl H. Catabolic effects and the influence on hormonal variables under treatment with Gynodian-Depot or dehydroepiandrosterone (DHEA) oenanthate. Maturitas 1981; 3:225–234.

117. Nestler JE, Barlascini CO, Clore JN, et al. Dehydroepiandrosterone reduces serum low density lipoprotein levels and body fat but does not alter insulin sensitivity in normal men. J Clin Endocrinol Metab 1988; 66:57–61.

118. Mortola JF, Yen SS. The effects of oral dehydroepiandrosterone on endocrine-metabolic parameters in postmenopausal women. J Clin Endocrinol Metab 1990; 71:696–704.

119. Usiskin KS, Butterworth S, Clore JN, et al. Lack of effect of dehydroepiandrosterone in obese men. Int J Obes 1990; 14:457–463.

120. Welle S, Jozefowicz R, Statt M. Failure of dehydroepiandrosterone to influence energy and protein metabolism in humans. J Clin Endocrinol Metab 1990; 71:1259–1264.

121. Morales AJ, Nolan JJ, Nelson JC, et al. Effects of replacement dose of dehydroepiandrosterone in men and women of advancing age. J Clin Endocrinol Metab 1994; 78:1360–1367.

122. Morales AJ, Haubrich RH, Hwang JY, et al. The effect of six months treatment with a 100 mg daily dose of dehydroepiandrosterone (DHEA) on circulating sex steroids, body composition and muscle strength in age-advanced men and women. Clin Endocrinol (Oxf) 1998; 49:421–432.

123. Villareal DT, Holloszy JO. Effect of DHEA on abdominal fat and insulin action in elderly women and men: a randomized controlled trial. JAMA 2004; 292:2243–2248.

124. Hernandez-Morante JJ, Milagro F, Gabaldon JA, et al. Effect of DHEA-sulfate on adiponectin gene expression in adipose tissue from different fat depots in morbidly obese humans. Eur J Endocrinol 2006; 155:593–600.

125. Porter DJ, Raymond LW, Anastasio GD. Chromium: friend or foe? Arch Fam Med 1999; 8:386–390.

126. Page TG, Southern LL, Ward TL, et al. Effect of chromium picolinate on growth and serum and carcass traits of growing-finishing pigs. J Anim Sci 1993; 71:656–662.

127. Mooney KW, Cromwell GL. Efficacy of chromium picolinate and chromium chloride as potential carcass modifiers in swine. J Anim Sci 1997; 75:2661–2671.

128. Mooney KW, Cromwell GL. Effects of dietary chromium picolinate supplementation on growth, carcass characteristics, and accretion rates of carcass tissues in growing-finishing swine. J Anim Sci 1995; 73:3351–3357.

129. Lindemann MD, Wood CM, Harper AF, et al. Dietary chromium picolinate additions improve gain: feed and carcass characteristics in growing-finishing pigs and increase litter size in reproducing sows. J Anim Sci 1995; 73:457–465.

130. Boleman SL, Boleman SJ, Bidner TD, et al. Effect of chromium picolinate on growth, body composition, and tissue accretion in pigs. J Anim Sci 1995; 73:2033–2042.

131. Myers MJ, Farrell DE, Evock-Clover CM, et al. Effect of recombinant growth hormone and chromium picolinate on cytokine production and growth performance in swine. Pathobiology 1995; 63:283–287.

132. Evock-Clover CM, Polansky MM, Anderson RA, et al. Dietary chromium supplementation with or without somatotropin treatment alters serum hormones and metabolites in growing pigs without affecting growth performance. J Nutr 1993; 123:1504–1512.

133. Bunting LD, Fernandez JM, Thompson DL Jr., et al. Influence of chromium picolinate on glucose usage and metabolic criteria in growing Holstein calves. J Anim Sci 1994; 72:1591–1599.

134. Hasten DL, Rome EP, Franks BD, et al. Effects of chromium picolinate on beginning weight training students. Int J Sport Nutr 1992; 2:343–350.

135. Grant KE, Chandler RM, Castle AL, et al. Chromium and exercise training: effect on obese women. Med Sci Sports Exerc 1997; 29:992–998.

136. Clancy SP, Clarkson PM, DeCheke ME, et al. Effects of chromium picolinate supplementation on body composition, strength, and urinary chromium loss in football players. Int J Sport Nutr 1994; 4:142–153.

137. Trent LK, Thieding-Cancel D. Effects of chromium picolinate on body composition. J Sports Med Phys Fitness 1995; 35:273–280.

138. Lukaski HC, Bolonchuk WW, Siders WA, et al. Chromium supplementation and resistance training: effects on body composition, strength, and trace element status of men. Am J Clin Nutr 1996; 63:954–965.

139. Bahadori B, Wallner S, Schneider H, et al. Effect of chromium yeast and chromium picolinate on body composition of obese, nondiabetic patients during and after a formula diet. Acta Med Austriaca 1997; 24:185–187.

140. Pasman WJ, Westerterp-Plantenga MS, Saris WH. The effectiveness of long-term supplementation of carbohydrate, chromium, fibre and caffeine on weight maintenance. Int J Obes Relat Metab Disord 1997; 21:1143–1151.

141. Walker LS, Bemben MG, Bemben DA, et al. Chromium picolinate effects on body composition and muscular performance in wrestlers. Med Sci Sports Exerc 1998; 30:1730–1737.

142. Campbell WW, Joseph LJ, Davey SL, et al. Effects of resistance training and chromium picolinate on body composition and skeletal muscle in older men. J Appl Physiol 1999; 86:29–39.

143. Volpe SL, Huang HW, Larpadisorn K, et al. Effect of chromium supplementation and exercise on body composition, resting metabolic rate and selected biochemical parameters in moderately obese women following an exercise program. J Am Coll Nutr 2001; 20:293–306.

144. Press RI, Geller J, Evans GW. The effect of chromium picolinate on serum cholesterol and apolipoprotein fractions in human subjects. West J Med 1990; 152:41–45.

145. Lee NA, Reasner CA. Beneficial effect of chromium supplementation on serum triglyceride levels in NIDDM. Diabetes Care 1994; 17:1449–1452.

146. Preuss HG, Grojec PL, Lieberman S, et al. Effects of different chromium compounds on blood pressure and lipid peroxidation in spontaneously hypertensive rats. Clin Nephrol 1997; 47:325–330.

147. Anderson RA. Nutritional factors influencing the glucose/insulin system: chromium. J Am Coll Nutr 1997; 16:404–410.

148. Anderson RA, Cheng N, Bryden NA, et al. Elevated intakes of supplemental chromium improve glucose and insulin variables in individuals with type 2 diabetes. Diabetes 1997; 46:1786–1791.

149. Evans GW, Bowman TD. Chromium picolinate increases membrane fluidity and rate of insulin internalization. J Inorg Biochem 1992; 46:243–250.

150. Stearns DM, Wise JP Sr., Patierno SR, et al. Chromium (III) picolinate produces chromosome damage in Chinese hamster ovary cells. FASEB J 1995; 9:1643–1648.

151. Stearns DM, Belbruno JJ, Wetterhahn KE. A prediction of chromium(III) accumulation in humans from chromium dietary supplements. FASEB J 1995; 9:1650–1657.

152. Anderson RA, Bryden NA, Polansky MM. Lack of toxicity of chromium chloride and chromium picolinate in rats. J Am Coll Nutr 1997; 16:273–279.

153. Vincent JB. The biochemistry of chromium. J Nutr 2000; 130:715–718.

154. McCarron DA, Morris CD, Henry HJ, et al. Blood pressure and nutrient intake in the United States. Science 1984; 224:1392–1398.

155. Zemel MB, Shi H, Greer B, et al. Regulation of adiposity by dietary calcium. FASEB J 2000; 14:1132–1138.

156. Zemel MB, Thompson W, Milstead A, et al. Calcium and dairy acceleration of weight and fat loss during energy restriction in obese adults. Obes Res 2004; 12: 582–590.

157. Zemel MB, Richards J, Milstead A, et al. Effects of calcium and dairy on body composition and weight loss in African-American adults. Obes Res 2005; 13: 1218–1225.

158. Zemel MB, Richards J, Mathis S, et al. Dairy augmentation of total and central fat loss in obese subjects. Int J Obes (Lond) 2005; 29:391–397.

159. Thompson WG, Rostad Holdman N, Janzow DJ, et al. Effect of energy-reduced diets high in dairy products and fiber on weight loss in obese adults. Obes Res 2005; 13:1344–1353.

160. Lappe JM, Rafferty KA, Davies KM, et al. Girls on a high-calcium diet gain weight at the same rate as girls on a normal diet: a pilot study. J Am Diet Assoc 2004; 104:1361–1367.

161. Lin YC, Lyle RM, McCabe LD, et al. Dairy calcium is related to changes in body composition during a two-year exercise intervention in young women. J Am Coll Nutr 2000; 19:754–760.

162. Davies KM, Heaney RP, Recker RR, et al. Calcium intake and body weight. J Clin Endocrinol Metab 2000; 85: 4635–4638.

163. Shapses SA, Heshka S, Heymsfield SB. Effect of calcium supplementation on weight and fat loss in women. J Clin Endocrinol Metab 2004; 89:632–637.

164. Shapses SA, Von Thun NL, Heymsfield SB, et al. Bone turnover and density in obese premenopausal women during moderate weight loss and calcium supplementation. J Bone Miner Res 2001; 16:1329–1336.

165. Barr SI. Increased dairy product or calcium intake: is body weight or composition affected in humans? J Nutr 2003; 133:245S–248S.

166. Bowen J, Noakes M, Clifton PM. Effect of calcium and dairy foods in high protein, energy-restricted diets on weight loss and metabolic parameters in overweight adults. Int J Obes (Lond) 2005; 29:957–965.

167. Nissen S, Sharp R, Ray M, et al. Effect of leucine metabolite beta-hydroxy-beta-methylbutyrate on muscle metabolism during resistance-exercise training. J Appl Physiol 1996; 81:2095–2104.

168. Kreider RB, Ferreira M, Wilson M, et al. Effects of calcium beta-hydroxy-beta-methylbutyrate (HMB) supplementation during resistance-training on markers of catabolism, body composition and strength. Int J Sports Med 1999; 20:503–509.

169. Lamboley CR, Royer D, Dionne IJ. Effects of beta-hydroxy-beta-methylbutyrate on aerobic-performance components and body composition in college students. Int J Sport Nutr Exerc Metab 2007; 17:56–69.

170. Ransone J, Neighbors K, Lefavi R, et al. The effect of beta-hydroxy-beta-methylbutyrate on muscular strength and body composition in collegiate football players. J Strength Cond Res 2003; 17:34–39.

171. Vukovich MD, Stubbs NB, Bohlken RM. Body composition in 70-year-old adults responds to dietary beta-hydroxy-beta-methylbutyrate similarly to that of young adults. J Nutr 2001; 131:2049–2052.

172. Nissen S, Sharp RL, Panton L, et al. Beta-hydroxy-beta-methylbutyrate (HMB) supplementation in humans is safe and may decrease cardiovascular risk factors. J Nutr 2000; 130:1937–1945.

173. Ronsard N. Cellulite: Those Lumps, Bumps, and Bulges You Couldn't Lose Before. New York: Beauty and Health Publishing Co., 1973.

174. Arner P. Adrenergic receptor function in fat cells. Am J Clin Nutr 1992; 55:228S–236S.

175. Arner P, Hellstrom L, Wahrenberg H, et al. Beta-adrenoceptor expression in human fat cells from different regions. J Clin Invest 1990; 86:1595–1600.

176. Lafontan M, Berlan M. Fat cell adrenergic receptors and the control of white and brown fat cell function. J Lipid Res 1993; 34:1057–1091.

177. Presta E, Leibel RL, Hirsch J. Regional changes in adrenergic receptor status during hypocaloric intake do not predict changes in adipocyte size or body shape. Metabolism 1990; 39:307–315.

178. Vernon RG. Effects of diet on lipolysis and its regulation. Proc Nutr Soc 1992; 51:397–408.

179. Greenway FL, Bray GA. Regional fat loss from the thigh in obese women after adrenergic modulation. Clin Ther 1987; 9:663–669.

180. Greenway FL, Bray GA, Heber D. Topical fat reduction. Obes Res 1995; 3(suppl 4):561S–568S.

181. Collis N, Elliot LA, Sharpe C, et al. Cellulite treatment: a myth or reality: a prospective randomized, controlled trial of two therapies, endermologie and aminophylline cream. Plast Reconstr Surg 1999; 104:1110–1114.

182. Richardson TP, Murphy WL, Mooney DJ. Selective adipose tissue ablation by localized, sustained drug delivery. Plast Reconstr Surg 2003; 112:162–170.

183. Neira R, Arroyave J, Ramirez H, et al. Fat liquefaction: effect of low-level laser energy on adipose tissue. Plast Reconstr Surg 2002; 110:912–922.

184. Lis-Balchin M. Parallel placebo-controlled clinical study of a mixture of herbs sold as a remedy for cellulite. Phytother Res 1999; 13:627–629.

185. Caruso MK, Pekarovic S, Raum WJ, et al. Topical fat reduction from the waist. Diabetes Obes Metab 2007; 9:300–303.

186. Mellinkoff S. Digestive system. Annu Rev Physiol 1957; 19:175–204.

187. Fernstrom JD. Role of precursor availability in control of monoamine biosynthesis in brain. Physiol Rev 1983; 63:484–546.

188. Wurtman RJ, Wurtman JJ. Carbohydrate craving, obesity and brain serotonin. Appetite 1986; 7(suppl):99–103.

189. Blundell JE, Leshem MB. The effect of 5-hydroxytryptophan on food intake and on the anorexic action of amphetamine and fenfluramine. J Pharm Pharmacol 1975; 27: 31–37.

190. Birdsall TC. 5-Hydroxytryptophan: a clinically-effective serotonin precursor. Altern Med Rev 1998; 3:271–280.

191. Weekley LB, Maher RW, Kimbrough TD. Alterations of tryptophan metabolism in a rat strain (Osborne-Mendel) predisposed to obesity. Comp Biochem Physiol A 1982; 72:747–752.

192. Ceci F, Cangiano C, Cairella M, et al. The effects of oral 5-hydroxytryptophan administration on feeding behavior in obese adult female subjects. J Neural Transm 1989; 76:109–117.

193. Cangiano C, Ceci F, Cascino A, et al. Eating behavior and adherence to dietary prescriptions in obese adult subjects treated with 5-hydroxytryptophan. Am J Clin Nutr 1992; 56:863–867.

194. Growdon JH, Melamed E, Logue M, et al. Effects of oral L-tyrosine administration on CSF tyrosine and homovanillic acid levels in patients with Parkinson's disease. Life Sci 1982; 30:827–832.

195. Avraham Y, Bonne O, Berry EM. Behavioral and neurochemical alterations caused by diet restriction: the effect of tyrosine administration in mice. Brain Res 1996; 732:133–144.

196. Hull KM, Maher TJ. L-tyrosine potentiates the anorexia induced by mixed-acting sympathomimetic drugs in hyperphagic rats. J Pharmacol Exp Ther 1990; 255: 403–409.

197. Hull KM, Maher TJ. L-tyrosine fails to potentiate several peripheral actions of the sympathomimetics. Pharmacol Biochem Behav 1991; 39:755–759.

198. Hull KM, Maher TJ. Effects of L-tyrosine on mixed-acting sympathomimetic-induced pressor actions. Pharmacol Biochem Behav 1992; 43:1047–1052.

199. Orentreich N, Matias JR., DeFelice A, et al. Low methionine ingestion by rats extends life span. J Nutr 1993; 123:269–274.

200. Epner DE, Morrow S, Wilcox M, et al. Nutrient intake and nutritional indexes in adults with metastatic cancer on a phase I clinical trial of dietary methionine restriction. Nutr Cancer 2002; 42:158–166.

201. Becker E, Jakober B, Luft D, al. Clinical and biochemical evaluations of the alga spirulina with regard to its application in the treatment of obesity. A double-blind crossover study. Nutr Rep Int 1986; 33:565–574.

202. Van Itallie TB. Dietary fiber and obesity. Am J Clin Nutr 1978; 31:S43–S52.

203. Krotkiewski M. Effect of guar gum on body-weight, hunger ratings and metabolism in obese subjects. Br J Nutr 1984; 52:97–105.

204. Kovacs EM, Westerterp-Plantenga MS, Saris WH, et al. The effect of addition of modified guar gum to a low-energy semisolid meal on appetite and body weight loss. Int J Obes Relat Metab Disord 2001; 25:307–315.

205. Walsh DE, Yaghoubian V, Behforooz A. Effect of glucomannan on obese patients: a clinical study. Int J Obes 1984; 8:289–293.

206. Cairella M, Marchini G. Evaluation of the action of glucomannan on metabolic parameters and on the sensation of satiation in overweight and obese patients. Clin Ter 1995; 146:269–274.

207. Hylander B, Rossner S. Effects of dietary fiber intake before meals on weight loss and hunger in a weight-reducing club. Acta Med Scand 1983; 213:217–220.

208. Porikos K, Hagamen S. Is fiber satiating? Effects of a high fiber preload on subsequent food intake of normal-weight and obese young men. Appetite 1986; 7:153–162.

209. Witkowska A, Borawska MH. The role of dietary fiber and its preparations in the protection and treatment of overweight. Pol Merkur Lekarski 1999; 6:224–226.

210. Pasman WJ, Saris WH, Wauters MA, et al. Effect of one week of fibre supplementation on hunger and satiety ratings and energy intake. Appetite 1997; 29:77–87.

211. Baron JA, Schori A, Crow B, et al. A randomized controlled trial of low carbohydrate and low fat/high fiber diets for weight loss. Am J Public Health 1986; 76: 1293–1296.

212. Rigaud D, Ryttig KR, Angel LA, et al. Overweight treated with energy restriction and a dietary fibre supplement: a 6-month randomized, double-blind, placebo-controlled trial. Int J Obes 1990; 14:763–769.

213. Solum TT, Ryttig KR, Solum E, et al. The influence of a high-fibre diet on body weight, serum lipids and blood pressure in slightly overweight persons. A randomized, double-blind, placebo-controlled investigation with diet and fibre tablets (DumoVital). Int J Obes 1987; 11 (suppl 1):67–71.

214. Rossner S, von Zweigbergk D, Ohlin A, et al. Weight reduction with dietary fibre supplements. Results of two double-blind randomized studies. Acta Med Scand 1987; 222:83–88.

215. Birketvedt GS, Aaseth J, Florholmen JR, et al. Long-term effect of fibre supplement and reduced energy intake on body weight and blood lipids in overweight subjects. Acta Medica (Hradec Kralove) 2000; 43:129–132.

216. Lee YP, Mori TA, Sipsas S, et al. Lupin-enriched bread increases satiety and reduces energy intake acutely. Am J Clin Nutr 2006; 84:975–980.

217. Lee KW, Song KE, Lee HS, et al. The effects of Goami No. 2 rice, a natural fiber-rich rice, on body weight and lipid metabolism. Obesity (Silver Spring) 2006; 14: 423–430.

218. Cani PD, Joly E, Horsmans Y, et al. Oligofructose promotes satiety in healthy human: a pilot study. Eur J Clin Nutr 2006; 60:567–572.

219. Thomson CA, Rock CL, Giuliano AR, et al. Longitudinal changes in body weight and body composition among women previously treated for breast cancer consuming a high-vegetable, fruit and fiber, low-fat diet. Eur J Nutr 2005; 44:18–25.

220. Maeda H, Yamamoto R, Hirao K, et al. Effects of agar (kanten) diet on obese patients with impaired glucose

tolerance and type 2 diabetes. Diabetes Obes Metab 2005; 7:40–46.

221. Birketvedt GS, Shimshi M, Erling T, et al. Experiences with three different fiber supplements in weight reduction. Med Sci Monit 2005; 11:PI5–PI8.

222. Gropper SS, Acosta PB. The therapeutic effect of fiber in treating obesity. J Am Coll Nutr 1987; 6:533–535.

223. Ryttig KR, Tellnes G, Haegh L, et al. A dietary fibre supplement and weight maintenance after weight reduction: a randomized, double-blind, placebo-controlled long-term trial. Int J Obes 1989; 13:165–171.

224. Quaade F, Vrist E, Astrup A. Dietary fiber added to a very-low caloric diet reduces hunger and alleviates constipation. Ugeskr Laeger 1990; 152:95–98.

225. Pasman WJ, Westerterp-Plantenga MS, Muls E, et al. The effectiveness of long-term fibre supplementation on weight maintenance in weight-reduced women. Int J Obes Relat Metab Disord 1997; 21:548–555.

226. Miller WC, Niederpruem MG, Wallace JP, et al. Dietary fat, sugar, and fiber predict body fat content. J Am Diet Assoc 1994; 94:612–615.

227. Alfieri MA, Pomerleau J, Grace DM, et al. Fiber intake of normal weight, moderately obese and severely obese subjects. Obes Res 1995; 3:541–547.

228. Han LK, Kimura Y, Okuda H. Reduction in fat storage during chitin-chitosan treatment in mice fed a high-fat diet. Int J Obes Relat Metab Disord 1999; 23:174–179.

229. Wuolijoki E, Hirvela T, Ylitalo P. Decrease in serum LDL cholesterol with microcrystalline chitosan. Methods Find Exp Clin Pharmacol 1999; 21:357–361.

230. Pittler MH, Abbot NC, Harkness EF, et al. Randomized, double-blind trial of chitosan for body weight reduction. Eur J Clin Nutr 1999; 53:379–381.

231. Guerciolini R, Radu-Radulescu L, Boldrin M, et al. Comparative evaluation of fecal fat excretion induced by orlistat and chitosan. Obes Res 2001; 9:364–367.

232. Kaats GR, Michalek JE, Preuss HG. Evaluating efficacy of a chitosan product using a double-blinded, placebo-controlled protocol. J Am Coll Nutr 2006; 25:389–394.

233. Mhurchu CN, Poppitt SD, McGill AT, et al. The effect of the dietary supplement, chitosan, on body weight: a randomised controlled trial in 250 overweight and obese adults. Int J Obes Relat Metab Disord 2004; 28: 1149–1156.

234. Rodgers S, Burnet R, Goss A, Phillips P, et al. Jaw wiring in treatment of obesity. Lancet 1977; 1:1221–1222.

235. Kark AE, Burke M. Gastric reduction for morbid obesity: technique and indications. Br J Surg 1979; 66:756–761.

236. Ross MW, Kalucy RS, Morton JE. Locus of control in obesity: predictors of success in a jaw-wiring programme. Br J Med Psychol 1983; 56(pt 1):49–56.

237. Ross MW, Goss AN, Kalucy RS. The relationship of panic-fear to anxiety and tension in jaw wiring for obesity. Br J Med Psychol 1984; 57(pt 1):67–69.

238. Garrow JS, Gardiner GT. Maintenance of weight loss in obese patients after jaw wiring. Br Med J (Clin Res Ed) 1981; 282:858–860.

239. Garrow JS, Webster JD, Pearson M, et al. Inpatient–outpatient randomized comparison of Cambridge diet versus milk diet in 17 obese women over 24 weeks. Int J Obes 1989; 13:521–529.

240. Pacy PJ, Webster JD, Pearson M. A cross-sectional cost/benefit audit in a hospital obesity clinic. Hum Nutr Appl Nutr 1987; 41:38–46.

241. Ramsey-Stewart G, Martin L. Jaw wiring in the treatment of morbid obesity. Aust N Z J Surg 1985; 55:163–167.

242. Simpson GK, Farquhar DL, Carr P, et al. Intermittent protein-sparing fasting with abdominal belting. Int J Obes 1986; 10:247–254.

243. Garrow JS. Morbid obesity: medical or surgical treatment? The case for medical treatment. Int J Obes 1987; 11(suppl 3):1–4.

244. Garrow JS. Treatment of morbid obesity by nonsurgical means: diet, drugs, behavior modification, exercise. Gastroenterol Clin North Am 1987; 16:443–449.

245. Garrow JS. Is it possible to prevent obesity? Infusionstherapie 1990; 17:28–31.

246. Garrow JS. The management of obesity. Another view. Int J Obes Relat Metab Disord 1992; 16(suppl 2):S59–S63.

247. Kirsch I, Montgomery G, Sapirstein G. Hypnosis as an adjunct to cognitive-behavioral psychotherapy: a meta-analysis. J Consult Clin Psychol 1995; 63:214–220.

248. Kirsch I. Hypnotic enhancement of cognitive-behavioral weight loss treatments: another meta-reanalysis. J Consult Clin Psychol 1996; 64:517–519.

249. Allison DB, Faith MS. Hypnosis as an adjunct to cognitive-behavioral psychotherapy for obesity: a meta-analytic reappraisal. J Consult Clin Psychol 1996; 64:513–516.

250. Johnson DL, Karkut RT. Participation in multicomponent hypnosis treatment programs for women's weight loss with and without overt aversion. Psychol Rep 1996; 79:659–668.

251. Johnson DL. Weight loss for women: studies of smokers and nonsmokers using hypnosis and multicomponent treatments with and without overt aversion. Psychol Rep 1997; 80:931–933.

252. Stradling J, Roberts D, Wilson A, et al. Controlled trial of hypnotherapy for weight loss in patients with obstructive sleep apnoea. Int J Obes Relat Metab Disord 1998; 22:278–281.

253. Haber CH, Nitkin R, Shenker IR. Adverse reactions to hypnotherapy in obese adolescents: a developmental viewpoint. Psychiatr Q 1979; 51:55–63.

254. Schoenberger NE. Research on hypnosis as an adjunct to cognitive-behavioral psychotherapy. Int J Clin Exp Hypn 2000; 48:154–169.

255. Cole AD, Bond NW. Olfactory aversion conditioning and overeating: a review and some data. Percept Mot Skills 1983; 57:667–678.

256. Wei Q, Liu Z. Effects of acupuncture on monoamine neurotransmitters in raphe nuclei in obese rats. J Tradit Chin Med 2003; 23:147–150.

257. Kwon YD, Lee JH, Lee MS. Increased temperature at acupuncture points induced by weight reduction in obese patients: a preliminary study. Int J Neurosci 2007; 117:591–595.

258. Mok MS, Parker LN, Voina S, et al. Treatment of obesity by acupuncture. Am J Clin Nutr 1976; 29:832–835.

259. Mazzoni R, Mannucci E, Rizzello SM, et al. Failure of acupuncture in the treatment of obesity: a pilot study. Eat Weight Disord 1999; 4:198–202.

260. Bahadori B, Wallner S, Wilders-Truschnig M, et al. Acupuncture as adjuvant therapy in obesity: effects on eating behavior and weight loss. Int J Obes Relat Metab Disord 2000; 24:S107.

261. Steiner R, Kupper N, Davis A. Obesity and appetite control: comparison of acupuncture therapies and behavior modification. Proceedings, International Forum on Family Medicine Education. Society of Teachers of Family Medicine, Kansas City, MO, 1983:313–326.

262. Cabioglu MT, Ergene N. Electroacupuncture therapy for weight loss reduces serum total cholesterol, triglycerides, and LDL cholesterol levels in obese women. Am J Chin Med 2005; 33:525–533.

263. Cabioglu MT, Ergene N. Changes in serum leptin and beta endorphin levels with weight loss by electroacupuncture and diet restriction in obesity treatment. Am J Chin Med 2006; 34:1–11.

264. Hsu CH, Hwang KC, Chao CL, et al. Effects of electroacupuncture in reducing weight and waist circumference in obese women: a randomized crossover trial. Int J Obes (Lond) 2005; 29:1379–1384.

265. Richards D, Marley J. Stimulation of auricular acupuncture points in weight loss. Aust Fam Physician 1998; 27(suppl 2):S73–S77.

266. Allison DB, Kreibich K, Heshka S, et al. A randomised placebo-controlled clinical trial of an acupressure device for weight loss. Int J Obes Relat Metab Disord 1995; 19:653–658.

267. Pittler MH, Ernst E. Complementary therapies for reducing body weight: a systematic review. Int J Obes (Lond) 2005; 29:1030–1038.

268. Schmidt JM, Ostermayr B. Does a homeopathic ultramolecular dilution of Thyroidinum 30cH affect the rate of body weight reduction in fasting patients? A randomised placebo-controlled double-blind clinical trial. Homeopathy 2002; 91:197–206.

269. Boozer CN, Nasser JA, Heymsfield SB, et al. An herbal supplement containing Ma Huang-Guarana for weight loss: a randomized, double-blind trial. Int J Obes Relat Metab Disord 2001; 25:316–324.

270. Coffey CS, Steiner D, Baker BA, et al. A randomized double-blind placebo-controlled clinical trial of a product containing ephedrine, caffeine, and other ingredients from herbal sources for treatment of overweight and obesity in the absence of lifestyle treatment. Int J Obes Relat Metab Disord 2004; 28:1411–1419.

271. Hackman RM, Havel PJ, Schwartz HJ, et al. Multinutrient supplement containing ephedra and caffeine causes weight loss and improves metabolic risk factors in obese women: a randomized controlled trial. Int J Obes (Lond) 2006; 30:1545–1556.

29

Is There a Future for Gene Therapy in Obesity?

SERGEI ZOLOTUKHIN

Division of Cellular and Molecular Therapy, Department of Pediatrics, Cancer and Genetics Research Complex, University of Florida, Gainesville, Florida, U.S.A.

INTRODUCTION

Obesity is an important health issue worldwide, particularly in the United States where the prevalence of obesity has increased substantially over the last two decades. In 2005, among the total U.S. adult population surveyed, 60.5% were overweight, 23.9% were obese, and 3.0% were extremely obese (1). Research has shown that obesity increases the risk of developing a number of conditions including type 2 diabetes mellitus (T2DM), hypertension, coronary heart disease, ischemic stroke, colon cancer, postmenopausal breast cancer, endometrial cancer, gallbladder disease, osteoarthritis, and obstructive sleep apnea.

In spite of a heavy burden imposed by the obesity epidemic and in the face of a massive effort from various pharmaceutical companies, no reliable weight-reducing drug is yet available. While many studies have highlighted the importance of environmental and behavioral modifications to treat obesity, little has been written about the possibility of genetic approaches. It is the intention of this author to summarize the advances in the area and to show that in this genomic age genetic therapy is a viable therapeutic strategy in treating obesity and its associated disorders.

UNDERSTANDING OBESITY: WHY WE GET FAT

At first glance, the rising rate of obesity seems to be simply a consequence of modern life's access to large amounts of palatable, high-calorie food with limited physical activity (2). On the other hand, the less susceptible part of the populace, exposed to the same environmental factors, remains lean and metabolically healthy; therefore indicating genetic makeup as essential component of body weight (BW) maintenance. So what "bears more weight": nature or nurture, genes or environment? Numerous studies have described complex environmental, behavioral, and genetic influences leading to a chronic imbalance favoring energy accumulation and excessive weight gain. But there is also growing evidence that suggests a significant contribution of epigenetic factors to the development of insulin resistance and obesity in childhood through adult life.

Genetic Factors: Human Obesity Gene Map

Progress in the human genome sequencing project and mapping of obesity genes have raised the possibility of selectively targeting this disease at the nucleic acid level. Figure 1 illustrates the exponential growth of the number of recently discovered genes associated with obesity. As of

Evolution in the status of the Human Obesity Gene Map

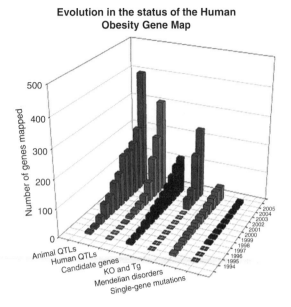

Figure 1 Evolution in the status of the human obesity gene map.

October 2005, 176 human obesity cases due to single gene mutations in 11 different genes have been reported, 50 loci related to Mendelian syndromes relevant to human obesity have been mapped to a genomic region, and causal genes or strong candidates have been identified for most of these syndromes (3). There are 244 genes that, when mutated or expressed as transgenes in the mouse, result in phenotypes that affect body weight and adiposity. The number of quantitative trait loci (QTLs) reported from animal models currently reaches 408. The number of human obesity QTLs derived from genome scans continues to grow, and there are 253 QTLs for obesity-related phenotypes from 61 genomewide scans. A total of 52 genomic regions harbor QTLs supported by two or more studies. The number of studies reporting associations between DNA sequence variation in specific genes and obesity phenotypes has also increased considerably, with 426 findings of positive associations with 127 candidate genes. A promising observation is that 22 genes are each supported by at least five positive studies. The obesity gene map shows putative loci on all chromosomes except Y (3).

The most common DNA sequence polymorphisms are single nucleotide polymorphisms (SNPs) occurring on average every 800 nucleotides across the genome. SNPs within the coding DNA sequence may be silent (when located in the third position of a codon) or may result in amino acid changes, the latter being implicated in mono-genic Mendelian disorders. In contrast, regulatory poly-morphisms occurring outside exonic regions have long been postulated to be important modulators of gene expression and evolutionary change (4). Regulatory poly-morphisms can be classified into two groups. The first are

cis-acting, acting on the copy of the gene present on that allele and typically present in or near the locus of the gene that it regulates. This may arise, for example, through the sequence change occurring in a regulatory DNA-binding site and altering the affinity with which a regulatory protein is recruited and hence how the gene is expressed. Alternatively, the regulatory polymorphism may be *trans*-acting, a polymorphism in one gene affecting the expression of another gene.

The expression level of a gene(s) could be considered a particular quantitative phenotype. At least 25% of the gene expression phenotypes differ significantly among the major populations studied (5). SNPs in coding regions of candidate genes do not always associate with susceptibility to complex multitrait diseases. Instead, in most cases, variability in gene expression is responsible for population differences in the prevalence of complex genetic diseases such as hypertension, obesity, and T2DM (6).

Other sequence polymorphisms include deletions and insertions of one or more nucleotides, rearrangements, and repeating sequences, which may be short tandemly repeated motifs of one to six nucleotides (microsatellites) or longer repeating "minisatellites." Such novel types of human genomic variability have been recently described as copy number variable regions (CNVRs), encompassing overlapping or adjacent deletions or insertions in DNA loci and covering a whopping 12% of the whole genome (7). These CNVRs contain hundreds of genes, disease loci, functional elements, and segmental duplications. Although it is too early to link obesity phenotype and CNVRs, the abundance of functional sequences of all types both within and flanking areas of copy number variation suggests that the contribution of CNVRs to such phenotypic manifestations is likely to be appreciable.

Recent progress in characterizing obesity-related genes, in and of itself, does not explain epidemic trends in recent history, for it is the environment not the human genome that undergoes dramatic changes.

Evolutionary Origins of Obesity

Our modern environment radically differs in many ways from the conditions that were present over most of human evolutionary history. An evolved physiological mecha-nism could be functioning precisely as it was designed to function, but because the environment has changed, the outcome may appear maladaptive. For example, humans may have evolved mechanisms designed to provide a survival advantage in times of a scarce food supply. Such mechanisms, collectively described as "thrifty gene," were designed to deal with the adaptive problem of food shortages. The "thrifty gene" hypothesis, proposed in 1962 by geneticist J. Neel, offers an explanation for the tendency of certain ethnic groups to be predisposed to obesity and diabetes (8). It postulates that certain genes in humans have evolved to maximize metabolic efficiency and food searching behavior and that in times of abundance these genes predispose their carriers to diseases caused by excess nutritional intake, such as obesity.

The alternative hypothesis by J.R. Speakman questions the adaptive attribute of the capacity to deposit enormous fat stores (9). Studies of wild animals suggest that stored body fat is actually regulated under stabilizing selection as part of a dynamic tradeoff between the risks of starvation, which promote fat storage, and the risks of predation, which promote leanness. Because early humans likely also faced these contrasting selective pressures, they probably also evolved a regulatory system (i.e., a lipostatic system) that not only promotes fat storage to avoid starvation but also prevents excessive fat storage to avoid predation (10). Several key events in human evolution have dramatically reduced the risks of predation. These events include the evolution of social behavior, the harnessing of fire, and the construction of tools and weapons. Under this release from constraint, it is feasible to imagine that target setpoints might have drifted upward at random because they had no selective consequences as long as actual body weights were constrained by limited food supply. This would remove the strong selection that imposed an upper limit on fat storage, but defense against energy deficits would still be strongly selected for. Several hundred generations later, when faced with the abundant lifestyle, the continued absence of strong selection on the lipostat target would result in a diversity of targets and the consequent diversity of body-fatness phenotypes that we presently observe.

Regardless of what was the actual evolutionary mechanism, the inevitable conclusion is that obesity results from a gene/environment interaction. Considerable numbers of individuals appear to have a maladaptive genetic predisposition to become obese, which is particularly expressed in the modern environment.

Environmental Factors: The Big Two and Other Causal Contributors

There is a consensus that recent environmental changes are almost certainly responsible for obesity epidemic. The most frequently mentioned factors include (i) food marketing practices and technology and (ii) institution-driven reductions in physical activity—the "Big Two" (11). A multitude of other environmental factors, coming into play during the last three decades, apparently contributed considerably into this trend (11). These factors include (i) sleep deprivation (12); (ii) endocrine disruptors (lipophilic, environmentally stable, and industrially produced

substances that can affect endocrine functions) (13); (iii) reduction in variability in ambient temperature (14); (iv) decreased smoking (15); (v) pharmaceutical iatrogenesis (weight gain induced by many psychotropic medications, anticonvulsants, antidiabetics, antihypertensives, steroid hormones contraceptives, antihistamines, protease inhibitors, and selective antidepressants) (11); (vi) changes in distribution of ethnicity and age (16); (vii) increasing gravida age (age of the first pregnancy) (17,18); (viii) intrauterine and intergenerational effects (19); (ix) greater body mass index (BMI), which is associated with greater reproductive fitness, yielding selection for obesity-predisposing genotypes (11,20); (x) assortative, nonrandom mating for adiposity trait (11,21); and (xi) composition of gut microbiome (22). Although the effect of any one of the above factors may be small, the combined effects appear to be significant. Of course, considering any environmental factor, it is important to be aware that such factors act in concert with individual genetic susceptibilities described in sections above.

Epigenetic Factors: Connecting Environment to Genes

If an "obesogenic" environment affects phenotype through genes, what is the molecular mechanism of this action? This question could be answered by investigating readily available animal models. The diet-induced obesity (DIO) rodent models, such as AKR/J, C57L/J, A/J, C3H/HeJ, DBA/2J, and C57BL/6J (23) mice, or Wistar (24) and DIO substrain of Sprague-Dawley rats (25) had been widely used as realistic models of human obesity. DIO models not only share a common polygenic mode of inheritance with many forms of human obesity (26,27), but these rodents also develop the metabolic syndrome with hypertension, insulin resistance, and hyperlipidemia (28–31). These are genetically homogenous (inbred) strains maintained in isolated colonies for hundreds of generations and, as such, would be expected to display a uniform response to environmental challenges. Indeed, when fed standard low-calorie chow, rodent from these inbred strains consistently maintain lean, insulin-sensitive phenotype. However, when fed a high-fat diet, they display differential metabolic adaptation: some animals remain lean and nondiabetic (diet-resistant) or lean and diabetic, but most become obese and diabetic (24,32,33). The differential metabolic adaptation of mice to a high-fat diet was shown to be associated with striking differences in gene expression patterns in the liver and skeletal muscles (32). The mechanisms triggering this differential adaptation are not presently known; however, data suggest that epigenetic modifications may play a significant role in the observed phenotypic diversity.

There are some mammalian alleles that display the unusual characteristic of variable expressivity in the absence of genetic heterogeneity. It has recently become evident that this is due to the activity of these alleles related to their epigenetic state. The epigenetic state is stochastic by nature, resulting in phenotypic mosaicism among cells (*variegation*) and also among individuals (*variable expressivity*) (34). The establishment of the epigenetic state occurs during early embryogenesis and is a probabilistic event that is influenced by whether the allele is carried on the paternal or maternal alleles. This parent-of-origin effect is classified as *genetic imprinting*. Classic imprinting involves the epigenetic silencing of one allele of a gene, based on the parent of origin, resulting in monoallelic expression. For instance, *Igf2* (insulin-like growth factor 2) is paternally expressed (or maternally imprinted); that is, the paternally inherited allele is active and the maternally inherited allele is inactive (35).

The interaction between imprinted genes and environmental factors could take place in at least two ways. First, inheritance of specific transcripts of imprinted genes, such as the placenta-specific *Igf2* transcript, could control the placental supply of nutrients available for fetal growth, irrespective of the maternal nutritional state (36). Secondly, imprinting of the genes themselves is controlled epigenetically by differential DNA methylation and chromatin modifications, which in turn can be modified by environmental factors such as nutrition. The latter effect is classified as *metabolic imprinting*. Metabolic imprinting reflects direct relationship between maternal nutritional state and fetal growth at the earliest stages of development. Mammalian alleles with such characteristics were termed *metastable epialleles* to distinguish them from traditional alleles (34). There is abundant evidence from genomic studies consistent with the hypothesis that metastable epialleles are the most promising candidate genes for transgenerational effects in response to rapid changes in the nutritional environment, such as those associated with the worldwide epidemic of metabolic syndrome, obesity, and T2DM (36–45).

Obesity Is a Chronic Condition

In the United States, the weight-loss industry is one of the fastest growing. It is nearly impossible to avoid pervasive advertisements promising clients "to achieve easy, effective, and affordable weight loss results." Unfortunately, attaining and subsequently maintaining lower weight is neither easy nor effective. Contrary to common belief, there is an emerging concept stating that obesity is a permanent, chronic condition (29,46) and, as such, will require chronic, perhaps a lifelong, treatment.

Although not universally accepted, the BW set-point hypothesis postulates that BW is regulated at a predeter-

mined, or preferred, level (set point) by a feedback control mechanism. It appears though that there is substantial difference in set-point maintenance in lean versus obese subjects: while lean subjects vigorously defend the low set point, obesity-prone subjects display a weight-gaining trend over the lifetime. This observation, along with considerable experimental data, lead to a hypothesis stating that obesity-predisposed individuals are born with a genetically raised threshold for sensing metabolic signals such as glucose, leptin, and insulin, which normally inhibit weight gain (29). Such a raised threshold may have been highly advantageous for survival when food was only intermittently available (thrifty gene).

Once the higher level of adiposity is attained, the obesity becomes irreversible because of the permanent changes established in the network of specialized "metabolic-sensing" neurons; in other words, the higher level of adiposity becomes "hard-wired" (29). Indeed, there is an abundance of experimental evidence supporting this notion (47–52). It is further postulated that changes become permanent because of intrinsic neural plasticity, which establishes new connections similar to those occuring during long-term memory formation and learning (53–55).

Temporal weight loss due to voluntary or experimentally imposed caloric restriction and chronic exercise is normally accompanied by profound drive to regain lost weight (56–60). A large body of evidence now suggests that a homeostatic feedback system defending peripheral adiposity is fundamental to this metabolic drive to regain lost weight. The feedback operates from peripheral tissues communicating to the central nervous system via neural, nutrient, and endocrine pathways integrating both satiety and adiposity signals (47,61–63). All these data corroborate our everyday experience, indicating that the effect of weight-lowering regimens last only as long as they are taken. But perhaps a new pharmacological drug will resolve this seemingly unsolvable problem.

TECHNICAL DEVELOPMENTS IN GENE THERAPY

Although many candidate obesity genes have been identified, tailoring treatment to a particular mutated gene target (pharmacogenomics) or to a particular patient (pharmacogenetics) (64) remains an elusive goal. New approaches in nonoral drug delivery, such as gene therapy, could substantially expand the "druggable" target pool as well as provide a treatment adjusted to a patient's genetic makeup. However, before these goals can be realized, two conditions must be met: (*i*) optimizations of methods of gene delivery and (*ii*) development of novel systems for the regulation of transgene expression.

Gene Delivery Vehicles

Excess adipose tissue accumulates over long periods of time, making obesity a chronic condition that discourages physical activity and energy expenditure, further promoting the vicious cycle of weight gain. If gene therapy is to be successful, the expression of a therapeutic transgene should be persistent for as long as the condition persists. Hence, the treatment should provide a long-term mode of transgene expression either through the integration into host cell chromosome or preferably via persistent episomal expression. Among current gene delivery systems, only viral vectors can fulfill this requirement.

Viruses are naturally evolved vehicles that efficiently transfer their genes into host cells. This ability makes them particularly useful for the delivery of therapeutic genes as engineered vectors. Viral vectors for gene transfer are the topic of several recent reviews (65,66), so the information provided here will highlight only recombinant adeno-associated virus (rAAV) vectors for the treatment of obesity and provide a rationale for the use of rAAV. For more complete information on the use of AAV in gene therapy, the reader is referred to a number of recent reviews (65,67–71).

There are three main reasons for AAV's attractiveness as a gene therapy vector: (i) lack of pathogenicity, (ii) ability to transduce differentiated cells, and (iii) a wide host range. Numerous preclinical studies and clinical trials (71,72) indicate that there is no detectable toxicity from the administration of rAAV. While some observed humoral immune responses to the AAV capsid, most studies indicate that cell-mediated immune responses to AAV are uncommon in the absence of adenovirus helper infection.

Unlike some viral vectors, rAAV leads to long-term transduction of cells due in part to its persistence as concatemerized episomes. This is particularly important in nonproliferating cells where episomal DNA is stable and not diluted by host cell division. Additionally, episomal persistence decreases the risk of insertional mutagenesis associated with random integration of vector DNA into the host genome.

Finally, the AAV vector repertoire has been substantially expanded with the recent isolation of several novel AAV serotypes (73,74). The natural abundance of AAV serotypes and their distinct cellular tropism contributes to the wide host range of AAVs and allows for incredible flexibility in vector design. For example, rAAV vectors based on serotypes 1, 7, and 8 have a transduction efficiency approaching 100% in muscle cells, and while all serotypes are effective in hepatocytes, rAAV8-based vectors display an astonishing "unrestricted" efficiency (75). Taking advantage of a serotype's structural relationship and diversity, investigators are able to exploit the

modular nature of AAV by combining vector components derived from different serotypes, thereby enhancing transduction of target cells or tissues. Using the processes dubbed "pseudotyping" (76), or "cross-packaging" (77), chimeric vectors are now constructed containing AAV2-derived terminal repeats harboring a transgene packaged into the capsids of other AAV serotypes. This greatly facilitates vector production and therapeutic screening, allowing same transgene cassette to be packaged in a "pseudotyped" vector for higher transduction efficiencies of target tissues. Another approach to improving transduction efficiency is the generation of chimeric rAAVs using a "transcapsidation" or "cross-dressing" technique, whereby the virion consists of a random mosaic of capsid proteins derived from two different AAV serotypes (78,79). This mosaic vector exhibits dual-binding characteristic of the parent viruses and, provided there is optimal stoichiometry of components, may display a synergistic effect on transduction (79).

The flexibility of the AAV virion is further demonstrated by the insertion of small peptides or protein ligands into the major component of the AAV capsid (VP3) with the goal of targeting tissues through cell-specific receptor/ligand interactions (80–87). Much larger proteins have been inserted at the N-terminus of VP2 capsid proteins for a similar purpose (71). In light of the rapid pace in developing "designer" AAV vectors, it seems reasonable to speculate that AAV vectors based on different serotypes and/or targeted to specific cell types will eventually be developed for clinical applications such as obesity.

Regulation of Gene Expression

The potentially lifelong consequences of gene therapy require that gene expression be reliably controlled. Over the years, many systems have been designed and successfully tested both in vitro and in vivo (88–91). Most of these systems rely on engineered transcription factors (TFs) binding to specific DNA sequences and resulting in induction or suppression of a transgene. In some cases, TF function can be controlled by a small organic compound capable of interacting with domains within TFs to induce allosteric conformational changes. Although very useful in the investigational setting, none of these systems have been utilized in gene therapy clinical protocols for the following reasons: (i) the inducer molecule had toxic (heavy-metal ion) or pleiotropic effects (glucocorticoid steroid) or had limited/restricted availability (synthetic dimerizers) (91); (ii) the gene encoding engineered TFs (activator/silencer) had to be introduced along with a therapeutic gene, thereby complicating the logistics of the treatment; (iii) chimeric TFs often induced immune response in the host organism (*tet* repressor-based systems); and (*iv*) no system has been designed to control the expression of endogenous genes within their own genetic context, i.e., under the control of its own promoter subject to the innate expression control and encoding multiple natural protein isoforms arising from an alternative splicing.

One of the alternative systems overcoming these limitations is based on RNA interference (RNAi). RNAi is a newly discovered mechanism for regulating gene expression where the presence of small fragments of double-stranded RNA (dsRNA) whose sequence matches a given gene interferes with the expression of that gene resulting in gene "knockdown." The effectors of the knockdown can be either small hairpin RNAs (shRNA) produced from RNA polymerase (pol) III promoters or micro-RNA-based shRNA expressed from pol II promoters (92). Small noncoding RNAs regulate gene expression at multiple levels including chromatin architecture, transcription, RNA editing, RNA stability, and translation.

RNAi was originally described in the nematode worm *Caenorhabditis elegans* as a cellular response to dsRNA, which initiates mRNA degradation in a sequence-specific manner (93). Subsequently, Tuschl and colleagues discovered that small interfering RNAs (siRNAs) of 21 nucleotides, normally generated from long dsRNA during RNAi, could be used to inhibit specific gene targets (94). Similarly, Caplen and coworkers have also reported the activity of siRNAs in somatic mammalian cells (95). Following these landmark observations, there have been numerous in vitro and in vivo studies supporting its therapeutic potential (96–99). Although efficient delivery of siRNAs remains a crucial challenge for transition from the laboratory to the clinic, there are a number of successful examples of vector-mediated siRNA delivery both in vitro and in vivo (100–105).

The application scope of RNAi has recently been expanded to incorporate dsRNA-induced gene activation by targeting noncoding regulatory regions in gene promoters. Li et al. had demonstrated long-lasting and sequence-specific induction of human genes E-cadherin, p21$^{WAF1/CIP1}$, and vascular endothelial growth factor A (106). Similarly, Janowski et al. observed induction of the expression of progesterone receptor gene and major vault protein (by 18-fold and 4-fold, respectively) with duplex RNAs of 21 residues targeting the respective promoter regions within chromosomal DNA (107).

Notably, RNAi, in general, does not provide extensive range of expression control, although for applications related to obesity this shortcoming does not seem to be critical. Rarely do people have mutations in single genes that result in severe obesity starting in infancy (e.g., congenital leptin deficiency or multiple melanocortin-4 receptor mutations) (3). Most often, weight gain and obesity result from only a small positive energy input

imbalance over extended periods of time. It is assumed that this imbalance could be attributed, at least in part, to allelic differences in expressions of hundreds of genes involved in metabolism that are of modest magnitude (typically, 1.5- to 2.0-fold) (108–110). It is then reasonable to assume that in most cases, save morbid obesity, the more prudent approach would be minor adjustments in genetic expression that might affect both caloric intake (food) and energy expenditure (resting metabolic rate), using strategies outlined in the next section.

GENERAL STRATEGIES IN GENE THERAPY FOR OBESITY

In the age of biotechnology, we have experienced unparalleled progress in gene delivery techniques and control of gene expression, but can we successfully apply these technologies to treat obesity? The general perception is that conventional gene therapy is not appropriate for multitrait disorder such as obesity. The argument is that even if one can achieve technical excellence in delivering and regulating genetic information in particular cell types or tissues, there are too many deregulated genes to balance, and that the subset of these genes are going to be different in each particular case of obesity anyway. Yet, the counterargument could be made that precisely because of the complex cumulative nature of this disorder manifesting in variable expressivity and variegation of many genes, one needs to modulate only limited number of shared pathways, or maybe even a single gene, as long as this particular gene occupies a key position in a crucial metabolic pathway. One might picture a recognizable energy scale balancing two cups with hundreds of genes combining for energy intake in one cup while as many genes acting together for energy expenditure in the opposite cup. To shift a balance in the desired direction, one needs to either "reduce the weight" in one cup by inhibiting the action of any gene in this pool or, conversely, induce the expression of any other gene in the opposite pool. In other words, regardless of the underlying causes, the treatment (gene target) could be a general one. In fact, Tiffin et al. has recently described a short list of such genes (111). The investigators reviewed seven independent computational disease gene prioritization methods and then applied them in concert to the analysis of 9556 positional candidate genes for T2DM and the related trait obesity. As a result, a list of nine primary candidate genes for T2DM and five genes for obesity had been generated (111). Two genes, lipoprotein lipase (LPL) and branched-chain α-keto acid dehydrogenase (BCKDHA), are common to these two sets.

What are the best gene targets among various genes associated with this complex disorder? In general, genes regulating anabolic pathways (inducing conservation and uptake of energy) and catabolic pathways (promoting energy expenditure and decreasing food intake) are legitimate targets. For example, to reduce BW, one would aim to downregulate the activity of the former (e.g., by utilizing siRNAs) and/or upregulate the latter (either by exogenous gene delivery or by control of endogenous gene). Furthermore, the mechanism of action of the targeted gene may require central (brain) or peripheral administration of a vector. The hypothalamus, a satiety center within the brain, is an attractive target because of its involvement in the integration of peripheral metabolic signals (see recent review in Ref. 61). In a clinical setting, however, the choice will most likely involve targeting peripheral organs involved in energy metabolism (gut, liver, muscle, or fat).

GENE TARGETS FOR OBESITY

The following selected list of genes does not represent a comprehensive catalog of potential targets but, rather, reflects only the contributing author's experimental data and bias. It is safe to assume that many more gene targets will be tested and, hopefully, applied in clinical practice in the future.

Leptin

In spite of the common manifestation of the disease, the reason for fat accumulation may be different among patients. In search of common denominator, researchers identified leptin—a protein hormone produced mostly by adipose tissue. Circulating leptin provides the brain with an indication of adipose mass for the purposes of regulating appetite and metabolism. Leptin works by inhibiting the actions of neuropeptide Y and agouti-related peptide and by increasing the actions of α-melanocortin-stimulating hormone.

It is believed that leptin cannot be used to treat obesity because most overweight patients develop peripheral as well as central leptin insensitivity/resistance. This opinion was substantiated when leptin replacement therapy was applied either peripherally or centrally (112,113). Under both treatment regimens, leptin initially mediated a very robust anorexigenic and weight-reducing effects, but then promoted the development of leptin resistance. Moreover, similar effects were documented in the rat brain exposed to the long-term elevated levels of leptin encoded by the rAAV vector (114–116). The exact mechanism of leptin resistance remains to be determined. Recent publications implicate downstream signaling cascades, such as signal transducer and activator of transcription and suppressor of cytokine signaling (SOCS-3), with downregulation of the leptin receptor Ob-Rb expression as partially responsible (51,116,117). Although SOCS-3 and Ob-Rb seem to be valid targets for gene therapy (via downregulating the former and upregulating the latter), attempting central nervous system regulation for the treatment of obesity is controversial.

Despite the problematic issues related to leptin resistance, two applications may be appropriate for peripheral administration of leptin gene therapy: (i) congenital leptin deficiency, a rare disorder of morbid obesity and (ii) lipodystrophic syndrome, an adiposopathy associated with low leptin levels. In both cases, clinical trials of leptin protein replacement therapy have been very successful. Leptin treatment of these patients improved metabolic abnormalities such as insulin resistance, hyperglycemia, hyperinsulinemia, dyslipidemia and hepatic steatosis (118). Intramuscular administration of rAAV encoding the leptin gene could provide long-term regulation of leptin expression (119) and replace daily injectable drug regimens. For most obese patients, however, leptin therapy does not represent a viable option, requiring the development of alternative strategies.

Neurocytokines

One strategy is to bypass the leptin signaling pathway altogether. This could be accomplished by utilizing ciliary neurotrophic factor (CNTF), a cytokine belonging to the interleukin 6 family. Acute treatment with CNTF reduced the obesity-related phenotype of *ob/ob* and *db/db* mice, which lack functional leptin and leptin receptor, respectively (120). Consistent with this finding, Lambert et al. (121) showed that CNTF can activate hypothalamic leptin-like pathways in DIO models that are unresponsive to leptin. Subsequently, a recombinant human variant of CNTF (rhvCNTF) has been tested in clinical trials for weight loss in obese adults (122).

Since CNTF is under investigation in clinical trials, studying the long-term effects of its action on the brain where it exerts anorexigenic effect is critical. This was accomplished in DIO rat models using centrally administered rAAV encoding CNTF, or leukemia inhibitory factor (LIF), another neurocytokine belonging to the interleukin 6 family (116). Using DNA microarray analysis of gene expression in the hypothalamus, the authors presented evidence that constitutive expression of cytokines in the brain evokes a state of perceived chronic inflammation leading to either temporal weight reduction (CNTF) or severe cachexia (LIF). Neither of these neurocytokines appears to fulfill the requirements of a sustained (CNTF) and safe (LIF) therapy. Because of development of CNTF tolerance, higher doses of the cytokine may be required to achieve persistent weight loss. However, high doses of

CNTF induce side effects (122,123). Furthermore, data from LIF-treated animals indicate that a potent JAK/ STAT inducer initiates pleiotropic processes in the brain that can trigger unwanted outcomes. These results convey a cautionary note regarding long-term use of neurocytokines in therapeutic applications.

AMP-Activated Protein Kinase

One of the genes activated downstream of leptin signaling in skeletal muscle is AMP-activated protein kinase (AMPK) (124), a "master switch" that mediates a majority of metabolic functions (125,126). AMPK is also the downstream effector of a protein kinase cascade that is switched on by increases in the AMP:ATP ratio. Once activated, AMPK switches on catabolic pathways that generate ATP while switching off ATP-consuming processes. AMPK appears to be a key regulator in controlling metabolism in response to diet and exercise. This enzyme also regulates food intake and energy expenditure at the whole body level by mediating the effects of hormones and cytokines such as leptin, adiponectin, and ghrelin.

In humans, the enzyme subunits are encoded by two or three genes, and all twelve combinations of α, β, and γ isoforms appear to be able to form complexes. Evidence of splice variants, especially of the $\gamma2$ subunit, has also emerged recently. This complex protein structure makes its upregulation via transgene vector delivery a difficult challenge, making AMPK unlikely as a direct gene therapy target. Modifying the upstream steps of the signaling cascade could provide an alternative approach.

Adiponectin

One example of upstream targeting of the AMPK signaling cascade was demonstrated by Shklyaev et al. who utilized rAAV-mediated peripheral delivery of adiponectin to counteract the development of DIO in rat model (127). Adiponectin (Acrp30) is a polypeptide hormone secreted by adipose tissue that shows insulin-sensitizing, anti-inflammatory, and antiatherogenic properties (128,129). In contrast to leptin, the expression of adiponectin is reduced in obese and diabetic mice (130), and plasma levels of Acrp30 are lower in obese compared with lean humans (131). Similarly, Acrp30 replenishment decreases body adiposity and improves insulin resistance in various models of obesity (132). The mechanism by which Acrp30 ameliorates insulin resistance and improves glucose metabolism remains obscure, but evidence suggests that Acrp30 increases fatty acid oxidation in muscle and liver and decreases hepatic glucose production (129,132–134).

The half-life of adiponectin is short, with 90% of the drug cleared in 3.3 half-lives ($T_{1/2}$, 4 hours). This fast turnover would require multiple daily injections of substantial doses to achieve the normal effective concentration found in serum (5–10 µg/mL). Because acute regulation of Acrp30 levels under normal conditions is modest, the hormone might be responsible for chronic adaptive responses, such as a increasing the β-oxidation of fatty acids. In light of adiponectin's pharmacokinetic properties, sustained transgene-mediated release of adiponectin may be the only effective method of achieving therapeutic levels. Curiously, in clinical studies involving Rimonabant, a selective cannabinoid-1 receptor (CB1) antagonist, one of the improved metabolic parameters was a significantly increased level of adiponectin (135). Is it conceivable that the therapeutic effect of the drug might be related, at least in part, to the improved adiponectin level?

To investigate the primary physiological role of Acrp30 in long-term studies, Shklyaev et al. employed gene therapy for the sustained peripheral expression of Acrp30 with rAAV (127). Remarkably, a single portal vein injection of rAAV-Acrp30 counteracted the development of DIO and ameliorated insulin resistance for 41 weeks. Experiments attempting to elucidate the mechanism of this sustained weight loss suggest that ectopically expressed adiponectin regulates hepatic lipogenesis and gluconeogenesis, dichotomizing downstream at the point of AMPK. More comprehensive studies of the mechanisms and safety of Acrp30 gene therapy are required, but these findings provide the groundwork for a candidate gene therapy treatment of obesity and T2DM.

Stearoyl-CoA Desaturase

Another gene linking peripheral leptin signaling and the activation of AMPK is stearoyl-CoA desaturase (SCD1), an important endoplasmic reticulum-bound enzyme that catalyzes the rate-limiting step in monounsaturated fatty acid synthesis, mainly oleate (C18:1) and palmitoleate (C16:1) (136). Leptin downregulates SCD1 expression in the liver, and SCD1 expression is induced in leptin-deficient *ob/ob* mice (137). Mice with targeted disruption of SCD1 have reduced adiposity, resistance to diet-induced weight gain, and increased insulin sensitivity (137,138). Furthermore, this mouse model demonstrates an increase in basal metabolic rate and an upregulation of genes encoding fatty acid oxidation enzymes. Conceivably, SCD1 gene disruption could be working through an AMPK-mediated decrease in hepatic malonyl-CoA levels, leading to the subsequent increase in carnitine acyltransferase activity and greater transport of fatty acids into mitochondria for β-oxidation (139). While gene therapy studies targeting the SCD1 are lacking, the current data in mouse models suggest SCD1 gene downregulation is an attractive target for gene therapy.

WNT-10B

Adipose tissue is derived from the embryonic mesenchyme. In adult organisms, a population of mesenchymal progenitor stem cells can be induced to multilineage differentiation including adipo-, osteo-, neuro-, and myogenesis. Surprisingly, even mature human adipocytes, when cultured in vitro, can dedifferentiate into fibroblasts, which on expansion can be turned into lipid-synthesizing adipocytes again (140). These facts demonstrate amazing flexibility and plasticity of adipose tissue, providing hope for a therapeutic, rather than surgical, reduction in fat mass.

At first glance, inhibition of adipogenesis is an inappropriate approach to antiobesity therapy. Indeed, enhanced adipogenesis cannot cause obesity (141). Adiposity represents increased energy storage, the result of an imbalance between energy intake and energy output. Blocking differentiation of preadipocytes into adipocytes does not alter this fundamental equation. Enhanced adipogenesis in obesity is the result of energy imbalance, not the cause. Adipocytes provide a safe place to store lipids; when these cells are absent, as in lipodystrophy, lipids accumulate in muscle, liver and other locations. This is believed to cause significant metabolic derangement, including insulin resistance and hepatosteatosis, which leads to cirrhosis (142).

Following this rationale, it appears that any therapy directed toward blocking adipocyte differentiation will be counterproductive. And yet, the in vivo experimental data obtained in this author's laboratory contradict conventional wisdom. Below is the description of the experiments conducted to upregulate the expression of a transgene Wnt10b in the skeletal muscle of DIO rats.

Recent studies have suggested that Wnt/β-catenin signaling plays a role in determining the fate of mesenchymal progenitor stem cells. Wnts are a family of paracrine and autocrine factors that regulate cell growth and differentiation (143). Constitutive activation of the canonical Wnt pathway favors myogenesis over adipogenesis (144). For preadipocytes to differentiate into adipocytes, Wnt signaling needs to be actively suppressed because sustained overexpression of Wnt10b blocks adipogenesis in 3T3-L1 preadipocytes (145). In vivo, transgenic expression of Wnt10b in adipocytes results in a 50% reduction in white adipose tissue (WAT) mass and total lack of brown adipose tissue (146). Furthermore, age-related deficiency of Wnt10b is associated with increased adipogenic potential of myoblasts (147). Finally, epidemiological data suggest a possible association of Wnt10 functional

mutation (C256Y) and obesity in humans (148), which shows that the Wnt–β-catenin pathway is an important regulator of adipogenesis in vivo.

In one study, the long-term metabolic consequences of the upregulated Wnt/β-catenin signaling in skeletal muscles of adult DIO rats had been investigated (134). The long-term expression of rAAV1-Wnt10b was tested after intramuscular injection in female DIO rats. Animals fed high-fat diet and treated with rAAV1-Wnt10b showed a sustained reduction of 16% in BW accumulation compared with controls, and expression of Wnt10b was accompanied by a reduction in hyperinsulinemia and triglycerides plasma levels, as well as improved glucose homeostasis. Magnetic imaging and resonance methods revealed that ectopic expression of Wnt10b resulted in a decrease in both global and muscular fat deposits in DIO rats. The long-range effect of locally expressed Wnt10b was also manifested through the increased bone mineral density. The detailed analysis of molecular markers revealed fibroblast growth factor-4 (FGF-4) and vascular endothelial growth factor (VEGF) as possible mediators of the systemic effect of Wnt10b transgene expression. These data demonstrate that altering Wnt/β-catenin signaling in the skeletal muscle of an adult animal invokes moderate responses with a favorable metabolic profile bringing the notion of alternative therapeutic modality in the treatment of obesity, diabetes, and osteoporosis.

Anorexigenic Gut Peptides

Obviously, the most straightforward and efficient way of BW maintenance could be achieved through voluntary reduction of consumed food. Mimicking postprandial satiety by modulation of circulating gastrointestinal hormones may provide an effective means of treating obesity (149). Several hormones released from the gastrointestinal tract act as peripheral appetite-regulating signals. Oxyntomodulin and peptide tyrosine–tyrosine (PYY) are synthesized within the gastrointestinal tract in specialized enteroendocrine cells, many of which cosecrete these hormones (150). After a meal, oxyntomodulin and PYY are released synchronously (151). The rapid rise of circulating hormone levels signals a change in energy status to the brain and also acts locally to enhance digestive processes. Within the gastrointestinal tract, oxyntomodulin delays gastric emptying and decreases gastric acid secretion (152); PYY increases ileal absorption, slows gastric emptying, and delays gallbladder and pancreatic secretion.

The weight loss that has been observed in animal models after repeated administration of oxyntomodulin and PYY has led to interest in developing these peptides as antiobesity therapies in humans. Indeed, preliminary studies have found that oxyntomodulin or PYY administration reduces food intake and body weight effectively in overweight human volunteers (153–155). Oxyntomodulin and PYY could, therefore, have important roles in the control of energy balance in humans: they acutely induce satiety in the healthy, postprandial state and decrease long-term food intake in disease conditions where the gut is unable to handle nutrients, for example, during infections or after bypass surgery (156–159).

In clinical trials of oxyntomodulin and PYY supplemental therapy, the peptides are administered via intravenous infusion or by subcutaneous injections three times daily 30 minutes before a meal. Obviously, this regimen requires significant effort and dedication on a patient's part. Alternatively, a gene transfer technology would mitigate the need for daily injections. Ideally, a gut peptides gene therapy protocol should emulate a natural regulation of peptide secretion, taking into account specific posttranslational modifications pathways. Oxyntomodulin, for example, is one of the products of the glucagon gene *GCG*, which is expressed in the intestine, pancreas, and central nervous system (160). Proglucagon is cleaved by prohormone convertases 1 and 2 into different breakdown products dependent on the tissue. In the pancreas, glucagon is the primary product. Within the gut and brain, posttranslational processing of proglucagon results in the production of glicentin, glucagon-like peptide-1 and -2. Glicentin (also known as enteroglucagon) is broken down to produce oxyntomodulin. It is reasonable, therefore, to put forward a strategy of designing a gene coding only for oxyntomodulin part of the whole *GCG* sequence, targeting the delivering vector to the endocrine L cells. In fact, such vectors had been constructed in this reviewer's laboratory and successfully used for in vivo targeting stem cells that were subsequently differentiated into several cell lineages in the small intestines in mice (A. Acosta, unpublished observation).

PYY, on the other hand, is synthesized and secreted into the circulation in two forms: PYY_{1-36} and the truncated form PYY_{3-36} (161). The truncated form is thought to be the biologically active satiety signal, which is the product of cleavage of the N-terminal tyrosine and proline residues from PYY_{1-36} by dipeptidyl peptidase 4 (162). It is possible, therefore, to design a gene encoding the whole PYY_{1-36} peptide and then utilize dipeptidyl peptidase 4 within a host endocrine L cell to process prepeptide into active form to be secreted in response to physiological stimuli. The ongoing clinical trials of gut peptides' supplemental therapy will undoubtedly pave the safest way to alternative therapeutic modality in the form of gene therapy, relieving patient from a burdensome treatment routine.

Fibroblast Growth Factors

Recently, select members of the FGF family have been described as potential new drug candidates to combat metabolic diseases (163). Specifically, FGF-19 (164,165) and FGF-21 (166,167) have demonstrated an ability to increase metabolism. Transgenic mice expressing either human FGF-19 or FGF-21 exhibit reduced adiposity and resistance to diet-induced metabolic disturbances. Moreover, both FGF-19 and FGF-21 significantly improve the overall metabolic state of diet-induced or genetically modified diabetic mice when the proteins are administered systemically over time. However, although FGF-19 and FGF-21 are similar in their metabolic activity, FGF-21 is free of the proliferative and tumorigenic effects (166–168) documented for some members of FGF family (including FGF-19). When administered daily for six weeks to diabetic rhesus monkeys, FGF-21 caused a dramatic decline in fasting plasma glucose, fructosamine, triglycerides, insulin, and glucagon (169). FGF-21 administration also led to significant improvements in lipoprotein profiles, including lowering of low-density lipoprotein cholesterol and raising of high-density lipoprotein cholesterol, beneficial changes in the circulating levels of several cardiovascular risk markers/factors, and the induction of a small but significant weight loss (169).

Obesity Gene Menu a La Carte

In the genomic age of biotechnology and bioinformatics, computational methods employ data from a variety of sources to identify the most likely candidate disease genes from vast gene sets. For example, Tiffin et al. utilized seven independent computational disease gene prioritization methods and then applied them in concert to the analysis of 9556 positional candidate genes for T2DM and the related trait obesity (111). The analysis exploited the premise that genes selected by the most independent methods are least likely to be false positives or artifacts of the type of approach used. This study generated a list of nine genes selected as potential T2DM genes: four of the nine genes were located in the mitochondrion (BCKDHA, OAT, ACAA2, ECHS1); some were involved in the metabolism of fatty acids (ACAA2, ECHS1, LPL), lipids (LPL and ACAA2), amino acids (BCKDHA and OAT), and glycogen and glucose (PRKCSH and PGM1). Using same approach, a total of five genes were selected as most likely candidate genes for obesity. Two of these, LPL and BCKDHA, overlap with the set of most likely T2DM candidates, and the additional three selected as candidates for obesity only are catalase, sialidase 1, and very low-density lipoprotein receptor (111).

Mitochondrial function also can impact on rates of metabolism (170). This is most evident in muscle, a metabolically flexible tissue that switches between carbohydrate and lipid as substrates to meet the energy demands (171). Indeed, impaired mitochondrial function that directs fatty acids toward storage, as opposed to oxidation, may contribute considerably to intramyocellular lipid accumulation, which has been linked to insulin resistance in obesity and T2DM in humans.

Microarray studies have also shown that expression of nuclear-encoded mitochondrial genes involved in oxidative phosphorylation is dysregulated in tissues obtained from humans with diabetes (172–175). Moreover, oxidative phosphorylation activity and mitochondrial bioenergetic capacity are both impaired in diabetic humans (176,177). Even in insulin-resistant but normoglycemic individuals (prediabetes), expression of oxidative genes and upstream regulators is decreased (175). Taken together, these data suggest that mitochondrial dysfunction, perhaps mediated in part via changes in nuclear-encoded mitochondrial gene expression and/or function, may be a primary candidate for the restoration of energy balance.

Mitochondrial dysfunction can be due to mutations/deletions in either nuclear genes encoding mitochondrial proteins or due to mutations or deletions in mitochondrial DNA (mtDNA). Human mtDNA is a circular molecule, 16,569 bp in size, and it codes for 13 polypeptides, 22 tRNAs and 2 rRNAs. Most of the proteins functioning in the mitochondria, however, are nuclear encoded, which makes them amenable to the regular gene transfer technology. On the other hand, mitochondria-encoded proteins (such as BCKDHA, OAT, ACAA2, and ECHS1) could not be replaced by utilizing regular gene transfer protocols. The current strategy to correct mtDNA mutations is to deliver a construct of the wild-type mitochondrial gene fused to a sequence encoding a mitochondrial targeting sequence into the nucleus, followed by nuclear cytosolic expression and subsequent import of the gene product into the mitochondria. This "indirect" approach to mitochondrial gene therapy is known as *allotopic* expression (178,179). Alternatively, the therapeutic gene could be introduced directly into the matrix of the mitochondrion. This strategy has been termed "direct" mitochondrial gene therapy (180,181). Yet another strategy involves an allotopic expression of DNA repair enzymes, such as human 8-oxoguanine DNA glycosylase/apurinic lyase downstream of the mitochondrial targeting sequence from manganese superoxide dismutase. Its overexpression in mitochondria had a protective effect against free fatty acids (FFA)-induced mtDNA damage and significantly reduced FFA-induced apoptosis (182). This approach explores the hypothesis that nitrous oxide–induced mtDNA damage generated after exposure to FFA initiates a cascade of processes that ultimately lead to mitochondrial dysfunction and apoptosis. Utilizing one common DNA repair enzyme (hOGG1) allows targeting and protecting the whole mitochondrial genome and all mitochondria-encoded genes including 22 tRNAs and 2 rRNAs.

CONCLUSION

The described list of potential obesity-related gene targets is not complete and will undoubtedly expand in the near future. At a first glance, the task of picking the most promising and efficient candidate target gene is overwhelming. It is the intent of this reviewer, however, to convey an encouraging message of optimism that is based on experimental evidence accumulated in the field in general and in the reviewer's laboratory in particular. Nevertheless, embracing gene-based therapeutics will require overcoming many obstacles. It will take a significant effort from the scientific community to educate public and physicians alike on the molecular mechanisms of obesity and diabetes while encouraging behavioral compliance with healthier food choices and promoting routine physical exercise.

ACKNOWLEDGMENT

I thank my colleague Dr. Kenneth Warrington for critically reading and discussing the manuscript.

REFERENCES

1. State-Specific Prevalence of Obesity Among Adults—United States, 2005. Available at: http://www.cdc.gov/mmwr/preview/mmwrhtml/mm5536a1.htm?s_cid=mm5536a1_e.
2. Ravussin E, Valencia ME, Esparza J, et al. Effects of a traditional lifestyle on obesity in Pima Indians. Diabetes Care 1994; 17:1067–1074.
3. Rankinen T, Zuberi A, Chagnon YC, et al. The human obesity gene map: the 2005 update. Obesity (Silver Spring) 2006; 14:529–644.
4. King MC, Wilson AC. Evolution at two levels in humans and chimpanzees. Science 1975; 188:107–116.
5. Spielman RS, Bastone LA, Burdick JT, et al. Common genetic variants account for differences in gene expression among ethnic groups. Nat Genet 2007; 39:226–231.
6. Knight JC. Regulatory polymorphisms underlying complex disease traits. J Mol Med 2005; 83:97–109.
7. Redon R, Ishikawa S, Fitch KR, et al. Global variation in copy number in the human genome. Nature 2006; 444:444–454.
8. Neel JV. Diabetes mellitus: a "thrifty" genotype rendered detrimental by "progress"? 1962. Bull World Health Organ 1999; 77:694–703; discussion 692–693.
9. Speakman JR. Obesity: the integrated roles of environment and genetics. J Nutr 2004; 134:2090S–2105S.
10. Mercer JG, Speakman JR. Hypothalamic neuropeptide mechanisms for regulating energy balance: from rodent models to human obesity. Neurosci Biobehav Rev 2001; 25:101–116.

11. Keith SW, Redden DT, Katzmarzyk PT, et al. Putative contributors to the secular increase in obesity: exploring the roads less traveled. Int J Obes (Lond) 2006; 30(11): 1585–1594.

12. Gangwisch JE, Malaspina D, Boden-Albala B, et al. Inadequate sleep as a risk factor for obesity: analyses of the NHANES I. Sleep 2005; 28:1289–1296.

13. Nilsson R. Endocrine modulators in the food chain and environment. Toxicol Pathol 2000; 28:420–431.

14. Westerterp-Plantenga MS, van Marken Lichtenbelt WD, Cilissen C, et al. Energy metabolism in women during short exposure to the thermoneutral zone. Physiol Behav 2002; 75:227–235.

15. Filozof C, Fernandez Pinilla MC, Fernandez-Cruz A. Smoking cessation and weight gain. Obes Rev 2004; 5:95–103.

16. Hedley AA, Ogden CL, Johnson CL, et al. Prevalence of overweight and obesity among US children, adolescents, and adults, 1999–2002. JAMA 2004; 291:2847–2850.

17. Mathews TJ, Hamilton BE. Mean age of mother, 1970–2000. Natl Vital Stat Rep 2002; 51:1–13.

18. Patterson ML, Stern S, Crawford PB, et al. Sociodemographic factors and obesity in preadolescent black and white girls: NHLBI's Growth and Health Study. J Natl Med Assoc 1997; 89:594–600.

19. Allison DB, Paultre F, Heymsfield SB, et al. Is the intrauterine period really a critical period for the development of adiposity? Int J Obes Relat Metab Disord 1995; 19:397–402.

20. Ellis L, Haman D. Population increases in obesity appear to be partly due to genetics. J Biosoc Sci 2004; 36:547–559.

21. Hebebrand J, Wulftange H, Goerg T, et al. Epidemic obesity: are genetic factors involved via increased rates of assortative mating? Int J Obes Relat Metab Disord 2000; 24:345–353.

22. Turnbaugh PJ, Ley RE, Mahowald MA, et al. An obesity-associated gut microbiome with increased capacity for energy harvest. Nature 2006; 444:1027–1131.

23. West DB, Boozer CN, Moody DL, et al. Dietary obesity in nine inbred mouse strains. Am J Physiol 1992; 262: R1025–R1032.

24. Chang S, Graham B, Yakubu F, et al. Metabolic differences between obesity-prone and obesity-resistant rats. Am J Physiol 1990; 259:R1103–R1110.

25. Levin BE, Dunn-Meynell AA, Balkan B, et al. Selective breeding for diet-induced obesity and resistance in Sprague-Dawley rats. Am J Physiol 1997; 273: R725–R730.

26. Stunkard AJ, Harris JR, Pedersen NL, et al. The body-mass index of twins who have been reared apart. N Engl J Med 1990; 322:1483–1487.

27. Bouchard C, Perusse L. Genetics of obesity. Annu Rev Nutr 1993; 13:337–354.

28. Triscari J, Nauss-Karol C, Levin BE, et al. Changes in lipid metabolism in diet-induced obesity. Metabolism 1985; 34:580–587.

29. Levin BE. Factors promoting and ameliorating the development of obesity. Physiol Behav 2005; 86:633–639.

30. Levin BE, Triscari J, Sullivan AC. Relationship between sympathetic activity and diet-induced obesity in two rat strains. Am J Physiol 1983; 245:R364–R371.

31. Dobrian AD, Davies MJ, Prewitt RL, et al. Development of hypertension in a rat model of diet-induced obesity. Hypertension 2000; 35:1009–1015.

32. de Fourmestraux V, Neubauer H, Poussin C, et al. Transcript profiling suggests that differential metabolic adaptation of mice to a high fat diet is associated with changes in liver to muscle lipid fluxes. J Biol Chem 2004; 279:50743–50753.

33. Burcelin R, Crivelli V, Dacosta A, et al. Heterogeneous metabolic adaptation of C57BL/6J mice to high-fat diet. Am J Physiol Endocrinol Metab 2002; 282: E834–E842.

34. Rakyan VK, Blewitt ME, Druker R, et al. Metastable epialleles in mammals. Trends Genet 2002; 18:348–351.

35. DeChiara TM, Robertson EJ, Efstratiadis A. Parental imprinting of the mouse insulin-like growth factor II gene. Cell 1991; 64:849–859.

36. Reik W, Constancia M, Fowden A, et al. Regulation of supply and demand for maternal nutrients in mammals by imprinted genes. J Physiol 2003; 547:35–44.

37. Constancia M, Kelsey G, Reik W. Resourceful imprinting. Nature 2004; 432:53–57.

38. Keverne EB. Genomic imprinting and the maternal brain. Prog Brain Res 2001; 133:279–285.

39. Plagge A, Gordon E, Dean W, et al. The imprinted signaling protein XL alpha s is required for postnatal adaptation to feeding. Nat Genet 2004; 36:818–826.

40. Curley JP, Barton S, Surani A, et al. Coadaptation in mother and infant regulated by a paternally expressed imprinted gene. Proc Biol Sci 2004; 271:1303–1309.

41. Dolinoy DC, Weidman JR, Waterland RA, et al. Maternal genistein alters coat color and protects Avy mouse offspring from obesity by modifying the fetal epigenome. Environ Health Perspect 2006; 114:567–572.

42. Waterland RA, Lin JR, Smith CA, et al. Post-weaning diet affects genomic imprinting at the insulin-like growth factor 2 (Igf2) locus. Hum Mol Genet 2006; 15:705–716.

43. Waterland RA, Jirtle RL. Early nutrition, epigenetic changes at transposons and imprinted genes, and enhanced susceptibility to adult chronic diseases. Nutrition 2004; 20:63–68.

44. Rakyan VK, Chong S, Champ ME, et al. Transgenerational inheritance of epigenetic states at the murine Axin (Fu) allele occurs after maternal and paternal transmission. Proc Natl Acad Sci USA 2003; 100:2538–2543.

45. Delrue MA, Michaud JL. Fat chance: genetic syndromes with obesity. Clin Genet 2004; 66:83–93.

46. Levin BE. Metabolic imprinting: critical impact of the perinatal environment on the regulation of energy homeostasis. Philos Trans R Soc Lond B Biol Sci 2006; 361:1107–1121.

47. MacLean PS, Higgins JA, Johnson GC, et al. Enhanced metabolic efficiency contributes to weight regain after weight loss in obesity-prone rats. Am J Physiol Regul Integr Comp Physiol 2004; 287:R1306–R1315.

48. Levin BE, Keesey RE. Defense of differing body weight set points in diet-induced obese and resistant rats. Am J Physiol 1998; 274:R412–R419.

49. Levin BE, Dunn-Meynell AA, Ricci MR, et al. Abnormalities of leptin and ghrelin regulation in obesity-prone juvenile rats. Am J Physiol Endocrinol Metab 2003; 285: E949–E957.

50. Levin BE, Dunn-Meynell AA. Reduced central leptin sensitivity in rats with diet-induced obesity. Am J Physiol Regul Integr Comp Physiol 2002; 283:R941–R948.

51. Levin BE, Dunn-Meynell AA, Banks WA. Obesity-prone rats have normal blood-brain barrier transport but defective central leptin signaling before obesity onset. Am J Physiol Regul Integr Comp Physiol 2004; 286: R143–R150.

52. Clegg DJ, Benoit SC, Reed JA, et al. Reduced anorexic effects of insulin in obesity-prone rats fed a moderate-fat diet. Am J Physiol Regul Integr Comp Physiol 2005; 288: R981–R986.

53. Levin BE, Hamm MW. Plasticity of brain alpha-adrenoceptors during the development of diet-induced obesity in the rat. Obes Res 1994; 2:230–238.

54. Levin BE. Diet cycling and age alter weight gain and insulin levels in rats. Am J Physiol 1994; 267:R527–R535.

55. Levin BE. Metabolic imprinting on genetically predisposed neural circuits perpetuates obesity. Nutrition 2000; 16:909–915.

56. Dulloo AG, Calokatisa R. Adaptation to low calorie intake in obese mice: contribution of a metabolic component to diminished energy expenditures during and after weight loss. Int J Obes 1991; 15:7–16.

57. Dulloo AG, Girardier L. Adaptive changes in energy expenditure during refeeding following low-calorie intake: evidence for a specific metabolic component favoring fat storage. Am J Clin Nutr 1990; 52:415–420.

58. Hill JO, Thacker S, Newby D, et al. Influence of food restriction coupled with weight cycling on carcass energy restoration during ad-libitum refeeding. Int J Obes 1988; 12:547–555.

59. Levin BE. The drive to regain is mainly in the brain. Am J Physiol Regul Integr Comp Physiol 2004; 287: R1297–R1300.

60. Levin BE, Dunn-Meynell AA. Chronic exercise lowers the defended body weight gain and adiposity in diet-induced obese rats. Am J Physiol Regul Integr Comp Physiol 2004; 286:R771–R778.

61. Woods SC, Benoit SC, Clegg DJ, et al. Clinical endocrinology and metabolism. Regulation of energy homeostasis by peripheral signals. Best Pract Res Clin Endocrinol Metab 2004; 18:497–515.

62. Niswender KD, Schwartz MW. Insulin and leptin revisited: adiposity signals with overlapping physiological and intracellular signaling capabilities. Front Neuroendocrinol 2003; 24:1–10.

63. MacLean PS, Higgins JA, Jackman MR, et al. Peripheral metabolic responses to prolonged weight reduction that promote rapid, efficient regain in obesity-prone rats. Am J Physiol Regul Integr Comp Physiol 2006; 290: R1577–R1588.

64. Weinshilboum R, Wang L. Pharmacogenomics: bench to bedside. Nat Rev Drug Discov 2004; 3:739–748.

65. Mah C, Byrne BJ, Flotte TR. Virus-based gene delivery systems. Clin Pharmacokinet 2002; 41:901–911.

66. Walther W, Stein U. Viral vectors for gene transfer: a review of their use in the treatment of human diseases. Drugs 2000; 60:249–271.

67. Tenenbaum L, Lehtonen E, Monahan PE. Evaluation of risks related to the use of adeno-associated virus-based vectors. Curr Gene Ther 2003; 3:545–565.

68. Grimm D, Kay MA. From virus evolution to vector revolution: use of naturally occurring serotypes of adeno-associated virus (AAV) as novel vectors for human gene therapy. Curr Gene Ther 2003; 3:281–304.

69. Sanlioglu S, Monick MM, Luleci G, et al. Rate limiting steps of AAV transduction and implications for human gene therapy. Curr Gene Ther 2001; 1:137–147.

70. McCarty DM, Young Jr SM, Samulski RJ. Integration of Adeno-Associated Virus (AAV) and Recombinant AAV Vectors. Annu Rev Genet 2004; 38:819–845.

71. Warrington KH, Jr., Herzog RW. Treatment of human disease by adeno-associated viral gene transfer. Hum Genet 2006; 119:571–603.

72. Kaplitt MG, Feigin A, Tang C, et al. Safety and tolerability of gene therapy with an adeno-associated virus (AAV) borne GAD gene for Parkinson's disease: an open label, phase I trial. Lancet 2007; 369:2097–2105.

73. Gao G, Alvira MR, Somanathan S, et al. Adeno-associated viruses undergo substantial evolution in primates during natural infections. Proc Natl Acad Sci U S A 2003; 100:6081–6086.

74. Gao GP, Alvira MR, Wang L, et al. Novel adeno-associated viruses from rhesus monkeys as vectors for human gene therapy. Proc Natl Acad Sci U S A 2002; 99:11854–11859.

75. Nakai H, Fuess S, Storm TA, et al. Unrestricted hepatocyte transduction with adeno-associated virus serotype 8 vectors in mice. J Virol 2005; 79:214–224.

76. Hildinger M, Auricchio A, Gao G, et al. Hybrid vectors based on adeno-associated virus serotypes 2 and 5 for muscle-directed gene transfer. J Virol 2001; 75: 6199–6203.

77. Rabinowitz JE, Rolling F, Li C, et al. Cross-packaging of a single adeno-associated virus (AAV) type 2 vector genome into multiple AAV serotypes enables transduction with broad specificity. J Virol 2002; 76:791–801.

78. Hauck B, Chen L, Xiao W. Generation and characterization of chimeric recombinant AAV vectors. Mol Ther 2003; 7:419–425.

79. Rabinowitz JE, Bowles DE, Faust SM, et al. Cross-dressing the virion: the transcapsidation of adeno-associated virus serotypes functionally defines subgroups. J Virol 2004; 78: 4421–4432.

80. Wu P, Xiao W, Conlon T, et al. Mutational analysis of the adeno-associated virus type 2 (AAV2) capsid gene and construction of AAV2 vectors with altered tropism. J Virol 2000; 74:8635–8647.

81. Muller OJ, Kaul F, Weitzman MD, et al. Random peptide libraries displayed on adeno-associated virus to select for targeted gene therapy vectors. Nat Biotechnol 2003; 21:1040–1046.

82. Girod A, Ried M, Wobus C, et al. Genetic capsid modifications allow efficient re-targeting of adeno-associated virus type 2. Nat Med 1999; 5:1052–1056.

83. Nicklin SA, Buening H, Dishart KL, et al. Efficient and selective AAV2-mediated gene transfer directed to human vascular endothelial cells. Mol Ther 2001; 4:174–181.

84. Shi W, Arnold GS, Bartlett JS. Insertional mutagenesis of the adeno-associated virus type 2 (AAV2) capsid gene and generation of AAV2 vectors targeted to alternative cell-surface receptors. Hum Gene Ther 2001; 12:1697–1711.

85. Grifman M, Trepel M, Speece P, et al. Incorporation of tumor-targeting peptides into recombinant adeno-associated virus capsids. Mol Ther 2001; 3:964–975.

86. Ried MU, Girod A, Leike K, et al. Adeno-associated virus capsids displaying immunoglobulin-binding domains permit antibody-mediated vector retargeting to specific cell surface receptors. J Virol 2002; 76:4559–4566.

87. Perabo L, Buning H, Kofler DM, et al. In vitro selection of viral vectors with modified tropism: the adeno-associated virus display. Mol Ther 2003; 8:151–157.

88. Zoltick PW, Wilson JM. Regulated gene expression in gene therapy. Ann N Y Acad Sci 2001; 953:53–63.

89. Weber W, Fussenegger M. Artificial mammalian gene regulation networks-novel approaches for gene therapy and bioengineering. J Biotechnol 2002; 98:161–187.

90. Weber W, Fussenegger M. Inducible gene expression in mammalian cells and mice. Methods Mol Biol 2004; 267:451–466.

91. Pollock R, Clackson T. Dimerizer-regulated gene expression. Curr Opin Biotechnol 2002; 13:459–467.

92. Zeng Y, Cai X, Cullen BR. Use of RNA polymerase II to transcribe artificial microRNAs. Methods Enzymol 2005; 392:371–380.

93. Fire A, Xu S, Montgomery MK, et al. Potent and specific genetic interference by double-stranded RNA in Caenorhabditis elegans. Nature 1998; 391:806–811.

94. Elbashir SM, Harborth J, Lendeckel W, et al. Duplexes of 21-nucleotide RNAs mediate RNA interference in cultured mammalian cells. Nature 2001; 411:494–498.

95. Caplen NJ, Parrish S, Imani F, et al. Specific inhibition of gene expression by small double-stranded RNAs in invertebrate and vertebrate systems. Proc Natl Acad Sci U S A 2001; 98:9742–9747.

96. Dorsett Y, Tuschl T. siRNAs: applications in functional genomics and potential as therapeutics. Nat Rev Drug Discov 2004; 3:318–329.

97. Sioud M. Therapeutic siRNAs. Trends Pharmacol Sci 2004; 25:22–28.

98. Caplen NJ. RNAi quashes polyQ. Nat Med 2004; 10:775–776.

99. Engels BM, Hutvagner G. Principles and effects of microRNA-mediated post-transcriptional gene regulation. Oncogene 2006; 25:6163–6169.

100. Berns K, Hijmans EM, Mullenders J, et al. A large-scale RNAi screen in human cells identifies new components of the p53 pathway. Nature 2004; 428:431–437.

101. Paddison PJ, Silva JM, Conklin DS, et al. A resource for large-scale RNA-interference-based screens in mammals. Nature 2004; 428:427–431.

102. Hosono T, Mizuguchi H, Katayama K, et al. Adenovirus vector-mediated doxycycline-inducible RNA interference. Hum Gene Ther 2004; 15:813–819.

103. Matta H, Hozayev B, Tomar R, et al. Use of lentiviral vectors for delivery of small interfering RNA. Cancer Biol Ther 2003; 2:206–210.

104. Tomar RS, Matta H, Chaudhary PM. Use of adeno-associated viral vector for delivery of small interfering RNA. Oncogene 2003; 22:5712–5715.

105. Wiznerowicz M, Szulc J, Trono D. Tuning silence: conditional systems for RNA interference. Nat Methods 2006; 3:682–688.

106. Li LC, Okino ST, Zhao H, et al. Small dsRNAs induce transcriptional activation in human cells. Proc Natl Acad Sci U S A 2006; 103:17337–17342.

107. Janowski BA, Younger ST, Hardy DB, et al. Activating gene expression in mammalian cells with promoter-targeted duplex RNAs. Nat Chem Biol 2007; 3:166–173.

108. Yan H, Yuan W, Velculescu VE, et al. Allelic variation in human gene expression. Science 2002; 297:1143.

109. Pastinen T, Sladek R, Gurd S, et al. A survey of genetic and epigenetic variation affecting human gene expression. Physiol Genomics 2004; 16:184–193.

110. Bray NJ, Buckland PR, Owen MJ, et al. Cis-acting variation in the expression of a high proportion of genes in human brain. Hum Genet 2003; 113:149–153.

111. Tiffin N, Adie E, Turner F, et al. Computational disease gene identification: a concert of methods prioritizes type 2 diabetes and obesity candidate genes. Nucleic Acids Res 2006; 34:3067–3081.

112. Halaas JL, Boozer C, Blair-West J, et al. Physiological response to long-term peripheral and central leptin infusion in lean and obese mice. Proc Natl Acad Sci U S A 1997; 94:8878–8883.

113. Ahima RS, Flier JS. Leptin. Annu Rev Physiol 2000; 62:413–437.

114. Scarpace PJ, Matheny M, Zhang Y, et al. Leptin-induced leptin resistance reveals separate roles for the anorexic and thermogenic responses in weight maintenance. Endocrinology 2002; 143:3026–3035.

115. Scarpace PJ, Matheny M, Zhang Y, et al. Central leptin gene delivery evokes persistent leptin signal transduction in young and aged-obese rats but physiological responses become attenuated over time in aged-obese rats. Neuropharmacology 2002; 42:548–561.

116. Prima V, Tennant M, Gorbatyuk OS, et al. Differential modulation of energy balance by leptin, ciliary neurotrophic factor, and leukemia inhibitory factor gene delivery: microarray deoxyribonucleic acid-chip analysis of gene expression. Endocrinology 2004; 145:2035–2045.

117. Munzberg H, Flier JS, Bjorbaek C. Region-specific leptin resistance within the hypothalamus of diet-induced obese mice. Endocrinology 2004; 145:4880–4889.

118. Gorden P, Gavrilova O. The clinical uses of leptin. Curr Opin Pharmacol 2003; 3:655–659.

119. Murphy JE, Zhou S, Giese K, et al. Long-term correction of obesity and diabetes in genetically obese mice by a single intramuscular injection of recombinant adeno-associated

virus encoding mouse leptin. Proc Natl Acad Sci USA 1997; 94:13921–13926.

120. Gloaguen I, Costa P, Demartis A, et al. Ciliary neurotrophic factor corrects obesity and diabetes associated with leptin deficiency and resistance. Proc Natl Acad Sci USA 1997; 94:6456–6461.

121. Lambert PD, Anderson KD, Sleeman MW, et al. Ciliary neurotrophic factor activates leptin-like pathways and reduces body fat, without cachexia or rebound weight gain, even in leptin-resistant obesity. Proc Natl Acad Sci U S A 2001; 98:4652–4657.

122. Ettinger MP, Littlejohn TW, Schwartz SL, et al. Recombinant variant of ciliary neurotrophic factor for weight loss in obese adults: a randomized, dose-ranging study. Jama 2003; 289:1826–1832.

123. Bok D, Yasumura D, Matthes MT, et al. Effects of adeno-associated virus-vectored ciliary neurotrophic factor on retinal structure and function in mice with a P216L rds/peripherin mutation. Exp Eye Res 2002; 74:719–735.

124. Minokoshi Y, Kim YB, Peroni OD, et al. Leptin stimulates fatty-acid oxidation by activating AMP-activated protein kinase. Nature 2002; 415:339–343.

125. Hardie DG. The AMP-activated protein kinase cascade: the key sensor of cellular energy status. Endocrinology 2003; 144:5179–5183.

126. Hardie DG. AMP-activated protein kinase: a master switch in glucose and lipid metabolism. Rev Endocr Metab Disord 2004; 5:119–125.

127. Shklyaev S, Aslanidi G, Tennant M, et al. Sustained peripheral expression of transgene adiponectin offsets the development of diet-induced obesity in rats. Proc Natl Acad Sci U S A 2003; 100:14217–14222.

128. Scherer PE, Williams S, Fogliano M, et al. A novel serum protein similar to C1q, produced exclusively in adipocytes. J Biol Chem 1995; 270:26746–26749.

129. Tsao TS, Lodish HF, Fruebis J. ACRP30, a new hormone controlling fat and glucose metabolism. Eur J Pharmacol 2002; 440:213–221.

130. Hu E, Liang P, Spiegelman BM. AdipoQ is a novel adipose-specific gene dysregulated in obesity. J Biol Chem 1996; 271:10697–10703.

131. Arita Y, Kihara S, Ouchi N, et al. Paradoxical decrease of an adipose-specific protein, adiponectin, in obesity. Biochem Biophys Res Commun 1999; 257:79–83.

132. Berg AH, Combs TP, Scherer PE. ACRP30/adiponectin: an adipokine regulating glucose and lipid metabolism. Trends Endocrinol Metab 2002; 13:84–89.

133. Yamauchi T, Kamon J, Waki H, et al. The fat-derived hormone adiponectin reverses insulin resistance associated with both lipoatrophy and obesity. Nat Med 2001; 7: 941–946.

134. Aslanidi G, Kroutov V, Philipsberg G, et al. Ectopic expression of Wnt10b decreases adiposity and improves glucose homeostasis in obese rats. Am J Physiol Endocrinol Metab 2007; 293(3):E726–736.

135. Despres JP, Golay A, Sjostrom L. Effects of rimonabant on metabolic risk factors in overweight patients with dyslipidemia. N Engl J Med 2005; 353:2121–2134.

136. Miyazaki M, Ntambi JM. Role of stearoyl-coenzyme A desaturase in lipid metabolism. Prostaglandins Leukot Essent Fatty Acids 2003; 68:113–121.

137. Cohen P, Miyazaki M, Socci ND, et al. Role for stearoyl-CoA desaturase-1 in leptin-mediated weight loss. Science 2002; 297:240–243.

138. Rahman SM, Dobrzyn A, Dobrzyn P, et al. Stearoyl-CoA desaturase 1 deficiency elevates insulin-signaling components and down-regulates protein-tyrosine phosphatase 1B in muscle. Proc Natl Acad Sci U S A 2003; 100: 11110–11115.

139. Dobrzyn P, Dobrzyn A, Miyazaki M, et al. Stearoyl-CoA desaturase 1 deficiency increases fatty acid oxidation by activating AMP-activated protein kinase in liver. Proc Natl Acad Sci U S A 2004; 101:6409–6414.

140. Tholpady SS, Aojanepong C, Llull R, et al. The cellular plasticity of human adipocytes. Ann Plast Surg 2005; 54:651–656.

141. Rosen ED, Macdougald OA. Adipocyte differentiation from the inside out. Nat Rev Mol Cell Biol 2006; 7:885–896.

142. Unger RH. Minireview: weapons of lean body mass destruction: the role of ectopic lipids in the metabolic syndrome. Endocrinology 2003; 144:5159–5165.

143. Cadigan KM, Nusse R. Wnt signaling, a common theme in animal development. Genes Dev 1997; 11:3286–3305.

144. Ross SE, Hemati N, Longo KA, et al. Inhibition of adipogenesis by Wnt signaling. Science 2000; 289: 950–953.

145. Bennett CN, Ross SE, Longo KA, et al. Regulation of Wnt signaling during adipogenesis. J Biol Chem 2002; 277:30998–31004.

146. Longo KA, Wright WS, Kang S, et al. Wnt10b inhibits development of white and brown adipose tissues. J Biol Chem 2004; 279:35503–35509.

147. Taylor-Jones JM, McGehee RE, Rando TA, et al. Activation of an adipogenic program in adult myoblasts with age. Mech Ageing Dev 2002; 123:649–661.

148. Christodoulides C, Scarda A, Granzotto M, et al. WNT10B mutations in human obesity. Diabetologia 2006; 49:678–684.

149. Stanley S, Wynne K, McGowan B, et al. Hormonal regulation of food intake. Physiol Rev 2005; 85:1131–1158.

150. Taylor RG, Beveridge DJ, Fuller PJ. Expression of ileal glucagon and peptide tyrosine-tyrosine genes. Response to inhibition of polyamine synthesis in the presence of massive small-bowel resection. Biochem J 1992; 286(pt 3): 737–741.

151. Anini Y, Fu-Cheng X, Cuber JC, et al. Comparison of the postprandial release of peptide YY and proglucagon-derived peptides in the rat. Pflugers Arch 1999; 438:299–306.

152. Schjoldager BT, Baldissera FG, Mortensen PE, et al. Oxyntomodulin: a potential hormone from the distal gut. Pharmacokinetics and effects on gastric acid and insulin secretion in man. Eur J Clin Invest 1988; 18:499–503.

153. Wynne K, Park AJ, Small CJ, et al. Subcutaneous oxyntomodulin reduces body weight in overweight and obese

subjects: a double-blind, randomized, controlled trial. Diabetes 2005; 54:2390–2395.

154. Wynne K, Bloom SR. The role of oxyntomodulin and peptide tyrosine-tyrosine (PYY) in appetite control. Nat Clin Pract Endocrinol Metab 2006; 2:612–620.

155. Batterham RL, Cowley MA, Small CJ, et al. Gut hormone PYY(3-36) physiologically inhibits food intake. Nature 2002; 418:650–654.

156. Besterman HS, Cook GC, Sarson DL, et al. Gut hormones in tropical malabsorption. Br Med J 1979; 2:1252–1255.

157. Naslund E, Gryback P, Hellstrom PM, et al. Gastrointestinal hormones and gastric emptying 20 years after jejunoileal bypass for massive obesity. Int J Obes Relat Metab Disord 1997; 21:387–392.

158. Holst JJ, Sorensen TI, Andersen AN, et al. Plasma enteroglucagon after jejunoileal bypass with 3:1 or 1:3 jejunoileal ratio. Scand J Gastroenterol 1979; 14:205–207.

159. Adrian TE, Savage AP, Bacarese-Hamilton AJ, et al. Peptide YY abnormalities in gastrointestinal diseases. Gastroenterology 1986; 90:379–384.

160. Tang-Christensen M, Vrang N, Larsen PJ. Glucagon-like peptide containing pathways in the regulation of feeding behaviour. Int J Obes Relat Metab Disord 2001; 25(suppl 5): S42–S47.

161. Grandt D, Schimiczek M, Beglinger C, et al. Two molecular forms of peptide YY (PYY) are abundant in human blood: characterization of a radioimmunoassay recognizing PYY 1-36 and PYY 3-36. Regul Pept 1994; 51:151–159.

162. Mentlein R, Dahms P, Grandt D, et al. Proteolytic processing of neuropeptide Y and peptide YY by dipeptidyl peptidase IV. Regul Pept 1993; 49:133–144.

163. Zhang X, Ibrahimi OA, Olsen SK, et al. Receptor specificity of the fibroblast growth factor family. The complete mammalian FGF family. J Biol Chem 2006; 281: 15694–15700.

164. Fu L, John LM, Adams SH, et al. Fibroblast growth factor 19 increases metabolic rate and reverses dietary and leptin-deficient diabetes. Endocrinology 2004; 145:2594–2603.

165. Tomlinson E, Fu L, John L, et al. Transgenic mice expressing human fibroblast growth factor-19 display increased metabolic rate and decreased adiposity. Endocrinology 2002; 143:1741–1747.

166. Kharitonenkov A, Shiyanova TL, Koester A, et al. FGF-21 as a novel metabolic regulator. J Clin Invest 2005; 115:1627–1635.

167. Wente W, Efanov AM, Brenner M, et al. Fibroblast growth factor-21 improves pancreatic beta-cell function and survival by activation of extracellular signal-regulated kinase 1/2 and Akt signaling pathways. Diabetes 2006; 55:2470–2478.

168. Huang X, Yu C, Jin C, et al. Forced expression of hepatocyte-specific fibroblast growth factor 21 delays initiation of chemically induced hepatocarcinogenesis. Mol Carcinog 2006; 45:934–942.

169. Kharitonenkov A, Wroblewski VJ, Koester A, et al. The metabolic state of diabetic monkeys is regulated by fibroblast growth factor-21. Endocrinology 2007; 148:774–781.

170. Lagouge M, Argmann C, Gerhart-Hines Z, et al. Resveratrol improves mitochondrial function and protects against metabolic disease by activating SIRT1 and PGC-1alpha. Cell 2006; 127:1109–1122.

171. Kelly DP, Scarpulla RC. Transcriptional regulatory circuits controlling mitochondrial biogenesis and function. Genes Dev 2004; 18:357–368.

172. Mootha VK, Lindgren CM, Eriksson KF, et al. PGC-1alpha-responsive genes involved in oxidative phosphorylation are coordinately downregulated in human diabetes. Nat Genet 2003; 34:267–273.

173. Antonetti DA, Reynet C, Kahn CR. Increased expression of mitochondrial-encoded genes in skeletal muscle of humans with diabetes mellitus. J Clin Invest 1995; 95:1383–1388.

174. Sreekumar R, Halvatsiotis P, Schimke JC, et al. Gene expression profile in skeletal muscle of type 2 diabetes and the effect of insulin treatment. Diabetes 2002; 51:1913–1920.

175. Patti ME, Butte AJ, Crunkhorn S, et al. Coordinated reduction of genes of oxidative metabolism in humans with insulin resistance and diabetes, Potential role of PGC1 and NRF1. Proc Natl Acad Sci U S A 2003; 100:8466–8471.

176. Simoneau JA, Kelley DE. Altered glycolytic and oxidative capacities of skeletal muscle contribute to insulin resistance in NIDDM. J Appl Physiol 1997; 83:166–171.

177. Kelley DE, He J, Menshikova EV, et al. Dysfunction of mitochondria in human skeletal muscle in type 2 diabetes. Diabetes 2002; 51:2944–2950.

178. Nakabeppu Y. Regulation of intracellular localization of human MTH1, OGG1, and MYH proteins for repair of oxidative DNA damage. Prog Nucleic Acid Res Mol Biol 2001; 68:75–94.

179. Zullo SJ. Gene therapy of mitochondrial DNA mutations: a brief, biased history of allotopic expression in mammalian cells. Semin Neurol 2001; 21:327–335.

180. D'Souza GG, Weissig V. Approaches to mitochondrial gene therapy. Curr Gene Ther 2004; 4:317–328.

181. Weissig V, Torchilin VP. Towards mitochondrial gene therapy: DQAsomes as a strategy. J Drug Target 2001; 9:1–13.

182. Rachek LI, Thornley NP, Grishko VI, et al. Protection of INS-1 cells from free fatty acid-induced apoptosis by targeting hOGG1 to mitochondria. Diabetes 2006; 55:1022–1028.

30

Prevention and Management of Dyslipidemia and the Metabolic Syndrome in Obese Patients

SCOTT M. GRUNDY

Center for Human Nutrition, University of Texas Southwestern Medical Center at Dallas, Dallas, Texas, U.S.A.

INTRODUCTION

The increasing prevalence of obesity in the United States and worldwide is a cause for great concern, both for the health of individuals and for national health care systems (1). The underlying causes of the obesity epidemic are largely the product of what might be called "progress" in human civilization. These include increased availability of inexpensive food, urbanization, and technological advances that promote sedentary lifestyles (see chap. 13). The combination of increased availability of food and lessened demand for physical activity produce the progressive increase in body weight of individuals throughout the world. The public health consequences of these changes are enormous and pose a challenge to health policy at every level. A fundamental question has emerged: *How do we approach the emerging epidemic of obesity?*

The medical and psychological complications to which obesity can contribute are far-reaching. Obesity can adversely affect many body systems as well as behavior. Immediate effects can be a decrease in self-respect, lack of social acceptance, and loss of a feeling of well-being. In the long term, obesity contributes to several chronic diseases that can shorten life. Among these are cardiovascular disease (CVD) and adult-onset (type 2) diabetes. Type 2 diabetes results in myriad secondary complications,

including heart failure, kidney failure, loss of limbs, and infections. Obesity also predisposes one to gallstones, sleep apnea, osteoarthritis, and various gynecological problems. Thus, among risk factors for chronic disease, obesity is near the top of the list (2).

PREVENTION OF OBESITY: THE ULTIMATE GOAL

A high priority for health care in our society is to prevent the development of mass population obesity. Prevention strategy is directed first toward factors leading to obesity in childhood, adolescence, and young adulthood. Nonetheless, prevention must extend into middle age and the later years, where changes in body composition accentuate the adverse effects of excess body fat. Once obesity becomes established, attention must turn to reducing excess weight as well as to preventing further weight gain. At this time too, medical intervention must aim to prevent the complications of obesity, particularly CVD and type 2 diabetes. This chapter will briefly address prevention of obesity in the general population and will then focus on the clinical management of overweight/obese patients, with particular attention to preventing medical complications.

In the approach to the problem of obesity, a clear distinction cannot be drawn between "prevention" and "treatment." Except when severe obesity is present, obesity per se does not cause physical limitation. Instead, associated medical problems usually develop insidiously over a period of many years. Once obesity is established, aims of management are twofold: (i) prevention of the medical complications and (ii) elimination of excess body fat. Unfortunately, clinical weight-reduction therapy has met with only limited success. Certainly, with therapy some obese patients will effectively lose weight, others will lose small amounts, and some will be able to prevent further weight gain, but still others will continue to gain weight. Efforts to achieve weight reduction are warranted, but in view of the limited success of weight reduction programs other than surgery, parallel intervention to prevent the complications of obesity must come into play.

COMPLICATIONS OF OBESITY AND THE METABOLIC SYNDROME

The complications of obesity—psychological, functional, and metabolic—are listed in Tables 1 and 2. In many social circles, obesity is not acceptable. Its presence, although common, still leads to social discrimination, followed by feelings of psychological inadequacy and guilt. If obesity is severe, it can impair mobility and musculoskeletal function. But the major health consequences of obesity lie in the metabolic sphere. The metabolic abnormalities induced by obesity frequently contribute to CVD, type 2 diabetes, fatty liver, gallstones, and polycystic ovary syndrome, among others (3–8).

Of particular importance for cardiovascular risk, obesity is almost always present in persons who manifest an aggregation of cardiovascular risk factors called the

Table 1 ATP III Classification of LDL, Total, and HDL Cholesterol (mg/dL)

LDL cholesterol—primary target of therapy	
<100	Optimal
100–129	Near optimal/above optimal
130–159	Borderline high
160–189	High
≥190	Very high
Total cholesterol	
<200	Desirable
200–239	Borderline high
≥240	High
HDL cholesterol	
<40	Low
≥60	High

Abbreviations: LDL, low-density lipoprotein; HDL, high-density lipoprotein.

Table 2 Classification of Major Nonlipid Risk Factors

Cigarette smoking (any smoking in past year)
Hypertension (BP ≥140/90 mmHg or on antihypertensive medication)
Low HDL cholesterol (40 mg/dL)[a]
Family history of premature CHD (CHD in male first-degree relative <55 yr, CHD in female first-degree relative (<65 yr)
Age (men ≥45 yr, women ≥55 yr)

[a]HDL cholesterol ≥60 mg/dL counts as a "negative" risk factor: its presence removes one risk factor from the total count.
Abbreviations: HDL, high-density lipoprotein; CHD, coronary heart disease.

metabolic syndrome (9–12). In the United States, this syndrome is emerging as a major contributor to CVD. In addition, it commonly precedes the development of type 2 diabetes (13). The metabolic syndrome typically consists of two underlying risk factors and five metabolic risk factors (14). Various combinations of these risk factors can occur in one individual to enhance cardiovascular risk.

The metabolic syndrome received increased emphasis as a major, multifaceted cardiovascular risk factor in the National Cholesterol Education Program's Adult Treatment Panel III (ATP III) report (14). ATP III chooses the term "metabolic syndrome" over others that have been used. Some of the other terms are "insulin resistance syndrome," "syndrome X" (or "metabolic syndrome X"), "multiple metabolic syndrome" or "dysmetabolic syndrome," and "deadly quartet."

ATP III favored "metabolic syndrome" because it is the most widely used and seems to apply most directly to clinical practice. Multiple metabolic syndrome and dysmetabolic syndrome are employed less frequently. Syndrome X offers some confusion with the cardiac syndrome X ("microvascular angina"); also, it does not point to a metabolic origin. Endocrinologists and diabetologists often prefer the "insulin resistance syndrome," which focuses on the common association between multiple risk factors and the presence of insulin resistance. On the other hand, that insulin resistance directly causes this syndrome has not been documented.

The causes of the metabolic syndrome have not been fully elucidated. Nonetheless, obesity and lack of physical activity are important underlying causes (9). The syndrome appears to arise in large part out of an overloading of tissues, particularly the liver and muscle, with lipid. With obesity, nonesterified fatty acids (NEFAs) are elevated; these excess NEFAs provide more energy substrate than is needed for normal metabolism. The accumulation of lipid in both liver and muscle contributes importantly to both insulin resistance and the metabolic syndrome. Beyond obesity and physical inactivity, however, genetic factors also are involved. The role of genetics is demonstrated by the variable expression of the metabolic syndrome in the presence of obesity and physical inactivity. Severity of the several risk factors of the syndrome varies widely among individuals and populations. The high prevalence of the metabolic syndrome, coronary heart disease (CHD), and type 2 diabetes in people of South Asian origin provides strong evidence that genetic factors play a role (15). Reasons for the increased CVD risk in persons with metabolic syndrome remain to be fully understood. The specific role of each risk factor has been difficult to determine. Even so, most of the risk factors associated with this syndrome appear to have atherogenic potential. Thus, the increased risk for CVD in patients with the metabolic syndrome almost certainly derives from multiple factors.

PUBLIC HEALTH APPROACHES TO PRIMARY PREVENTION OF OBESITY

Prevention of Childhood and Adolescent Obesity

Obesity in childhood and adolescence is increasing at an alarming rate (1) (see chap. 9). This increase appears to be largely due to social changes. Nowadays children generally do not walk to school. Compared with years past, less time is devoted to physical activity in school. After school, children have fewer opportunities for playing outside. Many go straight home and lock themselves in, waiting for parents to come home from work. At home, they settle down into chairs and watch television, and their consumption of snack food is very common. Internet "surfing" and video-game play commonly take time away from outside activities (16). The availability of cheap food enhances caloric intake. When busy parents return home at night, they often prefer eating out to preparing healthy meals at home. A trip for hamburgers or pizza typically provides both diversion and unneeded calories. All of these factors combine to promote weight gain in children and adolescents.

To reverse these trends, it will be necessary to bring about major changes in the behavior of society as well as individuals (17). New recreational facilities are needed to promote physical activity. Safe havens for physical play are required. Schools need to spend more time in teaching healthy life habits. Parents must be made aware of how to improve the household to reduce the tendency for weight gain in the family. School lunches should be modified to be less calorically dense as well as healthier. These social issues will require a concerted effort at local, state, and national levels.

The medical model for treatment of obesity in childhood so far has had only limited success. Reports of success in achieving weight loss through professional intervention for individual obese children have not been

encouraging. Thus, to deal with the problem of population childhood obesity, the social changes described above undoubtedly will be required.

Prevention of Obesity in Adults

Many people make it through adolescence without developing obesity. In fact, in our society, a great deal of weight gain typically occurs between ages 20 and 50 years. This gain is the result of several factors: decreasing physical activity, "stress" eating at both home and work, and for women, weight gain with pregnancy (18–20). The increase of body weight during young adulthood lays the foundation for the medical consequences of obesity.

Prevention of adult-onset obesity again must focus on social factors. Here, public education and enhanced awareness of the dangers of weight gain are needed. Many young adults are not yet tuned to the health drawbacks of obesity, and they fail to take precautions to avoid it at this stage. Consequently, a more intensive educational effort for this age range is required. Adults must restructure their lives to allow more time for exercise, to minimize use of "labor-saving devices," and to limit portion sizes of their food choices. Whether large-scale social changes beyond education can be brought into play to prevent obesity in adults is uncertain.

After age 50, many people do not gain further weight. Although weight gain can occur, overweight and obesity assume a new dimension in the later stages of life. Even when absolute weight does not increase, changes in body composition begin to accelerate. Foremost is decline in muscle mass (12,21,22). As a result, the ratio of adipose tissue to muscle usually is higher in older people than in middle age. This shifts the metabolic balance in ways that favor the development of insulin resistance and the metabolic syndrome (23–25). Loss of muscle mass is brought about in part by an increasingly sedentary lifestyle. In addition, metabolic changes that accompany aging, which are not well understood, probably play a role. In any case, loss of muscle mass makes older people more susceptible to the health consequences of obesity.

CLINICAL MANAGEMENT OF ADULTS WITH ESTABLISHED OBESITY

Clinical treatment of obesity in childhood and adolescence is beyond the scope of this chapter (see chap. 37). The Obesity Education Initiative (OEI) of the National Institutes of Health provides a reasonable approach to the management of adults with established obesity (3,4). Similar guidelines are available from other sources (4). The OEI report focused primarily on weight reduction strategies; although it indicated the need to evaluate coexisting risk factors, it did not directly recommend their management before instituting weight reduction. The ATP III report, on the other hand, placed a priority on initiating therapies for risk factors before dealing with the problem of obesity. ATP III contends that risk factors typically impart a more immediate risk to patients than does obesity itself; thus, risk factor control takes precedence in clinical management. The present chapter will attempt to integrate the OEI and ATP III reports so as to facilitate both weight reduction and treatment of metabolic risk factors. Both OEI and ATP III base their recommendations on available scientific evidence. They contain a large number of references and evidence tables. They are both available on the National Heart Lung and Blood Institute (NHLBI) Web site (26). The current chapter summarizes key features of these guidelines but does not detail the literature available in the reports. This literature can be obtained from the Web site or corresponding publications of the reports.

CLINICAL ASSESSMENT OF PERSONS WHO ARE OVERWEIGHT OR OBESE

Clinical management of overweight/obese patients includes identification of risk factors, among which are several body weight parameters and detection of comorbidities accompanying excess body weight (see chaps. 1 and 3).

Assessment of Risk Factors

Overall, the greatest danger of overweight/obesity is the development of CVD. Moreover, in the long term, obesity predisposes one to type 2 diabetes, which is itself a risk factor for CVD. ATP III provides a useful classification for lipid and nonlipid risk factors. These classifications are shown in Tables 1 and 2, respectively. In ATP III, estimates are made of a person's absolute risk using Framingham risk scoring, which is available through the NHLBI (27). This scoring estimates the 10-year risk for developing myocardial infarction or coronary death. It is based on absolute levels of the following risk factors: total cholesterol, high-density lipoprotein (HDL) cholesterol, blood pressure, smoking history, and age. Framingham scoring can be carried out by manual scoring or with a simple computer program, both of which are available on the NHLBI Web site. In addition, ATP III defines the metabolic syndrome for clinical practice according to five clinical features (Table 3). According to ATP III, three of five of these clinical features constitute a clinical diagnosis of the metabolic syndrome. In addition, however, it was recognized that there are other "hidden" metabolic risk factors. These are risk factors that are not routinely

Table 3 The Essential Features of the Metabolic Syndrome

Underlying risk factors
Obesity (especially abdominal obesity)
Physical inactivity
Metabolic risk factors
Atherogenic dyslipidemia
Elevated blood pressure
Insulin resistance + elevated plasma glucose
Prothrombotic state
Proinflammatory state

detected in clinical practice but could be identified with special testing. They include the following:

- Insulin resistance (with elevated plasma insulin)
- Prothrombotic state [with elevated plasma fibrinogen and plasminogen activator inhibitor-1 (PAI-1)]
- Proinflammatory state [with elevated high-sensitivity C-reactive protein (hs-CRP)]
- Fatty liver

Assessment for Underlying Risk Factors

Overweight/Obesity

Body mass index

According to the OEI report (3,4) (chap. 1), overweight is defined as a body mass index (BMI) of 25 to 29.9 kg/m² and obesity by a BMI of 30 kg/m². Several methods can be used to calculate total body fat: total body water, total body potassium, bioelectrical impedance, and dual-energy X-ray absorptiometry. However, in the clinical setting, BMI is the best indicator of body fat, and the BMI provides a more accurate measure of total body fat than does weight alone. Nonetheless, simply measuring body weight is a practical approach to monitor weight changes. A patient should be weighed with shoes off and clad only in a light robe or undergarments.
The BMI is calculated as follows:

$$BMI = weight\,(kg)\,divided\,by\,height\,squared\,(m^2)$$

To estimate BMI from pounds and inches use

$$[weight\,(lb)/height\,(in)^2] \times 703\,(1\,lb = 0.4536\,kg)\,(1\,in = 2.54\,cm = 0.0254\,m)$$

The relation between BMI and disease risk varies among individuals and among different populations. Highly muscular individuals often have a BMI placing them in an overweight category when body fat content is not high. Also, in very short persons (under 5 feet), high BMIs may not reflect a high body fat. In addition, susceptibility to risk factors at a given BMI varies among individuals. Some individuals may have risk factors in the absence of a high BMI; in these persons, genetic causes of risk factors may be predominant.

Clinical judgment must be used when interpreting BMI in situations where it may not be an accurate indicator of total body fat, e.g., the presence of edema, high muscularity, muscle wasting, or for very short people. The relationship between BMI and body fat content varies with age, sex, and possibly ethnicity (28) because of differences in factors such as composition of lean tissue, sitting height, and hydration state. For example, older persons often have less muscle mass and more fat for a given BMI than younger persons, women usually have more fat for a given BMI than men, and clinical edema gives erroneously high BMIs.

Waist circumference

Excess fat in the abdomen independently predicts risk factors and morbidity. Research has shown that the waist circumference correlates with the amount of fat in the abdomen, and thus is an indicator of the severity of abdominal obesity (Table 4). In ATP III (14), increased waist circumference was identified as a strong obesity-associated clinical correlate of the metabolic syndrome. "Waist" circumference (3,4) is used instead of "abdominal" circumference because it more accurately describes the anatomical site of measurement. Abdominal fat has three compartments: visceral, retroperitoneal, and subcutaneous. Some studies suggest that visceral fat is the most strongly correlated with risk factors, whereas others indicate that the subcutaneous component is the most highly correlated with insulin resistance. Regardless, the presence of increased total abdominal fat is considered to be an independent risk predictor even when the BMI is not markedly increased. Therefore, waist or abdominal circumference, as well as BMI, should be measured.

Although waist circumference and BMI are interrelated, waist circumference carries extra prediction of risk beyond that of BMI (3,4). Waist circumference measurement is particularly useful in patients who are categorized as normal or overweight on the BMI scale. At BMI > 35, waist circumference has little added predictive power of disease risk beyond BMI.

A high waist circumference carries increased risk for type 2 diabetes, dyslipidemia, hypertension, and CVD when a BMI falls between 25 and 34.9 kg/m². The

clinician should keep in mind that ethnicity- and age-related differences in body fat distribution can modify the predictive power of waist circumference. In general, and particularly in some populations (e.g., Asians), waist circumference is a better indicator of relative disease risk than BMI. Waist circumference in particular assumes greater value than BMI for estimating risk for obesity-related disease at older ages.

Physical Inactivity

Sedentary life habits are a major underlying risk factor for both CVD and type 2 diabetes (29,30). The detection of physical inactivity can be assessed in two ways: (*i*) by history and (*ii*) by detection of cardiovascular fitness. Since the recommendation for physical activity calls for 30 minutes of moderately intense activity daily, lesser amounts of activity constitute varying degrees of physical inactivity. Some investigators contend that quantitative measures of cardiovascular fitness through exercise testing provide a more reliable indication of physical activity status with respect to future cardiovascular risk; this advantage, however, has not been proven with certainty (31).

Detection of Comorbidities

Patients who are overweight or obese should be questioned for the presence of existing comorbidities (Table 5). When suspected, further diagnostic testing may be required. Diseases that are commonly present in overweight or

Table 4 Definition of Abdominal Obesity

Gender	Waist circumference
Men	≥102 cm (40 in)
Women	≥88 cm (35 in)

Table 5 Complications of Obesity

Development of risk factors
Hypertension
Dyslipidemia
Insulin resistance
Impaired fasting glucose
Risk factor-related chronic diseases
Coronary heart disease
Stroke
Type 2 diabetes
Comorbidities
Osteoarthritis
Some types of cancer (endometrial, prostate, colon)
Sleep apnea and other respiratory disorders
Gallstones
Menstrual irregularities and polycystic ovary syndrome
Complications of pregnancy
Stress incontinence
Psychological disorders (e.g., depression)
Fatty liver (rarely cirrhosis)
Impaired mobility (severe obesity)

obese persons are CHD, type 2 diabetes, gallstones, osteo-arthritis, and sleep apnea. Patients with severe obesity may also exhibit pulmonary disease and/or dysmobility. These conditions may require clinical intervention independent of risk factor management and weight reduction.

MANAGEMENT OF RISK FACTORS IN OVERWEIGHT OR OBESE PERSONS

In patients who are overweight or obese, clinical focus should be directed first to the risk factors associated with obesity. Most of these risk factors relate to CVD, but some may indicate an increased susceptibility to type 2 diabetes. Management of the metabolic risk factors that are characteristic of the metabolic syndrome will be discussed. However, consideration will be given first to management of elevated low-density lipoprotein (LDL) cholesterol, which is the prime risk factor for development of athero-sclerotic CHD.

Elevated LDL Cholesterol

Serum LDL cholesterol is the primary target of cholesterol-lowering therapy. Overweight and obesity contribute to elevations of LDL cholesterol. Moreover, at any given level of LDL cholesterol, the presence of obesity-induced metabolic syndrome raises the risk for CHD. For this reason, particular attention should be given to reducing LDL cholesterol levels in overweight or obese patients who are identified as having the metabolic syndrome. In this section, the key recommendations of ATP III for management of elevated LDL cholesterol levels will be summarized (14). These recommendations apply particularly to patients who are overweight or obese. The primary sequence of therapy in ATP III is to direct attention first toward elevated LDL cholesterol; the metabolic syndrome is a secondary target of therapy. In other words, the goals for LDL therapy are first achieved before turning to the risk factors of the metabolic syndrome. Of course, if cigarette smoking or categorical hypertension is present, intervention on these risk factors will be needed from the outset. After intervention on the major risk factors is established, attention can turn to control of the metabolic risk factors. The latter features weight reduction and increased exercise.

Therapeutic modalities for LDL cholesterol lowering include both nondrug and drug therapies. The former are designated *therapeutic lifestyle changes* (TLC). The components of TLC specifically directed toward LDL lowering are as follows:

• Reduced intakes of saturated fats (<7% of total calories) and cholesterol (<200 mg/day)

• Therapeutic options for enhancing LDL lowering, such as plant stanols/sterols (2 g/day) and increased viscous (soluble) fiber (10–25 g/day)

• Weight reduction

As the first step of TLC, intakes of saturated fats and cholesterol are reduced first to lower LDL cholesterol. To improve overall health, ATP III therapeutic diet generally corresponds to the recommendations embodied in the Dietary Guidelines for Americans, 2005. The ATP III also allows total fat to range from 25% to 35% of total calories provided saturated fats and *trans* fatty acids are kept low. A higher intake of total fat, mostly in the form of unsaturated fat, can help to reduce triglycerides and raise HDL cholesterol in persons with the metabolic syndrome. In accordance with the Dietary Guidelines, moderate physical activity is encouraged. After six weeks of reducing saturated fats and cholesterol, the LDL response is determined; if the LDL cholesterol goal has not been achieved, other therapeutic options for LDL lowering, such as plant stanol/sterols and viscous fiber, can be added. After maximum reduction of LDL cholesterol with dietary therapy, emphasis shifts to management of the metabolic syndrome and associated lipid risk factors (see below).

Several drugs are available for lowering lipids (Table 6). The major drugs available for LDL lowering are bile acid sequestrants and enzyme 3-hydroxy-3-methylglutaryl coenzyme A (HMG-CoA) reductase inhibitors (statins). Other drugs—nicotinic acid and fibrate—moderately lower LDL levels, but they primarily reduce triglycerides and raise HDL levels.

Table 7 defines LDL cholesterol goals and cutpoints for initiation of TLC and for consideration of drug therapy for persons with four categories of risk: (*i*) *high-risk patients* (CHD and CHD risk equivalents), (*ii*) *moderately high-risk* persons with *multiple* (2+) *risk factors* (10-year risk of 10–20%), (*iii*) *moderate-risk* persons with multiple (2+) risk factors (10-year risk of < 10%); and (*iv*) *lower-risk* persons with zero to one risk factor. The management of each group will be considered briefly.

High-Risk Patients: CHD and CHD Risk Equivalents

The high-risk category includes patients with established CHD and CHD risk equivalents. Established CHD includes a history of myocardial infarction, unstable angina, stable angina, and coronary artery procedures (coronary angioplasty, coronary bypass operation). CHD risk equivalents are present in (*i*) patients with clinical forms of noncoronary atherosclerotic disease (peripheral arterial disease, abdominal aortic aneurysm, and symptomatic carotid artery disease (carotid transient ischemic attacks and carotid strokes), (*ii*) patients with diabetes, and (*iii*) persons whose 10-year risk for CHD is estimated

Table 6 Drugs Affecting Lipoprotein Metabolism

Drug class, agents, and daily doses	Lipid/lipoprotein effects	Side effects	Contraindications	Clinical trial results
Bile acid sequestrants[a]	LDL C ↓15–30% HDL C ↑ 3–5% TG: No change or increase	Gastrointestinal distress Constipation Decreased absorption of other drugs	Absolute: dysbetalipoproteinemia TG >400 mg/dL Relative: TG >200 mg/dL	Reduced major coronary events and CHD deaths
HMG-CoA reductase inhibitors (statins)[b]	LDL C ↓18–55% HDL C ↑ 5–15% TG ↓ 20–50%	Myopathy Increased liver enzymes	Absolute: Active or chronic liver disease Relative: Concomitant use of certain drugs[c]	Reduced major coronary events, CHD deaths, need for coronary procedures, stroke, and total mortality
Nicotinic acid[d]	LDL C ↓ 5–25% HDL C ↑ 15–35% TG ↓ 20–50%	Flushing Hyperglycemia Hyperuricemia (or gout) Upper-GI distress Hepatotoxicity	Absolute: Chronic liver disease Severe gout Relative: Diabetes Hyperuricemia Peptic ulcer disease Absolute: Severe renal disease Severe hepatic disease	Reduced major coronary events and possibly total mortality
Ezetimibe	LDL C ↓ 15–25%	Rare allergic reactions		
Fibric acids[e]	LDL C ↓ 5–20% (may be increased in patients with high TG) HDL C ↑ 10–20% TG ↓ 10–50%	Dyspepsia Gallstones Myopathy		Reduced major coronary events. Increased non-CHD mortality (in 2/5 clinical trials)

[a]Cholestyramine (4–16 g), colestipol (5–20 g), and colesevelam (2.6–3.8 g).
[b]Lovastatin (20–80 mg), pravastatin (20–40 mg), simvastatin (20–80 mg), fluvastatin (20–80 mg), and atorvastatin (10–80 mg); standard starting doses of statins are lovastatin (40 mg), pravastatin (40 mg), simvastatin (20 mg), fluvastatin (40 mg), and atorvastatin (10 mg).
[c]Cyclosporine, gemfibrozil (or niacin), macrolide antibiotics, various antifungal agents, and cytochrome p-450 inhibitors.
[d]Immediate-release (crystalline) nicotinic acid (1.5–3 g), extended-release nicotinic acid (Niaspan) (1–2 g), sustained-release nicotinic acid (1–2 g).
[e]Gemfibrozil (600 mg b.i.d.), fenofibrate (200 mg), and clofibrate (100 mg b.i.d.).
Abbreviations: LDL C, low-density lipoprotein cholesterol; HDL C, high-density lipoprotein cholesterol; TG, triglyceride; CHD, coronary heart disease.

Table 7 LDL Cholesterol Goals and Cutpoints for Therapeutic Lifestyle Changes and Drug Therapy in Different Risk Categories

Risk category	LDL goal (mg/dL)	LDL level at which to start lifestyle changes[a] (mg/dL)	LDL level at which to consider drug therapy (mg/dL)
High risk (10-yr risk of >20%)[b]	<100	≥100	≥100
Moderately high risk (2+ risk factors and 10 yr risk of 10–20% or metabolic syndrome)	<130	≥130	≥130 (after dietary therapy)
Moderate risk (2+ risk factors; 10-yr risk of <10%)	<130	≥130	≥160 (after dietary therapy)
Lower risk (0–1 risk factor)	<160	≥160	≥190 (160–189 mg/dL: LDL-lowering drug optional)

[a]LDL level at which to initiate therapeutic lifestyle changes.
[b]This high-risk category includes patients with established CHD and CHD risk equivalents. Established CHD includes a history of myocardial infarction, unstable angina, stable angina, and coronary artery procedures (coronary angioplasty, coronary bypass operations). CHD risk equivalents are present in patients with clinical forms of noncoronary atherosclerotic disease [peripheral arterial disease, abdominal aortic aneurysm, and symptomatic carotid artery disease (carotid transient ischemic attacks and carotid strokes)], patients with diabetes, and persons whose 10-year risk for CHD is estimated to be >20% by Framingham risk scoring.
Abbreviations: LDL, low-density lipoprotein; CHD, coronary heart disease.

to be >20% by Framingham risk scoring. For high-risk patients with CHD and CHD risk equivalents, LDL-lowering therapy greatly reduces risk for major coronary events and stroke and yields highly favorable cost-effectiveness ratios.

The goal for LDL cholesterol is a level <100 mg/dL. Cholesterol-lowering drugs can be used to achieve this goal, but drug therapy should always be accompanied by dietary modification and control of other risk factors. For patients with the metabolic syndrome, the following principles should be followed:

- Initiate or intensify lifestyle and/or drug therapies specifically to achieve the goals for LDL-lowering therapy.
- Emphasize weight reduction and increased physical activity.
- Consider use of other lipid-modifying drugs (e.g., nicotinic acid or fibric acid) if the patient has elevated triglyceride or low HDL cholesterol. However, these drugs typically are add-on drugs to LDL-lowering drugs.
- For patients with established CVD or other forms of atherosclerotic diseases plus metabolic syndrome and/or diabetes, consideration should be given to reducing LDL-cholesterol levels to <70 mg/dL.
- Once the LDL-cholesterol goal is achieved, a secondary goal of therapy is to reduce non-HDL cholesterol to a level 30 mg/dL higher than the LDL-cholesterol goal.

Moderately High-Risk Patients: Multiple (2+) Risk Factors and a 10-Year Risk of 10% to 20%

In this category, the goal for LDL cholesterol is <130 mg/dL. The therapeutic aim is to reduce short-term risk as well as long-term risk for CHD. If baseline LDL cholesterol is ≥130 mg/dL, TLC is initiated and maintained for three months. If LDL remains ≥130 mg/dL after three months of TLC, consideration can be given to starting an LDL-lowering drug to achieve the LDL goal of <130 mg/dL. Use of LDL-lowering drugs at this risk level reduces CHD risk and is cost-effective. If the LDL falls to <130 mg/dL on TLC alone, TLC can be continued without adding drugs. In older persons (≥ 65 years), clinical judgment is required for determining how intensively to apply these guidelines; a variety of factors, including concomitant illness, general health status, and social issues may influence treatment decisions and may suggest a more conservative approach.

Moderate-Risk Patients: Multiple (2+) Risk Factors and a 10-Year Risk of Less Than 10%

Here the goal for LDL cholesterol also is <130 mg/dL. The therapeutic aim, however, is primarily to reduce longer-term risk. If baseline LDL cholesterol is ≥130 mg/dL, the TLC diet is initiated to reduce LDL cholesterol. If LDL is <160 mg/dL on TLC alone, it should be continued. LDL-lowering drugs generally are not recommended because the patient is not at high short-term risk. On the other hand, if LDL cholesterol is ≥160 mg/dL, drug therapy can be considered to achieve an LDL cholesterol <130 mg/dL; the primary aim is to reduce long-term risk. Cost-effectiveness is marginal, but drug therapy can be justified to slow development of coronary atherosclerosis and reduce long-term risk for CHD.

Lower-Risk Patients: 0 to 1 Risk Factor

Most persons with zero to one risk factor have a 10-year risk <10%. They are managed according to Table 4. The goal for LDL cholesterol in this risk category is <160 mg/dL. The primary aim of therapy is to reduce long-term risk. First-line therapy is TLC. If after three months of TLC, the LDL cholesterol is <160 mg/dL, TLC is continued. However, if LDL cholesterol is 160 to 189 mg/dL after an adequate trial of TLC, drug therapy is optional depending on clinical judgment. Factors favoring use of drugs include (i) a severe single risk factor (heavy cigarette smoking, poorly controlled hypertension, strong family history of premature CHD, or very low HDL cholesterol); (ii) multiple life-habit risk factors and emerging risk factors (if measured); (iii) 10-year risk approaching 10% (if measured). If LDL cholesterol is ≥190 mg/dL despite TLC, drug therapy should be considered to achieve the LDL goal of <160 mg/dL. The purpose of using LDL-lowering drugs in persons with zero to one risk factor and elevated LDL cholesterol (≥ 160 mg/dL) is to slow the development of coronary atherosclerosis, which will reduce long-term risk. This aim may conflict with cost-effectiveness considerations; thus, clinical judgment is required in patient selection for using drugs when LDL cholesterol remains ≥190 mg/dL after TLC. For persons whose LDL cholesterol levels are already below goal levels on first encounter, instructions for appropriate changes in life habits, periodic follow-up, and control of other risk factors are needed.

Metabolic Risk Factors (Metabolic Syndrome)

Atherogenic Dyslipidemia

Elevation of triglycerides and low levels of HDL are common in overweight and obese patients. They are especially common when patients have other risk factors of the metabolic syndrome (10–12). ATP III classification of serum triglycerides is shown in Table 8. In patients with atherogenic dyslipidemia (triglyceride ≥ 150 mg/dL, small LDL particles, and low HDL cholesterol (< 40 mg/dL)), a three-part therapeutic strategy is required. First, the LDL

Table 8 ATP III Classification of Serum Triglycerides (mg/dL)

<150	Normal
150–199	Borderline high
200–499	High
≥500	Very high

Abbreviation: ATP III, Adult Treatment Panel III.

cholesterol goal should be achieved (Table 6). Second, underlying risk factors—overweight/obesity and physical inactivity—should be treated as described later in this chapter. And third, consideration can be given to treatment of atherogenic dyslipidemia with drug therapy, particularly if lipid levels remain abnormal after an effort to achieve significant weight reduction. For patients who have high triglycerides (200–499 mg/dL), a secondary goal of cholesterol-lowering therapy is non-HDL cholesterol (total cholesterol minus HDL cholesterol). Non-HDL cholesterol consists of LDL + very low density lipoprotein (VLDL) cholesterol. When patients have a triglyceride level in the range of 200 to 499 mg/dL, the secondary goal of therapy is a non-HDL cholesterol level of 30 mg/dL above the LDL goal (Table 9). In some patients, the non-HDL cholesterol goal can be achieved by statin therapy, because statins lower both LDL cholesterol and VLDL cholesterol. Alternatively, a statin can be combined with either a fibrate or nicotinic acid. The use of combined drug therapy is particularly attractive when the HDL cholesterol level is low. Finally, it should be noted that when triglyceride levels are >500 mg/dL, the primary goal becomes to lower triglycerides to prevent the development of acute pancreatitis. The favored drug in this case is a fibrate (gemfibrozil or fenofibrate). Once the triglycerides are reduced to <500 mg/dL, consideration can then be given to adding an LDL-lowering drug. For patients with triglyceride >500 mg/dL, statin therapy is not indicated as the first drug; it will not effectively lower triglyceride levels.

Table 9 Comparison of LDL Cholesterol and Non-HDL Cholesterol Goals for Three Risk Categories

Risk category	LDL goal (mg/dL)	Non-HDL goal (mg/dL)
CHD and CHD risk equivalent (10-yr risk for CHD >20%)	<100	<130
Multiple (2+) risk factors and 10-yr risk of >20%	<130	<160
0–1 Risk factor	<160	<190

Abbreviations: HDL, high-density lipoprotein; LDL, low-density lipoprotein; CHD, coronary heart disease.

Elevated Blood Pressure

The National High Blood Pressure Education Program (NHBPEP) also recommends that lifestyle changes should be first-line therapy for elevated blood pressure. Recommendations for blood pressure are described in the Joint National Committee on Prevention, Detection, Evaluation, and Treatment of High Blood Pressure (JNC VI) report (32). These recommendations have been amplified recently by reports on the efficacy of the Dietary Approaches to Stop Hypertension (DASH) diet for reducing blood pressure (33). This diet resembles that for cholesterol control but places special emphasis on increased intakes of fruits and vegetables, higher potassium consumption, low sodium intakes, and alcohol restriction. Lifestyle therapies for blood pressure control also emphasize weight reduction and increased physical activity. All of these dietary recommendations apply equally well to patients with diabetes. Although the first-line approach to controlling elevated blood pressure is through lifestyle changes, many patients with high blood pressure will also require blood pressure-lowering drugs. Fortunately, a large number of safe and effective drugs are available for treatment of elevated blood pressure. It has been estimated that about 60 million Americans have high blood pressure, and a large fraction of these are overweight and have the metabolic syndrome. The magnitude of this problem thus is evident. Effective treatment of high blood pressure is required to reduce risk for stroke as well as heart attack.

Insulin Resistance, Impaired Fasting Glucose, and Type 2 Diabetes

Insulin resistance is present in most persons with the metabolic syndrome. Some investigators believe that insulin resistance is the underlying cause of the metabolic syndrome (34,35). In the final analysis, however, the causes of insulin resistance are also the causes of the metabolic syndrome (9). These include genetic predisposition, overweight/obesity, and physical inactivity. A genetic predisposition to insulin resistance appears to reside in abnormalities in the insulin-signaling pathway. Overweight/obesity and physical inactivity further impair insulin signaling. Treatment of the underlying causes of the metabolic syndrome thus is synonymous with "treatment of insulin resistance." Primary clinical therapy includes weight reduction and increased physical activity. Both have been shown to reduce insulin resistance and to mitigate the risk factors of the metabolic syndrome. In addition, there is a growing interest in the use of drugs to modify insulin resistance and to reduce risk accompanying the metabolic syndrome. One class of drugs includes the glitazones, which are peroxisome proliferator–activated receptor gamma (PPAR-γ) agonists. These drugs may have several actions, including suppression of release of NEFAs by adipose tissue (36). Although these agents are promising, they are associated with some side effects that at present limit their use to treatment of patients with clinical type 2 diabetes. They may, however, be a prototype for newer agents that are both more effective and safer and can be used to reduce insulin resistance in patients with the metabolic syndrome and who do not have frank diabetes. Metformin is another drug that reduces insulin resistance, and some investigators contend that it may be useful in some forms of insulin resistance, e.g., polycystic ovary syndrome (37,38).

A borderline-high glucose [impaired fasting glucose (IFG) (110–126 mg/dL)] is commonly associated with insulin resistance and the metabolic syndrome. Patients with borderline elevations of glucose are at increased risk for both CVD and type 2 diabetes. The goal in management of overweight or obese patients with IFG is twofold: to reduce risk for CVD and to delay the onset of diabetes. Therapeutic approaches to reduce insulin resistance may help to mitigate *all* the risk factors of the metabolic syndrome and thus reduce the risk for CVD. First-line therapies are weight reduction and increased physical activity. Therefore, all overweight or obese persons with IFG should be encouraged to lose weight and exercise more. One of the most important aims in the medical management of obese persons is to prevent the onset of adult-onset (type 2) diabetes.

A study being conducted by the National Institute of Diabetes and Digestive and Kidney Diseases (NIDDK) examines whether dietary or drug therapy can prevent the conversion of IFG into type 2 diabetes. The trial is the Diabetes Prevention Program (DPP), a major clinical trial comparing diet and exercise to treatment with metformin in 3234 people with impaired glucose tolerance, a condition that often precedes diabetes (39,40). Participants randomly assigned to intensive lifestyle intervention reduced their risk of getting type 2 diabetes by 58% (41). On average, this group maintained their physical activity at 30 min/day, usually with walking or other moderate exercise, and lost 5% to 7% of their body weight. Participants randomized to treatment with metformin reduced their risk of getting type 2 diabetes by 31%. Of the 3234 participants enrolled in the DPP, 45% are from minority groups that suffer disproportionately from type 2 diabetes: African-American, Hispanic-American, Asian-American, Pacific Island, and Native American ethnic groups. The trial also recruited other groups known to be at higher risk for type 2 diabetes, including individuals aged 60 and older, women with a history of gestational diabetes, and people with a first-degree relative with type 2 diabetes.

The use of drugs that reduce insulin resistance is particularly attractive for patients with borderline elevations of plasma glucose. It is possible that such drugs will forestall the development of type 2 diabetes. In fact, the DPP study described above indicated that one such drug, metformin, reduces the number of overweight persons who actually become diabetic. This study also started off with another drug, troglitazone, but hepatotoxicity led to discontinuation of this arm of the study. Other "glitazones" that are not hepatotoxic might be employed as an alternative to troglitazone for prevention of type 2 diabetes in patients with borderline-high glucose. These drugs are currently being used to treat the high blood glucose of some patients with established diabetes, but at present they are not approved for prevention of diabetes (42).

When the fasting plasma glucose exceeds 126 mg/dL on two occasions, a diagnosis of type 2 diabetes can be made. At this stage, risk for CVD, particularly CHD, is markedly increased. ATP III defined diabetes, especially type 2 diabetes, as a CHD risk equivalent. In patients with diabetes, the LDL cholesterol goal is a level <100 mg/dL. The goal for blood pressure control is a level <130/85 mmHg. The American Diabetes Association provides recommendations for control of plasma glucose (43). The goal for hemoglobin A_{1c} is a level <7%. One important approach to control of plasma glucose is to initiate weight reduction and increase physical activity. Thus, TLC, as outlined in this chapter, should be employed in all patients with type 2 diabetes.

Prothrombotic State

A tendency to form blood clots, which can result in coronary thrombosis (heart attack), is characteristic of the metabolic syndrome. Obese people are also more likely to have deep-vein thrombosis. The physician must decide whether to start chronic and low-dose aspirin therapy with the metabolic syndrome. If patients are properly selected, they can achieve a significant reduction in risk for heart attack and stroke (44).

Proinflammatory State

Obese persons also have a tendency to chronic inflammation in the arteries, causing plaque and heart attack. There are no proven ways to reduce this chronic inflammation. Hopes that vitamin E might reduce inflammation (45) have not been borne out in clinical trials (46).

UNDERLYING RISK FACTOR: OVERWEIGHT/OBESITY AND PHYSICAL INACTIVITY

These risk factors will be considered together because they are closely intertwined. In particular, management of physical inactivity is one therapy for obesity. Approaches to management of overweight/obesity include the following:

- Energy-restricted diets
- Increased physical activity
- Behavior modification
- Pharmacotherapy
- Surgical therapy

The first three are standard therapies. Pharmacotherapy and surgical therapy are reserved for special cases and are used mainly for more severe forms of obesity, particularly to control comorbidities. Theoretically, they could be considered for patients with type 2 diabetes, although they have not been thoroughly evaluated in such patients. The following approach to weight loss in overweight or obese persons at risk for CVD or type 2 diabetes is taken in large part from recommendations of the OEI report (3,4).

Energy-Restricted Diets

A decrease in energy intake is the most important dietary component of weight loss and maintenance. Low-calorie diets often reduce total body weight by an average of 8% over a period of six months. Included in this average are individuals who did not lose weight; thus a 10% loss is feasible. A decrease of 500 to 1000 kcal/day will produce a weight loss of 1 to 2 lb/wk, and a decrease of 300 to 500 kcal/day will produce a weight loss of ½ to 1 lb/wk.

The weight loss component of dietary therapy consists mainly of instructing patients on how to consume fewer calories. The key is a moderate reduction in caloric intake. This will achieve a slow but progressive weight loss. Caloric intake need be reduced only enough to maintain the desired weight. At this caloric intake, excess weight will gradually vanish. In practice, somewhat greater caloric deficits are generally used during active weight loss. Recommended dietary therapy for weight loss in overweight patients is a low-calorie diet (1000–1800 kcal/day). The low-calorie diet should be distinguished from a very low calorie diet (250–800 kcal/day). Very low calorie diets have generally failed to maintain weight loss over the long term. In fact, clinical trials reveal that low-calorie diets are as effective as very low calorie diets for producing weight loss after one year. Although more weight is initially lost with very low calorie diets, more is usually regained. Importantly, rapid weight reduction fails to allow for gradual acquisition of new eating behavior. Slower weight loss allows more time to adjust eating habits.

Follow-up of very low calorie diets reveals that patients are at increased risk of cholesterol gallstones. Low-calorie diets are more likely to be successful if a patient's food preferences are included. Certainly all the recommended dietary allowances should be met, even if a dietary supplement is needed. During low-calorie diet therapy, educational efforts should focus on the following topics: energy value of different foods; food composition—fats, carbohydrates (including dietary fiber), and proteins; reading nutrition labels to determine caloric content and food composition; new habits of purchasing (preference to low calorie) foods; food preparation and avoiding adding high-calorie ingredients during cooking (e.g., fats and oils); avoiding overconsumption of high-calorie foods (both high-fat and high-carbohydrate foods); maintenance of adequate water intake; reducing portion sizes; and limiting alcohol consumption.

The rate of weight loss generally diminishes by six months. Behavior therapy is helpful in addition to low-calorie diets. Frequent clinical visits during initial weight reduction will facilitate reaching the goals of therapy. During active weight loss, visits of once per month or more often with a health professional help to promote weight reduction. Weekly group meetings are low cost and can contribute favorable behavior changes. Adequate time must be made available to convey information, to reinforce behavioral and dietary messages, and to monitor the patient's response.

Increased Physical Activity

An increase in physical activity promotes weight loss through increased expenditure of energy and possibly through inhibition of food intake. Physical activity also helps to maintain a desirable weight and to reduce CHD risk beyond that produced by weight reduction alone. Several experts contend that a decrease in the amount of energy expended for work, transportation, and personal chores is a major cause of obesity in the United States. They note that total caloric intake has not increased over the last few decades; instead, the caloric imbalance leading to overweight and obesity is the result of a substantial decrease in physical activity and, consequently, a decrease in daily energy expenditure. This hypothesis is intriguing but not proven. Regardless, increased regular physical activity is the way to achieve this goal of augmenting daily energy expenditure.

Increased physical activity improves cardiorespiratory fitness, with or without weight loss. The latter improves the quality of life in overweight patients by improving mood, self-esteem, and physical function in daily activities. Physical activity reduces elevated levels of CVD risk factors, including blood pressure and triglycerides; increases HDL cholesterol; and improves glucose tolerance with or without weight loss. Furthermore, the more active an individual is, the lower the risk for CVD morbidity and mortality and diabetes. Physical activity apparently has a favorable effect on distribution of body fat. Several studies showed an inverse association between energy expenditure through physical activity and several indicators of body fat distribution. Only a few randomized controlled trials that tested the effect of physical activity on weight loss also measured waist circumference.

Many people live sedentary lives, have little training or skills in physical activity, and are difficult to motivate toward increasing their activity. For these reasons, starting a physical activity regimen may require supervision for many people. The need to avoid injury during physical activity is high. Extremely obese persons may need to start with simple exercises that can gradually be intensified. A decision must be made whether exercise testing for cardiopulmonary disease is needed before starting a physical activity regimen. This decision should be based on a patient's age, symptoms, and concomitant risk factors.

For most obese persons, physical activity should be initiated slowly. Initial activities may be walking or swimming at a slow pace. Gradually, the patients may engage in more strenuous activities, such as fitness walking, cycling, rowing, cross-country skiing, aerobic dancing, and rope jumping. Jogging provides a high-intensity aerobic exercise. If jogging is recommended, the patient's ability to do this must first be assessed because it can cause orthopedic injuries. Competitive sports, such as tennis and volleyball, can motivate people to exercise, but care must be taken to avoid injury, especially in older people. Because amounts of activity are functions of duration, intensity, and frequency, the same amounts of activity can be obtained in longer sessions of moderately intense activities (such as brisk walking) as can be obtained in shorter sessions of more strenuous activities (such as running). Daily walking is one good form of exercise, particularly for those who are overweight or obese. It is helpful to start by walking for 10-minute intervals, 3 day/wk. With this exercise, an additional 100 to 200 cal/day of physical activity can be used. Although other forms of physical activity are acceptable, walking at least 5 day/wk is to be recommended. With this exercise, an additional 100 to 200 cal/day of physical activity can be used. Although other forms of physical activity are acceptable, walking is particularly attractive because of its safety and accessibility.

Reducing sedentary time is another approach to increasing activity. Patients also should be encouraged to build physical activities into their lives. They should consider leaving public transportation one stop before the usual one, parking farther than usual from work or shopping, walking up stairs instead of taking elevators or escalators, gardening, and walking the dog every day. Of course, attention should be given to exercising in safe areas, e.g., community parks, gyms, pools, health clubs, an

area of the home, perhaps outfitted with a stationary bicycle or a treadmill. Helpful strategies include planning exercise in advance, budgeting necessary time, and documenting the duration and intensity of exercise.

Behavior Therapy

Behavioral strategies help to reinforce changes in diet and physical activity. Without new habits, long-term weight reduction is unlikely to succeed. Most people unfortunately return to baseline weights without continued behavior modification. Learning how to include behavior modification in weight reduction therapy is essential. Behavior therapy is designed to permanently alter eating and activity habits.

Behavior therapy is based on the following principles: (i) by changing eating and physical activity habits, it is possible to change body weight; (ii) patterns of eating and physical activity are learned behaviors that can be modified; and (iii) to change these patterns over the long term, the environment must be changed. Behavior therapies are designed to promote compliance with dietary therapy and/or increased physical activity; they are important components of weight loss therapy.

Various strategies of behavioral therapy can be employed. Therapies can be applied either on an individual basis or in groups. Group therapy is less expensive. Self-monitoring of eating and exercise and objectifying one's own behavior through observation and recording are all included in behavioral therapy. Patients should learn to record amounts and types of food consumed, the calorie values, and nutrient composition. Record keeping will add insight to personal behavior. Patients should record time, place, and feelings related to eating and physical activity. The following are several components of behavioral therapy.

(i) *Stress management.* Stress can trigger overeating that can be countered by stress management. Stress control employs coping strategies, meditation, and relaxation techniques.

(ii) *Stimulus control.* High-risk situations that promote incidental eating should be identified. Obese patients can learn to shop carefully for healthy foods, keep high-calorie foods out of the house, limit the times and places of eating, and consciously avoid situations in which overeating occurs.

(iii) *Problem solving.* Self-correction of problems includes identifying weight-related problems, generating possible solutions and choosing one, planning and implementing the healthier alternative, and evaluating the outcome of possible behavioral changes. Patients should reevaluate setbacks in behavior and learn from them.

(*iv*) *Contingency management.* Rewards for specific actions can help to change behavior. These rewards can either be verbal, social, or tangible (e.g., monetary). And they can come from the professional team or from the patients themselves.

(*v*) *Cognitive restructuring.* Unrealistic goals, inaccurate beliefs, and self-defeating thoughts and feelings often stand in the way of successful weight reduction.

(*vi*) *Social support.* A strong system of social support is an important component of weight loss therapy. Professionals should recruit family members, friends, or colleagues for assistance. Weight reduction support groups also can be used. A restructuring of family eating habits can also assist in therapy directed toward individuals. (Often, more than one family member is overweight, and thus several persons in the family may benefit from a modification of family eating habits.)

Weight Reduction Pharmacotherapy

The purpose of weight loss and weight maintenance is to reduce health risks. If weight is regained, health risks increase once more. The majority of persons who lose weight regain it, so the challenge to the patient and the practitioner is to maintain the weight loss. Because of the tendency to regain weight after weight loss, the use of long-term medication to aid in the treatment of obesity may be indicated in some carefully selected patients.

One weight loss drug is sibutramine. It has norepinephrine and serotonin effects (see chap. 18). Another agent, orlistat, has a different mechanism of action, namely the blockage of fat absorption (see chap. 19). A number of trials longer than six months have been done with these drugs. These drugs are effective but modest in their ability to produce weight loss. Net weight loss attributable to drugs generally has been reported to be in the range of 2 to 10 kg (4.4–22 lb), although some patients lost significantly more weight. It is not possible to predict how much weight an individual may lose. Most of the weight loss usually occurs in the first six months of therapy.

With sibutramine there is a tendency for increased blood pressure and pulse rate. People with a history of high blood pressure, CHD, congestive heart failure, arrhythmias, or stroke should not take sibutramine, and all patients taking the medications should have their blood pressure monitored on a regular basis. With orlistat, there is a possible decrease in the absorption of fat-soluble vitamins; overcoming this may require vitamin supplementation.

Given that adverse events may occur with drug therapy, it seems wise, until further safety data are available, to use weight loss drugs cautiously. Furthermore, drugs should be used only as part of a comprehensive program that includes behavior therapy, diet, and physical activity. Appropriate monitoring for side effects must be continued while drugs are part of the regimen. Patients will need to return for follow-up in two to four weeks, then monthly for three months, and then every three months for the first year after starting the medications. Drugs should be used only in the context of a long-term treatment strategy.

Weight Loss Surgery

Surgery is one option for weight reduction for some patients with severe and resistant obesity. The aim of surgery is to reduce net food intake. Generally weight loss surgery should be reserved for patients with severe obesity, in whom other therapies have failed, and who are suffering from the complications of obesity. Surgical interventions commonly used include gastroplasty, gastric partitioning, and gastric bypass. Treatment of clinically severe obesity involves an effort to create a calorie deficit sufficient to result in weight loss and reduction of weight-associated risk factors or comorbidities. Surgical approaches can result in substantial weight loss, i.e., from 50 kg (110 lb) to as much as 100 kg (220 lb) over a period of six months to one year. Compared with other interventions available, surgery has produced the longest period of sustained weight loss. Assessing both perioperative risk and long-term complications is important and requires assessing the risk/benefit ratio in each case. Patients whose BMI is >40 kg/m^2 are potential candidates for surgery because obesity severely impairs the quality of their lives. Less severely obese patients (BMI between 35 and 39.9 kg/m^2) may also be considered for surgery if they have comorbid conditions (e.g., sleep apnea, uncontrolled type 2 diabetes). In one study, patients with diabetes undergoing the surgical procedure had a decrease in mortality rate for each year of follow-up compared with nonsurgery patients. The major limitation of gastric surgery for obesity is the occurrence of side effects, which are various and occur either in the perioperative period or long term. Two recent papers document that bariatric surgery lengthens life (47,48).

SUMMARY

Obesity is emerging as one of the most serious health problems both in the United States and worldwide. It is the major reason why CVD will become the No. 1 killer of the 21st century and why the prevalence of diabetes threatens to triple over the next 30 years. Obesity is thus a health problem of the first magnitude and deserves increased attention in both public health and medical fields. Except for patients with severe obesity in whom excess body fat directly interferes with bodily functions (e.g., mobility or breathing), overweight/obesity should be viewed as an underlying risk factor for chronic diseases. Foremost among these are CVD and diabetes. Thus the clinical approach to overweight or obese patients requires that excess body weight be considered in the context of all risk factors. The intensity of clinical management of patients thus depends on the total risk profiles. This maximum holds for management of overweight/obesity as well as for other risk factors. Nonetheless, early intervention on underlying risk factors (overweight/obesity and physical inactivity) may forestall the development of other risk factors later in life.

REFERENCES

1. Ogden CL, Yanovski SZ, Carroll MD, et al. The epidemiology of obesity. Gastroenterology 2007; 132(6):2087–2102.
2. Poirier P, Giles TD, Bray GA, et al., and American Heart Association and Obesity Committee of the Council on Nutrition, Physical Activity, and Metabolism. Obesity and cardiovascular disease: pathophysiology, evaluation, and effect of weight loss: an update of the 1997 American Heart Association Scientific Statement on Obesity and Heart Disease from the Obesity Committee of the Council on Nutrition, Physical Activity, and Metabolism. Circulation 2006; 113(6):898–918.
3. Executive summary of the clinical guidelines on the identification, evaluation, and treatment of overweight and obesity in adults. Arch Intern Med 1998; 158(17): 1855–1867.
4. Clinical guidelines on the identification, evaluation, and treatment of overweight and obesity in adults—the evidence report. National Institutes of Health. Obes Res 1998; 6(suppl 2):51S–209S.
5. Shoelson SE, Herrero L, Naaz A. Obesity, inflammation, and insulin resistance. Gastroenterology 2007; 132(6): 2169–2180.
6. Bamba V, Rader DJ. Obesity and atherogenic dyslipidemia. Gastroenterology 2007; 132(6):2181–2190.
7. Parekh S, Anania FA. Abnormal lipid and glucose metabolism in obesity: implications for nonalcoholic fatty liver disease. Gastroenterology 2007; 132(6):2191–2207.
8. Giovannucci E, Michaud D. The role of obesity and related metabolic disturbances in cancers of the colon, prostate, and pancreas. Gastroenterology 2007; 132(6):2208–2225.
9. Grundy SM. Metabolic complications of obesity. Endocrine 2000; 13(2):155–165.
10. Grundy SM. Hypertriglyceridemia, insulin resistance and the metabolic syndrome. Am J Cardiol 1999; 83(9B): 25F–29F.
11. Grundy SM. Hypertriglyceridemia, atherogenic dyslipidemia and the metabolic syndrome. Am J Cardiol 1998; 81(4A):18B–25B.
12. Grundy SM. Small LDL, atherogenic dyslipidemia, and the metabolic syndrome. Circulation 1997; 95(1):1–4.
13. Haffner SM, Stern MP, Hazuda HP, et al. Cardiovascular risk factors in confirmed pre-diabetic individuals. Does the clock for coronary heart disease start tickling before the onset of clinical diabetes? JAMA 1990; 263(21): 2893–2898.
14. Executive Summary of the Third Report of the National Cholesterol Education Program (NCEP) Expert Panel on Detection, Evaluation, and Treatment of High Blood Cholesterol in Adults (Adult Treatment Panel III). JAMA 2001; 285(19):2486–2497.
15. Cappuccio FP. Ethnicity and cardiovascular risk: variations in people of African ancestry and South Asian origin. J Hum Hypertens 1997; 11(9):571–576.
16. Robinson TN. Television viewing and childhood obesity. Pediatr Clin North Am 2001; 48:1017–1025.
17. Dietz WH, Gortmaker SL. Preventing obesity in children and adolescents. Annu Rev Public Health 2001; 22:337–353.
18. DiPietro L. Physical activity in the prevention of obesity: current evidence and research issues. Med Sci Sports Exerc 1999; 31(11 suppl):S542–S546.
19. Schoeller DA. Balancing energy expenditure and body weight. Am J Clin Nutr 1998; 68(4):956S–961S.
20. Seidell JC. Obesity in Europe: scaling an epidemic. Int J Obes Relat Metab Disord 1995; 19(suppl 3):S1–S4.
21. Westerterp KR. Daily physical activity, aging and body composition. J Nutr Health Aging 2000; 4(4):239–242.
22. Seidell JC, Visscher TL. Body weight and weight change and their health implications for the elderly. Eur J Clin Nutr 2000; 54(suppl 3):S33–S39.
23. Ryans AS. Insulin resistance with aging: effects of diet and exercise. Sports Med 2000; 30(5):327–346.
24. Barzilai N, Gupta G. Interaction between aging and syndrome X: new insights on the pathophysiology of fat distribution. Ann N Y Acad Sci 1999; 892:58–72.
25. Paolisso G, Tagliamonte MR, Rizzo MR, et al. Advancing age and insulin resistance: new facts about an ancient history. Eur J Clin Invest 1999; 29(9):758–769.
26. National Heart Lung and Blood Institute. Available at: http://www.nhlbi.nih.gov.
27. National Heart Lung and Blood Institute. Available at: http://www.nhlbi.nih.gov/guidelines/cholesterol/profmats.htm.
28. Gallagher D, Heymsfield SB, Heo M, et al. Healthy percentage body fat ranges: an approach for developing guidelines based on body mass index. Am J Clin Nutr 2000; 72(3):694–701.
29. Nawaz H, Katz DL. American College of Preventive Medicine Practice Policy Statement. Weight management counseling of overweight adults. Am J Prev Med 2001; 21(1):73–78.
30. Epstein S, Sivarajan Froelicher ES, Froelicher VF, et al. Statement on exercise: benefits and recommendations for physical activity program for all Americans. Circulation 1996; 94:857–862.
31. Blair SN, Cheng Y, Holder JS. Is physical activity or physical fitness more important in defining health benefits? Med Sci Sports Exerc 2001; 33(6 suppl):S379–S399.
32. The sixth report of the Joint National Committee on prevention, detection, evaluation, and treatment of high blood pressure. Arch Intern Med 1997; 157(21):2413–2446.

33. Sacks FM, Svetkey LP, Vollmer WM, et al. Effects on blood pressure of reduced dietary sodium and the Dietary Approaches to Stop Hypertension (DASH) diet. Dash-Sodium Collaborative Research Group. N Engl J Med 2001; 344(1):3–10.

34. Reaven GM. Insulin resistance: a chicken that has come to roost. Ann N Y Acad Sci 1999; 892:45–57.

35. DeFronzo RA. Insulin resistance: a multifaceted syndrome responsible for NIDDM, obesity, hypertension, dyslipidaemia and atherosclerosis. Neth J Med 1997; 50(5):191–197.

36. Lebovitz HE, Banerji MA. Insulin resistance and its treatment by thiazolidinediones. Recent Prog Horm Res 2001; 56:265–294.

37. Norman RJ, Kidson WJ, Cuneo RC, et al. Metformin and intervention in polycystic ovary syndrome. Endocrine Society of Australia, the Australian Diabetes Society and the Australian Paediatric Endocrine Group. Med J Aust 2001; 174(11):580–583.

38. Kowalska I, Kinalski M, Straczkowski M, et al. Insulin, leptin, IGF-I and insulin-dependent protein concentrations after insulin-sensitizing therapy in obese women with polycystic ovary syndrome. Eur J Endocrinol 2001; 144(5):509–515.

39. Diabetes Prevention Program. Design and method for a clinical trial in the preventions of type 2 diabetes. Diabetes Care 1992; 22(4):623–634.

40. Diabetes Prevention Program. Baseline characteristics of the randomized cohort. Diabetes Care 2000; 23(11): 1619–1629.

41. Knowler WC, Barrett-Connor E, Fowler SE, et al., and Diabetes Prevention Program Research Group. Reduction in the incidence of type 2 diabetes with lifestyle intervention or metformin. N Engl J Med 2002; 346(6):393–403.

42. DREAM (Diabetes REduction Assessment with ramipril and rosiglitazone Medication) Trial Investigators, Gerstein HC, Yusuf S, Bosch J, et al. Effect of rosiglitazone on the frequency of diabetes in patients with impaired glucose tolerance or impaired fasting glucose: a randomised controlled trial. Lancet 2006; 368(9541):1096–1105.

43. American Diabetes Association. Clinical Practice Recommendations 2008. Summary of Revisions for the 2008 Clinical Practice Recommendations. Diabetes Care 2008; 31:S3–S4.

44. American Diabetes Association. Aspirin therapy in diabetes. Diabetes Care 1997; 20(11):1772–1773.

45. Devaraj S, Jialal I. Alpha tocopherol supplementation decreases serum C-reactive protein and monocyte interleukin-6 levels in normal volunteers and type 2 diabetic patients. Free Radic Bio Med 2000; 29(8):790–792.

46. Robinson I, de Serna DG, Gutierrez A, et al. Vitamin E in humans: an explanation of clinical trial failure. Endocr Pract 2006; 12(5):576–582.

47. Sjostrom L, Narbro K, Sjostrom CD, et al., and Swedish Obese Subjects Study. Effects of bariatric surgery on mortality in Swedish obese subjects. N Engl J Med 2007; 357(8):741–752.

48. Adams TD, Gress RE, Smith SC, et al. Long-term mortality after gastric bypass surgery. N Engl J Med 2007; 357(8):753–761.

31

Surgical Treatment and Comorbidities

HENRY BUCHWALD

Department of Surgery, University of Minnesota, Minneapolis, Minnesota, U.S.A.

INTRODUCTION

The surgical treatment of obesity, usually referred to as bariatric surgery, derived from the Greek word barrios for weight, originated in the 1950s. Today, this discipline is responsible for a major portion of the daily operating room schedules of most of the larger hospitals in the United States, both private and academic. Bariatric surgery is an example of metabolic surgery, which, together with extirpative and reparative surgery, represents the three principles of operative intervention. Metabolic surgery is defined as the manipulation of a normal organ or organ system to achieve a metabolic goal (1). More and more, the field of surgery has and is exploring metabolic surgical solutions for traditionally nonsurgical diseases, e.g., hyperlipidemia, diabetes, and obesity.

WHO IS A SURGICAL CANDIDATE?

The prevalence of obesity, in particular morbid or severe obesity, defined as a body mass index (BMI) ≥ 40 kg/m^2 or ≥ 35 kg/m^2 in the presence of significant comorbid conditions (2), in the United States and globally has been reviewed. The relative ineffectuality of nonsurgical therapy in this cohort has also been made evident. Should we, therefore, consider that the population for surgical treatment selection is composed of the 23 million estimated to be morbidly obese in the United States (3) and probably over 100 million worldwide (4–6)? We currently have trained surgeons, adequate facilities, and financial resources in the United States to operate on 1% to 2% of the morbidly obese (American Society for Metabolic and Bariatric Surgery, 2007, personal communication) and far less capability in the rest of the world (International Federation of Obesity Surgery, 2007, personal communication). Thus, who are the surgical candidates is not as relevant as asking how can we select the appropriate patients for bariatric surgery from the vast number of eligible individuals? This process will never be precise. The best we can do today is to construct and follow selection guidelines within the confines of geography, socioeconomic status, and availability of health care coverage. The two universal guidelines in use today are those set by the National Institutes of Health (NIH) in 1991 (2) and those of the American Society for Metabolic and Bariatric Surgery (ASMBS) of 2004 (7). These guidelines must be updated as the field of bariatric surgery evolves. The 1991 NIH guidelines are severely antiquated, being, among other shortcomings, limited to two procedures and making no mention of laparoscopic bariatric surgery.

EVOLUTION OF BARIATRIC SURGERY PROCEDURES

Historical Antecedents

When did surgeons enter into the history of obesity therapy? In the Talmud, it is told that Rabbi Eleazar underwent an operation where he was given a soporific potion and brought to a marble house, his abdomen was opened, and a number of baskets of fat were removed (8). Anecdotal references are made to Hua Toh, a third-century Chinese surgeon, who prescribed acupuncture in the pinna of the ear to reduce appetite and treat obesity and also to a fat removal procedure performed on the obese son of the Roman Consul, Lucius Apronius. It has also been rumored that Dr. John H. Kellogg (1852–1943), who with his brother William were pioneers of boxed grain cereals, removed a section of a patient's intestine when certain disease processes were not cured by a vegetarian diet. Weight loss by panniculectomy was practiced by 20th-century surgeons well before the introduction of bariatric surgery.

Classification

Bariatric surgery, as a type of metabolic surgery can be subdivided into four categories: malabsorptive procedures, malabsorptive/restrictive procedures, restrictive procedures, and others. The evolution of bariatric procedures and the emergence of new techniques is a function of the cost-benefit ratios for the various operative interventions. Factors to be considered in this ratio are the efficacy of weight loss (usually stated as percent excess weight loss in surgical reports), lasting weight loss obtained, operative mortality and perioperative morbidity, long-term mortality and morbidity, quality of life achieved, and financial burden of the procedure, as well as reversibility to provide a safe retreat from a potential iatrogenic catastrophe.

Malabsorptive Procedures

By the early 1950s, years of clinical observation had taught physicians that the shortened gut led to massive weight loss. Though he never published his procedure, Dr. Victor Henrikson of Gothenberg, Sweden, has often been credited for performing an intestinal resection specifically for the management of obesity in the early 1950s (9). In 1953, Dr. Richard L. Varco, of the Department of Surgery at the University of Minnesota, probably was the first to perform a jejunoileal bypass (10). This operation consisted of an end-to-end jejunoileostomy with a separate ileocecostomy for drainage of the bypassed segment (Fig. 1).

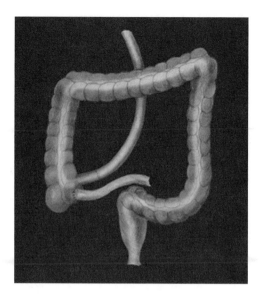

Figure 1 Varco (1953) and Kremen et al. (1954): Jejunoileal bypass with end-to-end jejunoileostomy with ileocecostomy. *Source*: From Ref. 142.

Varco did not publish his innovation, and the first publication on a jejunoileal bypass procedure, in 1954, is correctly credited to Kremen et al. (11).

In 1963, Payne et al. published the results of the first clinical program of massive intestinal bypass for the management of morbidly obese patients (12). They described bypassing nearly the entire small intestine, the right colon, and half of the transverse colon in 10 morbidly obese female patients, restoring intestinal continuity by an end-to-side anastomosis of the proximal jejunum to the mid-transverse colon. Although weight loss was dramatic, electrolyte imbalance, uncontrolled diarrhea, and liver failure proved prohibitive and required eventual reversal of the bypass, which led to a regaining of the previously lost weight (13).

There were several other modifications of the jejunoileal bypass and the eventual establishment of two operative techniques: the Payne and DeWind "14 to 4 inches" operation (13) and a return to the Varco and Kremen et al. procedure by Scott et al. (14), Salmon (15), and Buchwald and Varco (16). The Payne and DeWind procedure consisted of the anastomosis of the proximal 14 inches of jejunum end-to-side to the terminal 4 inches of ileum (Fig. 2). In the Scott et al., Salmon, and Buchwald and Varco procedures, the terminal ileum was divided with an end-to-end anastomosis to the proximal jejunum to prevent reflux, and the bypassed segment was drained into the transverse colon, the sigmoid colon, or the cecum, respectively.

There were many other modifications, none of them gaining popularity, and eventually the jejunoileal bypass itself was superseded and essentially ceased to be performed. For this procedure, the cost-benefit ratio of

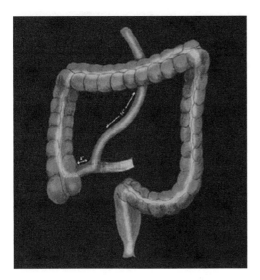

Figure 2 Payne and DeWind (1969): Jejunoileal bypass with 35 to 10 cm (14 to 4 inches) end-to-side jejunoileostomy. *Source*: From Ref. 142.

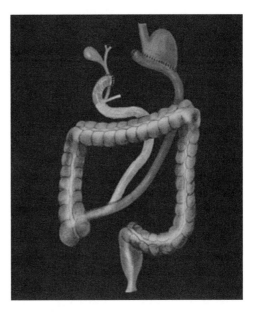

Figure 3 Scopinaro (1979): Biliopancreatic diversion. *Source*: From Ref. 142.

complications was too high to maintain it in the bariatric surgery armamentarium. The jejunoileal bypass was associated with diarrhea, electrolyte imbalance, gas-bloat syndrome, oxalate kidney stones, arthralgias, pustular eruptions, and mental disturbances. Many of these problems were attributed to the long segment of bypassed small intestine, where a stagnation of flow promoted the overgrowth of anaerobic bacteria and the elaboration of bacterial toxins.

Malabsorptive surgery, however, was far from eliminated from the scope of bariatric procedures, making a comeback in the 1970s and occupying a major role in bariatric surgery today. The key trait of the modern massive intestinal bypass procedures is that no limb of the small intestine is left without intraluminal flow. The enteric or Roux limb has the flow of food and the biliary or biliopancreatic limb contains the flow of bile and pancreatic juice.

In 1978, Lavorato et al. performed a standard end-to-side jejunoileal bypass; however, they anastomosed the proximal end of the bypassed segment of the small intestine to the gallbladder, thereby diverting bile into the bypassed limb (17). In 1981, Eriksson described a similar operation (18). These biliointestinal bypasses have not been widely performed, and the modern malabsorptive era began with the Scopinaro biliopancreatic diversion.

At present, thousands of biliopancreatic diversions have been performed, particularly in Italy, mainly by Dr. Scopinaro, beginning with his initial series of patients reported in 1979 (19). His current biliopancreatic diversion consists of a horizontal partial gastrectomy (leaving 200–500 mL of proximal stomach), closure of the duodenal stump, gastrojejunostomy with a 250-cm Roux limb,

and anastomosis of the long biliopancreatic limb to the Roux limb 50 cm proximal to the ileocecal valve, creating an extremely short common channel (20) (Fig. 3).

More than a decade later, the biliopancreatic diversion was modified into the duodenal switch in the United States and Canada. Hess and Hess, a father and son team in Ohio, the United States, deviated from the Scopinaro procedure by making a lesser curvature gastric tube (approximately 100 mL in volume) with a greater curvature gastric resection, preserving the pylorus, dividing the dudodenum with closure of the distal duodenal stump, and anastomosing the enteric limb to the postpyloric duodenum (21) (Fig. 4).

Marceau et al., in Canada, performed a similar operation but cross-stapled the duodenum distal to the duodenoileostomy without dividing it (22). The duodenum, however, unlike the stomach, does not tolerate cross-stapling, and these patients displayed disruption of the staple line with regaining of their weight. There have been several modifications of the Hess and Hess procedure, mostly in the lengths of the common channel, the enteric limb, and the biliopancreatic limb, and it has been performed by both open and laparoscopic surgical techniques.

Malabsorptive/Restrictive Procedures

Gastric restrictive procedures were introduced by Edward Mason. In the original Mason and Ito gastric bypass, the stomach was divided horizontally and a loop (not a Roux) gastrojejunostomy was created between the proximal gastric pouch and the proximal jejunum (23). The size of the

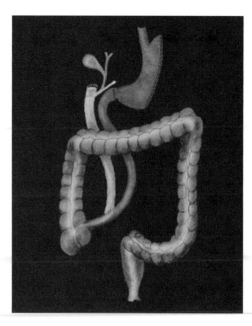

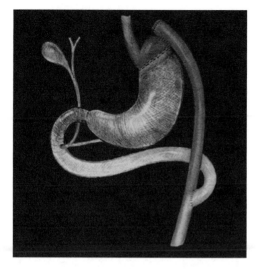

Figure 5 Griffen (1977): Gastric bypass with horizontal gastric stapling with Roux-en-Y gastrojejunostomy. *Source*: From Ref. 142.

Figure 4 Hess and Hess (1998): Biliopancreatic diversion with duodenal switch with division of the duodenum. *Source*: From Ref. 143.

upper pouch and the size of the stomach outlet dictate the restrictive aspect of the gastric bypass. Distention of this upper pouch by food causes the sensation of satiety by mechanisms as yet undetermined. The malaborptive aspect of the gastric bypass is inherent in the bypass of approximately 90% of the distal stomach, the duodenum, and varying lengths of jejunum.

Alden, in 1977, modified the Mason gastric bypass by the introduction of a horizontal staple line without gastric division and a loop gastrojejunostomy (24). That same year, the evolution to the modern gastric bypass was introduced by Griffen et al. with their Roux-en-Y gastro-jejunostomy in place of the loop gastrojejunostomy (25) (Fig. 5). The Roux gastric bypass has the advantage of avoiding tension on the gastrojejunostomy and of preventing bile reflux into the upper gastric pouch (26).

Over the next several years, variations of the Roux gastric bypass were described. Torres et al. stapled the stomach vertically rather than horizontally, a modification that in many hands has become the standard method for preparing the upper gastric pouch (27). Linner and Drew reinforced the gastrojejunal outlet with a fascial band (28). Torres and Oca again achieved a first with the modification of their vertical Roux nondivided gastric bypass and the creation of a long Roux limb for individuals who had failed their original procedure (29). Brolin et al. later popularized the long-limb Roux gastric bypass as a primary operation for the super obese (30). This operation was further modified and extensively employed by Nelson et al. at the Mayo Clinic (31). Salmon combined the distal

Roux gastric bypass with a vertical banded gastroplasty (32). And, finally, Fobi introduced two modifications combining a restrictive Silastic ring proximal to the gastrojejunostomy outlet of a standard gastric bypass (33,34). In the latter modification, Fobi divided the stomach and interposed the jejunal Roux limb between the gastric pouch and the bypassed stomach to ensure maintenance of the gastric division and avoidance of a gastro-gastric fistula.

In 1994, Wittgrove et al. reported the first cases of laparoscopic Roux gastric bypass (35). This event heralded the introduction of laparoscopic techniques into bariatric surgery and gave rise to the modern era where, worldwide, approximately 75% of bariatric surgery, at the time of this writing, is performed laparoscopically. The execution of the gastrojejunostomy has varied from the introduction of the end-to-end stapler endoscopically (35), the introduction of the end-to-end stapler intra-abdominally by Torre and Scott (36), and by the use of the side-to-side gastro-intestinal stapler intra-abdominally by Schauer and others (37). In 1999, Higa et al., to avoid the relatively high incidence of gastrointestinal anastomotic leaks in laparoscopic procedures, described a technique for hand-sewing the gastrojejunostomy laparoscopically (38).

Restrictive Procedures

In the 1970s and 1980s, bariatric surgery was simplified by the introduction of purely restrictive gastric operations. The restrictive procedures can be performed more rapidly than the gastric bypass and are more physiologic, since no part of the gastrointestinal tract is bypassed or rerouted.

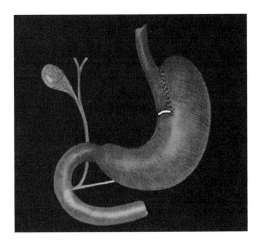

Figure 6 Laws (1981): Gastroplasty with Silastic ring vertical restriction. *Source*: From Ref. 142.

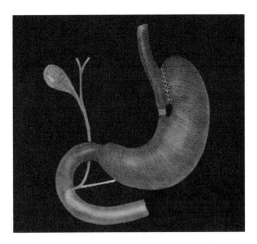

Figure 7 Mason (1982): Gastroplasty with Marlex® vertically banded outlet. *Source*: From Ref. 142.

The primary name in gastric restrictive surgery is, once again, Edward Mason who, in association with Printen, performed the first restrictive procedure in 1971 (39). They divided the stomach horizontally from lesser curvature to greater curvature, leaving a gastric conduit at the greater curvature—all performed without the benefit of stapling. This procedure was unsuccessful in maintaining weight loss, as was the modification by Gomez, in 1979, which utilized outlet reinforcement with a running suture (40). Two other modifications were equally unsuccessful, namely, the gastric partitioning operation by Pace et al. (1979) (41) and the total gastric cross-stapling with a gastrogastrostomy by LaFave and Alden (1979) (42).

In 1981, Fabito was the first to perform a vertical gastroplasty by employing a modified TA-90 stapler and reinforcing the outlet with seromuscular sutures (43). That same year, Laws was probably the first to use a Silastic ring as a permanent, nonexpandable support for the vertical gastroplasty outlet (44) (Fig. 6).

In 1980, Mason performed his last gastroplasty variation—the vertical banded gastroplasty (45). This procedure involved a novel concept, namely, making a window, a through-and-through perforation in both walls of the stomach, with the end-to-end stapling instrument just above the crow's foot on the lesser curvature. This window was used for the insertion of a standard TA-90 stapler to the angle of His to create a small, stapled vertical pouch. The lesser curvature outlet was banded with a 1.5-cm wide polypropylene (Marlex®) mesh collar through the gastric window and around the lesser curvature conduit (Fig. 7). In 1994, Hess and Hess (46) and, in 1995, Chua and Mendiola (47) performed the vertical banded gastroplasty laparoscopically.

In the last few years, gastric banding has become a dominant force in bariatric surgery operative technology and has fairly well displaced the stapled and banded

gastroplasty. It is the most utilized procedure in Europe and Australia and, though still second to gastric bypass, is gaining in popularity in the United States. Gastric banding is the least invasive of the gastric restrictive procedures: a small pouch and a small stoma are created by a band around the upper stomach, the stomach is not cut or crushed by staples, and no anastomoses are made.

In 1986, Kuzmak introduced the inflatable Silastic band connected to a subcutaneous port, which is used for the percutaneous introduction or removal of fluid to adjust the caliber of the gastric band (48) (Fig. 8). In 1992–1993, Broadbent et al. (49) and Catona et al. (50) were probably the first to perform gastric banding laparoscopically, and in 1993, Belachew et al. (51) and Forsell et al. (52) were the first to perform adjustable gastric banding laparoscopically. Niville et al. reported placing the posterior aspect of the band at the distal esophagus and thereby constructing an extremely small (virtual) anterior gastric pouch, which is the procedure advocated today (53). An important technique in universal use for the

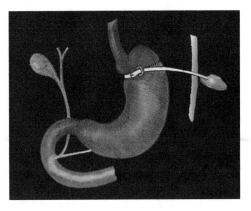

Figure 8 Kuzmak (1986): Gastric band with adjustable Silastic tubing and refill port. *Source*: From Ref. 143.

placement of the band today is the pars flaccida approach, more likely to prevent slippage and other complications than the perigastric approach of band placement. Cadiere et al. in 1999 reported the world's first laparoscopic gastric banding executed robotically (54).

The open surgery biliopancreatic diversion/duodenal switch procedures were being performed most successfully on both sides of the Atlantic in patients with super obesity (BMI $\geq$50 kg/m^2) and were, therefore, attempted laparoscopically with a resultant complication rate higher than expected. This led to the advocacy of a "two-stage" duodenal switch operation in these individuals, i.e., performing laparoscopically a greater curvature sleeve gastrectomy, waiting a year or so for weight loss, and reoperating laparoscopically to complete the duodenal switch. This first-stage sleeve gastrectomy is similar to the "Magenstrasse and Mill" operation popularized by Johnston et al. (55) and soon found advocates for use of a sleeve gastrectomy as a primary and only operation for morbid obesity. In the interval, however, relatively safe laparoscopic biliopancreatic diversion and duodenal switch procedures became feasible (56–58). At present, insufficient follow-up data are available to draw conclusions about the two-stage biliopancreatic diversion/duodenal switch or the use of the sleeve gastrectomy as a freestanding operation.

Other Procedures

In 1974, Quaade et al. described stereotactic stimulation and electrocoagulation of sites in the lateral hypothalmus (59). In three of five patients receiving unilateral electrocoagulation lesions, there was a statistically significant but transient reduction in caloric intake and a short-term reduction in body weight.

In the late 1990s, electrical stimulation of the stomach was introduced into the spectrum of bariatric procedures. The first innovator of this approach was Cigaina, who in an animal model was able to create gastric paresis and weight loss by antral electrical stimulation (60). An alternative stimulation approach to induce gastric paresis and satiety is vagal based (61). Several pacing systems are currently being tested in clinical trials.

Currently, there is experimental and clinical investigation to develop a nonrestrictive, nonmalabsorptive procedure for obesity, based on the induction of gut hormones that cause satiety and loss of appetite (62–64). Two such hormones are glucagon-like peptide-1 (GLP-1) and peptide YY (PYY), both normally elaborated by the L-type endocrine cells of the ileum. Segmental ileal transposition into the proximal jejunum could lead to the early release of GLP-1 and PYY and their subsequent action on the satiety centers of the hypothalmus. This effect has been termed the "ileal brake" phenomenon.

Other Approaches

Recent attention has been given to natural orifice procedures and natural orifice transluminal endoscopic surgery (NOTES). The simplest examples of this ultra noninvasive surgery is the endoscopic introduction of an intragastric balloon to create gastric fullness and hence satiety (65). This technique is in its developmental stage. Other endoscopic procedures include the establishment of a vertical banded gastroplasty (66) or a gastric pouch (67) with special instruments, as well as the placement of an intragastric mesh prosthesis (68) or duodenal sleeve (69).

With respect to NOTES and bariatric surgery, a field truly in its infancy, animal studies have been performed to create gastric bypasses transgastrically.

MATCHING THE PATIENT WITH THE PROCEDURE

Today, many bariatric surgeons perform only one bariatric operation—guided by their experience and technical skills. There are others, or surgical groups, however, who offer multiple operative procedures and believe that a specific patient may be best matched with a specific procedure. To this end, selection algorithms have been proposed but few have been put into practice. In 2002, I suggested such an algorithm (70) and it, too, has not been systematically tested. The final iteration of the algorithm is expressed as a flow diagram in Figure 9 and as an equation in Figure 10. In this construction, increasing BMI, age over 40, unfavorable gender, race, and body habitus, and significant comorbidities force the selection to the more durable operations with greater weight loss but with somewhat less safety. Others may argue with the selection of and weighting of these variables.

COMPLICATIONS

Mortality

There is a great interest in the mortality associated with bariatric surgery in the medical community, in the media, and, understandably, in the minds of morbidly obese patients. Operative mortality is dependent on several factors: (*i*) the skill of the bariatric surgeon; (*ii*) the available facilities of the institution in which the surgery is performed; (*iii*) the volume of procedures being performed and the stage in the "learning curve" of the surgeon and the institution; (*iv*) operative selection (laparoscopic adjustable gastric banding, vertical banded gastroplasty, gastric bypass, biliopancreatic diversion/duodenal switch); (*v*) patient selection with respect to age, gender, race, and body habitus; and (*vi*) the presence

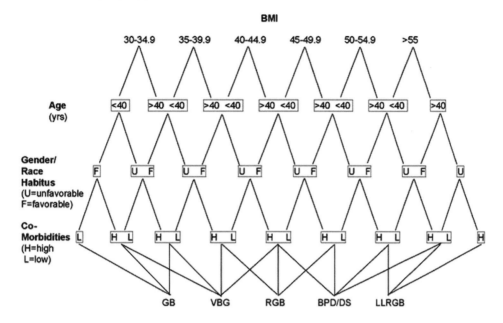

BMI = Body mass index; GB = Gastric band; VBG = Vertical banded gastroplasty; RGB = Roux gastric bypass;
BPD/DS = Biliopancreatic diversion/duodenal switch; LLRGB = Long-limb Roux gastric bypass

Figure 9 Flow diagram of a bariatric surgery patient selection algorithm taking into consideration preoperative BMI, age, gender/race/ habitus, and serious preoperative comorbidities. *Source*: From Ref. 70.

OC = 1.0 + BMI Number (1 to 6) ± 0.5 (age <40>) ± 0.5 (GRH, Favorable or Unfavorable) ± 1 (CoM, Low or High).

OC: GB = 0 to 3; VBG = 2 to 5; RGB = 3 to 6; BPD/DS = 4 to 7; LLRGB = 6 to 9.

Figure 10 Equation of a bariatric surgery patient selection algorithm utilizing the same preoperative variables as in Figure 9. *Source*: From Ref. 70.

of significant comorbidities such as diabetes, hyperlipidemia, hypertension, and obstructive sleep apnea.

A meta-analysis of outcomes in 22,094 patients with at least one of the four—type 2 diabetes, hyperlipidemia, hypertension, and obstructive sleep apnea—preoperative comorbidities showed a ≤30-day mortality of 0.1% for restrictive procedures (laparoscopic adjustable gastric banding and vertical banded gastroplasty), 0.5% for gastric bypass, and 1.1% for biliopancreatic diversion/ duodenal switch (71). In a more recent meta-analysis, the selection based only on mortality data, 85,048 patients were subjected to analysis in 3061 studies and 478 treatment arms (72). At baseline, the mean age was 40 years, BMI was 47.4 kg/m², 85% were females, and 11.5% had previous bariatric procedures. Meta-analysis of total mortality at ≤30 days was 0.28% (95% CI, 0.22–0.34) and total mortality at >30 days to 2 years was 0.35% (95% CI, 0.12–1.58). Mortality ≤30 days for all restrictive procedures was 0.30%, restrictive/malabsorptive (gastric bypass) 0.41%, and malabsorptive 0.76%. Subgroup analyses of ≤30-day mortality showed a male:female ratio of

4.74:0.13, with an 1.25% incidence in the superobese and 0.34% incidence in the elderly (≥65 years). As a rule, mortality rates declined over the years, as the number of procedures performed annually increased and operative experience accrued. Studies with larger cohorts reported lower mortality rates than those with smaller cohorts.

The results of this meta-analysis are in keeping with the figures from most of the multicentered data sets that have been reported in the literature (73–76). A recent survey by the Surgical Review Corporation is equally confirmatory of these findings, showing an in-hospital mortality for bariatric surgery of 0.14%, with 106 hospitals reporting with an average case load of 312 cases/yr (77). A notable exception in bariatric surgery mortality analyses is the 2005 article by Flum et al. (78). In this population-based study of Medicare beneficiaries, the authors found 2.0%, 2.8%, and 4.6% mortality for 30 days, 90 days, and 1 year, respectively, as well as higher mortality for individuals older than 65 years. Since all outcomes analyses findings are functions of the database and the methodology employed, these findings are complimentary and noncontradictory.

It is instructive to compare the mortality data for bariatric surgery with the population-based in-hospital mortality data compiled by Dimick and associates (79) for aortic aneurysms (3.9%), coronary artery bypass grafting (3.5%), craniotomy (10.7%), esophageal resections (9.9%), hip replacement (0.3%), pancreatectomy (8.3%), and pediatric heart surgery (5.4%)—all, with the

Table 1 Complications

Early complications	Late complications
Procedure independent	Procedure independent
Respiratory—airway obstruction, atelectasis, pneumonia	Ventral/incisional hernia
Wound infection	Internal hernia
Urinary tract infection	Intestinal obstruction—adhesions
Deep venous thrombosis and pulmonary embolism	
Prolonged ileus	Procedure specific
Intestinal obstruction—clot, internal hernia	Laparoscopic adjustable gastric banding
Early bleeding	Pouch dilation
Fistula	Pouch slippage/prolapse
Dehiscence and evisceration	Band erosion
Leak	Port migration/port or tube leakage
Peritonitis	Need for multiple adjustments
Sepsis and multiple organ failure	Vertical banded gastroplasty
	Food or capsule lodgment in band or ring
Procedure specific	Outlet obstruction/stenosis
Laparoscopic adjustable gastric banding	Ring slippage
Gastrointestinal perforation	Outlet dilation
Mechanical port and tubing failures	Staple line disruption
Gastric bypass	Gastric bypass
Acute gastric pouch dilation	Dumping syndrome
Biliopancreatic diversion/duodenal switch	Iron deficiency
Inhibited gastrointestinal motility	Vitamin B_{12} deficiency
	Staple line disruption and gastrogastric fistula
	Stricutre
	Stomal dilation
	Stomal ulcer
	Gastric remnant distention and rupture
	Biliopancreatic diversion/duodenal switch
	Diarrhea
	Foul flatulence
	Electrolyte abnormalities
	Vitamin and mineral deficiencies
	Anemia
	Bone demineralization
	Stomal ulcer
	Hypoproteinemia
	Liver failure

exception of hip replacement, exceeding that of the generally reported experience with bariatric surgery.

Early Complications

Procedure Independent

Bariatric surgery, procedure-independent early complications include respiratory problems (airway obstruction, atelectasis, pneumonia), wound infections, urinary tract infections, deep vein thrombophlebitis and pulmonary embolization, prolonged ileus, intestinal obstruction (clot, internal hernia), early bleeding, fistula formation, dehiscence and evisceration, intestinal leak, peritonitis

(usually secondary to leak), and sepsis and multiple organ failure (Table 1). These complications can occur after any major abdominal procedure, and their recognition and management are not within the scope of this chapter. While wound infections are less frequent following laparoscopic than open bariatric surgery, early bleeding and obstruction by clot or an internal hernia are more common after laparoscopic than open bariatric surgery, as are leaks. The best therapy for these complications is, of course, prevention, including the use of perioperative antibiotics and anticoagulation, lower extremities pumping and compression devices, respiratory toilet, and early ambulation. Certainly, there is no better prevention than good operative technique and judgment.

There are other, rare, nonspecific complications such as rhabdomyolysis involving the necrosis of the gluteal muscles and renal failure. This crush injury syndrome is a risk in the superobese who are on the operating room table for a prolonged period of time, and it is often fatal (80).

Procedure Specific

There are a few early procedure-specific complications (Table 1). With laparoscopic adjustable gastric banding it is possible to see gastrointestinal perforation, a technical error, and malfunctioning of the mechanical device's port and/or tubing (81). With biliopancreatic diversion/duodenal switch there may be a prolongation or inhibition of gastrointestinal motility, without any evidence of a specific site of obstruction, prolonging hospitalization for two to three days. This problem may be secondary to the longer operating time for these procedures or to the gastric resection component.

The most serious early procedure-specific complication is acute distal gastric pouch dilation after gastric bypass. If this problem is suspected, it can be definitively diagnosed by a CT scan, rather than by an ordinary abdominal X ray, since a fluid-filled structure not containing gas is poorly visualized on a flat X-ray plate. If this complication occurs, the distal pouch must be drained immediately to prevent gastric rupture. Drainage can usually be performed percutaneously by invasive radiology, without the need for a laparoscopic or open celiotomy. Localization of the distal gastric remnant for percutaneous drainage is facilitated by the intraoperative placement of a radio opaque marker attached to the gastric remnant and the abdominal wall.

Late Complications

Procedure Independent

The three main procedure-independent late complications of bariatric surgery are ventral/incisional hernias, internal hernias, and intestinal obstruction (Table 1).

The incidence of ventral or incisional hernias has been cited as high as 25% after open bariatric surgery, but usually is stated to be about 5% (82). Laparoscopic bariatric surgery ventral or port site hernias are uncommon but can be dangerous since the small size of the hernia opening is conducive to bowel entrapment, incarceration, and strangulation (83). On the other hand, internal hernia and intermittent or sustained bowel obstruction are far more common after laparoscopic than open surgery (83). This difference may be due to the relative paucity of adhesions after laparoscopic surgery and/or poor technical closure of potential internal hernia defects.

Adhesive intestinal obstruction, partial, intermittent, and complete, can occur after any abdominal cavity procedure. It is more common after open than laparoscopic bariatric surgery. In addition to the general diagnostic and therapeutic principles of management or bowel obstruction, the gastric bypass patient poses the extra danger of distal gastric remnant rupture (see above).

Procedure Specific

Laparoscopic adjustable gastric banding

The long-term complications of laparoscopic adjustable gastric banding are uniquely linked to this technology using a prosthetic, circumferential gastric band and its port and tubing (81). Pouch dilation usually refers to a band being too tight and leading to proximal band dilation, which, in turn, may cause esophageal dilation. Pouch slippage/prolapse refers to the band slipping down or the distal stomach protruding upward over the band, both resulting in an enlarged, malfunctioning, restricted upper gastric pouch. The Silastic band has been known to erode into the stomach wall and actually into the gastric lumen over time. The port and tubing can migrate, the port can flip over, and these parts may leak.

With global and regional learning curves and a universal conversion to the pars flaccida technique, the complication rate of laparoscopic adjustable gastric banding has decreased. We do not as yet know if over a prolonged period of time the procedure specific complications of this technique will diminish, remain constant, or increase.

The necessity for multiple adjustments, approximately six within the first year, can be viewed as an advantage, allowing for rest or off periods for special occasions and a guarantee for proper follow-up. These adjustments can also be viewed as an inconvenience and as a continuing reminder to the patient that the surgery was performed.

If a complication occurs, the surgeon can revise the laparoscopic adjustable gastric band or, since removal of the band is not difficult, replace it with another bariatric procedure (e.g., gastric bypass or biliopancreatic diversion/duodenal switch). Replacement with another purely restrictive procedure (i.e., vertical banded gastroplasty) is not advisable.

Vertical banded gastroplasty

The most common complication with vertical banded gastroplasty is lodgment of a food particle or a drug capsule in the purposely restricted gastroplasty orifice. If vomiting of all oral intake, including water, persists for over 24 hours, acute outlet obstruction is likely. Endoscopic removal of the foreign body is curative.

The outlet of a vertical banded gastroplasty can become chronically obstructive due to stenotic scarring, more often seen after the Mason procedure polypropylene mesh collar than the Silastic ring. On the other hand, the Silastic ring can slip inferiorly and cause obstruction by a ball-valving effect on the outlet lumen. Outlet dilation may also occur; possibly, this is not true dilation but improper original sizing at construction. Finally, staple line disruption is a complication and can cause a regaining of weight. These various complications of vertical banded gastroplasty are discussed and well covered by Jamieson (82).

Remedial vertical banded gastroplasty surgery consists of a redoing (restapling, rebanding) of the operation or, more to be recommended, conversion to a gastric bypass, long-limb gastric bypass, or biliopancreatic diversion/ duodenal switch.

Gastric bypass

The procedure-specific complications of gastric bypass have been well documented (83,84).

Gastric bypass is associated with the dumping syndrome, which some consider a benefit since it inhibits sweet eating. Especially, if they are not diligent about their supplementary vitamin intake, these patients can develop an iron deficiency and even an iron deficiency anemia; this is a finding most common in heavily menstruating women. Gastric bypass patients will not absorb adequate amounts of vitamin B_{12} and all require extra supplementation intramuscularly or orally to avoid the consequences of B_{12} insufficiency after a year or so postoperatively.

On the mechanical side, the gastrojejunostomy is subject to stricture, more commonly after laparoscopic than open surgery, as well as dilation and weight gain. Stomal ulceration with possible bleeding can occur. If proton pump blockers fail to control a stomal ulcer, anastomotic revision or even a distal gastrectomy may become necessary. A stapled gastric bypass without division of the upper pouch from the gastric remnant can be subject to staple line disruption; a divided pouch can form a gastrogastric fistula.

As has been discussed, distal small bowel obstruction can lead to reflux of intestinal contents into the gastric remnant, its distention, and eventual rupture. Again, immediate drainage of the gastric remnant is necessary.

Gastric bypass revisions consist of constructing a new gastric bypass, conversion to a long-limb gastric bypass, or conversion to a biliopancreatic diversion/duodenal switch. Rarely, construction of a vertical banded gastroplasty within a dilated upper gastric pouch or placement of a laparoscopic adjustable gastric band can be attempted.

Biliopancreatic diversion/duodenal switch

The procedure-specific complications of biliopancreatic diversion/duodenal switch have been well documented by Scopinaro (85) and Hess (86).

It is surprising that more patients with such a short common channel as is present after biliopancreatic diversion duodenal switch do not have diarrhea; however, this complication is infrequent. On the other hand, foul flatus is fairly prevalent. Both of these problems are easily managed with oral agents.

Electrolyte abnormalities, vitamin and mineral deficiencies, and anemia have all been reported but can be avoided by judicious supplement intake. Long-term bone demineralization is a threat following this malabsorptive procedure and bone mineral density should be monitored. Stomal ulcers are rare after the duodenal switch.

Patients selected for these procedures must have sound livers and not be alcoholics. They must be protein eaters and consume about 70 g of protein daily. If not, they can be subject to hypoproteinemia and, if unchecked, to liver failure and possible death.

A failed biliopancreatic diversion/duodenal switch for inadequate weight loss is most uncommon and can be treated by shortening of the common channel. A failed biliopancreatic diversion/duodenal switch for excess weight loss is also uncommon and can be treated by lengthening of the common channel.

Patient Failure

About 5% of patients will fail bariatric surgery therapy with no anatomic cause, i.e., a textbook perfect operative procedure by X-ray and endoscopic assessment; indeed, these individuals may subsequently fail revisional surgery. These patients can outeat the restrictive element of bariatric procedures by frequent meals, drinking calories, and eating comfort high-caloric foods; they can overwhelm the malabsorptive element of bypass procedures. Rarely does behavior modification or other medical therapy prove beneficial.

Most infrequently, there are patients with excellent weight results and anatomically competent procedures who demand a takedown and a return to their preoperative state, even if this entails regaining their weight. These examples of patient failure represent patient-selection failures; preoperative psychological evaluation and testing does not prevent this problem.

OUTCOMES

Weight Loss

In essence, every published series has cited its weight loss data. Possibly, the least biased assessments are obtained from global systematic reviews and meta-analyses, since selection bias for a meta-analysis is based on study method and quality and never on outcomes. Two global systematic reviews and meta-analyses with weight loss results have been performed: the first focused on four obesity comorbidity outcomes (type 2 diabetes, hyperlipidemia, hypertension, and obstructive sleep apnea) (71) and the second on type 2 diabetes (87). The

Table 2 Weight Loss—Systematic Review and Meta-analyses

Study (reference)	Study numbers			Weight loss (%EBWL)				
	Studies	Treatment groups	Patients	Overall	Laparoscopic adjustable gastric banding	Vertical banded gastroplasty	Gastric bypass	Biliopancreatic diversion/duodenal switch
Comorbidities study (71)	136	179	22,094	64.67	49.59	69.15	68.11	72.09
Diabetes study (87)	621	888	135,246	55.92	46.17	55.53	59.53	63.61

Abbreviation: %EBWL, percent excess body weight lost.

number of studies, treatment arms, and patients involved in each study, the overall weight loss (percent excess body weight loss), and the weight loss by procedure (laparoscopic adjustable gastric banding, vertical banded gastroplasty, gastric bypass, biliopancreatic diversion/duodenal switch) are given in Table 2. It is evident that the weight loss achieved is a function of the severity of the procedure and is reciprocal with respect to the previously discussed operative mortality. Thus, weight loss is progressive from laparoscopic adjustable gastric banding to vertical banded gastroplasty to gastric bypass to biliopancreatic diversion/duodenal switch.

These systematic review and meta-analytic data are for relatively short follow-up intervals. There are currently no comparable large, cumulative analyses of long-term (over five years) weight loss outcomes.

Nutrition and Metabolism

Discussion of the metabolic (88) and nutritional (89) outcomes in bariatric surgery are encyclopedic and fall into positive effects and negative outcomes. Energy metabolism subsequent to weight loss is more balanced. For example, fat is an insulator and an obese person burns fewer calories to maintain internal heat than a lean person and, thereby, increases caloric conversion to more adipose tissue. On weight loss, this individual will need to burn more calories for heat and, thereby, achieve a more homeostatic energy balance.

The purposely created malabsorption of bariatric surgery, either by diversion of food intake or limitation of digestive/absorptive surfaces can, as a function of the severity of the malabsorption, cause certain macronutrient (protein, essential fatty acids) and micronutrient (iron, calcium, zinc, magnesium, vitamins B_{12}, B_6, B_1, A, E, and K) deficiencies, as well as raise plasma homocysteine levels. The best preventive measure for these negative outcomes is appropriate selection of foods, especially those high in protein and with vitamin and mineral supplementation, with at least annual laboratory monitoring of all post-bariatric surgery patients for a lifetime.

Diabetes

As an outcome of the global epidemic of obesity, the prevalence of obesity-induced type 2 diabetes mellitus is in worldwide ascendancy. The marked amelioration, possibly "cure," of type 2 diabetes following bariatric surgery, in particular after gastric bypass, was articulated by Pories in 1995 in an article provocatively titled "Who would have thought it? An operation proves to be the most effective therapy for adult-onset diabetes mellitus" (90). This article inspired over 30 confirmative reports, including articles by Schauer et al. (91), Sugerman et al. (92), and the Swedish Obesity Subjects study (93).

In our 2004 comorbidities meta-analysis (71), we demonstrated complete resolution of type 2 diabetes in 77% of patients and resolution or improvement in 86%. These clinical findings were confirmed by reductions in the hemoglobin A_1c and fasting blood glucose levels. In our 2007 diabetes meta-analysis (87), 78% of patients had complete resolution of their diabetes and 87% had resolution or improvement. Again, there were corroborating declines in the hemoglobin A_1c and in the fasting blood glucose level. These changes were maintained for longer than two years. In both studies, weight loss and diabetes resolution was greatest for patients undergoing the greatest weight loss (biliopancreatic diversion/duodenal switch) and least for those undergoing the least weight loss (banding procedures).

An interesting phenomenon that has been observed is that the manifestation of type 2 diabetes can totally clear within days after a gastric bypass, before there is any significant weight loss (90,94,95). This finding would suggest that changes in the gut hormonal milieu following bypass of the distal stomach, duodenum, and proximal jejunum can influence the mechanism of type 2 diabetes. Substantiation of this hypothesis comes from the studies of Rubino et al. who demonstrated that a bypass of the duodenum and upper jejunum in lean diabetic rats would return them to euglycemia, even though they maintain normal weight (96). Further, Arguelles and associates recently reported a small series of lean diabetic patients who experienced remission of their diabetes with a modification of the Rubino procedure (97).

Hyperlipidemia

In the Swedish Obesity Surgery study (93), the incidence of hyperlipidemia was lower by 10-fold after two years in the surgery group in comparison with the control group. Similar findings have been reported by others (98–101). In the 1990 report of the Program on the Surgical Control of the Hyperlipidemias (POSCH), reductions in the levels of total (23%) and low-density lipoprotein cholesterol (38%), in association with an increase in high-density lipoprotein cholesterol (4%), after a surgical distal ileal malabsorptive procedure were described (102). In the 2004 outcomes meta-analysis, hyperlipidemia improved in 70% or more of patients (71).

Hypertension

The 2004 outcomes meta-analysis showed 62% resolution of hypertension and 79% resolution or improvement (71); this reduction was independent of the operative procedure performed. These findings have been repeated in several studies well reviewed by MacDonald and Pender (103). Decreases in systolic and diastolic blood pressure with a decrease in weight are well known (104–106). As a generalization, a decrease of 1% in body weight will decrease systolic blood pressure by 1 mmHg and diastolic blood pressure by 2 mmHg.

Obstructive Sleep Apnea

In the outcomes meta-analysis, improvement in obstructive sleep apnea was dramatic—over 80% (71). The extracted bariatric surgery literature is quite prolific on this subject. In association with the clinical findings, improvement in oxygen saturation, decreases in arterial carbon dioxide, and increases in arterial oxygen content have been demonstrated (107–109). These favorable physiologic changes in the blood contents, which in turn affect the neurologic pathways and cerebral centers responsible for respiration, are primarily the result of an increase in diaphragmatic excursion. This increase is brought about by a reduction in intra-abdominal pressure after successful bariatric surgery (110,111).

Other Comorbidities

The comorbidities of morbid obesity affect essentially every organ system: cardiovascular (hypertension, atherosclerotic heart and peripheral vascular disease with

Table 3 Effects on Comorbidities: Reversal or Improvement Proven

1. Type 2 diabetes
2. Hyperlipidemia
3. Hypertension
4. Obstructive sleep apnea
5. Cardiac function failure
6. Asthma
7 Back strain and disk disease
8. Weight-bearing osteoarthritis (hips, knees, ankles, feet)
9. Gastroesophageal reflux disease
10. Nonalcoholic fatty liver disease and cirrhosis
11. Stress incontinence
12. Polycystic ovarian syndrome
13. Intertriginous dermatitis
14. Pseudotumor cerebri
15. Depression

Source: From Ref. 143.

myocardial infarction and cerebral vascular accidents, peripheral venous insufficiency); respiratory (asthma, obstructive sleep apnea, obesity-hypoventillation syndrome); metabolic (type 2 diabetes, impaired glucose tolerance, dyslipidemia); musculoskeletal (back strain, disk disease, weight-bearing osteoarthritis of the hips, knees, ankles, and feet); gastrointestinal [cholelithiasis, gastroesophageal reflux disease, fatty metamorphosis of the liver (steatohepatitis), cirrhosis of the liver, hepatic carcinoma, colorectal carcinoma]; urinary (stress incontinence); endocrine and reproductive (polycystic ovary syndrome, increased risk for pregnancy and fetal abnormalities, male hypogonadism, and cancer of the endometrium, breast, ovary, prostate, and pancreas); dermatologic (intertriginous dermatitis); neurologic (pseudotumor cerebri, carpal tunnel syndrome); and psychologic (depression) (112,113). It is interesting to note how many carcinomas have been demonstrated to have an increased incidence in the presence of obesity.

The salutary effects of bariatric surgery on the comorbid conditions of obesity can be divided into those where reversal or improvement has essentially been proven (Table 3) and those where reversal or improvement can be reasonably presumed (Table 4).

Quality of Life

Quality of life needs to be differentiated from depression, and outcome of changes of quality of life can be analyzed as objective, perceived, and measured. Depression is a disease quite common in the obese and often mitigated by weight loss; yet, there are bariatric surgery patients with excellent weight loss and resolution of other comorbidities who continue to be depressed.

Table 4 Effects on Comorbidities: Reversal or Improvement Reasonably Presumed

1. Carcinoma: breast
2. Carcinoma: colon
3. Carcinoma: liver
4. Carcinoma: ovary
5. Carcinoma: pancreas
6. Carcinoma: prostate
7. Carcinoma: uterus
8. Cardiac and peripheral vascular disease
9. Carpal tunnel syndrome
10. Incidence of cerebrovascular accident
11. Incidence of cholelithiasis
12. Incidence of thrombophlebitis and pulmonary embolism
13. Obstetric and fetal complications

Source: From Ref. 143.

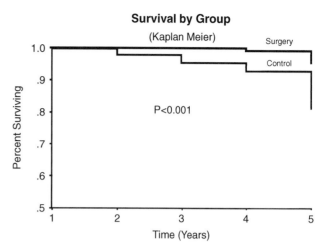

Figure 11 Bariatric surgery effect on longevity. *Source*: From Ref. 117.

When individuals lose more than 50% of their excess body weight, obtain resolution of debilitating comorbidities, and increase their ability to be active, exercise, and participate in work and social activities, the quality of life is objectively improved. And, for the most part, the post-bariatric surgery patients perceive these benefits as an improvement in their quality of life (114).

There are several instruments to measure quality of life, some specifically designed to be used in association with bariatric surgery (115,116). All of these analyses have demonstrated a dramatic improvement in the subjective quality of life after successful bariatric surgery. Changes in the quality of life tend to be linear and inversely proportional with the postoperative changes in the BMI.

Longevity

Since obesity per se reduces life expectancy and since most certainly many of the comorbidities of obesity also independently reduce life expectancy, it stands to reason that the marked weight reduction and reversal of comorbidities induced by bariatric surgery should increase longevity. Christou et al. published the first definitive major study to demonstrate this finding (117). This study showed a statistically significant 89% ($p < 0.001$) decrease in mortality at five years (control 6.17%, surgery 0.68%) with a risk ratio of 0.11 (0.04–0.27) (Fig. 11). These data were substantiated by four subsequent studies, well summarized by Dixon (118).

Costs

Insurance carriers claim that the costs for bariatric surgery are prohibitive—but this is the case only because they

cannot maintain their customer base long enough for the surgery to become profitable. Sampalis et al. have shown that the five-year health care utilization data for hospitalizations, hospital stay, and physician visits all indicate a greater use of health care facilities by obese controls in comparison with patients who had undergone bariatric surgery (119). Accounting for the initial cost for the operative procedure and hospital care, the costs for the obese control patients exceeded those for the bariatric patients before four years, with continued divergence thereafter (Fig. 12).

The literature on the financial benefits of bariatric surgery is quite substantial and has been well-reviewed by Martin, who states, "To-date, only bariatric surgery has been shown to treat any form of obesity in a truly cost-effective manner" (120).

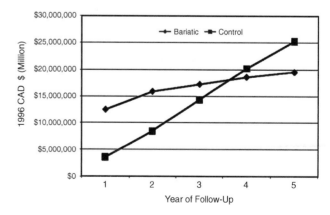

Figure 12 Bariatric surgery cost analysis. *Source*: From Ref. 119.

SPECIAL TOPICS

Surgery in the Elderly

The early mortality report by Flum et al. of Medicare beneficiaries raised doubts about bariatric surgery in the elderly, especially their data of a progressive fivefold increase in 90-day mortality for patients aged 75 years or more in comparison with those aged 65 to 74 years (78). On the other hand, in our 2007 mortality meta-analysis, being elderly, defined as $\geq$65 years, increased the 30-day mortality by only a modest amount—0.34% in comparison with 0.28% (72). All in all, the consensus on bariatric surgery for the elderly is favorable and would remove any upper age barrier for consideration of bariatric surgery (121,122).

Surgery in the Adolescent

Adolescent obesity is now one of the most common childhood disorders, with 4.7 million American adolescents having a BMI greater than the 95th percentile (123). Most of these adolescents do not respond to diet modification or exercise programs and attention is now turning toward surgery as a source of weight loss.

Adolescent bariatric surgery dates back to the 1970s (124) but has become more prevalent in the 21st century (125–131). This surgery is safe and results in significant weight loss. Proponents agree that bariatric surgery should involve a multidisciplinary approach including surgeons, pediatricians, dieticians, exercise therapists, and psychiatrists, as well as parents and other family members.

Body Contouring Postoperatively

Body contouring after bariatric surgery is not a luxury but often a necessity to achieve not only reasonable cosmetic results but also appropriate health care, e.g., huge abdominal folds can lead to back strain and fungal intertriginous dermatitis. Post-bariatric surgery skinfold procedures range from simple panniculectomies to upper, lower, and total body lifts—the latter a complex, anterior and posterior procedure that can involve 7 to 12 hours in the operating room (132,133).

Training of the Bariatric Surgeon

Bariatric surgery is expanding, hampered only by patient access restrictions posed by health care groups, insurance carriers, and often the ultimate payer organizations. Obviously, there is no lack of eager patients who meet current operative guidelines. If the cost-effectiveness of bariatric surgery becomes more universally appreciated and if carriers can alter their own business practices to realize a profit on the care of bariatric surgery patients, then the limiting factor in the number of bariatric procedures performed may well become the number of available trained bariatric surgeons. In 2003, a questionnaire was sent to the accredited surgery residency training programs and the accredited minimally invasive surgery fellowship programs in the United States. Of the 251 surgery residency training programs, 185 (73.7%) performed bariatric surgery, and of the 48 minimally invasive surgery fellowship programs, 43 (89.6%) performed bariatric surgery (134). These training exposures, however, do not result in a trained bariatric surgeon, and there are several programs available to train the bariatric surgeon in an academic setting (135) and in the community (136). Once trained, reasonable standards in bariatric surgery are maintained by the accreditation processes of the American Society for Metabolic and Bariatric Surgeon's Surgical Review Corporation (137) and the American College of Surgeons (138).

The Bariatric Surgery Multidisciplinary Team

The field of bariatric surgery has markedly changed in the past 50 years. Most strikingly, it has evolved from single or group practices, academic or community, often isolated by other members of the medical profession, to fairly large-scale endeavors based on a multidisciplinary team concept (139). Indeed, a specialized cadre of professionals has evolved in bariatric surgery consisting of the Allied Sciences (140) with their own representation and meetings within the ASMBS and the International Federation for the Surgery of Obesity. These changes in the field have enhanced patient care and provide the only reasonable means for following bariatric surgery patients for a lifetime.

CLOSURE

The future evolution of therapy for morbid obesity will include nonsurgical innovations: possibly new diets of noncaloric foods, newer methods of behavior modification, new and more effective drugs, hybridization of drugs and bariatric surgery, management of the intestinal flora that may facilitate caloric absorption, anti-etiologic/viral agents, and gene therapy. Strictly surgical innovations will, most certainly, consist of newer procedures to influence gastric and intestinal metabolism, possibly central nervous system or intravenous infusions of incretins by implantable pumps, and possibly hypothalamic stimulation and/or ablation. Whatever the next decade or so has in store for the treatment of morbid obesity, the literature will demonstrate that bariatric surgeons were there when there was no other effective therapy; at least for the present, morbid obesity is a surgical disease (141).

REFERENCES

1. Buchwald H, Varco RL, eds. Metabolic Surgery. New York: Grune and Stratton, 78.

2. NIH Consensus Statement. Gastrointestinal surgery for severe obesity. March 25, 1991; 9(1):1–20.

3. CDC/NHANES. Overweight and obesity: Obesity trends: U.S. Obesity Trends 1985–2005. Available at: http://www.cdc.gov/nccdphp/dnpa/obesity/trend/maps/index.htm. Accessed July 17, 2007.

4. Grummer-Strawn L, Hughes M, Kahn LK, et al. Obesity in women from developing countries. Eur J Clin Nutr 2000; 54:247–252.

5. International Union of Nutritional Sciences, The Global Challenge of Obesity and the International Obesity Task Force: The Global Epidemic of Obesity; Trends and Projections. Available at: Accessed July 17, 2007.

6. World Health Organization. Obesity and Overweight. Available at: http://www.who.int/dietphysicalactivity/publications/facts/obesity/en/. Accessed July 17, 2007.

7. Buchwald H, for the Consensus Conference Panel. Bariatric surgery for morbid obesity: health implications for patients, health professionals, and third-party payers. J Am Coll Surg 2005; 200:593–604.

8. Kottek SS. On health and obesity in Talmudic and Midrashic lore. Israel J Med Sci 1996; 32:509–510.

9. Henrikson V. Kan tunnfarmsresektion forsvaras som terapi mot fettsot? Nordisk Medicin 1952, 47, 744. Translation: Can small bowel resection be defended as therapy for obesity? Obes Surg 1994; 4:54.

10. Buchwald H, Rucker RD. The rise and fall of jejunoileal bypass. In: Nelson RL, Nyhus LM, eds. Surgery of the Small Intestine. Norwalk, CT: Appleton Century Crofts, 1987:529–541.

11. Kremen AJ, Linner LH, Nelson CH. An experimental evaluation of the nutritional importance of proximal and distal small intestine. Ann Surg 1954; 140:439–444.

12. Payne JH, DeWind LT, Commons RR. Metabolic observations in patients with jejunocolic shunts. Am J Surg 1963; 106:272–289.

13. Payne JH, DeWind LT. Surgical treatment of obesity. Am J Surg 1969; 118:141–147.

14. Scott HW, Sandstead HH, Brill AB. Experience with a new technic of intestinal bypass in the treatment of morbid obesity. Ann Surg 1971; 174:560–572.

15. Salmon PA. The results of small intestine bypass operations for the treatment of obesity. Surg Gynecol Obstet 1971; 132:965–979.

16. Buchwald H, Varco RL. A bypass operation for obese hyperlipidemic patients. Surgery 1971; 70:62–70.

17. Lavorato F, Doldi SB, Scaramella R. Evoluzione storica della terapia chirurgica della grande obesita. Minerva Med 1978; 69:3847–3857.

18. Eriksson F. Biliointestinal bypass. Int J Obes 1981; 5:437–447.

19. Scopinaro N, Gianetta E, Civalleri D. Biliopancreatic bypass for obesity: II. Initial experiences in man. Br J Surg 1979; 66:618–620.

20. Scopinaro N, Adami GF, Marinari GM, et al. Biliopancreatic diversion: two decades of experience. In: Deitel M, Cowan SM Jr., eds. Update: Surgery for the Morbidly Obese Patient. Toronto, Canada: FD-Communications Inc, 2000:227–258.

21. Hess DW, Hess DS. Biliopancreatic diversion with a duodenal switch. Obes Surg 1998; 8:267–282.

22. Marceau P, Biron S, Bourque R-A, Potvin M, et al. Biliopancreatic diversion with a new type of gastrectomy. Obes Surg 1993; 3:29–35.

23. Mason EE, Ito C. Gastric bypass in obesity. Surg Clin N Am 1967; 47:1345–1352.

24. Alden JF. Gastric and jejuno-ileal bypass: a comparison in the treatment of morbid obesity. Arch Surg 1977; 112:799–806.

25. Griffen WO, Young VL, Stevenson CC. A prospective comparison of gastric and jejunoileal bypass procedures for morbid obesity. Ann Surg 1977; 186:500–507.

26. McCarthy HB, Rucker RD, Chan EK, et al. Gastritis after gastric bypass surgery. Surgery 1985; 98:68–71.

27. Torres JC, Oca CF, Garrison RN. Gastric bypass: Roux-en-Y gastrojejunostomy from the lesser curvature. South Med J 1983; 76:1217–1221.

28. Linner JR, Drew RL. New modification of Roux-en-Y gastric bypass procedure. Clin Nutr 1986; 5:33–34.

29. Torres J, Oca C. Gastric bypass lesser curvature with distal Roux-en-Y. Bariatric Surg 1987; 5:10–15.

30. Brolin RE, Kenler HA, Gorman JH, et al. Long-limb gastric bypass in the superobese. A prospective randomized study. Ann Surg 1992; 21:387–395.

31. Nelson WK, Fatima J, Houghton SG, et al. The malabsorptive very, very long limb Roux-en-Y gastric bypass for super obesity. Surgery 2006; 140:517–522.

32. Salmon PA. Gastroplasty with distal gastric bypass: a new and more successful weight loss operation for the morbidly obese. Can J Surg 1988; 31:111–113.

33. Fobi MA. The surgical technique of the banded Roux-en-Y gastric bypass. J Obes Weight Reg 1989; 8:99–102.

34. Fobi MA. Why the operation I prefer is Silastic ring vertical banded gastric bypass. Obes Surg 1991; 1:423–426.

35. Wittgrove AC, Clark GW, Tremblay, LJ. Laparoscopic gastric bypass, Roux-en-Y: preliminary report of five cases. Obes Surg 1994; 4:353–357.

36. de la Torre RA, Scott JS. Laparoscopic Roux-en-Y gastric bypass: a totally intra-abdominal approach—technique and preliminary report. Obes Surg 1999; 9:492–497.

37. Schauer PR, Ikramuddin S, Gourash W, et al. Outcomes of laparoscopic Roux-en-Y gastric bypass for morbid obesity. Ann Surg 2000; 232:515–529.

38. Higa KD, Boone KB, Ho T. Laparoscopic Roux-en-Y gastric bypass for morbid obesity in 850 patients: technique and follow-up. Obes Surg 2000; 10:146 (abstr P34).

39. Printen KJ, Mason EE. Gastric surgery for relief of morbid obesity. Arch Surg. 1973; 106:428–431.

40. Gomez CA. Gastroplasty in morbid obesity. Surg Clin North Am 1979; 59:1113–1120.

41. Pace WG, Martin EW, Tetirick CE, et al. Gastric partitioning for morbid obesity. Ann Surg. 1979; 190:392–400.

42. LaFave JW, Alden JF. Gastric bypass in the operative revision of the failed jejuno-ileal bypass. Arch Surg. 1979; 114:438–444.

43. Fabito DC. Gastric vertical stapling. Read before the Bariatric Surgery colloquium, Iowa City, Iowa, June 1, 1981.

44. Laws HL, Piatadosi S. Superior gastric reduction procedure for morbid obesity. A prospective, randomized trial. Am J Surg 1981; 193:334–336.

45. Mason EE. Vertical banded gastroplasty. Arch Surg 1982; 117:701–706.

46. Hess DW, Hess DS. Laparoscopic vertical banded gastroplasty with complete transection of the staple-line. Obes Surg 1994; 4:44–46.

47. Chua TY, Mendiola RM. Laparoscopic vertical banded gastroplasty: the Milwaukee experience. Obes Surg 1995; 5:77–80.

48. Kuzmak LI. Silicone gastric banding: a simple and effective operation for morbid obesity. Contemp Surg 1986; 28:13–18.

49. Broadbent R, Tracy M, Harrington P. Laparoscopic gastric banding: a preliminary report. Obes Surg 1993; 3:63–67.

50. Catona A, Gossenberg M, La Manna A, et al. Laparoscopic gastric banding: preliminary series. Obes Surg 1993; 3:207–209.

51. Belachew M, Legrand M, Jacquet N. Laparoscopic placement of adjustable silicone gastric banding in the treatment of morbid obesity: an animal model experimental study: a video film: a preliminary report. Obes Surg 1993; 3:140 (abstr 5).

52. Forsell P, Hallberg D, Hellers G. Gastric banding for morbid obesity: initial experience with a new adjustable band. Obes Surg 1993; 3:369–374.

53. Niville E, Vankeirsblick J, Dams A, et al. Laparoscopic adjustable esophagogastric banding: a preliminary experience. Obes Surg 1998; 8:39–42.

54. Cadiere GB, Himpens J, Vertruyen M. The world's first obesity surgery performed by a surgeon at a distance. Obes Surg (England) 1999; 9:206–209.

55. Johnston D, Dachtler J, Sue-Ling HM, et al. The Magenstrasse and Mill operation for morbid obesity. Obes Surg 2003; 13:10–16.

56. Baltasar A, Bou R, Bengochea M, et al. Duodenal switch: an effective therapy for morbid obesity—intermediate results. Obes Surg 2001; 11:54–58.

57. Rabkin RA, Rabkin JM, Metcalf B, et al. Laparoscopic technique for performing duodenal switch with gastric reduction. Obes Surg 2003; 13:263–268.

58. Lee CM, Feng JJ, Cirangle PT, et al. Laparoscopic duodenal switch and sleeve gastrectomy procedures. In: Buchwald H, Pories W, Cowan GM Jr., eds. Surgical Management of Obesity. Philadelphia, PA: Elsevier, 2007: 267–277.

59. Quaade F, Vaernet K, Larsson S. Sterotaxic stimulation and electrocoagulation of the lateral hypothalamus in obese humans. Acta Neurochir (Wien) 1974; 30:1111–1117.

60. Cigaina V, Pinato G, Rigo V. Gastric peristalsis control by mono situ electrical stimulation: a preliminary study. Obes Surg 1996; 6:247–249.

61. Reddy R, Horovitz J, Roslin M. Chronic bilateral vagus nerve stimulation (VNS) changes eating behavior resulting in weight loss in a canine model. Surg Forum 2000; 51: 24–26.

62. Giralt M, Vergara P. Glucagonlike peptide-1 (GLP-1) participation in ileal brake induced by intraluminal peptones in rat. Dig Dis Sci 1999; 44:322–329.

63. Naslund E, Bogefors J, Skogar S, et al. GLP-1 slows solid gastric emptying and inhibits insulin, glucagon, and PYY release in humans. Am J Physiol 1999; 227:R910–R916.

64. Strader AD, Vahl TP, Jandacek RJ, et al. Weight loss through ileal transposition is accompanied by increased ileal hormone secretion and synthesis in rats. Am J Physiol Endocrinol Metab 2004; 288:E447–E453.

65. Mathus-Vliegen EM, Tytgat GN. Intragastric balloon for treatment-resistant obesity: safety, tolerance, and efficacy of 1-year balloon treatment followed by a 1-year balloon-free follow-up. Gastrointest Endosc 2005; 61:19–27.

66. Awan AN, Swain CP. Endoscopic vertical banded gastroplasty with an endoscopic sewing machine. Gastrointest Endosc 2002; 55:254–256.

67. Hu B, Chung SC, Sun LC, et al. Transoral obesity surgery: endoluminal gastroplasty with an endoscopic suture device. Endoscopy 2005; 37:411–414.

68. Feisher J, Rosen M, Farres H, et al. A novel endolaparoscopic intragastric partitioning for treatment of morbid obesity. Surg Laparosc Endosc Percutan Tech 2004; 14:243–246.

69. Malik A, Mellinger JD, Hazey JW, et al. Endoluminal and transluminal surgery: current status and future possibilities. Surg Endosc 2006; 20:1179–1192.

70. Buchwald H. A bariatric surgery algorithm. Obes Surg 2002; 12:733–746.

71. Buchwald H, Avidor Y, Braunwald E, et al. Bariatric Surgery: a systematic review and meta-analysis. JAMA 2004; 292:1724–1737.

72. Buchwald H, Estok R, Fahrbach K, et al. Trends in mortality in bariatric surgery: a systematic review and meta-analysis. Surgery, 2007; 142:621–635.

73. Zingmond DS, McGory ML, Ko CY. Hospitalization before and after gastric bypass surgery. JAMA 2006; 294:1918–1924.

74. Mason EE, Tang S, Renquist KE, et al. A decade of change in obesity surgery. National Bariatric Surgery Registry (NBSR) Contributors. Obes Surg 1997; 7:189–197.

75. Nguyen NT, Morton JM, Wolfe BM, et al. The SAGES Bariatric Surgery outcome inititiave. Surg Endosc 2005; 19:1429–1438.

76. Leffler E, Gustavsson S, Karlson BM. Time trends in obesity surgery 1987 through 1996 in Sweden—A population-based study. Obes Surg 2000; 10:543–548.

77. Pratt GM, McLees B, Pories WJ. The ASBS Bariatric Surgery Centers of Excellence program: a blueprint for quality improvement. SOARD 2006; 2:497–503.

78. Flum DR, Salem L, Elrod JAB, et al. Early mortality among Medicare beneficiaries undergoing bariatric surgical procedures. JAMA 2005; 294:1903–1908.

79. Dimick JB, Welch HG, Birkmeyer JD. Surgical mortality as an indicator of hospital quality. JAMA 2004; 292: 847–851.

80. Anthone G, Bostanjian D, Hamoui N, et al. Rhabdomyolysis of gluteal muscles leading to renal failure: a potentially fatal complciation of surgery in the morbidly obese. Obes Surg 2003; 13:302–305.

81. Belachew M. Laparoscopic adjustable gastric banding. In: Buchwald H, Pories W, Cowan GM Jr., eds. Surgical Management of Obesity. Philadelphia, PA: Elsevier, 2007: 158–166.

82. Jamieson AC. Vertical banded gastroplasty. In: Buchwald H, Pories W, Cowan GM Jr., eds. Surgical Management of Obesity. Philadelphia, PA: Elsevier, 2007:167–176.

83. Griffen WO Jr. Open Roux-en-y gastric bypass. In: Buchwald H, Pories W, Cowan GM Jr., eds. Surgical Management of Obesity. Philadelphia, PA: Elsevier, 2007:185–190.

84. Rogula T, Brethauer SA, Thodiyil PA, et al. Current status of laparoscopic gastric bypass. In: Buchwald H, Pories W, Cowan GM Jr., eds. Surgical Management of Obesity. Philadelphia, PA: Elsevier, 2007:191–203.

85. Scopinaro N, Papadia F, Marinari GM, et al. Biliopancreatic diversion. In: Buchwald H, Pories W, Cowan GM Jr., eds. Surgical Management of Obesity. Philadelphia, PA: Elsevier, 2007:239–251.

86. Hess DS. Biliopancreatic diversion with duodenal switch. In: Buchwald H, Pories W, Cowan GM Jr., eds. Surgical Management of Obesity. Philadelphia, PA: Elsevier, 2007:252–266.

87. Buchwald H, Estok R, Fahrbach K, et al. Effects of bariatric surgery on type 2 diabetes: a systematic review and meta-analysis. 2007 (in press).

88. Ikramuddin S. Energy metabolism and biochemistry of obesity. In: Buchwald H, Pories W, Cowan GM Jr., eds. Surgical Management of Obesity. Philadelphia, PA: Elsevier, 2007:29–33.

89. Dixon JB, O'Brien PE. Nutritional outcomes of bariatric surgery. In: Buchwald H, Pories W, Cowan GM Jr., eds. Surgical Management of Obesity. Philadelphia, PA Elsevier, 2007:357–364.

90. Pories WJ, Swanson MS, MacDonald KG, et al. Who would have thought it? An operation proves to be the most effective therapy for adult-onset diabetes mellitus. Ann Surg 1995; 222:339–352.

91. Schauer PR, Burguera B, Ikramuddin S, et al. Effect of laparoscopic Roux-en Y gastric bypass on type 2 diabetes mellitus. Ann Surg 2003; 238:467–484.

92. Sugerman HJ, Wolfe LG, Sica DA, et al. Diabetes and hypertension in severe obesity and effects of gastric bypass-induced weight loss. Ann Surg 2003; 237:751–756.

93. Sjostrom CD, Lissner L, Wedel H, et al. Reduction in incidence of diabetes, hypertension and lipid disturbances after intentional weight loss induced by bariatric surgery: the SOS Intervention Study. Obes Res 1999; 7:477–484.

94. Pories WJ, Albrecht RJ. Etiology of type II diabetes mellitus: role of the foregut. World J Surg 2001; 25:527–531.

95. Hickey MS, Pories WJ, MacDonald KG Jr., et al. A new paradigm for type 2 diabetes mellitus: could it be a disease of the foregut? Ann Surg 1998; 227:637–643.

96. Rubino F, Forgione A, Cummings DE, et al. The mechanism of diabetes control after gastrointestinal bypass surgery reveals a role of the proximal small intestine in the pathophysiology of type 2 diabetes. Ann Surg 2006; 244:741–749.

97. Arguelles-Sarmiento J, Barnal-Velasquez H, et al. Control of Type 2 diabetes mellitus in non-obese patients with stomach sparing duodeno-jejunal exclusion (SSDJE): Report of the first ten cases. Surg Obes Related Dis 2007 (in press).

98. Brolin RE, Kenler HA, Wilson AC, et al. Serum lipids after gastric bypass surgery for morbid obesity. Int J Obes 1990; 14:939–950.

99. Buffington CK, Cowan GSM, Hughes TA, et al. Significant changes in the lipid-lipoprotein status of premenopausal morbidly obese females following gastric bypass surgery. Obes Surg 1994; 4:328–335.

100. Cowan GSM Jr., Buffington CK. Significant changes in blood pressure, glucose, and lipids with gastric bypass surgery. World J Surg 1998; 232:987–992.

101. Gleysteen JJ. Results of surgery: long-term effects on hyperlipidemia. Am J Clin Nutr 1992; 55:591S–593S.

102. Buchwald H, Varco RL, Matts JP, et al. Effect of partial ileal bypass surgery on mortality and morbidity from coronary heart disease in patients with hypercholesterolemia. Report of the Program on the Surgical Control of the Hyperlipidemias (POSCH). New Engl J Med 1990; 323: 946–955.

103. MacDonald KG Jr., Pender JR. Resolution of bariatric comorbidities: hypertension. In: Buchwald H, Pories W, Cowan GM Jr., eds. Surgical Management of Obesity. Philadelphia, PA: Elsevier, 2007:371–376.

104. Dornfield TP, Maxwell MH, Waks AU, et al. Obesity and hypertension: long-term effects of weight reduction on blood pressure. Int J Obes 1985; 9:381–389.

105. Hypertension Prevention Treatment Group. The Hypertension Prevention Trial: three-year effects of dietary changes on blood pressure. Hypertension Prevention Trial Research Group. Arch Intern Med 1990; 150: 153–162.

106. Reisen E, Frohlich ED. Effects of weight reduction on arterial pressure. J Chronic Dis 1982; 33:887–891.

107. Nachmany I, Szold A, Klausner J, Abu-Abeid S. Resolution of bariatric comorbidities: sleep apnea. In: Buchwald H, Pories W, Cowan GM Jr., eds. Surgical Management of Obesity. Philadelphia, PA: Elsevier, 2007: 377–382.

108. Rajala R, Partinen M, Sane T, et al. Obstructive sleep apnea syndrome in morbidly obese patients. J Intern Med 1991; 230:125–129.

109. Rasheid S, Banasiak M, Gallagher SF, et al. Gastric bypass is an effective treatment for obstructive sleep apnea in patients with clinically significant obesity. Obes Surg 2003; 13:58–61.

110. Sugerman H, Windsor A, Bessos M, et al. Intra-abdominal pressure, sagittal abdominal diameter and obesity comorbidity. J Intern Med 1997; 24:71–79.

111. Weiner P, Walzman J, Weiner M, et al. Influence of excessive weight loss after gastroplasty for morbid obesity on respiratory muscle performance. Thorax 1998; 53: 39–42.

112. Buchwald H. Obesity comorbidities. In: Buchwald H, Pories W, Cowan GM Jr., eds. Surgical Management of Obesity. Philadelphia, PA: Elsevier, 2007:37–44.

113. Buchwald H, Ikramuddin S. Bariatric Surgery Primer CD-ROM, the American College of Surgeons. Released April 2004.

114. Hell E, Miller K. Social implications of obesity. In: Buchwald H, Pories W, Cowan GM Jr., eds. Surgical Management of Obesity. Philadelphia, PA: Elsevier, 2007: 52–56.

115. Ardelt E, Moorehead M. The validation of the Moorehead-Ardelt quality of life questionnaire. Obes Surg 1999; 9:132 (abstr).

116. Myers JA, Clifford JC, Sarker S, et al. Quality of life after laparoscopic adjustable gastric banding using the Baros and Moorehead-Ardelt Quality of Life Questionnaire II. J Soc Laparoendosc Surg 2006; 10:414–420.

117. Christou NV, Sampalis JS, Liberman M, et al. Surgery decreases long-term mortality, morbidity, and health care use in morbidly obese patients. Ann Surg 2004; 240: 416–424.

118. Dixon J. Survival advantage with bariatric surgery: report from the 10th International Congress on Obesity. Surg Obes Relat Dis 2006; 2:585–586.

119. Sampalis JS, Liberman M, Auger S, et al. The impact of weight reduction surgery on health-care costs in morbidly obese patients. Obes Surg 2004; 14:939–947.

120. Martin LF. Economic implications of obesity. In: Buchwald H, Pories W, Cowan GM Jr., eds. Surgical Management of Obesity. Philadelphia, PA: Elsevier, 2007:57–64.

121. Sosa JL, Pombo H, Pallavicini H, et al. Laparoscopic gastric bypass beyond age 60. Obes Surg 2004; 14: 1398–1401.

122. Sugerman HJ, DeMaria EJ, Kellum JM, et al. Effects of bariatric surgery in older patients. Ann Surg 2004; 240:243–247.

123. Epstein LH, Valoski A, Wong RR, et al. Ten-year follow-up of behavioral family-based treatment for obese children. JAMA 1990; 264:2519–2523.

124. Barnett SJ, Stanley C, Hanlon M, et al. Long-term follow-up and the role of surgery in adolescents with morbid obesity. Surg Obes Rel Dis 2005; 1:394–398.

125. Dolan K, Creighton L, Hopkins G, et al. Laparoscopic gastric banding in morbidly obese adolescents. Obes Surg 2003; 13:101–104.

126. Sugerman HJ, Sugerman EL, DeMaria EJ, et al. Bariatric surgery for severely obese adolescents. J Gastrointest Surg 2003; 7:102–108.

127. Abu-Abeid S, Gavert N, Klausner JM, et al. Bariatric surgery in adolescence. J Pediatr Surg 2003; 38:1379–1382.

128. Stanford A, Glascock JM, Eid GM, et al. Laparoscopic Roux-en-Y gastric bypass in morbidly obese adolescents. J Pediatr Surg 2003; 38:430–433.

129. Strauss RS, Bradley LJ, Brolin RE. Gastric bypass surgery in adolescents with morbid obesity. J Pediatr 2001; 138: 459–504.

130. Rand CS, Macgregor AM. Adolescents having obesity surgery: A 6-year follow-up. South Med J 1994; 87:1208–1213.

131. Garcia VF. Adolescent bariatric surgery. In: Buchwald H, Pories W, Cowan GM Jr., eds. Surgical Management of Obesity. Philadelphia, PA: Elsevier, 2007:315–323.

132. Buckley MC. Body contouring after massive weight loss. In: Buchwald H, Pories W, Cowan GM Jr., eds. Surgical Management of Obesity. Philadelphia, PA: Elsevier, 2007:325–333.

133. Boyd JB. Plastic surgery after rapid weight loss. General Surgery News, Obesity Care Special Edition Supplement 2007:74–81.

134. Buchwald H, Williams SE. Bariatric surgery training in the United States. SOARD 2006; 2:52–55.

135. Kaufman D, Kral JG. Academic training of bariatric surgeons. In: Buchwald H, Pories W, Cowan GM Jr., eds. Surgical Management of Obesity. Philadelphia, PA: Elsevier, 2007:397–400.

136. Flanagan L Jr. Practical training of the bariatric surgeon. In: Buchwald H, Pories W, Cowan GM Jr., eds. Surgical Management of Obesity. Philadelphia, PA: Elsevier, 2007: 401–405.

137. Surgical Review Corporation. Available at: http://www.surgicalreview.org/.

138. American College of Surgeons, Bariatric Surgery Center Network (BSCN) Accreditation Program. Available at: http://www.facs.org/cqi/bscn/.

139. Kendrick ML, Clark MM, Collazo-Clavell ML, et al. Multidisciplinary team in a bariatric surgery program. In: Buchwald H, Pories W, Cowan GM Jr., eds. Surgical Management of Obesity. Philadelphia, PA: Elsevier, 2007:425–431.

140. Walen ML. Allied science team in bariatric surgery. In: Buchwald H, Pories W, Cowan GM Jr., eds. Surgical Management of Obesity. Philadelphia, PA: Elsevier, 2007: 432–436.

141. Buchwald H. Is morbid obesity a surgical disease? General Surgery News, Obesity Care Special Edition Supplement 2007:9–15.

142. Buchwald H, Buchwald JN. Evolution of operative procedures for the management of morbid obesity 1950–2000. Obes Surg 2002; 12:705–717.

143. Buchwald H. Overview of bariatric surgery. J Am Coll Surg 2002; 194:367–375.

32

Swedish Obese Subjects: A Review of Results from a Prospective Controlled Intervention Trial

LARS SJÖSTRÖM

SOS Secretariat, Sahlgrenska University Hospital, Göteborg, Sweden

INTRODUCTION

The prevalence of obesity (BMI $\geq$ 30 kg/m^2) in the United States has doubled between 1980 and 2004 and is now over 30% (1,2). In fact, the obesity prevalence has increased in all parts of the world over the last 20 to 30 years (3). The majority of large and long-term epidemiological studies indicate that obesity is associated with increased mortality (4–10). The life span of severely obese persons is decreased by an estimated 5 to 20 years (11). Weight loss is known to be associated with improvement of intermediate risk factors for disease (12), suggesting that weight loss would also reduce mortality. However, the controlled interventional studies demonstrating that weight loss is in fact reducing mortality have been lacking. To date, most observational epidemiological studies have indicated that overall cardio-vascular mortality is increased after weight loss (13), even in subjects who were obese at baseline (14–16). This discrepancy concerning the effects of weight loss on risk factors as compared to mortality has been related to certain limitations inherent in observational studies, particularly the inability of such studies to distinguish intentional from unintentional weight loss. Thus, the observed weight loss might be the consequence of conditions that lead to death rather than the cause of increased mortality.

However, three observational epidemiological reports (17–19), all based on American Cancer Society data, have suggested that intentional weight loss is in fact associated with decreased mortality, though the information on intentionality was based on retrospective, self-reported data collected at baseline. Whether these weight losses before the baseline examination were maintained is unknown, as weight changes during the studies were not reported. Three retrospective cohort studies in obese subjects (20–22) and one in obese subjects with diabetes (23) have suggested that bariatric surgery may also result in a marked mortality reduction.

There has been a dramatic increase in the use of bariatric surgery during the past decade. In 2003, over 100,000 procedures were performed in the United States (24). However, until recently, it remained unclear whether the long-term weight loss induced by bariatric surgery has favorable effects on lifespan.

To ascertain the effects of intentional weight loss on mortality, controlled, prospective interventional trials are needed. In the Swedish Obese Subjects (SOS) trial, we used bariatric surgery to achieve weight loss, since such surgery was and still is the only technique available with proven long-term effects on weight loss.

OVERVIEW OF SOS

SOS Aims

The primary aim of SOS was to examine if intentional weight loss induced by bariatric surgery is associated with lower mortality as compared to conventional treatment in contemporaneously matched, obese controls. Several secondary aims, related to the effects of bariatric surgery on diabetes and other morbidity, risk factors, health-related quality of life (HRQL), and health economics were also defined. Finally, the genetics of obesity was an additional topic for research in the SOS trial.

Study Design and Baseline Description

The ongoing SOS project consists of four substudies:

- The *SOS Matching (or Registry) study* (n = 6905), from which patients were recruited to the SOS Intervention study.
- The *SOS Intervention study*, which consists of one surgical group (n = 2010) and one obese control group (n = 2037).
- The *SOS Reference study* (n = 1135), which is a small study on randomly selected subjects from the general population examined contemporaneously with and in the same way as subjects in the intervention trial.
- The *SOS sibpair study* (n = 768), consisting of weight-discordant sibs and their biological parents (25,26). These subjects were mainly recruited from the SOS registry and intervention studies, but also from other Swedish obesity studies such as the XENDOS study. The sibpair study will be used for a genome-wide scan using, among other variables, expression data from adipose tissue as phenotypes.

SOS Matching and Intervention Studies

The SOS (12,27,28) intervention trial is a prospective, matched, surgical interventional trial involving 4047 obese subjects. Patients were recruited over 13.4 years between September 1, 1987, and January 31, 2001. The follow-up duration is currently (September 2007) ranging from 6 to 20 years.

As a result of recruitment campaigns, 11,453 subjects sent standardized application forms to the SOS secretariat and 6905 completed a matching examination (the Matching/ Registry study). Among the pool of subjects examined, 2010 eligible subjects desiring surgery constituted the surgical group, and based on data from the matching examination, a contemporaneously matched control group (n = 2037) was created. The matching program used 18 matching variables, and the matching could not be influenced by the investigators (27).

A baseline examination for the surgical subjects and their matched controls was undertaken four weeks before surgery (Table 1).

The intervention began on the day of surgery for surgically treated subjects and their matched controls. Individual dates of all subsequent examinations and questionnaires (0.5, 1, 2, 3, 4, 6, 8, 10, 15, and 20 years) for surgically treated and control subjects were calculated based on the dates of operation. Inclusion criteria for the interventional study were age 37 to 60 years and BMI [weight (kg)/height (m^2)] of 34 kg/m^2 or more for men and 38 kg/m^2 or more for women. The BMI cutoffs corresponded to an approximate doubling in mortality rate in each gender as compared to mortality in the BMI range 20 to 25 kg/m^2 (29). Exclusion criteria, described elsewhere (27), were minimal and were aimed at obtaining an operable surgical group. Identical inclusion and exclusion criteria were used for the two treatment groups.

The Matching and the Intervention studies were undertaken at 480 primary health care centers and 25 surgical departments in Sweden. At each visit, measurements of weight, height, waist circumference, other anthropometric measures (Table 1), and blood pressure were obtained (27). Biochemical variables (Table 1) were measured at the matching examination, at the baseline examination (year 0 of the Intervention study), and at 2, 10, 15, and 20 years. Blood samples were obtained in the morning after a 10- to 12-hour fast and analyzed at the Central Laboratory of Sahlgrenska University Hospital (accredited according to European Norm 45001). The baseline questionnaire included self-reported information on previous myocardial infarction, stroke, and cancer, and questions designed to assess the likelihood of sleep apnea (30). Psychosocial variables (Table 1, bottom) were also evaluated (31). Subgroups have been examined for cardiovascular structure and function and with respect to genetic characteristics. For methodology, please see Methods of the reviewed studies below (32–44).

The surgically treated subjects underwent nonadjustable or adjustable banding (n = 376), vertical banded gastroplasty (n = 1369), or gastric bypass (n = 265) operations (45). For adjustable banding, the Swedish Adjustable Gastric Band (SAGB$^®$, Obtech Medical, Stockholm, Sweden) was used. The obese, contemporaneously matched controls received the customary nonsurgical obesity treatment for their given center of registration. No attempt was made to standardize the conventional treatment, which ranged from sophisticated lifestyle intervention and behavior modification to, in many practices, no treatment whatsoever.

All social security numbers from the SOS database were cross-checked against the Swedish Person and Address Register (SPAR) every year on November 1.

Table 1 Characteristics of the SOS Surgery and Control Groups at Inclusion

| | Inclusion examination | |
| | Surgery | Controls |
Variable	n, (%) or mean $\pm$ SD	n, (%) or mean $\pm$ SD
Total (n)	2010	2037
Males (n)	590	590
Females (n)	1420	1447
Postmenopausal women (%)	37.2	41.3
Age at examination (yr)	47.2 $\pm$ 5.9	48.7 $\pm$ 6.3
Daily smokers (%)	25.8	20.8
Diabetics (%)	10.7	11.4
Sleep apnea (%)	25.1	22.2
Lipid-lowering mediations (%)	1.8	1.6
Previous MI (n)	31	29
Previous stroke (n)	15	23
Previous stroke or MI (n)	46	49
Previous cancer (n)	24	21
Weight (kg)	121.0 $\pm$ 16.6	114.7 $\pm$ 16.5
Height (m)	1.69 $\pm$ 0.09	1.69 $\pm$ 0.09
BMI (kg/m^2)	42.4 $\pm$ 4.5	40.1 $\pm$ 4.7
Waist circumference (cm)	125.8 $\pm$ 11.0	120.2 $\pm$ 11.3
Hip circumference (cm)	127.1 $\pm$ 10.0	123.2 $\pm$ 10.0
Waist/hip ratio	0.99 $\pm$ 0.08	0.98 $\pm$ 0.07
Sagittal diameter (cm)	28.9 $\pm$ 3.7	27.4 $\pm$ 3.7
Neck circumference (cm)	43.7 $\pm$ 4.3	42.9 $\pm$ 4.29
Upper arm circumference (cm)	39.8 $\pm$ 3.8	38.7 $\pm$ 3.8
Thigh circumference (cm)	75.5 $\pm$ 7.5	73.4 $\pm$ 7.5
Systolic blood pressure (mmHg)	145.0 $\pm$ 18.8	137.9 $\pm$ 18.0
Diastolic blood pressure (mmHg)	89.9 $\pm$ 11.1	85.2 $\pm$ 10.7
Pulse pressure (mmHg)	55.2 $\pm$ 14.5	52.8 $\pm$ 13.0
Glucose (mmol/L)	5.45 $\pm$ 2.11	5.20 $\pm$ 1.92
Insulin (mU/L)	21.5 $\pm$ 13.7	18.0 $\pm$ 11.4
Triglycerides (mmol/L)	2.25 $\pm$ 1.54	2.02 $\pm$ 1.41
Total cholesterol (mmol/L)	5.86 $\pm$ 1.12	5.61 $\pm$ 1.06
HDL cholesterol (mmol/L)	1.20 $\pm$ 0.28	1.19 $\pm$ 0.29
Uric acid (μmol/L)	359.2 $\pm$ 79.8	352.3 $\pm$ 79.9
ASAT (μkat/L)	0.43 $\pm$ 0.23	0.39 $\pm$ 0.21
ALAT (μkat/L)	0.63 $\pm$ 0.39	0.56 $\pm$ 0.42
ALP (μkat/L)	3.12 $\pm$ 0.84	3.01 $\pm$ 0.87
Bilirubin (μmol/L)	9.51 $\pm$ 4.28	9.93 $\pm$ 5.27
Current health, scores	21.4 $\pm$ 6.10	22.7 $\pm$ 6.2
Monotony avoidance, scores	22.5 $\pm$ 5.1	22.6 $\pm$ 5.0
Psychasthenia, scores	23.9 $\pm$ 5.2	23.2 $\pm$ 5.3
Quantity of social support	6.02 $\pm$ 2.4	6.08 $\pm$ 2.45
Quality of social support	4.25 $\pm$ 1.32	4.28 $\pm$ 1.31
Stressful life events	2.49 $\pm$ 1.30	2.43 $\pm$ 1.28

Abbreviations: SOS, Swedish Obese Subjects; ASAT, aspartate aminotransferase; ALAT, alanine aminotransferase; ALP, alkaline phosphatase.
Source: Adapted from Ref. 28.

At several occasions, the SOS database has also been cross-checked against the Swedish Social Insurance System, Statistics Sweden, and the Swedish Hospital Discharge Register in order to obtain objective data on sick leave, disability pension, hospital care, and annual income for outcome and health economic studies.

SPAR provides current addresses and information on all deceased subjects. Social security numbers on all deceased subjects were cross-checked against the Swedish Cause of Death Register to obtain the official cause of death. In addition, all relevant case sheets and autopsy reports were adjudicated independently by two experienced clinicians blinded with respect to study arm. If the two examiners differed on a cause of death, a third, blinded physician also reviewed the case so that a final decision could be made. If the study-determined cause of death did not agree with the official cause, the study-determined cause of death was used.

For statistical procedures, please see the Method sections of the reviewed publications (12, 25–74).

The SOS Reference Study

The SOS reference study is a cross-sectional study of randomly selected individuals. The main purpose of the study was to create a reference sample to obese SOS subjects in genetic association studies and in comparative analyses of clinical conditions (see below).

Between August 1994 and December 1999, i.e., during the period when the major part of patients were included in the SOS intervention study, 524 men and 611 women were included in the SOS reference study. Body composition and biochemical characteristics of the SOS reference study have been published (46–49) and will not be further discussed in this review.

FINDINGS FROM SOS

Follow-Up Rates

In the recent publication on overall mortality, the vital status was known for all initial study participants except three: two who had requested to be deleted from the SOS database and one who had left the study and later obtained a secret social security number. The follow-up rate with respect to vital status on the date of analysis was thus 99.93%.

In the Intervention study, the participation rates of still living subjects at the 2-, 10-, and 15-year examinations ranged between 66% and 94%. The participation rate was 100% at the baseline examination.

Baseline Characteristics in the SOS Intervention Study

The matching procedure created two largely comparable groups, although the surgically treated subjects were on average 2.3 kg heavier ($p < 0.001$), 1.3 years younger ($p < 0.001$) and were smoking more frequently ($p < 0.001$) than the controls (28). The higher body weight of the surgery group was associated with higher values in several anthropometric measurements and in some biochemical variables (28).

Between the matching and baseline examinations, there was an increase in weight in the surgically treated patients (1.73 kg, $p < 0.001$) and a decrease in weight in the

control group (2.23 kg, $p < 0.001$). These diverging weight changes caused most variables to become significantly different between surgery and control groups at baseline (Table 1) (28). However, all observed baseline differences except three (age, thigh circumference, bilirubin) constituted survival disadvantages for the surgery group in univariate analyses (28).

In an early cross-sectional analysis of 450 men and 556 women from the Matching study of SOS, it was shown that as compared with randomly selected controls most cardiovascular risk factors were elevated in the obese (27). The exception was total cholesterol, which was similar in obese and nonobese males and lower in obese women as compared with reference women.

Risk factors have also been analyzed in relation to baseline body composition in 1083 men and 1367 women from the SOS Matching study (50). This analysis revealed one body compartment—risk factor pattern and one subcutaneous adipose tissue distribution—risk factor pattern. Within the first pattern, risk factors were positively and strongly related to an estimate of visceral adipose tissue mass and, more weakly, to subcutaneous adipose tissue mass. Some risk factors, such as glucose and triglycerides in men and insulin in women, were negatively related to lean body mass. In addition, the subcutaneous adipose tissue distribution was related to risk factors both when and when not taking the body compartments into account statistically. A preponderance of subcutaneous adipose tissue in the upper part of the trunk, as indicated by the neck circumference, was positively related to risk factors while the thigh circumference was negatively related to risk factors. These two risk factor patterns have also been observed longitudinally, i.e., changes in risk factors and changes in body composition and adipose tissue distribution are related (51) in the same way as in the cross-sectional observations (50).

Weight Changes in SOS

Figure 1 shows the weight changes for up to 15 years from baseline for control and surgery subgroups (28). The number of observations decreased over time, mainly owing to the 13-year-long recruitment period, but also due to dropout from examinations. In the control group, average weight change remained within ±2% over the observation period. In the three surgical subgroups, weight loss was maximal after 1 to 2 years (gastric bypass, 32% ± 8%; vertical banded gastroplasty 25% ± 9%; and banding, 20% ± 10%, mean ± SD). Weight increase was seen in all surgical subgroups in the following years, but the relapse curves leveled off after 8 to 10 years (Figure 1). After 10 years, the weight losses were 25% ± 11% (gastric bypass), 16% ± 11% (vertical

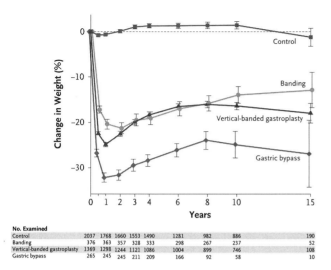

Figure 1 Mean percent weight change during the 15 first study years of the SOS intervention trial in the control group and the three surgical subgroups. I bars denote 95% CI. *Abbreviation*: SOS, Swedish Obese Subjects. *Source*: From Ref. 28.

banded gastroplasty) and 14% ± 14% (banding) compared with the baseline weight. After 15 years, the corresponding weight losses were 27% ± 12%, 18% ± 11%, and 13% ± 14%, respectively.

Effects of Weight Loss on Risk Factors

Two- and 10-year risk factor changes observed in the SOS trial were published in 2004 (Figures 2 and 3) (12). As illustrated in Figures 2 and 3, the 2- and 10-year recovery rates from diabetes, hypertriglyceridemia, low levels of HDL cholesterol, hypertension, and hyperuricemia were more favorable in the surgery group than in the control group, whereas recovery from hypercholesterolemia did not differ between the groups. The surgery group had lower 2- and 10-year incidence rates of diabetes, hypertriglyceridemia, and hyperuricemia than the control group, whereas differences between groups in the incidence of hypercholesterolemia and hypertension were not detectable.

A number of earlier SOS reports on risk factor changes have also appeared (51–54). In a 2-year report of 282 men and 560 women, pooled from the surgically treated group and the obese control group, risk factor changes were examined as a function of weight change (51). A 10-kg weight loss was enough to introduce clinically significant reductions in all traditional risk factors except total cholesterol. Preliminary calculations indicate that there is a fairly linear relationship between weight loss and risk factor improvement also over 10 years, although 15 to

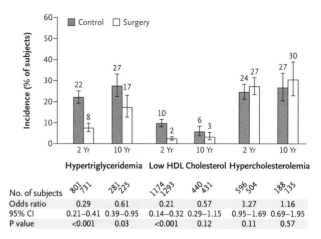

No. of subjects	801 731	281 225	1174 1293	440 431	596 504	188 135
Odds ratio	0.29	0.61	0.21	0.57	1.27	1.16
95% CI	0.21–0.41	0.39–0.95	0.14–0.32	0.29–1.15	0.95–1.69	0.69–1.95
P value	<0.001	0.03	<0.001	0.12	0.11	0.57

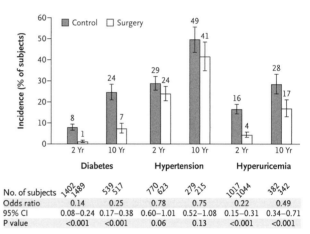

No. of subjects	1402 1489	539 517	770 623	279 215	1017 1044	382 342
Odds ratio	0.14	0.25	0.78	0.75	0.22	0.49
95% CI	0.08–0.24	0.17–0.38	0.60–1.01	0.52–1.08	0.15–0.31	0.34–0.71
P value	<0.001	<0.001	0.06	0.13	<0.001	<0.001

Figure 2 Incidence of diabetes, lipid disturbances, hypertension, and hyperuricemia over 2- and 10-year periods among surgically treated subjects and their obese controls in the SOS intervention study. Data are for subjects who completed 2 and 10 years of the study. The bars and the percentage values above the bars show unadjusted values for incidence. I bars represent the corresponding 95% CI. Below each panel, the odds ratios, 95% CI for the odds ratios and *p* values have been adjusted for gender, age, and BMI at the time of inclusion in the intervention study. *Abbreviation*: SOS, Swedish Obese Subjects. *Source*: From Ref. 12.

20 kg maintained weight loss is often required to achieve long-term risk factor improvements (Sjöström CD et al., to be published).

Effects of Weight Loss on the Cardiovascular System

In smaller subsamples of the SOS study, cardiac and vascular structure and function was examined at baseline and after 1 to 4 years of follow-up.

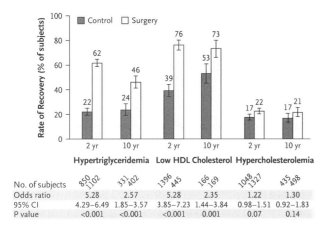

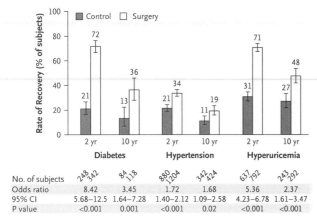

No. of subjects	850 1102	331 402	1396 445	166 169	1048 1327	435 498
Odds ratio	5.28	2.57	5.28	2.35	1.22	1.30
95% CI	4.29–6.49	1.85–3.57	3.85–7.23	1.44–3.84	0.98–1.51	0.92–1.83
P value	<0.001	<0.001	<0.001	0.001	0.07	0.14

No. of subjects	248 342	84 118	880 1204	342 424	637 792	243 292
Odds ratio	8.42	3.45	1.72	1.68	5.36	2.37
95% CI	5.68–12.5	1.64–7.28	1.40–2.12	1.09–2.58	4.23–6.78	1.61–3.47
P value	<0.001	0.001	<0.001	0.02	<0.001	<0.001

Figure 3 Recovery from diabetes, lipid disturbances, hypertension, and hyperuricemia over 2- and 10-year periods among surgically treated subjects and their obese controls in the SOS intervention study. Data are for subjects who completed 2 and 10 years of the study. The bars and the percentage values above the bars show unadjusted values for incidence. I bars represent the corresponding 95% CI. Below each panel, the odds ratios, 95% CI for the odds ratios and *p* values have been adjusted for gender, age, and BMI at the time of inclusion in the intervention study. *Abbreviations*: SOS, Swedish Obese Subjects; BMI, body mass index. *Source*: From Ref. 12.

At baseline, a surgically treated group ($n = 41$) and an obese control group ($n = 31$) were compared with a lean reference group ($n = 43$) (32,33). As compared to lean subjects, the systolic and diastolic blood pressure, left ventricular mass and relative wall thickness were increased in the obese while the systolic function (measured as left ventricular ejection fraction) and the diastolic function (estimated from the E/A ratio, i.e., the flow rate over the mitral valve "Early" in diastole divided by the flow rate late in diastole during the "Atrial" contraction) were impaired. After one year, all these variables had improved in the surgically treated group but not in the obese control group. When pooling the two obese groups and plotting left ventricular mass or E/A ratio as a function of quintiles of weight change, a "dose" dependency was revealed, i.e., the larger the weight reduction, the larger the reduction in left ventricular mass and the more pronounced the improvement in diastolic function. Unchanged weight was in fact associated with a measurable deterioration in diastolic function over one year.

In other small subgroups from SOS, heart rate variability from 24-hour Holter ECG recordings and 24-hour catecholamine secretion were examined (34). As compared with lean subjects, our baseline examinations in the obese indicated an increased sympathetic activity and a withdrawal of vagal activity at baseline. Both these disturbances were normalized in the surgically treated group but not in the control group after one year of treatment.

The intima-media thickness of the carotid bulb was examined by means of ultrasonography at baseline and after four year in the SOS intervention study (35). A randomly selected lean reference group matched for gender, age, and height was examined at baseline and after three years. The annual progression rate of the thickness was almost three times higher in the obese control group as compared to lean reference subjects ($p < 0.05$). In the surgically treated group, the progression rate was diminished. Although results from this small study group need to be confirmed in larger trials, this study offered the first data on hard endpoints after intentional weight loss.

We have also shown that the pulse pressure increases more slowly in the surgically treated group than in the obese control group after a mean follow-up of 5.5 years (54). In gastric bypass individuals, the pulse pressure in fact decreases. These observations are of interest since it has been shown that, at a given systolic blood pressure, a high pulse pressure is associated with increased arterial stiffness (55), increased intima-media thickness (75), and increased cardiovascular mortality (76). Thus pulse pressure changes (54) as well as ultrasonographic measurements (35) indicated that bariatric surgery may slow down the accelerated atherosclerotic process in the obese.

Further support for favorable effects on the atherosclerotic process was obtained in an analysis of effort-related calf pain. This symptom was much more common in 6328 obese subjects of the SOS matching study than in 1135 randomly selected subjects from the general population in the SOS reference study (men: OR = 5.0, women OR = 4.0, $p < 0.001$) (56). The six-year incidence of new cases of effort-related calf pain was lower in obese subjects undergoing bariatric surgery than in the conventionally treated control group (men: OR = 0.39, women: OR = 0.61, $p < 0.05$). Among subjects reporting symptoms at baseline, the six-year recovery rate was higher in the surgical group than in the control group (men: OR = 15.3, women: OR = 5.9, $p < 0.001$) (56).

Questionnaire data from 1210 surgically treated patients and 1099 obese SOS controls examined at baseline and after two years were analyzed with respect to various cardiovascular symptoms (57). At baseline, the two groups were comparable in most respects. After two years, dyspnea and chest discomfort were reduced in a much larger fraction of surgically treated as compared with controls. For instance, 87% of the surgically treated reported baseline dyspnea when climbing two flights of stairs while only 19% experienced such dyspnea at the two-year follow-up. In the obese control group, the corresponding figures were 69% and 57%, respectively ($p < 0.001$ for difference in change between groups).

Effects of Weight Loss on Sleep Apnea

Baseline sleep apnea was examined by means of a questionnaire in 1324 SOS men and 1711 SOS women (30,58). A high likelihood for sleep apnea was observed in 26% of obese men and in 9% of obese females. Sleep apnea was associated with WHO grade 4 daytime dyspnea, admission to hospital with chest pain, myocardial infarction, and elevations of blood pressure, insulin, triglycerides, and uric acid when adjusting for body fat, adipose tissue distribution, and other potential confounders (58). In addition, sleep apnea was also associated with increased psychosocial morbidity before and after these adjustments (30).

Sleep apnea has also been investigated in the SOS intervention study (57). A high likelihood for sleep apnea was observed in 23% of 1210 surgically treated cases at baseline but only in 8% after two years postsurgery. In the obese control group ($n = 1099$), the corresponding figures were 22% and 20%, respectively ($p < 0.001$ for difference in change between groups) (57). In a recent follow-up, these findings were confirmed, and it was also found that subjects reporting loss of obstructive sleep apnea had a lower two-year incidence of diabetes and hypertriglyceridemia, also after adjustment for baseline central obesity and weight change over two years (59).

Finally, a small experimental study in obese SOS patients demonstrated an association between sleep apnea, elevated catecholamine secretion, and elevated energy expenditure, particularly during sleep (60). Affected individuals were improved by means of nighttime treatment with continuous positive airway pressure (60).

Effects of Weight Loss on Joint Pain and Fracture Frequency

Self-reported work-restricting pain in the neck and back area and in the hip, knee, and ankle joints was more common in untreated obese men and women than in the general population as judged from the SOS matching and reference studies (ORs ranging from 1.7 to 9.9, $p < 0.001$)

(61). Obese women treated with bariatric surgery had a lower two- and six-year incidence of work-restricting pain in the knee and ankle joints than conventionally treated obese women (ORs 0.51–0.71). Recovery rates from baseline symptoms in knee and ankle joints for men, and in neck and back and in hip, knees, and ankle joints for women were higher after bariatric surgery than after conventional treatment (ORs 1.4–4.8) (61).

Preliminary data suggest that the fracture frequency is lower in individuals treated with bariatric surgery than in conventionally treated subjects (62).

Biliary Disease in the SOS Intervention and Reference Studies

Obese individuals had significantly higher prevalence of cholelithiasis and previous cholecystitis, cholecystectomies and pancreatitis than randomly selected subjects from the SOS reference study (63). BMI was related to biliary disease in both genders. Compared with conventional treatment, bariatric surgery was associated with increased incidence of biliary disease in men but not in women. Weight loss was associated with increased incidence of biliary disease in both genders (63).

Effects of Weight Loss on Lifestyle and HRQL

Physical inactivity was observed in 46% of the surgically treated before weight reduction but only in 17% after two years. Corresponding figures in the obese control group were 33% and 29%, respectively (p for difference in change < 0.001) (57). Later, we have found increased physical activity in the surgery group at each observation over the first 10 years of follow-up (12). Thus, physical inactivity does not only contribute to the development of obesity but obesity favors physical inactivity. This vicious cycle is broken by surgical treatment.

At baseline, the energy intake was slightly higher in the surgery group (2882 kcal/24 hr) than in the obese control group (2526 kcal/24 hr), while it was significantly lower in the surgery group over the first 10 years of follow-up (12).

Cross-sectional information from 800 obese men and 943 women of the SOS Matching study demonstrated that obese patients have a much worse health related quality of life (HRQL) than age-matched reference subjects (64). In fact, HRQL in the obese was as bad as, or even worse than, in patients with severe rheumatoid arthritis, generalized malignant melanoma, or spinal cord injuries. The measurements were performed with generic scales such as general health-rating index, hospital anxiety and depression scale (HAD), mood adjective checklist (MACL), and sickness impact profile in original or short form (31,64) and with more obesity specific instruments such as OP measuring obesity-related psychosocial problems (64) and Stunkard's three-factor eating questionnaire (77). All scales have been validated under Swedish conditions.

Stunkard's original findings based on the "three-factor eating questionnaire" (TFEQ) (77) (cognitive restraint, disinhibition, hunger) could not be replicated among 4377 obese SOS patients with respect to convergent and discriminative validity of the factors. Using multitrait/multi-item analysis and factor analysis, a short revised 18-item instrument has been constructed, representing the derived factors of cognitive restrain, uncontrolled eating and emotional eating (65).

In two- (66) and four-year (61) reports, results from all measuring instruments improved dose dependently, i.e., the larger the weight loss the more improvement of HRQL. In subjects with weight loss ≥25%, large effects were seen for obesity-related measures reflecting eating patterns and psychosocial problems and for general health and functional health domains such as ambulation, recreation, pastimes, and social interaction. Moderate effect sizes were observed for depressive symptoms (HAD-D), self-esteem and overall mood (MACL), while the effect on anxiety symptoms (HAD-A) were minor. In the obese control group only trivial effects were seen.

Over 10 years, the HRQL was significantly more improved in the surgery group as compared to the conventionally treated obese control group in the domains current health perception, social interaction, psychosocial functioning, and depression, whereas no significant differences between groups were found for overall mood and anxiety (68). The long-term results suggest that 10% weight loss within the surgery group is sufficient for favorable long-term effects of HRQL, a threshold that is achieved by two-thirds of surgical 10-year completers (68).

In summary, HRQL is very poor in obese subjects. Large (>25%) and moderate (10% to 25%) weight losses maintained over 4 to 10 years improve most aspects of HRQL.

Health Economical Consequences of Bariatric Surgery

In cross-sectional studies of SOS patients, it was shown that sick leave was twice as high and disability pension twice as frequent than in the general Swedish population independent of age and gender (69). The annual indirect costs (sick leave plus disability pension) attributable to obesity were estimated at Swedish crowns (SKr) 6 billion in Sweden, or US$1 million per 10,000 inhabitants per year.

The number of lost days due to sick leave and disability pension, the year before inclusion into the SOS interven-

tion, was almost identical in the surgically treated group and the obese control group (104 and 107 days, respectively) (70). The year after inclusion, the number of lost days was higher in the surgically treated group but, two to four years after inclusion, the lost days were lower in the surgically treated group. This was particularly evident in those individuals above the median age (46.7 years) (70).

Surgical obesity treatment is associated with higher hospital costs ($10,200) than conventional treatment ($2800) over six years (71). When adjusting for the surgical intervention as such ($4300) in the surgical group and conditions common after bariatric surgery in both groups ($2800 in surgically treated, $400 in controls), the remaining costs were not different in the two groups. These observations from 2002 indicated that the lag time between weight loss and improvement of hard endpoints requiring hospitalization was longer than six years. We now know that it took 13 study years until we obtained a significant effect on overall mortality (see below), but we have not yet had the possibility to examine the overall health economic data over 10 to 15 years.

At baseline, the fraction of individuals on medication for various conditions was usually higher in obese subjects of the SOS Intervention study (Int) than in lean randomly selected individuals of the SOS Reference study (Ref) (72). The fraction on medication for the following conditions was significantly different between groups: diabetes (Int 6.1%, Ref 0.7%9), CVD (Int 27.8%, Ref 8.2), pain (Int 10.8%, Ref 4.1%), while medications for the following conditions were not significantly different: asthma (Int 5.2%, Ref 2.3%), psychiatric disorders (Int 7.2%, Ref 4.6%), anemia (Int 1.3%, Ref 1.6%), gastrointestinal disorders (Int 4.4%, Ref 3.5%), all others (Int 20.5%, Ref 23.6%).

Among SOS intervention patients on medication at baseline, the fraction on medication dropped significantly more over six years in the surgically treated group than in the control group (72). In contrast, surgery did not significantly prevent the start of medication among those who had no medication at baseline. While the average cost per individual over six years was lower in the surgically than the conventionally treated obese control group regarding medication for diabetes and CVD, the costs were higher for anemia and gastrointestinal disorders. The total annual cost for all medication averaged over six years was not significantly different between surgically treated individuals (SKr 1386/yr, US$215) and obese control individuals (SKr 1261/yr, US$196). Again it must be stressed that we do not yet have 10 to 15 year data available for costs of medication.

In a separate study on CVD and diabetes medication, we found that a weight loss ≥10% was necessary to reduce the costs of medication among subjects with such treatment at baseline, while a ≥15% weight loss was required to prevent the initiation of a new treatment against the two conditions (73). The annual average cost over six years for medication against diabetes and CVD increased by SKr 463 (US$72) (96%) in subjects with weight loss <5%, and decreased by SKr 39 (US$6) (8%) with weight loss ≥15% (73).

Modern economists often use estimates of patients' willingness to pay for a given treatment as an expression of the degree of urgency. We measured the willingness to pay for an efficient obesity treatment at baseline and found it to be twice as high as the monthly salary of the participants (74). After inclusion, the willingness to pay for an efficient treatment increased markedly in the surgically treated group (unpublished observation).

Taken together, the direct plus indirect costs of surgical obesity treatment seem to be only marginally higher than conventional treatment over six years. Taking the reduced risk factors and the improved quality of life into account, the surgical approach seemed worthwhile already as based on six-year evaluations. As pointed out above, it is now urgent to repeat the health economic evaluations based on 10 to 15 year data in order to examine if the reduced incidence of hard endpoints translates into reduced costs. It should be stressed that our six-year evaluations are based on actually observed costs and are not the result of modeling from short-term observations as is usually the case in health economic studies.

Genetic Findings in SOS

Segregation analysis of the SOS cohort has indicated an age-dependent major gene effect explaining up to 34% of the BMI variance (36). This finding makes the SOS data promising for genetic association studies. So far, SOS results have demonstrated that variants in a number of genes, including the β_3-adrenergic receptor (37), Prader-Willi locus (38), mitochondrial DNA D-loop polymorphism (39), MC4 receptor (25), leptin (40), and UCP1 (41) are not important in "common" obesity.

Sequencing of the ghrelin gene revealed an Arg51Gln mutation found only in obese subjects (42). A Leu72Met mutation tended to associate with earlier onset of weight problems in obese carriers (42). In a larger study, the Arg51Gln was associated with lower levels of circulating ghrelin, but not with obesity (43). Met72 carrier status was more frequent among nonobese SOS subjects while obese Met72 carriers had lower prevalence of hypertension than obese noncarriers (43).

A novel T45G polymorphism in the adiponectin gene was equally common among obese and normal weight female SOS subjects (44). Although silent (i.e., resulting in no amino acid change), it was associated with serum cholesterol and waist circumference in the obese group,

possibly due to linkage disequilibrium with a nearby functional polymorphism. An IVS2 + G62T variant was equally prevalent in obese and control subjects, but obese GG homozygotes had higher blood glucose levels, and all six diabetics in this sample were in this group. Furthermore, this adiponectin gene polymorphism was associated with BMI, blood pressure, and sagittal diameter (44).

Spouse correlation in BMI declined over time among 8663 spouse pairs, suggesting that spouse similarity is the result of assortative mating, rather than the sharing of a common environment (26). Adult offspring of obesity concordant parents had the highest BMI, and an obesity prevalence being 20-fold higher than among offspring of nonobese parents. No environmental interaction could be detected in this study, which thus suggests that the globally observed increase in obesity prevalence may in part have a genetic etiology via assortative mating (26).

Surgical Complications in SOS

Five of the 2010 subjects who underwent surgery (0.25%) died postoperatively (within 90 days) (28). As reported elsewhere for 1164 patients (45), 151 individuals (13.0%) had 193 postoperative complications (bleeding 0.5%, thrombosis and embolism 0.8%, wound complications 1.8%, deep infections 2.1%, pulmonary complications 6.1%, other complications 4.8%). In 26 patients (2.2%), the postoperative complications were serious enough to require reoperation. The frequency of reoperations and/or conversions (excluding operations due to postoperative complications) among 1338 subjects followed for at least 10 years in November, 2005, was 31%, 21%, and 17% for those obtaining banding, vertical banded gastroplasty, and gastric bypass, respectively (28).

Effects of Bariatric Surgery on Overall Mortality

The effect of bariatric surgery on overall mortality in SOS was recently published (28). Figure 4 depicts the cumulative overall mortality over up to 16 years. Surgery was associated with an unadjusted hazard ratio (HR) of 0.76 relative to control (95% CI, 0.59 to 0.99, $p = 0.04$). Over the follow-up period, 129 subjects (6.3%) died in the control group and 101 (5.0%) in the surgery group.

The adjusted HR for treatment (surgery relative to controls) was similar when based on matching information (HR = 0.73, $p = 0.02$) and on baseline information (HR = 0.71, $p = 0.01$), although the two models did not use exactly the same variables (28). In both models, the strongest predictors were age and smoking, while the strongest univariate predictors were plasma triglycerides and blood glucose. By using multivariate models in an iterative way, it was possible to show that it took

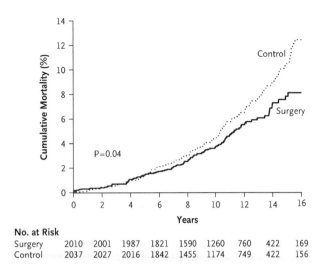

No. at Risk

Surgery	2010	2001	1987	1821	1590	1260	760	422	169
Control	2037	2027	2016	1842	1455	1174	749	422	156

Figure 4 Unadjusted cumulative mortality over 16 years among surgically treated subjects and their obese controls in the SOS intervention study. The hazard ratio for subjects who underwent bariatric surgery, as compared with control subjects, was 0.76 (95% CI, 0.59 to 0.99, $p = 0.04$), with 129 deaths in the control group and 101 in the surgery group. The statistical calculations were performed on all observations, i.e., up to 18 years of observation at the time of database analysis. *Abbreviation*: SOS, Swedish Obese Subjects. *Source*: From Ref. 28.

approximately 13 study years until the favorable effect of surgery became statistically significant.

There were 53 cardiovascular deaths in the control group and 43 in the surgery group (28). The most common cardiovascular causes of death were myocardial infarction, sudden death, and cerebrovascular damage. Cancer was the most common cause of noncardiovascular death. Lack of power made it impossible to estimate the risk reduction for specific causes of death.

Although we have found larger improvements in risk factors, left ventricular structure and function, and in HRQL with increasing weight loss, we failed to demonstrate a specific effect of the amount of weight loss on mortality. This may be related to lack of power but may also indicate that the favorable effect of bariatric surgery on mortality could be mediated by other mechanisms than weight loss. This possibility needs to be investigated.

Effects of Bariatric Surgery on the Incidence of Myocardial Infarction, Stroke, and Cancer

Current calculations indicate that the incidence rates of fatal plus nonfatal myocardial infarction and cancer are lower in the SOS surgery group than in the obese control group, while no significant differences between the two groups could be detected regarding the incidence of stroke.

CONCLUSIONS

The prevalence of obesity is high and increasing, and obesity is associated with a dramatically increased morbidity and mortality. Nonpharmacological conventional treatment at specialized obesity units may achieve, on average, a 5% weight loss over two to five years of follow-up. However, this is not enough to keep the risk factors down over long periods of time. As illustrated by the conventionally treated obese control group of SOS, nonpharmacological, obesity treatment at primary health care centers is not, on average, associated with any weight loss in the short or the long term. Unfortunately, most obese patients worldwide have no access to specialized obesity treatment.

Treatment with currently available antiobesity drugs results, on average, in 7% to 10% weight reduction over two to four years as compared with 4% to 6% in placebo groups (78–81). This is encouraging but more efficient drugs are clearly needed. So far, randomized drug trials lasting longer than four years have not been published.

Obese patients with prediabetes and type 2-diabetes deserves extra attention. It is more difficult to achieve conventional or pharmacologically induced weight loss in diabetic obese patients. Moreover, even when weight loss is achieved almost all patients relapse within a few years. Treatment with sulfonylureas or insulin causes weight increase. Thus, obesity not only causes diabetes but is also a complication of diabetes treatment. This vicious spiral must be broken.

Surgery is the only treatment of obesity resulting, on average, in more than 15% documented weight loss over 10 years. This treatment has dramatic positive effects on most but not on all cardiovascular risk factors over a 10-year period. It has excellent effects on established diabetes and prevents the development of new cases of diabetes. Large weight reductions achieved by surgery also improve left ventricular structure and function and slow down the atherosclerotic process as estimated from intima-media measurements and decreased prevalence of effort-related calf pain. Quality of life is markedly improved. Finally, and most importantly, overall mortality is reduced by surgery, as recently demonstrated by the prospective controlled SOS study (28) and by four retrospective cohort studies (20–23). Since all these positive effects are well documented and since direct and indirect costs for bariatric surgery treatment over six years seem to be only moderately higher than for conventional obesity treatment, surgical treatment must become attainable for many more obese individuals.

There is an urgent need for one specialized obesity center per approximately 500,000 inhabitants. At these centers, internists, surgeons, nurses, and dietitians would need to work full time with obese patients referred to them by general practitioners. The demand for such treatment is almost unlimited. Obese patients in a region with 500,000 inhabitants will generate at least 20,000 to 30,000 visits annually.

While waiting for more efficient antiobesity drugs, the surgical treatment of obesity must become more universally available. This author estimates that the real need is at least 500 to 1000 operations annually per 500,000 inhabitants in most Western countries even if the current visible demand for operations is lower. All obese patients with BMI ≥ 40 kg/m^2 need to be considered for bariatric surgery. However, a very large number of individuals with BMIs as low as 34 kg/m^2 will also benefit from surgical treatment. Finally, in the case of obese, diabetic, and prediabetic patients, the question must now be raised, if it can be considered *lege artis* not to offer surgical treatment for their obesity and associated metabolic disorders.

REFERENCES

1. Flegal KM. Epidemiologic aspects of overweight and obesity in the United States. Physiol Behav 2005; 86:599–602.
2. Ogden CL, Carroll MD, Curtin LR, et al. Prevalence of overweight and obesity in the United States, 1999–2004. JAMA 2006; 295:1549–1555.
3. World Health Organization. Obesity: Preventing and Managing the Global Epidemic. WHO/NUT/NCD/98.1 ed. Geneva: WHO, 1998.
4. Freedman DM, Ron E, Ballard-Barbash R, et al. Body mass index and all-cause mortality in a nationwide US cohort. Int J Obes Relat Metab Disord 2006; 30:822–829.
5. van Dam RM, Willett WC, Manson JE, et al. The relationship between overweight in adolescence and premature death in women. Ann Intern Med 2006; 145:91–97.
6. Price GM, Uauy R, Breeze E, et al. Weight, shape, and mortality risk in older persons: elevated waist-hip ratio, not high body mass index, is associated with a greater risk of death. Am J Clin Nutr 2006; 84:449–460.
7. Jee SH, Sull JW, Park J, et al. Body-mass index and mortality in Korean men and women. N Engl J Med 2006; 355:779–787.
8. Adams KF, Schatzkin A, Harris TB, et al. Overweight, obesity, and mortality in a large prospective cohort of persons 50 to 71 years old. N Engl J Med 2006; 355:763–778.
9. Yan LL, Daviglus ML, Liu K, et al. Midlife body mass index and hospitalization and mortality in older age. JAMA 2006; 295:190–198.
10. Sjöström L. Mortality of severely obese subjects. Am J Clin Nutr 1992; 55(suppl):516S–523S.
11. Fontaine KR, Redden DT, Wang C, et al. Years of life lost due to obesity. JAMA 2003; 289:187–193.
12. Sjöström L, Lindroos AK, Peltonen M, et al. Lifestyle, diabetes, and cardiovascular risk factors 10 years after bariatric surgery. N Engl J Med 2004; 351:2683–2693.
13. Higgins M, D'Agostino R, Kannel W, et al. Benefits and adverse effects of weight loss. Observations from the Framingham study. Ann Intern Med 1993; 119:758–763.
14. Cornoni-Huntley JC, Harris TB, Everett DF, et al. An overview of body weight of older persons, including the impact on mortality. The National Health and Nutrition Examination Survey I—Epidemiologic Follow-up Study. J Clin Epidemiol 1991; 44:743–753.
15. Pamuk ER, Williamson DF, Madans J, et al. Weight loss and mortality in a national cohort of adults, 1971–1987. Am J Epidemiol 1992; 136:686–697.
16. Pamuk ER, Williamson DF, Serdula MK, et al. Weight loss and subsequent death in a cohort of U.S. adults. Ann Intern Med 1993; 119:744–748.
17. Williamson DF, Pamuk E, Thun M, et al. Prospective study of intentional weight loss and mortality in never- smoking overweight US white women aged 40–64 years. Am J Epidemiol 1995; 141:1128–1141(erratum appears in Am J Epidemiol 1995; 142:369).
18. Williamson DF, Pamuk E, Thun M, et al. Prospective study of intentional weight loss and mortality in overweight white men aged 40–64 years. Am J Epidemiol 1999; 149:491–503.
19. Williamson D, Thompson T, Thun M, et al. Intentional weight loss and mortality among overweight individuals with diabetes. Diabetes Care 2000; 23:1499–1504.
20. Adams TD, Gress RE, Smith SC, et al. Long-term mortality following gastric bypass surgery. New Engl J Med 2007; 357:753–761.
21. Christou NV, Sampalis JS, Liberman M, et al. Surgery decreases long-term mortality, morbidity, and health care use in morbidly obese patients. Ann Surg 2004; 240:416–423, discussion 423–424.
22. Flum DR, Dellinger EP. Impact of gastric bypass operation on survival: a population-based analysis. J Am Coll Surg 2004; 199:543–551.
23. MacDonald KG, Jr., Long SD, Swanson MS, et al. The gastric bypass operation reduces the progression and mortality of non-insulin-dependent diabetes mellitus. J Gastrointest Surg 1997; 1:213–220.
24. Steinbrook R. Surgery for severe obesity. N Engl J Med 2004; 350:1075–1079.
25. Jacobson P, Ukkola O, Rankinen T, et al. Melanocortin 4 receptor sequence variations are seldom a cause of human obesity: the Swedish Obese Subjects, the HERITAGE family study, and a Memphis cohort. J Clin Endocrinol Metab 2002; 87:4442–4446.
26. Jacobson P, Torgerson JS, Sjostrom L, et al. Spouse resemblance in body mass index: effects on adult obesity prevalence in the offspring generation. Am J Epidemiol 2007; 165:101–108.
27. Sjöström L, Larsson B, Backman L, et al. Swedish obese subjects (SOS). Recruitment for an intervention study and a selected description of the obese state. Int J Obes Relat Metab Disord 1992; 16:465–479.
28. Sjöström L, Narbro K, Sjöström CD, et al. Effects of bariatric surgery on mortality in Swedish Obese Subjects. New Engl J Med 2007; 357:741–752.

29. Waaler H. Height, weight and mortality. The Norwegian experience. Acta Med Scand Suppl 1984; 679:1–56.

30. Grunstein RR, Stenlöf K, Hedner JA, et al. Impact of self-reported sleep-breathing disturbances on psychosocial performance in the Swedish Obese Subjects (SOS) study. Sleep 1995; 18:635–643.

31. Karlsson J, Sjöström L, Sullivan M. Swedish Obese Subjects (SOS)—an intervention study of obesity. Measuring psychosocial factors and health by means of short-form questionnaires. Results from a method study. J Clin Epidemiol 1995; 48:817–823.

32. Karason K, Wallentin I, Larsson B, et al. Effects of obesity and weight loss on left ventricular mass and relative wall thickness: survey and intervention study. BMJ 1997; 315:912–916.

33. Karason K, Wallentin I, Larsson B, et al. Effects of obesity and weight loss on cardiac function and valvular performance. Obes Res 1998; 6:422–429.

34. Karason K, Mölgaard H, Wikstrand J, et al. Heart rate variability in obesity and the effect of weight loss. Am J Cardiol 1999; 83:1242–1247.

35. Karason K, Wikstrand J, Sjöström L, et al. Weight loss and progression of early atherosclerosis in the carotid artery: a four-year controlled study of obese subjects. Int J Obes Relat Metab Disord 1999; 23:948–956.

36. Rice T, Sjöström CD, Perusse L, et al. Segregation analysis of body mass index in a large sample selected for obesity: the Swedish Obese Subjects study. Obes Res 1999; 7: 246–255.

37. Gagnon J, Mauriege P, Roy S, et al. The Trp64Arg mutation of the beta3 adrenergic receptor gene has no effect on obesity phenotypes in the Quebec Family Study and Swedish Obese Subjects cohorts. J Clin Invest 1996; 98: 2086–2093.

38. Perusse L, Wevrick R, Chagnon YC, et al. Lack of association between candidate genes for the Prader-Willi syndrome and obesity in the general population. Obes Res 1997; 5:30.

39. Rivera MA, Perusse L, Gagnon J, et al. A mitochondrial DNA D-loop polymorphism and obesity in three cohorts of women. Int J Obes Relat Metab Disord 1999; 23: 666–668.

40. Carlsson B, Lindell K, Gabrielsson B, et al. Obese (ob) gene defects are rare in human obesity. Obes Res 1997;5:30–35.

41. Gagnon J, Lago F, Chagnon YC, et al. DNA polymorphism in the uncoupling protein 1 (UCP1) gene has no effect on obesity related phenotypes in the Swedish Obese Subjects cohorts. Int J Obes Relat Metab Disord 1998; 22:500–505.

42. Ukkola O, Ravussin E, Jacobson P, et al. Mutations in the preproghrelin/ghrelin gene associated with obesity in humans. J Clin Endocrinol Metab 2001; 86:3996–3999.

43. Ukkola O, Ravussin E, Jacobson P, et al. Role of ghrelin polymorphisms in obesity based on three different studies. Obes Res 2002; 10:782–791.

44. Ukkola O, Ravussin E, Jacobson P, et al. Mutations in the adiponectin gene in lean and obese subjects from the Swedish Obese Subjects cohort. Metabolism 2003; 52:881–884.

45. Sjöström L. Surgical intervention as a strategy for treatment of obesity. Endocrine 2000; 13:213–230.

46. Larsson I, Lindroos AK, Peltonen M, et al. Potassium per kilogram fat-free mass and total body potassium: predictions from sex, age, and anthropometry. Am J Physiol Endocrinol Metab 2003; 284:E416–E423.

47. Larsson I, Berteus Forslund H, Lindroos AK, et al. Body composition in the SOS (Swedish Obese Subjects) reference study. Int J Obes Relat Metab Disord 2004; 28: 1317–1324.

48. Larsson I, Henning B, Lindroos AK, et al. Optimized predictions of absolute and relative amounts of body fat from weight, height, other anthropometric predictors, and age 1. Am J Clin Nutr 2006; 83:252–259.

49. Larsson I, Lindroos AK, Lustig TC, et al. Three definitions of the metabolic syndrome: relations to mortality and atherosclerosis. Metab Syndr Relat Disord 2005; 3:102–112.

50. Sjöström CD, Håkangård AC, Lissner L, et al. Body compartment and subcutaneous adipose tissue distribution—risk factor patterns in obese subjects. Obes Res 1995; 3:9–22.

51. Sjöström CD, Lissner L, Sjöström L. Relationships between changes in body composition and changes in cardiovascular risk factors: the SOS Intervention Study. Swedish obese subjects. Obes Res 1997; 5:519–530.

52. Sjöström CD, Lissner L, Wedel H, et al. Reduction in incidence of diabetes, hypertension and lipid disturbances after intentional weight loss induced by bariatric surgery: the SOS Intervention Study. Obes Res 1999; 7:477–484.

53. Sjöström CD, Peltonen M, Wedel H, et al. Differentiated long-term effects of intentional weight loss on diabetes and hypertension. Hypertension 2000; 36:20–25.

54. Sjöström CD, Peltonen M, Sjöström L. Blood pressure and pulse pressure during long-term weight loss in the obese: the Swedish Obese Subjects (SOS) intervention study. Obes Res 2001; 9:188–195.

55. Nichols WW, O'Rourke MF. McDonald's Blood Flow in Arteries. Philadelphia: Lea & Febiger, 1998.

56. Karason K, Peltonen M, Lindroos A, et al. Effort-related calf pain in the obese and long-term changes after surgical obesity treatment. Obes Res 2005; 13:137–145.

57. Karason K, Lindroos AK, Stenlöf K, et al. Relief of cardiorespiratory symptoms and increased physical activity after surgically induced weight loss. Results from the SOS study. Arch Int Med 2000; 160:1797–1802.

58. Grunstein RR, Stenlöf K, Hedner J, et al. Impact of obstructive sleep apnea and sleepiness on metabolic and cardiovascular risk factors in the Swedish Obese Subjects (SOS) study. Int J Obes Relat Metab Disord 1995; 19:410–418.

59. Grunstein R, Stenlöf K, Hedner J, et al. Two year reduction in sleep apnea symptoms and associated incidence after weight loss in severe obesity. Sleep 2007; 30:703–710.

60. Stenlöf K, Grunstein R, Hedner J, et al. Energy expenditure in obstructive sleep apnea: effects of treatment with continuous positive airway pressure. Am J Physiol 1996; 271: E1036–E1043.

61. Peltonen M, Lindroos A, Torgerson J. Musculosceletal pain in the obese: a comparison with a general population and long-term changes after conventional and surgical obesity treatment. Pain 2003; 104:549–557.

62. Lindroos AK, Lystig T, Torgerson JS, et al. Reduced rsik of fractures after obesity surgery – results from the SOS study. Int J Obes 2004; 28(suppl 1):182.

63. Torgerson JS, Lindroos AK, Näslund I, et al. Gallstones, gallbladder disease, and pancreatitis: cross-sectional and 2-year data from the Swedish Obese Subjects (SOS) and SOS reference studies. Am J Gastroenterol 2003; 98:1032–1041.

64. Sullivan M, Karlsson J, Sjöström L, et al. Swedish obese subjects (SOS)—an intervention study of obesity. Baseline evaluation of health and psychosocial functioning in the first 1743 subjects examined. Int J Obes Relat Metab Disord 1993; 17:503–512.

65. Karlsson J, Persson LO, Sjöström L, et al. Psychometric properties and factor structure of the Three-Factor Eating Questionnaire (TFEQ) in obese men and women. Results from the Swedish Obese Subjects (SOS) study. Int J Obes Relat Metab Disord 2000; 24:1715–1725.

66. Karlsson J, Sjöström L, Sullivan M. Swedish obese subjects (SOS)—an intervention study of obesity. Two- year follow-up of health-related quality of life (HRQL) and eating behavior after gastric surgery for severe obesity. Int J Obes Relat Metab Disord 1998; 22:113–126.

67. Sullivan M, Karlsson J, Sjöström L, et al: Why quality-of-life measures should be used in the treatment of patients with obesity. In: Björntorp P, ed. International Textbook of Obesity. Chichester: John Wiley and Sons, 2001: 485–510.

68. Karlsson J, Taft C, Rydén A, et al. Ten year trends in health related quality of life after surgical and conventional treatment for severe obesity: the SOS intervention study. Int J Obes (Lond.) 2007; 31:1248–1261.

69. Narbro K, Jonsson E, Larsson B, et al. Economic consequences of sick-leave and early retirement in obese Swedish women. Int J Obes Relat Metab Disord 1996; 20:895–903.

70. Narbro K, Ågren G, Jonsson E, et al. Sick leave and disability pension before and after treatment for obesity: a report from the Swedish Obese Subjects (SOS) study. Int J Obes Relat Metab Disord 1999; 23:619–624.

71. Ågren G, Narbro K, Jonsson E, et al. Cost of in-patient care over 7 years among surgically and conventionally treated obese patients. Obes Res 2002; 10:1276–1283.

72. Narbro K, Agren G, Jonsson E, et al. Pharmaceutical costs in obese individuals: comparison with a randomly selected population sample and long-term changes after conventional and surgical treatment: the SOS intervention study. Arch Intern Med 2002; 162:2061–2069.

73. Ågren G, Narbro K, Näslund I, et al. Long-term effects of weight loss on pharmaceutical costs in obese subjects. A report from the SOS intervention study. Int J Obes Relat Metab Disord 2002; 26:184–192.

74. Narbro K, Sjöström L. Willingness to pay for obesity treatment. Int J Technol Assess Health Care 2000; 16:50–59.

75. Boutouyrie P, Bussy C, Lacolley P, et al. Association between local pulse pressure, mean blood pressure, and large-artery remodeling. Circulation 1999; 100:1387–1393.

76. Franklin SS, Khan SA, Wong ND, et al. Is pulse pressure useful in predicting risk for coronary heart disease? The Framingham heart study. Circulation 1999; 100:354–360.

77. Stunkard AJ, Messick S. The three-factor eating questionnaire to measure dietary restraint, disinhibition and hunger. J Psychosom Res 1985; 29:71–83.

78. Sjöström L, Rissanen A, Andersen T, et al. Randomised placebo-controlled trial of orlistat for weight loss and prevention of weight regain in obese patients. European Multicentre Orlistat Study Group [see also editorial]. Lancet 1998; 352:167–172.

79. Torgerson JS, Hauptman J, Boldrin MN, et al. Xenical in the prevention of diabetes in obese subjects (XENDOS) study: a randomized study of orlistat as an adjunct to lifestyle changes for the prevention of type 2 diabetes in obese patients. Diabetes Care 2004; 27:155–161.

80. Despres JP, Golay A, Sjöström L. Effects of rimonabant on metabolic risk factors in overweight patients with dyslipidemia. N Engl J Med 2005; 353:2121–2134.

81. Stenlöf K, Rössner, S, Vercruysse, F, et al. Topiramate in the treatme.nt of obese subjects with drug-naive type 2 diabetes. Diabetes Obes Metab 2007; 9:360–368.

33

Laparoscopic Adjustable Gastric Banding

PAUL E. O'BRIEN

Centre for Obesity Research and Education, Monash University, The Alfred Hospital, Melbourne, Victoria, Australia

INTRODUCTION

The laparoscopic adjustable gastric band (LAGB) first appeared in the early 1990s as the fourth step in a process of development occurring over two decades. The setting was of an expanding epidemic of obesity. Preventive programs were not proving to be effective, nonsurgical treatments generally had only a mild and transient effect, and the range of existing surgical treatments were unacceptable to the majority of those with the disease and to their physicians. There was a major clinical need that was unfilled. The first step had been the development of fixed gastric banding procedures in the late 1970s. The second step was the introduction of an adjustable form of gastric banding in the 1980s, and the third step was the move to a laparoscopic approach to complex abdominal surgical procedures at the end of the 1980s.

Fixed Gastric Banding

Fixed gastric banding had been present since the late 1970s but had not provided sufficient effectiveness to become a standard therapy. The key attractions for fixed banding had been safety, lack of anatomical change, reversibility, and reduced invasiveness. The first procedure has been attributed to Wilkinson et al. in 1977 (1). They placed a strip of Marlex mesh around the upper stomach. Kolle from Oslo and Molina from Texas were the leading practitioners of the fixed banding techniques, and there was significant early involvement of surgeons in Sweden (2). The procedure was an important part of the Swedish Obese Subjects (SOS) study (3). However, problems including erosion, obstruction, inadequate weight loss, and maladaptive eating behaviors precluded widespread acceptance of the approach. In particular, with lack of adjustability, the band was either too tight and the patient had copious vomiting and maladaptive eating, or it was too loose, resulting in disappointing weight loss. Something better was needed.

Adjustable Gastric Banding

The concept of an adjustable gastric band was developed in a rabbit model by two Austrian surgical researchers, Szinicz and Schnapka, in 1982 (4). They created a silicone band with an inner balloon, connected by tubing to a subcutaneous port. Addition of saline to the port increased compression on the proximal stomach. The approach used in this animal model was brought into clinical practice by Lubomyr Kusmak of New Jersey in 1986 (5). He found that, when compared with a nonadjustable but otherwise similar silicone band that he had used since 1983, the patients had better weight loss and fewer complications. With the adjustable band, the group had lost 62.4% of excess weight compared with 49.4% at four years with the nonadjustable band.

An alternative device, based on the same concepts, was developed at about the same time by Dr. Forsell in Sweden (6). As these procedures required major open surgery, they did not divert attention from the more popular procedures of vertical banded gastroplasty and gastric bypass until the onset of the laparoscopic era of complex upper abdominal surgery, which began with laparoscopic cholecystectomy in 1989.

Laparoscopic Adjustable Gastric Banding

The first LAGB was the LAP-BAND® system (Allergan Health, Irvine, California, U.S.). Figure 1 shows the current version of this system.

This device was specifically designed for laparoscopic placement and was introduced into clinical practice by Mitiku Belachew from Huy, Belgium in September 1993 (7). Two key changes were made to the adjustable silicone gastric band of Kusmak to create the LAP-BAND. The first was use of a self-locking mechanism with a fixed, initial band circumference, which obviated the need for a tensioning clamp, and a pressure-measuring device that he called a gastrostenometer. Second, the inner balloon was

extended from being a side cushion on the ring of silicone to being an almost circumferential balloon, thereby augmenting the capacity for adjustment.

The Swedish adjustable gastric band (Obtech band®, Johnson and Johnson Endosurgery, Cincinnati, Ohio, U.S.) was introduced as a laparoscopic procedure in the mid 1990s (8), and subsequently, several other versions of the LAGB have been introduced, predominantly in Europe. There have now been over 1000 publications on the LAP-BAND system and a significant number on the Swedish band, but there have been no reports of outcomes, to my knowledge, for any of the alternative bands. At the time of writing, the LAP-BAND system is the only LAGB system approved for use in the United States. For convenience, we will use the abbreviation, LAGB, as a generic term.

The key features of the LAGB are illustrated in Figure 2.

There is an outer ring of silicone, and an inner balloon of silicone that fully covers the inner surface. The simple

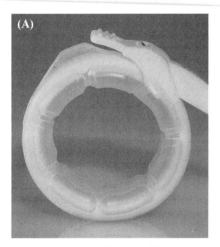

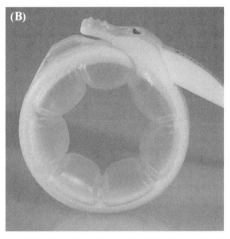

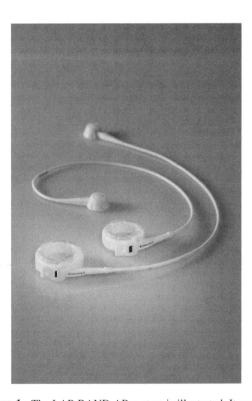

Figure 1 The LAP-BAND AP system is illustrated. It consists of a ring of silicone with an inner balloon and is placed around the cardia of the stomach just below the esophagogastric junction. The balloon connects via tubing to an access port that is placed on the left anterior rectus sheath. *Abbreviation*: AP, access port.

Figure 2 (**A**) A closer view of the LAP-BAND AP system showing the inner balloon that contains 3 mL of saline at its basal setting. (**B**) A further 4 mL has been added to the balloon to markedly reduce the area within the band.

but secure locking device can be reopened for repositioning or revision. With the addition of saline by injection into the access port, as shown in Figure 1, the area within the band is decreased, allowing progressive compression of the gastric cardia until an appropriate level of satiety is reached.

Because of the dual attractions of a controlled level of effect through adjustability and of laparoscopic placement without resection of gut or anastomoses, the LAGB procedure rapidly became the primary method of bariatric surgery across the world. This widespread acceptance occurred prior to adequate definition of optimal technique for placement or for follow-up care and adjustments and also prior to publication of any outcome data; so consequently, quite variable outcomes were initially encountered.

Because it was perceived as a safe, minimally invasive, and yet effective procedure, it led a resurgence of interest in bariatric surgery through the 1990s. In Australia, less than 400 bariatric procedures were performed in 1993. By 2003, the number exceeded 4000, nearly all being LAGB (9). A similar response was seen in Europe. The United States was a notable exception to this enthusiastic embrace as regulatory approval delayed the introduction of the LAGB until June 2001.

MECHANISMS OF ACTION

The range of bariatric surgical procedures currently available generate their effect through a variety of mechanisms. The narrow concept of a procedure being either restrictive or malabsorptive has fallen away with the improved understanding of the physiology of eating, appetite, satiety, the hormonal responses to food, and the absorption of nutrients. At least five mechanisms can now be demonstrated, including induction of satiety, restriction to food intake, diversion of food from the proximal gut, malabsorption of nutrients, and aversion to eating certain foods because of side effects. LAGB utilizes at least three of these mechanisms.

Induction of satiety is the principal mechanism of action of the LAGB. After LAGB, patients who are adequately adjusted will say they do not feel hungry. Their interest in food is reduced, and their appetite is less. They miss meals or forget to eat until well beyond the mealtime. This would not have happened before the LAGB placement.

To measure this feature in a controlled and objective way, we invited 17 patients, who were at least two years after LAGB placement and had achieved good weight loss, to undertake a blinded study (10). Two days before the test, there was a real or sham aspiration of the band. On the test day, after an overnight fast, each patient documented the state of hunger or satiety every 30 minutes for

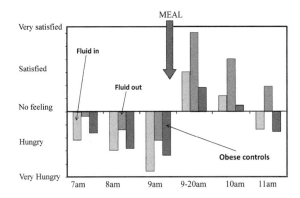

Figure 3 Satiety and adjustments. The figure shows the level of satiety is greater when fluid is placed in the band regardless of whether the person has eaten or not. This demonstrates the primary satiety-inducing effect of the LAGB. *Abbreviation*: LAGB, laparoscopic adjustable gastric band.

3 hours using a linear analogue scale. A standard meal was given midway through this period. The changes in the level of satiety are shown in Figure 3.

Note that at each time point prior to the meal, there is greater satiety with fluid present in the band compared with when fluid was absent—the latter being at a similar level of hunger to a control group of obese patients who did not have the LAGB. After the meal, there was increased satiety in all groups, but the difference between groups remained constant, indicating that the primary and dominant method of action is through satiety induction, not restriction and satiation associated with eating.

Early satiation is the second mechanism of action of the LAGB. A feeling of satiation is achieved after eating a small amount of food. Patients are encouraged to eat no more than three times per day and to eat a very small amount of food at each meal, about the amount of food that would fill half a glass. The presence of a restrictive effect enables them to do that.

Aversion is the final element. Eating red meat and fresh bread can be difficult. These, and less often other foods, tend to sit at the lower esophagus and can need to be regurgitated to give relief. Eating too rapidly or too large a volume leads to similar unpleasant episodes and helps the patients to become careful in their content and style of eating. Good education is the preferred approach to achieving good eating behaviors, but these reminders can reinforce the message.

LAGB TECHNIQUE I—SURGICAL PLACEMENT

Overview of the Procedure

Numerous variations to parts of the LAGB placement technique are practiced but a constant feature is that, at completion, the band is securely fixed across the cardia of the stomach. The procedure is performed on an outpatient basis or with an overnight stay. It is characterized by minimal tissue trauma with no dividing, stapling, resecting or anastomosing. The laparoscopic component of the technique takes between 10 and 20 minutes to complete. The author's current technique is briefly described.

Under full relaxant general anesthesia, four ports of 5-mm diameter and one port of 15-mm diameter are placed in the upper abdomen, generally to the left of the midline. The area of the left crus of the diaphragm is exposed by retraction of the gastric fundus, and a 1-cm length of peritoneum is opened. The pars flaccida of the lesser omentum is opened, and a 1-cm opening is made in the peritoneum on the posterior wall of the lesser sac just in front of the edge of the right crus of the diaphragm. A Lap-Band placer (Automated Medical Products, New Jersey, U.S.) is passed through this opening, across the dorsal surface of the upper stomach above posterior gastric recess of the lesser sac, and reappears at the area of dissection on the left crus. The band size is determined by measurement with the placer and that band is primed, introduced into the abdomen via the 15-mm port. The tubing and then the band are drawn around the cardia of the stomach, and the band is closed. A series of gastrogastric sutures across the band secure its position on the anterior cardia. The tubing is drawn out through the 15-mm port site and connected to an access port for subsequent adjustments. This access port is fixed by sutures to the left anterior rectus sheath.

The original technique for LAGB placement was described by Belachew (11). A number of significant changes in technique have occurred since that description, which have improved the effectiveness and reduced late adverse events. Table 1 lists some of the key changes that have been introduced in the 14 years since the initial LAGB was performed.

Several aspects of the technique deserve specific comment.

Laparoscopic Placement

The LAGB is specifically designed for laparoscopic placement. The band can be placed by open technique also, and occasionally this becomes necessary, usually due to the presence of a very large, fragile liver or copious amounts of intra-abdominal fat. Use of preoperative very low calorie diet in selected patients has reduced these challenges (12). Conversion to open placement should become necessary in less than 1 in 500 patients. The degree of visibility, and therefore, accuracy of placement and fixation are much greater with laparoscopic placement. Furthermore, there are fewer perioperative complications. Open placement is not an acceptable alternative. The operation requires prior experience with advanced

Table 1 Changes in Technique that have Occurred over the Initial 13 Years after Introduction of the LAGB

LAGB placement technique, 1994	Current technique, 2007
Place band 3 cm below esophagogastric junction	Band placed just below esophagogastric junction
Greater curve dissection above first of short gastric vessels	Greater curve dissection at the angle of His
Lesser curve dissection—perigastric path, often via the apex of lesser sac	Lesser curve dissection—pars flaccida path, above the lesser sac
Gastrostenometer used to determine initial balloon volume	Gastrostenometer not used. Band left empty initially
Anterior fixation—limited and central	Anterior fixation more extensive, from the greater curve to lesser curve
Gastrogastric sutures placed to fix band below a small gastric pouch (15–30 mL)	Gastrogastric sutures placed to fix band below a "virtual" pouch just below the esophagogastric junction
Access port placed within rectus abdominis	Access port placed on rectus abdominis
Adjustments performed in radiology with volume determined by barium study	Adjustments performed in office with volume determined by weight loss and symptoms

Abbreviation: LAGB, laparoscopic adjustable gastric band.

laparoscopic surgery, good laparoscopic skills, and comprehensive training.

Pars Flaccida or Perigastric Pathway

The perigastric pathway was the traditional pathway and generally served well but had the major flaw of permitting prolapse of the posterior wall of the stomach through the band. In a randomized controlled trial (RCT) of 200 patients (13), the pars flaccida approach was shown to be associated with significantly fewer revisional procedures for prolapse. Weight loss was equal. The pars flaccida approach is now recommended.

A potential disadvantage to the pars flaccida path has been the possibility of early postoperative obstruction to swallowing due to excess tissue within the band. The amount of fat included with the banded upper stomach is much more variable with the pars flaccida approach than with the perigastric approach. With too much fat present, transit of fluid across the band will be excessively delayed or stopped in the early days postoperatively. Particular attention needs to be given to the use of a calibration tube and the dissection of the lesser omental and perigastric fat to ensure the band is not too tight. The introduction of the LAP-BAND AP series has reduced this risk as the band is easily reopened at operation to dissect more of the lesser curve fat and it has a basal volume of 3 mL that could be removed in the event of delayed emptying in the postoperative phase.

Correct Positioning of LAGB at Gastric Cardia

The precise siting of the band at the top of the stomach is perhaps the most critical aspect of the operation. If the band is too high, it does not work properly, and if too low, it causes problems. The LAGB is a gastric band, not an esophageal band. The most important mechanism of its action is by inducing a feeling of satiety that is probably mediated, at least in part, by the vagal afferent receptors in the apex of the gastric cardia. The band needs to overlay this area to generate this response. There must be correct placement of the gastrogastric sutures as a part of the anterior fixation. The posterior aspect of the band is almost certainly around the distal esophagus as it runs along the line of the left crus. The anterior aspect, therefore, has to be fixed over the upper stomach to achieve the satiety-inducing effect.

Use of the Calibration Tube

The calibration tube has two important functions—enabling a check that the band is not too tight after closure and defining the line of the esophagogastric junction. Additionally, it can be helpful as an aspiration tube to empty the stomach of gas at the commencement of the operation. Failure to correctly identify the esophagogastric junction before fixing the band can result in persistence of a hiatal hernia and excessive stomach above the band.

Anterior Fixation

Correct anterior fixation is critical to set the band around the upper stomach and to prevent anterior prolapse. The first suture is the most important one. It must start near the greater curve. The placement above the band must be on the gastric wall just before the esophagogastric junction. If the first suture is placed correctly, the remaining sutures can be easily placed. The buckle of the band should not be included in the gastric wrap during anterior fixation as this could lead to band erosion.

Placement of the Access Port

Adjustability is the key to the LAGB's combination of effectiveness and gentleness, and this is facilitated by optimal placement of the access port. It should be placed on the anterior rectus sheath, not within or lateral to it. Office adjustment of the band is then used as an easy and cost-effective method of achieving the optimal tightness.

LAGB TECHNIQUE II— THE AFTERCARE PROGRAM

Clinical Consultation

The LAGB procedure is a process of care, not just an intervention. A major difference between LAGB and other bariatric procedures is the content and importance of the aftercare program. After gastric bypass, there is an ongoing need for nutritional assessment and advice and general supportive care, but the outcome from the procedure is set by the operation itself and cannot be altered a great deal by the nature of the follow-up. LAGB is quite different. The role of the operative procedure is to place the band correctly and safely. By itself, LAGB placement will not generate more than a modest and short-term weight loss. The diameter of the band is set such that, after the immediate perioperative phase, there is no significant effect of satiety or satiation without the adjustment. Correct eating, correct exercise and activity, and appropriate adjustments are the keys to an optimal outcome. A direct relationship has been shown between the frequency of follow-up visits and weight loss (14). An optimal follow-up program should be permanent, should be provided by a multidisciplinary team, and should represent a partnership between the health professionals and the patient.

The clinical consultation is at the center of the aftercare program. It involves review of health status, weight change, eating and exercise practices, and symptoms of possible band dysfunction. If an adjustment is required, the decision is made as a part of the clinical consultation and the procedure is incorporated into the episode of patient contact.

Recommended Schedule

The aftercare process begins with preoperative information, education, and discussion. Detailed patient information is now readily available (15), and all patients should be informed of the guidelines for eating and exercise and the importance of the follow-up process. This information is reinforced while they are in hospital and during the follow-up. The most important guidelines are summarized into a set of eight rules as shown in Table 2.

The initial postoperative visit usually occurs at four weeks with the initial adjustment occurring at that time. All adjustments occur in the office as a part of a clinical consultation. The need for an adjustment is determined by

Table 2 The Eight Golden Rules of LAGB Aftercare

1	Eat three or less meals per day.
2	Do not eat anything between meals.
3	Eat slowly and stop when no longer hungry.
4	Focus on nutritious foods.
5	Avoid calorie-containing liquids.
6	Exercise for at least 30 min every day.
7	Be active throughout the day.
8	Always keep in contact.

Abbreviation: LAGB, laparoscopic adjustable gastric band.

the rate of weight loss or weight status, the symptoms of inadequate induction of satiety (feeling hungry, looking for snacks between meals, focus on food), symptoms of inadequate restriction (eating easily, eating too great a volume of food), symptoms of excessive tightness or proximal gastric enlargement (restricted range of food; food sticking; reflux of food or fluid, particularly, at night; heartburn; vomiting; maladaptive eating behavior).

If the level of adjustment is insufficient, patients are said to be in the "yellow zone." They tend to get hungry, eat too easily or too much, and are not losing weight fast enough. They usually need more fluid added to the band. If they are in the "red zone," they are struggling with eating a normal range of food—they may have reflux, vomiting, or maladaptive eating with a tendency to consume liquid or slippery foods such as ice cream and chocolate in preference to healthy foods. There has been excessive adjustment or something is wrong. Normally, fluid needs to be removed.

If patients are in the "green zone," they are eating correctly, not experiencing much hunger through the day, happy to have three or less small meals per day, and are losing weight appropriately. This is the target for the adjustment process and the clinical consultation focuses largely on these symptoms, which guide us to the patient's position on the chart.

Adjustment Sequence

Each LAGB has its own schedule and limits. By way of illustration, my recommended adjustment schedule for the LAP-BAND AP Standard and AP Large is as follows:

1. A basal volume of 3 mL of normal saline is left in the band at the completion of placement. If there is excessive early postoperative restriction, some or all of this fluid can be removed. This has been very rarely necessary.
2. The first addition of more saline occurs at four weeks: 1 to 1.5 mL is added at this time, the volume being determined by the levels of satiety during the first four weeks.

3. Each patient is reviewed every two weeks initially. At each visit, there is a full clinical consultation, including review of weight loss and progress toward targets, discussion of the state of satiety, appetite and hunger, symptoms of excessive tightness, and general health issues. Additional saline in aliquots of 1 or 0.5 mL is added at these visits as appropriate for achieving the green zone.
4. As the green zone is approached, usually after two or four visits, the spacing of visits is increased to one month, then three months, and finally to six months.
5. All patients should be reviewed at least every six months permanently.
6. The typical final optimal volume for the APS band is 6 mL and for the APL is 9 mL. There is no set upper limit of volume. If the patient is getting hungry, not achieving nor maintaining the weight targets, and is not in the red zone, more fluid can be added.

Data Management

Tracking the patients and their progress and outcome is an essential part of the LAGB process of care. The number of patients being treated, the number of variables that should be tracked, and the need to have a summary of progress at each consultation make electronic management of the follow-up process absolutely necessary. A number of commercial systems are available. The author uses Lap-Base (www.lapbase.com), which has been specifically prepared to enable optimal follow-up of the bariatric surgical patient. Alternatives include RemedyMD and Exemplo. Each varies in the presence and ease of use of the important elements. The following features should be looked for as being of primary importance:

*   Patient demographics are linked to follow-up attendance so that minimal loss to follow-up should occur. Comprehensive follow-up is essential for all bariatric surgical patients, and we include loss to follow-up as one of our "failure" criteria because the most common reason they fail to come back is poor outcome and also because we have failed our patient if we are unable to follow them.
*   Weight targets—if we do not know where we are heading, we will not know when we arrive. In our practice, we set three targets—the first is to lose and maintain the loss of two-thirds of excess weight. If they achieve that, we set a second target of body mass index (BMI) of 27 kg/m^2, a cutoff for avoiding most of the comorbidities of obesity. The third target is normal weight, BMI of 25 kg/m^2, a target we can achieve with many of our adolescents but not so many adults.
*   Progress toward targets—as you see your patients, you should be able to see if they are on track to the

targets. It is a key component of decision making for adjustments.

- Investigational data, including all laboratory data but particularly video files of barium meals and endoscopic findings.
- Pooled data—to enable audit of outcome and data for research.

OUTCOMES AFTER LAGB

Outcomes can be measured by change in weight, health improvement, improvement in quality of life, and safety. All of these have been measured after LAGB but generally by observational study only.

Comparison with Nonsurgical Treatment

Comparison with observational studies of nonsurgical treatment (16) strongly suggests better weight loss with the LAGB. This has now been confirmed by a RCT (17). This study compared the outcomes of 60 mild-to-moderately obese adults (BMI 30–35 kg/m^2), half of whom had a program of optimal nonsurgical management and half had LAGB. Both groups were followed for two years. The LAGB group showed significant greater weight loss, greater resolution of the metabolic syndrome, and improvement in quality of life.

The incidence of adverse events was not different. Figure 4 shows the weight loss pattern over the two years expressed as percent of excess weight lost (EWL) with a loss at two years of 87% of excess weight or 21.6% of initial weight for the LAGB patients and a loss of 21% of excess weight or 5.5% of initial weight for the nonsurgical patients. We have continued to follow the surgical patients. At six years after randomization, all of the surgical group

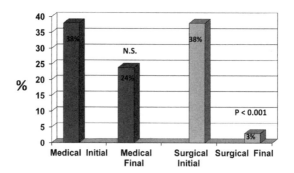

Figure 5 Reduction in the presence of the metabolic syndrome in the medical therapy group (38-24%, N.S.) and in the LAGB group (38-3%, $p < 0.001$) of the RCT. *Abbreviations*: LAGB, laparoscopic adjustable gastric band; RCT, randomized controlled trial.

are still in follow-up and show a durable effect with more than 80% of excess weight remaining lost.

This study was also the first RCT to show a significant difference between optimal medical care and weight loss induced by the LAGB. The metabolic syndrome, as defined by the ATP III criteria, was present in 15 of 40 (38%) of both groups at the commencement of the study. Figure 5 shows the change at the two-year point with a highly significant reduction in the surgical group and no significant reduction in the nonsurgical group.

Quality of life, measured with the Short Form 36, improved significantly in all eight subscores for the surgical group and in three of the subscores for the nonsurgical group.

Comparison with Other Bariatric Procedures

Numerous observational studies have been performed, and these have been subjected to several systematic reviews (18–21), which give comparison between LAGB and other procedures, principally gastric bypass. The systematic reviews by Chapman et al. (18) and Maggard et al. (19) examined safety and efficacy for up to three years after LAGB, Roux-en-Y gastric bypass (RYGB), and other procedures. The Buchwald et al. (20) review limited examination to studies that dealt with four specific comorbidities of obesity and reported weight loss at 12 months only. O'Brien et al. (21) reviewed all studies of LAGB, RYGB, and biliopancreatic diversion (BPD) that included at least 100 patients at commencement and had at least three years of follow-up data. They reported weight loss up to 10 years.

Safety

Perhaps the most attractive single feature of the LAGB is its safety. It has proved to be one of the safest of surgical

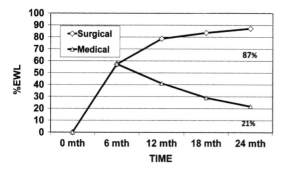

Figure 4 The pattern of loss of excess weight over a two-year period in two groups randomly allocated to optimal medical therapy (21% EWL) or LAGB (87% EWL). The difference is highly significant. *Abbreviations*: EWL, excess weight lost; LAGB, laparoscopic adjustable gastric band.

procedures, being 10 times safer than RYGB in terms of risk of dying (18,19) with an overall perioperative complication rate of 1% to 2%. The author has a clinical role with two large series—one of 4000 patients treated at the Centre for Bariatric Surgery in Melbourne, Australia, and of 8000 patients treated through the American Institute of Gastric Banding centered in Dallas, Texas, United States. There have been no deaths in these 12,000 LAGB patients, including all revisional operations. The perioperative complication rate is very low, being 1.8% in a prospective data collection on 700 LAGB patients (22). The Chapman systematic review identified an incidence of perioperative complications of 2.6%, to be compared with 29.9% for vertical banded gastroplasty (VBG) and 23.4% for RYGB (18).

Weight Loss

Medium term weight loss data

A summary of the weight loss after LAGB is provided in Tables 3 and 4. Most of the content of Table 3 is derived from a formal systematic review of the published literature of the three main bariatric procedures till September 2003 (21). Studies were included in the review if they included weight loss data for at least 100 patients and had follow-up of at least some of these for three years. Of a total of 1703 papers retrieved from the initial search, only 43 fulfilled the entry criteria of a minimum of three-year follow-up and at least 100 patients in the initial treatment. Eighteen studies of LAGB were included. Reports published since then that fulfill the original criteria have been added to the table. In summary, LAGB has achieved a weight loss of between 50% and 60% of excess weight by three years after surgery and has maintained a stable level of weight loss for up to 13 years.

Comparison with RYGB and BPD was made in the report, and a figure from that report (Figure 6) is provided. RYGB had a greater initial weight loss but by three years and beyond, there was no difference. There were fewer studies of BPD available, but this procedure did appear to generate a greater weight loss than either LAGB or RYGB. The difference at five years was statistically significant.

Long-term weight loss data

Very limited data are available for weight loss at 10 years and beyond. In Table 4, I have provided the current data on a personal unpublished series of 2053 patients (95% follow-up intact) with follow-up of up to 13 years. Outcomes up to three and, later, to seven years have been reported (22,44). Also included is a report by Miller et al. from Slazburg (45), providing data up to 12 years on 554 patients (90% follow-up intact) and a series by Favretti et al. from the University of Padua, Italy (46),

of 1791 patients (91% follow-up intact) with follow-up data extending to 12 years. Each series achieved a substantial and durable weight loss with a greater percent of EWL in the Austrian and Australian series than in Italy. After a steady state had occurred at about two years, the Italian series showed a mean excess weight loss over the next 10 years of 39% compared with a mean of approximately 62% in Salzburg and a mean of 51.1% in Australia. The basis for these differences is not clear.

The weight loss profile is significant. The initial weight loss occurs more slowly than is usually seen after gastric bypass or BPD. Maximum weight loss occurs at three or four years rather than one to two years. Once the maximum weight loss is achieved, current data indicate that the weight level remains relatively stable up to 13 years. These features reflect the benefit of adjustability. After initial placement there is no need for rapid weight loss but rather a gentle and progressive pattern controlled by the steady increments of saline added to the system. Once a new stable point of weight has occurred, the weight loss can be maintained and the recidivism of gastric bypass avoided by further small additions of saline.

Changes in the Comorbidities of Obesity

Type 2 diabetes

Treatment: Type 2 diabetes is the paradigm of an obesity-related disease. It is now present in more than 200 million people worldwide and increasing in parallel with the epidemic of obesity. There is a direct relationship between BMI and the risk of developing type 2 diabetes (47). Even modest weight loss has been shown to reduce the morbidity and mortality of the disease (48) and substantial weight loss through bariatric surgery is associated with full remission of the disease in 65% to 80% of patients (49).

The effect of weight loss on a range of health outcomes following LAGB was studied preoperatively and at one year postoperatively in 50 consecutive obese diabetic subjects from a cohort of 500 patients (50). The preoperative mean weight and BMI were 137 ± 30 kg and 48.2 ± 8 kg/m^2, respectively and at one-year 110 ± 24 kg and 38.7 ± 6 kg/m^2 (mean $\pm$ SD). There was significant improvement in all measures of glucose metabolism with remission of diabetes in 32 (64%) patients, major improvement of control in 13 (26%), and no change in five (10%). Mean preoperative HbA1c was $7.8\% \pm 3.2\%$ and $6.2\% \pm 2.7\%$ at one year ($p < 0.001$). Remission of diabetes was predicted by greater weight loss and a shorter history of diabetes. In association with the remission of diabetes, there were also increased insulin sensitivity and improved β-cell function. In association with weight loss, there were also significant improvements in fasting triglyceride, high-density lipoprotein cholesterol (HDL-C), hypertension, sleep, depression, appearance evaluation,

Table 3 Percent of Excess Weight Loss in Medium Term (3–8 Years) After LAGB

Author, yr (reference)	1	2	3	4	5	6	7	8
Belachew et al., 2002 (23), $n = 763$	40	50	55					
Ceelen et al., 2003 (24), $n = 625$	45.8	49.9	47.4					
Dargent, 2004 (25), $n = 1180$	49	56	57	57	54	49	50	
	(696)	(573)	(434)	(321)	(190)	(86)	(14	
Fox et al., 2003 (26), $n = 105$	61	75	72	60				
	(50)	(37)	(24)	(7)				
Frigg et al., 2004 (27), $n = 295$	40	46	47	54				
	(243)	(200)	(155)	(98)				
Greenslade et al., 2004 (28), $n = 273$	42.85	53.70	60.15	64	48			
Holloway et al., 2004 (29), $n = 504$	50	61	65					
	(489)	(469)	(469)					
Jan et al., 2005 (30), $n = 154$	38	45	56					
Mittermair et al., 2003 (31), $n = 454$			72					
O'Brien et al., 2002 (22), $n = 709$	47	52	53	54	57	57		
	(492)	(333)	(264)	(108)	(30)	(10)		
Steffen et al., 2003 (32), $n = 824$	29.5	41.1	48.7	54.5	57.1			
	(821)	(744)	(593)	(380)	(184)			
Suter et al., 2005 (33), $n = 180$	45	57.11	63.91					
	(178)	(171)	(172)					
Vertruyen, 2002 (34), $n = 543$	38	61	62	58	53		52	
	(405)	(372)	(261)	(123)	(52)		(15)	
Victorzon and Tolonen, 2002 (35), $n = 110$	45	52	53					
	(71)	(59)	(26)					
Weiner et al., 2003 (36), $n = 984$								59.3
								(100)
Zinzindohoue et al., 2003 (37), $n = 500$	42.8	52	54.8	62.15				
	(343)	(185)	(45)	(6)				
Biertho et al., 2005 (38), $n = 824$	29	41.5	47	51	55			
			(593)	(380)	(184)			
Ponce et al., 2005 (39), $n = 1014$	40.5	52.9	62	64.3				
	(668)	(240)	(68)	(12)				
Parikh et al., 2005 (40), $n = 749$	44	52	52					
	(640)	(376)	(90)					
Cottam et al., 2006 (41), $n = 181$	48	55	51					
Spivak et al., 2005 (42), $n = 500$	39	45	47					
	(290)	(143)	(81)					
Galvani et al., 2006 (83), $n = 470$	39	45	55					
Sarker et al., 2006 (43), $n = 409$	44.3	48	53					
	(105)	(61)	(20)					
Jan et al., 2005 (30), $n = 406$	34	39	39	35	49			
	(265)	(101)	(35)	(11)	(3)			
Mean percent of EWL	42.3	49.6	55.5	56.7	53.3	53	51	59.3
Sum of n	5756	4064	3330	1446	643	96	29	100
Weighted mean	41.7	51.9	54.4	54.3	55.2	49.8	51	59.3
Number of studies	22	22	23	11	7	2	2	1
Number of studies with n	15	15	16	10	6	2	2	1

Includes all studies where initial sample size >100 patients and follow-up of at least three years. The weighted mean is calculated on the data for each patient and so includes only those studies where n is provided.
Abbreviations: LAGB, laparoscopic adjustable gastric band; EWL, excess weight lost.

and health-related quality of life. Ponce et al. (51) reported very similar outcomes in 53 LAGB patients with type 2 diabetes with remission of the disease in 66% at 12 months and 80% at two years.

Four factors have been found to be significant predictors of remission—the amount of weight lost, shorter time with a diagnosis of diabetes, better preoperative β-cell function and lower preoperative fasting plasma glucose level.

Table 4 Published Studies and Personal Series Reporting Percent of Excess Weight Loss with Long-Term (>10 Years) Follow-Up

Years postoperative author (reference)	1	2	3	4	5	6	7	8	9	10	11	12	13
O'Brien,	51	57	53	52	52	52	50	51	47	50	46	53	59
n =	1382	1216	1192	880	687	541	399	295	206	104	45	28	14
Miller et al. (45)	42	59			68					65		62	
Favretti et al. (46)	40	44	41	39	37	37	36	38	39	35	38	49	
n =	1381	1198	1001	895	765	588	415	311	188	74	22	4	

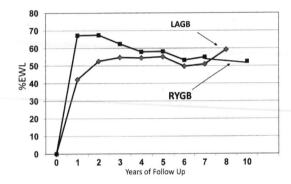

Figure 6 Comparison of the percent of EWL from a systematic review of all studies of LAGB and RYGB that include at least 100 patients at commencement and at least three years of follow-up. *Abbreviations*: EWL, excess weight lost; LAGB, laparoscopic adjustable gastric band; RYGB, Roux-en-Y gastric bypass.

Prevention: Patients with impaired fasting glucose are at high risk of developing type-2 diabetes. Weight loss after LAGB would be expected to prevent that progression. Table 5 shows the changes in markers of insulin resistance over a five-year period after LAGB. There is a substantial and durable improvement. No patient in this series or in a total series of over 2000 patients has presented with a new diagnosis of type 2 diabetes after LAGB, indicating a strong secondary preventive capacity.

Table 5 Changes in Markers of Insulin Resistance with Weight Loss

Time	N	Glucose (mmol/L)	HbA1c (%)	Insulin (μU/mL)
Preoperative	717	5.64	5.77	20.9
1 yr postoperative	451	5.13	5.37	10.9
2 year postoperative	251	5.04	5.28	11.4
3 year postoperative	137	5	5.21	9.6
4 year postoperative	73	4.84	5.2	9.4
5+ year postoperative	28	4.75	5.06	9.7

Hypertension

The prevalence of hypertension in severely obese patients is more than twice the community norm. We found an overall incidence of 33% compared with 14.6% for age- and sex-matched controls in the community. A relationship between weight loss and reduction in blood pressure has been known since the 1920s. A systematic review by the Cochrane Collaboration in 1998 (52) reported that modest weight loss of 3% to 9% body weight, achieved through dieting, was associated with a blood pressure decrease of systolic and diastolic pressures by about 3 mmHg. With substantial weight loss after LAGB, there is a much more impressive improvement. Of 147 consecutive patients with hypertension studied at 12 months after LAGB, 80 patients (55%) had normal blood pressure off therapy, 31% were improved, and 15% were unchanged (53). In a study of 189 hypertensive patients by Ponce et al. (51), there was resolution of hypertension (normal pressures, off therapy) in 60% at 12 months and 74% at two years.

Dyslipidemia

Dyslipidemia is an important comorbidity of obesity associated with a high incidence of coronary and vascular events (54). The changes in dyslipidemia in 515 severely obese patients have been studied before and up to four years after Lap-Band placement (55). Favorable changes in fasting triglycerides (TG), HDL-C, and total cholesterol (TC):HDL-C ratio were seen at one year, and there were further improvements in HDL-C and TC:HDL-C ratio in the second year. All improvements were maintained up to four years when BMI and weight were stable. Male sex, central obesity, elevated fasting glucose, and insulin resistance were found to be associated with less favorable lipid levels. TC and LDL-cholesterol did not correlate with measures of body shape or glucose metabolism. Dyslipidemia of obesity is related to weight distribution, insulin sensitivity, and impaired glucose tolerance. Improvement with weight loss is related to the fall in fasting glucose, improvement in insulin sensitivity, and extent of weight lost.

Asthma

The prevalence of asthma in obesity and the effects of weight loss on asthma were studied in a group of patients undergoing Lap-Band placement (56). A consecutive sample of 32 asthmatic patients were followed clinically and by a standard asthma severity score for at least 12 months after surgery, and any change in asthma was recorded.

The initial prevalence of doctor-diagnosed asthma was 24.6% (73 of 296 consecutive patients). This was significantly higher than the prevalence in the Australian community of 12% to 13% ($p < 0.001$). The 32 patients who were followed had a mean body weight of 125.2 kg (BMI = 45.7 kg/m^2) prior to operation and a weight of 89.3 kg (BMI = 32.9 kg/m^2) at follow-up. All 32 patients had a major clinical improvement in their asthma. The asthma severity score showed highly significant reduction from a mean preoperative scaled asthma severity score of 44.5 $\pm$ 16 to a score at follow-up of 14.3 $\pm$ 11. There were significant improvements in all aspects of asthma, including severity, daily impact, medications, hospitalization, sleep, and exercise. During the year preceding LAGB, 9 of these 32 patients had one or more admissions to hospital for acute asthma. No admissions were required during the 12-month follow-up. It is likely that mechanisms in addition to direct weight loss appear to play a part in this improvement such as prevention of gastroesophageal reflux as the benefit could be seen before substantial weight loss had occurred.

Gastroesophageal reflux disease

Gastroesophageal reflux is a common problem with an estimated prevalence in the community of around 20%, and 7% require daily medication. Obesity is regarded as an important contributing factor to the pathophysiology of gastroesophageal reflux, with a prevalence between 37% and 72% in obese patients (57–59).

A total of 450 consecutive preoperative patients have been studied looking for evidence of gastroesophageal reflux disease (GERD). Some diseases were present in 52% of the patients, well above the community norm of 20%. The prevalence of moderate disease (defined as daily symptoms requiring therapy) and severe disease (defined as requiring proton pump inhibitors $\pm$ other therapy) was 9.3% and 12.7%, respectively, giving a total prevalence for these groups of 21% (60).

The outcome of 82 patients who had moderate or severe disease was measured at one year following LAGB placement (60). The median age was 39 (range 23–58) with a male:female ratio of 5:43. Total resolution of all reflux symptoms occurred in 73 patients (89%), improvement in four (5%), no change in two (2.5%), and aggravation of symptoms in two (2.5%). Patients with severe and moderate symptoms had similar improvement. Resolution or improvement was reported to have occurred soon after surgery and before substantial weight loss.

The LAGB can also generate the symptoms of GERD with nocturnal reflux, dysphagia, and heartburn, if there is a mechanical obstruction through excessive tightening or the presence of prolapse or slippage. In two small series of patients having a Swedish adjustable gastric band, Ovrebo et al. (61) and Westling et al. (62) found that the band was implicated as a cause of gastroesophageal reflux. Patients often present with symptoms of heartburn as an early feature of prolapse. The reflux and heartburn are probably generated as much by the stasis of food and saliva in the lower esophagus rather than refluxed acid. Response to acid inhibition is often poor. The problem is corrected by establishing a more appropriate adjustment level or correcting the prolapse.

Sleep-disordered breathing

Sleep-disordered breathing (SDB), particularly in the form of obstructive sleep apnea (OSA) occurs in approximately 4% of men and 2% of women in the general population (63). Obesity, especially upper body obesity, is considered a major risk factor for OSA and clinical assessments, and sleep studies indicate a prevalence of OSA in morbid obesity (i.e., BMI > 40 kg/m^2) to be 42% to 48% in men and 8% to 38% in women (63).

Many studies have shown that there are major improvements in sleep disturbance and SDB in obese subjects associated with weight loss. These improvements are consistent for medical, dietary, and surgical methods of weight loss (64–67). Sleep disturbance understandably recurs with weight gain.

Three hundred and thirteen consecutive patients with severe obesity (BMI > 35 kg/m^2) completed a preoperative sleep questionnaire and a clinical assessment as a part of the preoperative evaluation prior to Lap-Band placement. A 12-month postoperative study was completed on 123 of these patients, which assessed the characteristics of sleep disturbance and changes in responses to weight loss (68). There was a high prevalence of significantly disturbed sleep in both men (59%) and women (45%), with women less likely to have had their sleep disturbance investigated. Observed sleep apnea was more common in men, but day sleepiness was not affected by gender. Waist circumference was the best clinical measure predicting observed sleep apnea. The group lost an average of 48% (SD 16) of excess weight by 12 months. There was a significant improvement in the responses to all questions at follow-up with habitual snoring reduced to 14% (preoperative 82%), observed sleep apnea 2% (33%), abnormal day sleepiness 4% (39%), and poor sleep quality 2% (39%). The sleep quality score changed markedly. Prior to surgery, 29% had poor quality sleep, and 28% had good quality sleep. These scores changed to 2% and 76%, respectively at one year after operation.

The beneficial finding of weight loss on sleep apnea has been confirmed by polysomnography (PSG) (69). A prospective study was conducted of 25 severely obese patients (17 men, 8 women; BMI 52.7 kg/m^2) with diagnostic PSG paired with biochemical and questionnaire studies, the first prior to LAGB and the second at least one year later. Subjects with a baseline apnea-hypopnea index (AHI) 425/hr were included, and all were stable on nasal continuous positive airway pressure (nCPAP).

The second PSG study was conducted 17.8 (range 12–42) months after surgery and mean weight loss was 50.1% of EWL (range 24–80%) and 45 kg (range 18–103 kg), respectively. There was a significant fall in AHI from 61.6734 to 13.4713, improved sleep architecture with increased REM and stage III and IV sleep, daytime sleepiness, as measured by Epworth Sleepiness Scale, of 13.8 to 3.8.

Twenty-one of 25 (84%) had ceased CPAP, and the remaining four were using lower pressures. There were also major improvements in the metabolic syndrome, quality of life (QOL), and body image, and there were fewer symptoms of depression ($p > 0.05$ for all).

Depression

The Beck Depression Inventory (BDI) (70) has been used for over 40 years as a measure of the characteristic attitudes and symptoms of depression. It has been validated and used in different ethnic groups, in subjects with coexistent medical conditions and in obese subjects (71–75).

In a consecutive study of 487 subjects before LAGB surgery (76), the mean BDI score was 17.7 ± 9.2, with approximately 25% in each category of normal, mild, moderate, and severe depressive illness. Higher scores were found in younger subjects, women, and those with poor body image. High BDI scores correlated with poor physical and mental quality of life measures. Weight loss was associated with a significant and sustained fall in BDI scores with a mean score of 7.8 ± 6.5 at one year and 9.6 ± 7.7 at four or more years after surgery. Greater falls in BDI score at one year were seen in women, those of younger age, and those with greater percent of EWL. Fall in BDI score correlated with improvement in appearance evaluation.

Change in Quality of Life

Severe obesity has a major impact on patients' physical, mental, psychosocial, and economic health. From the perspective of many patients, the improvement in quality of life is arguably the most important outcome to be achieved from a weight-reducing procedure.

Over a three-year period all patients attending for preoperative assessment ($n = 459$) or annual review after surgery ($n = 641$) completed the Medical Outcome Study Short Form 36 health survey (SF-36). The eight domain scores and physical component summary (PCS) and mental component summary (MCS) scores were calculated. Scores were analyzed in groups on the basis of time following surgery and compared with community normal (CN) values (77).

The preoperative scores were all markedly lower than the CN values for all eight domains, and all had lower scores than those in the community with severe medical conditions (78). All scores improved significantly after LAGB and remained similar to CN values up to four years after operation. Of the PCS and MCS scores, the preoperative impairment was greatest in the PCS score (36.8 ± 9.5 vs. CN 51.3 ± 8.3, $p < 0.001$) and improved the most with weight loss (52.4 at one year, 49.2 at four years).

Changes in Survival

The ultimate benefit of weight loss is improved survival. This has been measured in two studies of LAGB patients that have recently been published (46,79). Favretti et al. (46), in their study of the long-term outcomes of 1791 patients after LAP-BAND placement, performed a case-control study of 821 of these patients matched to 821 obese individuals who underwent a nonsurgical weight loss program. After adjusting for age, sex, and BMI, the relative risk of death in the surgical group was 0.38 (95% CI, 0.17–0.85). In a similar study of a Melbourne cohort, Peeters et al. (79) compared all-cause mortality in 966 Lap band patients between the ages of 37 and 60 and BMI >35 kg/m^2, with a similarly aged, obese population-based cohort. The surgical group had lost 23% of total body weight (57% of excess weight). After adjusting for patient years of follow-up, age, BMI, and sex, the surgical group had a 72% lower hazard ratio of death than the community control cohort (hazard ratio 0.28: 95% CI, 0.10–0.85). These two studies, which share many similarities of technique and outcome, show a 62% to 72% reduction in risk of death.

Late Complications After LAGB

Late adverse events have been relatively common but are proving to be avoidable with improved technique. There are three groups of problems: enlargements, erosion of the band into the stomach, and tubing and port problems.

Enlargements

The central feature of all enlargements—posterior prolapse, anterior prolapse, and symmetrical enlargement—is the pressure generated by eating. With correct placement of the band, there is only a virtual stomach present. A typical barium study after placement shows no actual volume reservoir. With eating, space needs to be created for the food before it transits the band into the stomach below. This will generate a force. The two key variables that determine the force are the volume of food present and the rapidity of eating. As the force seeks to create space, any weakness in fixation will be displayed.

Posterior prolapse was seen with the perigastric pathway of placing the band, which often passed across the upper reaches of the lesser sac (11). The smooth and extensive peritonealized posterior gastric surface was the most likely to slip under the stress of eating, creating a posterior slip. This greater level of posterior weakness protected any deficiency in the anterior fixation, and so anterior slips were relatively rare at that time. An RCT involving 200 LAGB patients (13) in which the perigastric pathway was compared with the pars flaccida pathway, which always places the band above the lesser sac, showed complete prevention of posterior prolapse by the pars flaccida approach.

With change to the pars flaccida approach, the posterior weakness was deleted and the next weakest link was shown to be the lateral, or less often the medial, aspect of the anterior fixation. Anterior prolapse became the common form of enlargement.

More recently, with the exercise of greater care in completing the anterior fixation, there is generally no weak area posteriorly or anteriorly. If the patient eats too big a volume or too rapidly or the adjustment is excessive, the force simply stretches what is there and, in time, a symmetrical enlargement develops. If there is too much stomach above the band from the time of the initial placement, as occurs with an unrecognized hiatal hernia, this enlargement occurs more readily.

The key steps to avoiding all forms of enlargement above the band are to ensure that all hiatal hernias are identified, reduced, and fixed at the time of initial LAGB placement; the pars flaccida pathway is used; complete anterior fixation is performed; and clear and repeated instruction is made to patients regarding eating behavior. They must eat three or less times a day, to take only a small amount at each meal (about the amount of food that would fit into half a glass, about 80 mL) and to eat it slowly, over a 15- to 20-minute period.

The incidence of this group of problems has decreased markedly with increasing experience (Table 6). In three cohorts of 600 patients treated by the author over a 10-year period, 32% of the first 600 patients have required a revisional procedure, 5.6% of the next 600, and 1.7% of the last 600. As time passes, more enlargements will present, but the rate of presentations per year of follow-up is significantly less than what occurred initially.

Table 6 Changing Incidence of Late Complications—Personal Series

	Prolapse	Erosions	Tubing/Port
1st 600 patients	194 (32.3%)	58 (9.9%)	94 (16%)
2nd 600 patients	88 (14.7%)	5 (0.9%)	69 (12%)
3rd 600 patients	10 (1.7%)	1	7 (1.2%)

Each of the forms of proximal gastric enlargement presents as a problem of stasis at the distal esophagus, the principal symptoms being reflux, especially at night, heartburn, vomiting, and food intolerance. Diagnosis is confirmed best by barium meal. If the symptoms persist in spite of removal of fluid from the band, the problem is treated by laparoscopic removal and replacement of the band along a new path above the previous one. It has proven to be a safe procedure, requiring no more than an overnight hospital stay, has rarely been associated with a second enlargement, and the patients' weight loss pattern remains on the track they were initially following.

Erosion of the band into the stomach

This was an uncommon problem (1–3%) in the early days of the LAGB and has now almost disappeared. The mechanism for the erosion is unclear. It can occur with different types of bands and appears not to be related to the amount of fluid added. Operative trauma can be a factor in those with early presentations but many erosions present at two or more years after LAGB placement. The author's experience with erosions is shown in Table 6 and indicates that it has become an uncommon event. It presents most commonly as a problem of lack of restriction and increased appetite. Diagnosis is made by gastroscopy, and the problem is treated by laparoscopic removal of the band and repair of the stomach, followed by replacement of the band at three or more months afterwards.

Tubing and port problems

A range of problems can arise from the access port and adjacent tubing. Most commonly, there have been breaks in the tubing at its junction with the metal connection to the port. Needlestick injury to the tubing, perforation of the tubing due to rubbing on a firm structure such as the anterior rectus sheath, and rotation of the port occur less frequently. The incidence of these problems is shown for our patients in Table 6. Diagnosis is confirmed by noting loss of fluid, on more than one occasion. Imaging with injected contrast has been unhelpful. It has been misleading in correctly identifying the site of leakage and is not recommended. Treatment is usually by replacement of the port as an outpatient procedure. The problem has become infrequent with improved design of the tubing-port interface.

INDICATIONS AND SELECTION FOR LAGB

Knowledge of outcomes should be the driver of indications and selection. As the strength of evidence improves, the ability to determine optimal application of LAGB will become clearer.

The correct selection of patients for bariatric surgery has always been a challenge. On the one hand, we would like to avoid operating on those in whom there is a significant chance that we can do more harm than good, either because the good outcomes—weight loss, improved health, improved quality of life—are likely to be modest or the bad outcomes—death or serious complications—are more probable. On the other hand, in recognizing the important benefits that weight loss provides to health, quality of life, and length of life, we should be reluctant to exclude someone from these benefits unless supported by strong evidence. Using the mantra of evidence-based medicine, we should "do what is known to be effective and not do what is known to be ineffective."

Predictors of Outcomes

An extensive database of 440 LAGB patients was studied to identify predictors of outcome (80). The percent of EWL at the end of one year was used as the outcome measure, and linear regression multivariate analysis was performed on the data to identify predictors of better or worse percent of EWL at one year.

There was one positive predictor. Those patients who consumed alcohol regularly had significantly better weight loss than the remainder. Those who consumed more than 100 g/wk of alcohol ($N = 71$) had lost 50.4% of their excess weight at 12 months compared with 45.4% EWL for those who consumed more than 20 g/wk ($N = 224$) and 40% EWL for the teetotalers ($N = 145$).

A number of negative predictors were identified. These included increasing age, increasing BMI, hyperinsulinemia, insulin resistance, and diseases associated with insulin resistance (type 2 diabetes, polycystic ovary syndrome), poor physical activity, high pain score, and poor general health. However, the differences in outcomes, although statistically significant, were small and when compared with the benefits that these patients achieved through the weight loss were judged insufficient to argue that the procedure should not be performed in those patients.

In this and other studies (81,82), several putative criteria were found to have no bearing on the outcome. These included gender, presence of mental illness such as depression and bipolar disorder, most comorbidities except those linked to insulin resistance, a past history of bariatric surgery, sweet-eating behavior, and the presence of superobesity (BMI > 50 kg/m^2).

Selection Criteria

The author uses the following four criteria for selection:

1. BMI greater than 30 kg/m^2. This is based on the findings of the RCT discussed above (17). For practitioners in the United States, the National Institute of Health criteria, established in 1991 on data from the 1980s and before, are generally required to be followed by the health insurers. These require the presence of a BMI of 40 kg/m^2 or a BMI of at least 35 kg/m^2 with two or more significant comorbidities. Outside United States, the practitioner should seek to decide on the basis of the current evidence of benefit and risk. The findings of the RCT and the data on safety and reversibility support the assessment of any obese individual for LAGB placement.

2. The presence of problems associated with the obesity. These may be medical, physical, psychosocial, or future health and life expectancy problems. There is no place for performing surgery because the physician believes there is a problem. Each patient must recognize that he or she has a problem and be seeking a solution.

3. A history of prolonged attempts at weight reduction by multiple means. We have not been specific about duration or numbers of methods tried but generally we are expecting that attempts have been made for five years or more.

4. A sense that the patients have an understanding of the role they must fulfill to ensure success and have realistic expectations of the potential outcomes, both positive and negative. They must recognize the partnership involved and agree to fulfill their role in that partnership (15).

Contraindications

(1) Absolute

- Mentally defective—unable to understand the rules of eating and exercise and therefore unable to fulfill the patient's part of the partnership
- Malignant hyperphagia—Prader-Willi syndrome
- Portal hypertension, due to high risk with perioperative and late postoperative bleeding in the region of the band
- Alcohol or drug addiction

(2) Relative

- Age
  There are currently no data supporting the treatment of children below the age of 14 years. Adolescent are treated if they understand and can fulfill their role in the partnership.

Without being fixed to any upper chronological age, there should be an increased skepticism of a favorable benefit-to-risk ratio for patients in their late 60s and into their 70s. The existing comorbidities create increased risk and are less likely to be reversible with weight loss. The extent of weight loss is likely to be more modest. The presence of serious levels of cardiovascular or pulmonary disease that is not expected to be improved by weight loss should be a contraindication to proceed in this group.

- Severe Immobility

Exercise and activity are key components of the weight loss process, and those who are unable to contribute in this area are not as likely to achieve a useful result.

KEY ATTRIBUTES OF THE LAGB

The LAGB has several particular attributes that potentially will enable it to overcome the community's resistance to bariatric surgery.

It is safe. It has proved to be remarkably safe for a major surgical procedure in a high-risk population.

It is effective. It is effective in achieving good weight loss, in leading to major improvements in health, in restoring quality of life, and in reducing the risk of premature death of obesity.

It is gentle. This gentleness can be seen in three particular ways. First, the operation does not generate major pain or disability. Day patient treatment or overnight stay is routine. Second, it is gentle in the follow-up phase because of the adjustability. This is the key to the long-term effectiveness. There is not the need to create excess tightness and excessive weight loss early as the adjustability permits smooth progression toward the weight goals. Fluid can be removed as well as added, enabling removal of restriction if desired, as with pregnancy, major illness or operation, or remote travel. The ability to provide further adjustments years after operation should provide a durability of weight loss that has not been available with the gastric stapling procedures. Third, it is easily reversible. There is no intention of reversing the procedure but it is highly probable that, within 15 to 20 years, better options for weight reduction will be available. Especially for the young and middle-aged, the ability to be able to turn to a new approach is potentially important and attractive.

CHALLENGES FOR THE FUTURE

Although the existing data show the procedure of LAGB to be safe, effective, and gentle, it still remains to be established whether the procedure will make an impact on the current epidemic of obesity. Three challenges must be overcome to achieve this. First, we need enough surgeons with good laparoscopic skills. The workload is immense, and optimal results will not occur with suboptimal technique. Second, we must have in place a system for good patient support and care to undertake the assessments and advice before operation and, most importantly, to provide the ongoing care, with adjustments and support, permanently after operation. The aftercare program is as important to the success of the LAGB as the surgical procedure. Third, we must continue to measure and to learn. The optimal techniques for LAGB and patient care after placement are still evolving. The sooner we can identify these and incorporate them into clinical practice, the more the LAGB will be broadly accepted, and the more the benefits of weight loss will be achieved across the community.

REFERENCES

1. Wilkinson LH, Pelosa OA, Milne RI. Gastric wrapping. In: Deitel M, ed. Surgery for Morbidly Obese Patients. Philadelphia, PA: Lea & Febiger, 1989:283–286.
2. Blackman L, Granstrom L. Initial (1 year) weight loss after gastric banding, gastroplasty and gastric bypass. Acta Chir Scand 1984; 150:63–67.
3. Sjostrom L, Lindroos AK, Peltonen M, et al. Lifestyle, diabetes, and cardiovascular risk factors 10 years after bariatric surgery. N Engl J Med 2004; 351:2683–2693.
4. Szinicz G, Schnapka G. A new method in the surgical treatment of disease. Acta Chir Austrica 1982; 14(suppl 43):p. 43.
5. Kuzmak LI. A review of seven years' experience with silicone gastric banding. Obes Surg 1991; 1:403–408.
6. Forsell P, Hallberg D, Hellers G. Gastric banding for morbid obesity: initial experience with a new adjustable band. Obes Surg 1993; 3:369–374.
7. Belachew M, Legrand MJ, Defechereux TH, et al. Laparoscopic adjustable silicone gastric banding in the treatment of morbid obesity. A preliminary report. Surg Endosc 1994; 8:1354–1356.
8. Forsell P, Hellers G. The Swedish Adjustable Gastric Banding (SAGB) for morbid obesity: 9 year experience and a 4-year follow-up of patients operated with a new adjustable band. Obes Surg 1997; 7:345–351.
9. O'Brien PE, Brown WA, Dixon JB. Obesity, weight loss and bariatric surgery. Med J Aust 2005; 183:310–314.
10. Dixon AF, Dixon JB, O'Brien PE. Laparoscopic adjustable gastric banding induces prolonged satiety: a randomized blind crossover study. J Clin Endocrinol Metab 2005; 90:813–819.
11. Belachew M, Legrand M, Vincenti V, et al. Laparoscopic placement of adjustable silicone gastric band in the treatment of morbid obesity: how to do it. Obes Surg 1995; 5:66–70.
12. Colles SL, Dixon JB, Marks P, et al. Preoperative weight loss with very-low-energy diet: quantitation of changes in liver and abdominal fat by serial imaging. Am J Clin Nutr 2006; 84:304–311.

13. O'Brien PE, Dixon JB, Laurie C, et al. A prospective randomized trial of placement of the laparoscopic adjustable gastric band: comparison of the perigastric and pars flaccida pathways. Obes Surg 2005; 15:820–826.

14. Shen R, Dugay G, Rajaram K, et al. Impact of patient follow-up on weight loss after bariatric surgery. Obes Surg 2004; 14:514–519.

15. O'Brien PE. The LAP-BAND Solution: A Partnership in Weight Loss. 1st ed. Melbourne: Melbourne University Publishing, 2007.

16. Glenny AM, O'Meara S, Melville A, et al, The treatment and prevention of obesity: a systematic review of the literature. Int J Obes Relat Metab Disord 1997; 21:715–737.

17. O'Brien PE, Dixon JB, Laurie C, et al. Treatment of mild to moderate obesity with laparoscopic adjustable gastric banding or an intensive medical program: a randomized trial. Ann Int Med 2006; 144:625–633.

18. Chapman AE, Kiroff G, Game P, et al. Laparoscopic adjustable gastric banding in the treatment of obesity: a systematic review. Surgery 2004; 135:326–351.

19. Maggard MA, Shugarman LR, Suttorp M, et al. Meta-analysis: surgical treatment of obesity. Ann Intern Med 2005; 142:547–559.

20. Buchwald H, Avidor Y, Braunwald E, et al. Bariatric surgery: a systematic review and meta-analysis. JAMA 2004; 292:1724–1737.

21. O'Brien PE, McPhail T, Chaston T, et al. Systemic review of medium term weight loss after bariatric operations. Obes Surg 2006; 16:1032–1040.

22. O'Brien PE, Dixon JB, Brown W, et al. The laparoscopic adjustable gastric band (Lap-Band): a prospective study of medium-term effects on weight, health and quality of life. Obes Surg 2002; 12:652–660.

23. Belachew M, Belva PH, Desaive C. Long-term results of laparoscopic adjustable gastric banding for the treatment of morbid obesity. Obes Surg 2002; 12:564–568.

24. Ceelen W, Walder J, Cardon A, et al. Surgical treatment of severe obesity with a low-pressure adjustable gastric band: experimental data and clinical results in 625 patients. Ann Surg 2003; 237:10–16.

25. Dargent J. Surgical treatment of morbid obesity by adjustable gastric band: the case for a conservative strategy in the case of failure-a 9-year series. Obes Surg 2004; 14:986–990.

26. Fox SR, Fox KM, Srikanth MS, et al. The Lap-Band system in a North American population. Obes Surg 2003; 13:275–280.

27. Frigg A, Peterli R, Peters T, et al. Reduction in co-morbidities 4 years after laparoscopic adjustable gastric banding. Obes Surg 2004; 14:216–223.

28. Greenslade J, Kow L, Toouli J. Surgical management of obesity using a soft adjustable gastric band. ANZ J Surg 2004; 74:195–199.

29. Holloway JA, Forney GA, Gould DE. The Lap-Band is an effective tool for weight loss even in the United States. Am J Surg 2004; 188:659–662.

30. Jan JC, Hong D, Pereira N, et al. Laparoscopic adjustable gastric banding versus laparoscopic gastric bypass for morbid obesity: a single-institution comparison study of early results. J Gastrointest Surg 2005; 9:30–41.

31. Mittermair RP, Weiss H, Nehoda H, et al. Laparoscopic Swedish adjustable gastric banding: 6-year follow-up and comparison to other laparoscopic bariatric procedures. Obes Surg 2003; 13:412–417.

32. Steffen R, Biertho L, Ricklin T, et al. Laparoscopic Swedish adjustable gastric banding: a five-year prospective study. Obes Surg 2003; 13:404–411.

33. Suter M, Giusti V, Worreth M, et al. Laparoscopic gastric banding: a prospective, randomized study comparing the Lapband and the SAGB: early results. Ann Surg 2005; 241:55–62.

34. Vertruyen M. Experience with Lap-band system up to 7 years. Obes Surg 2002; 12:569–572.

35. Victorzon M, Tolonen P. Intermediate results following laparoscopic adjustable gastric banding for morbid obesity. Dig Surg 2002; 19:354–358.

36. Weiner R, Blanco-Engert R, Weiner S, et al. Outcome after laparoscopic adjustable gastric banding-8 years experience. Obes Surg 2003; 13:427–434.

37. Zinzindohoue F, Chevallier JM, Douard R, et al. Laparoscopic gastric banding: a minimally invasive surgical treatment for morbid obesity: prospective study of 500 consecutive patients. Ann Surg 2003; 237:1–9.

38. Biertho L, Steffen R, Branson R, et al. Management of failed adjustable gastric banding. Surgery 2005; 137:33–41.

39. Ponce J, Paynter S, Fromm R. Laparoscopic adjustable gastric banding: 1014 consecutive cases. J Am Coll Surg 2005; 201:529–535.

40. Parikh MS, Fielding GA, Ren CJ. U.S. experience with 749 laparoscopic adjustable gastric bands: intermediate outcomes. Surg Endosc 2005; 19:1631–1635.

41. Cottam D, Atkinson J, Anderson A, et al. A case-controlled matched-pair cohort study of laparoscopic roux-en-Y gastric bypass and Lap-Band patients in a single US center with three year follow-up. Obes Surg 2006; 16:534–540.

42. Spivak H, Hewitt M, Onn A, et al. Weight loss and improvement of obesity-related illness in 500 U.S. patients following laparoscopic adjustable gastric banding procedure. Am J Surg 2005; 189:27–32.

43. Sarker S, Myers J, Serot J, et al. Three year follow up weight loss results for patients undergoing laparoscopic adjustable gastric banding at a major university medical center: does weight loss persist? Am J Surg 2006; 191:372–376.

44. O'Brien PE, Brown WA, Smith A, et al. Prospective study of a laparoscopically placed, adjustable gastric band in the treatment of morbid obesity. Br J Surg 1999; 86:113–118.

45. Miller K, Pump A, Hell E. Vertical banded gastroplasty versus adjustable gastric banding: prospective long-term follow-up study. Surg Obes Relat Dis 2007; 3:84–90.

46. Favretti F, Segato G, Ashton D, et al. Laparoscopic adjustable gastric banding in 1,791 consecutive obese patients: 12-year results. Obes Surg 2007; 17:168–175.

47. Colditz GA, Willett WC, Rotnitzky A, et al. Weight gain as a risk factor for clinical diabetes mellitus in women. Ann Intern Med 1995; 122:481–486.

48. Williamson DF, Thompson TJ, Thun M, et al. Intentional weight loss and mortality among overweight individuals with diabetes. Diabetes Care 2000; 23:1499–1504.

49. Dixon JB, Pories WJ, O'Brien PE, et al. Surgery as an effective early intervention for diabesity: why the reluctance? Diabetes Care 2005; 28:472–474.

50. Dixon JB, O'Brien P. Health outcomes of severely obese type 2 diabetic subjects 1 year after laparoscopic adjustable gastric banding. Diabetes Care 2002; 25:358–363.

51. Ponce J, Haynes B, Paynter S, et al. Effect of Lap-Band-induced weight loss on type 2 diabetes mellitus and hypertension. Obes Surg 2004; 14:1335–1342.

52. Mulrow CD, Chiquette E, Angel L, et al. Dieting to reduce body weight for controlling hypertension in adults. In: Cochrane Database of Systemic Reviews, 1998.

53. Dixon JB, O'Brien PE. Changes in comorbidities and improvements in quality of life after LAP-BAND placement. Am J Surg 2002; 184:S51–S54.

54. Lamarche B, Lemieux I, Despres JP. The small, dense LDL phenotype and the risk of coronary heart disease: epidemiology, patho-physiology and therapeutic aspects. Diabetes Metab 1999; 25:199–211.

55. Dixon JB, O'Brien PE. Lipid profile in the severely obese: changes with weight loss following Lap-Band surgery. Obes Res 2002; 10(9):903–910.

56. Dixon JB, Chapman L, O'Brien P. Marked improvement in asthma after Lap-Band surgery for morbid obesity. Obes Surg 1999; 9:385–389.

57. Hagen J, Deitel M, Khanna R, et al. Gastroesophageal reflux in the massively obese. Int Surg 1987; 72(1):1–3.

58. Lundell L, Ruth M, Sandberg N, et al. Dose massive obesity promote abnormal gastroesophageal reflux. Dig Dis Sci 1995; 40(8):1632–1635.

59. Naslund E, Granstrom L, Melcher A, et al. Gastro-oesophageal reflux before and after vertical banded gastroplasty in the treatment of obesity. Eur J Surg 1996; 162(4):303–306.

60. Dixon JB, O'Brien PE. Gastroesophageal reflux in obesity: the effect of lap-band placement. Obes Surg 1999; 9:527–531.

61. Ovrebo KK, Hatlebakk JG, Viste A, et al. Gastroesophageal reflux in morbidly obese patients with gastric banding or vertical banded gastroplasty. Ann Surg 1998; 228(1):51–58.

62. Westling A, Bjurling K, Ohrvall M, et al. Silicone-adjustable gastric banding: disappointing results. Obes Surg 1998; 8:467–474.

63. Kyzer S, Charuzi I. Obstructive sleep apnea in the obese. World J Surg 1998; 22:998–1001.

64. Kansanen M, Vanninen E, Tuunainen A, et al. The effect of a very low-calorie diet-induced weight loss on the severity of obstructive sleep apnea and autonomic nervous function in obese patients with obstructive sleep apnea syndrome. Clin Physiol 1998; 18:377–385.

65. Pasquali R, Colella P, Cirignotta F, et al. Treatment of obese patients with obstructive sleep apnea syndrome (OSAS): effect of weight loss and interference of otorhinolaryngoiatric pathology. Int J Obes 1990; 14:207–217.

66. Sugerman HJ, Fairman RP, Sood RK, et al. Long Term effects of gastric surgery for treating respiratory insufficiency of obesity. Am J Clin Nutr 1992; 55(2 suppl):597S–601S.

67. Charuzi I, Lavie P, Peiser J, et al. Bariatric surgery in morbid obesity sleep-apnea patients: short and long-term follow-up. Am J Clin Nutr 1992; 55(2 suppl):594S–596S.

68. Dixon JB, Schachter LM, O'Brien PE. Sleep disturbance and obesity: changes following surgically induced weight loss. Arch Intern Med 2001; 161:102–106.

69. Dixon JB, Schachter LM, O'Brien PE. Polysomnography before and after weight loss in obese patients with severe sleep apnea. Int J Obes (Lond) 2005; 29(9):1048–1054.

70. Beck AT, Ward CH, Mendelson M. An inventory for measuring depression. Arch Gen Psychiatry 1961; 4:516–571.

71. Rothschild M, Peterson HR, Pfeifer MA. Depression in obese men. Int J Obes 1989; 13:479–485.

72. Lustman PJ, Clouse RE, Griffith LS, et al. Screening for depression in diabetes using the Beck Depression Inventory. Psychosom Med 1997; 59:24–31.

73. Robinson BE, Kelley L. Concurrent validity of the Beck Depression Inventory as a measure of depression. Psychol Rep 1996; 79:929–930.

74. Gatewood-Colwell G, Kaczmarek M, Ames MH. Reliability and validity of the Beck Depression Inventory for a white and Mexican-American gerontic population. Psychol Rep 1989; 65:1163–1166.

75. Beck AT, Steer RA, Garbin MG. Psychometric properties of the Beck Depression Inventory: twenty-five years of evaluation. Clin Psychol Rev 1988; 8:77–100.

76. Dixon JB, Dixon ME, O'Brien PE. Depression in association with severe obesity: changes with weight loss. Arch Intern Med 2003; 163:2058–2065.

77. Dixon JB, Dixon ME, O'Brien PE. Quality of life after lap-band placement: influence of time, weight loss, and comorbidities. Obes Res 2001; 9:713–721.

78. McCallum J. The SF-36 in an Australian sample: validating a new, generic health status measure. Aust J Public Health 1995; 19:160–166.

79. Peeters A, O'Brien P, Laurie C, et al. Substantial intentional weight loss and mortality in the severely obese. Ann Surg 2007; 246(6):1028–1033.

80. Dixon JB, Dixon ME, O'Brien PE. Pre-operative predictors of weight loss at 1-year after Lap-Band surgery. Obes Surg 2001; 11:200–207.

81. Hudson SM, Dixon JB, O'Brien PE. Sweet eating is not a predictor of outcome after Lap-Band placement. Can we finally bury the myth? Obes Surg 2002; 12:789–794.

82. O'Brien P, Brown W, Dixon J. Revisional surgery for morbid obesity—conversion to the Lap-Band System. Obes Surg 2000; 10:557–563.

83. Galvani C, Gorodner M, Moser F, et al. Laparoscopic adjustable gastric band versus laparoscopic Roux-en-Y gastric bypass. Surg Endosc 2006; 20:934–941.

34

Evolving Surgical Therapy for Obesity

MICHAEL J. BARKER and WALTER J. PORIES

Department of Surgery, Brody School of Medicine, East Carolina University, Greenville, North Carolina, U.S.A.

THE OBESITY EPIDEMIC

There is no doubt that Americans are more obese than ever before. An increase in the total caloric consumption and a decrease in physical activity both at work and during leisure time have led to a staggering number of over-weight Americans. From the early 1960s to 2002, the percentage of overweight and obese Americans has increased from 44.8 and 13.3 to 65.2 and 31.1, respectively. Perhaps more frightening is the rise in childhood overweight, which rose from 4.2% to 15.8% during the same 40 years (1).

This epidemic is certainly not limited to the United States. The World Health Organization estimates that by 2015 there will be an astounding 2.3 billion overweight and 700 million obese persons worldwide (2).

In response to these trends, the National Institutes of Health in 1991 released a Consensus Statement on Gastrointestinal Surgery for Severe Obesity (3). After reviewing the available literature, a panel of experts recognized the failure of diets, exercise, behavioral modification and drugs in producing significant, sustained weight loss in the vast majority of severely obese patients. The panel went on to state that surgery is the only effective means of producing this weight loss and suggested that bariatric (weight loss) surgery be considered for all those with body

mass index (BMI) > 40 kg/m^2 or for those with a BMI ≥ 35 kg/m^2 with weight-related comorbidities.

Since this historic conference, the number of bariatric procedures performed in the United States has skyrocketed. Procedures developed during the infancy of bariatric surgery, such as the biliopancreatic diversion, gastric bypass, and vertical banded gastroplasty have evolved into the duodenal switch, laparoscopic gastric bypass, and laparoscopic adjustable gastric band. With this explosion has come an era of innovation, as surgeons search for a faster, safer, less invasive, and more effective treatment for obesity. According to the estimates of the American Society for Bariatric Surgery, approximately 176,000 bariatric operations were performed in the United States in 2006.

While there has been great success with established procedures such as the gastric bypass, duodenal switch, and even the adjustable gastric band, surgeons continue to search for safer, more effective procedures. This chapter will review several of the other surgical options for the management of obesity.

INTRAGASTRIC BALLOON

Intragastric balloons (IGBs) consist of air or liquid-filled shells that are inserted transorally and inflated inside the stomach lumen. These devices are generally placed under sedation with endoscopic assistance. The IGB was first described in 1982 when Nieben and Harboe proposed the device as a less invasive weight loss technique compared with the jejunal-ileal bypass, gastric bypass, and gastroplasty (4). The inspiration for the balloon was the observation that often the only complication of long-standing gastric bezoars was weight loss. The authors designed a 450-mL latex balloon, which was orally inserted and inflated with air. Their first series of five patients showed modest weight loss, but the technique was severely limited by the short life span of the balloons, averaging only 12 days.

The exact mechanism by which the IGB works is still unclear. The balloons may act as a space-occupying lesion, reducing the amount of food required to distend the stomach after a meal to produce satiety (5). The balloons may also work as an artificial bezoar, delaying gastric emptying of solid food and thus prolonging satiety. Several studies have documented this delay in emptying (6–9), but others have found no significant change (10,11).

Garren-Edwards Gastric Bubble

Other reports of balloon placements (12,13) followed soon after Nieben and Harboe's, and in 1985, the Garren-Edwards gastric bubble (GEGB) became the first IGB to be approved by the Food and Drug Administration (FDA). This device was a cylindrical balloon with a hollow center and filled with 200 mL of air. In theory, its design would allow liquids to easily pass but provides a partial obstruction to solid food, causing an early and prolonged sense of satiety. Initial optimism after its introduction in 1984 (14) led to the sale of approximately 20,000 devices during its first year of availability, with a market value of over $50,000,000 (15).

Unfortunately, the GEGB had been approved on the basis of rather limited clinical data, and as more devices were inserted, its shortcomings became evident. Numerous small, subsequent studies failed to reproduce the weight loss achieved by Garren (16–18). Several randomized double-blind studies showed no significant differences in weight loss between patients with the GEGB and those who underwent a sham procedure (19–21).

At the same time, as questions about the GEGB effectiveness surfaced, numerous reports of complications from the device were published (22–26), including gastric erosions, ulcers, bowel obstruction, Mallory-Weiss tears, and esophageal lacerations. These complications appeared at rates much higher (19,27) than reported in Garren's original paper, and soon the frenzy for the device subsided. The lack of reproducible effectiveness, combined with a high rate of complications, led to its withdrawal from the market in 1988.

Bioenterics IGB

On the basis of the failure of the GEGB, a consensus conference was held in 1987 at Tarpon Springs, Florida, to put forth guidelines for the development and use of subsequent devices (28). The panel recommended that further use of gastric balloons should only be allowed in controlled clinical trials. The panel also listed the qualities of the "ideal" IGB:

1. Efficacy
2. Adjustability
3. Durability, especially when subjected to the acid environment of the stomach
4. Low ulcerogenic and obstructive potential, with no edges or sharp ridges
5. Availability of a radiopaque marker for follow-up purposes

Although several studies using other balloons (29–31) were published in the decade following withdrawal of the GEGB from the market, the use of IGBs waned. Then, in the late 1990s, Inamed (formerly, BioEnterics, Santa Barbara, California, U.S.) introduced the BioEnterics intragastric balloon (BIB™) (32) (Fig. 1). This device meets all of the criteria for an "ideal intragastric balloon" in that it is smooth and seamless, resistant to stomach acid, has low obstructive potential, is adjustable, and has a radiopaque marker for identification on radiographic studies.

The BIB is placed transorally and inflated with 400 to 700 mL of saline under visualization with an endoscope. The manufacturer recommends that the balloon be left in place no longer than 180 days for fear of deflation and subsequent bowel obstruction. Recently, some centers have placed a mixture of saline and methylene blue into the BIB so that the patient's urine will turn green if the device ruptures, allowing retrieval before the deflated balloon can cause obstruction (33–35).

Initial studies using the BIB were promising (36,37), and a number of nonrandomized studies have shown good results (34,35,38–44) with excess weight loss (EWL) [defined as (original weight − final weight]/[(original weight − ideal weight)] in the range of 19% to 50% at six months. There are, however, few well-designed randomized, controlled studies (45,46) and only one has shown a difference between the BIB and sham treatment.

Despite the minimally invasive nature of the IGB, complications including ulcer, bowel obstruction, perforation, and even death (34,35,44) have been reported. The most common complication of the device is intolerance,

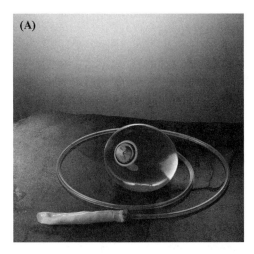

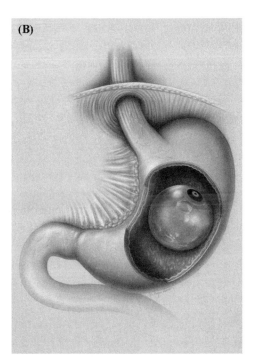

Figure 1 (**A**) The BIB™, Allergan Medical, Irvine, California, U.S. Deflated for insertion (*foreground*), and inflated. (**B**) The BIB inserted in the stomach. *Abbreviation*: BIB, Bioenterics intragastric balloon.

Table 1 Potential Indications for Use of Intragastric Balloons

Patients with BMI >40 kg/m^2 (or >35 kg/m^2 with comorbidities) prior to bariatric procedures or other surgery to reduce surgical risk
Patients with BMI >40 kg/m^2 (or >35 kg/m^2 with comorbidities) who are not candidates for bariatric surgery
Patients with BMI 30–39 kg/m^2 who have significant comorbidities and have failed a supervised weight loss program

Abbreviation: BMI, body mass index.

removal without second stage bariatric surgery would be followed by weight regain (48,49,51).

GASTRIC ELECTRICAL STIMULATION

The idea of using electrical stimulation of the stomach was first introduced by Cigaina in 1996 (52). In this study performed on swine, gastric stimulation caused decreased food intake and cyclical weight loss, while controls continued to gain weight. Although the potential application for the treatment of obesity was not immediately recognized, Cigaina reported the results of the first human trial to treat obesity in 2002 (53). Patients in this study had earlier satiety with less food intake and at 36-month follow-up had lost an average of 24% of their excess BMI.

Technique

The stomach has an intrinsic pacemaker, located in the proximal body along the greater curvature. There are two types of electrical activity that propagate through the stomach—slow waves and spikes. Slow waves in the human stomach are at a constant 3 cycles/min and travel distally with increasing velocity and amplitude (54). Spikes are more variable, and cause gastric contractions when superimposed on the slow waves (55).

Gastric electrical stimulation (GES) uses pulses of electricity, known as trains, which are produced by a generator implanted in the anterior abdominal wall. These pulses are delivered to the stomach through two to four electrical leads, usually placed along the lesser curve of the stomach, approximately 8 cm proximal to the pylorus. Placement may be accomplished via open or laparoscopic technique (56), which requires between three and five trocars. A seromuscular tunnel approximately 3 cm in length is fashioned for each lead. Endoscopy is performed to rule out violation of the mucosa, which may eventually lead to infection. A subcutaneous pocket is created for the generator and its battery. The

manifested by pain, nausea, and vomiting, which may necessitate removal of the device.

While the use of IGBs has met with limited success, there may be a place for them in the arsenal of the bariatric surgeon (Table 1). Since the device has a limited life span in the acid environment of the stomach, use of the IGB is probably best limited to short-term weight loss, such as preoperatively (47–50). Long-term use would necessitate repeated replacement of the balloon, as

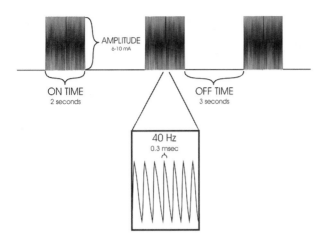

Figure 2 Gastric electrical stimulation. On time of each pulse is two seconds, followed by off time of three seconds. Pulses consist of amplitude of 6 to 10 mA for 0.3 milliseconds at a frequency of 40 Hz.

device is programmed using a computer via an external wand, much like a cardiac pacemaker.

The trains can be delivered in an antegrade (proximal to distal) or retrograde (distal to proximal) fashion and have even been shown to have similar effects when delivered to the duodenum (57). Although the settings for gastric stimulation can vary slightly, most pulses are delivered for 2 seconds ("on time") at a frequency of 40 Hz and amplitude of 6 to 10 mA and a pulse width of 300 microseconds (55) (Fig. 2). The on time is followed by an "off time" of 3 seconds, giving the stimulation a frequency of 12 cycles/min (2 seconds on, 3 seconds off, for a total of 5 seconds/cycle). These trains may interfere with the normal gastric waves, since they are significantly faster than the intrinsic 3 cycles/min.

Proposed Mechanisms of Action

Although the exact mechanism by which GES works is unknown, there are four main theories, which may explain its ability to cause weight loss.

Changes in Myoelectric Activity

As mentioned above, the stomach has rhythmic electrical activity. Normal response to a meal is an increase in amplitude of the slow wave with resultant increased contractility. In animals, GES has been shown to decrease the amplitude and frequency of slow waves and especially blunts the postprandial increase in activity (58). Similar findings have been reported in humans (59). GES has also been shown to entrain gastric slow waves (60).

Changes in Gastric Motor Function

During a meal, the stomach relaxes to allow food to be stored in a process called gastric accommodation. As the stomach distends, stretch receptors signal satiety centers in the brain via the vagus nerve. Gastric contractions in the form of peristaltic waves then propel the food distally to evacuate the stomach (55). GES decreases this normal accommodation by causing resting relaxation and thus distension of the stomach (61–63). This distension at rest may send a baseline satiety signal to the central nervous system (CNS), abolishing the impulse to feed again.

In addition to altering the resting state of the stomach, in animal studies, GES inhibits gastric contractions and peristalsis (64–66), delaying gastric emptying (64,67) and thus prolonging satiety after a meal. Studies in humans have shown similar results (68,69).

Influence on the CNS

Gastric stimulation may function by sending signals directly to the brain to influence feeding behavior, either via the vagus nerve or through other neural pathways. In rats, GES produces an excitatory effect on nucleus tractus solitarii neurons receiving input from the stomach via the vagus (70), increases the expression of oxytocin (an anorixigenic) neurons, and decreases the expression of orexin-containing (orixigenic) neurons (71). Also in rats, GES excites gastric distension sensitive neurons in the ventromedial hypothalamus (72). Interestingly, one human study showed that GES stimulates brain circuits similar to those shown to be involved in drug craving in addicts (73).

Hormonal Changes

Other investigators have postulated that gastric stimulation may affect the hormones, which influence hunger and feeding. Cigaina reported that GES in humans decreased the normal, postprandial response of cholecystokinin and somatostatin and decreased basal levels of glucagon-like peptide-1 and leptin (74).

Chen's group reported that GES blocks the effects of ghrelin in dogs, decreasing antral contraction and food intake in them (75), and in another canine study, the group reported that GES decreases plasma insulin and glucose (76).

Clinical Results

Although there remains much debate about the mechanism, there is growing evidence that GES may be effective in treating obesity. Multiple animal studies have shown decreased food intake (63,64,75,77,78) and weight loss (67,77,78). Similar effects on human food consumption (69,79) and weight loss (74,80,81) have been reported, but in small nonrandomized studies.

Cigaina reported a somewhat larger series of 65 patients in 2004, with a modest 20% EWL at 19 months with improvement in hypertension, reflux disease, and insulin sensitivity (82). Another larger nonrandomized study—Laparoscopic Obesity Stimulation Survey (LOSS)—was carried out in Europe and included 62 women and 29 men with average BMI of 41 kg/m^2. Mean EWL was 25% at two years and no severe complications were reported (83).

Other studies performed in the United States have yielded somewhat less encouraging results. The small nonrandomized DIGEST (Determining the efficacy and safety of an Innovative GastrointESTinal enzyme complex) trial consisted of a single group of patients, 26 women and four men with a mean BMI of 42 kg/m^2. There were no major complications or deaths, no lead dislodgements, and patients benefited from a 19% EWL at 14 months, although there were significant differences in results from the two participating centers (84).

The O-01 trial was a randomized, double-blind, placebo-controlled study consisting of 87 females and 16 males with a mean BMI of 46 kg/m^2. Patients were randomized to have their stimulator turned on or off for the first six months, at which time all were turned on. Stomach perforation that occurred in 20 patients was diagnosed by intraoperative endoscopy and leads replaced. Another 20 patients had postoperative lead dislodgments. There was no significant difference in weight loss between the groups at 6 or 12 months (84). A multicenter, double-blind, randomized trial known as Screened Health Assessment and Pacer Evaluation (SHAPE) was halted in late 2005 by the device manufacturer, Medtronic, Inc. (Minneapolis, Minnesota, U.S.—formerly, Transneuronix). The study failed to show a difference in weight loss at one year between the treatment and placebo groups.

The inability to reproduce the success of smaller studies in large randomized controlled trials has stalled the acceptance of GES as a mainstream treatment for obesity. As of this writing, no GES devices are approved by the FDA for the treatment of obesity, and its use is limited to investigational studies. While gastric stimulation may never reach widespread use, research in this area has led to a greater understanding of feeding and energy intake. Work continues on related topics, such as the role of the vagus nerve in obesity treatment.

SLEEVE GASTRECTOMY

As surgeons noticed a direct relationship between high BMI and complication rates, they began looking for ways to reduce the morbidity associated with operating on the "super" and "super super obese" (BMI >50 and >60 kg/m^2,

respectively). One solution was to perform operations in a "staged" manner, first performing a faster, less complicated, and thus safer procedure. Patients then return to the operating room months later for a definitive procedure, after significant weight loss has resulted in a lowering of their BMI and amelioration or elimination of their comorbidities.

Procedures proposed as these "first-stage" operations include the laparoscopic adjustable gastric band, the IGB, and the sleeve gastrectomy (SG). Also known as a "vertical" or "longitudinal" gastrectomy, SG is a purely restrictive, irreversible procedure, which was originally performed as part of the biliopancreatic diversion with duodenal switch. Chu and Gagner, in 2002, first proposed application of the staged approach to the operation (85).

Technique

A bougie is placed transorally down through the pylorus along the lesser curvature of the stomach. A linear stapler is then fired repeatedly along the bougie, from a point 6 to 10 cm proximal to the pylorus up to the angle of His. This creates a "gastric tube" on the basis of the lesser curve (Fig. 3). The size of the bougie used is variable, usually from 30 to 60 Fr, with some surgeons reporting better sustained weight loss with the creation of a smaller tube. This extremely long staple line has a relatively high incidence of bleeding and leaks, so many surgeons oversew, use staple line reinforcements, or tissue sealants to reduce this risk.

Clinical Results

SG as a separate procedure was initially intended to be the first stage, followed by either a biliopancreatic diversion

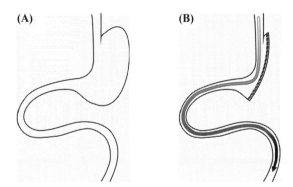

Figure 3 (**A**) Normal stomach. (**B**) The sleeve gastrectomy. Staple line is begun 6 to 10 cm proximal to the pylorus and continued to the angle of His. The staple firings are routinely performed alongside a bougie of 30 to 60 Fr size to size the gastric tube.

Table 2 Selected Publications on SG

Author (references)	Number of Patients	Preop BMI (kg/m²)	Female (%)	Bougie size (Fr)	EWL (%)	Follow-up (mo)	Morbidity (%)	Mortality (%)	Comments
Lee et al. (89)	216	49	80	32	59	12	4.6 major	0	
Cottam et al. (87)	126	65.3	53	46–50	46	12	8 major	0	36 patients underwent second stage LRYGBP
Hamoui et al. (90)	118	55	59		47.3	24	15.3	0.85	Only three cases performed laparoscopically
Han et al. (91)	60	37.2	87	48	83.3	12	3.6 overall	0	One patient underwent second stage BPD-DS
Silecchia et al. (92)	41	57.3	68	48	48.6	18	12.1	0	14 patients underwent second stage LBPD-DS
Himpens et al. (93)	40	39	78	34	66	36	5 major	0	
Roa et al. (94)	30	41.4	77	52	52.8	6	13.3 overall	0	
Langer et al. (95)	23	48.5	74	48	56	12			Three patients underwent second stage LRYGBP
Milone et al. (86)	20	68.8	35	60	35	6	5 overall	0	
Mognol et al. (96)	10	64	50	32	51	12	0	0	
Regan et al. (88)	7	63	43	60	33	11	35.7 overall	0	All underwent second stage LRYGBP

Abbreviations: SG, sleeve gastrectomy; EWL, excess weight loss; BMI, body mass index; BPD-DS, biliopancreatic diversion with duodenal switch; LBPD-DS, laparoscopic biliopancreatic diversion with duodenal switch; LRYGBP, laparoscopic Roux-en-Y gastric bypass.

with duodenal switch (85,86) or Roux-en-Y gastric bypass (87,88). As more of these procedures were performed and follow-up data became available, it became evident that many patients lost significant amounts of weight with the SG alone. Table 2 is a summary of published studies on SG.

Currently, there are no long-term data nor any randomized controlled trials to support the widespread use of SG as a stand-alone procedure. Initial results are certainly promising, but there is presently too little data to recommend this procedure as a primary bariatric operation. Table 3 lists the current potential indications for use of SG. While this procedure holds the most hope of any mentioned in this chapter, in our opinion, routine SG should only be performed as part of a clinical trial.

SUMMARY

The field of bariatric surgery has long been a bastion of improvement and innovation. While most new procedures (including those mentioned here) will eventually be abandoned, they still serve an important purpose. Lessons learned from these "failures" will continue to add to our knowledge of obesity and its treatment and will help shape the medical and surgical therapies of tomorrow.

Table 3 Potential Indications for Performing SG

As part of BPD-DS
As first stage operation in super obese, followed by RYGBP or BPD-DS
Patients with comorbidities making other procedures at higher risk for complications
    Steroid dependent
    Pre- or postorgan transplant
    Inflammatory bowel disease
    Anemia
    Malabsorptive disorders (celiac disease)
Intraoperative difficulty
    Large left hepatic lobe
    Massive intra-abdominal adiposity
"Rescue" procedure after primary surgical failure
    Laparoscopic adjustable gastric banding
    Resleeve after BPD-DS
Primary procedure (most controversial)

Abbreviations: SG, sleeve gastrectomy; BPD-DS, biliopancreatic diversion with duodenal switch; RYGBP, Roux-en-Y gastric bypass.

REFERENCES

1. National Center for Health Statistics. Health, United States, 2006: with Chartbook on Trends in the Health of Americans. Hyattsville, MD, 2006:279–284, 287–291.

2. Obesity and Overweight. Available at: http://www.who.int/ mediacentre/factsheets/fs311/en/index.html. Accessed May 2007.

3. Consensus Development Panel. Gastrointestinal surgery for severe obesity. Ann Intern Med, 1991; 115(12):956–961.

4. Nieben OG, Harboe H. Intragastric balloon as an artificial bezoar for treatment of obesity. Lancet 1982; 1(8265): 198–199.

5. Rigaud D, Trostler N, Rozen R, et al. Gastric distension, hunger and energy intake after balloon implantation in severe obesity. Int J Obes Relat Metab Disord 1995; 19(7):489–495.

6. Ziessman HA, Collen MJ, Fahey FH, et al. The effect of the Garren-Edwards gastric bubble on solid and liquid gastric emptying. Clin Nucl Med 1988; 13(8):586–589.

7. Velchik MG, Kramer FM, Stunkard AJ, et al. Effect of the Garren-Edwards gastric bubble on gastric emptying. J Nucl Med 1989; 30(5):692–696.

8. Bonazzi P, Pitrelli MD, Lorenzini I, et al. Gastric emptying and intragastric balloon in obese patients. Eur Rev Pharmacol Sci 2005; 9(5 suppl 1):15–21.

9. Mion F, Napoleon B, Roman S, et al. Effects of intragastric balloon on gastric emptying and plasma ghrelin levels in non-morbid obese patients. Obes Surg 2005; 15(4): 510–516.

10. Barkin JS, Reiner DK, Goldberg RI, et al. The effects of morbid obesity and the Garren-Edwards gastric bubble on solid phase gastric emptying. Am J Gastroenterol 1988; 83(12):1364–1367.

11. Mundt MW, Hausken T, Samsom M. Effect of intragastric barostat bag on proximal and distal gastric accommodation in response to liquid meal. Am J Physiol Gastrointest Liver Physiol 2002; 283:G681–G686.

12. Taylor TV, Pullan BR. Gastric balloons for obesity. Lancet 1982; 1(8274):750.

13. Percival W. The "balloon diet": a noninvasive treatment for morbid obesity: preliminary report on 108 patients. Can J Surg 1984; 27:135–136.

14. Garren M, Garren L, Giordano F. The Garren gastric bubble: an Rx for the morbidly obese. Endosc Rev 1984; 1:57–60.

15. Levine GM. Intragastric balloons: an unfulfilled promise. Ann Int Med 1988; 109(5):354–356.

16. Barkin JS, Reiner DK, Goldberg RI, et al. Effects of gastric bubble implant on weight change with and without compliance with a behavior modification program. Am J Gastroenterol 1988; 83(9):930–934.

17. Kirby DF, Wade JB, Mills PR, et al. A prospective assessment of the Garren-Edwards gastric bubble and bariatric surgery in the treatment of morbid obesity. Am Surg 1990; 56(10):575–580.

18. Kramer FM, Stunkard AJ, Spiegel TA, et al. Limited weight losses with a gastric balloon. Arch Intern Med 1989; 149(2):411–413.

19. Benjamin SB, Maher KA, Cattau EL, et al. Double blind controlled trial of the Garren-Edwards gastric bubble: an adjunctive treatment for exogenous obesity. Gastroenterology 1988; 95(3):581–588.

20. Meshkinpour J, Hsu D, Farivar S. Effect of gastric bubble as a weight reduction device: a controlled, crossover study. Gastroenterology 1988; 95(3):589–592.

21. Hogan RB, Johnston JH, Long BW, et al. A double-blind, randomized, sham-controlled trial of the gastric bubble for obesity. Gastrointest Endosc 1989; 35(5):381–385.

22. Benjamin SB. Small bowel obstruction and the Garren-Edwards gastric bubble: and iatrogenic bezoar. Gastrointest Endosc 1988; 34(6):463–467.

23. Patel NM. Gastric mucosal gouging during insertion of a Garren-Edwards gastric bubble. J Clin Gastroenterol 1987; 9(6):719–720.

24. Kirby DF, Mills PR, Kellum JM, et al. Incomplete small bowel obstruction by the Garren-Edwards gastric bubble necessitating surgical intervention. Am J Gastroenterol 1987; 82(3):251–253.

25. Fedotin MS, Ginsberg BW. Partial deployment of the Garren gastric bubble: a new complication. Am J Gastroenterol 1987; 82(5):470–471.

26. Zeman RK, Benjamin SB, Cunningham MB, et al. Small bowel obstruction due to Garren gastric bubble: radiographic diagnosis. AJR Am J Roentgenol 1988; 150(3): 581–582.

27. Ulicny KS, Goldberg SJ, Harper WJ, et al. Surgical complications of the Garren-Edwards gastric bubble. Surg Gyn Ob 1988; 166:535–540.

28. Schapiro M, Benjamin S, Blackburn G, et al. Obesity and the gastric balloon: a comprehensive workshop. Gastro Endosc 1987; 33(4):323–327.

29. Geliebter A, Melton PM, Gage D, et al. Gastric balloon to treat obesity: a double-blind study in nondieting subjects. Am J Clin Nutr 1990; 51:584–588.

30. Geliebter A, Melton PM, McCray RS, et al. Clinical trial of silicone-rubber gastric balloon to treat obesity. Int J Obes 1991; 15(4):259–266.

31. Marshall JB, Schreiber H, Kolozsi W, et al. A prospective, multi-center clinical trial of the Taylor intragastric balloon for the treatment of morbid obesity. Am J Gastroenterol 1990; 85(7):833–837.

32. Galloro G, DePalma GD, Catanzano C, et al. Preliminary endoscopic technical report of a new silicone intragastric balloon in the treatment of morbid obesity. Obes Surg 1999; 9(1):68–71.

33. Bernante P, Francini F, Zangrandi F, et al. Green urine after intragastric balloon placement for the treatment of morbid obesity. Obes Surg 2003; 13(6):951–953.

34. Doldi SB, Micheletto G, Perrini MN, et al. Intragastric balloon: another option for treatment of obesity and morbid obesity. Hepatogast 2004; 51:294–297.

35. Genco A, Bruni T, Doldi SB, et al. BioEnterics Intragastric Balloon: the Italian experience with 2,515 patients. Obes Surg 2005; 15:1161–1164.

36. Weiner R, Gutberlet H, Bockhorn H. Preparation of extremely obese patients for laparoscopic gastric banding by gastric-balloon therapy. Obes Surg 1999; 9(3): 261–264.

37. Loffredo A, Cappuccio M, DeLuca M, et al. Three years experience with the new intragastric balloon, and a preoperative test for success with restrictive surgery. Obes Surg 2001; 11(3):330–333.

38. Totte E, Hendrickx L, Pauwels M, et al. Weight reduction by means of intragastric device: experience with the

bioenterics intragastric balloon. Obes Surg 2001; 11(4): 519–523.

39. Evans JD, Scott MH. Intragastric balloon in the treatment of patients with morbid obesity. Br J Surg 2001; 88: 1245–1248.

40. Roman S, Napoleon B, Mion F, et al. Intragastric balloon for "non-morbid" obesity: a retrospective evaluation of tolerance and efficacy. Obes Surg 2004; 14(4):539–544.

41. Doldi SB, Micheletto G, Perrini MN, et al. Treatment of morbid obesity with intragastric balloon in association with diet. Obes Surg 2002; 12(4):583–587.

42. Busetto L, Segato G, DeLuca M, et al. Preoperative weight loss by intragastric balloon in super-obese patients treated with laparoscopic gastric banding: a case-control study. Obes Surg 2004; 14(5):671–676.

43. Sallet JA, Marchesini JB, Paiva DS, et al. Brazilian multicenter study of the intragastric balloon. Obes Surg 2004; 14(7):991–998.

44. Al-Momen A, El-Mogy I. Intragastric balloon for obesity: a retrospective evaluation of tolerance and efficacy. Obes Surg 2005; 15:101–105.

45. Mathus-Vliegen EMH, Tytgat GNJ. Intragastric balloon for treatment-resistant obesity: safety, tolerance, and efficacy of 1-year balloon treatment followed by a 1-year balloon-free follow-up. Gastro Endosc 2005; 61(1):19–27.

46. Genco A, Cipriano M, Bacci V, et al. BioEnterics Intragastric Balloon (BIB): a short-term, double-blind, randomized, controlled, crossover study on weight reduction in morbidly obese patients. Int J Obes 2006; 30:129–133.

47. Alfalah H, Philippe B, Ghazal F, et al. Intragastric balloon for preoperative weight reduction in candidates for laparoscopic gastric bypass with massive obesity. Obes Surg 2006; 16(2):147–150.

48. Melissas J, Mouzas J, Filis D, et al. The intragastric balloon—smoothing the path to bariatric surgery. Obes Surg 2006; 16:897–902.

49. Angrisani L, Lorenzo M, Borrelli V, et al. Is bariatric surgery necessary after intragastric balloon treatment. Obes Surg 2006; 16:1135–1137.

50. Spryopoulos C, Katsakoulis E, Mead N, et al. Intragastric balloon for high-risk super-obese patients: a prospective analysis of efficacy. Surg Obes Rel Dis 2007; 3:78–83.

51. Herve J, Wahlen CH, Schaeken A, et al. What becomes of patients one year after the intragastric balloon has been removed? Obes Surg 2005; 15(6):864–870.

52. Cigaina VV, Saggioro A, Rigo VV, et al. Long-term effects of gastric pacing to reduce feed intake in swine. Obes Surg 1996; 6(3):250–253.

53. Cigaina V. Gastric pacing as therapy for morbid obesity: preliminary results. Obes Surg 2002; 12:12S–16S.

54. Chen J, McCallum RW. Electrogastrography: Principles and Applications. New York, New York: Raven, 1995.

55. Chen J. Mechanisms of action of the implantable gastric stimulator for obesity. Obes Surg 2004; 14:S28–S32.

56. Shikora SA. Implantable gastric stimulation- the surgical procedure: combining safety with simplicity. Obes Surg 2004; 14:S9–S13.

57. Liu S, Hou X, Chen J. Therapeutic potential of duodenal electrical stimulation for obesity: acute effects on gastric emptying and water intake. Am J Gastroenterol 2005; 100:792–796.

58. Ouyang H, Yin J, Chen JDZ. Therapeutic potential of gastric electrical stimulation for obesity and its possible mechanisms: a preliminary canine study. Dig Dis Sci 2003; 48(4):698–705.

59. Lin Z, Denton S, Durham S, et al. Retrograde gastric electrical stimulation impairs gastric myoelectrical activity in patients with morbid obesity. Gastroenterology 2002; 122(4):A-326.

60. Xing J, Brody F, Rosen M, et al. The effect of gastric electrical stimulation on canine gastric slow waves. Am J Physiol Gastrointest Liver Physiol, 2003; 284:G956–G962.

61. Xing JH, Chen JDZ. Effects and mechanisms of long-pulse gastric electrical stimulation on canine gastric tone and accommodation. Neurogastroenterol Motil 2006; 18: 136–143.

62. Lei Y, Xing J, Chen JD. Effects and mechanisms of implantable gastric stimulation on gastric distension in conscious dogs. Obes Surg 2005; 15(4):528–533.

63. Ouyang H, Yin J, Chen JD. Gastric or intestinal electrical stimulation-induced increase in gastric volume is correlated with reduced food intake. Scand J Gastroenterol 2006; 41(11):1261–1266.

64. Xu X, Zhu H, Chen JDZ. Pyloric electrical stimulation reduces food intake by inhibiting gastric motility in dogs. Gastroenterology 2005; 128:43–50.

65. Ouyang H, Xing J, Chen JDZ. Tachygastria induced by gastric electrical stimulation is mediated via alpha- and beta-adrenergic pathway and inhibits antral motility in dogs. Neurogastroenterol Motil 2005; 17:846–853.

66. Zhu H, Chen JD. Implantable gastric stimulation inhibits gastric motility via sympathetic pathway in dogs. Obes Surg 2005; 15(1):95–100.

67. Yin J, Zhang J, Chen JD. Inhibitory effects of intestinal electrical stimulation on food intake, weight loss, and gastric emptying in rats. Am J Physiol Regul Integr Comp Physiol 2007; 293(1):R78–R82.

68. Yao S, Ke M, Wang Z, et al. Visceral sensitivity to gastric stimulation and its correlation with alterations in gastric emptying and accommodation in humans. Obes Surg 2005; 15(2):247–253.

69. Yao S, Ke M, Wang Z, et al. Retrograde gastric pacing reduces food intake and delays gastric emptying in humans: a potential therapy for obesity? Dig Dis Sci 2005; 50(9): 1569–1575.

70. Qin C, Sun Y, Chen JD, et al. Gastric electrical stimulation modulates neuronal activity in nucleus tractus solitarii in rats. Auton Neurosci 2005; 119(1):1–8.

71. Tang M, Zhang J, Xu L, et al. Implantable gastric stimulation alters expression of oxytocin- and orexin-containing neurons in the hypothalamus of rats. Obes Surg 2006; 16(6):762–769.

72. Sun X, Tang M, Zhang J, et al. Excitatory effects of gastric electrical stimulation on gastric distension responsive neurons in ventromedial hypothalamus (VMH) in rats. Neurosci Res 2006; 55(4):451–457.

73. Wang GJ, Yang J, Volkow ND, et al. Gastric stimulation in obese subjects activates the hippocampus and other regions

involved in brain reward circuitry. Proc Natl Acad Sci USA, 2006; 103(42):15641–15645.

74. Cigaina V, Hirschberg AL. Gastric pacing for morbid obesity: plasma levels of gastrointestinal peptides and leptin. Obes Res 2003; 11(12):1456–1462.

75. Yin J, Chen J. Inhibitory effects of gastric electrical stimulation on ghrelin-induced excitatory effects on gastric motility and food intake in dogs. Scand J Gastroenterol 2006; 41(8):903–909.

76. Xing JH, Lei Y, Ancha HR, et al. Effect of acute gastric electrical stimulation on the systemic release of hormones and plasma glucose in dogs. Dig Dis Sci 2007; 52:495–501.

77. Yin J, Chen JD. Retrograde gastric electrical stimulation reduces food intake and weight in obese rats. Obes Res 2005; 13(9):1580–1587.

78. Xing J, Brody F, Brodsky F, et al. Gastric electrical-stimulation effects on canine gastric emptying, food intake, and body weight. Obes Res 2003; 11(1):41–47.

79. Liu J, Hou X, Song G, et al. Gastric electrical stimulation using endoscopically placed mucosal electrodes reduces food intake in humans. Am J Gastroenterol 2006; 101:798–803.

80. D'Argent J. Gastric electrical stimulation as therapy of morbid obesity: preliminary results from the French study. Obes Surg 2002; 12:21S–25S.

81. Bohdjalian A, Prager G, Aviv R, et al. One-year experience with Tantalus: a new surgical approach to treat morbid obesity. Obes Surg 2006; 16:627–634.

82. Cigaina V. Long-term follow-up of gastric stimulation for obesity: the Mestre 8-year experience. Obes Surg 2004; 14:S14–S22.

83. Miller K, Hoeller E, Aigner F. The implantable gastric stimulator for obesity: an update of the European experience in the LOSS study. Treat Endocrinol 2006; 5(1):53–58.

84. Shikora SA, Storch K. Implantable gastric stimulation for the treatment of severe obesity: the American experience. Surg Obes Rel Dis 2005; 1:334–342.

85. Chu CA, Gagner M, Quinn T, et al. Two-stage laparoscopic bilio-pancreatic diversion with duodenal switch: an alternative approach to super-super morbid obesity. Surg Endosc 2002; 16:S069(abstr).

86. Milone L, Strong V, Gagner M. Laparoscopic sleeve gastrectomy is superior to endoscopic intragastric balloon as a first stage procedure for super obese patients. Obes Surg 2005; 15(5):612–617.

87. Cottam D, Qureshi FG, Mattar SG, et al. Laparoscopic sleeve gastrectomy as an initial weight loss procedure for high-risk patients with morbid obesity. Surg Endosc 2006; 20:859–863.

88. Regan JP, Inabnet WB, Gagner M, Pomp A. Early experience with two-stage laparoscopic Roux-en-Y gastric bypass as an alternative in the super-super obese patient. Obes Surg 2003; 13:861–864.

89. Lee CM, Cirangle PT, Jossart GH. Vertical gastrectomy for morbid obesity in 216 patients: report of two-year results. Surg Endosc 2007; 21(10):1810–1816.

90. Hamoui N, Anthone GJ, Kaufman HS, et al. Sleeve gastrectomy in the high-risk patient. Obes Surg 2006; 16(11):1445–1449.

91. Han SM, Kim WW, Oh JH. Results of laparoscopic sleeve gastrectomy (LSG) at 1 year in morbidly obese Korean patients. Obes Surg 2005; 15:1469–1475.

92. Silecchia G, Boru C, Pecchia A, et al. Effectiveness of laparoscopic sleeve gastrectomy (first stage of biliopancreatic diversion with duodenal switch) on co-morbidities in super-obese high-risk patients. Obes Surg 2006; 16(9):1138–1144.

93. Himpens J, Dapri G, Cadiere GB. A prospective randomized study between laparoscopic gastric banding and laparoscopic isolated sleeve gastrectomy: results after 1 and 3 years. Obes Surg 2006; 16:1450–1456.

94. Roa PE, Kaidar-Person O, Pinto D, et al. Laparoscopic sleeve gastrectomy as treatment for morbid obesity: technique and short-term results. Obes Surg 2006; 16(10):1323–1326.

95. Langer FB, Bohdjalalian A, Felberbauer FX, et al. Does gastric dilatation limit the success of sleeve gastrectomy as a sole operation for morbid obesity? Obes Surg 2006; 16:166–171.

96. Mognol P, Chosidow D, Marmuse JP. Laparoscopic sleeve gastrectomy as an initial bariatric operation for high-risk patients: initial results in 10 patients. Obes Surg 2005; 15(7):1030–1033.

35

Liposuction and Obesity

LUIGI FONTANA

Division of Geriatrics and Nutritional Sciences, Center for Human Nutrition, Washington University School of Medicine, St. Louis, Missouri, U.S.A., and Division of Food Science, Human Nutrition and Health, Istituto Superiore di Sanità, Rome, Italy

SAMUEL KLEIN

Division of Geriatrics and Nutritional Science and Center for Human Nutrition, Washington University School of Medicine, St. Louis, Missouri, U.S.A.

INTRODUCTION

Liposuction, also known as lipoplasty, liposculpture, and suction-assisted lipectomy, is a surgical procedure used to remove subcutaneous fat from specific body sites by using a suction vacuum. The procedure is most commonly performed on the buttocks, hips, thighs, and abdomen but is also frequently used to remove fat from under the chin, neck, breasts, knees, upper arms, calves, and ankles. Liposuction is the most common cosmetic surgical procedure performed in the United States. It is estimated that more than 400,000 persons undergo liposuction every year (1). Advances in liposuction technology now make it possible to remove considerable amounts of subcutaneous fat; in obese subjects, aspiration of ~14 kg of fat has been safely performed (2). The purpose of this chapter is to review the potential use of liposuction as a tool for treating obesity.

Attempts to remove subcutaneous fat by using surgical techniques are not new. In 1921, Charles Dujarrier, a French physician, removed adipose tissue from the legs of a dancer by using a uterine curette. Unfortunately, the procedure caused serious nerve and blood vessel injuries to one leg, which required amputation. The safer use of liposuction to remove subcutaneous fat began in 1974 when Giorgio Fischer, an Italian gynecologist, aspirated unwanted fat depots by using an open-ended curette-like instrument attached to a rudimentary suction apparatus (3). Several years later, two French plastic surgeons, Yves-Gerard Illouz and Pierre-Francois Fournier, improved the suction-assisted technique by using a blunt-tipped cannula (4), which reduced damage to nerves and blood vessels, thereby decreasing bleeding, neuropathic complications, recovery time, and postoperative discomfort. In addition, these physicians developed the "criss-cross," back and forth cannula motion of liposuction and the subcutaneous infusion of fluid, which are now commonly used to enhance fat aspiration. The era of modern liposuction began in 1985, when dermatologists Jeffrey Klein and Patrick Lillis incorporated the use of local anesthetics with epinephrine into the liposuction procedure (5,6). This new "tumescent liposuction" technique reduced pain and bleeding complications and permitted the safe removal of large volumes of fat by using local anesthesia alone.

Since then, new instruments and technical approaches continue to improve the cosmetic benefits and safety of liposuction surgery.

TECHNIQUES

In all liposuction procedures, fat is removed by inserting a cannula through a small skin incision and aspirating local subcutaneous fat by using mechanical suction. In some procedures, the cannula itself is used to mechanically break up adipose tissue architecture to facilitate aspiration, whereas in other procedures adipose tissue is emulsified by using laser or ultrasound instruments that disrupt fat cell membranes (7).

Many different types of liposuction procedures are currently performed. The tumescent liposuction technique is the most common procedure and involves injecting a saline solution containing lidocaine and epinephrine into the surgical area; the volume of injected fluid is three to four times greater than the amount of fat removed. This approach facilitates fat aspiration with minimal pain, bruising, and bleeding. Tumescent liposuction does not usually require more than a local anesthetic for pain control and can be performed as an outpatient procedure because general anesthesia is not used. The "super-wet" liposuction procedure involves injecting the same amount of the saline, lidocaine, and epinephrine solution as the amount of fluid aspirated. This procedure is associated with a lower risk of fluid overload, pulmonary edema, and congestive heart failure, but causes a greater blood loss, than the tumescent technique. "Power-assisted" liposuction involves the use of a specialized suction cannula that has a mechanized movement, making the procedure easier for the operator because of the decreased manual effort needed to perform the procedure (8). Recent technical innovations in liposuction involve disrupting subcutaneous fat cell membranes by using specialized cannulas that transmit ultrasonic, laser, or vibrational energy, which liquefies fat and facilitates aspiration with a small diameter cannula. Ultrasonic energy can also be applied by an external high-intensity, high-frequency source that transmits ultrasonic energy through the skin to rupture subcutaneous fat cell membranes (9).

MEDICAL COMPLICATIONS

The risk of having a complication after liposuction surgery is usually directly related to the amount of fat that is removed. Up to 3 kg of fat is considered the maximum amount that can be safely removed by liposuction as an outpatient procedure (10). Large volume liposuction (>5 L of aspirate containing >3–4 kg of fat) often requires an overnight hospital stay so that the patient can be monitored and given intravenous fluids to maintain plasma volume.

Minor complications of liposuction include skin irregularities, focal skin necrosis, seromas, hematomas, scarring, hyperpigmentation, and local edema. Major complications include the adverse consequences of anesthesia, such as respiratory depression and pulmonary aspiration, allergic reactions and toxicity to medications (e.g., lidocaine), thromboembolism, fat embolism, pulmonary edema because of excessive administration of intravenous fluids, visceral and vascular perforations, permanent nerve damage, excessive blood loss, hypothermia, severe wound infection, and life-threatening cardiac arrhythmias. Liposuction rarely causes death, and mortality is often associated with poor technique and inadequate medical management. The precise risk of death from liposuction surgery is not clear; reported mortality rates range from 0% to 0.02% (10–12).

BODY COMPOSITION AFTER LIPOSUCTION OR LIPECTOMY

Liposuction surgery can remove billions of adipocytes from selected adipose tissue depots. In addition, the procedure usually disrupts the connective tissue framework that supports adipocytes and other cells in adipose tissue. Although liposuction always decreases site-specific adipose tissue mass immediately after the procedure, the long-term effects of liposuction on body composition are less clear, particularly when there is a subsequent increase in body weight and fat mass.

Animal Models

Data obtained from studies conducted in animal models demonstrate variability in adipose tissue response to lipectomy (13). For example: (i) subcutaneous and epididymal adipose tissue lipectomy in hamsters and rodents caused a compensatory accumulation of intra-abdominal and retroperitoneal adipose tissue (14,15), (ii) subcutaneous and perirenal fat pad excision in rodents caused regeneration of lipectomized fat depots (16,17), and (iii) restitution of adipose tissue did not occur after lipectomy in rodents (18–20). In general, regeneration of the excised fat pad is rarely seen, and compensatory fat accumulation at other sites is common (13). The mechanism for adipose tissue regeneration after lipectomy probably involves differentiation of preadipocytes (15,21) and increased local lipoprotein lipase activity (21).

Human Subjects

Little information is available on adipose tissue regrowth after liposuction in human subjects. Liposuction damages blood vessels, nerves, and the fibrous network in subcutaneous fat, which causes scarring and lobular redistribution of remaining adipose tissue at the liposuction site (22). Data from case studies suggest that liposuction results in subcutaneous accumulation of fat in nonaspirated areas, particularly in breast, back, and arms, but does not result in fat reaccumulation in the aspirated areas (23–26). It is likely that the accumulation of fat after liposuction depends on whether patients gain weight. We have found that body fat mass and fat distribution remained unchanged for years after large volume liposuction in subjects who maintained their total body fat mass (B.S. Mohammed and S. Klein unpublished observations).

EFFECT OF LIPOSUCTION ON METABOLIC RISK FACTORS FOR CORONARY HEART DISEASE AND DIABETES

In theory, removal of subcutaneous fat by using liposuction surgery could have beneficial and/or adverse effects on metabolic risk factors for coronary heart disease (CHD) and diabetes. Moderate body fat loss in obese men and women, which occurs with as little as 5% body weight loss, simultaneously improves multiple metabolic risk factors for CHD, including blood pressure, insulin resistance, and plasma glucose, triglyceride, and high-density lipoprotein (HDL)-cholesterol concentrations (27,28). Therefore, it has been hypothesized that moderate body fat reduction induced by liposuction should have metabolic health benefits.

In contrast, it is possible that removal of a large amount of subcutaneous adipocytes decreases the ability of an important adipose tissue depot to store triglycerides so that weight gain after liposuction will cause harmful accumulation of triglycerides in nonexcised adipose tissue depots, such as visceral fat, and in other organs, such as liver, heart, and skeletal muscle. The presence of excess "ectopic" triglycerides in specific organs is associated with impaired metabolic function. For example, excess intrahepatic and intramyocellular triglyceride content is directly related to hepatic and skeletal muscle insulin resistance, increased very low density lipoprotein–triglyceride secretion, and dyslipidemia (29–32). In addition, a marked deficit in subcutaneous body fat, caused by lipoatrophy in both humans and animal models, results in severe insulin resistance, diabetes, dyslipidemia, and hepatic steatosis (33,34). Expanding subcutaneous fat mass by stimulating adipocyte differentiation with peroxisome proliferator–activated receptor-γ agonists (35) or adiponectin (36) or by adipose tissue transplantation (37) ameliorates or completely normalizes the metabolic abnormalities associated with lipoatrophy.

Animal Models

Data from studies conducted in rodents found that resection of large amounts of subcutaneous adipose tissue causes insulin resistance, manifested by increased serum insulin concentrations, increased homeostasis model assessment of insulin resistance (HOMA-IR) values, and decreased systemic insulin sensitivity (measured by intraperitoneal injection of insulin) (38–40). In addition, subcutaneous lipectomy in hamsters and ground squirrels increased serum triglyceride concentrations, liver fat content, and the ratio of intra-abdominal to subcutaneous fat masses (14,41). In contrast, surgical removal of visceral adipose tissue (epididymal and retroperitoneal depots) resulted in marked improvements in insulin action (42–47). However, visceral fat removed in these studies is not anatomically the same as visceral fat (omental and mesenteric depots) in humans, because epididymal and retroperitoneal fat drain directly into the systemic circulation, not into the portal vein (48). These data demonstrate that removal of different fat depots in rodents have distinct metabolic implications.

Human Subjects

Few studies have investigated the metabolic consequences of liposuction in obese men and women, and interpretation of the data is confusing, because of conflicting results from different studies. We are aware of 11 peer-reviewed, published studies that have evaluated the effect of liposuction alone on metabolic risk factors for CHD and diabetes in overweight and obese subjects (2,49–58) (Table 1). A total of ~ 252 overweight and obese subjects, almost exclusively women (only three male participants), participated in these studies. Liposuction was performed in one or more anatomical sites, including abdomen, hips, thighs, buttocks, and flanks. The average amount of fat removed in each study ranged from 1.3 (57) to 9.8 kg (2). Different outcome measures were used to evaluate the effect of liposuction on risk factors for CHD and diabetes, including blood pressure, insulin sensitivity (assessed by the hyperinsulinemic-euglycemic clamp procedure, intravenous glucose tolerance test, oral glucose tolerance test, HOMA-IR, and plasma glucose and insulin concentrations), plasma lipid profile (triglyceride, HDL-cholesterol and low-density lipoprotein cholesterol, and total cholesterol), and plasma inflammatory markers (cytokine/adipokine concentrations). The timing of postprocedure evaluations ranged from 2 weeks to 12 months after liposuction surgery. Although eight studies reported that subjects remained "weight stable" (49,53–58), the interpretation of metabolic outcomes might be confounded in the other three studies because of documented weight loss

Table 1 Summary of Results from Studies That Evaluated the Effect of Liposuction Surgery on Risk Factors for Coronary Heart Disease and Diabetes

First author, yr (reference)	Subjects treated with liposuction (n)	Age (range) (yr)	Initial BMI (range) (kg/m²)	Average amount of fat removed (kg)[c]	Timing of postliposuction study (wk)	Blood pressure	Insulin sensitivity Assessment	Insulin sensitivity Results	TG	HDL-C	Total or LDL-C	Plasma markers of inflammation
Enzi, 1979 (49)	14	45.7 ± 2.4	39.5	6.0 ± 0.5	3–5	NR	OGTT / IVGTT	NC / NC	NR	NR	NR	NR
Samdal, 1995 (50)	9[a]	44 (24–52)	30.1 (23.5–39)	~2.5	39–52	NR	OGTT	NC	↑	↑	NC	NR
Berntorp, 1998 (51)	10	51 (33–68)	36.9 (26.7–43.8)	NR	2–4	NR	Glucose / Insulin / HEC	NC / NC	NR	NR	NR	NR
Giese, 2001 (52)	14	39.4 ± 6.8	29.1 ± 2.3	6.1 ± 1.2	12	↓ SBP	HOMA	↑ / ↑	NC	NC	NC	NR
Gonzalez-Ortiz, 2002 (53)	6	29.3 ± 6.2	31.7 ± 1.7	~4	3–4	NR	Glucose / Insulin / IVGTT	↑ / NC / ↑	NC	NC	NC	→
Giugliano, 2004 (54)	30	37 ± 4.5	34 ± 2.7	2.7 ± 0.7	26	NR	HOMA	↑	NR	↑	NR	→
Klein, 2004 (2)	15	47.3 ± 10	37.3 ± 4.7	9.8 (13.8–5.4)	10–12	NC	HEC / Glucose / Insulin	NC / NC / NC	NC	NC	NC	NC
Robles-Cervantes, 2004 (55)	15	28.8	26.3 (25–28)	2.5 ± 1.1	3	NR	HOMA	NC	NR	NR	→	NR
D'Andrea, 2005 (56)	123	32–40	32.8 ± 0.8	5.0 ± 0.8	12	↓ SBP ↓ DBP	Glucose / Insulin / HEC	NC / ↓ / ↑	→	NR	→	→
Davis, 2006 (57)	15	34.5 ± 1.8	29.9 ± 0.8	1.3 ± 0.2	4	NR	HOMA / IVGTT	↑ / ↑	NC	NR	NR	NC
Hong, 2006 (58)	11[b]	27.3 (19–40)	23.8 ± 4.4	4.7 ± 0.9	8	NC	FBG / Insulin	NC / NC	NR	→	→	NC

Values are mean ± SEM for data reported from Refs. 49 and 57; all other values are mean ± SD.
Normal BMI (18.5–24.9 kg/m²) in [b]nine subjects.
[a]at least one subject; in [b]nine subjects. [c]Estimated as 70% of aspirate volume (51).
Abbreviations: HEC, hyperinsulinemic-euglycemic clamp procedure; IVGTT, intravenous glucose tolerance test; OGTT, oral glucose tolerance test; HOMA, homeostasis model assessment of insulin resistance; SBP, systolic blood pressure; DBP, diastolic blood pressure; TG, triglyceride; HDL-C, HDL-cholesterol; LDL-C, LDL-cholesterol; NR, not reported; NC, no change; ↓, decreased; ↑, increased.

that occurred after liposuction surgery was performed (50–52).

Among the eight studies that reported maintenance of body weight after liposuction, all eight reported some measure of insulin sensitivity, seven reported plasma lipid concentrations, five reported selected plasma cytokine concentrations, and three reported blood pressure values before and after liposuction (Table 1). The pattern of the metabolic responses to liposuction surgery was not consistent across studies. Some studies showed beneficial effects, some showed a mixed response, and some showed no change in metabolic outcomes: (*i*) insulin sensitivity: four found improvement (53,54,56,57) and four found no change (2,49,55,58); (*ii*) plasma lipids: three found improvement (54–56), one found mixed results with improvement and worsening in specific lipids (58), and three found no change (2,53,57); (*iii*) inflammatory markers: two found improvement (54,56) and three found no change (2,57,58); (*iv*) blood pressure: one found improvement (56) and two found no change (2,58). Although plasma HDL-cholesterol concentration decreased in one study (58), no other harmful metabolic effects of liposuction were detected.

The reason for the differences in metabolic outcomes between studies is not clear and is not explained by the amount of fat removed, the timing of the postliposuction studies, or the initial body mass index of the study subjects (Table 1). It is possible that beneficial effects were missed in the negative studies, because of the small number of study participants. The largest study that evaluated the effect of liposuction on metabolic risk factors for CHD and diabetes was conducted in 123 obese women and was able to detect as little as a 4% improvement in metabolic outcomes (56). It is also possible that lifestyle changes induced by the cosmetic benefits of liposuction resulted in "liposuction-independent" improvements in metabolic outcomes. Small changes in energy intake and negative energy balance, which are difficult to detect by history or body weight examination, can have considerable effects on plasma glucose and insulin concentrations and HOMA-IR values (59,60).

CONCLUSIONS

The effect of liposuction on metabolic risk factors for CHD and diabetes is not clear, because of the heterogeneity in results among published studies. The summation of current data do not support the notion that liposuction itself results in important metabolic benefits, because of the discrepancy in results between studies, no obvious pattern of metabolic outcome, and no relationship between the amount of fat removed and metabolic effects. However, this conclusion can change depending on the results

of future studies that carefully control body weight and fat mass after liposuction is performed. Nonetheless, liposuction can potentially have real benefits in obese patients by improving physical appearance, clothing choices, and self-confidence, and by making it easier to engage in regular physical activity and programmed exercise. Additional studies are needed to determine whether (*i*) liposuction can be used to stimulate and facilitate diet-induced weight loss; (*ii*) greater amounts of subcutaneous fat removal than previously reported improves metabolic outcomes; and (*iii*) weight gain after liposuction causes ectopic fat accumulation in liver, heart, and muscle and has adverse metabolic effects.

REFERENCES

1. The American Society for Aesthetic Plastic Surgery. Cosmetic Surgery National Data Bank 2006 Statistics. Available at: http://www.surgery.org/press/statistics-2006.asp. Accessed September 17, 2007.
2. Klein S, Fontana L, Young VL, et al. Effect of liposuction on insulin action and coronary heart disease risk factors. N Engl J Med 2004; 350:2549–2557.
3. Fischer G. First surgical treatment for modeling body's cellulite with three 5 mm incisions. Bull Int Acad Cosm Surg 1976; 2:35–37.
4. Illouz Y-G. History. In: Illouz Y-G, ed. Liposuction: The Franco-American Experience. Beverly Hills, CA: Medical Aesthetics, Inc., 1985:1–18.
5. Klein JA. Anesthesia for liposuction in dermatologic surgery. J Dermatol Surg Oncol 1988; 14:1124–1132.
6. Lillis PJ. Liposuction surgery under local anesthesia: limited blood loss and minimal lidocaine absorption. J Dermatol Surg Oncol 1988; 14:1145–1148.
7. Zocchi M. Ultrasonic liposculpturing. Aesthetic Plast Surg 1992; 16:287–298.
8. Katz BE, Maiwald DC. Power liposuction. Dermatol Clin 2005; 23(3):383–391.
9. de Souza Pinto EB, Abdala PC, Maciel CM, et al. Liposuction and VASER. Clin Plast Surg 2006; 33(1): 107–115.
10. Grazer F, de Jong R. Fatal outcomes from liposuction: census survey of cosmetic surgeons. Plast Reconstr Surg 2000; 105:436–446.
11. Yoho RA, Romaine JJ, O'Neil D. Review of the liposuction, abdominoplasty, and face-lift mortality and morbidity risk literature. Dermatol Surg 2005; 31(7 pt 1): 733–743.
12. Boni R. Safety of tumescent liposuction. Schweiz Rundsch Med Prax 2007; 96(27–28):1079–1082.
13. Mauer MM, Harris RB, Bartness TJ. The regulation of total body fat: lessons learned from lipectomy studies. Neurosci Biobehav Rev 2001; 25(1):15–28.
14. Weber RV, Buckley MC, Fried SK, et al. Subcutaneous lipectomy causes a metabolic syndrome in hamsters. Am J Physiol Regul Integr Comp Physiol 2000; 279(3): R936–R943.

15. Hausman DB, Lu J, Ryan DH, et al. Compensatory growth of adipose tissue after partial lipectomy: involvement of serum factors. Exp Biol Med (Maywood) 2004; 229(6):512–520.

16. Faust IM, Johnson PR, Hirsch J. Adipose tissue regeneration following lipectomy. Science 1977; 197:391–393.

17. Reyne Y, Nougues J, Vezinhet A. Adipose tissue regeneration in 6-month-old and adult rabbits following lipectomy. Proc Soc Exp Biol Med 1983; 174(2):258–264.

18. Harris RB, Hausman DB, Bartness TJ. Compensation for partial lipectomy in mice with genetic alterations of leptin and its receptor subtypes. Am J Physiol Regul Integr Comp Physiol 2002; 283:R1094–R1103.

19. Kral JG. Surgical reduction of adipose tissue in the male Sprague-Dawley rat. Am J Physiol 1976; 231:1090–1096.

20. Faust IM, Johnson PR, Hirsch J. Noncompensation of adipose mass in partially lipectomized mice and rats. Am J Physiol 1976; 231:539–544.

21. Roth J, Greenwood MR, Johnson PR. The regenerating fascial sheath in lipectomized Osborne-Mendel rats: morphological and biochemical indices of adipocyte differentiation and proliferation. Int J Obes 1981; 5(2):131–143.

22. Carpenada CA. Postliposuction histologic alterations of adipose tissue. Aesth Plast Surg 1996; 20:207–211.

23. Scarborough DA, Bisaccia E. The occurrence of breast enlargement in females following liposuction. Am J Cosmetic Surg 1991; 8:97.

24. Frew KE, Rossi A, Bruck MC, et al. Breast enlargement after liposuction: comparison of incidence between power liposuction versus traditional liposuction. Dermatol Surg 2005; 31:292–296.

25. Lambert EV, Hudson DA, Bloch CE, et al. Metabolic response to localized surgical fat removal in nonobese women. Aesthetic Plast Surg 1991; 15(2):105–110.

26. Yost TJ, Rodgers CM, Eckel RH. Suction lipectomy: outcome relates to region-specific lipoprotein lipase activity and interval weight change. Plast Reconstr Surg 1993; 92:1101–1108.

27. Wing RR, Koeske R, Epstein LH, et al. Long-term effects of modest weight loss in type II diabetic patients. Arch Intern Med 1987; 147:1749–1753.

28. Goldstein DJ. Beneficial health effects of modest weight loss. Int J Obes Relat Metab Disord 1992; 16:397–415.

29. Seppala-Lindroos A, Vehkavaara S, Hakkinen AM, et al. Fat accumulation in the liver is associated with defects in insulin suppression of glucose production and serum free fatty acids independent of obesity in normal men. J Clin Endocrinol Metab 2002; 87:3023–3028.

30. Gastaldelli A, Cusi K, Pettiti M, et al. Relationship between hepatic/visceral fat and hepatic insulin resistance in nondiabetic and type 2 diabetic subjects. Gastroenterology 2007; 133:496–506.

31. Sinha R, Dufour S, Petersen KF, et al. Assessment of skeletal muscle triglyceride content by (1)H nuclear magnetic resonance spectroscopy in lean and obese adolescents: relationships to insulin sensitivity, total body fat, and central adiposity. Diabetes 2002; 51:1022–1027.

32. Fabbrini E, Mohammed BS, Magkos F, et al. Alterations in free fatty acid and very low density lipoprotein kinetics in obese subjects with nonalcoholic fatty liver disease. Gastroenterology 2008; 134(2):424–431.

33. Simha V, Garg A. Lipodystrophy: lessons in lipid and energy metabolism. Curr Opin Lipidol 2006; 17(2): 162–169.

34. Reitman ML, Arioglu E, Gavrilova O, et al. Lipoatrophy revisited. Trends Endocrinol Metab 2000; 11:410–416.

35. Arioglu E, Duncan-Morin J, Sebring N, et al. Efficacy and safety of troglitazone in the treatment of lipodystrophy syndromes. Ann Intern Med 2000; 133:263–274.

36. Kim JY, van de Wall E, Laplante M, et al. Obesity-associated improvements in metabolic profile through expansion of adipose tissue. J Clin Invest 2007; 117(9):2621–2637.

37. Gavrilova O, Marcus-Samuels B, Graham D, et al. Surgical implantation of adipose tissue reverses diabetes in lipoatrophic mice. J Clin Invest 2000; 105:271–278.

38. Ishikawa K, Takahashi K, Bujo H, et al. Subcutaneous fat modulates insulin sensitivity in mice by regulating TNF-alpha expression in visceral fat. Horm Metab Res 2006; 38(10):631–638.

39. Palacios E, Pinon-Lopez MJ, Racotta IS, et al. Effect of lipectomy and long-term dexamethasone on visceral fat and metabolic variables in rats. Metabolism 1995; 44: 1631–1638.

40. Schreiber JE, Singh NK, Shermak MA. The effect of liposuction and diet on ghrelin, adiponectin, and leptin levels in obese Zucker rats. Plast Reconstr Surg 2006; 117(6):1829–1835.

41. Forger NG, Dark J, Stern JS, et al. Lipectomy influences white adipose tissue lipoprotein lipase activity and plasma triglyceride levels in ground squirrels. Metabolism 1988; 37:782–786.

42. Gabriely I, Ma XH, Yang XM, et al. Removal of visceral fat prevents insulin resistance and glucose intolerance of aging: an adipokine-mediated process? Diabetes 2002; 51(10):2951–2958.

43. Pitombo C, Araujo EP, De Souza CT, et al. Amelioration of diet-induced diabetes mellitus by removal of visceral fat. J Endocrinol 2006; 191(3):699–706.

44. Gabriely I, Barzilai N. Surgical removal of visceral adipose tissue: effects on insulin action. Curr Diab Rep 2003; 3:201–206.

45. Barzilai N, She L, Liu BQ, et al. Surgical removal of visceral fat reverses hepatic insulin resistance. Diabetes 1999; 48(1):94–98.

46. Kim YW, Kim JY, Lee SK. Surgical removal of visceral fat decreases plasma free fatty acid and increases insulin sensitivity on liver and peripheral tissue in monosodium glutamate (MSG)-obese rats. J Korean Med Sci 1999; 14(5):539–545.

47. Borst SE, Conover CF, Bagby GJ. Association of resistin with visceral fat and muscle insulin resistance. Cytokine 2005; 32(1):39–44.

48. Ho RJ, Meng HC. A technique for the cannulation and perfusion of isolated rat epididymal fat pad. J Lipid Res 1964; 5:203–209.

49. Enzi G, Cagnoni G, Baritussio A, et al. Effects of fat mass reduction by dieting and by lipectomy on carbohydrate

metabolism in obese patients. Acta Diabetol Lat 1979; 16(2):147–156.

50. Samdal F, Birkeland KI, Ose L, et al. Effect of large-volume liposuction on sex hormones and glucose- and lipid metabolism in females. Aesthetic Plast Surg 1995; 19(2): 131–135.

51. Berntorp E, Berntorp K, Brorson H, et al. Liposuction in Dercum's disease: impact on haemostatic factors associated with cardiovascular disease and insulin sensitivity. J Intern Med 1998; 243(3):197–201.

52. Giese SY, Bulan EJ, Commons GW, et al. Improvements in cardiovascular risk profile with large-volume liposuction: a pilot study. Plast Reconstr Surg 2001; 108(2):510–519.

53. Gonzalez-Ortiz M, Robles-Cervantes JA, Cárdenas-Camarena L, et al. The effects of surgically removing subcutaneous fat on the metabolic profile and insulin sensitivity in obese women after large-volume liposuction treatment. Horm Metab Res 2002; 34(8):446–449.

54. Giugliano G, Nicoletti G, Grella E, et al. Effect of liposuction on insulin resistance and vascular inflammatory markers in obese women. Br J Plast Surg 2004; 57(3):190–194.

55. Robles-Cervantes JA, Yanez-Diaz S, Cardenas-Camarena L. Modification of insulin, glucose and cholesterol levels in non-obese women undergoing liposuction: is liposuction metabolically safe? Ann Plast Surg 2004; 52(1):64–67.

56. D'Andrea F, Grella R, Rizzo MR, et al. Changing the metabolic profile by large-volume liposuction: a clinical study conducted with 123 obese women. Aesthetic Plast Surg 2005; 29(6):472–478.

57. Davis DA, Pellowski DM, Davis DA, et al. Acute and 1-month effect of small-volume suction lipectomy on insulin sensitivity and cardiovascular risk. Int J Obes (Lond) 2006; 30(8):1217–1222.

58. Hong YG, Kim HT, Seo SW, et al. Impact of large-volume liposuction on serum lipids in Orientals: a pilot study. Aesthetic Plast Surg 2006; 30(3):327–332.

59. Jazet IM, Pijl H, Frölich M, et al. Two days of a very low calorie diet reduces endogenous glucose production in obese type 2 diabetic patients despite the withdrawal of blood glucose-lowering therapies including insulin. Metabolism 2005; 54(6):705–712.

60. Henry RR, Scheaffer L, Olefsky JM. Glycemic effects of intensive caloric restriction and isocaloric refeeding in non-insulin-dependent diabetes mellitus. J Clin Endocrinol Metab 1985; 61(5):917–925.

36

Obesity and Binge Eating Disorder

JANET D. LATNER

Department of Psychology, University of Hawaii at Manoa, Honolulu, Hawaii, U.S.A.

G. TERENCE WILSON

Graduate School of Applied and Professional Psychology, Rutgers University, Piscataway, New Jersey, U.S.A.

BINGE EATING DISORDER

The American Psychiatric Association's (1994) *Diagnostic and Statistical Manual of Mental Disorders, Fourth Edition (DSM-IV)* lists anorexia nervosa and bulimia nervosa (BN) as the two best-characterized eating disorders (1). Patients who do not meet criteria for either anorexia nervosa or BN may be diagnosed as "eating disorder not otherwise specified" in the *DSM-IV* classification system. Binge eating disorder (BED), for which *DSM-IV* lists provisional diagnostic criteria, has been the most intensively researched disorder within the category of eating disorder not otherwise specified.

Individuals with anorexia nervosa are, by definition, underweight. Those with BN are typically within the healthy range [body mass index (BMI) between 20 and 25 kg/m^2]. Unlike BN, however, BED is significantly associated with obesity (2). Accordingly, in this chapter we focus on the analysis and treatment of obese patients with BED.

BED is characterized by recurrent uncontrolled binge eating. It is also typically associated with dysfunctional concerns about body weight and shape. BED is closely linked with obesity. Though relatively rare in the general community (2%), BED is common among patients attending hospital-based weight control programs (30%) (1,3,4). BED is also prevalent among obese patients presenting for other forms of treatment. On average, approximately 20% of bariatric surgery patients present with BED, though the exact figure varies depending on the assessment measure used (5–7) and is as high as 48% in some studies (8,9). Even among obese individuals who seek self-help treatment, 41% report binge eating at least once in the past month, and 17% report binge eating eight or more times in the past month (10).

CLINICAL CHARACTERISTICS OF BED

Although BED is common among obese patients presenting for treatment, patients with BED have been shown to differ from those without BED in numerous clinically significant ways. Those with BED exhibit greater eating pathology, body image disturbance, and general psychopathology. They also report poorer health-related quality of life and show abnormalities in certain physiological indicators of health. Even the actual health outcomes of people with BED may be impaired relative to people without BED, independent of BMI. The clinically significant differences between obese patients with and without

BED underscore the importance of research and clinical attention to this eating disorder.

Eating Disturbances

Extensive evidence has documented that obese individuals with BED have greater eating-related psychopathology than obese individuals without BED. This body of research has examined individuals with moderate and extreme obesity and those seeking treatment at eating disorder clinics, weight loss programs, and gastric bypass surgery centers. Among patients seeking treatment for weight loss, for example, scores on numerous items from the Eating Disorder Examination questionnaire (11) were higher among moderately obese individuals with BED than those without BED (12). These results have been replicated using various measures of eating pathology in multiple outpatient samples where obese BED patients have shown greater overall eating pathology than obese non-BED patients (13–17).

By comparing obese individuals with BED to obese patients without BED, these studies are able to conclude that the eating-related distress and psychopathology associated with BED does not stem from patients' obesity but from their binge eating. However, some studies have examined the relative contributions of obesity and binge eating using different methods. To examine the relative psychological burden conferred by obesity and binge eating, Barry and colleagues (18) compared obese and nonobese patients with BED. No differences were found on measures of bulimia and body dissatisfaction, and obese BED patients exhibited less psychopathology than nonobese BED patients on a measure of drive for thinness. Similarly, individuals with BED scored comparably on measures of eating pathology regardless of whether they were normal weight, overweight, obese, or extremely obese (19). Even though most studies of BED have included primarily moderately obese clinic samples, these findings suggest that even nonoverweight men and women with BED suffer similar eating-related psychopathology as obese BED patients.

On the other hand, some research studies have failed to find greater eating psychopathology in BED outpatients. Among obese women who were all presenting for treatment of their eating disorder, women with BED were compared to those with overeating episodes that did not involve a loss of control (20). Almost no differences in eating disorder symptoms or dieting history were found between binge eaters and controlled overeaters. However, all of these individuals were distressed enough about their eating pathology to seek specialized eating disorder treatment. This may account for the anomalous findings of this study compared with studies using community samples or obesity treatment samples or studies recruiting different samples (BED vs. non-BED) from different treatment centers (eating disorder clinics vs. weight loss centers).

Among extremely obese patients undergoing gastric bypass surgery, individuals with BED have been found to exhibit greater eating concern, shape concern, and disinhibition than those without BED. They also consumed greater amounts of a liquid meal during a 24-hour feeding test (21). This study also found that individuals with binge eating frequencies less than two per week but greater than one per week had elevated eating pathology relative to nonbinge eaters. Among morbidly obese medical outpatients, those with BED had higher scores on a measure of disinhibited eating, experienced an earlier onset of obesity, and were more likely to attribute their obesity to their eating habits (22).

Eating Patterns and Appetite

Research has suggested marked differences in the eating behavior of individuals with BED relative to non-BED weight-matched controls (23,24). For example, larger amounts of food and fat were consumed at test meals by obese BED than obese non-BED individuals (25). Obese individuals with BED ate more during the day than obese individuals without BED (14). BED patients also consumed significantly more calories and engaged in more feeding bouts on binge days than on nonbinge days, and they ate at a substantially faster rate during binge episodes than during nonbinge episodes (26). Overweight BED patients' energy intake during binge episodes exceeded both their own intake during nonbinge episodes and the intake of weight-matched controls instructed to binge eat (27). BED patients also consumed more energy from fat and less from protein than weight-matched controls when instructed to binge eat, as well as more dessert and snack foods. These eating disturbances are not reserved for binge episodes; BED patients also consumed more food than controls during nonbinge meals (27). BED patients have also been found to consume a higher percentage of calories from protein on nonbinge days than during binge episodes, which were typically high in carbohydrates (28).

These eating patterns reflect possible disturbances among BED patients in their experiences and their perceptions and signals of hunger and fullness. Disruptions in satiety could be a cause or consequence of binge eating. For example, binge eating may alter physiological or cognitive perceptions of appetite signals and lead to confusion of the perceptions of hunger and satiety (29). Deficits in satiety and other appetitive disturbances might help to maintain problematic eating patterns once they are established (30).

These appetitive disturbances may be linked to physiological abnormalities in neuropeptides that govern eating behavior. Ghrelin, a peptide hormone that stimulates hunger and food intake and normally decreases drastically after eating, was predicted to be greater in patients with BED relative to obese controls (31,32). However, fasting ghrelin was decreased in BED patients, suggesting that frequent binge eating may downregulate ghrelin levels. The finding is consistent with observations that binge eating can occur in the absence of hunger (1). The decline in ghrelin after meals, normally a signal for satiation, was also blunted in BED patients. However, these ghrelin levels approached normality after successful treatment of BED (31). Obese binge eaters have also been shown to have increased gastric capacity relative to obese individuals without BED (32,33). A larger stomach capacity necessitates a larger volume of food in the stomach to suppress food intake (34). This abnormality may severely inhibit gastric distension, which is usually involved in the development of fullness following food intake.

Body Image

Several studies have shown that individuals with BED had greater disturbances in body image than individuals without BED, even though both groups were obese. For example, among patients entering weight control treatment, obese binge eaters had greater body image disturbance than obese nonbinge eaters as measured by questions about self-evaluation of shape and weight, dissatisfaction with body weight, avoidance of seeing their body, and feeling and fearing fat (12). BED patients have shown similar weight and shape concerns to those of BN patients and higher concerns than anorexia nervosa patients and overweight controls; like other eating disordered patients, BED patients had elevated importance of shape and weight in self-evaluation. BMI level was unrelated to shape, weight, or eating concerns (35). In other samples, including obese individuals recruited from the general community and extremely obese surgery patients, individuals with BED have also demonstrated greater shape and weight concerns than those without BED (14,21). Other research has shown greater drive for thinness among individuals with BED compared with those without BED, despite similar levels of obesity (16,18).

Studies demonstrating differences in body image between BED and non-BED individuals have typically controlled for differences in body weight. This type of design makes it possible to conclude that the body image disturbance in BED individuals is not due to greater obesity on their part. Instead, the body dissatisfaction in these individuals may be a core attitudinal feature of the eating disturbance characterizing those with BED. However, although patients with and without BED often have similar mean BMIs at the time of assessment or presentation to treatment, they may have different weight histories or trajectories. Obese binge eaters have more severe and more unstable histories of obesity than nonbinge eaters, including heavier weight at their highest past weight (by 11 lb), greater frequency of having a BMI over 35 kg/m^2, earlier onset of overweight (age 16 vs. 20 years) and dieting (age 20 vs. 24 years), and greater frequency of having lost 20 lb or more (4,36). Johnsen and colleagues (37) documented the ages of overweight onset to be 18 and 25 years, respectively, for BED and non-BED obese community women. Other research has shown an even greater disparity in age of onset of obesity between BED and non-BED patients (age 16 vs. 25 years), along with a greater amount of weight ever lost during a single diet (15 vs. 10 kg) and greater percentage of life spent on a diet (15). Individuals with BED also reported that their parents binged significantly more than reported by individuals without BED; this may also be an important aspect of the history and development of patients' eating and weight patterns (15). Obese women with BED also have reported higher rates of maternal overweight than obese women without BED (37). Patients in most of these studies were engaged in weight control treatment. This suggests that although patients may have considered their presenting problem to be their obesity, the presence or absence of binge eating may still have distinguished them in less obvious weight-related ways, such as in the development of overweight.

Research on binge eating in children may also have implications for the early development of their weight problems. Among 6- to 10-year children with a BMI above the 85th percentile, those with binge eating (defined in this study as episodes of uncontrolled eating) were heavier and had more body fat than those without these eating episodes (38). Notably, children with binge eating were more likely to consider weight and shape to be of marked importance to their self-esteem (62% vs. 32%). It is possible that the earlier development of adiposity in binge eaters may be linked to their more acute body image disturbance.

Retrospective research also suggests that a history of frequent appearance-based teasing while growing up is associated with a higher frequency of binge eating among obese women with BED (39). Even those women with BED who were not obese showed a relationship between appearance-related teasing history and another form of eating disturbance, dietary restraint. As also suggested by Neumark-Sztainer et al. (40), the associates between teasing and eating disturbances even in nonoverweight women suggests a direct relationship between stigmatization and eating disturbances, regardless of weight status.

In a comparison of community women with BED, BN, other psychiatric disorders, and healthy controls, childhood obesity and negative comments made by family members about weight, shape, or eating were among the few risk factors that set the BED group apart from both the psychiatric and healthy control groups (41). These risk factors also characterized women with BN (42). Among Caucasian women, appearance-related discrimination before age 18 was more common in those with BED than in healthy or psychiatric controls (43). These different weight histories may be related to the body image disturbance documented in these patients. It is possible that earlier onset of obesity, familial obesity, more frequent yo-yo dieting, and greater history of weight-related and appearance-related teasing may have an impact on the development of these patients' negative body image.

An important question is whether extreme shape and weight concerns should be considered a defining component of BED and included as a criterion in future versions of the disorder's diagnostic classification. At present, individuals can meet criteria for BED whether or not they place exaggerated importance on their body shape and weight. Recent research has compared individuals with BED who do and do not consider shape or weight to be of supreme importance to their self-evaluation. In a community sample of women with BED, those with extreme shape and weight concerns (46%) were older, heavier, had greater eating pathology, poorer health-related quality of life, and were over three times more likely to have sought treatment for eating or weight problems, even though binge eating frequency did not differ between the groups. On most measures, women with BED without extreme shape or weight concerns were similar to obese nonbinge eaters (44). In a clinical sample of BED patients, 58% reported pathological overvaluation of shape and weight; these patients had significantly greater disturbances in eating pathology, mood, self-esteem, and body image (45), though BMI and binge frequency did not differ. Obese community women with BED without extreme shape and weight concerns resembled obese nonbinge eaters (44). Collectively, these findings suggest that a cognitive criterion of shape and weight overvaluation is a distinguishing and clinically significant feature of BED. As such, it deserves consideration as a possible new diagnostic criterion or as a diagnostic specifier.

General Psychopathology

Comparisons of obese individuals with and without BED have also typically demonstrated higher levels of general psychopathology among those with BED. As in studies of eating pathology, many of these samples have been drawn from clinical settings. First, using continuous measures of

negative affect such as the Beck Depression Inventory (46), multiple studies have found that obese binge eaters have higher levels of depression than obese patients without BED (13,17,47–49) and that depression scores are positively correlated with binge eating severity (50). Similar results have been found for measures of anxiety, self-esteem (17,48), and sleep quality and latency (51), which are more impaired in BED than non-BED patients. Greater depression and anxiety have also been demonstrated in overweight children with experiences of a loss of control over eating compared with overweight children without these experiences (38).

Other research has examined differences in continuous measures of general psychopathology such as the Symptom Checklist-90 (52). These studies have shown greater psychopathology among obese binge eaters than among nonbinge eaters on multiple domains, such as somatization, obsessive compulsive symptoms, hostility, paranoid ideation (53), interpersonal sensitivity (51), the tendency to outwardly express anger (13), and general symptom profile (17,49,53). The general symptom profile is also correlated with binge severity in individuals with BED (50). The depression and general psychopathology of BED patients are consistent across weight categories; these disturbances were not lower among nonobese than obese individuals with BED (19).

Some personality disturbances may also be more pronounced among binge eaters than nonbinge eaters (54). Among eating disorder patients with no comorbid Axis I disorders, self-directedness (viewing oneself as autonomous and integrated) and harm avoidance (carefulness, passivity, insecurity, and anxiety in reaction to stress) were lower in overweight women with BED than in overweight women without BED, although other temperament and character traits were similar between the groups (55). When examined with an interview-based, dimensional assessment of personality disorders, obese women with BED had significantly higher levels of personality disorder pathology than obese women without BED, including paranoid, schizotypal, antisocial, and borderline personality disorder traits (56).

Psychiatric diagnoses are also more prevalent among obese patients with BED than among obese controls. For example, lifetime prevalence rates for full-fledged Axis I disorders have been found to be more common among individuals with BED (37,47,57,58). The disturbances that were more common included current and past major depression, anxiety disorders, insomnia, and even suicidal ideation. BED women with high negative affect or a history of mood disorder might comprise a distinct subtype of BED. These individuals were characterized by greater distress, eating and weight concerns, social problems, psychopathology (e.g., anxiety and personality disorders), trauma and abuse history, and poorer self-esteem and response to treatment (59,60) than BED cases without mood disorders.

However, not all studies have found such differences; obese BED and non-BED patients did differ in eating pathology but not in general psychopathology, for example, as measured by continuous measures of depression (Beck Depression Inventory), general symptoms (Symptom Checklist-90), and diagnostic assessments (15). The authors of this study speculated that the mild degree of obesity and the low prevalence of the BED diagnosis (13 of 67 patients) in this weight loss treatment sample may have affected the results. At the other end of the weight spectrum, no differences in rates of Axis I psychiatric morbidity were found between BED and non-BED patients awaiting gastric bypass (21). Again, the small number of BED patients in this sample (9 of 37) may have limited the power of this study to detect differences in diagnostic prevalence rates.

Health-Related Quality of Life

Considering the impairments in mental health experienced by people with BED, it is not surprising that these individuals may have a poorer quality of life than their nonbinge eating counterparts. Several studies have documented differences in health-related quality of life between individuals with BED and weight-matched controls. Using the Medical Outcomes Study Short-Form Disability Scale (SF-36) (61), a measure of health-related quality of life, individuals seeking treatment for BED reported greater impairment in all domains relative to normative samples (based on previously published data). BED patients also showed impairments in several domains compared to individuals (also based on previously published data) seeking treatment for obesity (62). Domains that were impaired included mental health, emotional role functioning, social functioning, and vitality. The co-occurrence of both obesity and depression may have exacerbated quality of life: patients with BED who were obese were worse than those with BED who were not obese on physical quality of life, and depressed BED patients were worse than nondepressed BED patients on mental quality of life. In a direct comparison of extremely obese patients with or without BED who were awaiting gastric bypass surgery, the BED group had poorer functioning than the non-BED group in three domains of the SF-36: physical role functioning, emotional role functioning, and social functioning (21).

The impairments in quality of life may not be due solely to the comorbid psychiatric disorders that can accompany BED. In a large sample of primary care and obstetric and gynecologic patients, individuals with BED (as well as those with BN) had poorer mental health and general health perceptions and poorer physical, social, and role functioning than those without psychiatric disorders. These differences remained significant after co-occurring alcohol, anxiety, and mood disorders, and somatic symptoms were controlled statistically (57).

Other researchers have investigated the quality of life of individuals with BED using a measure of health-related quality of life that is specific to obesity, the impact of weight on quality of life (63). Obese patients with BED have demonstrated greater impairments in quality of life on this measure than obese patients without BED. These findings have extended to both moderately obese patients presenting for outpatient treatment (64) and extremely obese presurgery patients (65). Quality of life dysfunctions occurred in areas including work, sexual life, public distress, self-esteem, and total scores. On the other hand, Kolotkin and colleagues (49) found that BED was no longer independently associated with weight-specific quality of life after controlling for demographic variables, BMI, and psychological symptoms. The authors concluded that in this sample of patients in residential obesity treatment, the presence of depression and other psychological symptoms may have contributed more to quality of life than the presence of BED in itself.

Physical Health

BED may be associated with not only health-related quality of life but also certain physical health indices. Recent evidence suggests that obese binge eaters had higher morning basal cortisol and responded with greater increases in cortisol to a cold-pressor stress test than obese nonbinge eaters. Cortisol was related to abdominal fat only in those with BED; these abnormalities persisted even after treatment (66,67). Individuals with BED may also respond to stress in ways that affect cardiac health. Compared with non-BED obese participants, obese BED patients demonstrated a greater reduction in parasympathetic cardiac regulation during mental stress (68). This pronounced decrease in parasympathetic control of the heart during mental stress and the higher cortisol responses to the cold-pressor test suggest greater stress vulnerability in these patients. This vulnerability could ultimately impact health outcomes and, given the link between cortisol and adiposity in these patients, may be a cause or maintaining factor of their obesity, especially abdominal fat.

Are individuals with BED more likely to suffer from actual health problems than nonbinge eaters? Two large population-based studies have addressed this question. First, in a U.S. sample of twins, obese women with binge eating reported greater health dissatisfaction and higher rates of major medical disorders than obese women without binge eating (69). A Norwegian twin study further examined whether health problems are associated with

BED independent of obesity. Frequent binge eating in women was linked with early menarche, sleep difficulties, irritable bowel syndrome, and alcohol and smoking problems, but only early menarche and sleep problems remained significantly associated with BED when controlling for BMI. In males, the presence of frequent binge eating was associated with elevated neck, shoulder, back, and muscle pain, greater impairment due to physical health, alcohol and smoking problems, reliance on pain medication, and decreased exercise frequency. Notably, each of these associations was still significant after controlling for BMI (70,71).

Summary

In conclusion, BED is neither a variant of obesity with comorbid psychopathology nor merely a marker for psychopathology in some obese patients (72). Compared to weight-matched controls, BED is accompanied by greater disturbances in eating pathology, body image disturbance, and dysfunctional eating behavior. Beyond the impairment associated with obesity itself, BED is also linked with numerous forms of general psychopathology, including depression, anxiety, low self-esteem, sleep disorders, and personality disturbances. BED is also marked by impairments in physiological indicators of health, such as cardiac and cortisol functioning, health-related quality of life, and even certain measurable health outcomes, independent of BMI. More research is needed to examine the precise nature of the associations between BED, physical health, and obesity, as well as to identify the mechanisms of these relationships.

TREATMENT OF BINGE EATING DISORDER

A variety of treatments have been applied to overweight and obese patients with BED. Among these have been specialized psychological therapies, dietary and behavioral weight loss (BWL) programs, and different pharmacological treatments. There are four major targets in the treatment of obese patients with BED: (*i*) binge eating, (*ii*) specific eating disorder psychopathology (e.g., dysfunctional body shape and weight concerns), (*iii*) general psychopathology (e.g., comorbid depression), and (*iv*) obesity itself.

Specialized Psychological Therapies

In this section, we focus on the two most rigorously researched forms of psychological therapy for BED, namely, cognitive behavioral therapy (CBT) and interpersonal psychotherapy (IPT).

Cognitive Behavioral Therapy

CBT has been the most intensively studied form of psychological treatment of BED and has yielded the most consistently effective outcomes. Accordingly, the guidelines from the National Institute of Clinical Excellence (73) in the United Kingdom concluded that CBT is currently the treatment of choice for BED. This clinical recommendation was assigned a methodological grade of "A" indicating strong empirical support from randomized controlled trials.

Typically, controlled trials of CBT have shown substantial reductions in binge eating, with remission rates of roughly 60% or better, and reductions in specific eating disorder and general psychopathology. These changes are generally well maintained at a one-year follow-up. However, CBT does not produce clinically significant improvement in body weight. The overall pattern of findings can be illustrated with reference to a study by Wilfley et al. (74), one of the largest and best controlled in the literature. CBT was compared with IPT, both administered on a group basis. Both treatments were effective, with CBT producing remission rates of 79% and 59%, respectively, at posttreatment and one-year follow-up. Clinically significant reductions in body shape and weight concerns and associated psychiatric symptomatology were observed at follow-up. As in other studies, psychiatric comorbidity was notable. Of the CBT patients, 25% were diagnosed with current depression and 37% with an Axis II disorder. In a finding replicated in several other studies, Wilfley et al. (74) found that patients who had ceased binge eating had lost significantly more weight at follow-up (−2.4 kg) than those who did not. Indeed, the latter had gained weight (2.1 kg).

A common criticism of treatments for BED has been that they do not have specific effects. Whereas CBT is reliably more effective than a wait list control condition, it has been argued that all treatments—including BWL programs—are equally effective and that this compromises the diagnostic validity or utility of BED (72). The findings from the Wilfley et al. (74) study are consistent with this view. In contrast to BED, in the treatment of BN, CBT has been shown to be significantly more effective than IPT, at least in the short term (75). Nevertheless, more recent research has provided evidence of CBT-specific effects on treatment outcome.

First, CBT has been shown to be superior to pharmacological therapy. Grilo et al. (76) showed that individual CBT was significantly more effective than either fluoxetine or placebo in reducing binge eating. In this study, the remission rate for CBT plus placebo was 61% compared with 22% for fluoxetine. It should be noted, however, that fluoxetine did not prove superior to pill placebo (26%) in this study. Pharmacological treatment is discussed more fully below. In another study, consistent with the Grilo et al. (76) findings, Devlin et al. (77) found that adding CBT to BWL was more effective in reducing binge eating than combining fluoxetine with BWL, which had no additive effect.

Second, two well-controlled studies have recently shown that CBT is more effective than BWL in eliminating binge eating. Grilo et al. (78) compared CBT, BWL, and a sequential CBT plus BWL approach in obese patients with BED. In intent-to-treat (ITT) analyses at posttreatment, CBT had a significantly greater binge eating remission rate (60%) than BWL (31%). At the one-year follow-up the comparable rates were 51% and 36%, respectively. Predictably, at posttreatment weight loss in BWL (−2.6%) was greater than in CBT (−0.5%). At 12 months, the percentages were similar: CBT = −0.9% and BWL = 2.1%. One of the striking findings of this study was the disappointing outcome of the combined CBT + BWL group, which received 10 months of treatment as compared with 6 months for CBT and BWL alone. The posttreatment remission rate for binge eating was only 49%, less than that of CBT alone. Moreover, percentage weight loss was −2.6, the same as BWL alone. At the one-year follow-up, the percentage weight loss was a mere 1.5. Common clinical lore is that we should combine different treatments to achieve optimal effects. Indeed, as noted above, Devlin et al. (77) found that adding CBT to BWL did result in an improved outcome. The reasons for the discrepancy are not immediately obvious.

In Switzerland, Munsch et al. (79) compared 16 weekly sessions of CBT with BWL for obese patients with BED. In ITT analyses at posttreatment, consistent with the Grilo et al. (78) finding, CBT was significantly more effective than BWL in producing remission from binge eating. Similarly, BWL resulted in greater albeit modest weight loss than CBT. At a 12-month follow-up, differences between the two treatments were no longer statistically significant.

Guided Self-Help

CBT can also be administered in what has come to be called a "guided self-help" (CBTgsh) format. Fairburn (80) has developed a patient self-help version of the broader CBT approach, which is combined with a limited number of "therapy" sessions that can be delivered by health care providers of different degrees of expertise (81).

CBTgsh has yielded consistently positive findings in the treatment of BED (82). The National Institute of Clinical Excellence guidelines gave it a methodological grade of "B," recommending that it might be a good first-step treatment for many patients. More recently, two treatment outcome studies have provided significant support for CBTgsh. Grilo and Masheb (83) showed that CBTgsh was significantly more effective than a comparable

guided self-help program for weight loss per se based on the LEARN manual (84) and a control condition consisting of self-monitoring of eating designed to equate for the nonspecific influences of treatment. CBTgsh resulted in a 50% remission rate compared with less than 20% in either of the comparison conditions. Apart from demonstrating the value of a brief, focal treatment for binge eating, the superiority of CBTgsh over the self-help BWL treatment provides further evidence of the treatment-specific effects of CBT in general.

In a large, multisite study, Wilfley et al. (85) compared CBTgsh with IPT and BWL. Both IPT and BWL consisted of 20 sessions of individual treatment administered over a six-month period. CBTgsh comprised 10 sessions over this period, nine of which had a maximum duration of 25 minutes. Whereas IPT was administered by carefully trained and supervised doctoral-level clinical psychologists, CBTgsh was provided by beginning graduate students in clinical psychology with little therapeutic experience. The sample of BED patients ($n = 205$) were divided into patients characterized by high negative affect (HNA, a Beck Depression Inventory score above 18) or low negative affect (LNA, a Beck Depression Inventory score of 18 or lower). Previous research had shown that samples of BED patients could be reliably subtyped on this construct of negative affect (86), and it was predicted to be a moderator of treatment outcome.

At posttreatment, ITT analyses revealed no differences among the three treatments. The remission rates were as follows: IPT = 64%, BWL = 54%, and CBTgsh = 58%. Consistent with previous studies, BWL produced greater weight loss than either IPT or CBTgsh. Negative affect did not moderate outcome. However, over a 12-month follow-up negative affect did emerge as a significant moderator of treatment effects. Both IPT and CBTgsh were significantly more effective than BWL in reducing number of days on which binge eating occurred. In terms of remission from binge eating, IPT was significantly superior to BWL at six months. At no point did IPT differ from CBTgsh in terms of effectiveness in reducing binge eating.

Interpersonal Psychotherapy

Two randomized controlled trials have demonstrated that IPT is equivalent in efficacy to CBT in reducing binge eating and associated eating disorder specific and general psychopathology (74,87). A third study of IPT (85), summarized above, replicated the treatment's overall efficacy. In addition, it showed that IPT is superior to BWL—but not to CBTgsh—with high negative affect subset of BED patients over a 12-month follow-up.

A notable finding of this study was the low dropout rate in IPT—7% versus 28% and 30% for BWL and CBTgsh. Not only is IPT eminently acceptable to patients with

BED, but it is also relatively easy to train therapists in its administration. This is an advantage that it would enjoy over CBT, which is more technically complicated.

Summary

Specific effects of CBT on binge eating have been clearly documented in comparison with pharmacological and dietary/BWL interventions. It should be pointed out, however, that these differences are apparent at posttreatment rather than at longer-term follow-up. Finally, CBT has not been shown to be more effective than an alternative evidence-based psychological treatment. IPT is as effective as CBT in treating binge eating and associated psychopathology. Neither CBT nor IPT produces clinically significant weight loss.

It appears that CBTgsh can have effects comparable to those of full-fledged CBT and IPT administered by highly trained professionals. Moreover, CBTgsh is a robust treatment, proving as effective with high negative affect patients with significant psychiatric comorbidity as IPT. Its superiority over BWL with this subset of BED patients provides additional evidence for the specificity of CBT as a treatment approach. As with other psychological treatments, CBTgsh does not produce significant weight loss.

Behavioral Weight Loss

Some earlier studies of BWL for obesity included a questionnaire measure of binge eating and reported the successful reduction of binge eating (88). Similarly, severe caloric restriction in the form of a very low calorie diet (VLCD) was found to reduce binge eating in the short term (89). These and related findings on weight loss in obese binge eaters led some investigators to conclude that there might be no need for specialized therapies for obese binge eaters beyond that offered by standard BWL treatment (90). However, in their analysis of these studies, Wilfley et al. (2) pointed out several specific limitations of the research. The studies relied on a self-report measure (the Binge Eating Scale) (91) that does not assess binge eating frequency directly and has poor agreement with interview-based assessment (92). Therefore, whether the obese binge eaters in these studies were comparable to patients with a full and formal BED diagnosis is questionable.

Other earlier studies had compared weight loss outcome in obese patients with and without binge eating in BWL. The results were mixed. Gladis et al. (90) found that patients with BED actually lost more weight at posttreatment than did their non-BED counterparts, with no differences between the two groups in weight loss or regain during a one-year follow-up. Only 12 patients

diagnosed with BED were included in this analysis. Sherwood et al. (93) found that patients who were binge eating at baseline were more likely to drop out of treatment. Also in this study, binge eating, assessed using the problematic Binge Eating Scale, was a "weak prognostic indicator" (p. 485) of worse longer-term (18 months) outcome. A more recent study from Italy incorporated methodological improvements in a comparison of the outcome of obese patients with and without BED. Treatment consisted of a sequential therapy in which Fairburn's (80) CBT program was followed by BWL based on the LEARN manual (94). The BED diagnosis in this study was confirmed using the Eating Disorder Examination (95). Weight loss at posttreatment was less in the BED subgroup (mean = 7.7 kg) than the non-BED subgroup (mean = 11.1 kg).

The controlled comparisons of BWL with specialized psychological treatments (CBT and IPT) summarized above provide methodologically more rigorous evaluations of the efficacy of BWL in the treatment of obese patients with BED. In all four studies (78,79,83,85) BWL fared less well than the specialized psychological treatments even if they were administered in a guided self-help format. We conclude that there are more effective methods for treating binge eating in obese patients with BED and that this might be especially the case in that subset of patients with high negative affect or severe psychiatric comorbidity.

The foregoing studies that compared BWL with either CBT or IPT all included weight loss as a measure of outcome. Although BWL was significantly more effective than CBT or IPT, as noted above, the absolute amount of weight reduction was noticeably poor. Grilo et al. (78) reported a mean weight loss of −2.6% at six months posttreatment. The Wilfley et al. (85) findings revealed a mean loss of roughly half of the study's weight loss goal of 7%. Munsch et al. (79) noted that the weight loss in their BWL condition was "not of clinical relevance" (p. 111).

Whether the disappointing weight loss outcomes in these studies is attributable to the negative impact of BED itself or problems in the implantation of the particular BWL protocols cannot be answered at this point. Both Grilo et al. (78) and Wilfley et al. (85) demonstrated that BWL resulted in an increase in dietary restraint as would be predicted. However, the Munsch et al. (79) study found a decrease in dietary restraint in their BWL from pre- to posttreatment. This would arguably explain their poor weight loss outcome. (Parenthetically, it should be noted that the limited weight loss in the Devlin et al. (77) study might well be attributed to the nature of their BWL protocol. As the authors point out, it was a modified version of the LEARN manual that did not focus on caloric restriction to the degree more standard BWL interventions would.)

Several studies have examined the effect of VLCDs on obese patients with and without binge eating. Wadden et al. (96) concluded that there were no differences between the two groups in response to a 26-week combined behavior modification and VLCD treatment. However, the definition of binge eating in this study differed from that in *DSM-IV* (1). The criterion was a large amount of food. It was not necessary for each overeating episode to be accompanied by loss of control. As a result, it is likely that many of the patients classified as binge eaters were in fact overeaters who would not meet accepted criteria for BED. Telch and Agras (97), using a more conventional definition of binge eating, failed to show any difference in weight loss following VLCD treatment between obese patients with and without binge eating. Finally, De Zwaan et al. (65) reported that a combined VLCD and CBT treatment produced comparable weight loss in obese patients with and without BED diagnosed using the Structured Clinical Interview for Diagnosis. It should be pointed out that VLCDs have been shown to result in rapid relapse in follow-up evaluations with obese patients in general.

Summary

Contrary to the claim of some critics (98), weight loss treatment involving either moderate or severe caloric restriction does not trigger nor exacerbate binge eating (89,99). BWL, with or without a VLCD, reliably reduces binge eating in the short term. Whether obese patients with BED are less successful in losing weight than obese patients without this eating disorder when treated with BWL, or more likely to drop out of treatment, is still uncertain. Although recent trials have shown relatively poor results of BWL on weight reduction in obese BED patients, additional well-controlled studies with adequate follow-up are needed to reach a definitive conclusion.

Pharmacological Treatment

A variety of drugs have been used to treat BED in obese patients. Results of some early studies were interpreted as showing that BED is unusually responsive to pill placebos in the context of randomized controlled trials and that this was evidence for the nonspecificity of treatment response in these patients (72). However, subsequent research has demonstrated that the rate of placebo response in obese patients with BED is comparable to that in other psychiatric disorders such as depression (100).

Antidepressant Medication

Both tricyclics and selective serotonin reuptake inhibitors have been evaluated in randomized controlled trials. These drugs have typically resulted in a significantly greater reduction in binge eating than pill placebo (101). However, these findings must be tempered by a number of methodological limitations of the research base. Wilson et al. (102) summarized these as follows: "In general, pharmacological trials have been of relatively short duration, have used less stringent measures of outcome than the psychotherapy trials, have had higher dropout (an average 40% across studies), and have not reported follow-up data after medication discontinuation" (p. 210). It must be stressed that most studies of medication have relied on binge frequencies during the final week of treatment as opposed to the far more stringent and clinically meaningful demand of a 28-day period used in research on CBT and IPT (76).

Effects of antidepressant medication on body weight have been relatively minimal in existing short-term outcome studies (102). Moreover, as the American Psychiatric Association's *Practice Guideline for the Treatment of Eating Disorders* (101) cautions, long-term use of selective serotonin reuptake inhibitors has been associated with weight gain.

Antidepressant medication has fared less well when compared with an active treatment such as CBT. As noted above, Grilo et al. (76) found that CBT was significantly more effective than fluoxetine in producing remission from binge eating. The respective ITT remission rates were 22% for fluoxetine, 50% for fluoxetine plus CBT, and 61% for placebo plus CBT. Devlin et al. (77) found that whereas adding CBT to BWL enhanced treatment outcome, adding fenfluramine to BWL had little beneficial effect. A third study that compared CBT with fluoxetine (administered in an open-label format) found that CBT was more effective than the medication alone and that combining fluoxetine with CBT failed to increase treatment effects (103).

Grilo et al. (104) replicated findings from the treatment of BN (105,106) in demonstrating that rapid response to treatment is a clinically significant predictor of binge eating outcome. This finding is important given that no reliable predictors of treatment outcome of BED have been identified (73). Rapid response had different prognostic significance depending on the treatment. CBT patients without a rapid response showed a later pattern of continued improvement throughout treatment although it did not reach the very high levels of improvement achieved by the rapid responders. However, patients who did not show a rapid response to fluoxetine did not subsequently improve. The absence of rapid response to a selective serotonin reuptake inhibitor might indicate that treatment should be modified in some appropriate fashion (104). Apart from the practical clinical utility of this finding, the differing time courses and predictive significance of CBT versus fluoxetine provide further support for specific treatment effects.

Antiobesity Medication

Sibutramine is an FDA-approved appetite suppressant for the treatment of obesity. In a randomized controlled trial of BED, Appolinario et al. (107) showed that the drug was significantly more effective than placebo in reducing binge eating frequency over the course of treatment. Remission rates at posttreatment (based only on the 12th final week) were 40% for sibutramine and 27% for placebo. It is not clear whether this difference—or even the less informative rates based on only those who completed treatment (52% vs. 32%)—were statistically different. Sibutramine was significantly more effective in decreasing body weight (−7.4 kg) than placebo (+1.4 kg).

Orlistat (a lipase inhibitor) is the other currently FDA-approved antiobesity medication. Grilo et al. (108) found that combining orlistat with CBTgsh resulted in significantly better remission from binge eating at posttreatment (64%) compared with placebo plus CBTgsh (36%), but not at a three-month follow-up during which both medication and CBTgsh were discontinued (52% for both treatments). The combination of CBTgsh and orlistat resulted in significantly greater weight reduction at follow-up than CBTgsh plus placebo although the overall amount of weight lost was modest.

Topiramate, an anticonvulsant medication, has been evaluated in two randomized controlled trials. In the first study (109), the binge eating remission rates were 64% for topiramate versus 39% for the placebo group. Weight loss was 5.9 kg and 1.2 kg for the two conditions. A one-year open-label continuation of the study (110) is difficult to interpret, given that only 10 of the original 61 patients remained in the study. Adverse physical side effects, including cognitive problems and parathesias, resulted in roughly a third of patients dropping out.

A second, large multicenter trial (111) found similar results. Topiramate yielded a significantly greater ITT binge eating remission rate (58%) than placebo (29%). The drug also produced significantly more weight loss (−4.5 kg) than placebo (0.2 kg). Discontinuation rates in both treatment conditions were 30%.

Summary

Overall, current pharmacological treatments have been less effective than specialized psychological therapies in eliminating binge eating. The exception has been topiramate. Pharmacological treatments are also more intrusive and associated with a higher dropout rate. The major limitation of pharmacological treatments, however, is the absence of evidence of long-term treatment effects especially following discontinuation of medication. Sibutramine, orlistat, and topiramate have all resulted in successful weight reduction in short-term studies. Data on long-term effects are lacking.

Bariatric Surgery

BED and subthreshold problems with frequent binge eating are common among patients presenting for bariatric surgery (5,7,112). The presence of BED in these patients raises two important questions: (i) what effect does surgery have on binge eating behavior and (ii) is BED a negative prognostic indicator for the weight loss outcomes of surgery? It is possible that binge eating by presurgery patients could be a red flag, as uncontrolled bingeing on large amounts of food might persist after surgery and detrimentally affect its results. However, research on this issue, while somewhat mixed, suggests that this is not the case.

In prospective studies with follow-ups from 4 months (113) to 12 months (114) to 5.5 years (115), binge eating, which occurred at least weekly in 24% to 52% of patients, ceased following surgery. Diagnoses of BED decreased from 43% to 2% following biliopancreatic diversion (116) and from 48% to 0% following gastric bypass (9). A number of other recent studies have also documented dramatic decreases in binge eating (117,118) and demonstrated that binge eaters resemble nonbinge eaters on measures of eating disturbances following surgery (119).

It is possible that, in extremely obese patients presenting for surgery, binge eating and other symptoms may improve over time even without surgery. BED patients who had requested and received gastric bypass were compared with those who had requested but not received gastric bypass. Four and a half years after requesting treatment, weight loss was greater in patients who had received surgery, but both groups showed substantial decreases in BED as well as depressive symptoms (120). This finding is consistent with data suggesting a fluctuating natural course of BED over time in less obese individuals (121).

Numerous recent studies have addressed the question of whether binge eating influences weight outcome following surgery. A number of these studies have found no differences in weight loss between patients with and without presurgical binge eating. Follow-up lengths for studies finding that binge eating was not a prognostic indicator have ranged from 4 months (113), 6 months (118), 12 months (114,122,123), 16 months (9), and 18 months (119) to 5 years (115,124). It is even possible that a trend exists in the opposite direction: weight loss at 12 months after surgery tended to be greatest among severe binge eaters, compared with moderate binge eaters or nonbinge eaters (123). Sixteen months (on average) after surgery, presurgical binge eaters also tended to report more satisfaction with their surgery outcome than nonbinge eaters, and presurgical binge eating was a significant positive predictor of weight loss outcome (9). It is possible that when binge eating ceases following surgery, an important maintaining factor of these patients' obesity is discontinued, facilitating weight loss.

On the other hand, a few studies suggest that presurgical eating disturbances, including binge eating, may indeed predict outcome. Six months after gastric bypass, patients with presurgical binge eating lost a smaller percentage of their excess weight than nonbinge eaters (125). Hsu and colleagues (8) reported that the presence of presurgical eating disturbances was most likely to predict weight outcome after two years postsurgery, once weight regain begins. Studies on the postoperative eating patterns of patients at follow-up suggest that weight regain is more likely among those patients in whom eating disturbances are present at the time of follow-up (126–128). For example, in a postoperative assessment of patients between two and seven years after their surgery, current binge eating and other uncontrolled eating episodes were associated with greater weight regain (129). Thus, the assessment of binge eating preoperatively versus postoperatively may explain some of the discrepancy in findings. Long-term postoperative eating disturbances may or may not be related to preoperative eating behaviors.

Summary

Thus, though the evidence is mixed, the majority of research studies so far suggest that among extremely obese binge eaters, obesity surgery can reduce or eliminate binge eating episodes. Moreover, although postsurgical eating disturbances may be associated with concurrent poorer outcome or weight regain, presurgical binge eating does not appear to be a robust negative prognostic indicator for weight loss outcome following surgery.

CONCLUSION

CBT and IPT are currently the most effective therapies for treating binge eating, specific eating disorder psychopathology, and associated psychiatic problems. CBTgsh is a brief, cost-effective intervention that may be as effective as more complex psychological therapies such as CBT and IPT. As a focal, simplified form of full CBT, CBTgsh is more disseminable to a wider range of health care providers (81).

A limitation of these evidence-based psychological treatments is that they do not produce clinically significant reduction in body weight. BWL programs, with or without VLCDs, result in short-term weight loss. Maintenance of weight loss, however, is poor. Of course, this is the overriding problem of all dietary and behavioral treatments for obesity in general (99,130). If anything, obese patients with BED might respond even more poorly than obese patients without BED to treatments aimed at weight loss. Future research is needed to investigate ways of improving the weight loss outcomes of effective psychological treatments for BED.

Pharmacological therapies reduce binge eating—albeit not as successfully as CBT and IPT. Antiobesity drugs produce short-term weight loss. Evidence of long-term effects is lacking.

Bariatric surgery appears to result in dramatic reductions in binge eating in many cases. Binge eating in patients who are otherwise good candidates for surgery should not rule out their receiving surgery. However, the development of binge eating after surgical intervention should be closely monitored.

REFERENCES

1. American Psychiatric Association. Diagnostic and Statistical Manual of Mental Disorders. 4th ed. Washington, D.C.: American Psychiatric Press, 1994.
2. Wilfley DE, Wilson GT, Agras WS. The clinical significance of binge eating disorder. Int J Eat Disord 2003; 34(suppl):S96–S106.
3. Spitzer R, Williams JB, Gibbon M, et al. The structured clinical interview for DSM-III-R. Arch Gen Psychiatry 1992; 49:624–629.
4. Spitzer RL, Yanovski SZ, Wadden T, et al. Binge eating disorder: its further validation in a multisite study. Int J Eat Disord 1993; 13:137–153.
5. de Zwaan M, Mitchell JE, Howell LM, et al. Characteristics of morbidly obese patients before gastric bypass surgery. Compr Psychiatry 2003; 44:428–434.
6. Dymek-Valentine M, Rienecke-Hoste R, Alverdy J. Assessment of binge eating disorder in morbidly obese patients evaluated for gastric bypass: SCID versus QEWP-R. Eat Weight Disord 2004; 9:211–216.
7. Elder KA, Grilo CM, Masheb RM, et al. Comparison of two self-report instruments for assessing binge eating in bariatric surgery candidates. Behav Res Ther 2006; 44:545–560.
8. Hsu LKG, Sullivan SP, Benotti PN. Eating disturbances and outcome of gastric bypass surgery: a pilot study. Int J Eat Disord 1997; 21:385–390.
9. Latner JD, Wetzler S, Goodman E, et al. A prospective study of gastric bypass in a low income, inner city population: eating disturbances and weight loss. Obes Res 2004; 12:956–961.
10. Delinsky SS, Latner JD, Wilson GT. Binge eating and weight loss in a self-help behavior modification program. Obesity 2006; 14:1244–1249.
11. Fairburn CG, Beglin S. Assessment of eating disorders: interview or self-report questionnaire? Int J Eat Disord 1994; 16:363–3670.
12. Wilson GT, Nonas CA, Rosenblum GD. Assessment of binge eating in obese patients. Int J Eat Disord 1993; 13(1):25–33.
13. Fassino S, Leombruni P, Piero A, et al. Mood, eating attitudes, and anger in obese women with and without binge eating disorder. J Psychosom Res 2003; 54:559–566.

14. Allison KC, Grilo CM, Masheb RM, et al. Binge eating disorder and night eating syndrome: a comparative study of disordered eating. J Consult Clin Psychol 2005; 73:1107–1115.

15. Brody ML, Walsh BT, Devlin MJ. Binge eating disorder: reliability and validity of a new diagnostic category. J Consult Clin Psychol 1994; 62:159–162.

16. Fitzgibbon ML, Sanchez-Johnsen LAP, Martinovich Z. A test of the continuity perspective across bulimic and binge eating pathology. Int J Eat Disord 2003; 34:83–97.

17. Telch CF, Stice E. Psychiatric comorbidity in women with binge eating disorder: prevalence rates from a non-treatment-seeking sample. J Consult Clin Psychol 1998; 66: 768–776.

18. Barry DT, Grilo CM, Masheb RM. Comparison of obese patients with binge eating disorder and nonobese patients with binge eating disorder. J Nerv Ment Dis 2003; 191:589–594.

19. Didie ER, Fitzgibbon M. Binge eating and psychological distress: is the degree of obesity a factor? Eat Behav 2005; 6:35–41.

20. Antoniou M, Tasca GA, Wood J, et al. Binge eating disorder versus overeating: a failure to replicate and common factors in severely obese treatment seeking women. Eat Weight Disord 2003; 8:145–149.

21. Hsu LKG, Mulliken B, McDonagh B, et al. Binge eating disorder in extreme obesity. Int J Obes Relat Metab Disord 2002; 26:1398–1403.

22. Riener R, Schindler K, Ludvik B. Psychosocial variables, eating behavior, depression, and binge eating in morbidly obese subjects. Eat Behav 2006; 7:309–314.

23. Mitchell JE, Crow S, Peterson CB, et al. Feeding laboratory studies in patients with eating disorders: a review. Int J Eat Disord 1998; 24:115–124.

24. Walsh BT, Boudreau G. Laboratory studies of binge eating disorder. Int J Eat Disord 2003; 34(suppl):S30–S38.

25. Raymond NC, Bartholome LT, Lee SS, et al. A comparison of energy intake and food selection during laboratory binge eating episodes in obese women with and without a binge eating disorder diagnosis. Int J Eat Disord 2007; 40:67–71.

26. Rossiter EM, Agras WS, Telch CF, et al. The eating patterns of non-purging bulimic subjects. Int J Eat Disord 1992; 11:111–120.

27. Yanovski SZ, Leet M, Yanovski JA, et al. Food selection and intake of obese women with and without binge eating disorders. Am J Clin Nutr 1992; 56:979–980.

28. Rossiter EM, Agras WS, Telch CF, et al. The eating patterns of non-purging bulimic subjects. Int J Eat Disord 1992; 11:111–120.

29. Halmi KA, Sunday SR. Temporal patterns of hunger and fullness ratings and related cognitions in anorexia and bulimia. Appetite 1991; 16:219–237.

30. Walsh BT, Devlin MJ. Eating disorders: progress and problems. Science 1998; 280:1387–1390.

31. Geliebter A, Gluck ME, Hashim SA. Plasma ghrelin concentrations are lower in binge-eating disorder. J Nutr 2005; 135:132613–132630.

32. Geliebter A, Yahav EK, Gluck ME, et al. Gastric capacity, test meal intake, and appetitive hormones in binge eating disorder. Physiol Behav 2004; 81(5):735–740.

33. Geliebter A, Hashim SA. Gastric capacity in normal, obese, and bulimic women. Physiol Behav 2001; 74:743–746.

34. Geliebter A. Gastric distension and gastric capacity in relation to food intake in humans. Physiol Behav 1988; 44:665–668.

35. Wilfley DE, Schwartz MB, Spurrell EB, et al. Using the Eating Disorder Examination to identify the specific pathology of binge eating disorder. Int J Eat Disord 2000; 27:259–269.

36. Spitzer RL, Devlin MJ, Walsh BT, et al. Binge eating disorder: a multisite field trial of the diagnostic criteria. Int J Eat Disord 1992; 12:257–262.

37. Johnsen LA, Gorin A, Stone AA, et al. Characteristics of binge eating among women in the community seeking treatment for binge eating or weight loss. Eat Behav 2003; 3:295–305.

38. Morgan CM, Yanovski SZ, Nguyen TT, et al. Loss of control over eating, adiposity, and psychopathology in overweight children. Int J Eat Disord 2002; 31:430–441.

39. Jackson TD, Grilo CM, Masheb RM. Teasing history, onset of obesity, current eating disorder psychopathology, body dissatisfaction, and psychological functioning in binge eating disorder. Obes Res 2000; 8:451–458.

40. Neumark-Sztainer D, Falkner N, Story M. Weight-teasing among adolescents: correlations with weight status and disordered eating behaviors. Int J Obes 2002; 26: 123–1231.

41. Fairburn CG, Doll HA, Welch SL, et al. Risk factors for binge eating disorder: a community-based, case-control study. Arch Gen Psychiatry 1998; 55:425–432.

42. Fairburn CG, Welch SL, Doll HA, et al. Risk factors for bulimia nervosa: a community-based, case-control study. Arch Gen Psychiatry 1997; 54:509–517.

43. Striegel-Moore RH, Dohm FA, Pike KM, et al. Abuse, bullying, and discrimination as risk factors for binge eating disorder. Am J Psychiatry 2002; 159:1902–1907.

44. Mond JM, Hay PJ, Rodgers B, et al. Recurrent binge eating with and without the "undue influence of weight or shape on self-evaluation": implications for the diagnosis of binge eating disorder. Behav Res Ther 2007; 45: 929–938.

45. Hrabosky JI, Masheb RM, White MA, et al. Overvaluation of shape and weight in binge eating disorder. J Consult Clin Psychol 2007; 75:175–180.

46. Beck AT, Ward CH, Mendelson M. An inventory for measuring depression. Arch Gen Psychiatry 1961; 4: 561–571.

47. Fontenelle LF, Vltor Mendlowicz M, de Menezes GB, et al. Psychiatric comorbidity in a Brazilian sample of patients with binge-eating disorder. Psychiatry Res 2003; 15:189–194.

48. Jirik BP, Geliebter A. Gender comparisons in psychological characteristics of obese, binge eaters. Eat Weight Disord 2005; 10:e101–e104.

49. Kolotkin RL, Westman EC, Ostbye T, et al. Does binge eating disorder impact weight-related quality of life? Obes Res 2004; 1:999–1005.

50. Telch CF, Agras WS. Obesity, binge eating and psychopathology: are they related? Int J Eat Disord 1994; 15: 53–61.

51. Vardar E, Caliyurt O, Arikan E, et al. Sleep quality and psychopathological features in obese binge eaters. Stress Health 2004; 20:35–41.

52. Derogatis LR, Lipman RS, Covi L. SCL-90: an outpatient psychiatric rating scale-preliminary report. Psychopharmacol Bull 1973; 9:13–28.

53. Spitzer RL, Yanovski SZ, Wadden T, et al. Binge eating disorder: its further validation in a multisite study. Int J Eat Disord 1993; 13:137–153.

54. Wilfley DE, Friedman MA, Dounchis JZ, et al. Comorbid psychopathology in binge eating disorder: relation to eating disorder severity at baseline and following treatment. J Consult Clin Psychol 2000; 68(4):641–649.

55. Fassino S, Leombruni P, Piero A, et al. Temperament and character in obese women with and without binge eating disorder. Compr Psychiatry 2002; 43:431–437.

56. van Hanswijck de Jonge P, Van Furth EF, et al. The prevalence of DSM-IV personality pathology among individuals with bulimia nervosa, binge eating disorder and obesity. Psychol Med 2003; 33:1311–1317.

57. Johnson JG, Spitzer RL, Williams BW. Health problems, impairment and illnesses associated with bulimia nervosa and binge eating disorder among primary care and obstetric gynaecology patients. Psychol Med 2001; 31: 1455–1466.

58. Telch CF, Agras WS, Rossiter EM. Binge eating increases with increasing adiposity. Int J Eat Disord 1988; 7: 115–119.

59. Stice E, Agras WS, Telch CF, et al. Subtyping binge eating-disordered women along dieting and negative affect dimensions. Int J Eat Disord 2001; 30:11–27.

60. Peterson CB, Miller KB, Crow SJ, et al. Subtypes of binge eating disorder based on psychiatric history. Int J Eat Disord 2005; 38:273–276.

61. Ware J, Sherbourne C. The MOS 36-item Short-Form Health Survey (SF-36). Med Care 1992; 30:473–483.

62. Masheb RM, Grilo CM. Quality of life in patients with binge eating disorder. Eat Weight Disord 2004; 9: 194–199.

63. Kolotkin RL, Crosby RD, Kosloski KD, et al. Development of a brief measure to assess quality of life in obesity. Obes Res 2001; 9:102–111.

64. Rieger E, Wilfley DE, Stein RI, et al. A comparison of quality of life in obese individuals with and without binge eating disorder. Int J Eat Disord 2005; 37: 234–240.

65. de Zwaan M, Mitchell JE, Crosby RD, et al. Short-term cognitive behavioral treatment does not improve outcome of a comprehensive very-low-calorie diet program in obese women with binge eating disorder. Behav Ther 2005; 36:89–99.

66. Gluck ME, Geliebter A, Hung J, et al. Cortisol, hunger, and desire to binge eat following a cold stress test in obese women with binge eating disorder. Psychosom Med 2004; 66:876–881.

67. Gluck ME, Geliebter A, Lorence M. Cortisol stress response is positively correlated with central obesity in obese women with binge eating disorder (BED) before and after cognitive-behavioral treatment. Ann N Y Acad Sci 2004; 1032:202–207.

68. Friederich HC, Schild S, Schellberg D, et al. Cardiac parasympathetic regulation in obese women with binge eating disorder. Int J Obes 2006; 30:534–542.

69. Bulik CM, Sullivan PF, Kendler KS. Medical and psychiatric morbidity in obese women with and without binge eating. Int J Eat Disord 2002; 32:72–78.

70. Bulik CM, Reichborn-Kjennerud T. Medical morbidity in binge eating disorder. Int J Eat Disord 2003; 34(suppl): S39–S46.

71. Reichborn-Kjennerud T, Bulik CM, Sullivan PF, et al. Psychiatric and medical symptoms in binge eating in the absence of compensatory behaviors. Obes Res 2004; 12:1445–1454.

72. Stunkard AJ, Allison KC. Binge eating disorder: disorder or marker? Int J Eat Disord 2003; 34(suppl):S107–S116.

73. NICE. Eating disorders-core interventions in the treatment and management of anorexia nervosa, bulimia nervosa and related eating disorders. NICE Clinical Guideline No 9. London: NICE, 2004. Available at: http://www.nice.org.uk.

74. Wilfley DE, Welch RR, Stein RI, et al. A randomized comparison of group cognitive-behavioral therapy and group interpersonal psychotherapy for the treatment of overweight individuals with binge eating disorder. Arch Gen Psychiatry 2002; 59:713–721.

75. Agras WS, Walsh BT, Fairburn CG, et al. A multicenter comparison of cognitive-behavioral therapy and interpersonal psychotherapy for bulimia nervosa. Arch Gen Psychiatry 2000; 57:459–566.

76. Grilo CM, Masheb RM, Wilson GT. Efficacy of cognitive behavioral therapy and fluoxetine for the treatment of binge eating disorder: a randomized double-blind placebo-controlled comparison. Biol Psychiatry 2005; 57:301–309.

77. Devlin MJ, Goldfein JA, Petkova E, et al. Cognitive behavioral therapy and fluoxetine as adjuncts to group behavioral therapy for binge eating disorder. Obes Res 2005; 13:1077–1088.

78. Grilo CM, Masheb R, Brownell KD, et al. Randomized comparison of cognitive behavioral therapy and behavioral weight loss treatments for obese persons with binge eating disorder. 8th London International Eating Disorders Conference, March 29–31, 2007.

79. Munsch S, Biedert E, Meyer A, et al. A randomized comparison of cognitive behavioral therapy and behavioral weight loss treatment for overweight individuals with binge eating disorder. Int J Eat Disord 2007; 40(2): 102–113.

80. Fairburn CG. Overcoming Binge Eating. New York: Guilford Press, 1995.

81. Latner JD, Wilson GT. Continuing care and self-help in the treatment of obesity. In: Latner JD, Wilson GT, eds. Self-help for Obesity and Eating Disorders. New York: Guilford Press, 2007.

82. Grilo CM. Guided self-help for binge eating disorder. In: Latner J, Wilson GT, eds. Self-Help for Obesity and Binge Eating. New York: Guilford Press, 2007:73–91.

83. Grilo CM, Masheb RM. A randomized controlled comparison of guided self-help cognitive behavioral therapy and behavioral weight loss for binge eating disorder. Behav Res Ther 2005; 43:1509–1525.

84. Brownell KD. The LEARN Program for Weight Management. Dallas: American Health Publishing, 2000.

85. Wilfley DE, Wilson GT, Agras WS. Psychological Treatment of Binge Eating Disorder. Association for Behavioral and Cognitive Therapies, Chicago, IL, November 16–19, 2006.

86. Grilo CM, Masheb RM, Wilson GT. Subtyping binge eating disorder. J Consult Clin Psychol 2001; 69:1066–1072.

87. Wilfley DE, Agras WS, Telch CF, et al. Group cognitive-behavioral therapy and group interpersonal psychotherapy for the nonpurging bulimic individual: a controlled comparison. J Consult Clin Psychol 1993; 61:296–305.

88. Foster GD, Kendall PC, Wadden TA, et al. Psychological effects of weight loss and regain: a prospective evaluation. J Consult Clin Psychol 1996; 64:752–757.

89. National Task Force on the Prevention and Treatment of Obesity. Dieting and the development of eating disorders in overweight and obese adults. Int J Eat Disord 2000; 17:395–401.

90. Gladis MM, Wadden TA, Vogt R, et al. Behavioral treatment of obese binge eaters: do they need different care? J Psychosom Res 1998; 44:375–384.

91. Gormally J, Black S, Daston S, et al. The assessment of binge-eating severity among obese persons. Addict Behav 1982; 7:47–55.

92. Greeno CG, Wing RR, Marcus MD. How many donuts in a "binge"? Women with BED eat more but do not have more restrictive standards than weight-matched non-BED women. Addict Behav 1999; 24:299–303.

93. Sherwood NE, Jeffery RW, Wing RR. Binge status as a predictor of weight loss treatment outcome. Int J Obes 1999; 23:485–493.

94. Marchesini G, Natale S, Chierici S, et al. Effects of cognitive-behavior therapy on health-related quality of life in obese subjects with and without binge eating disorder. Int J Obes 2002; 26:1261–1267.

95. Fairburn CG, Cooper Z. The Eating Disorder Examination. 12th ed. In: Fairburn CG, Wilson GT, eds. Binge Eating: Nature, Assessment, and Treatment. New York: Guilford Press, 1993.

96. Wadden TA, Foster GD, Letizia KA. Response of obese binge eaters to treatment by behavior therapy combined with very low calorie diet. J Consult Clin Psychol 1992; 60:808–811.

97. Telch CF, Agras WS. The effects of a very low calorie diet on binge eating. Behav Ther 1993; 24:177–193.

98. Garner DM, Wooley SC. Confronting the failure of behavioral and dietary treatments of obesity. Clin Psychol Rev 1991; 6:58–137.

99. Wadden TA, Butryn ML, Byrne KJ. Efficacy of lifestyle modification for long-term weight control. Obes Res 2004; 12:151S–162S.

100. Jacobs-Pilipski MJ, Wilfley DE, Crow SJ, et al. Placebo response in binge eating disorder. Int J Eat Disord 2007; 40:204–211.

101. American Psychiatric Association. Practice Guideline for Treatment of Patients With Eating Disorders. 3rd ed. Washington, D.C.: American Psychiatric Press, 2006.

102. Wilson GT, Grilo C, Vitousek K. Psychological treatment of eating disorders. Am Psychol 2007; 62:199–216.

103. Ricca V, Mannucci E, Mezzani B, et al. Fluoxetine and fluvoxamine combined with individual cognitive-behavioral therapy in binge eating disorder: a one-year follow-up study. Psychother Psychosom 2001; 70:298–306.

104. Grilo CM, Masheb RM, Wilson GT. Rapid response to treatment for binge eating disorder. J Consult Clin Psychol 2006; 74:602–612.

105. Fairburn CG, Agras WS, Walsh BT, et al. Prediction of outcome in bulimia nervosa by early change in treatment. Am J Psychiatry 2004; 161:2322–2324.

106. Walsh BT, Sysko R, Parides MK. Early response to desipramine among women with bulimia nervosa. Int J Eat Disord 2006; 39:72–75.

107. Appolinario JC, Bacaltchuk J, Sichieri R, et al. A randomized, double-blind, placebo-controlled study of sibutramine in the treatment of binge eating disorder. Arch Gen Psychiatry 2003; 60:1109–1116.

108. Grilo CM, Masheb RM, Salant SL. Cognitive behavioral therapy guided self-help and orlistat for the treatment of binge eating disorder: a randomized, double-blind, placebo-controlled trial. Biol Psychiatry 2005; 57: 1193–1201.

109. McElroy SL, Arnold LM, Shapira NA, et al. Topiramate in the treatment of binge eating disorder associated with obesity: a randomized placebo-controlled trial. Am J Psychiatry 2003; 160:255–261.

110. McElroy SL, Shapira NA, Arnold LM, et al. Topiramate in the long-term treatment of binge-eating disorder associated with obesity. J Clin Psychiatry 2004; 65:1463–1469.

111. McElroy SL, Hudson JI, Capece JA, et al. Topiramate for the treatment of binge eating disorder associated with obesity: a placebo-controlled study. Biol Psychiatry 2007; 61:1039–1048.

112. Niego S, Kofman MD, Weiss JJ, et al. Binge eating in the bariatric surgery population: a review of the literature. Int J Eat Disord 2007; 40:349–359.

113. Kalarchian MA, Wilson GT, Brolin RE, et al. Effects of bariatric surgery on binge eating and related psychopathology. Eat Weight Disord 1999; 4:1–5.

114. White MA, Masheb RM, Rothschild BS, et al. The prognostic significance of regular binge eating in extremely obese gastric bypass patients: 124-month postoperative outcomes. J Clin Psychiatry 2006; 67:1928–1935.

115. Powers PS, Perez A, Boyd F, et al. Eating pathology before and after bariatric surgery: a prospective study. Int J Eat Disord 1999; 25:293–300.

116. Adami GF, Meneghelli A, Scopinaro N. Night eating and binge eating disorder in obese patients. Int J Eat Disord 1999; 25:335–338.

117. Boan J, Kolotkin RL, Westman EC. Binge eating, quality of life and physical activity improve after Roux-en-Y

gastric bypass for morbid obesity. Obes Surg 2004; 14:341–348.

118. Dymek-Valentine M, Rienecke-Hoste R, Alverdy J. Assessment of binge eating disorder in morbidly obese patients evaluated for gastric bypass: SCID versus QEWP-R. Eat Weight Disord 2004; 9(3):211–216.

119. Bocchieri-Ricciardi LE, Chen EY, Munoz D, et al. Presurgery binge eating status: effect on eating behavior and weight outcome after gastric bypass. Obes Surg 2006; 16:1198–1204.

120. Buddeberg-Fischer B, Klaghofer R, Krug L, et al. Physical and psychosocial outcome in morbidly obese patients with and without bariatric surgery: a 4 1/2-year follow-up. Obes Surg 2006; 16:321–330.

121. Fairburn CG, Cooper Z, Doll HA, et al. The natural course of bulimia nervosa and binge eating disorder in young women. Arch Gen Psychiatry 2000; 57:659–665.

122. Burgmer R, Grigutsch K, Zipfel S, et al. The influence of eating behavior and eating pathology on weight loss after gastric restriction operations. Obes Surg 2005; 15:684–691.

123. Malone M, Alger-Mayer S. Binge status and quality of life after gastric bypass surgery: a one-year study. Obes Res 2004; 12:473–481.

124. Busetto L, Segato G, De Luca M, et al. Weight loss and postoperative complications in morbidly obese patients with binge eating disorder treated by laparoscopic adjustable gastric banding. Obes Surg 2005; 15:195–201.

125. Green AE, Dymek-Valentine M, Pytluk S, et al. Psychosocial outcome of gastric bypass surgery for patients with and without binge eating. Obes Surg 2004; 14:975–985.

126. Hsu LKG, Betancourt S, Sullivan SP. Eating disturbances before and after vertical banded gastroplasty: a pilot study. Int J Eat Disord 1996; 19:23–34.

127. Larsen JK, Geenen R, van Ramshorst B, et al. Binge eating and exercise behavior after surgery for severe obesity: a structural equation model. Int J Eat Disord 2006; 39:369–375.

128. Burgmer R, Grigutsch K, Zipfel S et al. The influence of eating behavior and eating pathology on weight loss after gastric restriction operations. Obes Surg 2005; 15: 684–691.

129. Kalarchian MA, Marcus MD, Wilson GT, et al. Binge eating among gastric bypass patients at long-term follow-up. Obes Surg 2002; 12:270–275.

130. Jeffery RW, Drewnowski A, Epstein LH, et al. Long-term maintenance of weight loss: current status. Health Psychol 2000; 19(suppl):5–16.

37

Special Issues in Treatment of Pediatric Obesity

ROBERT E. KRAMER

Section of Pediatric Gastroenterology, Hepatology, and Nutrition, The Children's Hospital, University of Colorado School of Medicine, Aurora, Colorado, U.S.A.

STEPHEN R. DANIELS

Department of Pediatrics, The Children's Hospital, University of Colorado School of Medicine, Aurora, Colorado, U.S.A.

INTRODUCTION

The prevalence and severity of obesity in children and adolescents have been increasing over the past 15 years (1). This has been associated with increases in the prevalence of type 2 diabetes mellitus (2) and hypertension (3) among other adverse health outcomes. These trends have resulted in increased urgency regarding the prevention and treatment of obesity in young individuals to interrupt processes that are associated with increasing obesity and comorbidities in adulthood and possibly, a decrease in life expectancy (4).

In many ways, the treatment of obesity in children and adolescents is similar to that in adults; however, there are some important considerations in this younger population. There is a substantially smaller database regarding treatment of obesity in children and adolescents. This means that making evidence-based decisions is substantially more difficult. This is especially true for making decisions regarding the use of pharmacologic agents and bariatric surgery. Another important difference for children and adolescents is the fact that they are growing and developing. This means

that younger patients may be more vulnerable to side effects of different interventions. On the other hand, it may also mean that more modest targets for changing weight are acceptable. For example, in a growing child, maintenance of weight may lead to a decline in body mass index (BMI) as the child grows in height. It is also important to recognize that single cutpoints for BMI are not useful for children and adolescents because normal BMI changes with increasing age. This has resulted in the use of percentiles of BMI as the way to characterize adiposity in the clinical setting. The most recent recommendation is that children and adolescents between the 85th to 95th percentile be classified as overweight and that children at the 95th percentile and above be considered obese (5). In addition, recent studies have identified that the 99th percentile for BMI is a cutpoint above which the risk of comorbidities increases substantially (6). This may ultimately be important in making decisions regarding the intensity of treatment in young patients. In the subsequent sections, we present treatment approaches of obesity for children and adolescents and highlight areas of difference between pediatric and adult patients.

OBESITY ISSUES BY AGE

Infant/Toddler

Overview

In general, infancy and early childhood are not considered as times during development when treatment of obesity is most important. As shown by Whitaker et al., the risk of adult obesity is less strong when overweight is present early in life, particularly if the parents are not overweight, compared with overweight later in childhood or adolescence (7). On the other hand, there is increasing epidemiologic evidence that nutrition and weight gain early in life have great importance for future weight gain and obesity (8,9). For these reasons, clinical issues early in life are more likely to be focused on prevention rather than treatment of obesity.

Traditionally, overweight in patients younger than two years has been evaluated using weight for height rather than BMI percentiles. This is in part because BMI percentiles are not readily available for this age group. There are no accepted cutpoints for defining obesity using weight for height; however, higher percentiles and crossing to higher percentiles with increasing age are a concern.

Calorie restriction in children younger than two years is generally not recommended because of rapid growth and development. An important caveat is whether healthcare providers determine from the diet history that a patient is ingesting a far greater number of calories than would be required for normal growth. It may also be useful to evaluate from which food sources those extra calories arise so that an intervention can be devised.

If extreme obesity is found early in life, especially if height growth is impaired, a genetic or syndromic form of obesity such as Prader-Willi should be considered. This should lead to referral to a geneticist or other provider experienced in these forms of obesity for further evaluation and treatment. In addition, genetic counseling for families may be warranted.

Role of Physical Activity

It is difficult to be prescriptive about physical activity in this age group. However, parents can be counseled on ways to encourage increased physical activity and decreased sedentary time. Parents should be aware that experiences early in life, with physical activity, may provide important modeling for future activity patterns. Television watching should be discouraged for the first 12 months of life. However, in practical terms, this may be difficult in families with multiple children of different ages. Parents should not allow children to have television in their bedrooms. In addition, television watching during meals should be discouraged.

Role of Infant Nutrition

Breast-feeding has been a nutritional area of potential interest. Several studies have suggested that breast-feeding may be associated with a lower risk for future obesity (10,11). This could be due to a number of factors, including the fact that breast-feeding may allow the infant and mother to regulate intake based more on hunger cues than on other factors. However, this relationship could also be due to the confounding effect that mothers who breast-feed are more likely to promote other healthful behaviors for the infant, including those related to diet and physical activity throughout life. In addition, not all studies of breast-feeding have shown a protective effect against obesity development (12,13). Further research is needed for better understanding.

Adiposity Rebound

Another issue during the first few years of life is the phenomenon of BMI rebound. This is a time during development when BMI reaches nadir and begins to increase. This usually happens between age four and six years. An earlier age at BMI rebound has been associated with an increased risk of future obesity, independent of the level of BMI at the age of rebound (14,15). Earlier BMI rebound is also associated with increased risk of diabetes in adulthood (16). The mechanism of BMI rebound is not known. It is also not known whether clinical intervention can lead to BMI rebound at a later age and a reduction in the risk for obesity. Further, research is needed to evaluate the clinical relevance for BMI rebound.

The role of sleep

There is a growing body of evidence linking sleep deprivation to metabolic changes that increase subsequent risk for obesity and diabetes. Mechanistically, these changes have been hypothesized to occur through increase in appetite (17,18), impairment of growth hormone secretion due to decreased non–rapid eye movement sleep (19,20), decreased energy expenditure (21), and increased cortisol levels (22). Several cohort studies in young children, ages five to seven years, have been performed that illustrate an increased risk of obesity in children with decreased amount of sleep, ranging from less than 10 to 10.5 hours per night (23–25). In a Japanese cohort of 8274 children, odds ratios increased in a dose-dependent fashion with decreasing sleep, ranging from 1.49 in those with 9 to 10 hours per night to 2.87 in those with less than eight hours per night (25). The long-term effects of these early alterations in sleep on metabolism require further research; however, the study by Reilly demonstrated that short sleep duration at age three independently increased the risk of obesity at age seven (24).

Intervention

Patterns of diet and physical activity are established early in life and may persist during childhood, adolescence, and young adulthood. The early patterns are often reinforced by parents and are established at an age when parents have substantial control over the home environment with respect to availability of food, patterns of eating, and patterns of physical activity. Thus, intervention early in life has the potential for long-lasting effects. This emphasizes the importance of nutrition and activity counseling as part of primary well-child care. It would be optimum if infants or young children at the highest risk of future obesity could be identified. This would allow for targeted intervention that would be the most cost-effective investment of resources. Unfortunately, the current state of knowledge does not allow such prediction with certainty, nor is it certain which interventions would be most likely to be successful in prevention or treatment of obesity.

School Age/Preadolescent

Overview

Review of the most recent data from the National Health and Nutrition Examination Survey (NHANES) through 2004 estimates the prevalence of obesity, defined as a BMI > 95th percentile, as 18.8% in children between the ages of 6 and 11. This data continues the trend observed in previous NHANES surveys, having increased from 16.3% in 2002 and 15.1% in 2000 (1). The number of obese school-aged children in the United States is therefore more than 4 million (26). This obesity prevalence is even higher in the non-Hispanic black population and Mexican-American population of children aged 6 to 11, where it was found to be 22.0% and 22.5%, respectively. With an additional 37.2% of children with a BMI between 85% and 95%, more than 11.8 million of the nation's estimated 21 million children between the ages of 6 and 11 are either overweight or obese.

Role of the School Environment

There has been a growing awareness of the important role the school environment plays in both development and prevention of pediatric obesity. Much of this attention has been focused on the nutritional value of school lunches, availability of competitive foods within schools, and diminishing frequency of physical education. The National School Lunch Program was established in 1946 and currently provides free or reduced-cost lunch to more than 29 million students per day in the United States. Although federal guidelines exist that establish the

minimal acceptable nutritional value of these meals, specific choices about what items are offered to students is primarily determined by individual school districts. The federal guidelines require that an individual student's intake has no more than 30% of calories from fat, less than 10% of calories from saturated fat, and provide one-third of the recommended dietary allowance (RDA) for vitamin A, vitamin C, iron, calcium, protein, and total calories. Although these broad macronutrient guidelines follow the conventional recommendations, concern still exists regarding the nutritional value of the individual food items offered on these school menus and whether the food choices made by a given child still conform to these guidelines.

The role of competitive foods available to students is yet another controversial topic, pitting the nutritional interests of children against the financial needs of many public schools. These competitive foods, also termed Foods of Minimal Nutritional Value (FMNV), which may be offered in vending machines, snack carts or sold a la carte in cafeterias, are exempt from the U.S. Department of Agriculture (USDA) standards required for school breakfasts and lunches. With the growing recognition that these competitive foods may be contributing to the current obesity epidemic in children, many school districts are now imposing additional restrictions, as part of the federally mandated Wellness policies that all schools were required to have in place by 2006. A survey of the nation's largest school districts showed that by 2004, 39% had adopted a policy that in some way restricted competitive foods, with most being directed at restriction of soft drinks (63%) and vending machines (95%) (27). Nevertheless, 89.5% of schools surveyed by the Centers for Disease Control and Prevention (CDC) in the 2004 School Health Profiles offered competitive foods to students, with 95.4% of those offering sugar-sweetened beverages and only 44.5% offering fruits or vegetables (28).

With increased pressure on school systems to validate academic achievement of students through the use of standardized testing, paired with limited budgets, there has been a steady decrease in the frequency and quality of physical education programs in public schools. U.S. Department of Education statistics verify that the mean number of days of physical education class for elementary school students is 2.4/wk. In fifth grade students, physical education classes at least twice per week were associated with a 39% decreased risk for childhood overweight and a 46% decreased risk of obesity (29). School-based interventions designed to increase physical activity have shown success in improving BMI (30), and those states with more stringent physical education requirements for their schools do have increased physical activity among students (31).

The implications of the obesogenicity of the school environment on obesity treatment in this age group are myriad. On an individual level, there may be limited changes that can be made to this environment, where the child obviously spends a large proportion of his or her time. Nevertheless, examination of the specific school factors contributing to excessive weight, while counseling the child and family on the potential pitfalls of the school environment, is often invaluable in initiating a lifestyle modification program. Despite the federally mandated parameters for school meals, having the child bring lunch to school rather than purchasing it may be protective, as buying lunch was shown in one study to increase obesity risk by 39% (29). Eating breakfast at home may also be beneficial. Restricting access to competitive foods at school by sending children to school without money may also be an effective strategy. Encouragement of active participation in physical education classes and implementation of a program of walking or riding to and from school, when feasible, are additional methods that are useful in this age group. Clearly from the standpoint of advocacy, as well as obesity prevention, there are many more interventions that are worth pursuing. Adequate funding for public schools, allowing them to provide structured, well-designed physical education classes, appropriate playgrounds, and facilities for active play and the financial independence from competitive food sale revenue, is a key goal. Furthermore, a uniform definition of competitive foods, as well as federally mandated minimal nutritional requirements for all foods offered to students, is sorely needed.

Developmental Aspects

When addressing overweight and obesity issues in the school-aged child, the developmental capabilities of the child must shape the approach of the caregiver. It is important to recognize the developmental issues occurring during this time, typically referred to as the latency period, between the ages of 6 and 11. During latency, children are beginning to construct their social identity: trying to understand who they really are and how others see them (32). Intellectually, they become able to categorize themselves into various recognizable groups that help them to form their social identity. They are developing the ability to reason logically and can conceptualize relational differences in mass, size, and weight. For the overweight child, these new cognitive abilities may enable greater feelings of isolation and recognition of the stigmatization of being overweight. Erickson defined this stage of development as one of "industry versus inferiority" in which children try to develop a belief in their own ability by performing and competing within a peer group (28,33). The overweight child faces consistent challenges in this struggle to

measure up to peers, reflected in the negative attitudes toward obesity offered by adults and children alike. Evidence suggests that the stigmatization of obese school-aged children by their peers, originally reported in the classic study by Richardson in 1961 (34), has worsened over a 40-year period. In the replicated study, when subjects were asked to rank who they liked best, 49.4% ranked the obese child last among a series of six drawings depicting children with various physical deformities (35). These negative attitudes are internalized within the context of the developing social identity of the latency phase, further damaging self-esteem. Sensitivity toward these developmental issues is vital if the caregiver is to engage the child in a discussion of obesity and lifestyle modification without "defining the child" as being inferior or inept.

Instead, focus should be maintained on the child's positive attributes, regarding what achievements he or she has been able to attain in relation to peers. It may be beneficial to point out how common a problem obesity has become among children of this age group and to stress that the motivation to make lifestyle changes should be driven by improvement in health rather than the necessity to make the child appear "like everybody else." Developmentally, the child is now able to understand the concept of reversibility as well as past and present. Thus, the child can understand that changing past behavior that brought about obesity can reverse this state for the future.

Attainment of these new developmental milestones allows the school-aged child to be engaged as an active participant in a lifestyle modification program on a level not possible in a child younger than seven. In many aspects, this is an ideal time to initiate a treatment regimen, since their ability to participate is far greater than the younger age group, yet the degree of supervision and parental control over the environment is still far greater than is commonly the case among adolescents. Furthermore, the degree of obesity, maladaptive behaviors, and related comorbidities are much less pronounced than in their adolescent counterparts.

Television

It has been determined that children now spend more time watching television, videotapes, and video games than any other activity other than sleeping (36). Between the ages of 2 and 17, the average American child watches more than three years of television (37). This pattern of sedentary activity is strongly implicated in the obesity epidemic through a number of epidemiologic studies. First, hours of television viewing has been found to have an inverse relationship to both physical activity (38,39) and physical fitness (40,41). Additionally, television viewing has been found to adversely impact intake of dietary fat and calories (42,43). Having a television in the bedroom has been found to result in watching significantly more hours of TV per week (17.4 ± 0.5 vs. 12.8 ± 0.3) and having a greater risk of overweight (odds ratio 1.31, CI 1.01–1.69), even in preschool children (44). Reduction in television viewing has, therefore, been proposed as an effective target for obesity prevention in children. This strategy was successfully utilized in Robinson's 1999 randomized controlled trial of a school-based educational program designed to decrease television and videotape viewing among third and fourth grade students from two public elementary schools. Results demonstrated a significant decrease in the television viewing of the intervention group to approximately two-thirds of baseline levels. More importantly, compared with the control group, there was a significant relative decrease in the BMI, triceps skinfold thickness, waist circumference, and waist-to-hip ratio, with the greatest effect among those with more adiposity (45).

Besides the direct effect of television in decreasing energy expenditure of children during viewing, TV and other media, shape their conceptions about their own body image. Development of gender identity is an important component of the overall social identity constructed during the latency phase outlined above. This process entails the child identifying himself or herself as either male or female and defining the criteria of both the masculine and feminine personas. Initially, much of the social context for defining these roles is derived from the child's parents. Increasingly, however, the child looks to outside sources to consolidate these ideas further. Not surprisingly, television and other media outlets have a profound influence in framing these concepts in many children. Children, who now spend more time watching TV and other media than ever before, are bombarded with images of large-breasted yet waif-thin women and thin, extremely muscular men. Not surprisingly, the amount of exposure to soap operas, music videos, and movies has been correlated with the degree of body image dissatisfaction and desire to be thin (28,46). The growing gap between what our society idealizes as the proper shape of a woman and the reality of what most women truly look like is reflected in the fashion industry. The typical fashion model twenty-five years ago was just 8% thinner than the typical women, but by 1999 that gap had risen to 23% (47). This influence may result in pathologic responses in those trying to conform to the ideals portrayed in the media. A startling example of the power of this influence was illustrated in Becker's study, which demonstrated increased rates of eating disorders among native Fijians adolescent females after the introduction of television in 1995. Prior to this media exposure, eating disorders in this population were essentially nonexistent (48).

Additional concerns about television exposure and its influence on obesity stems from the direct marketing of food products to children. A study by Connor examined standardized viewing blocks of programming on three different networks aimed at children. Results showed that the average 30-minute block of programming had 1.4 food advertisements, more than half of which were directed at children, with the majority promoting fast food restaurants or sugar-sweetened cereal (49). A multinational study, in 10 different countries, found a correlation of 0.85 between the prevalence of childhood obesity and the number of "obesogenic" advertisements per 20-hour block of children's programming. In this study, the United States was the leader in the prevalence of obesity and the number of obesogenic advertisements, defined as those promoting sweet or fatty foods or those promoting sedentary behaviors, such as toys, computer games, movies, or music (50). The efficacy of this advertising is likely due, in part, to the inability of children to comprehend the intent of advertising and, in many cases, to differentiate the advertisements from the actual programming (51). This data and similar studies have led some countries to restrict or ban advertising aimed directly at children, considering them a vulnerable population.

Beverage Intake

Excessive caloric intake from beverages is an important contributing factor in the development of obesity across all age groups. In the school-aged child, however, it becomes particularly important, as maladaptive consumption patterns initiated in early childhood may become further entrenched by behavioral modeling observed in peers while in the school setting. In addition, the school environment is often the first setting in which the child has both the exposure to additional sugar-sweetened beverages as well as relative autonomy to make beverage selection choices. Thus, it is a critical period in managing this potential risk factor for the development of obesity. Fruit juice consumption has been implicated as being associated with childhood obesity as well as short stature (52,53). Data comparing energy intake from sweetened beverage consumption in children between 1977 and 2001 showed an increase of 135%, coupled with an increase of total energy intake of 4.2% (54). Fruit drink consumption, specifically, increased significantly in terms of mean serving size (13.1 oz/serving to 18.9 oz/serving) and in its percent of total daily calorie intake by 89% (1.8–3.4%).

The relationship between milk intake and the development of obesity is less defined. The study by Nielsen of changes in beverage intake between 1977 and 2001 (54) demonstrates a decrease in the number of servings of milk per day (3.46 vs. 2.75), the mean serving size (15.4 vs. 13.6 oz/serving) and the percent of total calorie intake due to milk (13.2–8.3%) in children 2 to18 years of age. Nevertheless, current federal nutritional guidelines advocate 1% of skim milk for children greater than two years of age (55). A study of 1938 low-income preschool children, however, revealed that 75% of the children drank whole milk exclusively, with only 6.9% drinking skim or 1% milk (56). Black race and Hispanic ethnicity were both found to be independently associated with consumption of whole milk; both the groups demonstrated to have higher prevalence of pediatric obesity. The strongest predictor of type of milk consumed by the child was parental belief about which type of milk is healthiest for children, suggesting that interventions targeting parental education will be important to change behavior. If an intervention were successful in changing milk consumption from whole milk to 1%, it would decrease energy intake from milk by 34% (0.63–0.42 kcal/mL). Obviously the effect size of this type of intervention on an individual basis will depend on the quantity of milk consumed per day. Bearing in mind, however, that in most cases obesity is the result of small, sustained overconsumption of calories over a prolonged period, these small decreases may achieve a large effect on health and nutrition if initiated at an early age.

Adolescent

Overview

Review of NHANES data on adolescents through 2004 shows increases in obesity similar to other age groups. Obesity prevalence in children of 12 to 19 years of age has significantly increased from 14.8% in 2000 to 16.7% in 2002 to 17.4% in 2004. Again, this prevalence is even higher among non-Hispanic blacks (21.8%) but has been decreasing in adolescent Mexican-Americans, from 23.2% in 2000 to 21.1% in 2002 to 16.3% in 2004. Nevertheless, the odds ratio of Mexican-American children being obese, compared with a non-Hispanic white child, was 1.73 for males and 1.56 for females. For non-Hispanic blacks, the odds ratio was 1.13 for males and 1.46 for females. There was also an increasing risk of obesity associated with age, as the odds ratios for obesity in adolescents versus those of two- to five-year-olds were 1.56 for males and 1.50 for females. Using the most recent U.S. Census data from 2000 with more than 32 million children between the ages of 12 and 19 years, this amounts to at least 5.6 million obese and 11 million overweight adolescents in the United States.

Discrimination and Impact on Quality of Life

The psychosocial implications of obesity within Western culture are profound, impacting nearly every aspect of life. Despite the fact that obesity prevalence among children and adults continues to increase, bias and prejudice against those suffering from obesity continues unabated. Adolescence is traditionally characterized by psychosocial difficulties in relating to one's peers, even without the added challenge of this negative obesity bias. In Swallen's analysis of health-related quality of life in 4827 adolescents, obesity was associated with an increased odds ratio of reporting impairment within the areas of general health (2.17) and functional limitations (1.81) compared with nonobese peers. Interestingly, significant impairment in psychosocial quality of life for the obese adolescents was only seen in the younger 12- to 14-age group, with increased odds ratios of depression (3.04), low self-esteem (3.47), and poor school and social functioning (2.33), without significant effects at older ages of 15 to 20 (57). The pervasive effects of increasing weight on perceived quality of life in children has led to the development and validation of a specific measure, the impact of weight on quality of life-kids (IWQOL-Kids) to measure this impact and track changes over time (58).

Within the realm of sexual development, there is ample evidence of the negative impact that overweight and obesity has on desirability and sexual activity. Studies in both adolescents and adults have shown the obese to be viewed as less attractive (59), date less often (60), have fewer sexual partners (61), and a decreased sexual quality of life (62). Surprisingly, this sexual stigmatization of the obese is shared even by those who are themselves overweight or obese (63). The societal bias against obesity, however, is not merely confined to peer and romantic relationships. Long-term educational and economic disadvantages to obese adolescents have been demonstrated as well, with decreased college acceptance rates (64), less financial support from parents of obese daughters (65), and increased poverty rates (66).

Developmental Aspects/Lack of Parental Control

The developmental issues taking place in the adolescent phase primarily revolve around the consolidation of the various aspects of the autonomous, gender, sexual, peer, and social identities into one comprehensive "overall" or emancipated identity (32). This process is greatly influenced by the physical changes brought on by puberty, which generally compels the adolescent to pay more attention to their bodies. This increased body awareness engenders both internal responses as well as external perceptions about how others are viewing these physical changes. These influences help develop the adolescent's body image. The implications obesity may have on these developmental processes are profound. During this phase, adolescents are already becoming better able to reconcile their concept of an "ideal self" with more realistic ambitions and ideals. The negative consequences of the societal obesity bias, as outlined above, may frame these more "realistic" views of the identity and body image, perhaps creating the roots for a subsequent eating disorder.

While these developmental changes may place the obese child at greater risk of psychologic comorbidity, there are numerous aspects that allow the adolescent patient to be a more insightful and motivated candidate for an obesity treatment program. Having the interest and motivation of the adolescent is absolutely critical at this stage, as the parental influence on the child's environment is typically lower than at any other time. It is at this stage that adolescents often struggle to demonstrate their own views and opinions as separate from that of their parents, further limiting the impact parents may have as part of a weight loss program. Nevertheless, it is during adolescence that children enter into what Piaget termed the "formal cognitive phase" of development, where they become more adept at logical thinking and rational thought (67). Whereas in the latency period, children are preoccupied with the present, during adolescence there is a growing appreciation for how their own thoughts may affect their future. They can process information about the past, present, and the future to use in addressing problems or issues. There is also a growing awareness that their own actions are not always under their direct conscious control and that there may be unconscious issues that account for their behavior (32). The astute clinician will integrate these developmental aspects into their care of the obese adolescent, to engage them on a level they were not previously capable of. With this greater degree of insight into the contributing factors involved in their own obesity and the implications these insights may have for the individual's own future, the adolescent may be in a more appropriate position to make the behavioral changes necessary to be successful in an obesity program.

Development and Treatment of Comorbidities

With increasing age, the prevalence of obesity-related comorbid conditions increases as well. It is therefore incumbent upon the clinician caring for these patients to be vigilant in screening for these commonly associated conditions and be prepared to either initiate treatment or refer the patient to an appropriate pediatric subspecialist. For most of these comorbidities, the preferred treatment is significant weight loss through lifestyle and behavior modification. For those patients who are unwilling or unable to achieve adequate weight loss to sufficiently control these comorbidities, the risks and benefits of adjunctive pharmacotherapy must be carefully weighed. Use of these agents in children has not been nearly as well defined as in adults; however, there is increasing experience among pediatric practitioners forced to deal with the consequences of the growing obesity epidemic.

Type 2 diabetes mellitus

The prevalence of type 2 diabetes in children has seen a dramatic rise in recent years. Pinhas-Hamiel et al. documented a 10-fold increase in the number of pediatric type 2 diabetes patients diagnosed from 1982 to 1994 (2). Like obesity itself, the increase in diabetes was particularly pronounced among minority groups. In addition, it is estimated that 2 million adolescents in the United States, and more than 16% of overweight teens have prediabetes (68). The long-term implications of this rapid increase in children are not known. However, type 2 diabetes is a condition with serious morbidity and mortality when diagnosed in adults. The logical presumption would be that the sequelae would become even more significant with disease onset in childhood. A study by Panzram found a 17-year loss in life expectancy if diabetes was diagnosed by age 14 (69).

Prior to development of frank diabetes, the intermediate steps of impaired glucose tolerance and impaired fasting glycemia are typically noted and often classified as "prediabetes." These patients may typically have serum glucose and glycosylated hemoglobin levels within normal limits. Specific categorization for fasting plasma glucose define normal as below 100 mg/dL, impaired fasting glycemia as between 100 and 125 mg/dL, and levels greater than 125 mg/dL as being consistent with a provisional diagnosis of diabetes. For oral glucose tolerance testing, a two-hour postload glucose of less than 140 mg/dL is defined as normal, between 140 and 199 mg/dL is defined as impaired glucose tolerance, and greater than 200 mg/dL is defined as provisional diabetes (70). Another useful indicator of impaired carbohydrate metabolism is the homeostasis model assessment of insulin resistance (HOMA-IR) (71). The HOMA-IR utilizes the fasting insulin and glucose to calculate an index of insulin resistance, which correlates closely with more costly and invasive measures of insulin resistance, such as the hyperinsulinemic-euglycemic clamp (72). The HOMA is calculated by dividing the product of the fasting insulin level (in $\mu U/mL$) and glucose level (in mg/dL) by 402. The cutoff value to define insulin resistance in adults has been defined as 2.5 (71). In adolescent patients, however, cutoff values of HOMA-IR have not been well established. Utilizing oral glucose tolerance tests as the standard, Keskin et al. established a cutoff point of 3.16 in adolescents to define insulin resistance (72). The higher cutoff in adolescents is likely a reflection of the transient influence of puberty in increasing insulin resistance (73). Applying this cutoff to data from the NHANES from 1999 to 2002, Lee et al. found the prevalence of insulin resistance in adolescents to be 18% in normal weight, 42% in overweight, and 75% in obese subjects (74).

Treatment of type 2 diabetes in adolescents remains highly individualized and must account for the severity of illness, the developmental stage, the socioeconomic status of the family, and the patient's historical adherence/compliance with treatments up to that point. The base of the treatment pyramid should rest upon a foundation of diet and activity modification, although these are rarely adequate to achieve glycemic control. Pharmacotherapy is typically required, including insulin therapy, oral antidiabetic agents, or combination therapy. Oral agents offer the advantage of simplicity and improved compliance compared with injected insulin. Of the oral insulin-sensitizing agents, metformin is the most commonly prescribed with proven safety and efficacy in children (75). For those with severe disease, insulin therapy will be most effective in rapidly regaining glycemic control (76). Specific dosing and treatment strategies utilizing the various insulin analogs are beyond the scope of this chapter. However, multicenter studies aimed at determining the optimal treatment regimen for type 2 diabetes in children are ongoing (77).

The use of oral insulin-sensitizing agents such as metformin for prediabetes or insulin resistance remains more controversial. Srinivasan et al. demonstrated significant reduction in weight, BMI, and measures of insulin resistance with metformin at a dose of 1 g b.i.d., compared with placebo in a double-blind crossover trial of 28 obese children (78). Larger studies will be needed to determine if early treatment with metformin for obese adolescents with isolated insulin resistance has long-term benefits in terms of improving weight loss and decreasing progression to type 2 diabetes and other comorbidities.

Dyslipidemia and atherosclerosis

It has now been well established that the atherosclerotic disease process may begin in childhood and track into adulthood. The Pathobiological Determinants of Atherosclerosis in Youth (PDAY) study was the first autopsy study of adolescents and young adults to find that the extent of atherosclerotic lesions correlated directly to risk factors such as hyperlipidemia and hypertension (79). A subsequent autopsy study in children, as part of the Bogalusa Heart Study, was able to demonstrate characteristic atherosclerotic lesions in the coronary arteries of children as young as 10, with fatty streaks present in up to 50% and fibrous plaques in 8% of those studied. The degree of atherosclerosis was proportional to the number of risk factors present, including increased BMI, elevated blood pressure, elevated total cholesterol, low-density lipoprotein (LDL) cholesterol, and triglycerides (80). As in adults, this relationship between dyslipidemia and atherosclerosis argues for treatment of lipid abnormalities to delay or prevent premature cardiovascular disease.

In 1992, a consensus report from the National Cholesterol Education Program established guidelines for screening and management of dyslipidemia in children and adolescents (81). These guidelines were limited by the relative lack of adequate placebo-controlled trials of lipid-lowering agents in children. Since that time, however, there have been several studies documenting the safety and efficacy of a variety of 3-hydroxy-3-methyl-glutaryl coenzyme A (HMG CoA) reductase inhibitors in adolescents, including lovastatin (82–84), simvastatin (85), pravastatin (86,87), and atorvastatin (88). Although these studies were performed in patients with familial hypercholesterolemia, safety and efficacy were similar to adult studies involving obese patients with secondary dyslipidemia. There has been no evidence of adverse effects on growth or development. The primary adverse events noted were mildly elevated liver aminotransferases, typically not significantly greater than placebo or less than twice the upper limit of normal. Elevated creatinine phosphokinase levels and myopathy have also been described in adults receiving HMG CoA reductase inhibitor therapy. Dosing for these studies ranged from 10- to 40-mg/day, with reduction in total cholesterol from 17% to 31%, reduction in LDL from 17% to 41%, increase in high-density lipoprotein (HDL) from 2% to 11% (with one study showing a decrease of 23%) and change in triglycerides from +9% to 18%. Although long-term studies are needed to further demonstrate the safety of these agents in children, they are generally considered the first-line pharmacologic therapy for adolescent hyperlipidemia and have pediatric labeling from the Food and Drug Administration (FDA).

Other agents that have been shown to be effective in adolescents have been bile acid–binding resins [cholestyramine (89,90) and colestipol (91,92)], niacin (93), and fibrates (94). Generally, bile acid-binding agents in children are limited by poor palatability and compliance and may potentially increase triglyceride levels. Although they may cause gastrointestinal upset and decrease fat-soluble vitamin levels, they are not systemically absorbed and are considered safe. Niacin therapy in children was complicated by a high prevalence of adverse effects, including abdominal pain, flushing, vomiting, headache, and elevated aminotransferases, resulting in 38% of subjects discontinuing therapy. Fibrates primarily act to lower triglycerides and are less likely than the statins to elevate liver aminotransferases. They may cause gastrointestinal upset, cholelithiasis, myopathy, or rhabdomyolysis.

In 2007, the American Heart Association published a revised set of guidelines regarding pharmacologic therapy of dyslipidemia in children and adolescents, which are as follows, adapted from McCrindle et al. (88):

1. Screening should be performed with a fasting lipid profile in those with a positive family history or with overweight/obesity, along with other aspects of the metabolic syndrome (insulin resistance, diabetes, hypertension, central adiposity).

2. Consider therapy for children ≥ 10 years (and post-menarche in females) who have failed a 6- to 12-month trial of therapy with a low-fat/low-cholesterol diet.

3. Consider therapy for LDL ≥ 190 mg/dL or LDL ≥ 160 mg/dL, with either a family history of premature cardiovascular disease or with more than two other risk factors present in the child.

4. Treatment goals are ideally LDL ≤ 110 mg/dL, or minimally LDL ≤ 130 mg/dL.

5. For those meeting criteria for treatment, statin drugs are recommended as the first line of therapy.

6. Additional factors that may warrant consideration of therapy below an LDL of 190 mg/dL or earlier than 10 years of age include male gender, strong family history of premature cardiovascular disease, presence of low HDL/high triglycerides/small dense LDL, overweight/obese, metabolic syndrome, hypertension, smoking or passive smoke exposure, presence of increased risk markers such as elevated C-reactive protein, lipoprotein (a), homocysteine.

The Council also recommended further study to examine the long-term safety and efficacy of lipid-lowering drug therapy in children and adolescents.

Nonalcoholic fatty liver disease

In 1980, Ludwig published the first description of a form of liver disease in which there were histopathologic changes, including hepatic steatosis, inflammation, and fibrosis. This entity was termed nonalcoholic steatohepatitis (NASH) and has been associated with obesity, type 2 diabetes, and hyperlipidemia (95). Subsequently, this term was broadened to nonalcoholic fatty liver disease (NAFLD) to include the entire spectrum of this disorder from simple steatosis through to steatohepatitis, with associated inflammatory and fibrotic changes. Current estimates of the prevalence of this form of liver disease in children are startling. In an autopsy study of children who died of unrelated causes, Schwimmer et al. found a population prevalence of fatty liver disease in children of 9.6%, with a 38% prevalence in obese children (96). Therefore, with greater than 5.6 million obese adolescents in the United States, prevalence of NAFLD in this population may be as high as 2.1 million. On the basis of adult cross-sectional studies of NAFLD showing cirrhosis on liver biopsy in up to 14% of subjects (97), pediatric cirrhosis cases could total as high as 300,000. This would be an unprecedented epidemic of pediatric liver disease and have tremendous implications for pediatric and adult liver transplantation.

Screening for NAFLD remains problematic. The most common presentation is with asymptomatic elevation of liver transaminases, most specifically alanine aminotransferase (ALT), in the 1.5 to 4 times the upper limit of normal range. Hepatic ultrasound has been used as a noninvasive screening test for NAFLD, demonstrating increased echogenicity due to fatty infiltration of the liver. Ultrasound, however, is unable to discriminate simple steatosis from more advanced fibrotic lesions found in steatohepatitis. Elevated HOMA scores of insulin resistance and uric acid levels have also been found to be independently associated with NAFLD in adults (98) and children (99). With the increasing prevalence of obesity in children, attributing increased transaminases in all obese patients to NAFLD risks missing alternative etiologies of liver disease in this age group. Therefore, screening for viral hepatitis, autoimmune hepatitis, Wilson's disease, and alpha 1 antitrypsin deficiency should be considered as well. For cases with persistent elevation of transaminases for greater than six months, percutaneous liver biopsy provides greater sensitivity and specificity than ultrasound and can help exclude other causes of liver disease.

Treatment guidelines for NAFLD have yet to be established. Lavine performed the first study to document the efficacy of antioxidant vitamin E treatment in decreasing transaminases in children with NAFLD (100). Without liver biopsies, however, to follow the degree of inflammation, it is difficult to assess whether vitamin E truly changes the natural history of this disease. Bile acid supplementation has been proposed to be a potential therapy for NAFLD; however, a review of the pooled published adult literature on the subject failed to find any significant benefit (101), as did the one pediatric study (102). With the strong link between insulin resistance and NAFLD, much interest has focused on the use of insulin-sensitizing agents for treatment. A small study of 10 pediatric patients with NAFLD treated with metformin 500 mg b.i.d. for six months demonstrated significant reduction in ALT level and percent liver fat measured by MR spectroscopy (103). A large prospective study of metformin in children is underway as part of the NASH Clinical Research Network.

Metabolic syndrome

The metabolic syndrome has been defined as a clustering of physiologic risk factors that in concert confer an increased risk for the development of type 2 diabetes and atherosclerotic cardiovascular disease. The ability to predict increased risk for morbidity is arguably even more critical in the evaluation of pediatric patients than it is in adults. The prevalence of the metabolic syndrome among U.S. adolescents has been estimated to be 6.4%, with a prevalence as high as 32.1% in obese teens, based on data from the 1999–2000 NHANES. This would correspond to more than 2 million affected adolescents in the United States alone (104).

Yet the defining criteria for the metabolic syndrome in the adolescent age group remain elusive and controversial.

The adult criteria have been well established, with two primary recognized definitions, from the National Cholesterol Education Program Adult Treatment Panel III and from the International Diabetes Federation. The Adult Treatment Panel (ATP) guidelines require three of the five following criteria: central adiposity (defined as a waist circumference $\geq$102 cm in men and $\geq$88 cm in women), high systolic or diastolic blood pressure (defined as systolic $\geq$130 mmHg or diastolic $\geq$85 mmHg), decreased HDL cholesterol (defined as <40 mg/dL in men and <50 mg/dL in women), increased triglycerides (defined as >150 mg/dL) and elevated glucose levels (defined as $\geq$100 mg/dL). The International Diabetes Federation (IDF) criteria are similar, with the exception that they require that elevated waist circumference be one of the three criteria necessary and use different cutoff points than the ATP ($\geq$94 cm in men and $\geq$80 cm in women) for waist circumference. The cutoff points for the other parameters are identical.

To date, there has not been a universally accepted set of criteria to define adolescent metabolic syndrome. Many have proposed utilizing the same basic diagnostic parameters but altering cutoff points to correspond with age- and gender-specific percentiles, typically at the 90th percentile. Others have developed pediatric cutoff points by taking data from population-based studies of children and extrapolating curves that correspond to the ATP and IDF cutoffs for adults (105). Recently, the IDF has published a set of guidelines to define the metabolic syndrome in children of 10 to 16 years of age. All must have evidence of central adiposity, defined as a waist circumference $\geq$ the 90th percentile for age and gender. They must then meet at least two of the following four criteria: triglycerides $\geq$150 mg/dL, HDL-cholesterol <40 mg/dL, systolic blood pressure $\geq$130 mmHg or diastolic blood pressure $\geq$85 mmHg, or serum glucose >100 mg/dL, or known type 2 diabetes. For adolescents of 16 years or older, the adult IDF criteria can be used. The IDF advised against making a diagnosis of metabolic syndrome in children younger than 10 years but recommended close follow-up of these same parameters for children with a waist circumference above the 90th percentile and with a positive family history.

In the clinical setting, beyond the challenge of deciding which set of diagnostic criteria to use in defining the metabolic syndrome in adolescents, controversy exists over the validity of applying this model to children. Specifically, Goodman et al. documented the instability of the diagnosis of metabolic syndrome in 1098 adolescents with repeated measures over a three-year period. They found that subjects initially diagnosed with metabolic syndrome lost the diagnosis on follow-up assessment of 49% to 56% of the time, depending upon which set of diagnostic criteria were used to define the disease (106).

This significant degree of within-subject variability over time in this age group questions the validity and utility of the metabolic syndrome in adolescents. Certainly, in considering pharmacologic therapy for treatment of metabolic syndrome in teens, one must keep this variability in mind. Metformin therapy has been used in adults with the metabolic syndrome, but placebo-controlled trials in adolescents are lacking.

Hypertension

Unlike adults, the definition of hypertension in the pediatric population is not based on cutoff values directly associated with increased risk of adverse cardiovascular events, but rather on population studies of blood pressure distribution in normal children. It is known in adults that at a blood pressure above 120/80, the increased risk of adverse events begins to accrue (107); however, in children significant elevation of blood pressure begins with either a systolic or diastolic blood pressure above the 90th percentile for age, gender, and height. Specific percentile curves for blood pressure have been published, delineating the 50th, 90th, 95th, and 99th percentiles (108). The limitations of using a single blood pressure measurement, taken in the office setting, to classify or diagnose hypertension have been well documented, especially in children (109). Current guidelines therefore recommend that elevated blood pressure be documented on at least three occasions, using an appropriate cuff size, before labeling a child as hypertensive. Ambulatory monitoring of blood pressure has also been advocated for this reason. Elevated blood pressure has been classified by percentile into prehypertension ($\geq$90th and $\leq$95th percentile or $\geq$120/80 in adolescents), hypertension ($\geq$95th percentile), stage 1 hypertension (95th to 99th percentile + 5 mmHg) and stage 2 hypertension ($\geq$99th percentile + 5 mmHg) (108).

After diagnosing hypertension in a child, identification of any underlying etiology should be sought. For the majority of obese pediatric patients, elevated blood pressure is the result of primary hypertension, which is often associated with a number of other risk factors such as positive family history, hyperlipidemia, insulin resistance/diabetes, and obstructive sleep apnea. Nevertheless, screening for renal disease as a cause of secondary hypertension is indicated for any child with persistent elevation in BP $\geq$95th percentile. The extent of this evaluation should be individualized, depending on the age of the patient and severity of the elevation, but could potentially include blood urea nitrogen (BUN)/creatinine, electrolytes, urine culture, urinalysis, complete blood count (CBC), and renal ultrasound.

Treatment is usually centered around lifestyle modification with weight reduction, with pharmacologic treatment reserved for those with either stage 2 hypertension, secondary hypertension, evidence of end-organ damage, symptomatic hypertension, or diabetes. Pharmacologic treatment may also be considered for those with persistent hypertension despite an adequate trial of therapeutic lifestyle changes. Specific changes that have been validated in adult trials are increase in fruit, vegetable, and low-fat dairy intake (110), sodium restriction (111), increased physical activity (112), and weight reduction (113). For those patients meeting criteria for initiation of pharmacologic therapy, monotherapy with a single agent should be initiated, with a goal of decreasing BP to <95th percentile. There are an increasing number of approved medications for management of pediatric hypertension, and accepted classes include angiotensin-converting enzyme (ACE) inhibitors, calcium channel blockers, diuretics, β-blockers and angiotensin receptor blockers. ACE inhibitors and angiotensin receptor blockers are both contraindicated in pregnancy and must be used with reliable contraception in sexually active females of childbearing age. Once treatment is initiated, patients should be reevaluated every two to four weeks until adequate control has been reached. If control is not achieved, the dose should be increased until control is achieved or the maximum dose is reached. If control is still not achieved, addition of a second, complementary agent should be considered. Further studies are needed to develop guidelines on endpoints of therapy and to directly compare efficacy of different therapies in specific classes of patients.

Polycystic ovary syndrome

Menstrual irregularity is a commonly encountered complaint in obese adolescent females, and care must be taken to differentiate normal irregularity associated with the recent onset of menarche from polycystic ovary syndrome (PCOS). A careful menstrual history is important to determine if irregular menses have been occurring since menarche or if there ever was an intervening period of regular menstruation that subsequently became perturbed. PCOS is a heterogenous disorder characterized by hyperandrogenism, chronic anovulation, and polycystic ovaries on ultrasound. It is commonly associated with acne, hirsutism, obesity, metabolic syndrome, infertility, and menstrual dysfunction (114). Patients with PCOS are at increased risk for type 2 diabetes and insulin resistance is suspected to be involved in its pathogenesis.

Diagnostic criteria for PCOS remain controversial, with two commonly proposed definitions (115,116). The first, from the 1990 National Institutes of Health (NIH) criteria, necessitates both chronic anovulation as well as clinical or biochemical evidence of hyperandrogenism. The second, from the 2003 Rotterdam criteria, is somewhat less stringent, requiring at least two of the following: polycystic ovaries, chronic anovulation, and clinical or biochemical evidence of hyperandrogenism. These guidelines become further complicated by the lack of consensus regarding the definition of each of these criteria. Clinical assessment of

hyperandrogenism can be regarded as subjective assessment of acne, hirsutism, and/or female pattern alopecia. Although hirsutism is present in about 60% of patients with PCOS, its prevalence differs among various ethnic groups (117). Similarly acne is typically deemed an unreliable indicator. The alopecia is more commonly found in older women, and therefore, not as helpful in the assessment of obese adolescents. Biochemical determination of hyperandrogenism has limitations as well, with no universally accepted assay. Most commonly, elevation in total serum testosterone is used, although biochemical testing may fail to identify PCOS in 20% to 40% of patients, and many commercial assays have not been validated for women (118). Alternatively, plasma luteinizing hormone (LH) levels are elevated while follicle-stimulating hormone (FSH) levels are normal, resulting in an elevated LH:FSH ratio, usually greater than two to three. The definition of chronic anovulation is more straightforward, with either less than eight menses per year or more than three consecutive months without menses in the absence of pregnancy. Polycystic ovaries on ultrasound are an obvious defining characteristic, but assessment of ovarian cysts has been limited to transvaginal ultrasound where more than 12 follicles between 2 and 9 mm are identified. For the more commonly utilized transabdominal ultrasound, assessment of follicles, especially in obese females, is unreliable, and therefore, ovarian volume of >10 mL has been defined as diagnostic of PCOS (119).

Baseline prevalence of PCOS, using the NIH criteria, is between 6.5% and 8%, with up to 66% of PCOS patients either overweight or obese (120). Treatment strategies for PCOS include lifestyle changes, oral contraceptives, and insulin-sensitizing agents such as metformin. Even modest reduction in weight has been shown to restore ovulation in 71% of obese PCOS patients (121). Oral contraceptives are the most commonly prescribed treatment for PCOS. However, their use in obese patients remains controversial due to their propensity to decrease insulin sensitivity and exacerbate dyslipidemia (122). Conversely, metformin was shown in a meta-analysis to induce ovulation in 46% of PCOS patients (123). Uncontrolled studies of metformin in adolescents with PCOS have shown modest but significant improvement in BMI, dyslipidemia, insulin resistance, and anovulation (124–126). Further study is needed to better define this disorder in adolescents and develop an evidence base to more effectively guide treatment.

OBESITY IN SPECIAL POPULATIONS

Acquired Brain Injury/CNS Malignancy

Obesity secondary to hypothalamic injury has been well documented in children as a consequence of acute lymphoblastic leukemia (127,128) and cranial irradiation for malignancy (129,130). The ventromedial hypothalamus (VMH) is responsible for receiving hormonally mediated signals from the periphery regarding caloric intake, macronutrient composition, and adipose stores to impact satiety and feeding behavior. Receptors for insulin, leptin, and ghrelin modulate the activity of neurons producing neuropeptide Y and agouti-related protein to promote feeding behavior and of neurons that produce cocaine and amphetamine regulated transcript and α-melanocyte-stimulating hormone (α-MSH) to promote satiety. Thus, damage to the VMH may induce obesity by interfering with these satiety signals, with the development of secondary hyperinsulinemia (131). Alternatively, others have postulated that excessive insulin secretion in response to meals due to decreased VMH inhibition of vagal stimulation on pancreatic β-cells results in increased adipose storage of energy and obesity (132). The somatostatin analog octreotide has been proposed as a potential therapy for excessive weight gain associated with hypothalamic injury, due to its inhibitory effect on insulin release from β-cells. Small, open-label, and placebo-controlled trials of octreotide in pediatric patients with hypothalamic obesity have demonstrated efficacy in stabilizing weight gain, with good tolerance (133,134). Although a limited trial of topiramate in adults with acquired brain injury showed efficacy in those with binge-eating characteristics, no trials have been performed in the pediatric population of brain-injured patients (135).

Genetic Syndromes

A variety of genetic syndromes have been found to be commonly associated with morbid obesity and these patients often are particularly challenging to treat. These are discussed in chapter 3.

Psychiatric Illness

Depression

Clinical depression is a relatively common condition, with a 12-month prevalence of 6.7% in the U.S. adult population. It is associated with significant morbidity and mortality (136). Reported prevalence and incidence of depression within the pediatric population varies greatly depending on the age group studied and the criteria used to make the diagnosis. Overall, the prevalence of depression in childhood has been estimated at 2%, with rates as high as 9% reported for adolescents (137). The morbidity and mortality of clinical depression in children are significant. Perhaps the most concerning of these is the risk of suicide, which is the third leading cause of death in children older than 10 years (138). Not surprisingly, the majority of suicide victims suffer from major depression

around the time of death (139). Children and adolescents with depression have a risk up to 7.7% to commit suicide in future years and have a fivefold increased risk for suicide attempts (140).

The relationship between depression and obesity in both adults and children has not been clarified. In adolescent females, obese and nonobese subjects were screened for depression and anxiety, only to find that obese adolescent females had "normative discontent" but no significant depression or anxiety (141). Other studies, however, have documented a significant association between obesity and depression in children and adolescents, with rates of depression ranging from 23% to 32% (142–144). A cross-sectional study of 3101 adolescents found that those above the 90th percentile in their depression scores were twice as likely to be obese (145).

A number of plausible theories exist to explain the association of obesity and depression, and it is quite likely that many, if not all, are involved in some patients at some point in time. In contrast to reactive depression following stigmatization of the obese child, decreases in activity, medications, illicit drug or alcohol use, excessive sleep, and anhedonia in the depressed patient may be mechanisms by which depression may lead to obesity. Nevertheless, alterations in appetite and satiety are symptoms common to both disorders and may offer a compelling explanation for their observed comorbidity. As a result, simultaneous pharmacologic treatment of depression and obesity remains an attractive strategy.

Serotonin has long been known to be closely involved in the regulation of feeding behavior and satiety, and a number of medications that alter serotonin metabolism have been studied as potential therapies for weight loss, in addition to depression. Currently, among serotonin selective reuptake inhibitors (SSRIs), FDA-approved pharmacologic therapy for depression in adolescents is limited to fluoxetine. High-dose fluoxetine was shown in a small study of morbidly obese adult patients awaiting bariatric surgery to result in greater weight loss than in control patients and prompted almost a third of them to postpone surgery by at least six months (146). Other studies have shown modest efficacy of fluoxetine for weight loss in obese adults with diabetes (147,148). In clinical practice, numerous other antidepressant medications are used to treat childhood depression, despite lack of specific FDA approval. Other SSRIs have been generally associated with greater likelihood of weight gain compared with fluoxetine, although no clinical trials have directly compared the effect of various antidepressants on weight in either adults or children. Newer, more highly SSRIs such as escitalopram have been proposed to be more effective for weight loss (149), but clinical trials have not demonstrated any proven benefit over placebo (150). Sibutramine, a serotonin and noradrenaline reuptake inhibitor originally developed as an antidepressant, has been studied in adults and adolescents as an appetite-suppressant and has shown efficacy over placebo (151,152). Its efficacy for treatment of childhood depression, however, has not been studied. In both depressed and nondepressed adults, the serotonin, dopamine, and norepinephrine reuptake inhibitor bupropion has been shown to result in increased weight loss compared with placebo (153,154) but has not yet been studied in the pediatric population.

For children with severe psychiatric morbidity, it may often be necessary to address their psychopathology with appropriate family and individual psychotherapy before attempting to engage them in a comprehensive weight loss program. The psychologic damage that may occur from half-hearted attempts and subsequent failure of a weight loss regimen may result in significant weight gain and decreased success rates for future weight loss trials. Prompt referral and close cooperation with psychiatric caregivers is vital in the treatment of this challenging subgroup of patients.

Schizophrenia

Obesity has already been well established as a commonly encountered comorbidity in patients with schizophrenia (155). Treatment of schizophrenia, however, has been associated with even greater prevalence of obesity due to the effects of antipsychotic medications (156). Newer, atypical antipsychotics, such as risperidone and olanzapine, are being more used in pediatric patients due to their decreased risk of extrapyramidal side effects and greater efficacy in controlling psychiatric symptoms. Unfortunately, they have also been associated with even greater risk of obesity. A prospective study by Ratzoni et al. directly compared weight gain among 50 adolescents with schizophrenia, schizoaffective disorder, or conduct disorder started on treatment with olanzapine, risperidone, or haloperidol over a 12-week period (157). The olanzapine group had the greatest weight gain of 7.2 ± 6.3 kg, followed by risperidone at 3.9 ± 4.8 kg and haloperidol at 1.1 ± 3.3 kg. Risk factors for increased weight gain with antipsychotics are low initial BMI, a history of obesity in the patient's father, and female gender with low concern about weight gain. Treatment for antipsychotic-induced weight gain should focus on prevention, with initiation of lifestyle modification measures at the time medications are first prescribed. Alternatively, for those who have already developed excessive weight gain due to these medications, consideration should be given to switching agents to something more weight neutral, such as ziprasidone (158).

Binge Eating Disorder

Binge eating disorder (BED) has been described as the most common of all eating disorders and has been clearly associated with obesity. BED shares the primary characteristic of uncontrolled periods of eating with bulimia nervosa but differs in that there are no compensatory behaviors, such as purging or excessive exercising. Use of adult criteria to define BED in children and adolescents is controversial. A modified, broader definition of BED in adolescents has been proposed by Marcus and Kalarchian (159). These criteria define BED as having

A. recurrent episodes of binge eating, with both of the following:
   1. Food-seeking behavior in the absence of hunger
   2. A sense of lack of control over eating
B. binge episodes associated with at least one of the following:
   1. Food seeking in response to a negative affect, such as sadness or boredom
   2. Food seeking as a reward
   3. Sneaking or hiding food
C. persistence of symptoms for at least three months
D. eating tendency not associated with regular use of compensatory behavior, such as purging, fasting, or excessive exercise.

Growing evidence indicates that BED may develop from two distinctive phenotypes. The first, which typically presents at a later age, is characterized by the onset of binge eating following the initiation of dieting. The second, which typically has an earlier onset, is characterized by the onset of binge eating before the initiation of dieting, reported in 33% to 55% of adult BED patients (160,161). This group tended to have onset of binge eating between 11 and 13 years of age and had greater evidence of psychiatric disturbance. Epidemiologic studies of BED have shown a variable prevalence of binge eating, with one showing 30% in obese adolescent girls between 14 and 16 (162), while another showed a prevalence of those meeting BED criteria at 5.3% in overweight children 6 to 10 years of age (163). Binge episodes were reported in 36.5% of 126 children in an obesity residential treatment program, supporting the notion that binge eating is common in overweight children and adolescents (164).

Treatment of BED, like other eating disorders, requires special consideration and a multidisciplinary approach is preferred. Adjunctive pharmacologic therapy is often used and studies have shown efficacy of antidepressants, centrally acting appetite suppressants, and anticonvulsants. Comorbid psychopathology is not a prerequisite for use of pharmacologic therapy in BED. If present, however, the type of psychopathology may help guide the choice of therapy, with those having depression being prescribed antidepressants and those having bipolar disorder with anticonvulsants. Appetite suppressants such as sibutramine may be considered for those unresponsive to the other agents. Nevertheless, SSRIs are the most well-established therapies for BED (165). Further research is needed regarding pharmacologic treatment for BED among adolescents.

TREATMENT STRATEGIES FOR PEDIATRIC OBESITY

Multidisciplinary Approach

Overview

The most recent guideline for treatment of childhood obesity were constructed by an expert panel of the American Medical Association and published by Barlow (5). They recommend that treatment of overweight children be approached using a staged or stepped method that takes into account the child's age, BMI percentile, obesity related comorbidities, and the weight status of parents.

In this schema, stage 1 care should be implemented by the primary care physician and includes behavioral counseling with a focus on dietary habits and physical activity. This early intervention focuses on reduction of intake of sugar-sweetened beverages, consuming five or more servings of fruit and vegetables daily, limiting meals outside the home, eating breakfast daily, reducing screen time to less than two hours per day, and encouraging one hour or more of physical activity daily. This intervention should be implemented over a three- to six-month period. If there is little or no improvement based on this approach, then stage 2 intervention is warranted.

Stage 2 recommendations can also be performed in a primary care office setting but may be improved by involvement of allied health professionals such as dietitians trained in behavioral pediatric weight management. This stage includes a more structured approach to diet and activity behaviors. This intervention should be carried out over a three- to six-month period with a goal of weight maintenance or a loss of up to 1 lb/wk. If stage 2 is unsuccessful, stage 3 intervention may be considered.

Stages 3 to 4 include a comprehensive multidisciplinary approach to weight management. Stage 3 may occur in a primary care setting with appropriate referrals. Stage 3 intervention includes even more regimented and aggressive behavioral therapy, often directed by a pediatric psychologist or dietitian trained in behavior modification approaches. Often the approach, which is more labor-intensive, involves setting one behavior goal at a time and then moving on to additional goals once the initial favorable behavior has been established. For adolescents, this stage should involve individual approaches to behavior changes and skill building around decision making. For younger children, the focus is often on the parents and

may involve teaching parenting skills, which can be applied to diet and activity behaviors in the child.

The behavioral approach in stage 3 should also include self-monitoring (or family monitoring) of behaviors and stronger behavioral support, which includes setting specific behavioral goals and rewarding accomplishment of those goals. Rewards should be structured in a way to be positive reinforcement but should not be overly expensive. This can include opportunities for time spent with a parent or with friends and should not include food.

The goal of stage 3 is weight maintenance with continued growth or weight loss at a rate of 1 to 2 lb/wk. If there is no improvement in weight or BMI after three to six months and, particularly, if the patient is in higher BMI percentiles (99th percentile and above) or has comorbidities related to obesity, then stage 4 should be implemented.

Stage 4 should usually occur in a referral setting and should be delivered by a multidisciplinary team. The team should include pediatric physicians with training and experience in weight management, dietitians, exercise physiologists, pediatric psychologists, and may include a pediatric bariatric surgeon. Other disciplines that may be included are social workers, physical therapists, and occupational therapists. This team must also have ready access to pediatric subspecialists who can evaluate and treat comorbid conditions related to obesity. This would include endocrinologists (diabetes), pulmonary medicine specialists (sleep apnea), cardiologists (hypertension, dyslipidemia), gastroenterologists (nonalcoholic fatty liver disease), orthopedic surgeons, and neurologists. Pediatric psychiatrists may also be needed for patients with established psychopathology.

Stage 4 is the most intensive therapeutic approach used and is reserved for the most severely affected patients. This stage may include implementation of special diets, including very low-calorie diets, which require more intensive medical monitoring. Stage 4 may also include the use of pharmacologic agents and bariatric surgery. However, even with more aggressive treatment, behavior therapy should remain as an important component of the treatment plan. In stage 4, standard clinical protocols for patient selection, evaluation, and treatment should be in place. Mechanisms for evaluation of the treatment protocol and quality improvement should also be included.

It should be recognized that the development of pediatric obesity has a variety of important components, including the overall environment, the home environment, family behavioral dynamics, peer behavioral influences, and individual behavioral issues. Treatment paradigms at all four stages should address all of these to some extent. Perhaps the most important focus, especially for younger patients, is the home environment and family dynamics. This requires a family-based approach to therapy. If treatment is focused only on an individual child and his or her behaviors, then success is much less likely. Parents must understand the environmental factors that influence diet and physical activity behaviors. Intervention in a family context may be difficult because changing behaviors related to diet and physical activity often requires that everyone in the family make substantial changes. It may also be important for treatment team members to identify saboteurs who are not helping or who are actively working against the treatment plan.

This staged approach should be applicable to almost all pediatric patients. However, patients with physical or mental disabilities may require additional support. Unfortunately, at present, there is a limited base of evidence on which to design therapy for such patients.

Pharmacologic Treatment

Overview

There are fewer data regarding the safety and efficacy of pharmacologic treatment of obesity in pediatric compared with adult patients. This is important because, historically, the use of pharmacologic agents to treat obesity in adults has been complicated by less than optimum efficacy with the potential for substantial and, in some cases, unpredicted side effects. Thus, few pharmacologic agents are approved to treat obesity in adolescents and, in general, pharmacologic treatment of pediatric obesity is considered more in the realm of research than in routine clinical practice. Drugs that are approved for obesity treatment in adults are potentially available for off-label use in pediatric patients, but they should only be used with caution.

The most recent expert committee recommendations on the prevention, assessment, and treatment of child and adolescent overweight and obesity has developed a staged approach to the treatment of obesity in pediatric patients (5). Pharmacologic agents are reserved for use in tertiary care intervention. This would include a center with a multidisciplinary team, including a physician, nurse, dietitian, behavioral counselor, and an exercise specialist, all with experience in the treatment of pediatric obesity.

The expert panel recommended two medications for which there are some data in adolescent patients: sibutramine and orlistat (5). The FDA has approved orlistat for use in patients of 12 years and older. The FDA has approved the use of sibutramine in patients 16 years of age and older. Any use of medication to treat pediatric obesity should be combined with intensive behavioral treatment to reduce calorie consumption and increase physical activity. Without such combined intervention, it

is unlikely that the pharmacologic intervention will have a long-term effect.

Orlistat

Orlistat is an inhibitor of enteric lipase, which results in fat malabsorption. In individuals consuming a diet of approximately 30% of calories from fat, orlistat will result in a reduction of fat absorption of 30% (166). Orlistat is not systemically absorbed and does not have an effect on systemic lipases.

The major side effects of orlistat are gastrointestinal and result from fat malabsorption and steatorrhea. When dietary fat intake is low, orlistat is generally well tolerated with minimal side effects. As fat intake increases, increased side effects may be seen. These side effects include abdominal cramps, flatulence, fecal incontinence, and oily spotting.

Orlistat has been shown to improve weight management in obese adolescents compared with behavioral therapy alone. Chanoine et al. performed a randomized, double-blind, placebo-controlled clinical trial of orlistat in 539 obese adolescents aged 12 to 16 years (167). They found that BMI decreased by 0.55 kg/m^2 in the group who received orlistat compared with an increase of 0.31 kg/m^2 in the placebo group ($p < 0.01$) after 54 weeks of treatment. Compared with 15.7% of the placebo group, 26.5% of participants taking orlistat had a 5% or higher decrease in BMI. Dual energy X-ray absorptiometry demonstrated that these differences were due to decreases in fat mass in the group who received orlistat.

Side effects were more common in the orlistat group. Mild-to-moderate adverse events related to the gastrointestinal tract occurred in 9% to 50% of the orlistat group compared with 1% to 13% of the placebo group (167). Unfortunately, the side effects of orlistat may be more limiting in adolescents compared with adults in the clinical setting. Studies have shown that one of three adolescents who are prescribed orlistat is not compliant because of unpleasant gastrointestinal side effects (168).

Orlistat is now available in a low dose over the counter. The use of this new and more readily available formulation by adolescents remains to be determined. Orlistat should be taken with each meal. This may limit its utility in school-aged children and could potentially lead to disadvantageous patterns of eating in adolescents who do not want to take the medication at lunchtime at school.

Sibutramine

Sibutramine is a nonselective reuptake inhibitor that is most potent for serotonin and norepinephrine. It also blocks the reuptake of dopamine. As an agent for weight management, sibutramine appears to work most through the suppression of appetite. Sibutramine can cause vasoconstriction and has been associated with increased heart rate and blood pressure. In adults, the increase in heart rate and blood pressure has not been ameliorated by weight loss (169). In adults, sibutramine has been approved for an interval of treatment of two years.

The largest study of sibutramine in adolescents was published by Berkowitz et al. (152). In this study, 498 participants aged 12 to 16 years with a BMI at least two units greater than the 95th percentile were randomly allocated to treatment with sibutramine combined with behavioral therapy or placebo with behavioral therapy. In this study, 76% of the subjects in the sibutramine group and 62% of subjects in the placebo group completed the study. The sibutramine group had greater improvement in BMI (2.9 kg/m^2) than the placebo group (0.3 kg/m^2) ($p < 0.001$). A BMI reduction of $\geq 5\%$ and $\geq 10\%$ occurred in 62.3% and 38.89 of subjects treated with sibutramine, respectively, compared with 18.1% and 5.5% of subjects treated with placebo. The group treated with sibutramine also had greater improvements in triglycerides, HDL-cholesterol and insulin.

The side effects observed in adults were also evaluated in this study (152,170). Tachycardia was significantly more prevalent in the sibutramine group. None of the other adverse events, including hypertension (11% in the sibutramine group vs. 8% in the placebo group), were statistically and significantly more common in the sibutramine group compared to the placebo group. Overall, adverse events led to withdrawals in 6.3% of participants on sibutramine compared with 5.4% of participants in the placebo group. Increased blood pressure led to withdrawal in 1.4% of subjects in the sibutramine group compared to 0% in the placebo group.

In a subsequent analysis of the cardiovascular effects of sibutramine, small mean decreases in blood pressure and heart rate were seen in both the sibutramine and placebo groups (170). At the end of the study, the average systolic blood pressure had decreased 2.1 mmHg in both groups, diastolic blood pressure decreased 0.1 mmHg in the sibutramine group compared with 1.1 mmHg in the placebo group. From this analysis it appears that sibutramine may have the same direct cardiovascular effects in obese adolescents as seen in adults, but these effects may be balanced by the reduction in BMI associated with use of sibutramine.

Metformin

Metformin has not been approved for use in weight management. However, because it improves insulin resistance, some have advocated its use in patients judged to be at risk of type 2 diabetes mellitus. In studies related to type 2 diabetes, the use of metformin has been associated with weight loss (170). However, the mechanism through which metformin impacts weight is unclear. Its use is associated with decreased appetite in some patients. In studies of prevention of type 2 diabetes in adults who were at risk, metformin was effective in reducing the incidence of diabetes; however, the lifestyle intervention was even more effective (171). Orchard et al. found similar results for the metabolic syndrome (172).

It should be emphasized that the pediatric studies for all of these pharmacologic agents have been short term. In adults, the treatment effect associated with these agents appears to diminish over time and is eliminated completely with discontinuation of medication. This may result in rebound weight gain and ultimately increased BMI. No long-term data are available on either safety or efficacy in adolescents and studies have not included younger children. In addition, no studies have been performed that compare one pharmacologic agent to another, and studies have not been powered to see if agents may be more effective in one population versus another. For these reasons, pharmacologic agents should only be used after failure of behaviorally focused lifestyle intervention. If they are used, they should be used with close follow-up of the patient and with caution.

Bariatric Surgery

Bariatric surgery has become an accepted modality for treatment of severe obesity in adults (174). This has led to serious discussion regarding whether surgical approaches to obesity might also be acceptable for massively obese children and adolescents. However, there has been a relatively small evidence base on which to determine the safety, efficacy, and the most appropriate patients as well as the procedures for the population of young, severely obese patients. From a theoretical perspective, numerous clinical and ethical issues arise. Children and early adolescents are still growing. There has been concern that growth and sexual maturation in adolescents might be adversely affected by bariatric surgical procedures. In addition, pediatric patients younger than 18 years cannot provide consent for clinical interventions. This is in part a legal issue but also arises because cognitive development may not be sufficient for such patients to make a rational decision. This means that parents must provide consent, while adolescent patients can only provide assent. It has not been clear how to gauge the level of understanding of the potential risks and benefits of bariatric surgery for either parents or their adolescent offspring. It is not always easy to assess the motivation for pursuing bariatric surgery or the level of understanding that will provide the optimum postoperative behavior change to maximize the long-term efficacy and minimize potential adverse effects. Adolescents may have difficulty with adherence to regimens of vitamins and appropriate approaches to diet (174). There has also been concern about the psychologic issues in the aftermath of bariatric surgery. It has been documented that the quality of life of severely obese children and adolescents is likely to be low (175). However, it remains unknown whether bariatric surgery will appropriately improve quality of life for adolescents. It is not known how adolescents will respond to the changing body habitus that may occur with bariatric surgery. It is also not clear whether this will improve social interaction and integration. There is also uncertainty about whether severely obese adolescents, who may have previously been marginalized socially (176), will have the appropriate social skills to deal with such body changes. It is not known what level and type of psychologic and social support is needed for the adolescent and other family members to ensure a smooth and healthy transition after surgery. Adolescents are prone to risk-taking behaviors. Will such behaviors increase in the wake of bariatric surgery? How should health professionals and family members approach such risk taking that could include drinking alcohol, smoking cigarettes, taking illicit drugs, and high-risk sexual activity that could result in sexually transmitted diseases or pregnancy? It is with these background uncertainties that clinical decisions regarding adolescent bariatric surgery must be made.

The current recommendations for eligibility of adolescents for bariatric surgery are relatively conservative (177). These guidelines are primarily for the gastric bypass procedure and include adolescents who have completed growth in height and who have tried and failed at serious behavioral and/or pharmacologic attempts at weight management over at least a 6- to 12-month period. A patient with a BMI of 40 to 50 kg/m^2 can qualify if a major comorbid condition such as type 2 diabetes or severe obstructive sleep apnea is associated with his or her obesity. A patient with a BMI of 50 kg/m^2 or greater will qualify with less severe comorbidities, including hypertension, dyslipidemia, psychosocial distress, and interference of obesity in daily activities. All patients and their families must also undergo evaluation to determine their understanding of the procedure, potential risks and benefits, and their commitment to the behavioral changes in diet and physical activity that will be necessary in the postoperative period.

Given the numerous clinical issues regarding bariatric surgery in young patients, such procedures should only be performed in centers with experienced surgeons and a team that includes a dietitian, behavioral therapist, exercise physiologist, and pediatric/adolescent medicine. Appropriate training for pediatric surgeons performing bariatric surgery should ideally be obtained at a large bariatric center where adequate experience can be developed with suitable patient numbers. Because of the significant learning curve in performing these operations and providing proper postoperative management, patient care

may be best served by consolidating these procedures in a few specialized pediatric centers. Because bariatric surgery is not a cure for obesity, but rather a tool to be used in treatment, long-term follow-up is needed to ensure optimal success. In addition, adolescent bariatric surgical centers should maintain appropriate clinical databases from which lessons about the procedures can be learned and quality improvement can be initiated.

At the present time there are two main potential surgical options, the Roux-en-Y gastric bypass and the adjustable gastric band procedure. However, the device currently used for gastric banding has not been approved by the FDA for use in patients younger than 18 years. Both approaches have been shown in preliminary studies to result in weight loss in adolescents (178,179). Gastric bypass has been shown to result in substantial weight loss and resolution of comorbidities in adolescents (179).

Nadler et al. have published results in adolescent patients, aged 13 to 17 years, using adjustable gastric banding (178). Fifty-three patients received the operation, 41 were female, the mean age was 15.9 years, and the mean initial BMI was 47.6 kg/m^2. The percent of excess weight lost was 37.5% at six months, 62.7% at 12 months, and 48.5% at 18 months follow-up postoperatively. There were no intraoperative complications, but two patients had slipping of the band that required laparoscopic repositioning, and one patient developed a wound infection. There were some postoperative dietary complications, including iron deficiency in four patients and hair loss in five patients. One patient had nephrolithiasis and cholelithiasis postoperatively.

Abu-Abeid et al. reported on 11 patients aged 11 to 17 years who underwent adjustable gastric band surgery (180). They found that mean BMI was reduced from 46.6 to 32.1 kg/m^2 at a mean follow-up of 23 months postoperatively, with few complications in their experience. Dolan et al. reviewed experience in seven adolescents after receiving the adjustable gastric band (181). In their analysis, BMI was reduced from 44.7 kg/m^2 preoperatively to 30.2 kg/m^2 after 24 months of follow-up postoperatively.

Retrospective studies have also been published regarding the gastric bypass operation in adolescents. Sugerman et al. reported on 33 severely obese adolescents with a mean age of 16 years and a mean BMI of 52 kg/m^2 (range 38–91) who underwent the procedure (182), following some of the patients as long as 14 years after their surgery. The majority of patients had substantial and sustained weight loss after the procedure. However, nine patients had subsequent weight regain. Sugerman et al. were not able to identify factors related to weight regain. In their series, there were surgical complications in 13 patients and there were two sudden deaths at one and five years postoperatively.

Strauss et al. presented results on 10 adolescents younger than 17 years who underwent gastric bypass surgery

(183). The mean weight at surgery was 148 kg. They found that 9 of 10 adolescents had weight loss in excess of 30 kg with a mean weight loss of 53.6 kg. All obesity-related comorbid conditions were resolved. There were some nutritional problems, including five patients who had iron deficiency anemia and three who had folate deficiency. One patient required total parenteral nutrition for protein calorie malnutrition with vitamin A and D, iron, and zinc deficiency. Two patients had cholelithiasis. Inge et al. reported on the results of 40 adolescents who underwent gastric bypass at a mean age of 17 years and with a mean BMI of 56 kg/m^2 (184). They found that BMI changed from a mean of 56 to 39 kg/m^2 over the first six months of follow-up representing a 30% reduction. Body composition analysis at one year after surgery indicated that the ratio of fat to lean mass loss was 5:1, suggesting good preservation of lean body mass during weight loss. All of those studies taken together demonstrate substantial short-term weight loss in almost all patients. Limited longer-term follow-up suggests that regain of weight could be a problem for some patients. Better understanding of that phenomenon is needed.

Perioperative and postoperative risks are important for adolescent patients undergoing bariatric surgery. These risks should not be minimized because, while some are rare, they can be life threatening. Patients and their families must understand and accept the potential for these risks prior to undergoing the procedure. The mortality rate for bariatric surgical procedures is thought to be similar for adolescents and adults, approximately 0.5% for gastric bypass and 0.1% for gastric banding (185). Causes of death include anastomotic leaks with peritonitis and pulmonary embolism. In adults, lack of experience on the part of the surgeon or the supporting program, severe obesity (BMI $\geq$ 50 kg/m^2) and coexisting morbidity have been found to be factors that increase the risk of mortality (185,186). It is clear that these factors are likely to also be quite relevant to adolescent bariatric surgery, however, supportive specific data are lacking. Postoperative complications are often gastrointestinal but may also be due to nutritional and particularly vitamin insufficiency especially for procedures with a malabsorptive component, such as the gastric bypass operation. Deficiency of iron, folate, and vitamin B12 can occur as a result of the malabsorptive aspect of gastric bypass. Beriberi is a complication reported in adolescents, which is a particular concern (187). This complication can be avoided, but requires routine adherence with vitamin supplements. Adolescent compliance with this regimen has been reported to be quite low (6). Dehydration can also occur when adolescents fail to drink adequate fluids. This often occurs because postoperatively they must drink small amounts frequently. This may be difficult in some settings for adolescents, such as during the school day.

The most appropriate criteria for adolescents to be acceptable for bariatric surgery remain unclear. Availability of gastric banding with potentially lower perioperative risk, the ability to adjust the band or even remove it, and without a malabsorptive component raises the question regarding the appropriateness of intervention with that device at an earlier age or at a lower BMI threshold in pediatric patients. Recent research has suggested that the 99th percentile for BMI is a cutpoint at which the risk of comorbidity increases substantially (6). This may help to provide an evidence base on which to make these important decisions.

It should also be clear that new research is needed to better understand the best weight management strategies for severely overweight children and adolescents. This should include clinical databases with long-term follow-up of patient outcomes. It should also include randomized controlled clinical trials to compare outcomes in head-to-head comparisons of different treatment strategies. Until such data are available, there will be uncertainty regarding the best approach for individual patients, including the likely long-term success and risks.

REFERENCES

1. Ogden CL, Carroll MD, Curtin LR, et al. Prevalence of overweight and obesity in the United States, 1999–2004. JAMA 2006; 295(13):1549–1555.
2. Pinhas-Hamiel O, Dolan LM, Daniels SR, et al. Increased incidence of non-insulin-dependent diabetes mellitus among adolescents. J Pediatr 1996; 128(5 pt 1):608–615.
3. McNiece KL, Poffenbarger TS, Turner JL, et al. Prevalence of hypertension and pre-hypertension among adolescents. J Pediatr 2007; 150(6):640–644.
4. Olshansky SJ, Passaro DJ, Hershow RC, et al. A potential decline in life expectancy in the United States in the 21st century. N Engl J Med 2005; 352(11):1138–1145.
5. Barlow SE. Expert committee recommendations on the prevention, assessment and treatment of child and adolescent overweight and obesity: summary report. Pediatrics 2007; 120 (suppl 4):S164–S192.
6. Freedman DS, Mei Z, Srinivasan SR, et al. Cardiovascular risk factors and excess adiposity among overweight children and adolescents: the Bogalusa Heart Study. J Pediatr 2007; 150(1):12–17.
7. Whitaker RC, Wright JA, Pepe MS, et al. Predicting obesity in young adulthood from childhood and parental obesity. N Engl J Med 1997; 337(13):869–873.
8. Stettler N, Zemel BS, Kumanyika S, et al. Infant weight gain and childhood overweight status in a multicenter, cohort study. Pediatrics 2002; 109(2):194–199.
9. Stettler N, Stallings VA, Troxel AB, et al. Weight gain in the first week of life and overweight in adulthood: a cohort study of European American subjects fed infant formula. Circulation 2005; 111(15):1897–1903.

10. Gillman MW, Rifas-Shiman SL, Camargo CA Jr, et al. Risk of overweight among adolescents who were breastfed as infants. JAMA 2001; 285(19):2461–2467.

11. von Kries R, Koletzko B, Sauerwald T, et al. Breast feeding and obesity: cross sectional study. BMJ 1999; 319(7203):147–150.

12. Li L, Parsons TJ, Power C. Breast feeding and obesity in childhood: cross sectional study. BMJ 2003; 327 (7420):904–905.

13. Burdette HL, Whitaker RC, Hall WC, et al. Breastfeeding, introduction of complementary foods, and adiposity at 5 y of age. Am J Clin Nutr 2006; 83(3):550–558.

14. Whitaker RC, Pepe MS, Wright JA, et al. Early adiposity rebound and the risk of adult obesity. Pediatrics 1998; 101(3):E5.

15. Rolland-Cachera MF, Deheeger M, Guilloud-Bataille M, et al. Tracking the development of adiposity from one month of age to adulthood. Ann Hum Biol 1987; 14(3): 219–229.

16. Bhargava SK, Sachdev HS, Fall CH, et al. Relation of serial changes in childhood body-mass index to impaired glucose tolerance in young adulthood. N Engl J Med 2004; 350(9):865–875.

17. Simon C, Gronfier C, Schlienger JL, et al. Circadian and ultradian variations of leptin in normal man under continuous enteral nutrition: relationship to sleep and body temperature. J Clin Endocrinol Metab 1998; 83(6):1893–1899.

18. Dzaja A, Dalal MA, Himmerich H, et al. Sleep enhances nocturnal plasma ghrelin levels in healthy subjects. Am J Physiol Endocrinol Metab 2004; 286(6):E963–E967.

19. Van Cauter E, Copinschi G. Interrelationships between growth hormone and sleep. Growth Horm IGF Res 2000; 10(suppl B):S57–S62.

20. Van Cauter E, Leproult R, Plat L. Age-related changes in slow wave sleep and REM sleep and relationship with growth hormone and cortisol levels in healthy men. JAMA 2000; 284(7):861–868.

21. Briones B, Adams N, Strauss M, et al. Relationship between sleepiness and general health status. Sleep 1996; 19(7):583–588.

22. Spiegel K, Leproult R, Van Cauter E. Impact of sleep debt on metabolic and endocrine function. Lancet 1999; 354 (9188):1435–1439.

23. von Kries R, Toschke AM, Wurmser H, et al. Reduced risk for overweight and obesity in 5- and 6-y-old children by duration of sleep—a cross-sectional study. Int J Obes Relat Metab Disord 2002; 26(5):710–716.

24. Reilly JJ, Armstrong J, Dorosty AR, et al. Early life risk factors for obesity in childhood: cohort study. BMJ 2005; 330(7504):1357.

25. Sekine M, Yamagami T, Handa K, et al. A dose-response relationship between short sleeping hours and childhood obesity: results of the Toyama Birth Cohort Study. Child Care Health Dev 2002; 28(2):163–170.

26. U.S. Bureau of the Census. Census 2000 Summary File 1; 1990 Census of Population, General Population Characteristics, United States (1990 CP-1-1). Washington, D.C.: U.S. Bureau of the Census, 2000.

27. Greves HM, Rivara FP. Report card on school snack food policies among the United States' largest school districts in 2004–2005: room for improvement. Int J Behav Nutr Phys Act 2006; 3:1.

28. Centers for Disease Control and Prevention (CDC), Competitive foods and beverages available for purchase in secondary schools—selected sites, United States, 2004. MMWR Morb Mortal Wkly Rep 2005; 54(37):917–921.

29. Veugelers PJ, Fitzgerald AL. Prevalence of and risk factors for childhood overweight and obesity. CMAJ 2005; 173(6):607–613.

30. Sallis JF, McKenzie TL, Conway TL, et al. Environmental interventions for eating and physical activity: a randomized controlled trial in middle schools. Am J Prev Med 2003; 24(3):209–217.

31. Cawley J, Meyerhoefer C, Newhouse D. The impact of state physical education requirements on youth physical activity and overweight. Health Econ 2007; 16(12): 1287–1301.

32. Gemelli R. Normal Child and Adolescent Development. London: American Psychiatric Press, Inc., 1996.

33. Erikson E. Childhood and Society. New York: Norton, 1963.

34. Richardson SA, Goodman N, Hastorf AH. Cultural uniformity in reaction to physical disabilities. Am Soc Rev 1961; 26:241–247.

35. Latner JD, Stunkard AJ. Getting worse: the stigmatization of obese children. Obes Res 2003; 11(3):452–456.

36. Annenberg Public Policy Center, 1997. Available at http://annenbergpublicpolicycenter.org/Downloads/Media_and_Developing_Child/Media_and_TV_in_the_Home/19990628_Media_House_report.pdf.

37. Robinson TN. Does television cause childhood obesity? JAMA 1998; 279(12):959–960.

38. Robinson TN, Hammer LD, Killen JD, et al. Does television viewing increase obesity and reduce physical activity? Cross-sectional and longitudinal analyses among adolescent girls. Pediatrics 1993; 91(2):273–280.

39. DuRant RH, Baranowski T, Johnson M, et al. The relationship among television watching, physical activity, and body composition of young children. Pediatrics 1994; 94 (4 pt 1):449–455.

40. Pate RR, Corbin CB, Simons-Morton BG, et al. Physical education and its role in school health promotion. J Sch Health 1987; 57(10):445–450.

41. Tucker LA. The relationship of television viewing to physical fitness and obesity. Adolescence 1986; 21(84):797–806.

42. Robinson TN. Television advertising for health. Pediatr Ann 1995; 24(2):73–78.

43. Taras HL, Sallis JF, Patterson TL, et al. Television's influence on children's diet and physical activity. J Dev Behav Pediatr 1989; 10(4):176–180.

44. Dennison BA, Erb TA, Jenkins PL. Television viewing and television in bedroom associated with overweight risk among low-income preschool children. Pediatrics 2002; 109(6):1028–1035.

45. Robinson TN. Reducing children's television viewing to prevent obesity: a randomized controlled trial. JAMA 1999; 282(16):1561–1567.

46. Tiggemann M, Pickering AS. Role of television in adolescent women's body dissatisfaction and drive for thinness. Int J Eat Disord 1996; 20(2):199–203.

47. Kilbourne J. Deadly Persuasion: Why Women Must Fight the Addictive Power of Advertising. New York: Free Press, 1999.

48. Becker AE, Burwell RA, Gilman SE, et al. Eating behaviours and attitudes following prolonged exposure to television among ethnic Fijian adolescent girls. Br J Psychiatry 2002; 180:509–514.

49. Connor SM. Food-related advertising on preschool television: building brand recognition in young viewers. Pediatrics 2006; 118(4):1478–1485.

50. Lobstein T, Dibb S. Evidence of a possible link between obesogenic food advertising and child overweight. Obes Rev 2005; 6(3):203–208.

51. Schlosser E. Your Trusted Friends. Fast Food Nation. New York: HarperCollins Publishers, Inc., 2002:31–57.

52. Dennison BA, Rockwell HL, Baker SL. Excess fruit juice consumption by preschool-aged children is associated with short stature and obesity. Pediatrics 1997; 99(1):15–22.

53. Dennison BA, Rockwell HL, Nichols MJ, et al. Children's growth parameters vary by type of fruit juice consumed. J Am Coll Nutr 1999; 18(4):346–352.

54. Nielsen SJ, Popkin BM. Changes in beverage intake between 1977 and 2001. Am J Prev Med 2004; 27(3):205–210.

55. U.S. Department of Health, 2000. Healthy People 2010, 2000. Available at: http://www.healthypeople.gov/Document/HTML/uih/uih_1.htm. Accessed September 2007.

56. Dennison BA, Erb TA, Jenkins PL. Predictors of dietary milk fat intake by preschool children. Prev Med 2001; 33(6):536–542.

57. Swallen KC, Reither EN, Haas SA, et al. Overweight, obesity, and health-related quality of life among adolescents: the National Longitudinal Study of Adolescent Health. Pediatrics 2005; 115(2):340–347.

58. Kolotkin RL, Zeller M, Modi AC, et al. Assessing weight-related quality of life in adolescents. Obesity (Silver Spring) 2006; 14(3):448–457.

59. Chen EY, Brown M. Obesity stigma in sexual relationships. Obes Res 2005; 13(8):1393–1397.

60. Halpern CT, Udry JR, Campbell B, et al. Effects of body fat on weight concerns, dating, and sexual activity: a longitudinal analysis of black and white adolescent girls. Dev Psychol 1999; 35(3):721–736.

61. Nagelkerke NJ, Bernsen RM, Sgaier SK, et al. Body mass index, sexual behaviour, and sexually transmitted infections: an analysis using the NHANES 1999–2000 data. BMC Public Health 2006; 6:199.

62. Kolotkin RL, Binks M, Crosby RD, et al. Obesity and sexual quality of life. Obesity (Silver Spring) 2006; 14(3):472–479.

63. Latner JD, Stunkard AJ, Wilson GT. Stigmatized students: age, sex, and ethnicity effects in the stigmatization of obesity. Obes Res 2005; 13(7):1226–1231.

64. Canning H, Mayer J. Obesity: its possible effect on college acceptance. N Engl J Med 1966; 275:1172–1174.

65. Crandall CS. Do parents discriminate against their heavy-weight daughters? Pers Soc Psychol Bull 1991; 21:724–735.

66. Gortmaker SL, Must A, Perrin JM, S et al. Social and economic consequences of overweight in adolescence and young adulthood. N Engl J Med 1993; 329(14):1008–1012.

67. Piaget J. Intellectual evolution from adolescence to adulthood. Hum Dev 1972; 15:1–12.

68. ADA Factsheet. Total Prevalence of Diabetes and Pre-Diabetes. American Diabetes Association, 2007. Available at: diabetes.org/diabetes-statistics/prevalence.jsp. Accessed August 16, 2007.

69. Panzram G. Mortality and survival in type 2 (non-insulin-dependent) diabetes mellitus. Diabetologia 1987; 30(3):123–131.

70. Craig ME, Hattersley A, Donaghue K. ISPAD Clinical Practice Consensus Guidelines 2006-2007. Definition, epidemiology and classification. Pediatr Diabetes 2006; 7(6):343–351.

71. Matthews DR, Hosker JP, Rudenski AS, et al. Homeostasis model assessment: insulin resistance and beta-cell function from fasting plasma glucose and insulin concentrations in man. Diabetologia 1985; 28(7):412–419.

72. Keskin M, Kurtoglu S, Kendirci M, et al. Homeostasis model assessment is more reliable than the fasting glucose/insulin ratio and quantitative insulin sensitivity check index for assessing insulin resistance among obese children and adolescents. Pediatrics 2005; 115(4):e500–e503.

73. Moran A, Jacobs DR Jr, Steinberger J, et al. Insulin resistance during puberty: results from clamp studies in 357 children. Diabetes 1999; 48(10):2039–2044.

74. Lee JM, Okumura MJ, Davis MM, et al. Prevalence and determinants of insulin resistance among U.S. adolescents: a population-based study. Diabetes Care 2006; 29(11):2427–2432.

75. Moon RJ, Bascombe LA, Holt RI. The addition of metformin in type 1 diabetes improves insulin sensitivity, diabetic control, body composition and patient well-being. Diabetes Obes Metab 2007; 9(1):143–145.

76. Copeland KC, Becker D, Gottschalk M, et al. Type 2 diabetes in children and adolescents: Risk factors, diagnosis and treatment. Clinical Diabetes 2005; 23(4):181–185.

77. The TODAY Study Group, . Treatment options for type 2 diabetes in adolescents and youth: a study of the comparative efficacy of metformin alone or in combination with rosiglitazone or lifestyle intervention in adolescents with type 2 diabetes. Pediatr Diabetes 2007; 8(2):74–87.

78. Srinivasan S, Ambler GR, Baur LA, et al. Randomized, controlled trial of metformin for obesity and insulin resistance in children and adolescents: improvement in body composition and fasting insulin. J Clin Endocrinol Metab 2006; 91(6):2074–2080.

79. Relationship of atherosclerosis in young men to serum lipoprotein cholesterol concentrations and smoking. A preliminary report from the Pathobiological Determinants of Atherosclerosis in Youth (PDAY) Research Group. JAMA 1990; 264(23):3018–3024.

80. Berenson GS, Srinivasan SR, Bao W, et al. Association between multiple cardiovascular risk factors and atherosclerosis in children and young adults. The Bogalusa Heart Study. N Engl J Med 1998; 338(23):1650–1656.

81. American Academy of Pediatrics. National Cholesterol Education Program: Report of the Expert Panel on Blood Cholesterol Levels in Children and Adolescents. Pediatrics 1992; 89(3 pt 2):525–584.

82. Clauss SB, Holmes KW, Hopkins P, et al. Efficacy and safety of lovastatin therapy in adolescent girls with heterozygous familial hypercholesterolemia. Pediatrics 2005; 116(3):682–688.

83. Lambert M, Lupien PJ, Gagne C, et al. Treatment of familial hypercholesterolemia in children and adolescents: effect of lovastatin. Canadian Lovastatin in Children Study Group. Pediatrics 1996; 97(5):619–628.

84. Stein EA, Illingworth DR, Kwiterovich PO Jr., et al. Efficacy and safety of lovastatin in adolescent males with heterozygous familial hypercholesterolemia: a randomized controlled trial. JAMA 1999; 281(2):137–144.

85. de Jongh S, Ose L, Szamosi T, et al. Efficacy and safety of statin therapy in children with familial hypercholesterolemia: a randomized, double-blind, placebo-controlled trial with simvastatin. Circulation 2002; 106(17):2231–2237.

86. Knipscheer HC, Boelen CC, Kastelein JJ, et al. Short-term efficacy and safety of pravastatin in 72 children with familial hypercholesterolemia. Pediatr Res 1996; 39(5): 867–871.

87. Wiegman A, Hutten BA, de Groot E, et al. Efficacy and safety of statin therapy in children with familial hypercholesterolemia: a randomized controlled trial. JAMA 2004; 292(3):331–337.

88. McCrindle BW, Ose L, Marais AD. Efficacy and safety of atorvastatin in children and adolescents with familial hypercholesterolemia or severe hyperlipidemia: a multicenter, randomized, placebo-controlled trial. J Pediatr 2003; 143(1):74–80.

89. McCrindle BW, O'Neill MB, Cullen-Dean G, et al. Acceptability and compliance with two forms of cholestyramine in the treatment of hypercholesterolemia in children: a randomized, crossover trial. J Pediatr 1997; 130(2):266–273.

90. Tonstad S, Knudtzon J, Sivertsen M, et al. Efficacy and safety of cholestyramine therapy in peripubertal and prepubertal children with familial hypercholesterolemia. J Pediatr 1996; 129(1):42–49.

91. Tonstad S, Ose L. Colestipol tablets in adolescents with familial hypercholesterolaemia. Acta Paediatr 1996; 85(9):1080–1082.

92. McCrindle BW, Helden E, Cullen-Dean G, et al. A randomized crossover trial of combination pharmacologic therapy in children with familial hyperlipidemia. Pediatr Res 2002; 51(6):715–721.

93. Colletti RB, Neufeld EJ, Roff NK, et al. Niacin treatment of hypercholesterolemia in children. Pediatrics 1993; 92(1):78–82.

94. Wheeler KA, West RJ, Lloyd JK, et al. Double blind trial of bezafibrate in familial hypercholesterolaemia. Arch Dis Child 1985; 60(1):34–37.

95. Ludwig J, Viggiano TR, McGill DB, et al. Nonalcoholic steatohepatitis: Mayo Clinic experiences with a hitherto unnamed disease. Mayo Clin Proc 1980; 55(7):434–438.

96. Schwimmer JB, Deutsch R, Kahen T, et al. Prevalence of fatty liver in children and adolescents. Pediatrics 2006; 118(4):1388–1393.

97. Angulo P. Nonalcoholic fatty liver disease. N Engl J Med 2002; 346(16):1221–1231.

98. Fenkci S, Rota S, Sabir N, et al. Ultrasonographic and biochemical evaluation of visceral obesity in obese women with non-alcoholic fatty liver disease. Eur J Med Res 2007; 12(2):68–73.

99. Sartorio A, Del Col A, Agosti F, et al. Predictors of non-alcoholic fatty liver disease in obese children. Eur J Clin Nutr 2007; 61(7):877–883.

100. Lavine JE. Vitamin E treatment of nonalcoholic steatohepatitis in children: a pilot study. J Pediatr 2000; 136(6): 734–738.

101. Orlando R, Azzalini L, Orando S, et al. Bile acids for non-alcoholic fatty liver disease and/or steatohepatitis. Cochrane Database Syst Rev 2007; (1):CD005160.

102. Vajro P, Franzese A, Valerio G, et al. Lack of efficacy of ursodeoxycholic acid for the treatment of liver abnormalities in obese children. J Pediatr 2000; 136(6):739–743.

103. Schwimmer JB, Middleton MS, Deutsch R, et al. A phase 2 clinical trial of metformin as a treatment for non-diabetic paediatric non-alcoholic steatohepatitis. Aliment Pharmacol Ther 2005; 21(7):871–879.

104. Duncan GE, Li SM, Zhou XH. Prevalence and trends of a metabolic syndrome phenotype among U.S. adolescents, 1999–2000. Diabetes Care 2004; 27(10):2438–2443.

105. Jolliffe CJ, Janssen I. Development of age-specific adolescent metabolic syndrome criteria that are linked to the Adult Treatment Panel III and International Diabetes Federation criteria. J Am Coll Cardiol 2007; 49(8): 891–898.

106. Goodman E, Daniels SR, Meigs JB, et al. Instability in the diagnosis of metabolic syndrome in adolescents. Circulation 2007; 115(17):2316–2322.

107. Chobanian AV, Bakris GL, Black HR, et al. Seventh report of the Joint National Committee on Prevention, Detection, Evaluation, and Treatment of High Blood Pressure. Hypertension 2003; 42(6):1206–1252.

108. National High Blood Pressure Education Program Working Group on High Blood Pressure in Children and Adolescents. The fourth report on the diagnosis, evaluation, and treatment of high blood pressure in children and adolescents. Pediatrics 2004; 114(2 suppl):555–576.

109. Stergiou GS, Yiannes NJ, Rarra VC, et al. White-coat hypertension and masked hypertension in children. Blood Press Monit 2005; 10(6):297–300.

110. Sacks FM, Svetkey LP, Vollmer WM, et al. Effects on blood pressure of reduced dietary sodium and the Dietary Approaches to Stop Hypertension (DASH) diet. DASH-Sodium Collaborative Research Group. N Engl J Med 2001; 344(1):3–10.

111. Vollmer WM, Sacks FM, Ard J, et al. Effects of diet and sodium intake on blood pressure: subgroup analysis of the DASH-sodium trial. Ann Intern Med 2001; 135(12): 1019–1028.

112. Whelton SP, Chin A, Xin X, et al. Effect of aerobic exercise on blood pressure: a meta-analysis of randomized, controlled trials. Ann Intern Med 2002; 136(7):493–503.

113. He J, Whelton PK, Appel LJ, et al. Long-term effects of weight loss and dietary sodium reduction on incidence of hypertension. Hypertension 2000; 35(2):544–549.

114. Norman RJ, Dewailly D, Legro RS, et al. Polycystic ovary syndrome. Lancet 2007; 370(9588):685–697.

115. Azziz R. Controversy in clinical endocrinology: diagnosis of polycystic ovarian syndrome: the Rotterdam criteria are premature. J Clin Endocrinol Metab 2006; 91(3): 781–785.

116. Franks S. Controversy in clinical endocrinology: diagnosis of polycystic ovarian syndrome: in defense of the Rotterdam criteria. J Clin Endocrinol Metab 2006; 91(3):786–789.

117. Conway GS, Honour JW, Jacobs HS. Heterogeneity of the polycystic ovary syndrome: clinical, endocrine and ultrasound features in 556 patients. Clin Endocrinol (Oxf) 1989; 30(4):459–470.

118. Chang WY, Knochenhauer ES, Bartolucci AA, et al. Phenotypic spectrum of polycystic ovary syndrome: clinical and biochemical characterization of the three major clinical subgroups. Fertil Steril 2005; 83(6):1717–1723.

119. Balen AH, Laven JS, Tan SL, et al. Ultrasound assessment of the polycystic ovary: international consensus definitions. Hum Reprod Update 2003; 9(6):505–514.

120. Azziz R, Woods KS, Reyna R, et al. The prevalence and features of the polycystic ovary syndrome in an unselected population. J Clin Endocrinol Metab 2004; 89(6): 2745–2749.

121. Huber-Buchholz MM, Carey DG, Norman RJ. Restoration of reproductive potential by lifestyle modification in obese polycystic ovary syndrome: role of insulin sensitivity and luteinizing hormone. J Clin Endocrinol Metab 1999; 84(4):1470–1474.

122. Vrbikova J, Cibula D. Combined oral contraceptives in the treatment of polycystic ovary syndrome. Hum Reprod Update 2005; 11(3):277–291.

123. Lord JM, Flight IH, Norman RJ. Metformin in polycystic ovary syndrome: systematic review and meta-analysis. BMJ 2003; 327(7421):951–953.

124. Glueck CJ, Aregawi D, Winiarska M, et al. Metformin-diet ameliorates coronary heart disease risk factors and facilitates resumption of regular menses in adolescents with polycystic ovary syndrome. J Pediatr Endocrinol Metab 2006; 19(6):831–842.

125. Nazari T, Bayat R, Hamedi M. Metformin therapy in girls with polycystic ovary syndrome: a self-controlled clinical trial. Arch Iran Med 2007; 10(2):176–181.

126. De Leo V, Musacchio MC, Morgante G, et al. Metformin treatment is effective in obese teenage girls with PCOS. Hum Reprod 2006; 21(9):2252–2256.

127. Didi M, Didcock E, Davies HA, et al. High incidence of obesity in young adults after treatment of acute lymphoblastic leukemia in childhood. J Pediatr 1995; 127 (1):63–67.

128. Nysom K, Holm K, Michaelsen KF, et al. Degree of fatness after treatment for acute lymphoblastic leukemia in childhood. J Clin Endocrinol Metab 1999; 84(12):4591–4596.

129. Sklar CA, Mertens AC, Walter A, et al. Changes in body mass index and prevalence of overweight in survivors of childhood acute lymphoblastic leukemia: role of cranial irradiation. Med Pediatr Oncol 2000; 35(2):91–95.

130. Craig F, Leiper AD, Stanhope R, et al. Sexually dimorphic and radiation dose dependent effect of cranial irradiation on body mass index. Arch Dis Child 1999; 81(6):500–504.

131. Sklar CA. Craniopharyngioma: endocrine sequelae of treatment. Pediatr Neurosurg 1994; 21(suppl 1):120–123.

132. Jeanrenaud B. An hypothesis on the aetiology of obesity: dysfunction of the central nervous system as a primary cause. Diabetologia 1985; 28(8):502–513.

133. Lustig RH, Hinds PS, Ringwald-Smith K, et al. Octreotide therapy of pediatric hypothalamic obesity: a double-blind, placebo-controlled trial. J Clin Endocrinol Metab 2003; 88(6):2586–2592.

134. Lustig RH, Rose SR, Burghen GA, et al. Hypothalamic obesity caused by cranial insult in children: altered glucose and insulin dynamics and reversal by a somatostatin agonist. J Pediatr 1999; 135(2 pt 1):162–168.

135. Dolberg OT, Barkai G, Gross Y, et al. Differential effects of topiramate in patients with traumatic brain injury and obesity—a case series. Psychopharmacology (Berl) 2005; 179(4):838–845.

136. Kessler RC, Chiu WT, Demler O, et al. Prevalence, severity, and comorbidity of 12-month DSM-IV disorders in the National Comorbidity Survey Replication. Arch Gen Psychiatry 2005; 62(6):617–627.

137. Birmaher B, Ryan ND, Williamson DE, et al. Childhood and adolescent depression: a review of the past 10 years. Part I. J Am Acad Child Adolesc Psychiatry 1996; 35(11): 1427–1439.

138. Hoyert DL, Arias E, Smith BL, et al. Deaths: final data for 1999. Natl Vital Stat Rep 2001; 49(8):1–113.

139. Shaffer D, Gould MS, Fisher P, et al. Psychiatric diagnosis in child and adolescent suicide. Arch Gen Psychiatry 1996; 53(4):339–348.

140. Weissman MM, Wolk S, Goldstein RB, et al. Depressed adolescents grown up. JAMA 1999; 281(18):1707–1713.

141. Wadden TA, Foster GD, Stunkard AJ, et al. Dissatisfaction with weight and figure in obese girls: discontent but not depression. Int J Obes 1989; 13(1):89–97.

142. Britz B, Siegfried W, Ziegler A, et al. Rates of psychiatric disorders in a clinical study group of adolescents with extreme obesity and in obese adolescents ascertained via a population based study. Int J Obes Relat Metab Disord 2000; 24(12):1707–1714.

143. Csabi G, Tenyi T, Molnar D. Depressive symptoms among obese children. Eat Weight Disord 2000; 5(1):43–45.

144. Wallace WJ, Sheslow D, Hassink S. Obesity in children: a risk for depression. Ann N Y Acad Sci 1993; 699: 301–303.

145. Richardson LP, Garrison MM, Drangsholt M, et al. Associations between depressive symptoms and obesity during puberty. Gen Hosp Psychiatry 2006; 28(4):313–320.

146. Dolfing JG, Wolffenbuttel BH, Hoor-Aukema NM, et al. Daily high doses of fluoxetine for weight loss and

improvement in lifestyle before bariatric surgery. Obes Surg 2005; 15(8):1185–1191.

147. Gray DS, Fujioka K, Devine W, et al. A randomized double-blind clinical trial of fluoxetine in obese diabetics. Int J Obes Relat Metab Disord 1992; 16(suppl 4): S67–S72.

148. Daubresse JC, Kolanowski J, Krzentowski G, et al. Usefulness of fluoxetine in obese non-insulin-dependent diabetics: a multicenter study. Obes Res 1996; 4(4):391–396.

149. Schaller JL, Rawlings DB. Escitalopram in adolescent major depression. Med Gen Med 2005; 7(1):6.

150. Szkudlarek J, Elsborg L. Treatment of severe obesity with a highly selective serotonin re-uptake inhibitor as a supplement to a low calorie diet. Int J Obes Relat Metab Disord 1993; 17(12):681–683.

151. Weintraub M, Rubio A, Golik A, et al. Sibutramine in weight control: a dose-ranging, efficacy study. Clin Pharmacol Ther 1991; 50(3):330–337.

152. Berkowitz RI, Fujioka K, Daniels SR, et al. Effects of sibutramine treatment in obese adolescents: a randomized trial. Ann Intern Med 2006; 145(2):81–90.

153. Anderson JW, Greenway FL, Fujioka K, et al. Bupropion SR enhances weight loss: a 48-week double-blind, placebo-controlled trial. Obes Res 2002; 10(7):633–641.

154. Jain AK, Kaplan RA, Gadde KM, et al. Bupropion SR vs. placebo for weight loss in obese patients with depressive symptoms. Obes Res 2002; 10(10):1049–1056.

155. Allison DB, Fontaine KR, Heo M, et al. The distribution of body mass index among individuals with and without schizophrenia. J Clin Psychiatry 1999; 60(4):215–220.

156. Green AI, Patel JK, Goisman RM, et al. Weight gain from novel antipsychotic drugs: need for action. Gen Hosp Psychiatry 2000; 22(4):224–235.

157. Ratzoni G, Gothelf D, Brand-Gothelf A, et al. Weight gain associated with olanzapine and risperidone in adolescent patients: a comparative prospective study. J Am Acad Child Adolesc Psychiatry 2002; 41(3):337–343.

158. McDougle CJ, Kem DL, Posey DJ. Case series: use of ziprasidone for maladaptive symptoms in youths with autism. J Am Acad Child Adolesc Psychiatry 2002; 41(8):921–927.

159. Marcus MD, Kalarchian MA. Binge eating in children and adolescents. Int J Eat Disord 2003; 34(suppl):S47–S57.

160. Grilo CM, Masheb RM. Onset of dieting vs. binge eating in outpatients with binge eating disorder. Int J Obes Relat Metab Disord 2000; 24(4):404–409.

161. Spurrell EB, Wilfley DE, Tanofsky MB, et al. Age of onset for binge eating: are there different pathways to binge eating? Int J Eat Disord 1997; 21(1):55–65.

162. Berkowitz R, Stunkard AJ, Stallings VA. Binge-eating disorder in obese adolescent girls. Ann N Y Acad Sci 1993; 699:200–206.

163. Morgan CM, Yanovski SZ, Nguyen TT. Loss of control over eating, adiposity, and psychopathology in overweight children. Int J Eat Disord 2002; 31(4):430–441.

164. Decaluwe V, Braet C, Fairburn CG. Binge eating in obese children and adolescents. Int J Eat Disord 2003; 33(1):78–84.

165. Carter WP, Hudson JI, Lalonde JK, et al. Pharmacologic treatment of binge eating disorder. Int J Eat Disord 2003; 34(suppl):S74–S88.

166. Mittendorfer B, Ostlund RE Jr., Patterson B, et al. Orlistat inhibits dietary cholesterol absorption. Obes Res 2001; 9(10):599–604.

167. Chanoine JP, Hampl S, Jensen C, et al. Effect of orlistat on weight and body composition in obese adolescents: a randomized controlled trial. JAMA 2005; 293(23): 2873–2883.

168. Ozkan B, Bereket A, Turan S, et al. Addition of orlistat to conventional treatment in adolescents with severe obesity. Eur J Pediatr 2004; 163(12):738–741.

169. James WP, Astrup A, Finer N, et al. Effect of sibutramine on weight maintenance after weight loss: a randomised trial. STORM Study Group. Sibutramine Trial of Obesity Reduction and Maintenance. Lancet 2000; 356(9248): 2119–2125.

170. Daniels SR, Long B, Crow S, et al. Cardiovascular effects of sibutramine in the treatment of obese adolescents: results of a randomized, double-blind, placebo-controlled study. Pediatrics 2007; 120(1):e147–e157.

171. Lustig RH, Mietus-Snyder ML, Bacchetti P, et al. Insulin dynamics predict body mass index and z-score response to insulin suppression or sensitization pharmacotherapy in obese children. J Pediatr 2006; 148(1):23–29.

172. Knowler WC, Barrett-Connor E, Fowler SE, et al. Reduction in the incidence of type 2 diabetes with lifestyle intervention or metformin. N Engl J Med 2002; 346(6): 393–403.

173. Orchard TJ, Temprosa M, Goldberg R, et al. The effect of metformin and intensive lifestyle intervention on the metabolic syndrome: the Diabetes Prevention Program randomized trial. Ann Intern Med 2005; 142(8): 611–619.

174. Maggard MA, Shugarman LR, Suttorp M, et al. Meta-analysis: surgical treatment of obesity. Ann Intern Med 2005; 142(7):547–559.

175. Rand CS, Macgregor AM. Adolescents having obesity surgery: a 6-year follow-up. South Med J 1994; 87(12): 1208–1213.

176. Schwimmer JB, Burwinkle TM, Varni JW. Health-related quality of life of severely obese children and adolescents. JAMA 2003; 289(14):1813–1819.

177. Strauss RS, Pollack HA. Social marginalization of overweight children. Arch Pediatr Adolesc Med 2003; 157(8): 746–752.

178. Inge TH, Krebs NF, Garcia VF, et al. Bariatric surgery for severely overweight adolescents: concerns and recommendations. Pediatrics 2004; 114(1):217–223.

179. Nadler EP, Youn HA, Ginsburg HB, et al. Short-term results in 53 US obese pediatric patients treated with laparoscopic adjustable gastric banding. J Pediatr Surg 2007; 42(1):137–141.

180. Apovian CM, Baker C, Ludwig DS, et al. Best practice guidelines in pediatric/adolescent weight loss surgery. Obes Res 2005; 13(2):274–282.

181. Abu-Abeid S, Gavert N, Klausner JM, et al. Bariatric surgery in adolescence. J Pediatr Surg 2003; 38(9):1379–1382.

182. Dolan K, Creighton L, Hopkins G, et al. Laparoscopic gastric banding in morbidly obese adolescents. Obes Surg 2003; 13(1):101–104.

183. Sugerman HJ, Sugerman EL, DeMaria et al. Bariatric surgery for severely obese adolescents. J Gastrointest Surg 2003; 7(1):102–107.

184. Strauss RS, Bradley LJ, Brolin RE. Gastric bypass surgery in adolescents with morbid obesity. J Pediatr 2001; 138(4): 499–504.

185. Inge TH, Daniels SR, Garcia VF. Bariatric Surgical Procedures in Adolescents. In: Ashcroft KW, Holcomb GW, Murphy JP, eds. Pediatric Surgery. Philadelphia, PA: Elsevier, Sanders, 2005:1116–1125.

186. DeMaria EJ. Bariatric surgery for morbid obesity. N Engl J Med 2007; 356(21):2176–2183.

187. Nguyen NT, Paya M, Stevens CM, et al. The relationship between hospital volume and outcome in bariatric surgery at academic medical centers. Ann Surg 2004; 240(4):586–593.

188. Towbin A, Inge TH, Garcia VF, et al. Beriberi after gastric bypass surgery in adolescence. J Pediatr 2004; 145(2): 263–267.

38

Weight Loss Clinics: Range of Capabilities, Benefits, Risks, and Costs

KEN FUJIOKA

Nutrition and Metabolic Research and Center for Weight Management, Department of Diabetes and Endocrinology, Scripps Clinic, La Jolla, California, U.S.A.

INTRODUCTION

When it comes to choosing a weight loss clinic, overweight to morbidly obese patients have many options. A patient could approach his primary care physician for treatment, or the treating physician could refer the patient to a weight loss clinic, if such a coverage exists in the patient's health insurance network. In addition, a patient could simply join any of the numerous commercial weight loss programs.

Such a large group of diverse weight loss programs can be divided into those that provide a visit with a physician and those that do not. Commercial weight loss programs that are based on a low-calorie diet (LCD), such as Jenny Craig, NutriSystem, and Weight Watchers, generally do not retain a physician on staff.

Another type of weight loss program, very low calorie diets (VLCDs), typically utilizes a calorie level of less than 800 cal/day. Examples of VLCDs include Health Management Resources (HMR), Optifast, and Medifast. Follow-up with a physician is recommended for patients on a VLCD for safety reasons (1), and subsequently the majority of these patients are seen in a medical office.

Weight loss medication-dispensing clinics became popular in the 1990s, dispensing "phen-fen," an inexpensive combination of phentermine and fenfluramine.

Physician-supervised, weight loss medication–dispensing clinics dispensed the medication directly to the patient, as opposed to giving a prescription through which the medication could be obtained at a pharmacy. In addition, weight loss medication–dispensing clinics typically do not accept health insurance, operating as "cash-only" clinics.

Multispecialist weight loss centers dedicated to obesity treatment, such as the Center for Weight Management at Scripps Clinic in San Diego, the Comprehensive Weight Control Program at New York's Presbyterian Hospital, and the Center for Weight and Eating Disorders at the University of Pennsylvania, usually are associated with a large medical group, hospital, or university. In such programs, specialists in many disciplines are available to patients: A registered dietitian provides a nutritional program, a psychologist assists with lifestyle changes and psychological issues, and a physician assists with weight loss medications or medical issues. Some centers have surgeons available for patients who are appropriate for bariatric surgery.

Although many types and combinations of weight loss clinics are available to patients, this chapter will discuss the range of capabilities, costs, risks, and benefits of four: commercial nonmedical weight loss programs, VLCD medical clinics, weight loss medication–dispensing clinics, and multispecialist weight loss centers.

COMMERCIAL NONMEDICAL WEIGHT LOSS PROGRAMS

Four popular commercial weight loss programs in North America are Jenny Craig, NutriSystem, LA Weight Loss, and Weight Watchers, although numerous commercial weight loss programs exist. These programs consist of patients undergoing a diet and, to a varying degree, lifestyle changes. Patients are usually seen weekly, either meeting as a group or one-on-one with a counselor. Food may be provided to the patients for the week, or the program might provide a menu with recipes or a system to count calories, giving the patients the opportunity to choose what they eat, but ensuring that they eat appropriate amounts (2–4).

Most dietary regimens are designed to produce approximately 1 to 2 lb of weight loss per week, with a caloric deficit of 750 kcal; thus, most diets are in the range of 1200 to 1800 kcal/day. The major difference among these programs is how the patients obtain their food. Many programs, including Weight Watchers, have patients buy food and prepare meals according to a diet plan. Foods are given a point value to guide the patient to make correct choices of food in appropriate amounts. Low-calorie foods are assigned a low score or low number of points and high-calorie foods are given a higher score or more points. Patients are thus able to eat most foods, but learn portioning with high-calorie foods and that low-calorie foods can be eaten more liberally.

In other programs, including Jenny Craig and Nutri-System, participating patients buy a majority of prepared and packaged food directly from the commercial program. Commonly called meal replacements, this prepared food can be as simple as a liquid shake or bar, or a hot meal that can be prepared in a microwave oven. Patients usually obtain this prepared food weekly from the weight loss program, eliminating much of the decision of what or how much to eat. If the patients follow the diet, then they will come close to attaining a 750-cal deficit per day.

Evidence exists that programs that provide meal replacements can result in significant weight loss above that achieved with a standard caloric-restriction diet, in which the patients choose and prepare their own food (5–8). A meta-analysis by Heymsfield and colleagues indicates that patients lost on average 7% to 8% of their body weight using meal replacements, compared with a group of patients who lost 3% to 7% of their bodyweight by dieting conventionally (7). Comparing these two methods of dieting after one year yielded a difference of approximately 2.5 kg. It remains unclear, however, whether meal replacements are superior to a highly structured diet plan prepared by the patients themselves. A six-month study comparing meal replacements with a highly structured dietary plan with

weigh-ins every two weeks showed similar weight loss (9.4% and 9.3%, respectively) between the groups.

Access to commercial weight loss programs can also be obtained through the Internet, as Web-based diet sites have become a rather recent means of access weight loss. Many nonmedical commercial programs provide this option (3–4), and many commercial as well as noncommercial Web sites exist (9–11). In a randomized controlled study comparing eDiets.com, a commercial, Internet-based weight loss program, with *The LEARN Program for Weight Control* (12), a standard weight loss manual, patients on the Internet-based weight loss program lost 1.1% of their weight at 52 weeks, compared with a 4% weight loss in patients using the weight loss manual (13). Although in this particular study the amount of weight lost was statistically lower in patients on the Internet-based program, two more recent studies of noncommercial, Web-based weight management reported better results, with weight loss ranging from 3% to 5% for patients on a Web-based program (14–15). Further research is needed to determine how Web-based dieting compares with programs in which patients physically attend meetings or physician or counselor visits.

In addition to providing a diet for the patient, most commercial weight loss programs offer other services to help with weight loss. Many programs offer group or individual support on a weekly basis and, depending on the program, behavior modification is usually attempted, although to varying degrees depending on the program. Patients who participate in these programs are usually encouraged to exercise but methods of actual counseling vary. Some programs offer participants group or individual exercise sessions; in other programs, patients purchase exercise CDs or DVDs.

Nonmedical weight loss programs accept participants with body mass indexes (BMIs) ranging from overweight to morbidly obese, and many programs will accept patients with comorbid disease, provided the patient's physician has given permission. Patients with severe comorbid diseases such as renal failure, liver failure, diabetes that is difficult to control despite insulin use, or congestive heart failure, and patients on blood thinners such as warfarin sodium (Coumadin, Bristol-Myers Squibb, Princeton, New Jersey, U.S.) are not routinely recommended for participation in nonmedical weight loss programs.

These programs usually incorporate some sort of maintenance, which may require an additional fee—for example, the expense of the weekly meetings. Little data exist on weight maintenance in commercial programs. In one review, Weight Watchers participants maintained weight loss of 3.2% over a two-year period (16,17), and in a Canadian study with a follow-up of 5 to 11 years, 29.1% of patients maintained a weight loss of 5% of their initial weight (18).

Simply getting patients to the maintenance stage is difficult because of very low retention rates. In a study of 60,164 patients participating in a Jenny Craig program, retention dropped steadily over a year, with retention rates of 73% at 4 weeks, 42% at 13 weeks, 22% at 26 weeks, and 6.6% at 52 weeks (19). Patients who completed a year of the program averaged a weight loss of 15.6%, but only 6.6% of patients who started the program completed the year. Multiple reasons exist for why patients are unable to stay in these programs, and it is suspected that a majority of other programs have a similar retention rate.

Costs

Patients usually pay some type of initial fee at the start of the program, which can vary from $30 for a program like Weight Watchers to hundreds of dollars for other programs (20,21). The initial starting fee is usually followed by a weekly or monthly fee (Table 1).

One of the popular programs, LA weight loss, was not able to give a cost for a three- or six-month program. For a 5-ft 9-in, 190-lb male who presented with a desire to lose weight, the initial fee was "$700 to $800." This entailed a 78-week program and additional weekly costs of approximately $11. The patient asked if there were less expensive programs or programs that were not as long and was told this was the only available option.

Prices vary according to the cost and availability of prepared foods and counseling. The price of food can vary from $11 to $15 per day, and weekly meeting fees may also be incurred: The price of a support group and/or counselor is approximately $10 to $15 per weekly meeting, depending on the structure of the payment plan.

In some programs, patients are encouraged to buy additional items to aid in weight loss, such as exercise equipment, various nutritional supplements and motivational

CDs or DVDs. These additional products vary widely in price and may be mandatory.

Risks

The risks of these programs are minimal; the only potential medical risk is gallstone formation during weight loss, which is a minimal risk with diets of more than 1200 kcal and at least 20 g of fat per day (22,23). Subsequently, when advising patients on selection of a weight loss program, this author recommends having at least 20 g of fat in the dietary program.

Potential risks to patients on medications for chronic diseases related to obesity exist. With weight loss, patients on diabetic medications will experience a drop in blood sugar (6) and will need medications adjusted accordingly. Most nonmedical commercial programs require that patients with diabetes inform their physician of their intention to participate in a particular weight loss program. For patients on diabetes medications, most programs require a letter from a physician granting permission to participate in the program. For patients who take insulin, programs such as Jenny Craig require a screening from a corporate dietitian to ensure that follow-up with the patient is completed and that he/she understands the risks associated with losing weight while on insulin.

Patients taking hypertension medications, as well as patients taking blood thinners such as Coumadin (warfarin sodium tablets, Bristol-Myers Squibb Co., Princeton, New Jersey, U.S.), are also at risk for adverse events during weight loss. As patients change their diet and lose weight, the adjustment of medications becomes important; subsequently, a patient's physician must be involved in nonmedical commercial weight loss programs. If the patient's physician is unwilling or unable to follow and make necessary adjustments during a patient's participation in a weight loss program, then the patient's participation in a nonmedical commercial weight loss program is not recommended.

Participation in a nonmedical commercial weight loss program is also not recommended for patients with severe illness, such as heart failure, renal failure, or liver failure. Certain diets (for example, normal- to high-protein diets) can cause problems with the diseased organ. In addition, the need to adjust medications in this type of patient exists, but is made difficult due to the fact that drug elimination often is compromised.

A financial risk also exists. With a retention rate of 42% (19) at three months, paying for six months of treatment up front indicates that more than half of patients who enroll in the program could pay for services that are never received. It is recommended by this author that

Table 1 Estimated Program Costs for Commercial and Organized Self-Help Weight Loss Programs

Program	Initial costs	Weekly costs	Required food costs	Typical cost over 6 mo
Jenny Craig	$200	none	$75/wk	$2200
Weight Watchers	$30	$12/wk	None	$318
NutriSystem	none	None	$325/mo	$2000
LA Weight Loss	$88	$7/wk	none	Cannot determine[a]

[a]Unable to determine the six-month cost of LA Weight Loss because participants are asked to pay weekly until they reach their goal weight. A fee is charged for those who withdraw from the program before reaching their goal weight but they are reimbursed for unused visits.
Source: From Ref. 17.

patients do not pay up front more that three months in advance. The author visited (as a potential patient) many of these nonmedical commercial weight loss programs and noted the "hard sell" atmosphere of some of the programs.

Benefits

In terms of starting patients on a weight loss program, most of these programs are successful. Generally speaking, these programs are conveniently located close to either a patient's place of employment (Weight Watchers actually will start a program at a work facility if enough people are willing to participate) or to the patient's home (often times located in a local shopping mall), thus making it easy for a patient to attend regularly.

It remains unknown, however, how efficacious and cost-effective these programs are. In a systematic review of major commercial weight loss programs in the United States, Tsai and Wadden cite a complete lack of controlled trials (17). With the exception of one Weight Watchers trial showing approximately 3% weight loss at the end of two years, the evidence of the efficacy of these programs is suboptimal. In a more recently conducted controlled randomized trial of a multifaceted commercial program, patients participating in the program lost approximately 7% more weight than patients in the control group (8). It appears that meal replacements and a highly structured weight loss program can result in reasonable weight loss, but the costs may be prohibitive for many patients. With the exception of Weight Watchers, most highly structured programs can cost thousands of dollars.

MEDICAL CLINICS USING VLCDs

Commercial medically supervised weight loss programs became popular in the 1980s. At that time, few physicians prescribed weight loss medications, and, subsequently, a popular method of weight loss was with VLCDs. Well-known American television talk show host Oprah Winfrey, who battled with her weight, was noted on her daily show to be losing weight. Winfrey's announcement that she had lost 67 lb using a liquid diet resulted in the height of popularity of VLCDs. The scene was dramatized with the depiction of Winfrey pulling a wagon of 67 lb of fat across the television stage, a representation of her 67-lb weight loss (24).

Many medically supervised commercial weight loss programs use VLCDs as a main method of weight loss; some popular examples include Optifast and HMR. By definition, a VLCD is a diet consisting of fewer than 800 cal. With their relatively low level of caloric intake, these diets are intended for patients with a BMI of greater than

30 kg/m^2, and participants should be medically supervised (1,25).

Medically supervised weight loss programs employ VLCDs for multiple reasons. The first reason is economic: Much of the program's income results from the sale of the liquid VLCD directly to the patient or to the physician, who then sells it to the patient.

Additionally, medically supervised weight loss programs employ VLCDs because of the desire for simple and rapid weight loss. Typical LCDs provide a weight loss of 0.4 to 0.5 kg/wk, for a total of 6 to 8 kg over 12 to 16 weeks of treatment. The average weight loss of a VLCD is 1.5 to 2.5 kg/wk, resulting in 20 kg of weight loss over 12 to 16 weeks (1). Patients find simplicity in drinking a shake or eating a bar several times a day while losing weight rapidly.

Similar to commercial nonmedical programs, the amount and intensity of behavior modification, exercise, and counseling vary depending on the medically supervised program. Data indicate that programs that use lifestyle changes (behavior modification, exercise, and dietary instruction) have better results at one year than a VLCD alone, but at five years, weight loss of patients who are taught lifestyle changes may be similar to that of patients who are not instructed in lifestyle changes (26).

In medically supervised weight loss programs, patients are seen weekly and are supplied with a weekly VLCD liquid supplement. Blood chemistry is taken monthly (27). If a patient is on a VLCD of fewer than 800 cal or has a medical problem that requires monitoring, the weekly visit may include a visit with a physician. Many programs' weekly groups are led by a health care provider, and many of these medically supervised programs also offer standard LCDs with meal replacements, thus reducing the need for intensive medical management of the patient.

With the current trend toward programs that are available on the Internet, situations may exist in which patients are not monitored medically when they are participating in a VLCD or have a chronic disease requiring medical attention during weight loss.

Because patients with medical problems are followed by a physician, the range of potential patients is much larger for medically supervised programs (compared with nonmedically supervised programs). Participation in a weight loss program for a patient with diabetes can result in improvement in blood sugar control, often necessitating a decrease or withdrawal of diabetic medications (28). Patients with hyperlipidemia, hypertension, or diabetes are good candidates for VLCDs and would be safe using them under medical supervision (28). The known benefit of weight loss for patients with chronic medical diseases indicates that medically supervised weight loss clinics will enroll patients with chronic disease.

Risks

Several risks of medically supervised weight loss programs exist. Problems can result with the VLCD itself or with the medical diseases that patients may have when they initially begin the program.

Many medically supervised programs offer both LCDs and VLCDs. If a patient is on an LCD of 1200 to 1500 cal, then the risks are low. The risks discussed in this section apply only to patients participating in a VLCD and to patients with chronic diseases who are participating in either VLCDs or LCDs.

To understand the risks, it is important to know the macronutrients in the liquid VLCDs. Liquid VLCDs are typically high in protein, low in carbohydrates, and include at least 10 g of fat per day. By definition, putting a patient on a VLCD is putting a patient into starvation; patients eat fewer calories than they need and subsequently lose weight. In addition to losing fat, patients can lose protein. For medical reasons, this protein loss should be minimized. Ensuring that patients receive adequate protein and amount of calories is important. In most of these programs, patients eat between 420 and 800 cal/day (1). At a caloric intake of 500 to 800, it appears participants receive a minimum of 45 to 75 g of protein per day (Table 2).

Several studies indicate VLCDs produce a weight loss of 25% lean tissue (protein) and 75% fat tissue (29), an acceptable ratio of loss of lean tissue to loss of fat tissue. Diets with a caloric intake of more than 400 cal and protein intake of more than 50 g/day should maintain this ratio (30), resulting in a low risk of protein and/or calorie malnutrition when patients are compliant with the dietary prescription.

Protein quality is important, demonstrated in its implication as the cause of sudden death in a cluster of patients on VLCDs in the 1970s (31–34). Patients were dying because of secondary complications related to participating

in a VLCD of poor protein quality, which resulted in the development of cardiac problems. In recent years, VLCDs containing high-quality biologic proteins have been found to have a low potential for amino acid deficiency or myocardial protein depletion (35–37).

The fat content of VLCDs is important for several reasons. A theoretical risk of a deficiency of essential fatty acids exists. Fortunately, this risk is usually not an issue; patients are losing fat and liberating essential fatty acids that can meet their needs (30).

More of an issue is the risk of gallstones; an adequate amount of fat in a VLCD may prevent them. Obese patients are at risk for cholesterol gallstones because their bile is saturated with cholesterol. The risk increases during rapid weight loss secondary to super saturation of the bile with cholesterol (38), but after weight loss, the risk is reduced to normal. Two studies following gallstone formation by ultrasound determined that the intake of 10 or 12 g of fat can decrease the risk of gallstones (38,39). When a VLCD with 3 g of fat was applied over a three-month period, 54% of patients developed ultrasound evidence of gallstones; no patients receiving 12 g of fat per day over a three-month period developed ultrasound evidence of gallstones. If a patient receives at least 10 g of fat per day, the risk of gallstones is reduced. In a study of maximal emptying of the gallbladder during VLCD participation, data showed that a single dose of 10 g of fat per day was optimal (38).

Electrolyte abnormalities are common in the beginning of a VLCD, when fluid loss is highest. A decrease in potassium and magnesium can occur, but these are easily replaced if not initially available in the VLCD. Many physicians prescribe a daily supplement of potassium to correct low potassium levels. For patients on certain hypertensive medications, potassium levels can be increased (angiotensin-converting enzyme inhibitors) or decreased (non-potassium sparing diuretics) based on the needs of the individual, medical decision making is often necessary (40).

During participation in a VLCD or any type of starvation, gout attacks are common and are considered a predisposing factor (41). Gout attacks can be difficult to treat, and if a patient does not respond to standard treatment, he/she may be required to switch from a VLCD to an LCD diet or halt dieting altogether until the gout is under control. When a patient has a gout attack, uric acid–lowering agents should not be started, although they can be used prophylactically before starting a weight loss program in a difficult-to-control gout patient. Standard nonsteroidal anti-inflammatory agents (NSAIDs) and anti-gout medications may be utilized during weight loss to keep gout attacks from occurring. NSAIDs should be the first-line therapy, unless contraindications exist (42).

Table 2 Macronutrients and Costs[a] of VLCDs

	Optifast 800	HMR 800[b]
Calories (per serving)	160	170
Protein (per serving)	14	16
Carbohydrates (per serving)	20	22
Fat (per serving)	3	2
Initial cost[c]	$270	$270
Monthly costs[d]	$180–$400	$180–$400
Meal replacement/month	$380	$300–$375

[a]Initial costs and monthly costs can vary depending on the program.
[b]HMR's VLCD is 500 to 1000 cal/day.
[c]History and physical exam.
[d]Includes lifestyle counseling, laboratories, and physician visits.
Abbreviation: VLCD, very low calorie diets.

Patients who are not recommended for placement on a VLCD include those with unstable cardiac disease, systemic infections, cerebral vascular disease, renal disease, or hepatic disease. Patients with a history of certain psychiatric disorders, such as bulimia nervosa or anorexia nervosa, should not be permitted to participate in a VLCD. Patients with major depression, major psychiatric illnesses, or who are on various psychotropic medications are also at high risk for medical as well as worsening of psychiatric problems and thus are not recommended to participate in a VLCD. Lastly, patients who have type 1 diabetes requiring insulin have the potential for ketoacidosis and should not attempt to participate in a VLCD (1).

Costs

In general, VLCDs are expensive relative to LCDs (Table 2), a result of the medical costs associated with VLCDs. Cost for items such as an initial history, physical exam, and laboratory values can easily reach $500, depending on the extent of the initial workup. Medical items such as electrocardiograms (EKGs), blood draws, and physician visits may be partially covered by health insurance, but these types of procedures are needed regularly and will put monthly payments (most programs require payment up front every four weeks) in the range of $200 to $400. Some programs provide the patients with an invoice of typically covered medical procedures (e.g., blood draw or EKG), and the patients can then submit to their insurance company for possible partial compensation. Meal replacements are typically not covered by insurance, and the liquid diet or bars generally cost $10 to $13 per day, similar to nonmedical commercial LCDs.

Benefits

Losing weight through a medically monitored clinic that offers a VLCD can have many benefits, particularly for the obese patient with comorbidities such as diabetes, hypertension, low high-density lipoprotein (HDL) cholesterols, and high triglycerides. VLCDs have proven beneficial for the majority of comorbidities of obesity, and no data indicate that commercial VLCD programs are any less beneficial. In patients participating in a VLCD, diabetes and glucose control show impressive improvement. Participation in a VLCD reduces hepatic glucose output, increases insulin action in the liver, increases insulin action in the peripheral tissues, and enhances insulin secretion (28,43,44). Blood pressure in hypertensive patients who participate in a VLCD can improve by 8% to 13% (28,45–48). Lipids improve with a drop in triglycerides and, in the long term, an increase in HDL and a

decrease in triglycerides can be expected (1,44,47–50). Such metabolic benefits are numerous and outweigh the risks associated with VLCD use. The biggest risk of VLCD participation for the diabetic patient is hypoglycemia, which can occur with any weight loss in patients with diabetes on medications such as insulin and sulphonureals. Hypoglycemia appears to be particularly problematic in these patients who are participating in a VLCD; fortunately, an experienced weight management physician can anticipate this and adjust the patient's medications before the VLCD is started.

When comparing the benefits of a program offering VLCDs with programs offering LCDs, debate exists regarding long-term benefits (1,17,51). In a randomized trial of a VLCD versus an LCD, slightly more weight was lost in patients participating in the VLCD, although this was not statistically significant at one year (51). There was a slight tendency to see less in the way of side effects with the LCD versus the VLCD. The differences were not statistically significant. All the adverse events were mild and generally transient.

Patients may start and stop a VLCD program, stopping after weight loss but returning after regaining weight to try to lose weight again. Although a patient may lose weight with each attempt, this weight cycling could be considered a risk for deleterious effects on blood pressure, lipids, or blood sugar. Contrary to this, in a retrospective study of patients who had restarted a VLCD program, at least once no such deleterious effect was discovered (52). Surprisingly, the patient's lipids were, in fact, lower at each restart. Data show that VLCDs have the potential to provide long-term benefits to the obese patients with diabetes, despite any weight regain (28).

In conclusion, VLCD programs offer many benefits, particularly when they include a comprehensive program and lifestyle. Costs can be an obstacle for many patients, particularly those who cannot receive partial insurance coverage. Controlled trials are needed to assess the efficacy and cost-effectiveness of these programs (17).

MEDICATION-DISPENSING WEIGHT LOSS CLINICS

The use of phentermine and fenfluramine, commonly known as phen-fen, for weight loss increased dramatically in the mid-1990s (53). Phen-fen usage brought about an impressive increase in the number of medication-dispensing weight loss clinics.

These clinics, which made phen-fen available as well as dispensed it, were usually physician-supervised. The majority of the medications were dispensed from the clinic itself, although a patient could be given a prescription to obtain medications at a pharmacy. Despite a rather dramatic fall in phentermine usage at the end of 1997, phentermine and other weight loss medications are still sold through these clinics.

An Internet search of medical weight loss clinics identifies at least a dozen in any major city (54). A vast majority of these programs advertise the use of weight loss medications, nutritional supplements, and diet programs. A majority of the Web pages of these medical clinics that this author visited feature testimonials, including what appear to be before and after pictures, of patients who have participated in the program, as well as pictures of women with supermodel-like figures (55–57), often emphasizing the abdominal region with a tape measure around the waist.

Typical weight loss medications advertised by medication-dispensing clinics include phentermine; Bontril (phendimetrazine, Carnrick Laboratories Inc., Cedar Knolls, New Jersey, U.S.); Tenuate (diethylpropion hydrochloride, Sanofi-Aventis, Bridgewater, New Jersey, U.S.); Meridia (sibutramine hydrochloride monohydrate, Abbott Laboratories, North Chicago, Illinois, U.S.); and Xenical (orlistat, Roche, Basel, Switzerland). Phentermine, the most commonly prescribed medication in these types of clinics, is inexpensive, and has been available for nearly 50 years. Many discount drug stores sell phentermine for $18 per month's supply (58). Medication-dispensing weight loss clinics often buy phentermine in bulk and sell the medication directly to the patient. Phendimetrazine and diethylpropion hydrochloride are also dispensed in this manner. Sibutramine and orlistat are less commonly used because both are still under patent as well as are more expensive than other available weight loss medications. Subsequently, patients are often given a prescription for sibutramine and orlistat, as opposed to the clinic dispensing them.

The majority of medication-dispensing weight loss clinics also use supplements, such as vitamins (including B vitamin injections) and "fat metabolizers." Some clinics' Web sites use comments such as "scientifically proven" or "proven results" to describe the supplements or diet plan.

In the past, the Federal Trade Commission (FTC) has tried to alert consumers to deceptive advertising (59). In the early 1990s, for example, a chain of weight loss clinics operating in California, Nevada, Texas, Georgia, and Virginia and featuring a supplement known as growth hormone releasers came under FTC investigation. The FTC charged that the clinics misled consumers by falsely advertising that through the clinics' "medically safe" program consumers can adjust their metabolism and lose up to 1.5 lb/day without exercise or strict dieting (59). Most medication-dispensing clinics do not practice deceptive advertising, although some claims can be difficult to believe.

The types of patients who present to these clinics vary, but patients are usually female and suffer from simple obesity. Because these sites are run by physicians, patients who have comorbidities can enter these programs, although patients with complicated medical histories or multiple comorbid problems typically do not participate in these programs for fear that the medications or supplements will exacerbate existing medical problems (60).

The range of weight loss treatments is extensive; in addition to medications and nutritional supplements, diets and meal replacements are also offered. Some medication-dispensing clinics offer other therapies, such as body wraps, mesotherapy, and injections of human choriongonadoptric hormone (hCG).

Little has been published regarding these weight loss clinics. In one peer-reviewed article, patients participating in a commercial medication-dispensing weight loss clinic were seen by a nurse between two and five times per week and were followed for 12 months (61). For patients who completed the program, weight loss at the end of 12 months was 10% to 11%; the dropout rate, however, was between 55% and 85% at 12 months. The study followed patients who were given a prescription for a weight loss medication, however, which is not the norm for that particular clinic; as verified by the study's author, the majority of patients seen in that clinic receive phentermine. In the study author's experience, the one-year weight loss was similar or slightly better to weight loss with phentermine.

Risks

Risks of weight loss medications can be significant, and the safety of obesity drugs historically has been poor (62). The two approved long-term weight loss medications, sibutramine and orlistat, have reasonable safety records; serious adverse events were not associated with these drugs despite several reviews, although continued research and follow-up is recommended (63–65).

As discussed earlier, phentermine is the most commonly prescribed drug by medication-dispensing clinics; currently, more phentermine is prescribed than sibutramine and orlistat combined (53). Unfortunately, little safety data have been published on phentermine because it was approved in the 1950s. The approval process in the 1950s was very different from our current standards, both the number of patients studied and the rigorous nature of studying FDA-approved medications have changed dramatically. Phentermine is currently approved for short-term use, although in clinical practice, it is used much longer.

When medications are dispensed directly to the patient, without the involvement of a prescription or pharmacist, the dispensing physician serves the role of pharmacist as well as prescribing doctor (66). The physician may not have access to patient information, such as what medications the patient may already be taking, and subsequently a drug-drug interaction is possible. When a physician is dispensing weight loss medications, the physician should understand all potential problems as well as inform the patient of these problems.

The risk of administering weight loss medications to patients who are not truly obese also exists. In this author's experience over the last 10 years as an expert witness for the state of California (expert opinion on the appropriate use of weight loss medications), the most common departure from the standard of care was a physician prescribing or administering weight loss medications to patients who were not obese or had BMIs of less than 27 kg/m^2.

True of all weight loss clinics, the risk of spending money on placebo-induced weight loss exists. Patients may pay for supplements, vitamins, or other treatments that may not have scientific basis for weight loss.

The risk of "placebo therapies" that do not have proven benefit also exists with medication-dispensing weight loss clinics. For example, hCG injections are commonly given in medication-dispensing clinics. hCG is a hormone produced in large quantities during pregnancy and obtained from the urine of pregnant women. In the 1950s, British physician A.T.W. Simeons popularized a reducing diet known as "curra romana," which consisted of daily injections of 125 IU intramuscular of hCG and 500 cal/day (67). The diet was meant to facilitate weight loss in particular parts of the body (hips, belly, and thighs) and decrease hunger (68,69). Several randomized controlled trials and meta-analysis, however, have shown hCG shots are no more efficacious than the diet alone (67–69).

Costs

The majority of medication-dispensing clinics do not accept health insurance, and subsequently the majority of costs are paid by the patient. Costs vary tremendously depending on what services or weight loss treatments are provided. Initial costs vary the most: Some clinics offer specials, making the initial visit or consultations free, while others charge for extensive hormonal and metabolic workups that include various laboratory blood draws and EKGs.

Typical costs for a medical visit and a week's supply of weight loss medications (usually phentermine) range from $35 to $65, although the medical visit may not include a one-on-one visit with a physician. Vitamin injections, most commonly vitamin B, cost an additional $20/wk, and hCG injections cost an additional $50 to $55 per week.

Meal replacements, VLCD liquid beverages, and meal replacement bars were comparable to costs of such items in noncommercial and VLCD medical clinics. Some medication-dispensing clinics carry their own brand of meal replacements; others use available, established meal replacements.

Benefits

Weight loss in obese patients has numerous benefits, as previously noted. Weight loss medications can be prescribed for patients participating in a program that is medically supervised, which may make significant weight loss attainable. Patients who regularly visit a physician during weight loss may also benefit with regard to management of comorbid diseases and medications.

Unfortunately, little is known regarding the patient benefits for those who attend medication-dispensing clinics. Little published peer-reviewed data exist.

A significant percentage of the physicians who operate these clinics are bariatricians and belong to the American Society of Bariatric Physicians (ASBP). The mission statement of ASBP states that members will establish and maintain practice guidelines, and a certifying exam is required before membership is granted. The organization's quarterly journal, the *Bariatrician*, is peer-reviewed (70), according to the ASBP Web site. The journal, however, is not indexed in Medline or Web of Knowledge, and may not be peer-reviewed in the classic sense typical of most indexed journals.

Because there is so little information on the benefits of weight loss achieved through medication-dispensing programs, no conclusion can be drawn regarding their risks or benefits.

MULTISPECIALTY WEIGHT LOSS CLINICS

Multispecialty weight loss clinics are obesity management programs staffed by highly qualified specialists from each of the different disciplines that make up obesity treatment. Such clinics employ a registered dietitian to teach proper nutrition, a psychologist to implement behavioral changes, and a physician to handle medical issues. Many programs also feature an exercise physiologist, and some of the more comprehensive programs have a surgeon on staff, providing the option of bariatric surgery.

To meet the needs of their large patient base, multispecialty clinics are associated with large medical groups, hospitals, or universities, and are usually located in large cities. A large percentage of the patients participating in these programs are referred by physicians within a medical group or community physicians associated with a university or hospital. It is not uncommon for a large medical group such as Kaiser or Scripps Clinic to have ownership of the multispecialty obesity clinic. The same is true for large universities and hospitals.

The expertise of the physicians conducting the program is typically very high due to several factors. Many programs associated with a teaching hospital have fellowship or postgraduate training in obesity management, and many attending physicians and psychologists have trained in obesity management. In addition, many programs conduct ongoing research in the form of clinical trials, and much of the literature in obesity management is published by these programs.

Patients who participate in multispecialty weight loss clinics vary from patients with no comorbidities who need to lose 20 to 30 lb to patients who are super morbidly obese (having a BMI of greater than 50) and who have difficult-to-manage comorbidities. Serious and often difficult-to-treat comorbidities typically seen in these clinics include insulin-dependent diabetes, renal failure, liver failure, and congestive heart failure. In addition, multispecialty weight loss clinics also accommodate super morbidly obese patients who are too large to fit on an operating table and subsequently need to lose weight before a surgical procedure.

Patients who participate in multispecialty clinics have incomes ranging from upper to lower, and some clinics honor medical insurance or workers' compensation cases and state-funded medical plans.

Services provided by these clinics range from simple (the use of one health care provider) to multidisciplinary (for complex cases). For example, if a patient has a BMI of 25 kg/m^2 and needs to lose 20 lb, then that patient might work one-on-one with a dietitian. However, a morbidly obese patient with recently diagnosed diabetes may require a full workup by a physician, group behavior modification, a VLCD, and weight loss medications.

Because of the dramatic rise in the number of patients undergoing bariatric surgery, many multispecialty programs are associated with a bariatric surgeon group or have a bariatric surgeon on staff. An increasing number of insurance companies require a documented six-month medical attempt at weight loss before covering surgery, and, subsequently, multispecialty groups often perform this part of the preparation for bariatric surgery candidates. Recent findings indicate that many post-gastric bypass patients are at high risk for nutritional and metabolic problems, such as nutritional deficiencies, medical problems, and weight regain, and many multispecialty clinics assist post-gastric bypass patients with these issues (71).

When appropriate, weight loss medications are used in many multispecialty clinics; in this setting, the patient is given a prescription, which is filled at a pharmacy.

Similar to other programs, the diet of a multispecialty clinic can range from regular patient-prepared food to meal replacements or VLCDs. Much of the dietary coun-

seling is done by dietitians, and all multispecialty programs offer lifestyle counseling, either individually or in a group setting.

Costs

Costs vary widely for participants in multispecialty programs because many honor medical insurance. Initial visits and physical exams can cost from $150 to $270, and a laboratory workup can cost $50 to several hundred dollars, depending on its extent. For obese patients who have no related comorbid disease, the possibility exists that the initial visit or laboratory workup cost will not be covered. For patients who have a comorbid disease related to obesity, who are morbidly obese, or who have a flexible medical spending account, most, if not all, of the initial visit and laboratory workup costs are covered. Typical comorbid or medical conditions that are covered by insurance are diabetes mellitus, metabolic syndrome, sleep apnea, abnormal cholesterols, and hypertension. Table 3 lists some of the International Classification of Diseases (ICD)-9 codes that are often covered by medical insurance.

Costs for group and individual therapy and/or behavior modification are usually not covered by insurance. Most programs charge a nominal fee for group lifestyle counseling, typically costing $240 to $350 for 10 to 12 group sessions. Most groups meet weekly, although some meet every other week, and almost all of the programs surveyed charge $20/wk for group participation or brief one-on-one visits. A few multispecialty clinics offer six-month programs at a cost of $1200 to $1500. The six-month program includes visits with all appropriate specialties and weekly weigh-ins. Similar to other programs, costs of meal replacements, VLCD beverages, high-protein bars, and vitamins are not covered, although costs of these items are similar to other programs.

Table 3 List of ICD-9 Codes of Common Obesity Related Medical Problems Used in Billing of Medical Insurance Companies[a]

Code	Medical problem
250.0	Diabetes
790.21	Impaired fasting glucose
272.0	Hypercholesterolemia
780.53	Sleep apnea
401.9	Hypertension
278.01	Morbid obesity
277.7	Dysmetabolic syndrome

[a]This list is not meant to be all-inclusive and coverage can vary for different insurances.
Abbreviation: ICD, International Classification of Diseases.

Weekly or monthly physician visits may be covered by medical insurance for patients with comorbid disease or morbid obesity. The coverage of medications depends on the insurance company and medical diagnosis. Morbidly obese patients have a good chance of having weight loss medications paid for by medical insurance. Economically speaking, weight loss medications are much less expensive than bariatric surgery, for which morbidly obese patients qualify. A medical insurance company is more likely to cover weight loss medications if the patient is enrolled in a program that offers lifestyle changes and diet than if the patient is not enrolled in such a program. For a patient to receive coverage for weight loss medications, physicians often are required to fill out a prior authorization request (PAR) (61), which asks the patient's BMI, related comorbidities, and questions the patient's participation in a lifestyle program. Insurance companies use the PAR to determine a patient's eligibility for coverage of weight loss medications.

In programs offering bariatric surgery, as much as one-third of patients pay out-of-pocket or cash for bariatric surgery (laparoscopic adjustable gastric band or gastric bypass). Table 4 lists the cost of these surgical procedures. In the current trend, multispecialty clinics offer both the adjustable gastric band as well as the gastric bypass surgeries. Many insurance companies prefer to have provider relationships with multispecialty centers that demonstrate expertise, so that the insurance company is confident in the abilities of the physicians and the bariatric surgery team.

Risks

Risks of going to a multispecialty clinic are similar to those of both medical and nonmedical commercial programs. As calories are further restricted (LCDs vs. VLCDs), the risk of gallstones and side effects such as fatigue, constipation, cold intolerance, electrolyte abnormalities, and hair loss increases (1). Medications have their own risks, and these are discussed in other chapters.

The average BMI of patients presenting to a multispecialty clinic can be high, particularly in clinics that offer bariatric surgery. Many patients weigh in excess of 400 lb when initially presenting to these clinics. These super morbidly obese patients face risks related to their much higher weights (72), and simple things, such as undergoing

Table 4 Costs of Bariatric Surgery[a]

Procedure	Cost
Laprascopic adjustable gastric band	$16,500–$22,000
Gastric bypass	$21,000–$26,000

[a]Costs typically include the pre- and postsurgical care and hospitalization.

a diagnostic imaging study, are more difficult because a morbidly obese patient will not fit in the scanner or on the imaging table. Most magnetic resonance imaging (MRI) or computed axial tomography (CAT) scanners have weight limits of 400 to 450 lb. In the author's experience, referrals for these patients to lose weight to undergo a MRI or CAT scan are not uncommon. These patients will benefit from weight loss, although other risks will require management.

Patients in multispecialty clinics tend to have multiple comorbid problems, and will be of higher risk accordingly (73). Some of the more common risks are difficult-to-control blood pressures and blood sugars, cardiac arrhythmias, pulmonary emboli, and skin infections. Multiple comorbid diseases usually indicate the use of more medications, which will need to be adjusted as the patient loses weight. During weight loss, the risk of a blood pressure or blood sugar that is too low is increased, making frequent adjustment of a patient's antihypertensive and diabetic medications necessary.

Multispecialty clinics are often a "last resort" for patients who have failed weight loss programs in the past. Expectations will be high, and the risk of not meeting these expectations is very real (74,75). Currently, a method that produces dramatic weight loss in each and every patient does not exist.

Benefits

Published data on the benefits of a multispecialty clinic are difficult to find. Few of these types of clinics exist, and very rarely are studies conducted to prove the benefits of these clinics. Still, studies conducted by multispecialty clinics show that multiple treatment modalities are more effective than using a single treatment option (76). In a study comparing weight loss with a medication to weight loss from group lifestyle counseling and to the combination of these approaches, data indicate that the combination of these approaches was the most efficacious, resulting in significantly more weight loss than either approach alone (76) (Fig. 1).

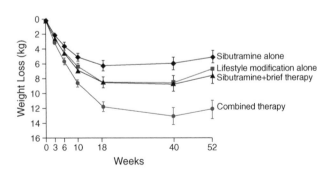

Figure 1 Additive effects of a weight loss medication with lifestyle modification. *Source*: From Ref. 76.

Table 5 List of Multispecialty Clinics in the United States[a]

Scripps Clinic Center for Weight Management
  San Diego, California 92130
University of Pennsylvania's Center for Weight and Eating
  Disorders:
  Philadelphia, Pennsylvania 19104
Washington University Weight Management Program
  Washington University School of Medicine
  St. Louis, Missouri 63110
Pennington Biomedical Research Center (Research Only)
  Louisiana State University System
  Baton Rouge, Louisiana 70808
Comprehensive Weight Control Program at New York's
  Presbyterian Hospital
  New York, New York 10021
Center for Nutrition and Metabolic Disorders
  University of Nevada School of Medicine
  Reno, Nevada 89557-0046
Solutions for Life™, Via Christi Regional Medical Center
  Wichita, Kansas 67208
UCLA Risk Factor Obesity Clinic
  Los Angeles, California 90095-1742
University of Iowa Carvar College of Medicine
  Iowa City, Iowa 52242
Wellness Institute, Northwestern Memorial Hospital
  Chicago, Illinois 60611
George Washington University Weight Management Program
  Washington D.C. 20037-3077>

[a]This list is not complete. Many other multispecialty clinics exist in the United States and internationally.

This is the basic premise of the multispecialty clinics: Optimal results are possible through the availability of all potential treatment options and various combinations of treatments.

From an organizational and logistics standpoint, it is a benefit to have various medical personnel housed in one place. Having an appropriate health care provider for instruction within a specialty also provides a potential benefit with regard to cost-effectiveness; for example, it is more cost-effective for a dietitian to offer dietary instruction, as opposed to a physician offering dietary instruction. In addition to increasing the cost-effectiveness, it may also increase the quality of care; in a similar scenario of appropriate use of nurse management in diabetics, the care actually improved (77).

If a multispecialty center offers bariatric surgery, then the number of patients who undergo follow-up also increases. In studies of successful weight loss after bariatric surgery, better outcomes were achieved with increased follow-up (78). The nature of a multispecialist center increases the amount of preliminary and follow-up visits, as patients are required to see multiple specialists as opposed to one physician.

Bariatric surgical centers with a low volume of bariatric cases have higher morbidities and mortalities (79,80). Multispecialty centers that perform surgery can accommodate high volumes of bariatric patients because a large number of morbidly obese patients present to these clinics. In a typical clinic receiving 100 new patients per month, more than 20 patients will be considering bariatric surgery and will qualify for the procedure. This translates into 15 to 20 surgeries per month, which is above the minimum established for a Center of Excellence (COE) designation for a bariatric surgical program (81).

Because multispecialty clinics tend to work by referral and tend to accommodate the needs of larger communities, they are not available in all areas. For the medically complicated patient, a multispecialty clinic can be a good referral source. Table 5 is a list of some of the multispecialty clinics available in the United States.

REFERENCES

1. National Task Force on the Prevention and Treatment of Obesity, National Institutes of Health. Very low-calorie diets. JAMA 1993; 270(8):967–974.
2. http://jennycraig.com. Accessed April 24, 2007.
3. www.weightwatchers.com. Accessed April 24, 2007.
4. www.nutrisystem.com. Accessed April 24, 2007.
5. Hannum SM, Carson L, Evans EM, et al. Use of portion-controlled entrees enhances weight loss in women. Obes Res 2004; 12(3):538–546.
6. Metz JA, Stern JS, Kris-Etherton P, et al. A randomized trial of improved weight loss with prepared meal plan in overweight and obese patients: impact on cardiovascular risk reduction. Arch Intern Med 2000; 160(14):2150–2158.
7. Heymsfield SB, van Mierlo CA, van der Knaap HC, et al. Weight management using meal replacements strategy: meta and pooling analysis from six studies. Int J Obes Relat Metab Disord 2003; 27(5):537–549.
8. Rock CL, Bilge P, Flatt SW, et al. Randomized trial of a multifaceted commercial weight loss program. Obesity 2007; 15:939–949.
9. www.ediets.com. Accessed May 3, 2007.
10. www.webmd.com. Accessed May 3, 2007.
11. www.mayoclinic.com. Accessed May 3, 2007.
12. Brownell KD. The LEARN Program for Weight Control. 7th ed. Dallas, Texas: American Health Publishing Company, 1998.
13. Womble LG, Wadden TA, McGuckin BG, et al. A randomized controlled trial of a commercial internet weight loss program. Obes Res 2004; 12(6):1011–1018.
14. Rothert K, Strecher VJ, Doyle LA, et al. Web-based weight management programs in an integrated health care setting: a randomized, controlled trial. Obesity (Silver Spring). 2006; 14(2):266–272.
15. Tate DF, Jackvony EH, Wing RR. A randomized trial comparing human e-mail counseling, computer-automated tailored counseling, and no counseling in an Internet

weight loss program. Arch Intern Med 2006; 166(15): 1620–1625.

16. Heshka S, Anderson JW, Atkinson RL, et al. Weight loss with self-help compared with a structured commercial program: a randomized trial. JAMA 2003; 289(14): 1792–1798.

17. Tsai AG, Wadden TA. Systematic review: an evaluation of major commercial weight loss programs in the United States. Ann Intern Med 2005; 142(1):56–66.

18. Gosselin C, Cote G. Weight loss maintenance in women 2 to 11 years after participation in a commercial program: a survey. BMC Womens Health 2001; 1(1):2.

19. Finley CE, Barlow CE, Greenway FL, et al. Retention rates and weight loss in a commercial weight loss program. Int J Obes (Lond) 2007; 31(2):292–298.

20. Tsai AG, Wadden TA, Womble LG, et al. Commercial and self-help programs for weight control. Psychiatr Clin N Am 2005; 28(1):171–192.

21. Witherspoon B, Rosenzweig M. Industry-sponsored weight loss programs: description, cost, and effectiveness. J Am Acad Nurse Pract 2004; 16(5):198–205.

22. Erlinger S. Gallstones in obesity and weight loss. Eur J Gastroenterol Hepatol 2000; 12(12):1347–1352.

23. Heshka S, Spitz A, Nunez C, et al. Obesity and risk of gallstone development on a 1200 kcal/d (5025Kj/d) regular food diet. Int J Obes Relat Metab Disord 1996; 20(5):450–454.

24. Oprah regrets her 1988 liquid diet. Available at: http://www.usatoday.com/life/people/2005-11-16-oprah-liquid-diet_x.htm. Accessed May 3, 2007.

25. National Institutes of Health. Clinical Guidelines on the Identification, Evaluation, and Treatment of Overweight and Obesity in Adults: The Evidence Report. Rockville, Maryland: National Institutes of Health, 1998:1–228.

26. Wadden TA, Sternberg JA, Letizia KA, et al. Treatment of obesity by very low calorie diet, behavior therapy, and their combination: a five-year perspective. Int J Obes 1989; 13(suppl 2):39–46.

27. Anderson JW, Grant L, Gotthelf L, et al. Weight loss and long-term follow-up of severely obese individuals treated with an intensive behavior program. Int J Obes (Lond) 2007; 31(3):488–493.

28. Henry RR, Gumbiner B. Benefits and limitations of very-low-calorie diet therapy in obese NIDDM. Diabetes Care 1991; 14(9):802–823.

29. Van Gaal LF. Dietary treatment of obesity. In: Bray GA, Bouchard C, James WPT, eds. Handbook of Obesity. New York, NY: Marcel Decker, 1978:875–890.

30. Saris WH. Very-low-calorie diets and sustained weight loss. Obes Res 2001; 9(suppl 4):295S–301S.

31. Centers for Disease Control. Liquid protein diets. Public Health Service report EPI-78-11-2. Atlanta, Georgia, 1979.

32. Sours HE, Frattali VP, Brand CD, et al. Sudden death associated with very low calorie diet weight reduction regimens. Am J Clin Nutr 1981; 34(4):453–461.

33. Isner JM, Sours He, Paris AL, et al. Sudden, unexpected death associated in avid dieters using the liquid-protein-modified-fast diet. Observations in 17 patients and the role of the prolonged QT interval. Circulation 1979; 60(6): 1401–1412.

34. Frank A, Graham C, Frank S. Fatalities on the liquid-protein diet: an analysis of possible causes. Int J Obes 1981; 5(3):243–248.

35. Atkinson RL, Kaiser DL. Non-physician supervision of a very-low-calorie diet. Results in over 200 cases. Int J Obes 1981; 5(3):237–241.

36. Amatruda JM, Biddle TL, Patton ML, et al. Vigorous supplementation of a hypocaloric diet prevents cardiac arrhythmias and mineral depletion. Am J Med 1983; 74(6): 1016–1022.

37. Phinney SD, Bistrian BR, Kosinski E, et al. Normal cardiac rhythm during hypocaloric diets of varying carbohydrate content. Arch Intern Med 1983; 143(12):2258–2261.

38. Gebhard RL, Prigge WF, Ansel HJ, et al. The role of gallbladder emptying in gallstone formation during diet-induced rapid weight loss. Hepatology 1996; 24(3): 544–548.

39. Festi D, Colecchia A, Orsini M, et al. Gallbladder motility and gallstone formation in obese patients following very low calorie diets. Use it (fat) to lose it (well). Int J Obes Relat Metab Disord 1998; 22(6):592–600.

40. Drug Facts and Comparisons. 2007 ed. St. Louis, Missouri: Wolters Kluwer Health, 2007.

41. Gout and predisposing factors. Available at: http:www.uptodateonline.com. Accessed May 3, 2007.

42. Kasper DL, Braunwald E, Fauci A, et al. Harrison's Principles of Internal Medicine. Chap. 167, 16th ed. Alexandria, VA: McGraw Hill Medical, 2004.

43. Atkinson RL, Kaiser DL. Effects of calorie restriction and weight loss on glucose and insulin levels in obese humans. J Am Coll Nutr 1985; 4(4):411–419.

44. Kelley DE, Wing R, Buonocore C, et al. Relative effects of calorie restriction and weight loss in non-insulin-dependent diabetes mellitus. J Clin Endocrinol Metab 1993; 77(5): 1287–1293.

45. Atkinson RL. Low and very low calorie diets. Med Clin North Am 1989; 73(1):203–215.

46. Hoffer LJ, Bistrian BR, Young VR, et al. Metabolic effects of very low calorie weight reduction diets. J Clin Invest 1984; 73(3):570–758.

47. Hong K, Li Z, Wang HJ, et al. Analysis of weight loss outcomes using VLCD in black and white overweight and obese women with and without metabolic syndrome. Int J Obes (Lond) 2005; 29(4):436–442.

48. Pekkarinen T, Takala I, Mustajoki P. Weight loss with a very-low-calorie diet and cardiovascular risk factors in moderately obese women: one-year follow-up study including ambulatory blood pressure monitoring. Int J Obes Relat Metab Disord 1998; 22(7):661–666.

49. Harder H, Dinesen B, Astrup A. The effect of a rapid weight loss on lipid profile and glycemic control in obese type 2 diabetic patients. Int J Obes Relat Metab Disord 2004; 28(1):180–182.

50. Lantz H, Peltonen M, Agren L, et al. Intermittent versus on-demand use of a very low calorie diet: a randomized 2-year clinical trial. J Intern Med 2003; 253(4):463–471.

51. Rossner S, Flaten H. VLCD versus LCD in long-term treatment of obesity. Int J Obes Relat Metab Disord 1997; 21(1):22–26.

52. Li Z, Hong K, Wong E, et al. Weight cycling in a very low-calorie diet programme has no effect on weight loss velocity, blood pressure, and serum lipid profile. Diabetes Obes Metab 2007; 9(3):379–385.

53. IMS Health. National Prescription Audit Plus 7™, years 1997–2003. Extracted March 2004, NPA Plus™ Therapeutic Category Report, December 1966.

54. Medical weight loss clinics. Available at: http://www.google.com/search. Accessed April 8, 2007.

55. www.4Weightclinics.com. Accessed April 8, 2007.

56. www.sobobamedspa.com/. Accessed April 8, 2007.

57. www.lindora.com. Accessed April 8, 2007.

58. Costco and Wal-Mart retail prices of phentermine in California, March 2007 (unpublished data).

59. FTC News Release, September 19, 1990. Available at: http://www.ftc.gov/opa/1997/03/dietcase.htm. Accessed May 3, 2007.

60. Review of 200 patients presenting for weight loss at the Center for Weight Management. Unpublished data, Scripps Clinic, 2002–2003.

61. Risser JA, Vash PD, Nieto L. Does prior authorization of sibutramine improve medication compliance or weight loss? Obes Res 2005; 13(1):86–92.

62. Greenway FL, Caruso MK. Safety of obesity drugs. Expert Opin Drug Saf 2005; 4(6):1083–1095.

63. Li Z, Maglione M, Tu W, et al. Meta-analysis: pharmacologic treatment of obesity. Ann Intern Med 2005; 142(7):532–546.

64. Ryan DH. Use of sibutramine and other noradrenergic and serotonergic drugs in the management of obesity. Endocrine 2000; 13(2):193–199.

65. Ioannides-Demos LL, Proietto J, Tonkin AM, et al. Safety of drug therapies used for weight loss and treatment of obesity. Drug Saf 2006; 29(4):277–302.

66. Guidebook to Laws Governing the Practice of Medicine by Physicians and Surgeons. 5th ed. Department of Consumer Affairs, Medical Board of California, 1996.

67. Rabe T, Richter S, Kiesel L, et al. Risk-benefit analysis of a hCG-500 kcal reducing diet (cura romana) in females. Geburtshilfe Frauenheilkd 1987; 47(5):297–307.

68. Theeuwen I, Assendelft WJ, Van Der Wal G. The effect of human chorionic gonadotropin (HCG) in the treatment of obesity by means of the Simeons therapy: a criteria-based meta-analysis. Br J Clin Pharmacol 1995; 40:237–243.

69. Shetty KR, Kalkhoff RK. Human chorionic gonadotropin (HCG) treatment of obesity. Arch Intern Med 1977; 137:151–155.

70. American Society of Bariatric Physicians. Available at: www.asbp.org. Accessed May 3, 2007.

71. Fujioka K. Follow-up of nutritional and metabolic problems after bariatric surgery. Diabetes Care 2005; 28(2):481–484.

72. Abou-Nukta F, Alkhoury F, Arroyo K, et al. Clinical pulmonary embolus after gastric bypass surgery. Surg Obes Relat Dis 2006; 2(1):24–28.

73. Fujioka K, Toussi RH, Brunson ME, et al. Health care utilization before and after bariatric surgery, the managed care experience. Obes Res 2001; 9(3):O123 (abstr).

74. Foster GD, Wadden TA, Vogt RA, et al. What is a reasonable weight loss? Patients' expectations and evaluations of obesity treatment outcomes. J Consult Clin Psychol 1997; 65(1):79–85.

75. Wadden TA, Womble LG, Sarwer DB, et al. Great expectations: "I'm losing 25% of my weight no matter what you say." J Consult Clin Psychol 2003; 71(6):1084–1089.

76. Wadden TA, Berkowitz RI, Womble LG, et al. Randomized trial of lifestyle modification and pharmacotherapy for obesity. N Eng J Med 2005; 353(20):2111–2120.

77. Phylis-Tsimikas A, Heaton S, Springer S, et al. Nurse management improves care in a managed-care setting. Diabetes 2000; 40(1):190 (abstr).

78. Fielding GA, Ren CJ. Laparoscopic adjustable gastric band. Surg Clin North Am 2005; 85(1):129–140.

79. Flum DR, Salem L, Elrod JA, et al. Early mortality among Medicare beneficiaries undergoing bariatric surgical procedures. JAMA 2005; 294(15):1903–1908.

80. Maggard MA, Shugarman LR, Suttorp M, et al. Meta-analysis: surgical treatment of obesity. Ann Intern Med 2005; 142(7):547–559.

81. American Society for Bariatric Surgeons qualifications for Center of Excellence status for 2007. Available at: http://www.asbs.org, www.surgicalreview.org. Accessed April 8, 2007.

39

Economic Aspects of Obesity

PING ZHANG and RUI LI

Division of Diabetes Translation, National Center for Disease Prevention and Health Promotion,
Centers for Disease Control and Prevention, Atlanta, Georgia, U.S.A.

INTRODUCTION

Obesity is not only a health but also an economic issue. Economic aspects of obesity cover a wide spectrum, ranging from the economic causes and consequence of obesity to the economics measures to prevent and manage obesity. In this chapter, we focus on two aspects of the economics of obesity: the economic cost of obesity and the cost-effectiveness of different interventions used to treat obesity. For each aspect, we begin with a brief description of the research method used and then summarize the major findings and their policy implications. Finally, we discuss future research.

ECONOMIC COSTS OF OBESITY

Methods to Estimate the Cost of Obesity

The cost-of-illness (COI) method is historically the most common method used to estimate the total economic cost of obesity. With the COI method, the total economic cost of obesity is grouped into three components: the direct, indirect, and intangible costs. The direct cost is further grouped into direct medical and nonmedical costs.

Direct Medical Cost

The direct medical cost of obesity includes the cost associated with treatment of obesity and medical expenditures for diseases for which excess body weight is a risk factor, such as type 2 diabetes and hypertension. Direct medical costs include expenditures to reduce body weight that are paid by a health care system, such as medications and surgical procedures. Treatment costs not paid by the health care system, such as exercise equipment, are not considered direct medical costs. Not all medical expenditures spent on treating obesity-related diseases are attributable to obesity because obesity is only one of many causes for these conditions. Only the proportion of the total expenditure in which obesity is the primary cause is accounted for in the computation of medical expenditures for obesity. The total medical expenditure of an obesity-related disease such as type 2 diabetes represents the value of health care resources used to diagnose and treating the disease, including hospital inpatient care, physician inpatient care, physician outpatient visits, emergency department outpatient visits, nursing home care, hospice care, rehabilitation care, specialists' and other health professionals' care, diagnostic tests, prescription drugs, and medical supplies.

The direct nonmedical cost includes the expense of health education efforts to maintain a healthy lifestyle and the expense of preventing and treating obesity, which is not paid by health care system, such as special diet and exercise equipments for losing weight, transportation, and the patients' time involved in the treatment. The direct nonmedical cost is normally paid by the individual.

However, few obesity cost studies include this component in deriving estimations for the total direct cost of obesity.

Indirect Cost

Indirect costs are the value of time that obese persons lose from employment or other productive activities because of mortality or morbidity. In addition, indirect costs include the value ascribed to time lost from work, housekeeping, etc., by family members or friends who transport, visit, and care for treating obesity and its attributed diseases, although this component of the cost is often excluded from the indirect cost estimates of obesity.

The human capital approach is the most commonly used method to estimate the indirect costs of obesity. This approach measures the indirect COIs in terms of market valuation of lost wage earnings from morbidity and mortality. For those who stay at home, the loss in productivity is measured by the value of lost household services, which is imputed on the expected earning if such services are performed by service workers such as maids and cooks. Indirect costs due to morbidity are the value of time lost as measured by wage earnings from decreased productivity while on the job and from the number of missed workdays as a result of obesity and its related diseases. Indirect costs due to mortality are the value of future income lost due to obesity-related premature death. The human capital approach excludes the value of leisure time and volunteer work that are not reflected in earnings from the indirect cost estimates.

"Intangible costs of obesity" refers to costs associated with the pain and suffering of obesity itself and those diseases for which obesity is an attributable factor. Because of the difficulty of assigning a monetary value to both physical and physiological suffering, this component of the cost has not been included in the total cost of obesity.

Prevalence-Based Vs. Incidence-Based Estimates

The COI method has been used to derive two sets of estimates related to the economic costs of obesity: the prevalence-based and incidence-based estimates. The prevalence-based (or annual cost) approach measures the direct and indirect costs, which accrue during a base year because of all existing (or prevalent) cases of obesity in that year. If a person died prematurely in the base year because of obesity and its contributed diseases, the loss in future productivity is also included. The loss in future productivity is estimated as the present discounted value of future earnings expressed in the base year.

Two main approaches have been used to derive the prevalence-based direct medical cost: epidemiological and econometric approach. The former is also referred to as the attributable risk approach. Using this approach, the total medical cost of obesity is the sum of medical costs across all diseases that are attributable to obesity. The cost of obesity from a disease such as diabetes is estimated by multiplying the population-attributable fraction (PAF) to the total direct medical cost of that disease. The PAF is calculated by using information on the prevalence rate of obesity and the unadjusted relative risk of an obesity-related disease for people who are obese, compared with those who have a normal body weight. The total medical cost of each obesity-related disease used in studies based on the attributable risk approach is obtained from the published studies rather than being estimated directly by the authors of those studies.

The econometric approach estimates the difference in costs between a cohort of the obese population and a cohort of the population with normal body weight. Regression analysis is used to adjust the difference of the two cohorts in demographic characteristics (e.g., sex, age, race, geographic location) and the presence of other chronic conditions. The incremental cost of obesity is the difference in costs incurred by each of the two cohorts, adjusting for those factors that affect the medical expenditures. Both the mean difference approach and a multistage regression approach are used to derive the incremental costs, where the former compares the mean costs incurred by each of the two cohorts to determine the incremental difference and the latter uses a multiple-stage regression technique (usually two stages). The multistage regression approach is most appropriate when there are many persons with zero expenditure and a few with very high costs. The approach involves estimating the likelihood of an individual receiving any care and then the excess cost if care is received. The incremental cost of the disease is measured by comparing the regression estimate with the disease dummy variable turned on to the regression estimate with the disease dummy variable turned off. The total medical cost of obesity using this approach is estimated as the product of the incremental cost per case of obesity and the number of obese persons.

The incidence-based (or lifetime cost) approach measures the present value of the lifetime costs of all new cases of obesity that occurred during the given base year. Incidence-based costs require knowledge of the diseases that obesity contributes to, the likely courses of those diseases and their durations, survival rates, onset and patterns of medical care to treat them, and the impact of obesity on employment. Incidence-based estimates are generally more difficult to estimate than prevalence-based estimates. However, the incidence-based approach is more useful for comparing the effects of alternative interventions to prevent, treat, or manage obesity. However, because of its complexity, few cost estimates related to obesity are incidence-based cost estimates.

Study Perspective

Economic costs of obesity have also been conducted from several different perspectives: costs to society, to health care system, to businesses, to government, and to patients and their families. Each perspective includes slightly different costs, thus provides useful information about the costs to the particular group. For example, the health care system perspective is concerned with only the direct medical care costs of obesity while the governmental perspective focuses on the specific governmental share. The societal perspective is the most comprehensive perspective, in which all direct medical costs and indirect costs for all members of the society are included.

Limitation of the COI Study

The economic cost of obesity measures the amount of resources that would be saved if obesity were eliminated. While such estimates can reveal the magnitude of obesity as an economic problem, they are limited in informing policy makers how to allocate resources. Allocating resources for a high-cost illness or condition that is not necessarily responsive to treatment by current medical technology may not be an efficient use of resources. In contrast, investing in a condition that presents a low cost to society and tends to be fully amenable to low-cost prevention can lead to health gains and better use of health care resources. Without an understanding of the benefits (or health outcomes) gained, it is not possible to assess whether or not resources should be spent on treating or preventing obesity.

Current Estimates on the Cost of Obesity

Prevalence-Based Cost Estimates

Aggregate direct medical costs for a nation or region

Numerous studies have attempted to estimate costs of obesity in different countries with most of the studies conducted in the United States. Thompson and Wolf (1) summarized the result from these studies published before 2001. We added the studies after 2001 and present all the estimates in Table 1.

The estimated cost of obesity in the United States ranged from $26.6 to $70 billion, which represents between 5% and 7% of annual health care expenditures. In other countries, the estimated costs as a percentage of total health care expenditures are lower than that of the United States, ranging from 2% to 4%. All studies used the epidemiological approach to derive their estimates with the exception of a study by Finkelstein et al. (2), which used the econometric approach. Differences in both the obesity criteria used and the number of obesity-related

diseases have contributed to the variation in cost estimates among studies.

There is no consensus on the proportion of the total direct medical cost associated with each individual disease. Wolf and Colditz (3) reported that approximately 63% of the direct cost was from type 2 diabetes, 14% from coronary heart disease (CHD), 8% from osteoarthritis, 6% from hypertension, and less than 10% from other diseases. In comparison, Sander and Bergemann (4) estimated that 34% of the total cost was attributable to hypertension, 22% to myocardial infarction, 20% to stroke, 14% to type 2 diabetes, and 11% to the obesity treatment. However, all studies indicated that majority of the total cost is due to treating obesity-related complications rather than obesity itself. For example, of the €2.03 billion direct medical costs associated with obesity in Germany in 2001, only €216 million or 11% of the total was due to the obesity-related additional physician visits and drug expenses.

Direct medical costs at individual patient level

Obese persons have a higher total health care expenditure than those with a normal body weight. Thompson et al. (5) examined the relation of current body mass index (BMI) to health care utilization over a nine-year period among adults in a health maintenance organization in Portland, Oregon. They reported that compared with persons with a normal body weight (BMI 20 to 24.9 kg/m^2), obese persons (BMI $\geq$ 30 kg/m^2) spent 36% more for medical care. Quesenberry et al. (6) reported that for all persons aged 20 years and older, the total medical cost was 25% greater for those with BMI of 30 to 34.9 kg/m^2 and 44% greater for those with BMI of 35 kg/m^2 and above compared with those of normal weight. Three studies (2,7,8) using nationally representative data showed that the additional per capita health care expenditure for obese persons was 36% to 37%, relative to those with normal body weight.

The degree of additional medical cost increases with the severity of obesity. Andreyeva et al. (9) reported that relative to a normal body weight, a BMI of 30 to 35 kg/m^2, 35 to 40 kg/m^2, or over 40 kg/m^2 was associated with a 25%, 50%, or 107% increase in health care expenditure, respectively, among a national representative sample of 54- to 69-year-old Americans. Using data for 16,262 adults from the 2000 U.S. Medical Expenditure Panel Survey, Arterburn et al. (10) reported that per capita health care expenditures for morbidly obese adults (BMI over 40 kg/m^2) were 81% greater than normal-weight adults, 65% greater than overweight adults, and 47% greater than adults with class I obesity (BMI 30–34.9 kg/m^2).

Obese individuals have a higher cost across all types of health services. Compared with individuals of normal weight (20 kg/m^2 $\leq$ BMI $\leq$ 24.9 kg/m^2), Quesenberry et al. (6) estimated that individuals who were moderately

Table 1 Direct Medical Costs of Obesity in Different Countries

Author(s), yr	Country and yr of costs	BMI (kg/m²) cut points	Diseases included	Absolute amount	Percentage of total health care expenditure
Colditz, 1992	United States, 1986	≥29	Type 2 diabetes, hypertension gallbladder disease, colon cancer, breast cancer, cardiovascular disease	$39.3 billion	5.5%
Wolf and Colditz, 1994	United States, 1990	≥29	Type 2 diabetes, hypertension gallbladder disease, cancer, coronary heart disease, musculoskeletal disease	$45.8 billion	6.8%
Wolf and Colditz, 1996	United States, 1993	≥29	Type 2 diabetes, hyperbaton gallbladder disease, coronary heart disease	$22.6 billion	—
Wolf and Colditz, 1998	United States, 1996	≥29	Type 2 diabetes, hypertension gallbladder disease, endometrial cancer, colon cancer, breast cancer, coronary heart disease, osteoarthritis	$51.6 billion	5.7%
Colditz, 1999	United States, 1995	≥30	Type 2 diabetes, hypertension gallbladder disease, endometrial cancer, colon cancer, breast cancer, coronary heart disease	$70.0 billion	7%
Finkelstein et al., 2003	United States, 1998	≥30	Both obesity-related and non-obesity-related diseases[a]	$47.5 billion	5.3%
Segal et al., 1994	Australia, 1989	≥30	Type 2 diabetes, hypertension gallbladder disease, colon cancer, breast cancer, coronary heart disease	A$395 million	2%
Levy et al., 1995	France, 1992	≥27	Hypertension dyslipidemias, gallbladder disease, endometrial cancer, colon cancer, breast cancer, osteoarthritis, myocardial infarction, gout, genitourinary cancer	FF 11.9 billion	2%
Sander and Bergemann, 2003	Gemany, 2001	≥30	Type 2 diabetes, hypertension, myocardial infarction, stroke	€1.34 billion	—
Birmingham et al., 1999	Canada, 1997	≥27	Type 2 diabetes, hypertension, stroke, coronary heart disease, hyperlipidemias, pulmonary embolism, gallbladder disease postmenopausal breast cancer, endometrial cancer, colorectal cancer	Can$1.8 billion	2.4%
Pereira et al., 2000	Portugal, 1996	≥30	Osteoarthritis, type 2 diabetes, hypertension, hyperlipidemias, cardiovascular disease, gallbladder disease, arthropathies, colon cancer, breast cancer, endometrial cancer, obesity	PTE 46.2 billion	3.5%
Swinburn et al., 1997	New Zealand, 1991	≥30	Type 2 diabetes, hypertension, hyperlipidemias, coronary heart disease, gallbladder disease, colon cancer, breast cancer	NZ$135 million	2.5%

[a]Using regression approach, including excess expenditures from both obesity-related and non-obesity-related diseases.

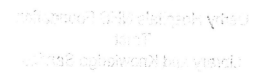

obese (30 kg/m^2 ≤ BMI ≤ 34.9 kg/m^2) or severely obese (BMI ≥ 35 kg/m^2) had 14% and 25% more physician visits, respectively. Thompson et al. (11) found that obese adults (BMI ≥ 30 kg/m^2) had 38% more visits to primary care physicians. Quesenberry et al. (6) reported that moderately and severely obese individuals have 34% and 74%, respectively, more inpatient days than those of normal weight. Thompson et al. (11) reported that obese individuals averaged 48% more inpatient days per year. They also reported that individuals with a BMI greater than 30 kg/m^2 had 1.84 times the annual number of pharmacy dispensations, including six times the number for diabetes medication and 3.4 times for cardiovascular medications (11).

The excess medical cost associated with obesity varies by age group. However, there is no consensus on how the excess cost changes with age. Quesenberry et al. (6) reported that the total medical costs including both inpatient and outpatient care increased first and then decreased, independent of the level of the obesity. For example, relative to persons with normal body weight (BMI 20–24.9 kg/m^2), individuals with BMI of 35 kg/m^2 and greater had a total additional cost of 48% for the 20- to 39-years age group, 72% for the 40- to 59-years group, and 38% for the 60- to 74-years group. The total medical cost for the oldest age group was actually lower (47% lower) than for those who had a normal body weight. In comparison, Wee et al. (12) found that health care expenditure associated with obesity was not significant for those younger than 35 years and then become aggressively higher as age increased. Thompson et al. (11) estimated that the cost ratios of individuals with BMI 30 kg/m^2 and greater relative to those with BMI of 20 to 24.9 kg/m^2 were 1.36 for those aged 35 to 44 years, 1.1 for those aged 45 to 54 years, and 1.50 for those aged 55 to 64 years. Different study populations may have contributed the different results across studies. Health care costs associated with obesity also vary according to race. Wee et al. (12) reported that health care expenditures related to higher BMI rose dramatically among white adults but not among blacks.

Indirect cost to society

The indirect cost of obesity was estimated at $47.6 billion in 1995 or 48% of the total economic cost of obesity that year in the United States (3) and at €2.2 billion or 51% of the total cost in 2001 in Germany (4). Both studies derived their estimates using the same epidemiological approach as used for deriving the direct medical cost. The proportion of the total indirect cost attributable to each obesity-related disease varies by country. In the United States, the major contributor was chronic heart disease (48%), followed by type 2 diabetes (17.5%), and osteoarthritis (17.1%). In Germany, myocardial infarction constituted 50% of the indirect cost, followed by stroke (21%), hypertension (18%), and type 2 diabetes (9%).

Costs to employers

Obesity also has a substantial financial impact on employers in terms of health care expenditure and excess sick leave and disability. Wang et al. (13) analyzed medical claim data for 175,000 General Motor employees from 1996 to 1997 and reported that medical charges for the very obese employee (BMI ≥ 40 kg/m^2) were 69% higher than those with normal weight (BMI 18.5–24.9 kg/m^2). Burton et al. (14) reported that obese employees (defined as BMI ≥ 27.8 kg/m^2 for men and BMI ≥ 27.3 kg/m^2 for women) in a larger firm located in Chicago had a mean three-year health care cost of $6822 in 1996, compared with $4496 for nonobese employees. Finkelstein et al. (15) reported that obese men or women (BMI ≥ 30 kg/m^2) spent $392 to $1591 or $1071 to $1395, respectively, more than those with normal BMI (18.5–24.9 kg/m^2). The increase in cost was not only the result of higher cost for each health claim but reflected the great number of health claim in comparison with nonobese employees.

Obese employees also miss more workdays and are more likely to be disabled than nonobese employees. Burton et al. (14) reported that obese employees used, on average, more than twice as many sick leave days as their normal-weight counterparts (i.e., 8.45 vs. 3.73 day/yr). When the sum of sick day absences over the six-year study period was converted to costs, the obese employee cost $863 (or $144/yr) more than a nonobese employee. Finkelstein et al. (15) reported that obese male employees (BMI ≥ 35 kg/m^2) missed about two more days of work than normal-weight men per year. In comparison, female employees with BMI 35 to 40 kg/m^2 and BMI ≥ 40 kg/m^2 missed about three and eight more days, respectively, than female employees with BMI ≥ 18 to 24.9 kg/m^2. Colditz (16) estimated that in 1994, there was a total of 58.5 million work-lost days in the United States, amounting to approximately $5.7 billion. Narbro et al. (17) reported that obese Swedish women (BMI 28 to 68 kg/m^2) were more than twice as likely to receive disability pensions compared with nonobese women (12% vs. 5%). In a study of Swedish men, Mansson (18) also found that obese persons had a relative risk of 2.8 in receiving disability pensions, compared with normal-weight men.

Adding the medical and nonmedical cost, the total cost of obesity imposed on employers is substantial. Thompson et al. (11) estimated the cost to U.S. business due to mild-to-severe obesity in 1994 was $12.7 billion, including $7.7 billion on health insurance expenditures, $2.4 billion on paid sick leave, $1.8 billion on life insurance, and $800 million on disability insurance. Finkelstein (15) reported that for obese male employees, the total cost to employers ranged from \$460 to \$2030 a year, and for female obese employees, the costs were between \$1370 and \$2485 a year. The cost of obesity at a firm with 1000 employees was estimated to be \$285,000/yr. The costs were highly skewed to the heaviest group among the three groups of obesity (BMI 30–34.9 kg/m^2, 35–39.9 kg/m^2, and $\geq$ 40 kg/m^2), which represented 3% of the employed population but accounted for 21% of the total cost.

Costs to obese individuals and their families

The cost of obesity to individuals and their families can be measured in both monetary and nonmonetary terms. The nonmonetary cost is the cost associated with a shorter life expectancy and lower health-related quality of life (HRQOL) as a result of obesity. Flegal et al. (19) estimated there were 111,909 premature deaths attributable to obesity in the United States in 2002. Forty-year-old female nonsmokers lost 7.1 years and 40-year-old male nonsmokers lost 5.8 years of life expectancy because of obesity (20). Fontaine and Braofsky (21) reviewed the studies that examined the impact of obesity on HRQOL among obese individuals and concluded that (*i*) obese persons reported significant decrements on HRQOL, (*ii*) the degree of the impairment rose with the level of obesity, (*iii*) obesity appeared to affect the physical health aspect of HRQOL more than the mental health aspect, and (*iv*) pain appeared to be an important comorbid condition that, in and of itself, produced significant reduction in HRQOL among obese persons. Both obesity and obesity-related diseases contributed to the lower HRQOL.

Obesity imposes several monetary costs on obese persons and their families. First, some direct medical costs are paid by individuals. There are great variations in the fraction of the total medical cost privately paid by individuals between countries and among individuals within a country because of different ways to finance the health care and individuals' ability to pay. Finkelstein et al. (2) estimated that about 14% of the direct medical costs of obesity were privately paid in 1998 in the United States. This translated into a total of at least \$3.8 billion or an annual average of \$125 per obese person. Second, individuals also pay for most, if not all, of the expenses for weight management and control. The Centers for Disease Control and Prevention (22) estimated that 17.2 million Americans (7% of the adult population) used nonprescription weight loss products during 1996 through 1998. In 2000, consumers spent an estimated \$34.7 billion on weight-loss products and programs (23). This expenditure included books, videos and tapes, low-calorie foods and drinks, sugar substitutes, meal replacements, prescription drugs, over-the-counter drugs, dietary supplements, medical treatments, commercial weight-loss chains, and other products or services related to weight loss or weight maintenance. Thirdly, obese persons are more likely to

be unemployed, work in low-paid jobs, and earn less than their lean counterparts because of job discrimination. Evidence from previous research showed that this negative impact is more pertinent for women than for men. Sarlio-Lahteenkorva et al. (24) reported that obese women were 2.5 times more likely to report long-term unemployment and to have higher rates of poverty than normal-weight women. Pagan and Davila (25) showed that women who were obese were largely excluded from high-paying managerial/professional and technical occupations and were present at a higher proportion in relatively low-paying occupations. Within similar occupations, obese women may earn less than normal-weight women do. The effect of weight on women's wages may differ by race. White women who were obese (BMI $\geq$ 30 kg/m^2) earned 17% less than did white women of normal weight (19 kg/m^2 < BMI < 25 kg/m^2) (26). An increase of two standard deviations in body weight was associated with a 7% decrease in wages among white women (27). However, no significant effect was found between body weight and wage rates among black women (26,27). The negative impact of obesity on earning for men is less clear. While most studies showed no relationship between earnings and body weight, others reported both negative and positive relationships. Finally, an obese person may also pay a higher health insurance or life insurance premium than a lean counterpart but there have been no studies to estimate the magnitude of those higher payments.

Incidence-Based Cost Estimates

In spite of higher annual medical costs, it is still not clear that they translate into higher lifetime costs because obese individuals have a shorter life expectancy. Thompson et al. (28) estimated the lifetime cost of treating five obesity-related diseases (hypertension, hypercholesterolemia, type 2 diabetes, CHD, and stroke) at various BMI levels for different sex and age groups. Relative to a BMI of 22.5 kg/m^2, the lifetime higher costs for persons with a BMI of 32.5 kg/m^2 ranged from \$8600 to \$11,200 and for those with a BMI of 37.5 kg/m^2 from \$14,500 to \$17,100, depending on age and sex. The age group with the highest cost was 45 to 54 years for men and 55 to 64 years for women. There was no clear pattern for the lifetime cost by gender. Gorsky et al. (29) simulated the excess medical cost for a period of 25 years for a cohort of 10,000 40-year-old U.S. women and found that the average additional cost per person reached \$5300. Allison et al. (30) reported that 4.3% of lifetime costs are attributable to obesity.

Summary and Conclusions

The COI method has been the dominant approach used to estimate the economic cost of obesity up to date. The COI method has been used to derive two sets of cost estimates related to obesity: prevalence-based and incidence-based estimates. Applying the COI approach, the economic cost of obesity consists of direct medical costs, direct non-medical costs, and indirect costs. Two methods have been used to estimate the direct medical costs and indirect costs of obesity: epidemiological and econometric approaches. Earlier studies tended to use the former method while the more recent studies tended to use the latter method. No studies have estimated the direct nonmedical cost and some components of the indirect cost, such as loss in productivity by caregivers, nor the cost of preventing obesity.

Several conclusions could be drawn based on the studies we reviewed. First, the economic burden imposed by obesity was substantial, in all countries for which the COI studies of obesity were conducted. At the national level, the direct medical cost represents 2% to 7% of the total health care expenditure. At the individual level, an obese person spent about 36% more on health care expenditure than a normal-weight individual. There is a great consistency across studies in these cost estimates. Second, the health care expenditure attributable to obesity was borne by multiple entities: national health system, private health insurers, and obese persons themselves and their families. The exact distribution of the burden varies across countries and among individuals within countries, depending on the health care finance system, insurance reimbursement policies, and employment benefit and welfare policies. In the United States, Finkelstein (14) estimated that of the total medical spending attributable to obesity, in 1998, about half was paid by the public Medicare and Medicaid program, 35% paid by private insurers, and 15% was paid by individual and their family. Finally, obesity also imposed a large economic burden on employers and obese individuals and their families. The high economic burden associated with obesity implies that more investment is needed to identify effective interventions for the prevention and control of obesity.

There are a number of limitations for previous studies. First, few studies were able to include all components of the costs and all of obesity-attributable diseases. Thus, current estimates of obesity may underestimate the "true" economic burden of obesity. On the other hand, there was a large variation on the numbers of obesity-related diseases included in the cost estimates, ranging from 4 to 10. Thompson and Wolf (1) reported that there was a strong evidence and consensus on only six medical conditions (CHD, type 2 diabetes, hypertension, gallbladder disease, endometrial cancer, and osteoarthritis of the knee). Including fewer or more diseases led to under- or overestimating the cost attributable to obesity. Second, the BMI criteria used to define obesity differed across studies. Studies from the United States used the criteria developed by

the National Center for Health Statistics (BMI $\geq$ kg/m^2) while those from Europe used the WHO obesity criteria (BMI $\geq$ 30 kg/m^2). Both the inconsistency in the number of diseases included and the definition of obesity have contributed to the difference in cost estimates and made comparison across the studies difficult.

Most economic studies on the cost of obesity focus on estimating the economic burden at a given time, using the prevalence-based approach. Only three studies were designed to derive an incidence-based cost estimate. While the prevalence estimate is useful to document the economic burden of obesity, such estimates are less useful in evaluating intervention options related to preventing and controlling obesity. In addition, current incidence-based estimates may well underestimate the true economic burden of obesity (1) and the cost-effectiveness of interventions for treating obesity.

COST-EFFECTIVENESS OF OVERWEIGHT AND OBESITY INTERVENTIONS

Methods Used to Evaluate the Cost-Effectiveness of the Intervention

Cost-effectiveness analysis is the most widely used method to evaluate the economic efficiency of obesity interventions to date. It is an analytic tool in which the costs and effects of a program and at least one alternative are calculated and presented in a ratio of incremental cost to incremental effect. The cost-effectiveness ratio (CER) of intervention A versus intervention B is the difference in costs divided by the difference in health outcomes between the two interventions, where the difference in costs is the cost of intervention B minus the cost of intervention A, and the difference in health outcomes is the health outcome of intervention B minus the health outcome of intervention A.

The cost consequence of the intervention is always measured in monetary terms. In comparison, the health outcome can be measured in physical units, such as number of pounds of body weight lost or number of life years gained. When the health outcome is measured by a quality of life–adjusted measure, such as quality-adjusted life year (QALY), the cost-effectiveness analysis is referred to a cost-utility analysis.

Figure 1 illustrates the way in which the cost-effectiveness analysis can aid decisions on health care resource allocation. In comparing the effectiveness and cost of two interventions, B and A, four combinations are possible. The four quadrants in the figure represent those four possibilities. The lower-right quadrant shows that compared to intervention A, intervention B has a better outcome at a lower cost, thus the intervention clearly should be adopted. This is the most desirable of the four

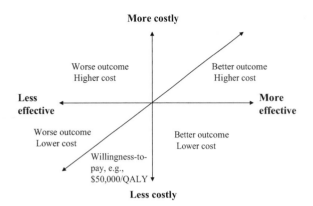

Figure 1 A framework of applying cost-effectiveness analysis for adding resource allocation decisions.

but probably the least-often achieved in practice. The upper-right quadrant represents a scenario in which intervention B has a better outcome but at a higher cost, thus the acceptability of intervention B depends on the extent to which the health outcome is improved and the cost increased. This is the most likely case when we decide whether a newer or better intervention or drug becomes available. The upper-left quadrant is the scenario in which intervention B has a worse health outcome at an even higher cost than intervention A. In this case, intervention B should be rejected. This is least desirable of the four. The lower-left quadrant represents the scenario that intervention B results in a worse outcome at lower cost. The decision on whether to adopt intervention B depends on how much benefit is forfeited and whether and how the available resources are used.

The willingness-to-pay (WTP) line (Fig. 1) represents how much a particular society is willing to pay for a health outcome resulting from a particular intervention. If the health outcome is measured in terms of QALYs, the line represents how much the society is willing to pay for one QALY. The line divides the upper-right and lower-left quadrants where the decision on adopting the intervention is inconclusive into two zones. The WTP line represents the "acceptable threshold" of cost-effectiveness of an intervention, below which the intervention is considered acceptable, and above which the interventions is not considered acceptable by the society.

Although there is no consensus on what this acceptable threshold should be, several thresholds have been proposed. In the United States, a figure of $50,000/QALY has been frequently quoted for many years as being cost-effective. Hirth et al. (31) retraced the origin of this $50,000/QALY and concluded that it was based on the "dialysis standard," the purported annual cost per QALY to Medicare program for patients with chronic renal failure. In Canada, Laupacis et al. (32) proposed that evidence for adoption of an intervention was strong if the

CER was, in Canadian dollars, $20,000/QALY, moderate if it was between $20,000/QALY and $100,000/QALY, and weak if it exceeded $100,000/QALY. In the United Kingdom, the National Institute for Health and Clinical Excellence, an independent body that decides which drugs should be available in the National Heath Services in England and Wales, has adopted a cost-effectiveness threshold range of £20,000 to £30,000/QALY since its inception in 1999 (33).

Current Evidence on the Cost-Effectiveness of Overweight and Obesity Interventions

We searched PubMed using key words "cost-effectiveness" and "obesity" for articles on the cost-effectiveness of obesity interventions published between 1997 and 2007. We included both original studies and review articles and placed no restriction on the country setting. Sixteen articles were selected. We reported all CERs in the 2005 U.S. dollar ($) and converted non-U.S. currencies into U.S. dollars using the annual average exchange rate at the cost year for which the CER was based on. We inflated the U.S. dollar at other years into year 2005 values using the consumer price index. If a study did not contain information on which year was used to calculate the cost, we assumed the dollar year was one year prior to the publication date. The articles were grouped into tables by types of intervention, including physician counseling and commercial weight loss programs, behavioral intervention, pharmaceutical therapies, and surgical interventions.

Cost-Effectiveness of Behavioral Interventions

Physician counseling and commercial weight loss programs

A physician's weight loss advice was associated with both fewer calories and fat intake and more exercise to lose weight in the United States (34). Segal et al. (35) estimated the cost-effectiveness of general practitioner's advice on weight loss and lifestyle changes in two hypothetical Australian populations: one with BMI > 27 kg/m², cardiovascular disease risk factors, and impaired glucose tolerance (IGT), and the other a mixed population with both IGT and normal glucose tolerance (NGT) (Table 2). The intervention was defined as healthy lifestyle advice provided by specially recruited primary care physicians, supported by printed material, up to eight visits in 12 months. The data on both cost and effectiveness used in the study were based on a review of literature. The authors reported that the intervention cost $864 per life year gained (LYG) among persons with IGT and $2340/LYG among the mixed population with IGT and NGT from a health system perspective.

Table 2 Cost-Effectiveness of Physician Counseling and Commercial Weight Loss Programs

Study	Study type	Study population	Intervention	Comparison	Perspective	Time horizon	Benefits included	CERs (original)	CERs (2005 U.S. dollars)
Physician counseling Segal et al., 1998, Australia	CEA	BMI >27 kg/m², IGT, or mixed IGT and NGT	General practitioner advice	No intervention	Health system	25 yr	Diabetes	$700–$1700 (1997)	$964–$2340 per LYG
Commercial weight loss programs									
Yates et al., 2006, Australia	CBA	Obese adults	Weight Watchers™ for 3 mo	No intervention	Societal	20 yr		$488 per new enrollee (2005)	$488 per new enrollee
Tsai et al., 2006, United States	Not a formal CEA	U.S. population	Nonmedical commercial weight loss programs	No intervention	Patients	3–6 mo		NA, Weight Watchers™ cost $167/3 mo, Jenny Craig™ cost $1249/3 mo	
		Obese or with chronic diseases such as diabetes	Medically supervised proprietary programs	No intervention				NA, Cost between $840–$2100/3 mo	
		U.S. population	Internet-based and self-help programs	No intervention				NA, Free or cost less than $100/3 mo	

Abbreviations: CEA, cost-effectiveness analysis; CBA, cost-benefit analysis; CER, cost effectiveness ratio; BMI, body mass index; IGT, impaired glucose tolerance; NGT, normal glucose tolerance; LYG, life year gained.

Few high-quality studies have been conducted to assess the cost-effectiveness of commercial and organized self-programs for weight loss to date. Yates and Murphy (34) conducted a cost-benefit analysis of weight management strategies from the Australian health system perspective. They used a program such as Weight Watchers™ for three months to illustrate benefits and costs. Assuming a 10% cure rate for obesity per enrollee, they estimated that the benefit per new enrollment from avoiding treatment costs for diseases related to overweight and obesity was $690. The cost per new enrollment of the weight loss program was $202. The net benefit per new enrolment was $488.

Tsai and Wadden (37) systematically reviewed the costs and effectiveness of major commercial weight loss programs in the United States. They found that among all nonmedical commercial weight loss programs, only Weight Watchers™ tested its efficacy in a large, multisite, randomized controlled trial. Those who regularly attended the program lost approximately 5% of initial weight within three to six months. Medically supervised proprietary programs such as Health Management Resources and OPTIFAST are often used by obese persons with chronic diseases such as diabetes. The authors suggest that individuals who completed a comprehensive program providing a low-calorie diet or very low calorie diet (VLCD) could expect to lose approximately 15% to 25% of initial weight during three to six months of treatment, 7% at three years, and 5% at four years. However, these results did not include those who did not complete treatment or declined to participate in follow-up assessment and were excluded from the analysis, a substantial percentage. Minimal evidence existed to recommend the use of commercial Internet-based interventions and the use of the best-known organized self-help programs, which typically used an online "virtual dietitian" program and physical activity seminars.

Regarding the cost of the commercial weight loss programs, Tsai and Wadden (2006) (35) reported that the medically supervised proprietary program was the most expensive because of the physician monitoring. The estimated costs of a three-month program of Health Management Resources or OPTIFAST ranged from $1700 to $2100. Medifast/Take Shape for Life was cheaper, but the cost was still $840 for three months. Among the nonmedical commercial weight loss programs, Jenny Craig™ was costly because of the company's prepackaged meals, about $1300 for three months. Weight Watchers™ was much less expensive, costing only $167 per three months. Internet-based commercial weight loss programs and self-help programs were even less expensive, less than $100 per three months or free.

Without a formal cost-effectiveness analysis, Tsai and Wadden (35) compared the benefit with the cost of each commercial weight loss programs and concluded that Weigh Watchers™ might be cost-effective because of its demonstrated effectiveness and the moderate cost. Medically supervised programs were expensive, but achieved more weight loss than Weight Watchers™ in the best scenario. It may be appropriate in selected cases, such as patients with severe obesity or other complications, in which more aggressive weight loss and medical care is warranted, as well more intensive physician monitoring. Although there is insufficient evidence for the effectiveness of weight loss of inexpensive self-help programs and Internet-based programs, they are potentially cost-effective if the weight loss goal can be achieved.

Comprehensive diet, exercise, and lifestyle modification

The Diabetes Prevention Program (DPP) study was a large randomized clinical trial to test whether diet and exercise or oral diabetes drug metformin could prevent or delay type 2 diabetes among persons who were overweight and had IGT. Eligible participants were randomly assigned to one of the three interventions: standard lifestyle recommendation plus metformin, standard lifestyle recommendation plus placebo, or an intensive lifestyle intervention program mainly through diet and physical activity. The trial results showed that 50% of the participants in the lifestyle-intervention group had achieved the goal of weight loss of 7% or more by 24 weeks and 38% had a weight loss of at least 7% at the end of the study. The incidence of diabetes was 58% lower in the lifestyle-intervention group than in the control group. The DPP group (36) analyzed the cost-effectiveness of lifestyle intervention within the three-year clinical trial period. From a health system perspective, the CER of intensive lifestyle intervention was $19,000 per case of diabetes prevented or $39,074/QALY gained. From a societal perspective, the DPP lifestyle intervention cost $32,156 per case of diabetes prevented or $67,720/QALY gained at the end of the 2.8-year follow-up period (36)(Table 3).

Four studies (37–39) analyzed the long-term cost-effectiveness of the DPP intensive lifestyle intervention in either 30 years or a lifetime, compared with standard lifestyle intervention or no intervention. The study by Eddy et al. (37), conducted in the United States, compared the cost-effectiveness of the DPP-intensive lifestyle intervention to no intervention and reported that, assuming its effect persisted beyond the three-year trial period, the intervention would reduce the risk of developing diabetes by 15%. From a societal perspective, the CER was $78,000/QALY. From a perspective of 100,000 member-managed care organizations and considering the effect of member turnover, the CER was 177,329/QALY.

Herman et al. (38) found the cost-effectiveness of intervention was $1400/QALY from a health care perspective and $10,885/QALY from a societal perspective in the United States.

Comparing the standard lifestyle recommendations from the health system or a single payer's perspective, Palmer et al. (2004) (39) reported that in Australia and other four European countries (France, Germany, Switzerland, and the United Kingdom), intensive lifestyle change was cost-saving in terms of LYG, except in the United Kingdom, where the CER was $7600/LYG. Caro et al. (40) reported cost-savings from intensive lifestyle intervention for primary prevention of diabetes in Canada over 10 years.

The intensive lifestyle intervention used in the clinical trial was an individual-based intervention. The intervention was more likely to be conducted in a group setting if implemented in the "real" world. Assuming that the intervention was conducted in a group of 10, the cost of lifestyle intervention per person would decrease from about $2700 to about $650 per participant over a three-year period. Under this scenario, the intensive lifestyle intervention would be cost-saving from a health system perspective (38) or cost $14,880/QALY gained from a societal perspective (37).

A U.K. study (41) estimated the cost-effectiveness of lifestyle intervention as in the Finnish Diabetes Prevention Study among middle-aged overweight people with IGT. The intervention group was given detailed dietary recommendations by dietitians and was asked to undertake moderate exercise for at least 30 min/day. Control subjects received oral and written information about diet and exercise at a baseline visit. At the end of the sixth year, the risk of diabetes was significantly reduced by 58% in the intervention group. For 100 people, 3.6 more QALYs were gained, and based on unit costs of health care calculated for the United Kingdom in 2001, the direct medical cost among intervention group was $39,770 more than the no-intervention group. From the health system perspective, the incremental cost-utility ratio was $10,979/QALY.

Segal et al. (33) simulated the cost-effectiveness of intensive diet and behavioral modification in seriously obese persons with IGT or a mixed population with IGT and NGT, or in women with previous gestational diabetes who now have IGT or mixed group of IGT and NGT in Australia. The intensive diet and behavioral modification included a low- or very low calorie diet combined with counseling and nutrition advice, delivered by a multidisciplinary team with a two- to three-year follow-up. For all seriously obese persons with IGT only, the intensive diet and behavioral modification was cost-saving, for a mixed group with IGT and NGT, the intervention cost $2622/LYG. For women with IGT who previously had gestational diabetes, the intensive lifestyle modification cost $1246/LYG, and for the mixed group with IGT and NGT, the intervention cost $2346/LYG.

Segal et al. (33) also simulated the cost-effectiveness of group behavioral modification for overweight and obese

men in working places. The group behavior modification for men was achieved by five to six group sessions aimed at reduction in waist size through change in diet and increased physical activity, using an empowerment philosophy. They reported cost-saving for both the IGT-only group and the mixed group from Australian health system's perspective. Another intervention targeting the Australian general population, a media campaign with community support for weight loss among obese adults, was also cost-saving.

Roux et al. (42) evaluated the cost-effectiveness of weight loss interventions in a cohort of 10,000 healthy 35-year-old overweight and obese women in the United States. The interventions were: (i) diet only; (ii) diet and pharmacotherapy using orlistat; (iii) diet and exercise; and (iv) diet, exercise, and behavior modification. Behavioral modification consisted of a one-hour cognitive therapy counseling session led by a psychologist every other week. The comparison group received routine primary care. Comparing with routine primary care group, the average undiscounted marginal QALY gains in the intervention groups ranged from 1.55 to 4.92 months depending on the intervention. The diet, exercise, and behavior modification intervention dominated all the other interventions. Comparing with routine primary care, the combination of diet, exercise, and behavior modification cost $71,547/LYG or $14,915/QALY gained.

Pharmacological Therapy

Orlistat

Orlistat, a potent inhibitor of pancreatic lipases, is an important aid in obtaining and maintaining weight loss. The cost-effectiveness of orlistat was evaluated within and following the clinical trial. O'Meara et al. (43) did a review on the economic evaluation of orlistat. They reported the results of a cost-utility analysis conducted by Foxcroft and Ludders (44) on the basis of data from three double-blind randomized clinical trials. A two-year orlistat plus a hypocaloric-diet treatment produced an additional 3% to 4% of initial body weight reduction, and 11.5 % more patients in the orlistat group achieved at least 5% loss of initial body weight over two years, compared with the placebo group in which persons were treated with a hypocaloric diet alone (17.5% vs. 6%). Related to the placebo treatment, treating 100 obese persons with orlistat for two years would result in an increase in direct medical costs of $58,750 and a gain of QALY of 1.601. It yielded a CER of $36,912/QALY gained (Table 4).

Lamotte et al. (45) and Maetzel et al. (46) analyzed the cost-effectiveness of orlistat treatment plus standard antidiabetic care compared with standard diabetic care alone in overweight or obese people with type 2 diabetes in

Table 3 Cost-Effectiveness of Lifestyle Interventions

Study	Study type	Study population	Intervention	Comparison	Perspective	Time horizon	CERs (original)	CERs (2005 U.S. dollars)
Segal et al., 1998, Australia	CEA	Seriously obese, with IGT, or mixed population with IGT and NGT	Intensive diet and behavioral modification	No intervention	Health system	25 yr	$1900/LYG (1997)	$2622/LYG
		Women with previous gestational diabetes, now IGT only, or mixed group of IGT and NGT	Intensive diet and behavioral modification	No intervention	Health system	25 yr	$900/LYG for IGT only $1700/LYG for mixed group of IGT and NGT (1997)	$1242/LYG for IGT only $2346/LYG for mixed group of IGT and NGT
		Overweight and obese men, with IGT, or mixed group of IGT and NGT	Group behavior modification for men				Cost saving	Cost saving
		Australian general population, obese adults	Media campaign with community support for weight loss				Cost saving	Cost saving
Palmer et al., 2004, Australia, France, Germany, Switzerland, United Kingdom	CEA CUA	Mean age 50.6 years, mean body weight 94.2 kg, mean BMI 34 kg/m²	Intensive lifestyle change through diet and exercise	Standard lifestyle advice	Health system	Lifetime	Cost saving except in United Kingdom United Kingdom: £6381/LYG (2002)	Cost saving, except in United Kingdom United Kingdom: $7600/LYG,
DPP, 2004, United States	CUA	Mean age 50.6 years, mean body weight 94.2 kg, mean BMI 34 kg/m²	Intensive lifestyle change through diet and exercise	Standard lifestyle recommendations	Health system	2.8 yr	$15,655 per case of diabetes prevented, or $31,512/QALY Group intervention: $8982/QALY (2000)	$19,000 per case prevented, or $39,074/QALY Group intervention: $11,138/QALY
					Societal		$31,512 per case prevented, or $51,582/QALY saved Group intervention: $29,052/QALY	$32,156 per case prevented, or $67,720/QALY saved Group intervention: $36,024/QALY

Study	Type	Population	Intervention	Comparison	Perspective	Time horizon	Results	Results
Caro et al., 2004, Canada	CEA	With IGT, all Caucasian in the base model, all race in the sensitivity analysis	Intensive lifestyle modification through diet and exercise	No intervention	Health system	10 yr	Can $749/LYG (2000)	$629/LYG
Avenell et al., 2004 (43), United Kingdom	CUA	522 middle-aged overweight Finnish people with IGT	Detailed dietary recommendations and follow-up meetings with dietitian and supervised exercise sessions	Oral and written information about diet and exercise at a baseline visit	Health system	6 yr	£13,389/QALY (2001)	$10,979/QALY
Eddy et al., 2005, United States	CUA	Mean age 50.6 yr, mean body weight 94.2 kg, mean BMI 34 kg/m²	Intensive lifestyle modification through diet and exercise	No intervention	Societal; A 100,000-member health plan	30 yr	$62,600/QALY (2000) Group intervention: $12,000/QALY $143,000/QALY Group intervention: $27,000/QALY	$78,000/QALY Group intervention: $14,880/QALY $177,329/QALY Group intervention: $33,480/QALY
Herman et al., 2005, United States	CUA	Mean age 50.6 yr, mean body weight 94.2 kg, mean BMI 34 kg/m²	Intensive lifestyle modification through diet and exercise	Standard lifestyle recommendations	Health system	Lifetime	$1100/QALY (2000)	$1400/QALY Group intervention: cost saving
Roux et al., 2006, United States	CUA	Healthy, nonpregnant 35-year-old overweight and obese women	Weight loss interventions, consisting of diet, exercise, behavior modification, and/or pharmacotherapy	Routine primary care	Societal Societal	Lifetime	$8800/QALY Diet, exercise and behavior modification–dominated diet only, diet and pharmacotherapy, diet and exercise. Comparing with routine care, $60,390/LYG, $12,640/QALY (2001)	$10,885/QALY $71,547/LYG $14,915/QALY

Abbreviations: CEA, cost-effectiveness analysis; CUA, cost-utility analysis; IGT, impaired glucose tolerance; CER, cost effectiveness ratio; NGT, normal glucose tolerance; LYG, life year gained; QALY, quality-adjusted life year; BMI, body mass index; DPP, Diabetes Prevention Program.

Table 4 Cost-Effectiveness of Pharmaceutical Treatment for Weight Loss

Study	Study type	Study population	Intervention	Comparison	Perspective	Time horizon	CERs (original)	CERs (2005 U.S. dollars)
Orlistat treatment								
O'Meara et al., 2001, United Kingdom (Review)	CUA	Overweight and obese	2-yr orlistat treatment	Diet	Health system	2 yr	£45881/QALY (1998)	$36,912/QALY
Lamotte et al., 2002, Belgium	CEA	Obese patients with type 2 diabetes, with/without hypertension or hypercholesterolemia	2-yr orlistat treatment plus usual antidiabetic care	Usual antidiabetic care mainly through diet	Health system	10 yr	For obese people without AHT and without hypercholesterolemia: €19,986/LYG obese with hypercholesterolemia: €7407/LYG obese with AHT: €7388/LYG obese with hypercholesterolemia and AHT: €3462/LYG (2000)	For obese people without AHT and without hypercholesterolemia: $23,783/LYG obese with hypercholesterolemia: $8814/LYG obese with AHT: $8792/LYG obese with hypercholesterolemia and AHT: $4120/LYG
Martzel et al., 2002, United States	CEA	Overweight or obese patients with type 2 diabetes and no preexisting complications	2-yr orlistat treatment plus standard antidiabetic care and weight management	Standard antidiabetic care and weight management	Health system	11 yr	$8327 per event-free LYG under the assumption of drug effect lasting for 3 yr $23,574 per event-free LYG under the assumption of drug effect lasting for 1 yr (2001)	$9826 per event-free LYG under the assumption of drug effect lasting for 3 yr $27,817 per event-free LYG under the assumption of drug effect lasting for 1 yr
Lacy et al., 2005, Ireland	CUA	Obese patients without diabetes, BMI ≥ 28 kg/m²	1-yr orlistat treatment in combination with a 12-mo dietary program	Dietary program alone	Health system	11 yr	€16,945/QALY(2003)	$16,283/QALY
Heraman et al., 2005, Sweden	CUA	Age > 18 yr, BMI ≥ 30, without diabetes Be able to lose 2.5 kg during 1 mo	1-yr orlistat treatment plus diet	1-yr weight management program based on diet only	Health care system	10 yr	SEK13,125/QALY, 2003	$1767/QALY

Sibutramine treatment

Study	Type	Population	Intervention	Comparator	Perspective	Time horizon	Results	Results
O'Meara et al., 2002, United Kingdom (Review)	CUA	A 1000 hypothetical cohort, BMI > 30 kg/m², free of comorbidities and complications at the start of the modeling period	1-yr sibutramine treatment combined with a dietary and exercise program	A dietary and exercise program and placebo	Health system	5 yr	Benefits for weight loss alone, £19,000/QALY (United Kingdom, 1999) — Benefits for diabetes incidence reduction alone, £77,000/QALY; Benefits for CHD reduction alone, £42,000/QALY; Benefits for all three endpoints together, £10,500/QALY	Benefits for weight loss alone, $15,207/QALY — Benefits for diabetes incidence reduction alone, $61,600/QALY; Benefits for CHD reduction alone, $33,600/QALY; Benefits for all three endpoints together, $8400/QALY
Wareen et al., 2004, United Kingdom, United States	CUA	20% male, mean age 42 yr, mean BMI 32.7 kg/m²	1-yr sibutramine treatment combined with diet and lifestyle advice	Diet and lifestyle advice in primary care	Health system	5 yr	£4780/QALY in United Kingdom, $9299/QALY in United States (2000)	$3920/QALY in United Kingdom, $11,531/QALY in United States
Brennan et al., 2006, Germany	CUA	Obese patients without comorbidities at baseline	1-yr sibutramine treatment in combination with the best nonpharmacological practice aimed at changing lifestyle for weight reduction	The best nonpharmacological practice alone	Health system	5 yr	Benefit including weight loss alone, €29351/QALY (2003) — Benefit including weight loss and reduced incidence of diabetes and reduced risk of CHD, $13706/QALY; Assuming weight regain by 0.668/yr, $51027/QALY	Benefit including weight loss alone, $28204/QALY — Benefit including weight loss and reduced incidence of diabetes and reduced risk of CHD, $13,158/QALY; Assuming weight regain by 0.668/yr, $48,986/QALY

Abbreviations: CEA, cost-effectiveness analysis; CUA, cost-utility analysis; CER, cost effectiveness ratio; IGT, impaired glucose tolerance; NGT, normal glucose tolerance; LYG, life year gained; QALY, quality-adjusted life year; AHT, arterial hypertension; BMI, body mass index; DPP, Diabetes prevention program; CHD, coronary heart disease.

Belgium and the United States beyond the trial period. The study population for the study by Lamotte (45) consisted of obese Belgian patients with type 2 diabetes but without micro- or macrovascular complications. The study assumed that five years after the two-year orlistat trial, almost all weight was regained. The analysis took a patient's perspective and estimated both the incremental cost and benefits over a period of 10 years. Treating 100 patients without arterial hypertension and without hypercholesterolemia for two years would yield a health gain of 8 life years and CER of $23,783/LYG. The corresponding estimates would be 20.4 life years and $8792/LYG for patients with hypercholesterolemia and 47.4 LYG and $4120/LYG for patients with hypercholesterolemia plus arterial hypertension, respectively.

Using meta-analysis of four placebo-controlled randomized trials, Maetzel et al. (46) estimated the cost-effectiveness of a two-year orlistat treatment with standard type 2 diabetes management compared with standard diabetes management alone among overweight or obese patients with type 2 diabetes in the United States. Under the assumption that the treatment effect persisted over three years, treating 100 patients with orlistat for two years would result in 13 more micro- and macrovascular event-free years over a period of 11 years and the cost per event-free years gained was $9826. Under the assumption that the treatment effect persisted for only one year after the treatment stopped, at the end of 11 years, the treatment yielded five more event-free years and CER of $27,817 per event-free LYG.

Lacey et al. (47) studied the cost-effectiveness of a one-year orlistat treatment in combination with diet treatment compared with diet treatment alone among overweight or obese adults without diabetes in Ireland. It was assumed that patients achieved their maximum weight loss at 12 months and regained their original weight at a uniform rate over the following three years. The main clinical outcome was type 2 diabetes prevented due to weight loss, subsequent life years gained, and QALYs gained. Results showed that after one year, the orlistat group had lost 11.6% of initial body weight compared with 7.9% in the diet alone group, treating 100 persons with orlistat plus diet would lead to seven more diabetes-free life years or nine more QALYs at an additional cost of $45,888 over the 11-year modeling period compared with diet treatment alone. From a health system perspective, the incremental cost per QALY gained was £16 283.

Hertzman (48) analyzed the cost-effectiveness of orlistat in a one-year weight management program similar with Lacey's study among overweight and obese patients without type 2 diabetes in Sweden. At month 3, 48.9% of the treatment group study participants had lost 5% of initial weight, compared with 26.3% in the control group. Subjects treated with orlistat had a weight loss of 15.5% at

month 12 compared with 7.9% for patients on diet only. The clinical outcomes included changes in incidence of obesity-related diseases including type 2 diabetes, hypertension, and hyperlipidemia, and QALYs related to obesity and the diseases. Over a 10-year period, assuming a three-year sustainability of the weight loss effect from orlistat, the incremental gain in QALY was 3.04 at an additional cost of $5187 for 100 average orlistat-treated patients. The CER was $1767/QALY.

Sibutramine

Sibutramine is a weight loss drug that inhibits the reuptake of the neurotransmitters involved in the control of food intake. In Europe, sibutramine was restricted in those patients who were unsuccessful at losing weight and were maintaining weight loss with diet and exercise alone, and the prescription is continued only in responders who lose 2 kg after one month and 5% of their initial weight after three months. Continuation of the treatment is limited to 12 months.

A review study from the United Kingdom (49) reported that one-year sibutramine use produced 4.1 to 4.8 kg more weight loss compared with the placebo group. No published economic evaluations were identified in the United Kingdom at that time. O'Meara et al. reported the economic evaluation results from an unpublished study submitted by the drug manufacturer. Benefits included in the study were weight loss, reduction of diabetes incidence, and reduction of CHD. The CERs of using sibutramine for treating obese people without comorbidities for one year varied by the type of health benefit included, $15,207/QALY by including weight loss alone, $61,600/QALY by including diabetes alone, and $33,600/QALY by including CHD alone. If all three benefits were considered, sibutramine treatment cost only $8400/QALY. Again, this analysis assumed that the benefit of a one-year sibutramine treatment would last four years.

A newer study by Warren et al. (50) conducted a cost-effectiveness study of sibutramine in the treatment of obesity in the United Kingdom and the United States, with a healthy overweight and obese population. Intervention was a 12-month sibutramine treatment combined with diet and lifestyle advice. The control group received only diet and lifestyle advice in a primary care setting. The health benefits included in the study were risk reductions for CHD and diabetes and quality of life gained due to weight loss itself. On the basis of a one-year Smith and Goulder study (51), responders to sibutramine treatment experienced a mean weight loss of 10 kg compared with the placebo group who experienced a mean weight loss of 2 kg over the 12-month period. At month 50, the treatment group regained weight to the level consistent with the natural history growth rate at month 18. In the United Kingdom, over the five-year study period, 0.64

more nonfatal CHD events, 0.32 more CHD-related deaths, and 1.54 more incident cases of diabetes were avoided in the sibutramine group compared with the comparison group. Taking into account all three benefits, the total marginal QALYs gained in 1000 patients was 58.95. The cost per QALY gained was $3920. In the United States, at the end of the fifth year, 0.44 more nonfatal CHD events, 0.23 more CHD-related deaths, and 2.01 more incident cases of diabetes were avoided, the marginal QALYs gain of 1000 patients were 46.79. The cost per QALY gained was $11,530 when taking into account all three benefits.

Brennan et al. (52) assessed the cost-effectiveness of a one-year sibutramine treatment in combination with lifestyle intervention for weight loss versus lifestyle intervention alone for obese patients without comorbidities at baseline in Germany, on the basis of data derived from five clinical trials. The study assumed the health benefit would last up to four years after the one-year treatment. Under the best scenario, at year 1, the sibutramine group lost 5.5 kg more than the placebo group. Treating 1000 persons with sibutramine resulted in 30 more QALYs at an extra total cost of €900,000, which was translated into in a CER of $28,204/QALY if only the benefit of weight loss is considered. The treatment resulted in a gain of 51.5 more QALYs at an additional cost of $677,914 if the additional benefit of reduced incidence of diabetes and reduced risk of CHD is considered. This yields an incremental CER of $13,158/QALY gained. The model was sensitive to the magnitude of weight regain used under each scenario. Using a mean rate weight regain of 0.668, the CER increased to $48,986/QALY gained.

Surgical Interventions

There are two types of weight loss surgical procedures: restrictive procedures and malabsorption procedures. The restrictive procedures are done mainly to reduce the size of the stomach using a gastric band, staples, or both. The specific restrictive operations included gastric binding (GB, adjustable or not adjustable) and vertical banded gastroplasty (VBG). The malabsorptive procedures involve reducing stomach size and bypassing the duodenum. The two most used malabsorptive procedures include Roux-en-Y and resectional gastric bypass (GBP) and biliopancreatic diversion with or without duodenal switch. The frequency of each procedure performed varies by country. The cost-effectiveness of several surgical procedures has been evaluated.

Gastric binding

Ackroyd et al. (53) studied the cost-effectiveness of adjustable gastric binding (AGB) versus conventional treatment of obesity in patients with BMI $\geq$ 35 kg/m^2

and type 2 diabetes in Germany, France, and the United Kingdom. There was no standard for conventional therapy. According to health technology assessment (HTA) reports or author's opinion, the therapy was defined as follow-up monitoring of a second year of medically guided diet after failure of at least one prior year of well-conducted medical treatment on obesity. The clinical effectiveness included BMI reduction and reversing the glucose back to "normal." Five years after the surgery, AGB reduced BMI by 13.2 kg/m^2 and the prevalence of type 2 diabetes by 50%, and an extra 1.34 QALY was gained. The procedure resulted in cost-saving in Germany of $1972 per patient and in France of $2477 per patient. In the United Kingdom, AGB surgery cost $871 more per patient than the conventional treatment, which led to CER of $833/QALY gained.

Clegg et al. (54) assessed the cost-effectiveness of three surgical procedures—adjustable silicone gastric banding (ASGB), VBG, Roux-en-Y gastric bypass (RYGBP)—compared with conventional treatment (nonsurgical management) for obesity treatment, using a computer simulation model. The nonsurgical management was not defined clearly but consisted of physician counseling and VLCDs. The effectiveness of costs of different surgical treatments and nonsurgical management were based on the systematic review conducted by the authors. The cohort had an average age of 40 years, and 90% were women. Average body weight was 135 kg, and average BMI was 45 kg/m^2. Benefits included improving quality of life by avoiding secondary disease such as diabetes, hypertension, asthma, and arthropathy. They also included gains from avoiding diabetes on the basis of an assumption of 10% prevalence of diabetes among the morbidly obese. The study did not assume any change in life expectancy. For all surgical procedures, the benefit of the weight loss would last five years and the benefit of reducing diabetes incidence would last to the eighth year. The effectiveness data of the different surgical procedures were drawn from a literature review. For ASGB, the authors assumed an initial weight loss of 20% of original weight, but that weight loss continued up to a loss of 33% of the original weight by year 5. They also assumed that weight loss for patients in the nonsurgical management group was very modest. After 20 years of the surgery, ASGB surgery gained an additional 0.45 QALY per patient and cost an additional £3831 per patient, resulting in a cost of $7017 per QALY gained, compared to the nonsurgical management (Table 5).

Vertical banded gastroplasty

Van Gemert and colleagues (55) compared VBG with no treatment for 21 morbidly obese patients. They found that VBG resulted in a gain of 12 QALYs in a lifelong scenario, in a productivity gain of $3677/yr, and saved

Table 5   Cost-Effectiveness of Surgery for Weight Loss

Study	Study type	Study population	Intervention	Comparison	Perspective	Time horizon	CERs (original)	CERs (2005 U.S. dollars)
Martin et al., 1995, United States	CEA	Morbidly obese	RYGBP	Medical therapy (VLCD)	unclear	2–6 yr	Not formally calculated, Surgical treatment cost $250–$750 per pound of weight loss, Medial therapy cost $100–$1600 per pound of weight loss (1994)	Surgical treatment cost $383–$1140 per pound of weight loss Medial therapy cost $153–$2448 per pound of weight loss
Chua et al., 1995, United States	Cost-minimization	Morbidly obese	Laparoscopic VBG	Open RYGBP	unclear	Hospital stay for surgery	No CERs reported Average hospital charge for laparoscopic VBG was $12,800 compared with $16,700 for open RYGBP (1994)	Average hospital charge for laparoscopic VBG was $19,584 compared with $25,551 for open RYGBP
Segal et al., 1998, Australia	CEA	Seriously obese, BMI > 40 kg/m^2 or 45 kg excess weight, seriously obese with IGT	GBP surgery plus prior to counseling and 12 mo active follow-up	No treatment	health system	25 yr	$3300/LYG for obese patients with IGT $8900/LYG for mixed group of obese patients with IGT and NGT (1997)	$4554/LYG for obese patients with IGT $12,282/LYG for mixed group of obese patients with IGT and NGT
Van Gemert, et al., 1999, United States	CEA	Morbidly obese patients	VBG surgery	No treatment	unclear	Lifetime	Cost saving (1998)	Cost saving

Nguyen et al., 2001, United States	Not a formal CEA	155 patients with BMI between 46 and 60 kg/m²	Laparoscopic GBP surgery	Open GBP surgery	unclear	1 yr	Not formally provided Costs were not significantly different, laparoscopic procedure resulted in significant greater weight loss as well as QALYs gained at recovery	$7017/QALY
Clegg et al., 2002, United Kingdom (Review)	CUA	Average age of 40-yr, 90% were female, average body weight of 135 kg, average BMI 45 kg/m²	ASGB surgery	Nonsurgical treatment		20 yr after surgery	£8527/QALY (2001)	
			VBG surgery	Nonsurgical treatment			£10,237/QALY	$8394/QALY
			GBP surgery	Nonsurgical treatment			£6289/QALY	$51.57/QALY
			ASGB	VBG			£6176/QALY	$5064/QALY
			GBP	VBG			£742/QALY	$608/ QALY
			ASGB	GBP			£256,856/QALY	$210,621/QALY
Ackroyd et al., 2006, Germany, France, United Kingdom	CUA	BMI ≥ 35 kg/m², with type 2 diabetes	GBP surgery	Conventional nonsurgical therapy		5 yr	Cost saving in France and Germany £1517/ QALY in United Kingdom (2005)	Cost saving in France and Germany $833/ QALY in United Kingdom
			AGB surgery	Nonsurgical treatment			Cost saving in France and Germany £1929/ QALY in United Kingdom (2005)	$1060/QALY

Abbreviations: CEA, cost-effectiveness analysis; CUA, cost-utility analysis; CER, cost effectiveness ratio; RYGBP, Roux-en-Y gastric bypass; GBP, gastric bypass; IGT, impaired glucose tolerance; NGT, normal glucose tolerance; LYG, life year gained; QALY, quality-adjusted life year; BMI, body mass index; VLCD, very low calorie diet; ASGB, adjustable silicone gastric banding; VBG, vertical banded gastroplasty; AGB, adjustable gastric banding.

$5224 to $5325/QALY, compared with no treatment. The study took a societal perspective and included costs of productivity loss from obesity. However, costs of obesity related comorbidities were not included.

Clegg (54) compared VBG to nonsurgical treatment over a 20-year period and reported that after 20 years of the surgery, treating 100 patients with the intervention led to a gain of 26 QALYs, and $218,345 more in direct health care cost compared with nonsurgical treatment. The net cost per QALY gained was $8394. The study assumed that VBG patients lost 25% of their weight in the first year but regained 2% of their original weight in each subsequent year.

Gastric bypass procedure

Ackroyd (53) evaluated the cost-effectiveness of GBP in patients with BMI ≥ 35 kg/m^2 and type 2 diabetes, related to conventional treatment of obesity, in Germany, France, and the United Kingdom. In this paper, patients who began with type 2 diabetes but had a reduction in blood glucose to normal levels after the surgery treatment were considered nondiabetic. By the fifth year following the surgery, GBP reduced a patient's BMI on average by 16.1 kg/m^2, decreased type 2 diabetes prevalence by 50%, and gained an extra 1.03 QALYs, compared with the conventional treatment. From a payer perspective, the GBP surgery saved $4040 per patient in Germany and $3598 per patient in France compared with the conventional treatment. In the United Kingdom, over the five years, the cost for GBP surgery was $1118 more than the conventional treatment, but the incremental CER of GBP surgery was quite small, $833/QALY gained.

Martin et al. (56) compared RYGBP with VLCD treatment in the obese population. They estimated the average cost of per pound lost from the two therapies. The surgical therapy cost between $383 and $1140 and VLCD cost $153 to $2448 for a follow-up of two to six years for 1 lb lost. Since all nonsurgical patients' treatment regained the weight lost after seven years, the authors concluded that surgical treatment appears to be more cost-effective in producing and maintaining weight loss.

Segal et al. (34) estimated the cost-effectiveness of GBP surgery among patients with BMI greater than 45 kg/m^2 in Australia compared with nonintervention. The surgery cost $12,282/LYG in a general population with 10% IGT and 90% NGT. The CER would drop to $4554 if the procedure was restricted to persons with IGT only.

Clegg et al. (54) reported RYGBP cost $5157/QALY gained. Performing the surgery among 100 patients with the intervention led to a gain of 45 QALYs, and $154,011 more in the direct health care cost compared with the nonsurgical treatment. The study assumed that RYGBP reduced 36% of the original weight in the first year and the weight loss was maintained over time.

Relative cost-effectiveness of different surgical procedures

Chua and Mendiola (57) compared laparoscopic VBG with open RYGBP in the obese population. The laparoscopic VBG had a short length of hospital stay but a longer operating time. Average hospital charges for the laparoscopic VBG was $19,584 compared with $29,551 for open RYGBP. However, the study was a retrospective study and did not include the effectiveness of comparison procedures in terms of weight loss and complications.

The relative cost-effectiveness of three types of surgical procedures—RYGBP, VBG and ASGB—were compared by Clegg et al. (54). The total net costs of treating morbid obesity per person (>20 years) through surgical procedures varied from $7894 for VBG to $8005 for RYGBP and $8852 for ASGB. Treating 100 patients resulted in QALYs of 1149 from VBG, of 1167 for RYGBP, and of 1168 for ASGB. The RYGBP had a net cost per QALY of $608 compared with VBG. The ASGB cost $5064/QALY gained compared with VGB and $210,621/QALY compared with the RYGBP. On the basis of these results, the RYGBP seems the most cost-effective procedure in terms of cost per QALY gained.

Nguyen et al. (58) evaluated the cost-effectiveness of laparoscopic GBP surgery compared with open GBP surgery. The clinical outcomes included complications during and after surgery, as well as the patient's quality of life at 1, 3, 6, and 12 months following surgery. The study considered direct medical hospital costs and indirect costs related to time lost from work. Result from this study indicated that laparoscopic surgery had higher operating costs but short hospital stays. There was no statistically significant difference in direct hospital cost, indirect cost, or total cost between the two procedures. Complications rates were also not statistically different although quality of life was higher at various interim points during the year following the surgery for laparoscopic relative to open GBP surgery. Since the laparoscopic surgery resulted in fewer intensive care unit stays, shorter hospital stays, faster recovery, and earlier return to work than did the open surgery without additional costs, the laparoscopic GBP surgery may be more cost-effective compared with open GBP surgery.

Summary and Conclusions

Cost-effectiveness analysis can be a very useful tool to determine the relative economic efficiency of various interventions used for treating overweight and obesity. Information provided by the cost-effectiveness studies can aid clinical and public health decision on how to allocate limited health care resources. The cost-effectiveness of many different interventions used to reduce body weight has been evaluated in a number of developed countries.

Interventions studied included weight loss strategies at different obese level and treatment stages. For example, intensive lifestyle intervention through diet and exercise are compared with standard lifestyle recommendation or no intervention, combining weight loss drugs such as orlistat and sibutramine and a dietary and exercise program among respondents, surgery for morbidly obese patients compared with no treatment, or medical therapy mainly through low-calorie diet and weight loss medications.

A number of conclusions can be drawn on the basis of the results from the cost-effective studies. First, the robustness of the evidence for cost-effectiveness of weight loss interventions is diverse. Strong evidence exists for making a firm conclusion on weight loss through intensive lifestyle intervention. A number of good quality cost-effectiveness studies based on large multicenter clinical trials such as DPP and the Finnish study consistently demonstrated that the intensive lifestyle intervention was both effective and cost-effective in reducing body weight among overweight or obese persons with IGT. Evidence for the cost-effectiveness of orlistat is also robust and consistent among at least four good quality studies. Evidence for the cost-effectiveness of sibutramine is relatively weak, but still strong enough to allow us draw a conclusion. Evidence of cost-effectiveness of obesity surgery is not very strong, mainly because of the lower quality of the study. Of the seven studies we included, three of them (56–58) are not strict cost-effectiveness analyses and do not report CERs. One study (33) used a simulation model with model parameters obtained from published literature or assumptions when the needed data were not available. Evidence on the cost-effectiveness of weight loss through physician counseling or commercial weight loss programs is the weakest. Only one study (33) simulated physician counseling in Australia, and the quality of the study was low. The study on the cost-effectiveness of the commercial weight loss programs is low in quality because of the large number of assumptions used in the study.

A second conclusion is that the CERs of most of the interventions are under $30,000/QALY gained or LYG. They are far below the $50,000/QALY criteria for recommendation for adoption. The CERs are also comparable to the Canadian $20,000/QALY and the United Kingdom threshold of £20,000 to £30,000 (1999) per QALY. Thus, the interventions for weight loss and obesity treatment in general are very cost-effective. Combined with the robustness of the evidence of the cost-effectiveness for the interventions, we conclude that losing weight through intensive lifestyle modification such as diet and exercise and adding orlistat and sibutramine into a diet and exercise program are clearly a good use of resources. Surgical treatment for people who are morbidly obese (BMI > 40 kg/m^2) or have a BMI >35 kg/m^2 with significant comorbid conditions appears cost-effective compared with nonsurgical management. GBP seems a more cost-effective procedure than GB (adjustable or not adjustable) and VBG in terms of cost per QALY gained. Regarding the two surgical procedures, the laparoscopic surgery may be more cost-effective than open surgery for GBP surgery. Physician counseling and commercial weight loss programs are potentially cost-effective and should be confirmed by further studies.

Third, health benefits and costs included in the studies are very diverse. As we described in the COI studies for obesity section, most obesity costs are not from obesity treatment itself, but from treating obesity-related diseases. The total number and specific type of diseases included differs by study. Most of the studies included the benefit of preventing or delaying type 2 diabetes, but some studies included an additional benefit of reduction in CHD as a result of weight loss from obesity treatments. The cost-effectiveness of an intervention also varies greatly because of medical costs saved from different diseases. For example, Brennan et al. (52) reported that when only the benefit of weight loss was included, sibutramine treatment cost $28,204/QALY gained, but the treatment cost $13,158/QALY gained when additional benefits from reduction in the incidence of diabetes and risk of CHD were included.

FUTURE RESEARCH

In this chapter, we focused on two issues related to the economics aspect of obesity: the economic burden of obesity and the cost-effectiveness of interventions used for intentional weight loss and obesity treatments. The economic burden of obesity on society as a whole is substantial. The direct medical cost attributable to obesity accounted for 2% to 7% of the total health care expenditure in the developed countries. Obesity also imposed a large financial burden on employers, private business, private insurers, public health care and pension system, as well as obese individuals themselves and their families.

Obesity has reached pandemic proportions throughout the world. The International Obesity Task Force estimated 300 million people around the world are obese (BMI > 30 kg/m^2). The obese population from the developed world will continue to increase in the next two decades. Crude projections, extrapolated from existing data, suggest that by the year 2025 levels of obesity could be as high as 45% to 50% in the United States and between 30% and 40% in Australia, England, and Mauritius (59). In addition, as income has increased, overweight and obesity have become a public health problem in the developing countries. For example, in Egypt, 70% of women and 48% of men are overweight or obese. In Morocco, 40% of the population was overweight in 2004, and in Kenya, 12%. In Brazil and Colombia, the prevalence of overweight and obesity was around 40%—a level comparable to that found in a number of European countries (60). This worldwide increase in the prevalence of obesity implies that the future economic burden of obesity will increase.

COI studies can be valuable tools for promoting attention to the economic burden imposed by obesity and are a crucial first step in the economic evaluation of prevention interventions. Future economic studies should focus on filling information gap in the following areas. First, all studies on the economic burden of overweight and obesity reviewed in this chapter are from the developed world. Future research should pay special attention to documenting the economic burden of overweight and obesity in developing countries. Overweight and obesity is already a significant public health problem for some developing countries and will become a public health problem soon for the rest of the developing region. The economic consequences of the increase in overweight and obesity need to be understood and assessed to support advocacy activities and to help define public policies to stop or reverse this trend. Second, besides documenting the economic burden of obesity, future studies should provide information that can be used for addressing a particular health policy. For example, a recent study by Finkelstein et al. (2) examined who pays for obesity treatment in the United States and reported that the government pays for about 50% of the health care costs associated with persons who are obese or overweight. These findings clarify the debate over whether obesity is a personal or societal issue and provide a clear motivation for government to try to reduce the costs of obesity. Finally, majority of the economic studies related to costs of obesity in developed countries have been focusing on estimating the economic burden at a given time using prevalence approach. Only three studies have been designed to get an incidence-based cost estimate. Incidence-based cost estimates are more useful in evaluating intervention options related to preventing and control obesity. In addition, current incidence-based estimates may well underestimate the true economic burden of obesity (1). Thus, more incidence-based cost studies are needed.

Previous analysis on the cost-effectiveness of different approaches to reducing body weight in the overweight and obese population can provide valuable information for public and clinical decisions. Future studies should focus on filling in the current information gap and improving the quality of the study quality. More studies are needed to evaluate the cost-effectiveness of physician counseling and commercial and self-organized weight loss programs. This is because comprehensive lifestyle intervention was cost-effective in achieving weight loss, but the conclusion was based on the assumption that effectiveness from trials could be achieved. It is still a question on how to translate the

research into practice. Counseling by physicians and other trained health providers might be the first step to achieve this and studies demonstrated some effectiveness of these counseling services on lifestyle change among patients. In addition, it would be difficult and expensive for health providers alone to supervise and monitor these kinds of programs. Commercial and organized self-programs might be more cost-effective ways for comprehensive lifestyle interventions. Unfortunately few cost-effectiveness studies have investigated this area.

Second, a major problem in synthesizing the literature is the high degree of difference among studies in their research perspective and their calculation of costs and benefits. These differences make the comparisons between the interventions impossible. To standardize the methods of cost-effectiveness studies, an expert panel of the U.S. Public Health Services (61) has developed specific recommendations that should result in research findings that are more comparable. By addressing these recommendations, the usefulness of cost-effectiveness studies would be greatly enhanced.

Finally, to conduct sound research on the cost-effectiveness of interventions, data on both effectiveness and cost should be collected systematically, especially alongside clinical trials. Although this requirement poses a challenge, researchers should view economic evaluation as a critical component of clinical trials.

REFERENCES

1. Thompson D, Wolf AM. The medical-care cost burden of obesity. Obes Rev 2001; 2:189–197.
2. Finkelstein EA, Fiebelkorn IC, Wang G. National medical spending attributable to overweight and obesity: how much, and who's paying? Health Aff (Millwood) 2003; Suppl Web Exclusives:W3-219–W3-226.
3. Wolf AM, Colditz GA. Current estimates of the economic costs of obesity in the United States. Obes Res 1998; 6: 97–106.
4. Sander B, Bergemann R. Economic burden of obesity and its complications in Germany. Eur J Health Econ 2003; 4(4):248–253.
5. Thompson D, Brown JB, Nichols GA, et al. Body mass index and future health-care costs: a retrospective cohort study. Obes Res 2001; 9:210–218.
6. Quesenberry CP, Caan B, Jacobson A. Obesity, health services use, and health care costs among members of a health maintenance organization. Arch Intern Med 1998; 158:466–472.
7. Thorpe KE, Florence CS, Howard DH, et al. The impact of obesity on rising medical spending. Health Aff (Millwood) 2004; Suppl Web Exclusives:W4-480–W4-486.
8. Sturm R. The effects of obesity, smoking, and drinking on medical problems and costs. Health Aff 2002; 21(2): 245–253.

9. Andreyeva T, Sturm R, Ringel JS. Moderate and severe obesity have large differences in health care costs. Obes Res 2004; 12(12):1936–1943.

10. Arterburn DE, Maciejewski ML, Tsevat J. Impact of morbid obesity on medical expenditures in adults. Int J Obes (Lond) 2005; 29(3):334–339.

11. Thompson D, Edelsberg J, Kinsey KL, et al. Estimated economic costs of obesity to U.S. business. Am J Health Promot 1998; 13(2):120–127.

12. Wee CC, Phillips RS, Legedza AT, et al. Health care expenditures associated with overweight and obesity among US adults: importance of age and race. Am J Public Health 2005; 95(1):159–165.

13. Wang F, Schultz AB, Musich S, et al. The relationship between National Heart, Lung, and Blood Institute Weight Guidelines and concurrent medical costs in a manufacturing population. Am J Health Promot 2003; 17(3):183–189.

14. Burton WN, Chen CY, Schultz AB, et al. The economic costs associated with body mass index in a workplace. J Occup Environ Med 1998; 38(9):786–792.

15. Finkelstein E, Fiebelkorn C, Wang G. The costs of obesity among full-time employees. Am J Health Promot 2005; 20(1):45–51.

16. Colditz GA. Economic costs of obesity and inactivity. Med Sci Sports Exerc 1999; 31(suppl 11):S663–S667.

17. Narbro K, Jonsson E, Larsson B, et al. Economic consequences of sick-leave and early retirement in obese Swedish women. Int J Obes Relat Metab Disord 1996; 20(10):895–903.

18. Månsson NO, Eriksson KF, Israelsson B, et al. Body mass index and disability pension in middle-aged men—nonlinear relations. Int J Epidemiol 1996; 25(1):80–85.

19. Flegal KM, Graubard BI, Williamson DF, et al. Excess deaths associated with underweight, overweight, and obesity. JAMA 2005; 293(15):1861–1867.

20. Peeters A, Barendregt JJ, Willekens F, et al. Obesity in adulthood and its consequences for life expectancy: a lifetable analysis. Ann Intern Med 2003; 138(1):24–32.

21. Fontaine KR, Barofsky I. Obesity and health-related quality of life. Obes Rev 2001; 2:173–182.

22. Blanck HM, Khan LK, Serdula MK. Use of nonprescription weight loss products: results from a multistate survey. JAMA 2001; 286(8):930–935.

23. Bryant J. Fat is a $34 billion business. Atlanta Business Chronicle (September 24, 2001), citing research by Marketdata Enterprises, Inc.

24. Sarlio-Lahteenkorva S, Lahelma E. The association of body mass index with social and economic disadvantage in women and men. Int J Epidemiol 1999; 28:445–449.

25. Pagan JA, Davila A. Obesity, occupational attainment and earnings. Soc Sci Q 1997; 78(3):757–770.

26. Averett S, Korenman S. Black-white differences in social and economic consequences of obesity. Int J Obes Relat Metab Disord 1999; 23(2):166–173.

27. Cawley J. What explains race and gender differences in the relationship between obesity and wages? Gender Issues 2003; 21(3):30–49.

28. Thompson D, Edelsberg J, Colditz GA, et al. Lifetime health and economic consequences of obesity. Arch Intern Med 1999; 159(18):2177–2183.

29. Gorsky RD, Pamuk E, Williamson DF, et al. The 25-year health care costs of women who remain overweight after 40 years of age. Am J Prev Med 1996; 12(5):388–394.

30. Allison DB, Zannolli R, Narayan KMV. The direct health care costs of obesity in the United States. Am J Public Health 1999; 89:1194–1199.

31. Hirth RA, Chernew ME, Miller E, et al. Willingness to pay for a quality-adjusted life year: in search of a standard. Med Decis Making 2000; 20:332–342.

32. Laupacis A, Feeny D, Detsky AS, et al. How attractive does a new technology have to be to warrant adoption and utilization? Tentative guidelines for using clinical and economic evaluations. Can Med Assoc J 1992; 146:473–478.

33. Segal L, Dalton AC, Richardson J. Cost-effectiveness of the primary prevention of non-insulin dependent diabetes mellitus. Health Promot Int 1998; 13:197–209.

34. Yates J, Murphy C. A cost benefit analysis of weight management strategies. Asia Pac J Clin Nutr 2006; 15 (suppl):74–79.

35. Tsai AG, Wadden TA. Systematic review: an evaluation of major commercial weight loss programs in the United States. Ann Intern Med 2005; 142:56–66.

36. Diabetes Prevention Program Research Group. Reduction in the incidence of type 2 diabetes with lifestyle intervention or metformin. N Engl J Med 2002; 346(6):393–403.

37. Eddy DM, Schlessinger L, Kahn R. Clinical outcomes and cost-effectiveness of strategies for managing people at high risk for diabetes. Ann Intern Med 2005; 143:251–264.

38. Herman WH, Hoerger TJ, Brandle M, et al. The cost-effectiveness of lifestyle modification or metformin in preventing type 2 diabetes in adults with impaired glucose tolerance. Ann Intern Med 2005; 142:323–332.

39. Palmer AJ, Roze S, Valentine WJ, et al. Intensive lifestyle changes or metformin in patients with impaired glucose tolerance: modeling the long-term health economic implications of the diabetes prevention program in Australia, France, Germany, Switzerland, and the United Kingdom. Clin Ther 2004; 26:304–321.

40. Caro JJ, Getsios D, Caro I, et al. Economic evaluation of therapeutic interventions to prevent Type 2 diabetes in Canada. Diab Med 2004; 21:1229–1236.

41. Avenell A, Broom J, Brown TJ, et al. Systematic review of the long-term effects and economic consequences of treatments for obesity and implications for health improvement. Health Technol Assess 2004; 8(21):1–182

42. Roux L, Kuntz KM, Donaldson C, et al. Economic evaluation of weight loss interventions in overweight and obese women. Obesity 2006; 14(6):1093–1106.

43. O'Meara S, Riemsma R, Shirran L, et al. A rapid and systematic review of the clinical effectiveness and cost-effectiveness of orlistat in the management of obesity. Health Technol Assess 2001; 5(18):1–81.

44. Foxcroft D, Ludders J. Orlistat for the treatment of obesity. Southampton: Wessex Institute for Health Research and Development, 1999. Report No. 101:1–49.

45. Lamotte M, Annemans L, Lefever A, et al. A health economic model to assess the long-term effects and cost-effectiveness of orlistat in obese type 2 diabetic patients. Diabetes Care 2002; 25:303–308.

46. Maetzel A, Ruof J, Covington M, et al. Economic evaluation of orlistat in overweight and obese patients with type 2 diabetes mellitus. Pharmacoeconomics 2003; 21:501–512.

47. Lacey LA, Wolf A, O'shea D, et al. Cost-effectiveness of orlistat for the treatment of overweight and obese patients in Ireland. Int J Obes (Lond) 2005; 29(8):975–982.

48. Hertzman P. The cost effectiveness of orlistat in a 1-year weight-management programme for treating overweight and obese patients in Sweden: a treatment responder approach. Pharmacoeconomics 2005; 23(10):1007–1020.

49. O'Meara S, Riemsma R, Shirran L, et al. The clinical effectiveness and cost-effectiveness of sibutramine in the management of obesity: a technology assessment. Health Technol Assess 2002; 6(6):1–97.

50. Warren E, Brennan A, Akehurst R. Cost-effectiveness of sibutramine in the treatment of obesity. Med Decis Making 2004; 24(1):9–19.

51. Smith IG, Goulder MA. Randomised placebo-controlled trial of long-term treatment with sibutramine in mild to moderate obesity. J Fam Pract 2001; 50(6):505–512.

52. Brennan A, Ara R, Sterz R, et al. Assessment of clinical and economic benefits of weight management with sibutramine in general practice in Germany. Eur J Health Econ 2006; 7(4):276–284.

53. Ackroyd R, Mouiel J, Chevallier JM, et al. Cost-effectiveness and budget impact of obesity surgery in patients with type-2 diabetes in three European countries. Obes Surg 2006; 16(11):1488–1503.

54. Clegg AJ, Colquitt J, Sidhu MK, et al. The clinical effectiveness and cost-effectiveness of surgery for people with morbid obesity: a systematic review and economic evaluation. Health Technol Assess 2002; 6(12):1–153.

55. Van Gemert WG, Adang EM, Kop M, et al. A prospective cost-effectiveness analysis of vertical banded gastroplasty for the treatment of morbid obesity. Obes Surg 1999; 9(5):484–491.

56. Martin LF, Tan T-L, Horn JR, et al. Comparison of the costs associated with medical and surgical treatment of obesity. Surgery 1995; 118:599–607.

57. Chua TY, Mendiola RM. Laparoscopic vertical banded gastroplasty: the Milwaukee experience. Obes Surg 1995; 5:77–80.

58. Nguyen NT, Goldman C, Rosenquist CJ, et al. Laparoscopic versus open gastric bypass: a randomized study of outcomes, quality of life, and costs. Ann Surg 2001; 234(3):279–289.

59. The Global Challenge of Obesity and the International Obesity Task Force. Available at: http://www.iuns.org/features/obesity/obesity.htm. Accessed March 12, 2008.

60. Health First Europe-Obesity. Available at: http://www.iotf.org/popout.asp?linkto=http://www.fao.org/FOCUS/E/obesity/obes1.htm. Accessed March 12, 2008.

61. Gold MR, Siegel JE, Russell LB, et al, eds. Cost-Effectiveness in Health and Medicine. New York Oxford University Press, 1996.

40

Government's Evolving Role: Nutrition, Education, Regulation, Monitoring, and Research

CATHERINE E. WOTEKI

Scientific Affairs, Mars, Incorporated, McLean, Virginia, U.S.A.

SAMIRA S. JONES

Department of Nutrition, University of California, Davis, California, U.S.A.

M.R.C. GREENWOOD

Departments of Nutrition and Internal Medicine, University of California, Davis, California, U.S.A.

INTRODUCTION

Over the last 25 years, the obesity epidemic has reached detrimental proportions in the United States, and more recently it has emerged as an international public health problem. Increases in prevalence of obesity and overweight in both adults and children have been observed in many countries worldwide (1–5). The surge in rates of obesity has caused global and domestic agencies to respond with multilevel efforts, ranging from research to search for genetic and environmental factors that predispose individuals to obesity, to public policy changes. Evidence has shown that environmental factors such as diet and inactivity interact with at least several genes resulting in excessive fat storage (6–9). The concept that much of the world now lives in an "obesifying" environment and that the remainder of the world may aspire to this lifestyle is widely accepted and the rising rates of obesity in developing countries seem to support this belief (2,5). Concomitantly, nearly all countries—developed and developing—are experiencing increasing prevalence of obesity in children of all ages (10). Internationally, the World Health Organization (WHO) estimates that there are over a billion overweight adults with at least 300 million meeting the criteria for "clinically obese." This rising obesity prevalence coexists in countries that also have undernutrition (4). Because overweight and obesity are associated with increased risk for diabetes, cardiovascular disease, hypertension, stroke, and some cancers, the WHO is rallying the international community to implement a "Global Strategy on Diet, Physical Activity and Health" (11). The WHO's policy guidance to member countries is the basis of recent legislative initiatives and other actions in many countries and will be further discussed later in this chapter.

By and large, governments have been slow to respond to the data chronicling that an obesity epidemic has been under way and gathering momentum for an entire generation. Governments' responses to obesity have been complicated by the fact that until very recently their major policy focus has been on providing enough food, particularly to those of low income, and that obesity was viewed as a personal failing largely intractable to treatment. Initially, the public response was to blame obesity on gluttony and sloth, two of the cardinal sins, and thus government action was not appropriate. Later, as data from public surveys amassed and research identified obesity as a risk factor for chronic diseases, governments provided information about the roles of diet and exercise in maintaining healthy weight through a variety of different routes. More recently, attention is focusing on other levers that government can wield through regulatory agencies to change the environment to make it easier for people to make healthy food choices and to expend energy in daily activities (12). Throughout this 25-year period, governments have supported research to identify effective treatments and to develop intervention programs to prevent obesity. This chapter reviews the history of the government response to the obesity epidemic in the United States and globally, a history of avoiding action through blaming the victim, searching for treatments, trying to motivate public action through teaching, and tinkering with legislation to encourage desirable behaviors.

THE U.S. HISTORY IN ADDRESSING OBESITY

Obesity is now recognized as a leading public health concern in the United States with prevalence rates increasing dramatically since the 1970s (1,13,14). Much of the impetus for government action stems from the recognition that obesity is responsible for the development of at least 300,000 preventable deaths, although this number is being constantly revised. In addition, well over $100 billion in annual health costs were incurred in the United States in 2004 (15,16).

No single government agency "owns" the obesity problem, and no single entity exists to coordinate the government response. A number of U.S. government agencies play key roles in addressing the obesity epidemic: the Department of Health and Human Services (DHHS), which includes the Centers for Disease Control and Prevention (CDC), the Food and Drug Administration (FDA), the National Institutes of Health (NIH), and the Office of the Surgeon General; the United States Department of Agriculture (USDA), which administers the food assistance programs and substantial nutrition education efforts; and the President's Council on Fitness and Health. The Department of Defense and the Veterans Administration also have significant interests in stemming the obesity epidemic to maintain defense forces in peak health and to contain costs in providing health care for veterans.

The Institute of Medicine (IOM) of the National Academies of Sciences in response to requests from Congress and executive agencies has conducted several important policy studies and recommended policy and program initiatives (3,15,17). Additionally, several foun-

dations, including the Robert Wood Johnson Foundation (RWJ), the Kaiser Family Foundation (KFF), and William J. Clinton Foundation, have developed an interest in obesity prevention (18–20). The obesity epidemic may have first been recognized in the United States but in some ways, other governments, especially in the European Union, have taken more of a direct legislative active approach. This was stimulated in part by the WHO working with professional societies such as the International Association for the Study of Obesity, which seeks to form alliances to develop worldwide effective strategies to address the growing problem (21).

The history of how this patchwork approach arose in the United States to a nutrition-related national health crisis is long. The science of nutrition evolved late in the 19th century, and prior to that the U.S. government had little engagement in matters of diet and health. During the 40 years between 1880 and 1920 frequently referred to as the "golden age of public health," the federal government created the NIH in 1887, the Cooperative Extension Service in 1914 as part of the USDA, and issued the first dietary guidance pamphlet titled "Food for Young Children" in 1916 (22–24). This document focused on children's dietary needs and sets the theme for what would be the focus of most government nutrition advice for the next half century—getting enough food in the right amounts to prevent nutrient deficiency diseases. To help keep the population healthy during World War I, the U.S. Food Administration published the first food guide, the *Five Food Groups—What the Body Needs* (23–25). When milk supplies fell and prices rose, priority was given to children by the Children's Bureau to allocate milk and other food supplements to the poor and people on limited incomes to assist them in preparing an adequate diet (26,27).

During the 1930s, the Great Depression produced food shortages and poor health. The U.S. government shouldered more responsibility to ensure food availability through farm programs to increase production and stabilize prices through welfare and food assistance programs (24). The USDA began buying and distributing surplus agricultural commodities as food relief in 1930, thus carrying out its stated purpose when created in 1862, which was to promote the full range of American agricultural products and advise consumers about food choices (23,24,28,29). The U.S. Agricultural Act was amended in 1933 to permit surplus commodity purchases of food for donation to child nutrition and school lunch programs, and in 1935, the Social Security Act authorized grants to United States for nutrition services to mothers and children called the Food Distribution Program (24,30). This program was later adopted as an experimental Food Stamp Program in 1939 (24). As the Depression subsided and the country was entering World War II in 1941, President Roosevelt's administration requested that the Food and Nutrition Board establish the first Recommended Dietary Allowances to guide the procurement of food for the population (31). After the war, additional policy and governmental efforts continued to emphasize getting enough food, especially to children, and the National School Lunch Program was established in 1946 and the Special Milk Program in 1954 (24,32).

The United States entered an era of food surplus and after World War II, indulgent food behaviors became more customary and people experienced the metabolic response of the body, storing the additional energy as fat. The Framingham Study of Coronary Heart disease risk factors, which began in 1949 and other studies found that excess body weight was a risk factor for developing several chronic diseases (33–35). In 1949, the Mutual Life Insurance Company published "desirable" and "ideal" weight-for-height tables derived from its database of insured persons with the longest life spans (33). In 1959, these tables were revised to reflect the results of the Build and Blood Pressure Study of 1959 and later in 1983 to reflect results of the 1979 Build Study (33,36–38). Although they were widely used, the tables were frequently criticized because of the demographics of the population from which the data were drawn. People who could afford life insurance were typically young to middle-aged, Caucasian, and middle to upper income, and therefore, the data were not representative of the U.S. population.

Although the scientific evidence relating excess body weight to increased risk of chronic diseases continued to mount during the 1960s and 1970s, the U.S. government's attention was still focused on providing adequate nutrition to those with limited access to food (24). President Lyndon Johnson outlined the "War on Hunger" Program, and Congress (spearheaded by a select committee on nutrition and human needs) passed the Food Stamp Act in 1965 providing surplus foods to needy families, amended the Older Americans Act to establish congregate dining and home-delivered meals to older Americans, and enacted the Child Nutrition Act establishing the School Breakfast Program in 1966 (24,39–42). The first national food consumption survey was fielded in 1965 (43). The country began funding professional dietetic training programs in 1966; the Department of Health, Education, and Welfare, which later became the Department of Health and Human Services, drafted a report on hunger and malnutrition among various U.S. poverty groups, and recommendations were made about the role nutrition has in human reproduction between 1968 and 1970 (24,44).

In 1969, President Nixon convened the first and only White House Conference on Nutrition (45). While most of the conference agenda focused on the nutritional needs and shortfalls of vulnerable population groups—children, the poor, the elderly—the Conference did recognize the role of obesity as a risk factor for chronic diseases.

However, the whole section on obesity was very short and emphasized the need to prevent obesity in children due to both physical and psychological problems they encounter (45). The recommendations ranged from studying self-help groups such as TOPS (Take off Pounds Sensibly) to research on new drugs and etiologies and changes to school lunch programs (46). Most of the conference recommendations that were acted on related to improving food assistance programs. The Secretary of Agriculture established the Food and Nutrition Service to coordinate and administer federal food assistance programs. The Special Supplementary Food Program for Women, Infants, and Children was established in 1972. To improve information about the health and nutritional status of the U.S. population, the National Center for Health Statistics conducted the first National Health and Nutrition Examination Survey (NHANES I) in 1971–1974 (32). By 1979, the United States sponsored over 350 programs in agricultural support, nutrition services and training, food intake and food fortification and assistance, food and nutrition research, and food and nutrition education, but little funding on obesity prevention (24).

During the mid-1970s, overconsumption of fat, cholesterol, sugar, salt, and alcohol emerged as dietary factors contributing to chronic disease (24). Congress became impatient with the lack of attention being paid to the emerging scientific data and in 1977 published the *Dietary Goals for the U.S.* (47) and the USDA followed in 1979 with *Building a Better Diet—Five Food Groups* (24). This began a slow shift in dietary advice from "eat more" to "eat less" based on emerging scientific consensus on the relationship between diet and health (24,29). Goaded to action, the Surgeon General published *Healthy People: the Surgeon General's Report on Health Promotion and Disease Prevention* in 1979, and USDA and DHHS in response to the public's need for authoritative, consistent guidance on diet and health and through a collaborative effort issued the first edition of *Nutrition and Your Health: Dietary Guidelines for Americans* in 1980 (23,24,48) with a second edition in 1985. Examples of major U.S. policies on the prevention of obesity through diet and exercise can be found in Table 1.

A major innovation in public health policy was introduced when in the early 1980s the U.S. DHHS began setting specific objectives for health improvement. The first set of health objectives created in 1979 and published in 1980 titled *Promoting Health/Preventing Disease: Objectives for the Nation* included 17 nutrition objectives to be achieved by 1990 and found in Table 2 (49).

Two pivotal reports published during the 1980s identified that obesity prevalence was increasing to epidemic proportions—*Nutrition Monitoring in the United States*, a report of the Joint Nutrition Monitoring and Evaluation Committee in 1986 and the 1988 *Surgeon General's Report on Nutrition and Health* (24,50).

Table 1 Examples of Major Policy Guidelines Published by U.S. Government Agencies and Health Organizations for Prevention of Obesity Through Diet, Exercise, or Both

Yr	Organization
1952	American Heart Association: Food for Your Heart
1965	American Heart Association: Diet and Heart Disease
1968	American Heart Association: Diet and Heart Disease
1970	White House Conference on Food, Nutrition, and Health
1971	American Diabetes Association: Principles of Nutrition and Dietary Recommendations
1974	National Institutes of Health: Obesity in Perspective
1974	American Heart Association: Diet and Coronary Heart Disease
1977	National Institutes of Health: Obesity in America
1977	U.S. Senate Select Committee on Nutrition and Human Needs: *Dietary Goals for the United States, 2nd Edition*
1978	American Heart Association: Diet and Coronary Heart Disease
1979	National Cancer Institute: Statement on Diet, Nutrition, and Cancer
1979	American Diabetes Association: Principles of Nutrition and Dietary Recommendations
1980	U.S. Department of Agriculture and U.S. Department of Health and Human Services: Dietary Guidelines for Americans
1980	U.S. Public Health Service Surgeon General's Office: Healthy People: Promoting Health/Preventing Disease—Objectives for the Nation
1984	American Cancer Society: Nutrition and Cancer: Cause and Prevention
1985	National Institutes of Health: Consensus Development Conference Statement
1985	U.S. Department of Agriculture and U.S. Department of Health and Human Services: *Dietary Guidelines for Americans, 2nd Edition*
1986	American Heart Association: Dietary Guidelines for healthy American adults
1986	American Diabetes Association: Nutritional Recommendations and Principles
1988	U.S. Department of Health and Human Services: *The Surgeon General's Report on Nutrition and Health*
1988	American Heart Association: Dietary Guidelines for Healthy American Adults
1988	National Heart, Lung and Blood Institute: National Cholesterol Education Program
1989	National Research Council: diet and health: Implications for Reducing Chronic Disease Risk
1990	U.S. Department of Agriculture and U.S. Department of Health and Human Services: *Dietary Guidelines for Americans, 3rd Edition*
1990	U.S. Public Health Service Surgeon General's Office and U.S. Department of Health and Human Services: *Healthy People 2000: National Health Promotion and Disease Prevention Objectives*
1991	American cancer Society: Guidelines on diet, Nutrition, and Cancer
1993	National Heart, Lung, and Blood Institute: National Cholesterol Education Program
1994	American Diabetes Association: Nutrition Principles for the Management of Diabetes and Related Complications
1995	U.S. Department of Agriculture and U.S. Department of Health and Human Services: *Dietary Guidelines for Americans, 4th Edition*
1996	American Heart Association: Dietary Guidelines for Healthy American Adults
1996	American Cancer Society: Guidelines on Diet, Nutrition, and Cancer Prevention
1996	American Diabetes Association: Nutrition Recommendations and Principles
1997	American Heart Association: Guide to Primary Prevention of Cardiovascular Diseases
1997	World Cancer Research Fund and American Institute for Cancer Research: Food, Nutrition and the Prevention of Cancer: A Global Perspective
1999	American Heart Association: Preventive Nutrition: Pediatrics to Geriatrics
2000	U.S. Department of Agriculture and U.S. Department of Health and Human Services: *Dietary Guidelines for Americans— MyPyramid, 5th Edition*
2000	U.S. Public Health Service Surgeon General's Office and U.S. Department of Health and Human Services—*Healthy People 2010 Objectives*
2003	U.S. Department of Health and Human Services, Office of the Secretary—President's Steps to a Healthier U.S.

Source: Updated from Figure 1 in Ref. 66.

Despite that, throughout the 1980s, the major theme of nutritional advice to the American population focused on dietary variety, maintaining an ideal body weight for disease prevention, inclusion of starch and fiber in the diet and limiting intake of sugar, fat, cholesterol, salt, and alcohol (23,24). The NIH issued new dietary guidance pertaining to chronic disease prevention through the National Cancer Institute (NCI) and the National Heart, Blood, and Lung Institute (NHBLI). The NCI developed the *Cancer Control Nutrition Objectives for the Nation: 1985–2000* in 1986 and the *Dietary Guidelines for Cancer Prevention* in 1988, and NHLBI developed the National

Table 2 Progress of Healthy People 1990, 2000, and 2010 Objectives Related to Obesity

Yr	Objective/benchmarks	Baseline (%)	Status (%)	Explanation	Met/not met
Healthy People: Promoting Health/Preventing Disease: Objectives for the Nation (1990 Objectives) (96,97)					
1986	**Objective M: Nutrition**				
	Objective c: The prevalence of significant overweight (120% of "desired" weight) among the U.S. adult population should be decreased to 10% of men and 17% of women, without nutritional impairment.[a] (baseline data from 1971–1974 NHANES I, status data from 1976–1980 NHANES II due lack of other data)				
	(a) Men	14	26.3	Increased	Not met
	(b) Women	24	29.6	Increased	Not met
	Objective d: By 1990, 50% of the overweight population should have adopted weight loss regimens, combining an appropriate balance of diet and physical activity. (baseline data unavailable)				
	(a) Males	N/A	25	N/A	N/A
	(b) Females	N/A	30	N/A	N/A
	Objective k: By 1990, 90% of adults should understand that to lose weight people must either consume foods that contain fewer calories or increase physical activity or both. (baseline data unavailable)	N/A	74	N/A	N/A
	Objective N: Physical Activity				
	Objective a: By 1990, the proportion of children and adolescents ages 10 to 17 participating regularly in appropriate physical activities, particularly cardiorespiratory fitness programs which can be carried into adulthood, should be greater than 90%. (baseline data unavailable)	N/A	66	N/A	N/A
1990	*Objective c*: By 1990, the proportion of adults 18–64 participating regularly in vigorous physical exercise should be greater than 60%.	35	41	Increased	Not met
	Objective d: By 1990, 50% of adults 65 years and older should be engaging in appropriate physical activity, e.g., regular walking, swimming or other aerobic activity. (baseline data from 1975)	35	10–20	Decreased	Not met
Healthy People 2000: National Health Promotion and Disease Prevention Objectives (98)					
1994–95	**Objective: Nutrition**				
	2.3: Reduce overweight to a prevalence of no more than 20% among people aged 20 and older (20–74 years) and no more than 15% among adolescents aged 12–19[b].				
	• People 20–74 years	26	35	Increased	Not met
	• Adolescents 12–19 years	15	24	Increased	Not met
	2.3a: Reduce overweight to a prevalence of no more than 25% among low-income women aged 20 and older.	37	47	Increased	Not met
	2.3b: Reduce overweight to a prevalence of no more than 30% among black women aged 20 and older.	44	52	Increased	Not met
	2.3c: Reduce overweight to a prevalence of no more than 25% among Hispanic women aged 20 and older.	33	35	Increased	Not met
	2.3d: Reduce overweight to a prevalence of no more than 30% among American Indians and Alaskan Natives.	29	43	Increased	Not met
	2.3e: Reduce overweight to a prevalence of no more than 25% among people with disabilities[c].	36	40	Increased	Not met
	2.3f: Reduce overweight to a prevalence of no more than 41% among women with high blood pressure.	50	N/A	N/A	

(Continued)

Table 2 Progress of Healthy People 1990, 2000, and 2010 Objectives Related to Obesity (*Continued*)

Yr	Objective/benchmarks	Baseline (%)	Status (%)	Explanation	Met/not met
	2.3g: Reduce overweight to a prevalence of no more than 35% among men with high blood pressure.	39	N/A	N/A	
	2.3h: Reduce overweight to a prevalence of no more than 25% among Mexican-American men.	30	37	Increase	
	2.7: Increase to at least 50% the proportion of overweight people aged 12 and older who have adopted sound dietary practices combined with regular physical activity to attain an appropriate body weight.				
	• Overweight males aged 18 years and over	25	15	Increase	50
	• Overweight females aged 18 years and over	30	19	Increase	50
	2.7a: Increase to at least 24% the proportion of overweight Hispanic males aged 18 and older who have adopted sound dietary practices combined with regular physical activity to attain an appropriate body weight.	15	13	Increase	24
	2.7b: Increase to at least 22% the proportion of overweight Hispanic females aged 18 and older who have adopted sound dietary practices combined with regular physical activity to attain an appropriate body weight.	13	16	Increase	22
	Objective: Physical Activity and Fitness				
	1.3: Increase to at least 30% the proportion of people aged 6 and older who engage regularly, preferably daily, in *light to moderate* physical activity for at least 30 minutes per day. People aged 18–74 years				
	• 5 or more times per week	22	23	Increased	Not met
	• 7 or more times per week	16	16	No change	Not met
	1.3a: Hispanic 18 years and over 5 or more times per week	20	22	Increase	Not met
	1.4: Increase to at least 20% the proportion of people aged 18 and older and to at least 75% the proportion of children and adolescents aged 6–17 who engage in *vigorous* physical activity that promotes the development and maintenance of cardiorespiratory fitness 3 or more days per week for 20 or more minutes per occasion.				
	• Children and adolescents 6–17 years	59	64	Increased	Not met
	• People aged 18 years and older	12	16	Increased	Not met
	1.4a: Lower-income people 18 years and over	7	14	Increased	Not met
	1.4b: Blacks 18 years and over				
	1.4c: Hispanics 18 years and over	14	14	No change	Not met
	1.5: Reduce to no more than 15% the proportion of people aged 6 and older who engage in no leisure-time physical activity. People 18 years and over	24	23	Decreased	Not met
	1.5a: Reduce to no more than 22% the proportion of people aged 65 years and older who engage in no-leisure time physical activity.	43	27	Decreased	Not met
	1.5b: Reduce to no more than 20% the proportion of people with disabilities and older who engage in no-leisure time physical activity.	35	29	Decreased	Not met
	1.5c: Reduce to no more than 17% the proportion of low-income people aged 18 years and older (annual family income less than $20,000) who engage in no-leisure time physical activity.	32	28	Decreased	Not met
	1.5d: Reduce to no more than 20% the proportion of Blacks aged 18 years and older who engage in no-leisure time physical activity.	28	28	No change	Not met

Yr	Objective/benchmarks	Baseline (%)	Status (%)	Explanation	Met/not met
	1.5e: Reduce to no more than 25% the proportion of Hispanics aged 18 years and older who engage in no-leisure time physical activity.	34	31	Decreased	Not met
	1.5f: Reduce to no more than 21% the proportion of American Indian/Alaskan Natives aged 18 years and older who engage in no-leisure time physical activity.	29	23	Decreased	Not met
	1.7 Increase to at least 50% the proportion of overweight people aged 12 and older who have adopted sound dietary practices combined with regular physical activity to attain an appropriate body weight.				
	• Overweight male 18 years and over	25	15	Decreased	Not met
	• Overweight females 18 years and over	30	19	Decreased	Not met
	a. Overweight Hispanic male 18 years and over	15	13	Decreased	Not met
	b. Overweight Hispanic females 18 years and over	13	16	Increased	Not met

Healthy People 2010 Objectives: Objectives for Improving the Health

Yr	Objective/benchmarks	Baseline (%)	Status (%)	Explanation	Met/not met
2005	**Objective 19: Nutrition and Overweight**				
	19-1: Increase the proportion of adults (20 years and older) who are at a healthy weight to 60%.	42	33	Decreased	Not met
	19-2: Reduce the proportion of adults (20 years and older) who are obese to 15%.	23	15	Decreased	Not met
	19-3: Reduce the proportion of children and adolescents (6–19 years) who are overweight and obese to 5%.	11	16	Increased	Not met
	Objective 22: Physical Activity and Fitness				
	22-1: Reduce the proportion of adults (18 years and older) who engage in no leisure-time activity to 20%.	40	40	No change	Not met
	22-2: Increase the proportion of adults who engage regularly, preferably daily, in moderate physical activity for at least 30 minutes per day 5 or more days per week or vigorous physical activity for at least 20 minutes per day 3 or more days per week to 50%.	32	30	Decreased	Not met
	22-3: Increase the proportion of adults who engage in vigorous physical activity that promotes the development and maintenance of cardio-respiratory fitness 3 or more days per week to 30%.	23	22	Decreased	Not met
	22-6: Increase the proportion of adolescents who engage in moderate physical activity for at least 30 minutes on 5 or more of the previous 7 days to 35%.	27	27	No change	Not met
	22-7: Increase the proportion of adolescents who engage in vigorous physical activity that promotes cardiorespiratory fitness 3 or more days per week for 20 or more minutes per occasion to 85%.	65	64	Decreased	Not met

[a]Overweight status was assessed using the 1976–1980 NHANES II defined as BMI greater than or equal to 27.8 for males and 27.3 for females. Severe overweight was defined as BMI greater than or equal to 31.1 for males and 32.3 for females, where these values are equal to the 95th percentile for 20 to 29 years males and females.

[b]For people aged 20 and older, overweight is defined as body mass index (BMI) equal to or greater than 27.8 for men and 27.3 for women. For adolescents, overweight is defined as BMI equal to or greater than 23 kg/m^2 for males aged 12 to 14 years, 24.3 kg/m^2 for males aged 15 to 17 years, 25.8 kg/m^2 for males aged 18 to 19 years, 23.4 kg/m^2 for females aged 12 to 14 years, 24.8 kg/m^2 for females aged 15 to 17 years, and 25.7 kg/m^2 for females aged 18 to 19 years.

[c]People with disabilities are people who report any limitations in activity due to chronic conditions.

Abbreviation: NHANES, National Health and Nutrition Examination Survey.

Source: From Refs. 96–98.

Cholesterol Education Program Guidelines in 1987 (24,51).

Throughout the 1990s, new government advisory materials continued to be released to help the general public understand what constitutes an appropriate weight for height and how to choose a health-promoting diet. These included the 1990, 1995, 2000, and 2005 Dietary Guidelines for Americans in which the 1990 issue was the first to address attaining a healthy weight (52–55). In 1993, the NHLBI released the updated National Cholesterol Education Program guidelines, which emphasized the importance of a "healthy" weight for the prevention of cardiovascular disease, and in 1998 *Clinical Guidelines on the Identification, Evaluation, and Treatment of Overweight and Obesity in Adults* (56,57). These governmental materials were also accompanied by statements and recommendations of professional and medical societies and the IOM (Table 1).

Healthy People 2000, the Public Health Service (PHS) ten-year plan, released in 1990 had two prominent goals intended to reduce the prevalence and consequences of obesity in the United States by 2000. They were to (*i*) reduce the prevalence of overweight to no more than 20% of adults and 15% of adolescents and (*ii*) increase to 50% the proportion of overweight peoples of ages 12 and older who have adopted sound dietary practices combined with regular activity to attain an appropriate body weight (58).

By 2000, it was abundantly clear that these goals were not met and that the obesity situation had become progressively worse as shown in Table 2. Thus, when the next set of guidelines for Healthy People 2010 was formulated and released, the goals were modified to reflect this reality (59). The 2000 goal was "to reduce the prevalence of overweight to no more than 20% of the U.S. population," but in the 2010 goal the wording was reversed to "increase to 60%" of those who had a healthy weight, leaving a remaining 40% of the population overweight. Consequently, in this decade, the PHS conceded that not only had the previous advice failed to have an impact but because the obesity problem was much worse than before, even a "goal" of only 20% of the population being overweight, was considered impractical. These are compelling statistics that have led to a variety of "calls to action" and an increasing referral to an "obesity epidemic" by national governmental agencies (60). This use of an "epidemic" analogy has raised public awareness of the consequences of the increasing prevalence of obesity in adults, adolescents, and younger children setting the stage for new policy actions and frameworks.

This decade has also been characterized by an increasing awareness of obesity prevalence as a global issue and has stimulated considerable activity in nongovernmental organizations and in professional societies.

THE EVOLVING ROLE OF INTERNATIONAL ORGANIZATIONS

Two international organizations have played very significant roles related to food and health policy. Both the Food and Agricultural Organization (FAO) and the WHO were formed as the United Nations began its work and their constitutions date to 1945 and 1946, respectively (11,61).

The FAO arose from a meeting in Hot Springs, Virginia, in 1943 in which 44 governments who resolved to commit to founding a permanent organization for food and agriculture. The FAO has as its primary mandate, a role in reducing hunger and achieving food security for all. It strives to "raise levels of nutrition, improve agricultural productivity, better the lives of rural populations and contribute to the growth of the world economy" (61). In the 2002 Food Summit, 179 countries and the European Commission reaffirmed commitment to reducing the number of hungry individuals by half in 2015 (61). Over the decades, the FAO has remained focused on the reduction of hunger and has had noted successes in some areas of the world where obesity is now beginning to rise. Overall, its mission related to hunger reduction has remained the main focus as recently as 2002. Obesity, food production, and trade issues may emerge as priority at the FAO as the obesity epidemic has its effects in countries previously classified as having low food security.

Juxtaposed, since its founding, WHO has had a much more expansive definition of health and well-being that was, in some ways, ahead of the public health concerns of the time in the United States. The United States, as noted in the earlier section of the chapter, was focused on the elimination of disease rather than the promotion of health in the 1940s (Fig. 1).

Thus, it should be noted that WHO and the international partners involved had an early lead on what has become a modern contemporary understanding of the importance of health promotion as well as the need to control disease. Over the decades, the WHO has published many reports on topics such as AIDS, child and maternal health, emerging diseases, and the impact of natural disasters on health. In the 1990s, the WHO turned attention to obesity and held or was involved in expert and technical meetings to document the increasing health challenges posed by increases in obesity on a global scale. WHO has now become very active in documenting and addressing the obesity epidemic and used the term "globesity" (4,11,21). The WHO has noted that in developing countries a double public health burden exists in that both undernutrition and obesity may coexist. As the distribution of body mass indices (BMIs) shifts upward in these countries, there are additional issues. For example, when people who were undernourished in early life become obese later in life, the severity of the accompanying comorbidities may be greater (2,8,10).

Today, WHO hosts what is probably the best international Web site on obesity statistics: www.who.int/dietphysicalactivity/publications/facts/obesity/en/. On this site one can follow the international dimensions of the problem and conduct national comparative analyses. According to the WHO data, by 2015, 2.3 billion adults will be overweight and 700 million will be obese. In

Constitution of the World Health Organization

The States Parties to this Constitution declare, in conformity with the Charter of the United Nations, that the following principles are basic to the happiness, harmonious relations, and security of all peoples:

- Health is a state of complete physical, mental and social well-being and not merely the absence of disease or infirmity.
- The enjoyment of the highest attainable standard of health is one of the fundamental rights of every human being without distinction of race, religion, political belief, economic or social condition.
- The health of all peoples is fundamental to the attainment of peace and security and is dependent upon the fullest co-operation of individuals and States.
- The achievement of any State in the promotion and protection of health is of value to all.
- Unequal development in different countries in the promotion of health and control of disease, especially communicable disease, is a common danger.
- Healthy development of the child is of basic importance, the ability to live harmoniously in a changing total environment is essential to such development.
- The extension to all peoples of the benefits of medical, psychological and related knowledge is essential to the fullest attainment of health.
- Informed opinion and active co-operation on the part of the public are of the utmost importance in the improvement of the health of the people. Governments have a responsibility for the health of their peoples which can be fulfilled only by the provision of adequate health and social measures.

Figure 1   The 1946 Statement of Principles in the WHO Constitution.

addition, WHO launched the new WHO Child Growth Standards in 2006, which include BMI charts for infants and children up to five years of age. The WHO readily notes that there is no standard international definition of childhood obesity, but this latest endeavor may well accelerate the effort to provide such information.

Accompanying the substantial effort, work by the WHO to document the obesity epidemic is the policy framework presented in the Global Strategy on Diet, Physical Activity and Health, which was adopted by the World Health Assembly in 2004. This document is a powerful statement about what is at stake as the impact of noncommunicable diseases is felt internationally. The strategy document makes the point that there has been a major shift in the causes of death in both developed and, now, developing countries. As of 2001, 60% of the 56 million deaths were attributed to noncommunicable diseases as was 47% of the global burden of disease. Most of this morbidity and mortality was also attributed to factors typically associated with overweight and obesity (2,3,14,15,62–67). The strategy has provided a rallying force for coordinated national efforts to control obesity, promote "healthier choices," regulate food products and advertising, and increase physical fitness. In the recent past, considerable legislative activity at both the national and international level has begun. Some examples of this activity are detailed in subsequent sections. It is too early to predict the successful implementation or impact of these proposed policies on the obesity epidemic, but it seems highly likely that efforts to legislate for "better health" will continue to influence both

the funding for obesity research and the type and level of interventions necessary to prevent its inexorable growth, especially in children.

ROLE OF FOUNDATIONS AND PRIVATE ORGANIZATIONS—NEW STAKEHOLDERS

As the obesity epidemic has captured both media and political interest, it has also become a focal point for the work of private foundations and nonprofit groups. One of the largest programs was recently announced by the RWJ Foundation. The program will award $500 million over five years to fight childhood obesity (19,67). The goal is to reverse the epidemic in the United States by 2015. When compared with the relatively low NIH and CDC investments for national obesity research, the impact of private foundations characterized by large programs, such as this one, could begin to surpass the national governmental programs (66). In addition, these foundations may have an increasingly larger policy role.

The increasing impact of private foundations on policy was recently illustrated when the RWJ foundation supported an independent evaluation of efforts to implement Arkansas Act 1220, which mandated a comprehensive approach to addressing childhood obesity in public schools (67,68). This effort was followed by a research study on the BMIs of children in Arkansas and reported that the state had halted the progression of childhood obesity (19). If proven sustainable, such efforts are likely to be models for other state programs.

The RWJ Web site further notes that the foundation is working with the Alliance for a Healthier Generation, which is a partnership between the American Heart Association and the William J. Clinton Foundation to improve nutrition, physical activity, and staff wellness in schools nationally. In addition, RWJ has engaged in substantial advocacy and education efforts with the National Governors Association, the National Conference of State Legislators, and the U.S. Conference of Mayors.

The Alliance for a Healthier Generation announced in 2006 its first industry agreement as part of its Healthy Schools Program (20). The voluntary guidelines capped the number of calories per container at 100 and were to be implemented prior to the 2009–2010 school year. In addition, a goal of at least half of all beverages in high school was to be water, no-calorie, and low-calorie selections. As is noted further in this chapter, much stronger guidelines have been proposed in multiple legislations and also by the IOM in their recently released report titled, "Nutrition Standards for Foods in Schools" (69).

Another private foundation that has had a considerable impact in the policy arena is the KFF. A major focus of their work has been on the impact of television advertising to children in the United States. In March of 2007, the foundation released a report titled "Food for Thought," which notes that government agencies and advisory bodies have had difficulty in obtaining the data needed to accurately assess the impact of television advertising on children's eating behavior and on the rise in childhood obesity (70). The study they presented was the largest ever conducted and used over 1600 hours of programming in contrast to previous studies that typically used 40 to 50 hours of sample 20. The study concluded that children of all ages are exposed to substantial food and beverage advertising, that 8- to 12-year-olds watch more television and may be the group most affected, and that of the 8854 food advertisements reviewed, there were none for fruits and vegetables. Additionally, only 15% of the advertisements currently depicted an active lifestyle (70). The foundation has produced work in this area for many years, and according to their Web site foundation representatives, they have frequently testified in legislative hearings. The study and previous work have been cited in numerous policy circles.

While foundations may have their own agenda and do not have to set priorities with the same constraints that federal and state agencies may have, it is also true that they are not subject to the same political pressure that federal agencies such as DHHS, USDA, and CDC occasionally must face. In addition, as in the case of RWJ and the Clinton Foundation, they are free to directly engage consumers, industry participants, and individual scientists and to form coalitions both educational and financial to further their work. Thus, it is reasonable to expect that these "new entrants" into the funding and policy arena will have a progressively more important voice, as their work is known by both governmental and nongovernmental agencies. They also frequently have more freedom to publicize their results and can take an advocacy role that is not possible for government agencies. There are many other private players and foundations that are engaging in obesity prevention, including individual large employers and other foundations. For example, the Chagnon Foundation collaborated with the Quebec government to match $200 million for a total of $400 million to promote healthy lifestyle practices and prevent problems connected to weight over 10 years (71). A challenge for the future will be to assess the collective impact of this distributed private effort.

OPTIONS FOR ACTION: TREATMENT OR PREVENTION?

Many other chapters in this volume have concentrated on the available treatments for existent obesity. In short, while there are an array of diet and exercise programs that have been promoted and numerous efforts to find a suitable pharmaceutical solution, our treatments to date are only modestly successful and recidivism is high. In extreme cases of obesity, surgical solutions have been promoted and the age at which surgery is being considered has moved downward. Substantial risks remain, and in a few, poorly understood cases, the surgery does not lead to sufficient weight loss. The frustrations faced by health professionals in the obesity treatment area are immense and include a continuing battle over governmental classification of obesity as a disease and whether obesity treatment and/or prevention are covered by insurance plans.

Most current obesity experts emphasize the importance of even modest weight loss in mitigating the risk factors associated with diabetes and cardiovascular disease. They stress slow but consistent weight loss and steadily increasing physical activity. Such advice is rarely welcomed by overweight and obese individuals who are seeking "quick" solutions and who often have unrealistic expectations of the rate of weight loss and a limited ability to understand and implement portion control (8,10,13). Such unrealistic expectations make them susceptible to products advertising rapid weight loss and "silver bullets." Many of the products that prey on these obese individuals have no scientific basis for their claims. These products do not require FDA approval and may be harmful. Most consumers do not know this and falsely believe that they are proven to be safe (72). A recent article has shown that many physicians also are unaware that the products have not been approved for safety and efficacy (73). Thus, one area of policy work has focused on removing such products from the market (72). The FTC also has studied the issue and developed a Web site (www.ftc.gov/) that helps to identify claims that are likely to be misleading (74,75).

With such limited options for successful reversal of obesity once established, it should be no surprise that much effort is now being directed at prevention of obesity. In addition, programs to encourage increased physical activity are evolving in many countries and within individual states.

CURRENT DIRECTION OF GOVERNMENT ACTIONS: BLAME, TREAT, TEACH, OR TINKER

The evolution of governmental policy has moved from an earlier position that obesity was an individual problem related to individual choice (BLAME the individual) to the multiple decadal search for treatments (TREAT the patient) combined with educational efforts (TEACH people how to eat and lead a healthier lifestyle), to one where there is an active search for incentives and policy levers that can have population impact (TINKER with policies to provide incentives or threats). While most professionals in the obesity field no longer blame the individual, it is not uncommon to hear recommendations in policy circles that are, in effect, "name and shame" pressure tactics used to force ingredient changes in foods or to blame corporations or companies for the unhealthy consequences of providing high sugar or high fat foods. The regulation of food advertising content is contentious, with constitutional overtones, because there is public support, and the U.S. Constitution does permit the regulation of misleading messages directed toward young people (76).

A plethora of new legislation to regulate the international food industry is currently underway, although the effectiveness of such regulation is in much dispute. In addition, as the long-term impact of the obesity epidemic is recognized as a threat to national economic health as well as to individual health, policy research, which includes the economic impact of obesity and its attendant effect on national competitiveness, is becoming increasingly salient. In any case, rarely have we seen such coordinated and concentrated efforts, perhaps only paralleled by the efforts in the United States to decrease smoking and its attendant health effects or encourage seat belt use. The next decade promises to be one of accelerated public health policy activity, and it is unclear what will work and in which environments governmental policies can be most useful.

Currently, both internationally and nationally, much effort is directed toward prevention of obesity, especially in children. Thus, one sees an increasing array of efforts and accompanying legislation to regulate advertising to children, change the school food environment, specify which foods are "healthy choices," and promote physical activity. In addition, legislation or task forces to explore other avenues to influence behavior ranging from building code and urban planning changes, to tax incentives for corporations and individuals to maintain a healthy body weight, to taxing foods with high fat or sugar content are emerging on many fronts. Most of these efforts could be classified as tinkering with existing programs or environments to make consistent but incremental changes.

Examples of Tinkering with Advertising Regulations

With respect to the advertising of food and food products to children in the United States, in January 2007, new rules decreed by the Federal Communications Commission (FCC) regarding TV broadcasting of advertising for Web sites came into force (77). The new rules state that during programs aimed at children aged 12 and younger, cable and broadcast operators may not display addresses for Web sites that contain any links to commercial content. Subsequently, the FCC established a task force on "Media and Childhood Obesity: Today and Tomorrow" with members of the U.S. Congress and hosts a Web site (http://www.fcc.gov/obesity/) as a public information resource (78).

On February 2, 2007, the U.S. DHHS and the Ad Council formed a coalition with the film studio Dream-Works Animation SKG to launch a series of new public service advertisements (PSAs) designed to help address childhood obesity (79). As part of the ongoing "Small Steps" campaign, designed to prevent childhood obesity and encourage families to lead healthier lifestyles, the new PSAs use characters from the movie *Shrek*. Children are encouraged to engage in physical activity by slogans such as "be a player: get up and play an hour a day," which will complement existing PSAs geared toward promoting healthy diets. The advertisements will appear on TV and outdoor billboards. Online advertisements will direct children and families to the DHHS's newly redesigned Web site on healthy lifestyles (www.HealthierUS.gov). The Small Steps Web site also includes new material related to the new advertisements (www.smallstep.gov/index.html). Concomitantly, on June 1, 2007, the FTC published the study "Children's Exposure to TV Advertising in 1977 and 2004: Information for the Obesity Debate." This study compared data from the 2004 television programming season and the FTC's 1978 Children's Advertising Rule-making, and found television food advertising to children of ages 2 to 11 years has decreased by approximately 9% (www.ftc.gov/) (80).

An international example of action to impact childhood obesity includes the Committee of Advertising Practice, the body responsible for writing the United Kingdom nonbroadcast advertising code, which published the new rules for food and soft drink product advertisements to children (81). The rules came into force in July 2007. The new rules state that (*i*) marketing communications should not condone or encourage poor nutritional habits or an unhealthy lifestyle in children, (*ii*) marketing communications should not directly advise or ask children to buy or to ask their parents or other adults to make enquiries or purchases, and (*iii*) marketing communications should neither try to sell to children by directly appealing to emotions such as pity, fear, or self-confidence nor suggest that having the advertised product somehow confers superiority, for example, making a child more confident, clever, popular, or successful.

Standards have been established by various childhood obesity experts in the area of marketing communications addressed to children (3,19,70,74). These communications should avoid "high pressure" and "hard sell" techniques, and they should neither directly urge children to buy or persuade others to buy nor suggest that children could be bullied, cajoled, or otherwise put undue pressure to acquire the advertised item. Furthermore, products and prices should not be presented in marketing communications in a way that suggests children or their families can easily afford them. Other regulations advise that marketing communications addressed to or targeted directly at children should not actively encourage them to eat or drink at or near bedtime, to eat frequently throughout the day, or to replace main meals with confectionery or snack foods. Except those for fresh fruit or fresh vegetables, food or drink advertisements that are targeted directly at preschool or primary school children through their content should not include promotional offers. Marketing communications featuring a promotional offer linked to food products of interest to children should avoid creating a sense of urgency or encouraging the purchase of excessive quantities for irresponsible consumption. These communications should not seem to encourage children to eat or drink a product only to take advantage of a promotional offer: the product should be offered on its merits, with the offer as an added incentive. Marketing communications featuring a promotional offer should ensure a significant presence for the product. Fresh fruit or vegetable products are exempt from this restriction. Marketing communications for collection-based promotions should not seem to urge children or their parents to buy excessive quantities of food. Communications should not encourage children to eat more than they otherwise would, except those for fresh fruit or fresh vegetables. Food or drink advertisements that are targeted directly at preschool or primary school children through their content should not include licensed characters or celebrities popular with children. Marketing communications should not give a misleading impression of the nutritional or health benefits of the product as a whole. Except those for fresh fruit or fresh vegetables, food or drink advertisements that are targeted directly at preschool or primary school children through their content should not include nutrition or health claims. Finally, marketing communications should not disparage good dietary practice or the selection of options, such as fresh fruit and vegetables that accepted dietary opinion recommendations should form part of the average diet.

In March 2007, the Canadian parliament's Standing Committee on Health tabled a report calling on the federal government to take immediate action in response to levels of childhood obesity, including action on food advertising aimed at children (82). Nonetheless, although the report was tabled, the Committee presented 13 recommendations for the federal government, including one titled "Control of Children's Food Advertising," which recommended that the government (*i*) assess the effectiveness of self-regulation as well as the effectiveness of prohibition in the province of Quebec, in other Canadian jurisdictions, as well as in Sweden, (*ii*) report on the outcomes of these reviews within one year, (*iii*) explore methods of regulating advertising to children on the Internet, and (*iv*) collaborate with the media industry, consumer organizations, academics, and other stakeholders as appropriate.

The Australian Communications and Media Authority (ACMA) announced a review of the standards for children's television programs, first introduced in 1990 (83). The review—expected to last between 12 and 18 months—will include issues such as the amount of children's programs TV broadcasters must screen each year and food advertising. Initially, ACMA indicated it would conduct a program of research in 2006 that will inform the review and assist in the development of a discussion paper. The discussion paper on children's TV standards will be released for public comment later during the year (2007) and industry, parents, teachers, as well as other interested parties will be invited to respond.

In February 2007, the South Korean Government outlined a set of measures aimed at restricting the population's exposure to high fat, salt, and sugar (HFSS) foods (84). The new rules include a ban on "fast-food" advertising on television before 9 PM and on the Internet and a ban of HFSS food promotion in school cafeterias. The advertising ban on fast food will take effect from 2008 and will be expanded in 2010 to include all foods containing high levels of sugar and fat. The government will determine permissible standards for fat and sugar content later this year. Similarly, these actions are also being implemented in the United Kingdom (85).

In contrast, in May 2007, Mexico's Parliament Economy Committee rejected a Senate Bill proposing restrictions on cereal, snack food, and soft drink advertising targeted at children (86,87). Members of the Committee voted against the Bill arguing that it would have jeopardized thousands of food industry jobs without representing a balanced response to childhood obesity.

Another significant development is that the WHO Global Strategy Secretariat plans to develop a draft working plan on marketing recommendations, which will propose timing, approval process, presentation, and so on. Also, in November 2006, the WHO released its report summarizing the WHO Forum and Technical Meeting that took place in Oslo, Norway, in May 2006 (88). The report suggests wide-ranging policy restrictions to be imposed at the national level ranging from a ban during prime-time television to a complete ban on all advertising to children. In addition to these recommendations, the report set out the case for the WHO to pursue an International Code of Practice on Food Marketing. Recommendations for policy changes or TINKERING were not confined to television advertising but include school food policies and some indications of changes in tax policies.

Examples of Tinkering with School Diets and Food Labeling

In March 2007, the U.S. Senate Agricultural Committee and the U.S. House of Representatives Committee on Education and Labor held a hearing to discuss nutrition issues in schools. The "Child Nutrition Promotion and School Lunch Protection Act 2006" was referred to the committees (89). The stated goal of the Act is to "improve the nutrition and health of schoolchildren by updating the definition of 'food of minimal nutritional value' to conform to current nutrition science" and is sponsored by several senators, including Senate Agriculture Committee Chairman Tom Harkin (D-IA), Senator Lisa Murkowski (R-AK), and Senator Hillary Rodham Clinton (D-NY). To understand the Act it is necessary to appreciate that for a school food service program to receive federal reimbursements, school meals served by that program must meet science-based nutritional standards established by Congress and the Secretary of Agriculture and that foods sold individually outside the school meal programs (including foods sold in vending machines, a la carte or snack lines, school stores, and snack bars) are not required to meet comparable nutritional standards. Thus, this is an effort to revise the definition of "food of minimal nutritional value" to apply to all foods sold (*i*) outside the school meal programs, (*ii*) on the school campus, and (*iii*) at any time during the school day. In revising the definition, legislation instructs the Secretary to consider

a. both the positive and negative contributions of nutrients, ingredients, and foods (including calories, portion size, saturated fat, trans fat, sodium, and added sugars) to the diets of children;

b. evidence concerning the relationship between consumption of certain nutrients, ingredients, and foods to both preventing and promoting the development of overweight, obesity, and other chronic illnesses;

c. recommendations made by authoritative scientific organizations concerning appropriate nutritional standards for foods sold outside the reimbursable meal programs in schools; and

d. special exemptions for school-sponsored fund-raisers (other than fund-raising through vending machines, school stores, snack bars, a la carte sales, and any other exclusions determined by the Secretary), if the fundraisers are approved by the school and are infrequent within the school (89).

Across the United States, action is occurring at the local and state level. For example, a new law in New York City effective from July 2007 requires that calorie counts be posted next to prices in some chain restaurants (76,90). Similar laws are under consideration in at least 20 states as well (76).

In September 2006, the South Korean government introduced requirements for food companies to disclose all ingredients on food packages, but restaurants were excluded (84). Under the new measures, major fast food restaurants will now be obliged to list ingredients and additives on food packaging, beginning in 2010. The relevant authorities will designate schools and areas within 200 m of them as being Green Food Zones, in which the sale of unhealthy foods such as fast food and carbonated drinks will be banned. Elementary schools will also be required to expand education on healthy food and nutrition. The Korean Food and Drug Administration will also require food producers to list amounts of trans fats on packages beginning in December 2007, aiming to reduce the amount of trans fats to below 1% in all foods by 2010 (84).

On May 30, 2007, the European Commission adopted a White Paper on "A Strategy for Europe on Nutrition, Overweight and Obesity Related Health Issues" (91). The paper "stresses the importance of enabling consumers to make informed choices, ensuring that healthy options are available, and calls upon the food industry to work on reformulating recipes, in particular to reduce levels of salt and fats." Another area of focus is the benefits of physical activity and the necessity to encourage Europeans to exercise more. The Commission's preference, at this stage is "to keep the existing voluntary approach at the European Union level due to the fact that it can potentially act quickly and effectively to tackle rising overweight and obesity rates". The Commission will assess this approach and the various measures taken by industry in 2010 and determine whether other approaches are also required. The Commission proposes to explore new actions which include "a revision of nutrition labeling, programs to promote the consumption of fruit and vegetables, a White Paper on Sport and a study to explore the potential of food re-formulation to improved diet" (91). On another front there is evidence that, at least in some political circles, tax policy is also being considered.

Examples of Tinkering with Tax Policy

In the United States, a bipartisan bill, The Healthy Workforce Act 2007, introduced by Senator Tom Harkin and Senator Gordon Smith proposes awarding tax credits to companies that provide programs to help employees to "eat better, exercise, manage stress, and quit smoking" (92).

In Germany in May 2007, Ursula Heinen, the government spokesperson on nutrition and consumer protection, told the German newspaper Bild am Sonntag of potential plans to raise the tax on HFSS foods from 7% to 19% (93). This is not currently a government policy, but may be supported by a number of parliamentarians both within the governing coalition between the *Christlich Demokratische Union Deutschlands* or Christian Democratic Union and the Social Democratic Party (SPD) and in opposition parties. Under the current rules, all foods are taxed at a 7% lower rate of the value added tax (VAT). The full rate of VAT (19%) is presently levied on beverages. Elvira Drobinski-Weiss, the SPD's health expert, apparently stated that "an unhealthy lifestyle should also be made financially unattractive" (94).

In Norway, it was reported that Norway's Ministry of Health is currently examining a new "personal health strategy proposal" that would introduce higher rates of VAT on high-sugar products in order to discourage consumption (95). The proposal would reduce VAT on fresh fruit and vegetables from 12.5% to 0%. The VAT on sugar-rich foods and beverages would rise from 25% to 50%. The government will explore the possibilities of economic incentives, including taxes on chocolate and sweets as well as supporting incentives (presumably for healthy products) (95). Fiscal policies are among the measures recommended in the WHO global strategy, and the reduction of consumption of HFSS products is one of the aims of the Nordic Council of Ministers' work in this area.

SUMMARY

As the alarm associated with recognition that the obesity epidemic has become increasingly compelling, the role of government, at the federal, state, and even local level has become more activist. As the case is made that overweight and obesity is "everybody's business," we can expect to see an increasing interest among politicians, community activists, media, and business leaders. This will inevitably lead to some concern that the problem is too important to "leave to the scientists and doctors," and researchers in the field can expect to see their research become both more important and subjected to increased scrutiny. The sequence of "blame, treat, teach, and tinker" is likely to take on some new nuances. For example, there is still a danger that "blaming the individual" will resurface with new insurance and other policies that penalize individuals for exceeding BMI guidelines. The continuous search for effective treatments (TREAT) will keep pressure on government agencies and insurance companies to reclassify preventive treatment and treatment of the already obese. In addition, individual desperation and the desire for a "silver bullet" will continue to encourage the "bilking" of a gullible public with purported treatments that have no scientific validity. One can expect that over the next years, at least in the United States, most of the food security programs will be reexamined both for their effectiveness and for the food consumption patterns that they encourage (TEACH). In addition, many organizations, both governmental and nongovernmental, are developing age appropriate curriculum to help teach healthy choices and behaviors to children and families. Perhaps, the regulatory area (TINKER) will be the most interesting to watch as there is little evidence to document the impact and effectiveness of the multitude of proposed rules and regulations, and serious research is surely warranted here.

ACKNOWLEDGMENT

In our survey of the current national and international regulatory environment, we had access and permission to use the Web site provided by the Advertising Education Forum, which tracks regulatory issues on an ongoing basis. We thank them for their help.

REFERENCES

1. Ogden CL, Carroll MS, Curtin LR, et al. Prevalence of overweight and obesity in the United States, 1999–2004. JAMA 2006; 295:1549–1555.
2. Davey RC. The obesity epidemic: too much food for thought? Br J Sports Med 2004; 38:360–363.
3. Institute of Medicine National Academy of Sciences. Preventing Childhood Obesity—Health in the Balance. 1st ed. Washington, D.C.: National Academies Press, 2005.
4. World Health Organization. Obesity: Preventing and Managing the Global Epidemic (research). Geneva: WHO, 1998.
5. Hill JO, Wyatt HR, Reed GW, et al. Obesity and the environment: where do we go from here? Science 2003; 299:853–855.
6. Mutch DM, Clement K. Unraveling the genetics of human obesity. PLoS Genet 2006; 2(12):e188.

7. Johnson RL, Williams SM, Spruill IJ. Genomics, nutrition, obesity and diabetes. J Nurs Scholarsh 2006; 38:11–18.

8. Lowe MR. Self-regulation of energy intake in the prevention and treatment of obesity: is it feasible? Obes Res 2003; 11(suppl):44S–59S.

9. U.S. Food and Drug Administration Center for Food Safety and Applied Nutrition. Calories Count: Report of the Working Group on Obesity (research). Washington, D.C.: U.S. FDA CFSAN, 2004.

10. Lau DC, Douketis JD, Morrison KM, et al. 2006 Canadian clinical practice guidelines on the management and prevention of obesity in adults and children (research summary, Ontario). CMAJ 2007; 176(8):S1–S13.

11. World Health Organization. Global Strategy on Diet, Physical Activity, and Health. Provisional Agenda Item. Geneva: World Health Organization, 2004. Report No. A57/9.

12. Mello MM, Studdert DM, Brennan TA. Obesity—the new frontier of public health law. N Engl J Med 2006; 354: 2601–2610.

13. Latner JD. Self-help for obesity and binge eating. Nutr Today 2007; 42:81–85.

14. Flegal KM, Carroll MD, Kuczmarski RJ, et al. Overweight and obesity in the United States: prevalence and trends, 1960–1994. Int J Obes Relat Metab Disord 1998; 22:39–47.

15. Institute of Medicine National Academy of Sciences. Progress in Preventing Childhood Obesity–How Do We Measure Up? 2nd ed. Washington, D.C.: National Academies Press, 2007.

16. Townsend MS. Obesity in low-income communities: prevalence, effects, a place to begin. J Am Diet Assoc 2006; 106:34–37.

17. Institute of Medicine National Academy of Sciences. Weighing the Options—Criteria for Evaluating Weight-Management Programs. 1st ed. Washington, D.C.: National Academy Press–Library of Congress, 1995.

18. Kaiser Family Foundation. Survey on Childhood Obesity (summary). San Jose: San Jose Mercury News & Kaiser Family Foundation, 2004.

19. Robert Wood Johnson Foundation. Balance: A Report on State Action to Promote Nutrition, Increase Physical Activity and Prevent Obesity (summary). Princeton: Robert Wood Johnson Foundation, 2006. Report No. 3.

20. William J Clinton Foundation AfaHG. Healthy Schools Program Receives $20 Million Expansion Grant. Little Rock, AR, 2007:1.

21. International Obesity Taskforce. Global Strategies to Prevent Childhood Obesity: Forging a Societal Plan That Works (research report). London: IASO, 2006.

22. Hunt CL. Food for Young Children. Washington, D.C.: USDA Farmer's Bulletin, 1916.

23. Davis C, Saltos E. Dietary recommendations and how they have changed over time. In: America's Eating Habits: Changes and Consequences. Washington, D.C.: Economic Research Service, United States Department of Agriculture, 1999. Agriculture Information Bulletin No. 750:33–50.

24. Office of the Surgeon General. The Surgeon General's Report on Nutrition and Health. In: U.S. Department of Health and Human Services PHS, ed. 1st ed. Rockville, MD: Government Printing Office, 1988:1–81.

25. Hunt CL, Atwater HW. How to select foods: I. What the body needs. Washington, D.C.: U.S. Farmer's Bulletin, 1917.

26. Egan MC. Public health nutrition services: issues today and tomorrow. Am Diet Assoc 1980; 77:423–427.

27. Hunt CL. A Week's Food for an Average Family. Washington, D.C.: USDA Farmer's Bulletin 1228, 1921:25.

28. Hunt CL. Good Proportions in the Diet. Washington, D.C.: USDA Farmer's Bulletin 1313, 1923:18.

29. Nestle M. Editorial: the politics of dietary guidance—a new opportunity. Am J Public Health 1994; 84:713–715.

30. Stiebeling HK, Ward M. Diets at Four Levels of Nutrition Content and Cost. Washington, D.C.: USDA Circular No. 296, 1933:59.

31. Federal Security Agency. Proceedings of the National Nutrition Conference for Defense. In: National Nutrition Conference for Defense. Washington, D.C., 1941.

32. U.S. Senate Select Committee on Nutrition and Human Needs. The role of the federal government in human nutrition research. Washington, D.C.: U.S. Government Printing Office, 1976.

33. Office of the Surgeon General: The Surgeon General's Report on Nutrition and Health. In: U.S. Department of Health and Human Services PHS, ed. The Surgeon General's Report on Nutrition and Health. Vol. 1. 1st ed. Rockville, MD: Government Printing Office, 1988:275–309.

34. Garrison RJ, Castelli WP. Weight and thirty-year mortality of men in the Framingham Study. Ann Intern Med 1985; 103:1006–1009.

35. Hubert HB, Feinleib M, McNamara PM. Obesity as an independent risk factor for cardiovascular disease: a 26 year follow-up of participants in the Framingham Heart Study. Circulation 1983; 67:968–977.

36. Metropolitan Life Insurance Company. New Weight Standards for Men and Women. Chicago, IL: Statistical Bulletin, 1959:1–4.

37. Society of Actuaries. Build and Blood Pressure Study, 1959. Chicago, IL: Society of Actuaries, 1960.

38. Society of Actuaries and Association of Life Insurance Medical Directors of America. Build Study, 1979. Chicago, IL: Society of Actuaries, 1980.

39. Citizen's Board of Inquiry into Hunger and Malnutrition in the United States. Hunger, U.S.A. Boston: Beacon Press, 1968.

40. U.S. Department of Agriculture. A Brief History of the Food Stamp Program. 2006. Available at http://www.fns. usda.gov/fsp/rules/Legislation/about_fsp.htm.

41. USDA Food and Nutrition Service, Special Nutrition Programs. Evaluation of the School Breakfast Program Pilot Project: Findings from the First Year of Implementation United States Specail Report No. CN-02-SBP. October 2002. Washington, DC.

42. U.S. Department of Agriculture Food and Nutrition Service. School Breakfast Program-History. 2007. Available at: http://www.fns.usda.gov/cnd/Breakfast/AboutBFast/ProgHistory.htm.

43. National Research Council. National Survey Data on food consumption: Uses and Recommendations. Washington, D.C.: National Academy Press, 1984.

44. U.S. Department of Health, Education, and Welfare. Ten State Nutrition Survey 1968–70. In: Administration HSaMH, ed. Washington, D.C.: Government Printing Office, 1972.

45. U.S. White House 1969 Conference Members of President Richard Nixon. White House Conference on Food, Nutrition, and Health Final Report (research summary recommendations). Washington, D.C.: U.S. Government Printing Office, 1970.

46. U.S. White House Conference Members of President Richard Nixon. White House Conference on Food, Nutrition, and Health Final Report—Section 2 Obesity (research summary recommendations). Washington, D.C.: U.S. Government Printing Office, 1970.

47. U.S. Senate Select Committee on Nutrition and Human Needs. Dietary Goals for the United States. In: Congress U, ed. 2nd ed. Washington, D.C.: Government Printing Office, 1977.

48. U.S. Department of Agriculture and U.S. Department of Health and Human Services. Nutrition and Your Health: Dietary Guidelines for Americans. 1st ed. Washington, D.C.: U.S. Government Printing Office, 1980.

49. U.S. Department of Health and Human Services. Healthy people—promoting health/preventing disease: objectives for the nation. In: Service PH, ed. Healthy People Objectives. 1st ed. Washington, D.C.: Government Printing Office, 1980:200.

50. U.S. Department of Health and Human Services and U.S. Department of Agriculture. Nutrition Monitoring in the United States: A progress report from the Joint Nutrition Monitoring Evaluation Committee. Progess Report of Research. Hyattsville, MD: National Center for Health Statistics, 1986. DHHS Publication No. (PHS) 86-1255.

51. National Cancer Institute. Cancer Control Objectives for the Nation: 1985–2000. Bethesda, MD: NCI, 1986. NCI Monographs No. 2.

52. U.S. Department of Agriculture and U.S. Department of Health and Human Services. Nutrition and Your Health: Dietary Guidelines for Americans. 3rd ed. Washington, D.C.: U.S. Government Printing Office, 1990.

53. U.S. Department of Agriculture and U.S. Department of Health and Human Services. Nutrition and Your Health: Dietary Guidelines for Americans. 4th ed. Washington, D.C.: U.S. Government Printing Office, 1995.

54. U.S. Department of Agriculture and U.S. Department of Health and Human Services. Nutrition and Your Health: Dietary Guidelines for Americans. 5th ed. Washington, D.C.: U.S. Government Printing Office, 2000.

55. U.S. Department of Agriculture and U.S. Department of Health and Human Services. Dietary Guidelines for Americans. 6th ed. Washington, D.C.: U.S. Government Printing Office, 2005.

56. National Heart, Lung, and Blood Institute. Clinical Guidelines on the Identification, Evaluation, and Treatment of Overweight and Obesity in Adults: The Evidence Report Research report. Bethesda, MD: National Institutes of Health 1998. Report No. 98-4083.

57. National Heart, Lung, and Blood Institute. National Cholesterol Education Program Guidelines. Bethesda, MD: National Institutes of Health, 2007.

58. U.S. Department of Health and Human Services. Healthy people 2000: national health promotion and disease prevention objectives. In: DHHS PHS, ed. Healthy People Objectives. 2nd ed. Washington, D.C.: Government Printing Office, 1990.

59. U.S. Department of Health and Human Services. Healthy people 2010 objectives: objectives for improving health. In: DHHS PHS, ed. Healthy People Objectives. 3rd ed. Washington, D.C.: Government Printing Office, 2000:300.

60. Office of the Surgeon General. The Surgeon General's Report Call to Action to Prevent and Decrease Overweight and Obesity. In: U.S. Department of Health and Human Services PHS, ed. 2nd ed. Rockville, MD: Government Printing Office, 2001.

61. Food and Agricultural Organization. History of the FAO, 2007. Available at: www.fao.org.

62. Allison DB, Fontaine KR, Manson JE, et al. Annual deaths attributable to obesity in the United States. JAMA 1999; 282:1530–1538.

63. Anderson PM, Butcher KF. Childhood obesity: trends and potential causes. Future Child 2006; 16:19–45.

64. Crosson FJ, Kessler DA, L R. Childhood obesity: an epidemic is gripping California and the nation. How did we get here and what do we do now? New York Times 2006 January 2006, sect. 1–24.

65. Fontaine KR, Redden DT, Wang C, et al. Years of life lost due to obesity. JAMA 2003; 289:187–193.

66. Nestle M, Jacobson MF. Halting the obesity epidemic: a public health policy approach. Public Health Rep 2000; 115:12–24.

67. Robert Wood Johnson Foundation. Childhood obesity. In: Obesity Strategy. Princeton, 2007.

68. An Act to Create A Child Health Advisory Committee. In: Arkansas Act 1220 of the 84th General Assembly. State of Arkansas 84th General Assembly, ed., 2003:1–5.

69. Institute of Medicine National Academy of Sciences. Nutrition Standards for Foods in Schools—Leading the Way Toward Healthier Youth. 1st ed. Washington, D.C.: National Academies Press, 2007.

70. Kaiser Family Foundation. Food for Thought: Television Food Advertising to Children in the United States. Research. Menlo Park: Henry J. Kaiser Family Foundation, 2007.

71. Press Communications Secretary to the Quebec Minister of Health and Social Services. La Loi instituant le Fonds pour la promotion des saines habitudes de vie est adoptée à l'unanimité. "The Law Instituting the Funds for Promotion Healthy Practices of Life was Adopted Unanimously." Item 1046, 2007.

72. Greenwood M. Help not hype: Getting real about weight loss. Obes Manage 2007; 3:11–21.

73. Ashar BH, Rice TN, SD S. Physician's understanding of the regulation of dietary supplements. Arch Intern Med 2007; 167:966–969.

74. U.S. Federal Trade Commission. Weight-Loss Advertising: An Analysis of Current Trends. Federal Trade Commission Staff Report, 2002.

75. U.S. Federal Trade Commission. Red Flag: Bogus Weight Loss Claims, 2003.

76. Gostin LO. Law as a tool to facilitate healthier lifestyles and prevent obesity. JAMA 2007; 297:87–90.

77. Advertising Educational Foundation. FCC Ok's Kids TV Compromise. In: AEF Newsletter, 2006. Available at: www.aef.com.

78. Advertising Educational Foundation Forum. New FCC rules come into force In: AEF Newsletter. Available at: www.aeforum.org. Accessed January 2007.

79. The Ad Council. Obesity Prevention. 2006. Available at: www.adcouncil.org.

80. U.S. Federal Trade Commission. Children's Exposure to Television Advertising. 2007. Available at: www.ftc.gov/.

81. Committee of Advertising Practice. The British Code of Advertising, Sales Promotion and Direct Marketing. U.K., 2005:1–40.

82. House of Commons Canada. Healthy Weights for Healthy Kids: Report of the Standing Committee on Health. Ottawa: Canadian Congress 38th Parliament, 1st Session, March 2007.

83. Australian Communications and Media Authority. Children's Television Standards Review. In: ACMA, 2007.

84. Advertising Educational Foundation Forum. South Korea: Government restricts food advertising. In: AEF Latest News, 2007. Available at: www.aeforum.org.

85. Kreifels T, Blain J. Food Safety Update. UK: Junk food TV advertising ban comes into force. Freshfields Bruckhaus Deringer, 2007:4.

86. News Post India. Mexican Lawmakers Worry About Obesity. New Delhi, India, August 18, 2007:3.

87. Advertising Educational Foundation Forum. Mexican Senate Rejects Restrictions on Food Advertising to Children Over alleged pressure by the Food Industry In: AEF Newsletter, May 2007. Available at: www.aeforum.org.

88. World Health Organization Regional Office for Europe. The challenge of obesity in the WHO European Region and strategies for response (summary). Copenhagen, 2007. Available at: http://www.euro.who.int/eprise/main/who/InformationSources/Publications/Catalogue/20070220.

89. U.S. Senate Agricultural Committee. Child Nutrition Promotion and School Lunch Protection Act of 2006.

90. New York City Department of Health and Mental Hygiene Board of Health. Notice of adoption of an amendment (81.08) to article 81 of the New York City Health Code. In: Health DoHaMHBo, ed. NYC. Available at: http://www.nyc.gov/html/doh/downloads/pdf/public/notice-adoption-hc-art81-08.pdf 2006:1–7.

91. Commission of the European Communities. A Strategy for Europe on Nutrition, Overweight and Obesity related health issues (research report). Brussels: European Commission, 2007. Report No. 279.

92. Healthy Workforce Act of 2007. In: 110th Congress SB 1753 Internal Revenue Code 1986. 1st ed. 2007:1–15.

93. Advertising Educational Foundation Forum. Germany: Parliamentarians discuss higher taxes for HFSS food AEF News, 2007.

94. German Federal Ministry of Health and German Federal Ministry of Food Agriculture and Consumer Protection. Reports from the Working Groups. In: Health GFMo, ed. Prevention for Health. Nutrition and Physical Activity—A Key to Healthy Living. Bandeweiler, Germany, 2007:1–16.

95. EACA. Tax levels may rise on high-sugar food and drink. EACA Monthly April 2007, Sect. 1–10.

96. McGinnis JM, Lee PR. Healthy people 2000 at mid decade. JAMA 1995; 273:7.

97. McGinnis JM, Richmond JB, Brandt EN, et al. Health progress in the United States: results of the 1990 objectives for the nation. JAMA 1992; 268:8.

98. U.S. Department of Health and Human Services NCfHS. Healthy People 2000 Midcourse Review, 1998–99. In: Center for Disease Control and Prevention NCfHS, ed. 1st ed. Hyattsville: DHHS, NCHS, 1999:200.

Index